Medical pharmacology

PRINCIPLES AND CONCEPTS

Medical
pharmacology

PRINCIPLES AND CONCEPTS

Andres Goth, M.D.

Professor of Pharmacology and Chairman of the Department,
The University of Texas Health Science Center at Dallas,
Southwestern Medical School,
Dallas, Texas

TENTH EDITION

with 112 illustrations

The C. V. Mosby Company

ST. LOUIS • TORONTO • LONDON   1981

MOSBY

1906 **75** 1981
YEARS

A TRADITION OF PUBLISHING EXCELLENCE

Editor: John E. Lotz
Manuscript editor: Mary Dolan
Design: Diane Beasley
Production: Margaret Bridenbaugh

TENTH EDITION

Copyright © 1981 by The C. V. Mosby Company

Previous editions copyrighted 1961, 1964, 1966, 1968, 1970, 1972,
1974, 1976, 1978
Printed in the United States of America

The C. V. Mosby Company
11830 Westline Industrial Drive, St. Louis, Missouri 63141

Library of Congress Cataloging in Publication Data

Goth, Andres.
    Medical pharmacology.

    Includes bibliographies and index.
    1. Pharmacology.   I. Title.
RM300.G65   1981   615′.7   81-2861
ISBN 0-8016-1949-1   AACR2

GW/VH/VH   9 8 7 6 5 4 3 2 1   01/B/087

Contributors

BURNELL R. BROWN, Jr., M.D., Ph.D.

Professor and Chairman, Department of Anesthesiology, University of Arizona School of Medicine, Tucson, Arizona

GREGORY G. DIMIJIAN, M.D.

Clinical Assistant Professor of Pharmacology and Psychiatry, The University of Texas Health Science Center at Dallas, Southwestern Medical School, Dallas, Texas

PARKHURST A. SHORE, Ph.D.

Professor of Pharmacology, The University of Texas Health Science Center at Dallas, Southwestern Medical School, Dallas, Texas

ELLIOT S. VESELL, M.D.

Evan Pugh Professor and Chairman, Department of Pharmacology, Pennsylvania State University College of Medicine, Hershey, Pennsylvania

Preface

The tenth edition of *Medical Pharmacology* stresses medically relevant aspects of the action and uses of drugs. Pharmacology has been expanding not only with the discovery of new drugs, but also with the development of important concepts that must be learned by the student and the practicing physician. These concepts are becoming so important that without them rational therapeutics is impossible.

Because of these developments, the tenth edition of this book has been more extensively revised and enlarged than any previous editions. Several new chapters have been added and others greatly expanded. For example, much more space had to be devoted to drug-receptor interactions and pharmacokinetics.

I have been fortunate to obtain the help of several contributors. Dr. Burnell R. Brown, Jr. wrote a new chapter on general anesthetics. Dr. Parkhurst A. Shore modified extensively the chapters on adrenergic drugs and psychopharmacological agents. His chapter, "General Aspects of Psychopharmacology," is entirely new. Dr. Elliot S. Vesell contributed new chapters on pharmacogenetics and the effects of age, diet, and disease on drug responses or drug disposition. In addition, Dr. Vesell made many suggestions for extensive changes in the chapter on pharmacokinetics. Dr. Gregory G. Dimijian, a previous contributor, revised his chapter on contemporary drug abuse.

Although the tenth edition of *Medical Pharmacology* has necessarily become somewhat more extensive and complex than the previous editions, every effort has been made to keep it readable and straightforward. It emphasizes understanding rather than complete coverage of the literature, and it is not a collection of review articles. Nevertheless, the reader will find a sufficient number of recent reviews listed at the end of various chapters to provide extensive documentation if the need arises.

Andres Goth

Contents

SECTION THREE   **Psychopharmacology**

SECTION FOUR   **Depressants and stimulants of the central nervous system**

Medical pharmacology

PRINCIPLES AND CONCEPTS

CHAPTER 1

Introduction

Chemical agents not only provide the structural basis and energy supply of living organisms but also regulate their functional activities. The interactions between potent chemicals and living systems contribute to the understanding of life processes and in addition provide effective methods for the treatment, prevention, and diagnosis of many diseases. Chemical compounds used for these purposes are *drugs*, and their actions on living systems are referred to as *drug effects*.

Pharmacology deals with the properties and effects of drugs or, in a more general sense, with the interactions of chemical compounds and living systems. It is a discipline of biology and is closely related to other disciplines, particularly physiology and biochemistry.

Despite the considerable overlap among the various disciplines of biology, pharmacology is unique in dealing primarily with the mechanism of action of biologically active substances.

Although its specific aim is to define the biological activity of chemical compounds, pharmacology also contributes greatly to knowledge of living systems. This contribution to the understanding of life processes is valuable to biological sciences in general and to medicine in particular. An understanding of drugs is necessary for the diagnosis, prevention, and treatment of disease. Some aspects of pharmacology are of remote relevance to the study of medicine. To emphasize this distinction, the title *Medical Pharmacology* was chosen for this book.

There are several fields of study that may be considered subdivisions of pharmacology or disciplines related to it.

Pharmacodynamics is the study of drug effects and the handling of drugs by the body. This aspect of pharmacology is perhaps nearest to a basic science of medicine.

Emphasis on mode of action of chemical compounds distinguishes pharmacology from some of the other basic sciences of medicine. As used in medicine, the term *pharmacology* is essentially synonymous with pharmacodynamics.

Chemotherapy is that subdivision of pharmacology which, according to the definition first proposed by Paul Ehrlich, deals with drugs that are capable of destroying invading organisms without destroying the host.

Pharmacy is concerned with the preparation and dispensing of drugs. Today

SUBDIVISIONS OF PHARMACOLOGY AND RELATED DISCIPLINES

1

the physician seldom has the need to prepare or dispense drugs. Even the pharmacist has very little to do with the preparation of drugs; most of them are manufactured by large companies. The pharmacist may provide useful services, however, as a member of the health team having special knowledge about drug preparations.

Therapeutics is the art of treatment of disease. *Pharmacotherapeutics* is the application of drugs in the treatment of disease.

Toxicology is the science of poisons and poisonings. Although toxicology may be viewed as a special aspect of pharmacology, it developed into a separate discipline for a variety of reasons. Forensic and environmental medicine requires the services and knowledge of toxicologists with special training in drug identification and poison control.

HISTORICAL DEVELOPMENT OF PHARMACOLOGY

Although no detailed discussion will be attempted, it should be pointed out that the history of pharmacology can be divided into two periods. The early period goes back to antiquity and is characterized by empiric observations in the use of crude drugs. It is interesting that even primitive people could discover relationships between drugs and disease. The use of drugs has been so prevalent throughout history that Sir William Osler stated (1894) with some justification that "man has an inborn craving for medicine."

In contrast to this ancient period, modern pharmacology is based on experimental investigations concerning the site and mode of action of drugs. The application of the scientific method to studies on drugs was initiated in France by François Magendie and was expanded by Claude Bernard (1813-1878). The name of Oswald Schmiedeberg (1838-1921) is commonly associated with the development of experimental pharmacology in Germany, and John Jacob Abel (1857-1938) played a similar role in the United States.

The growth of pharmacology was greatly stimulated by the rise of synthetic organic chemistry, which provided new tools and new therapeutic agents. More recently, pharmacology has benefited from developments of other basic sciences and in turn has contributed to their growth.

One of the most dynamic areas of pharmacological research is that which deals increasingly with drug receptors and important new developments; for example, the discovery of the endorphins was made possible by the existence of drug receptors being recognized. There are those who feel that one of the basic functions of pharmacology is to map out drug receptors in the body.

Some of the greatest changes in medicine that have occurred during the last few decades are directly attributable to the discovery of new drugs. Progress in this field has not been without its problems, however. Success in the search for new therapeutic agents has not been matched by equal expertise in the evaluation of their clinical safety and efficacy. Furthermore, the practicing physician has not always been prepared for some of the new drugs whose clinical use requires considerable understanding of basic principles. Nevertheless, in the recent history of pharmacology the many successes more than make up for the problems created by drugs.

There are several reasons for considering pharmacology one of the increasingly important basic sciences of medicine. Some of these are obvious; others are not yet generally recognized.

Large numbers of drugs are used in the practice of medicine. They cannot be applied intelligently or even safely without some understanding of their mode of action, side effects, toxicity, and metabolism. As powerful new drugs are introduced, adequate pharmacological knowledge on the part of the physician becomes mandatory. Pharmacological terms and concepts are used so commonly in the clinical journals that a physician without a good grounding in the subject would find it difficult to read and understand the current medical literature.

Pharmacology is taught in medical schools for other reasons. As a basic science it contributes important concepts to the understanding of various functions in health and disease. In research, drugs are used increasingly as chemical tools for elucidating basic mechanisms. Also, drugs are being utilized more frequently for diagnostic purposes.

Pharmacology is also important in medicine because of the commercial influences that are exerted on the physician in the selection of drugs. A good understanding of the principles of pharmacology should provide the physician with a critical attitude and the ability to evaluate rationally the claims made for various new drug preparations.

Finally, it is increasingly recognized that numerous functions in the body are regulated by endogenous compounds which interact with specific receptors. Many commonly used drugs mimic or oppose the action of these endogenous compounds or alter their metabolism. When viewed in this light, pharmacology is not only the scientific basis of drug therapy but also is a basic science of medicine, which contributes to our understanding of how the body functions in health and disease.

PLACE OF PHARMACOLOGY IN MEDICINE

Problem 1-1. In view of the importance of pharmacology in the practice of medicine and the current preoccupation with adverse drug reactions, why is there so little time devoted to it in the medical curriculum? The answer seems to lie in the interdisciplinary nature of the subject and in tradition. Because of its interdisciplinary nature, many areas of pharmacology could be taught in other courses. On the other hand, as has been pointed out by the Nobel Laureate Carl Cori,[1] information on drugs can be taught by experts in various disciplines, but an organized course outside a medical school pharmacology department is difficult.

Tradition is an obstacle to the adequate teaching of pharmacology. It is believed by many medical educators that students will learn about drugs "later," perhaps in residency training or as they pick up information when they need it in their practice. Many critical physicians will admit, however, that what they pick up "later" is some practical information essential for therapeutics but not much basic knowledge of pharmacology, which is often badly needed.

Although pharmacology is concerned with drug effects in all species of animals, in medicine there is increasing interest in clinical pharmacology, which concerns itself with pharmacological effects in human beings.

There are many reasons for this increasing interest. Results of pharmacological studies on animals sometimes cannot be applied to human beings because of species variations in the response to the drug or in its metabolism. Clinical pharmacology also provides scientific methods for the determination of usefulness, potency, and toxicity of new drugs in humans.

CLINICAL PHARMACOLOGY

Pharmacological knowledge essential for good medical practice includes not only the findings of clinical pharmacology but also those principles and concepts generally derived from animal experiments, which are necessary for thorough understanding of drug effects. Without these principles and concepts, rational therapeutics is impossible.

REFERENCE

1 Cori, C. C.: The call of science, Annu. Rev. Biochem. **38**:1, 1969.

SECTION ONE

General aspects of pharmacology

CHAPTER 2

Drug-receptor interactions

Most drugs exert their potent and specific effects in the body by forming a bond, generally reversible, with some cellular constituent. This cellular constituent is the *receptor*. Drugs that interact with a receptor and elicit a response are termed *agonists;* compounds that interact with receptors preventing the action of agonists are referred to as *specific antagonists*.

The existence of receptors for a drug in cells can be deduced from (1) relationships between structure and activity in a homologous or congeneric series, (2) quantitative studies on agonist-antagonist pairs, and (3) selective binding of radioactive drugs to isolated cells or membranes.

The role of a receptor is to recognize a chemical signal and to discriminate between such a signal and other molecules. The drug-receptor interaction is then coupled to an effector mechanism to provide an appropriate cellular response. The presence of receptors at an anatomical site determines the selective nature of many drug effects. For example, acetylcholine when applied directly to a motor end-plate produces an action potential. When the same drug is applied a short distance from the end-plate, it has no effect.[11]

Not all drug actions are mediated by receptors. Volatile anesthetics, metal chelating agents, or osmotic diuretics exert effects that are not mediated by specific receptors. On the other hand, drugs of the autonomic nervous system, the opiate narcotics, and most antipsychotic drugs act on specific receptors.

RECEPTOR THEORY

The *receptor concept* was first proposed by Langley in 1878[12] and was used extensively by Paul Ehrlich in his studies on chemotherapy. Investigating the opposing actions of pilocarpine and atropine on salivary section, Langley hypothesized the presence of some substance in the nerve endings or glands with which the drugs may combine. To Ehrlich, receptors were groups of protoplasmic macromolecules with which drugs could combine *reversibly* or *irreversibly*.

According to current concepts,[27] there are several types of drug receptors. Type I receptors are on the external surface of the plasma membrane of target cells. They interact with drugs that mimic or block the actions of autonomic mediators, such as catecholamines and some peptide hormones and releasing factors. Type II receptors are located in the cytoplasm of target cells and combine with drugs that mimic or block the actions of steroid hormones. The drug-receptor combination may be modi-

7

fied and translocated to the nucleus where it may regulate the concentration of a specific messenger ribonucleic acid (RNA) and, ultimately, the synthesis of proteins. Type III receptors are in the cell nucleus, the thyroid hormone being the best example of a drug that interacts with nuclear receptors.

The binding forces in the drug-receptor interaction are represented by covalent bonds, ionic and hydrogen bonds, and van der Waals bonds. Covalent bonds, because of their high binding energy provide essentially irreversible effects. If the drug is an antagonist, such as phenoxybenzamine, the covalent bond formation results in noncompetitive antagonism. Ionic bonds are important because most drugs contain cationic and anionic groups. Consequently the pH may influence their interaction with receptors. The van der Waals bond is a weak interaction between dipoles. Although the bond energy is only about 0.5 kcal per mole—compared with 100 kcal per mole for the covalent bond—van der Waals bonds are very important in drug-receptor interactions for several reasons. First of all, the binding forces are summed over a large number of interacting atoms. Secondly, since drugs and receptors "fit" in three-dimensional space, the critical role of interatomic distances allows the receptor to discriminate between the specific drug and a related compound having a different conformation. Finally, the relatively weak van der Waals bond allows for reversible interactions and drug effects of short duration.

DRUG-RECEPTOR INTERACTIONS

The basic requirement for a receptor is the ability to discriminate signal from noise.[27] To receive the signal the receptor must have an affinity for the drug. At the same time, receptors must have specificity, in other words, an appropriately low affinity for less active drugs.

Affinity is quantitated by studying the dose-response relationship between a drug and a receptor, using one of several methods. In systems in which only dose and response can be determined, the log dose is plotted against the response (Fig. 2-1). In such studies, the dose of a drug that produces a response which is 50% of the maximum is referred to as ED_{50}.

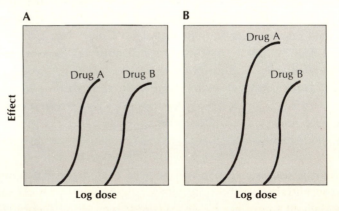

FIG. 2-1. Log dose-response curves illustrating difference between potency and efficacy. **A,** Drug *A* is much more potent than drug *B,* but both have the same maximal effect. **B,** Drug *A* is not only more potent but also has a greater efficacy. It produces a higher peak effect than drug *B.*

With newer methods, usually requiring radioactive drugs, the relationships between free and specifically bound drugs can be quantitated, and much additional useful information can be obtained.

The binding of a drug (D) and a receptor (R) can be represented as follows:

$$[D] + [R] \xrightarrow{k_1} [DR]$$

The rate at which they combine is described by the rate constant k_1. Since most drug-receptor interactions are reversible, it is also true that

$$[DR] \xrightarrow{k_2} [D] + [R]$$

At equilibrium the rates of the forward and backward reactions are equal and

$$k_1[D][R] = k_2[DR]$$

The concept of K_d emerges if the above equation is rewritten:

$$\frac{[D][R]}{[DR]} = \frac{k_2}{k_1} = K_d$$

K_d is the equilibrium dissociation constant, and it is related to affinity. In the above equation, if half of the receptors are combined with a drug, the concentrations of R and DR are equal and will be canceled. It follows then that under those conditions $K_d = D$. This means that the free concentration of drug necessary to saturate 50% of the receptors equals the K_d. If this concentration is low, affinity is high.

Affinity and intrinsic activity

In the model described before, the magnitude of a response is a function of the number of receptors occupied. *Affinity* is the tendency of a drug to form a combination with the receptor.

It is known, however, that there are *partial agonists*, which act on the same receptor as a full agonist but which cannot produce the same maximal effect regardless of concentration. Also, a drug may not only have a higher affinity than another compound but also may produce a higher maximal effect (Fig. 2-1). Therefore, the response not only is a function of the concentration of the drug-receptor complex, but also depends on what is termed *intrinsic activity*[2] or efficacy.[22] This concept may be defined as the capacity to stimulate for a given receptor occupancy.

An agonist is a drug that has affinity for a receptor and that has intrinsic activity. A competitive antagonist has affinity for the receptor but lacks significant intrinsic activity.

Rate models of drug action

In the foregoing discussion it has been implied that response to a drug is proportional to the concentration of the drug-receptor complex. There are some observations that are difficult to explain by this receptor occupation theory. For example, some drugs stimulate first and then act as antagonists. Nicotine does this in ganglionic transmission.

It is conceivable[8] that the response to a drug is not dependent on the *concentration* of the drug receptor complex but on the *rate* of drug-receptor combinations. Furthermore, the receptor and the rate constants may be altered by the initial drug action. Initial stimulation followed by block as in the case of nicotine would be explained by such alterations of the receptor and the rate constants for association and dissociation.

Drugs that do not act on specific receptors

The biological activity of anesthetics, hypnotics, and alcohol depends not on drug-receptor interactions but on the *relative saturation* at some cellular phase (Ferguson's principle).[7] Whenever chemically unrelated drugs give the same effect at the same relative saturation, they are unlikely to act on specific receptors. It is more probable that by reaching a certain level of saturation at some cellular site (the so-called biophase) they hinder some metabolic function.[7]

Receptor regulation

The response to drugs depends on the number of the receptors. This number may be affected by the continued presence of the drug. Generally, receptors that activate adenyl cyclase, α receptors for catecholamines, and insulin receptors tend to decrease in number or undergo down-regulation with continued administration of the drugs. This phenomenon is sometimes referred to as *desensitization* or *tachyphylaxis*. Although there is great interest in this form of down-regulation, it should be pointed out that most drugs can be administered repeatedly or continuously over periods of hours without much densensitization occurring. Furthermore, only agonists produce homologous down-regulation.

There are a few examples of increased receptor numbers produced by certain hormones. For example, the thyroid hormone increases the number of β receptors in the myocardium, which fits with the clinical impression of an increased sensitivity of hyperthyroid individuals to catecholamines.

Receptor-related diseases

There is great interest in the role of receptor changes in certain diseases. In myasthenia gravis, practically all patients have antibodies to acetylcholine receptors present in the motor end-plate. In some forms of insulin-resistant diabetes, there are antibodies to insulin receptors. Other interesting examples of receptor-related diseases are testicular feminization (androgen insensitivity), familial hypercholesterolemia (decrease in "receptors" for low density lipoproteins), and a number of endocrine diseases that may depend on receptor insensitivity rather than on hormonal deficiencies.

QUANTITATIVE ASPECTS OF DRUG POTENCY AND EFFICACY

A drug is said to be potent when it has great biological activity per unit weight. When the dose of a drug is plotted on a logarithmic scale against a measured effect, a sigmoid curve is obtained, usually referred to as a log *dose-response* curve. Any point on such a curve could indicate the potency of a drug, but for comparative purposes, the dose that gives 50% of the total or maximal effect is most often selected. This dose is the ED_{50}, or effective dose$_{50}$. In Fig. 2-1, drugs A and B produced parallel dose-response curves. The ED_{50} of drug B may be 10 times greater than that of drug A. As a consequence, it may be said that drug A is 10 times as potent as drug B. *It is essential to realize that potencies are compared on the basis of doses that produce the same effect and not by comparing the magnitudes of effects elicited by the same dose.*

A clinically important example of a potency relationship very similar to that given in Fig. 2-1, *A*, is given by the diuretic drugs chlorothiazide and hydrochlorothiazide. One hundred milligrams of hydrochlorothiazide given orally to a patient promotes a significant increase in the urinary output of sodium chloride. It takes about 1 g of chlorothiazide to achieve the same effect. As a consequence, one may say that hydrochlorothiazide is 10 times as potent as chlorothiazide.

Fig. 2-1, *B*, illustrates another property of a drug that should not be confused with potency. Drug A is not only 10 times as potent as drug B, but it also has a higher maximum or "ceiling" of activity. The maximum effect is commonly referred to as *efficacy*, or *power*, and is illustrated by the following example.

Chlorothiazide as well as hydrochlorothiazide has a definite "ceiling" of activity. Two grams of chlorothiazide will exert the maximal effect. Furosemide, however, has not only greater potency than chlorothiazide but also a higher ceiling. It can cause the excretion of a larger percentage of the total amount of sodium chloride filtered by the glomeruli. Consequently, furosemide not only is more *potent* than chlorothiazide but also has greater *efficacy*, or power.

Potency and efficacy are often confused in medical terminology. Potency alone is an overrated advantage in therapeutics. If drug A is 10 times as potent as drug B but has no other virtues, this means only that the patient will take smaller tablets. Pharmaceutical companies often emphasize that a drug is more potent than some other drug. This in itself has little importance to the physician. On the other hand, if the drug has a greater efficacy, it may accomplish things that are unattainable with a less efficacious compound.

Parallel shifts in the log dose-response curve may be attributed to varying affinities, whereas variations in the maximal height of the curves are expressions of varying intrinsic activities, or efficacies. In Fig. 2-1, *B*, drug B is less potent than drug A and has less affinity for the receptor. The relative actions of chlorothiazide, hydrochlorothiazide, and furosemide discussed previously are examples of the differences between potency and efficacy.

An agonist is a drug that has affinity and efficacy. It interacts with receptors and elicits a response. Acetylcholine is a good example of an agonist. However, if a log dose-response curve to acetylcholine is obtained in the presence of atropine (an antagonist), it will be found that atropine has no effects of its own but that it shifts the log dose-response curve of acetylcholine to the right.

Atropine is viewed as competing with acetylcholine for the same receptors; in other words, the antagonist has affinity but lacks efficacy. This is an example of *competitive* or *surmountable* antagonism. The key feature of this kind of antagonism

GRAPHIC PRESENTATION OF AFFINITY, INTRINSIC ACTIVITY, AND EFFICACY

AGONIST, ANTAGONIST, AND PARTIAL AGONIST

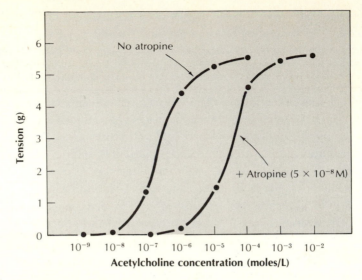

FIG. 2-2. Effect of acetylcholine on tension development of guinea pig ileum. Atropine, a competitive antagonist, caused a parallel shift of the log dose-response curve.

is *parallel displacement of the log dose-response curve to the right without a shift in the maximum* (Fig. 2-2).

Somewhere between pure agonists and pure antagonists are the drugs termed partial agonists. They have affinity and some efficacy but may antagonize the action of other drugs that have a higher efficacy.

NONCOMPETITIVE ANTAGONISM
In the case of atropine and acetylcholine the antagonist and agonist were competing for the same receptor, as evidenced by the parallel shift in the log dose-response curve without a shift in the maximum. In some instances the antagonist may combine irreversibly with the receptor or a portion of the receptor, in which case increasing the concentration of the agonist will never fully overcome the inhibition. The net effect will be a decrease in the maximum height of the log dose-response curve, which is interpreted to reflect a decrease in the number of drug-receptor complexes.

QUANTITATION OF DRUG ANTAGONISM
The potency of an antagonist may be measured by several methods. One of the earliest, the measurement of pA2, was introduced by Schild.[20] The value of pA2 is the negative logarithm of the concentration of an antagonist, which necessitates doubling the concentration of the agonist to obtain the same response as in the absence of the antagonist. For example, the pA2 for diphenhydramine as determined on histamine contractions of the guinea pig ileum is approximately 8. This means that a concentration of 10^{-8} M diphenhydramine necessitates the doubling of the concentration of histamine in order to obtain the same concentration.

Problem 2-1. How is the potency of an antagonist related to its pA2 value? Clearly, the higher the pA2, the more potent the antagonist. If instead of measuring pA2 the value of pA10 is measured, would it be greater or smaller than the pA2?

For other methods of expressing drug antagonism, the reader should consult the review of Gaddum.[9]

Problem 2-2. What is the role of receptors in causing the opposite effects of the same drug in different organs? For example, acetylcholine relaxes vascular smooth muscle but causes contraction of intestinal or bronchial smooth muscle. Are the receptors different? This is not likely since the same antagonist, atropine, blocks all of these effects. It seems that the drug-receptor interaction only initiates or triggers a series of events, the final outcome of which is built into the system beyond the receptor.

REFERENCES

1 Albert, A.: Selective toxicity, ed. 3, New York, 1965, John Wiley & Sons, Inc.

2 Ariëns, E. J.: Molecular pharmacology, the mode of action of biologically active compounds, vol. 1, New York, 1964, Academic Press, Inc.

3 Burger, A., and Parulkar, A. P.: Relationship between chemical structure and biological activity, Annu. Rev. Pharmacol. 6:19, 1966.

4 Clark, A. J.: General pharmacology. In Heffter, A., editor: Handbunch der experimentellen Pharmakologie, vol. 4, Berlin, Springer-Verlag.

5 Croxatto, R., and Huidobro, F.: Fundamental basis of the specificity of pressor and depressor amines in their vascular effects, Arch. Int. Pharmacodyn. 106:207, 1956.

6 Cuatrecasas, P.: Membrane receptors, Annu. Rev. Biochem. 43:169, 1974.

7 Ferguson, J.: Use of chemical potentials as indices of toxicity, Proc. R. Soc. Biol. 127:387, 1939.

8 Furchgott, R. F.: Receptor mechanisms, Annu. Rev. Pharmacol. 4:21, 1964.

9 Gaddum, J. H.: Drug antagonism, Pharmacol. Rev. 9:211, 1957.

10 Gourley, D. R. H.: Basic mechanisms of drug action, Fortschr. Arzneimittelforsch. 7:11, 1964.

11 Katz, B.: Microphysiology of the neuromuscular junction. The chemoreceptor function of the motor end-plate, Bull. Johns Hopkins Hosp. 102:296, 1958.

12 Langley, J. N.: On the mutual antagonism of atropin and pilocarpin, having especial reference to their relations in the sub-maxillary gland of the cat, J. Physiol. 1:339, 1878.

13 Mautner, H. G.: The molecular basis of drug action, Pharmacol. Rev. 19:107, 1967.

14 Michaelis, L., and Menten, M. L.: Die Kinetik der Invertinwirkung, Biochem. Z. 49:333, 1913.

15 Paton, W. D. M.: A theory of drug action based on the rate of drug-receptor combination, Proc. R. Soc. Biol. 154:21, 1961.

16 Paton, W. D. M.: Receptors as defined by their pharmacological properties. In Porter, R., and O'Connor, M., editors: Molecular properties of drug receptors, Ciba Foundation Symposium, London, 1970, J. & A. Churchill.

17 Pauling, L.: A molecular theory of general anesthesia, Science 134:15, 1961.

18 Pert, C. B., and Snyder, S. H.: Opiate receptor: demonstration in nervous tissue, Science 179:1011, 1973.

19 Porter, C. G., and Stone, C. A.: Biochemical mechanisms of drug action, Annu. Rev. Pharmacol. 7:15, 1967.

20 Schild, H. O.: pA, a new scale for the measurement of drug antagonism, Br. J. Pharmacol. Chemother. 2:189, 1947.

21 Schild, H. O.: Introduction. In de Jonge, H., editor: Quantitative methods in pharmacology, Amsterdam, 1961, North-Holland Publishing Co.

22 Stephenson, R. P.: A modification of receptor theory, Br. J. Pharmacol. 11:379, 1956.

23 Triggle, D. J.: Chemical aspects of the autonomic nervous system, New York, 1965, Academic Press, Inc.

24 Waud, D. R.: Pharmacological receptors, Pharmacol. Rev. 20:49, 1968.

REVIEWS

25 Albert, A.: Relations between molecular structure and biological activity: stages in the evolution of current concepts, Annu. Rev. Pharmacol. 11:13, 1971.

26 Ariëns, E. J., and Beld, A. J.: The receptor concept in evolution, Biochem. Pharmacol. 26:913, 1977.

27 Baxter, J. D., and Funder, J. W.: Hormone receptors, N. Engl. J. Med. 301:1149, 1979.

28 Burgen, A. S. V.: Receptor mechanisms, Annu. Rev. Pharmacol. 10:7, 1970.

29 Flier, J. S., Kahn, R., and Roth, J.: Receptors, antireceptor antibodies and mechanisms of in-

sulin resistance, N. Engl. J. Med. **300**:413, 1979.

30 Hurwitz, L., and Suria, A.: The link between agonist action and the response in smooth muscle, Annu. Rev. Pharmacol. **11**:303, 1971.

31 Jacobs, S., and Cuatrecasas, P.: Cell receptors in disease, N. Engl. J. Med. **297**:1383, 1977.

32 Lefkowitz, R. J.: Direct binding of adrenergic receptors: biochemical, physiologic, and clinical implications, Ann. Intern. Med. **91**:450, 1979.

33 Overstreet, D. H., and Yamamura, H. I.: Receptor alterations and drug tolerance, Life Sci. **25**:1865, 1979.

34 Porter, R., and O'Connor, M., editors: Molecular properties of drug receptors, Ciba Foundation Symposium, London, 1970, J. & A. Churchill.

35 Snyder, S. H.: Receptors, neurotransmitters and drug responses, N. Engl. J. Med. **300**:465, 1979.

CHAPTER 3

Pharmacokinetic principles in the use of drugs

Pharmacokinetics is the study of the time course of absorption, distribution, metabolism, and excretion of drugs and their metabolites in the intact organism. For the complexities of pharmacokinetics to be understood, it is necessary to appreciate present concepts concerning the passage of drugs across body membranes.

In order for a drug to reach its site of action it must pass across various body membranes. This can be seen in Fig. 3-1, which depicts the general handling of a drug in the body. Absorption, capillary transfer, penetration into cells, and excretion are basic examples of the passage of drugs across body membranes.

PASSAGE OF DRUGS ACROSS BODY MEMBRANES

Because of its lipoid nature, the cell membrane is highly permeable to lipid-soluble substances. Since the cell is also easily penetrated by water and other small lipid-insoluble substances such as urea, it is postulated that the lipid membrane has pores or channels that allow passage of lipid-insoluble molecules of small dimensions.[32]

In addition to the passive movement of many substances across body membranes, it is necessary to postulate more complex processes for the passage of glucose, amino acids, and some inorganic ions and drug substances. A simplified summary of the various types of passage across body membranes follows:

1. Passive transfer
   a. Simple diffusion
   b. Filtration
2. Specialized transport
   a. Active transport
   b. Facilitated diffusion
   c. Pinocytosis

The essential features of these transfer mechanisms will be described briefly.

Simple diffusion is characterized by the rate of transfer of a substance across a membrane being directly proportional to the concentration gradient on both sides of the membrane. Both lipid-soluble substances and lipid-insoluble molecules of small size may cross body membranes by simple diffusion. *Filtration* is spoken of when a porous membrane allows the bulk flow of a solvent and the substances dissolved in it,

Passive transfer

15

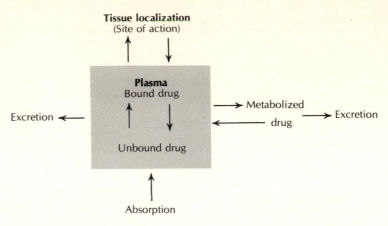

FIG. 3-1. Absorption and fate of a drug. (Modified from Brodie, B. B.: Clin. Pharmacol. Ther. **3:**374, 1962.)

except for those of large size. The glomerular membrane of the kidney is a good example of a filtering membrane.

A special situation exists in the case of partly ionized drugs, since cell membranes are more permeable to the nonionized form of a given drug than to its ionized form because of the greater lipid solubility of the nonionized form. As a consequence, the passage of many drugs into cells and across other membranes becomes a function of the pH of the internal environment and the pK_a of the drug.

The concept of pK_a is derived from the Henderson-Hasselbalch equation. For an acid:

$$pK_a = pH + Log \frac{\text{Molecular concentration of nonionized acid}}{\text{Molecular concentration of ionized acid}}$$

For a base:

$$pK_a = pH + Log \frac{\text{Molecular concentration of ionized base}}{\text{Molecular concentration of nonionized base}}$$

It follows from these equations that, when a substance is half-ionized and half-nonionized at a certain pH, its pK_a is equal to this pH. In other words, a substance is half-ionized at a pH value that is equal to its pK_a.

Although these concepts may seem academic, they have become of great importance in explaining a number of clinically important facts. For example, weak acids such as salicylic acid ($pK_a = 3$) are well absorbed from the stomach, whereas weak bases such as quinine ($pK_a = 8.4$) are not absorbed until they reach the less acidic intestine. The influence of urinary pH on the excretion of salicylic acid and phenobarbital represents another example of the dependence of diffusion on the pK_a of drugs.[34]

The pK_a values for a number of acidic and basic drugs are listed in Table 3-1. It should be remembered that for acidic drugs the lower the pK_a, the stronger the acid, whereas for basic drugs the higher the pK_a, the stronger the base.

TABLE 3-1. pK_a values for some weak acids and bases (at 25° C)

Weak acids	pK_a	Weak bases	pK_a
Salicylic acid	3.00	Reserpine	6.6
Aspirin	3.49	Codeine	7.9
Sulfadiazine	6.48	Quinine	8.4
Barbital	7.91	Procaine	8.8
Boric acid	9.24	Ephedrine	9.36
		Atropine	9.65

TABLE 3-2. Effect of pH on the ionization of salicylic acid (pK_a 3)

pH	Percent nonionized
1	99.0
2	90.9
3	50.0
4	9.09
5	1.00
6	0.10

The relationships between pH, pK_a, and ionization of an acidic drug are illustrated in Table 3-2, using salicylic acid as an example.

Specialized transport

The passage of many substances into cells and across body membranes cannot be explained simply on the basis of diffusion of filtration. For example, compounds may be taken up against a concentration gradient, great selectivity can be shown for compounds of the same size, competitive inhibition can occur among substances handled by the same mechanism, and in some instances metabolic inhibitors can block the transport processes.

To explain these phenomena the existence of specific *carriers* in membranes has been postulated.[37] *Active transport* is spoken of when, in addition to many other criteria, substances are moving against a concentration or electrochemical gradient. *Facilitated diffusion* is a special form of carrier transport that has many of the characteristics of active transport, but the substrate does not move against a concentration gradient. The uptake of glucose by cells is an example of facilitated diffusion. *Pinocytosis* refers to the ability of cells to engulf small droplets. This process may be of some importance in the uptake of large molecules.

PRINCIPLES OF PHARMACO-KINETICS

Studies on drug distribution, absorption, and excretion led to the concept that the body may be treated as if it consisted of different compartments. A drug is transferred from one compartment to another in conformance with first-order kinetics. The simplest model, the "one-compartment model," assumes that after administration drugs are homogeneously distributed throughout the tissues and fluids of

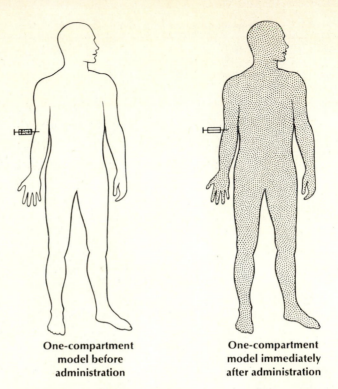

One-compartment
model before
administration

One-compartment
model immediately
after administration

FIG. 3-2. One-compartment model before and after drug administration. (From Dvorchik, B. H., and Vesell, E. S.: Clin. Chem. **22**:868, 1976.)

the body (Figs. 3-1 and 3-2). In this model the *apparent volume of distribution* (V_d) is determined, using the following equation:

$$V_d = \frac{\text{Amount of drug in the body}}{\text{Concentration of drug in plasma}}$$

In determining the apparent volume of distribution, it is not implied that the concentration of the drug in various tissues is the *same* as in plasma. It is assumed, however, that changes in plasma concentrations reflect changes in tissue concentrations. If a drug is concentrated in some tissues, its apparent volume of distribution may be very large, even greater than total body water.

In most instances both the absorption and elimination of drugs take place according to an exponential decay curve (Fig. 3-3). This exponential process follows first-order kinetics; in other words, a constant fraction of the drug is absorbed or eliminated per unit time. The time required for 50% completion of the process is known as the *half-time*, or $t_{1/2}$, which is independent of the concentration of the drug. Measurement of the half-time may be understood by examining Fig. 3-3. It can be calculated that it requires four half-times for the exponential processes to become 94% complete. Thus, it takes more than four half-times for the drug to be completely eliminated.

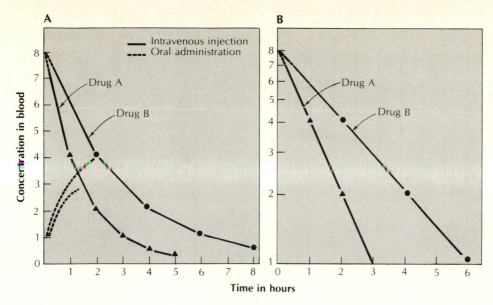

FIG. 3-3. Schematic representation of drug disappearance curves and biological half-life. The y axis is on the arithmetic scale in **A** and on the logarithmic scale in **B**. Drug *A* has a biological half-life of 1 hour. The biological half-life of drug *B* is 2 hours.

In a few instances elimination is a zero-order process, that is, the same quantity of drug is eliminated per unit time. The best example is alcohol, and it is assumed that the saturation of the metabolizing enzymes is responsible for the deviation from first-order kinetics. In other cases, the rate of elimination may be dose related, so that small doses are handled by first-order kinetics, but as the dose is increased half-times become prolonged. Examples of drugs that show dose-related elimination are aspirin and phenytoin.

Two-compartment open model

The single-compartment model just discussed assumes an instantaneous and homogeneous distribution of drugs throughout the body. This is obviously an oversimplification. A *two-compartment open model* describes more adequately the observed changes in the concentration of drugs in the body (Figs. 3-4 and 3-5).[42]

The two-compartment model envisions the existence of a small central compartment and a larger peripheral compartment. Although no specific anatomical spaces are implied, the central compartment usually corresponds to the blood volume and the extracellular fluid volume of highly perfused organs. The peripheral compartment consists of more poorly perfused tissues, such as skin, fat, and muscle.

It is assumed further that drugs enter the central compartment and are eliminated from that compartment, although some reversible transfer occurs to the peripheral compartment that acts as a reservoir.[42]

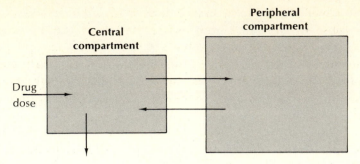

FIG. 3-4. Diagram of two-compartment open model. (Modified from Greenblatt, D. J., and Koch-Weser, J. Reprinted, by permission. From The New England Journal of Medicine **293:**702, 1975.)

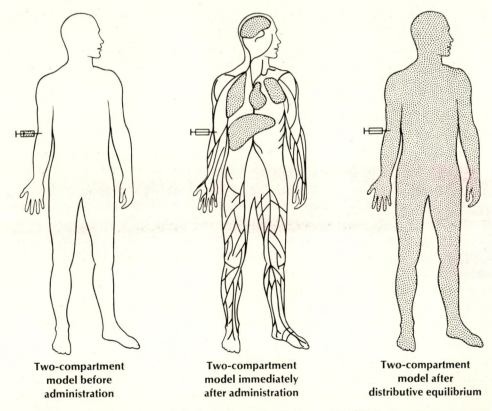

Two-compartment
model before
administration

Two-compartment
model immediately
after administration

Two-compartment
model after
distributive equilibrium

FIG. 3-5. Two-compartment model. (From Dvorchik, B. H., and Vesell, E. S.: Clin. Chem. **22:** 868, 1976.)

ABSORPTION   The process whereby a drug is made available to the fluids of distribution is referred to as absorption. The rate of this process depends on the method of administration, solubility, and other physical properties of the drug.

Drugs are administered by the oral route in many different forms—solutions, suspensions, capsules, and tablets with various coatings. When the drug is not in solution, its rate of absorption will be the net result of the two processes[21]: the process of solution and the absorption process itself. The solution process can be altered by pharmaceutical manipulations, thus influencing the absorption rate, but the absorption process is a basic characteristic of the membranes of the gastrointestinal tract.

In general, the absorption of drugs from the gastrointestinal tract can be explained by simple diffusion across a membrane having the characteristics of a lipoid structure with water-filled pores. Simple diffusion does not account for the uptake of sugars and other nutrients, in which case absorption can only be explained in terms of active mechanisms. A useful principle, derived from experimental data, is that the limiting membrane is permeable to nonionized lipid-soluble forms of drugs and less permeable to the ionized form. This principle has considerable predictive value.

Weak acids such as salicylates and barbiturates are largely nonionized in the acidic gastric contents and are therefore well absorbed from the stomach. Such weak bases as quinine or ephedrine and highly ionized quaternary amines such as tetraethylammonium are not significantly absorbed from the stomach. Alkalinization of gastric contents would be expected to decrease absorption of weak acids from the stomach and increase that of weak bases.

Absorption from the small intestine is similar in principle to that from the stomach, except that the pH of intestinal contents is usually 6.6. Interestingly, drug distribution studies between plasma and small intestinal fluid would indicate a possible pH value of 5.3 for the area just adjacent to the intestinal absorbing membrane. Weakly acidic and weakly basic drugs are well absorbed from the small intestine, but highly ionized acids and bases are not well absorbed. Special mechanisms exist for the absorption of sugars, amino acids, and compounds related to normal nutrients. Some inorganic ions such as sodium and chloride are well absorbed despite the fact that they are in the ionic form.

In the oral cavity the oral mucosa also appears to behave as a lipid pore membrane, and drugs may be absorbed on sublingual administration.[35] Nitroglycerin is usually administered in this manner.

Drug effects on gastric emptying may greatly affect absorption. For example, chloroquine has a much higher LD_{50} when given by mouth to rats than after its direct administration into the intestine. This difference is a consequence of inhibition of gastric emptying by chloroquine.[33]

When injected intravenously, a drug is rapidly distributed in the various compartments of the body.

The rate of absorption following subcutaneous or intramuscular injection depends largely on two factors: solubility of the preparation and blood flow through the area. Suspensions or colloidal preparations are absorbed more slowly than aqueous solu-

Absorption from the gastrointestinal tract

Absorption with parenteral administration

tions. Advantage is taken of this fact in many instances when prolonged absorption is desirable. For example, protamine is added to insulin to form a suspension and thereby decrease the rate of absorption from the subcutaneous depot site. The various injectable penicillin suspensions are good examples of prolonging the action of a therapeutic agent by slowing its absorption.

The blood flow through a tissue has much to do with the speed of absorption of a drug from its site of injection. Absorption from a subcutaneous site may be very slow in the presence of peripheral circulatory failure. This has been observed in the subcutaneous administration of morphine to patients in shock. Similarly, the greater blood flow per unit weight of muscle is responsible for the more rapid absorption of drugs from this tissue than from subcutaneous fat.

Certain practical consequences of these facts may be of real clinical importance. Cooling an area of injection will slow absorption, a desirable effect if an excessive dose has been inadvertently injected or if untoward reactions begin to develop in an unusually susceptible patient. On the other hand, massage of the site of injection will speed up absorption.

Clinical pharmacology of absorption: bioavailability

Drugs used in medicine seem to fall into three categories from the standpoint of absorption. Some are completely absorbed, some are not absorbed significantly, and still others are partially absorbed. Examples of well-absorbed drugs are most sulfonamides, digitoxin, aspirin, and barbiturates. Drugs not absorbed significantly include streptomycin, neomycin, and kanamycin. Examples of partially or variably absorbed drugs are penicillin G, certain digitalis glycosides, and dicumarol.

Drugs that are incompletely and variably absorbed present a problem to the physician, since dosage cannot be used as a guide to adequacy of treatment. In this situation it is helpful to monitor the concentration of the drug in the blood or to carefully follow a characteristic effect of the drug.

The dosage form of the drug has a great influence on absorption. Solutions are absorbed most rapidly and coated tablets most slowly. Enteric-coated tablets are commonly used to provide a sustained level of the drug in the body, but despite the popularity of this dosage form, it cannot be considered a predictable method of administering drugs. There are great individual variations in gastric emptying and rate of dissolution of such preparations. They may even be eliminated unchanged in the feces.

Bioavailability

There is much current interest in observations indicating that various preparations of the same drug administered orally may give different serum concentrations. The term *bioavailability* has been defined as the relative absorption efficiency of a test dosage form relative to a standard oral or intravenous preparation.[12]

The most popular mode of drug administration is the oral route. After oral administration, the area under blood drug concentration–time curve (AUC) reflects the amount of drug that reaches the systemic sampling site. The ratio of $AUC_{oral}/AUC_{intravenous}$ is a measure of the bioavailability of the drug after oral administration.[40]

When administered orally, drugs must pass through the intestinal wall and ordinarily must traverse the liver before reaching the systemic sampling site. Even with complete gastrointestinal absorption a fraction of the dose may not reach the sampling site because of metabolism within gut or liver. This concept is referred to as "first-pass" effect and is important for such drugs as imipramine, lidocaine, meperidine, nortriptyline, phenacetin, propranolol, and others.[40]

"First-pass" effect

Once a drug reaches the plasma, its main fluid of distribution, it must pass across various barriers to reach its final site of action. The first of these barriers is the capillary wall. Through processes of diffusion filtration,[19] most drugs rapidly cross the capillary wall, which has the characteristics of a lipid membrane with water-filled pores. Lipid-soluble substances diffuse through the entire capillary endothelium, whereas lipid-insoluble drugs pass through pores, which represent a fraction of the total capillary surface. The capillary transfer of lipid-insoluble substances is inversely related to molecular size. Large molecules such as dextran are transferred so slowly that they can be used as plasma substitutes.

DISTRIBUTION OF DRUGS IN THE BODY

There are several factors that contribute to the unequal distribution of drugs in the body. Some of these are (1) binding to plasma proteins, (2) cellular binding, (3) concentration in body fat, and (4) the blood-brain barrier.

Factors contributing to the unequal distribution of drugs

The *binding of drugs to plasma proteins* creates a higher concentration of the drug in the blood than in the extracellular fluid. It also provides a depot, since the bound portion of the drug is in equilibrium with the free form. As the unbound fraction is excreted or metabolized, additional amounts are eluted from the protein. Protein binding prolongs the half-life of a drug in the body, since the bound fraction is not filtered through the renal glomeruli and is not exposed to processes of biotransformation until freed.

The protein-bound fraction of a drug is generally inactive until it becomes free. Thus the protein-bound fractions of sulfonamides and penicillins exert no chemotherapeutic effect. The protein responsible for binding is usually albumin, although globulins may be very important in relation to the binding of some hormonal agents and drugs.

The binding capacity of proteins is not unlimited. Once it become saturated, a sudden increase in toxicity may occur with further administration of some drugs. In hypoalbuminemia, toxic manifestations to drugs may appear as a consequence of deficiency in the binding protein.[26]

Drugs may influence the protein binding of other substances or drugs. Thus salicylates decrease the binding of thyroxine to proteins.[38] The binding of bilirubin to albumin may be inhibited by a variety of drugs such as sulfisoxazole or salicylates, the free bilirubin thereby becoming ultrafiltrable.[22]

Binding to plasma protein influences not only the biological activity of drugs but also their distribution. A highly protein-bound drug could displace another and increase its pharmacological activity and toxicity and changes its distribution.[1] Fatal kernicterus has occurred in premature infants who were given sulfisoxazole.[22] The sulfonamide displaced bilirubin from plasma protein and thereby promoted the penetration of the bile pigment into the brains of the infants. Recent studies[1] indicate that sulfinpyrazone can increase the concentration of sulfonamides in the fetus by a similar mechanism of displacement on plasma proteins of the mother. Other examples of drug interactions based on displacement in protein binding will be discussed in Chapter 63.

The *cellular binding* of drugs is usually a result of an affinity for some cellular constituent. The high concentration of the antimalarial drug quinacrine (Atabrine) in the liver or muscle is probably caused by the affinity of this drug for nucleoproteins.

The short duration of action of certain drugs such as the thiobarbiturate intravenous anesthetics has been explained on the basis of the rapid uptake by the brain, followed by a rapid decrease as the concentration of the drug in the blood falls.[7]

The *blood-brain barrier* represents a unique example of unequal distribution of drugs.[4] Even if injected intravenously, many drugs fail to penetrate into the central nervous system, the cerebrospinal fluid, or the aqueous humor as rapidly as into other tissues. Known exceptions to this principle are the neurohypophysis and the area postrema.

The capillaries in the central nervous system (CNS) are enveloped by glial cells, which represent a barrier to many water-soluble compounds, although they are permeable to lipid-soluble substances. Thus quaternary amines penetrate the CNS poorly, but the general anesthetics do so with ease.

A fact of great importance in medicine is the change in the permeability of various barriers produced by inflammation. In the early days of penicillin therapy it was known that the administration of large doses to normal persons failed to produce detectable levels of the antibiotic in the cerebrospinal fluid. It was found, however, that penicillin would penetrate into the spinal fluid of patients with meningitis.

Although many drugs do not penetrate the cerebrospinal fluid well, they can move efficiently in the reverse direction when administered by intracisternal injection.[31] Perhaps they are removed from the cerebrospinal fluid by filtration across the arachnoid villi. In addition, the choroid plexus is capable of pumping out certain substances from the cerebrospinal fluid, for example, penicillin.[44]

The passage of drugs into *milk* may be explained by diffusion of the nonionized, nonprotein-bound fraction. Since most drugs are weak electrolytes, they will appear in varying amount in milk and may exert adverse effects on the breast-fed infant. When taken in larger than average doses by the mother, atropine, bromides, anthraquinones, metronidazole, and ergot alkaloids may cause intoxication in the breast-fed infant. On the other hand, the following drugs appear in milk only in small quantities and are generally of no clinical significance for the infant[13]: morphine, codeine, phenolphthalein, tolbutamide, quinine, and salicylates. Large doses of drugs in general should not be administered to the mother who is breast-feeding her child without considering the possible danger to the infant.[13]

The most important route of excretion for most drugs is the kidney. Many drugs are also excreted into bile, but they are then usually recycled through the intestine, making this route quantitatively unimportant. Excretion of drugs into milk may have some significance for the breast-fed child[13] but is not an important avenue of excretion for the mother. Elimination of drugs through the lungs, salivary and sweat glands, and feces is important only in special cases to be discussed under individual drugs.

Two major mechanisms are involved in the renal handling of drugs: glomerular filtration with variable tubular reabsorption and tubular secretion. The half-life of a drug in the body will be influenced also by such extrarenal factors as plasma protein binding, the existence of tissue depots and, most importantly, by the rate of drug metabolism.

The usual situation is that the drug is filtered through the glomeruli and partially reabsorbed by the tubules. Since water is reabsorbed to a much greater extent than are most drugs, the concentration of drugs in the urine is most frequently greater than in plasma.

A study of the excretion of weak electrolytes has revealed an interesting connection between the pH of urine and renal handling of these drugs.[11,19] Generally, drugs that are bases are excreted to a greater extent if the urine is acid, whereas acid compounds are excreted more favorably if the urine is alkaline. The magnitude of this pH dependence is influenced also by the dissociation constant of a given drug. To explain these results it has been postulated that the undissociated fraction is reabsorbed more readily than the ionic form of a drug. This thesis is favored by the known lipid solubility of undissociated electrolytes.[31]

A practical application of this knowledge has been proposed in the treatment of phenobarbital poisoning.[34] Since phenobarbital is a weak acid having a pK_a of 7.3, its dissociation is greatly influenced by changes in pH at levels obtainable in mammalian urine. Alkalinization of the urine by the administration of sodium bicarbonate causes a significant increase in the excretion of phenobarbital.

Since urine is normally acid, the excretion of weakly acid drugs by renal handling alone would require a very long time. Fortunately, drug metabolism tends to transform these into stronger acids, thereby increasing the percentage of the ionic forms and hindering their tubular resorption.

In addition to glomerular filtration with passive tubular reabsorption, the renal tubule can actively secrete organic anions and cations. Examples of organic anions are aminohippurate sodium, iodopyracet (Diodrast), phenol red, and penicillin; examples of organic cations are tetraethylammonium, mepiperphenidol (Darstine), and N-methylnicotinamide. These active secretory processes may also handle other anions and cations such as salicylic acid, quinine, and tolazoline (Priscoline).[27] Competition for active tubular secretion exists among the various anions and cations.

Drugs that, in addition to undergoing glomerular filtration, are also secreted by the tubules, such as penicillins, have a very short half-life. Efforts have been made to inhibit the process of tubular secretion by such drugs as probenecid, which

EXCRETION OF DRUGS

was specifically developed for this purpose. Usually, however, it is simpler to prolong the half-life of drugs by slowing their absorption. This is the reason for the development of many penicillin preparations that are absorbed slowly following intramuscular injection.

DRUG DISAPPEARANCE CURVES

The final net effect of absorption, excretion, distribution, and drug metabolism can be described in the form of drug disappearance curves, using blood or tissue concentration data.

A careful examination of Fig. 3-3 and most other drug disappearance studies indicates that they follow an *exponential decay* curve.

Nonlinear pharmacokinetics and interindividual variations

Many drug disappearance curves are not as smooth as the hypothetical ones shown in Fig. 3-3. There are several reasons for nonlinearity. The limited capacity of drug-metabolizing enzymes may lead to increased half-times with increasing doses or plasma concentrations. For example, increasing the dose of aspirin from 0.5 to 1.0 g every 8 hours may delay the steady state from 2 days to 1 week.[15]

Interindividual variations may also be considerable.[41] Drugs such as desipramine, dicumarol, and phenylbutazone may vary greatly in regard to half-life or steady state plasma concentrations, although the patients are receiving the same dosage regimen.[41]

Implications of exponential drug disappearance curve

The frequency of drug administration to patients is often dependent on the biological half-life of the drug. This is always the case when a sustained blood level of the drug is desirable. For example, the sulfonamides should be used in such a manner that a sustained blood level is achieved. The frequency with which various members of the sulfonamide group of drugs is administered depends then on the biological half-life. The $t_{1/2}$ of sulfisoxazole in man is 8 hours, whereas that of sulfamethoxypyridazine is 34 hours. It is not unexpected, then, that the former is administered orally every 4 hours and the latter every 24 hours. The delay in absorption after oral administration is the main reason why these drugs are administered more frequently than could be predicted from their half-life.

Occasionally the physician wishes to obtain a steadily rising blood or tissue level of a drug until a certain effect is achieved. Quinidine is sometimes given orally every hour for several doses until atrial fibrillation stops. In this case the physician deliberately creates drug cumulation by giving quinidine more frequently than would be justified on the basis of its $t_{1/2}$.

Failure to appreciate the exponential nature of drug disappearance can lead to erroneous ideas in therapeutics. For example, if a drug has a short duration of action, doubling the dose will not double the duration of its effect.

DOSAGE SCHEDULES AND PHARMACO-KINETICS

Drugs may be administered in a single dose or in a repetitive fashion. Fig. 3-6 shows a drug concentration curve following a single intravenous administration. From such a curve it is possible to calculate the apparent volume of distribution, since the total amount of drug is known and blood concentration can be extrapolated

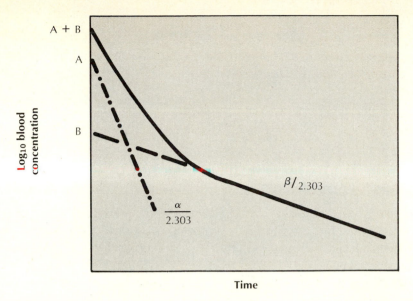

FIG. 3-6. Logarithm of drug concentration in blood plotted against time (solid line) after intravenous administration of a drug whose disposition can be described by a two-compartment model. Broken line (----) represents extrapolation of terminal *(B)* phase. The line · -· - · - was obtained by method of residuals. (From Dvorchik, B. H., and Vesell, E. S.: Clin. Chem. **22:** 868, 1976.)

to zero time. The ratio of these figures gives the apparent volume of distribution.

If the drug is administered orally in a single dose, the curve will have an ascending limb, a peak, and a descending limb. Variations in absorption and elimination may greatly influence the concentration curve reflecting changes in the peak effect, the time required for achieving the peak effect, and the duration of action of the drug.

Repetitive dosing

If a drug is given repetitively at intervals shorter than the time necessary for its complete elimination, it will accumulate in the body. As stated before, more than four half-times are required for complete clearance. A typical plot of the concentration of a drug in blood after repetitive oral administration of equal doses at equal time intervals is depicted in Fig. 3-7. It may be seen that the drug concentration rises until it reaches a *plateau*. In addition the curve shows *fluctuations*.

The plateau concentration is reached in little more than four half-times. More precisely, in four half-times a concentration equal to 94% of the maximum is reached. The time required to reach the plateau depends *only* on the elimination half-time. The maximal concentration of the drug at the plateau level depends on the maintenance dose and the elimination half-time. The maintenance dose is the amount of drug administered at each dosage interval.

It is useful to compare the maximal drug concentration reached after a single dose with that obtained after repetitive dosage. If a drug is administered at intervals equal to its elimination half-time, its concentration at the plateau will be about 1.5

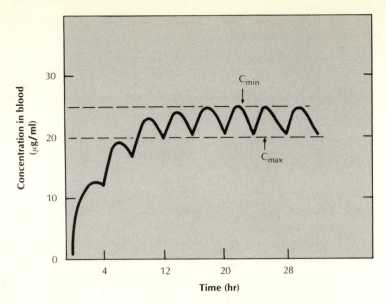

FIG. 3-7. Plot of concentration of a drug in blood after repetitive oral administration of equal doses at equal time intervals. (From Dvorchik, B. H., and Vesell, E. S.: Clin. Chem. **22:**868, 1976.)

times that reached after a single dose. Many drugs are administered at intervals shorter than their elimination half-time. If a drug has a half-time of 7 days and it is administered once a day, it will take more than 28 days (four half-times) to reach a plateau concentration.

The fluctuations in drug concentration depend on the maintenance dose, the dose interval, and the elimination half-time. Frequent administration of a drug tends to minimize fluctuations in the drug concentration, since the ratio of dosage interval/half-time is decreased.

As shown in Fig. 3-7 repetitive administration of equal doses of a drug will produce a desired plateau concentration, which may require many hours or days, depending on the elimination half-time. In many clinical situations, the physician does not consider such a long wait desirable and administers an *initial loading dose*, followed by a maintenance dose. This is usually done with digitalis glycosides, which have a long half-time of elimination. In this case, the initial loading dose is larger than the maintenance doses.

The importance of fluctuations depends on the drug and on the clinical situation. With some drugs, such as penicillin, large fluctuations are quite acceptable, whereas with the sulfonamides sustained blood levels are necessary to achieve a therapeutic objective. Impaired renal function has an important effect on dosage of drugs that are cleared by the kidney. In this situation, either the dose must be decreased or the dose interval must be increased with corresponding changes in drug concentrations.

Total body clearance of a drug, which results from all processes of elimination, may be determined by the following equation:

Total body clearance

$$\text{Clearance} = (V_c)(k_e) = \text{Dose/AUC}$$

(where V_c is the apparent volume of distribution, k_e is the rate constant for the overall elimination of drug from the body, and AUC is the area under the blood concentration curve)

Problem 3-1. A sleeping medication has a half-life of 1 hour. It is administered in a dose of 100 mg, and the patient wakes up when only 12.5 mg remain in the body. How many hours will the patient sleep? If 200 mg of the same drug is administered, how much longer will the patient sleep? The answer can be found by examining Fig. 3-3. Doubling the dose simply adds one half-life to the duration of sleep.

In general, if a drug has a short duration of action, the following methods are available for prolonging its action:

1. Frequent administration. Most sulfonamides are administered every 4 hours.
2. Slowing absorption. Enteric coating and other pharmaceutical maneuvers can accomplish this.
3. Interfering with renal excretion. Probenecid blocks the excretion of penicillin.
4. Inhibiting drug metabolism. Allopurinol was originally developed for blocking the metabolic degradation of mercaptopurine.

REFERENCES

1 Anton, A. H., and Rodriguez, R. E.: Drug induced change in the distribution of sulfonamides in the mother rat and its fetus, Science **180**:974, 1973.
2 Bakay, L.: The blood-brain barrier, Springfield, Ill., 1956, Charles C Thomas, Publisher.
3 Barlow, C. F.: Clinical aspects of the blood-brain barrier, Annu. Rev. Med. **15**:187, 1964.
4 Brodie, B. B., and Hogben, C. A. M.: Some physicochemical factors in drug action, J. Pharm. Pharmacol. **9**:345, 1957.
5 Cserr, H. F.: Blood-brain barrier in vertebrates, Fed. Proc. **26**:1024, 1967.
6 Doluisio, J. T., and Swintosky, J. V.: Drug partitioning. III. Kinetics of drug transfer in an in vitro model for drug absorption, J. Pharm. Sci. **54**:1594, 1965.
7 Goldstein, A., and Aronow, L.: The duration of action of thiopental and pentobarbital, J. Pharmacol. Exp. Ther. **128**:1, 1960.
8 Gosselin, R. E.: Kinetics of pinocytosis, Fed. Proc. **26**:987, 1967.
9 Gutman, A. B., Yü, T. F., and Sirota, J. H.: A study, by simultaneous clearance techniques, of salicylate excretion in man. Effect of alkalinization of the urine by bicarbonate administration: effect of probenecid, J. Clin. Invest. **34**:711, 1955.
10 Hogben, C. A. M., Schanker, L. S., Tocco, D. J., and Brodie, B. B.: Absorption of drugs from the stomach. II. The human, J. Pharmacol. Exp. Ther. **120**:540, 1957.
11 Hogben, C. A. M., Tocco, D. J., Brodie, B. B., and Schanker, L. S.: On the mechanism of intestinal absorption of drugs, J. Pharmacol. Exp. Ther. **125**:275, 1959.
12 Huffman, D. H., and Azarnoff, D. L.: Absorption of orally given digoxin preparations, J.A.M.A. **222**:957, 1972.
13 Knowles, J. A.: Excretion of drugs in milk—a review, J. Pediatr. **66**:1068, 1965.
14 Levy, G.: Dose dependent effect in pharmacokinetics. In Tedeschi, D. H., and Tedeschi, R. E., editors: Importance of fundamental principles in drug evaluation, New York, 1968, Raven Press.
15 Levy, G., and Tsuchiya, T.: Salicylate accumulation kinetics in man, N. Engl. J. Med. **287**:430, 1972.
16 Mark, L. C., Kayden, H. J., Steele, J. M., Cooper, J. R., Berlin, I., Rovenstine, E. A., and Brodie, B. B.: The physiological disposi-

tion and cardiac effects of procaine amide, J. Pharmacol. Exp. Ther. **102:**5, 1951.

17 Mayer, S. E., Maickel, R. P., and Brodie, B. B.: Kinetics of penetration of drugs and other foreign compounds into cerebrospinal fluid and brain, J. Pharmacol. Exp. Ther. **127:**205, 1959.

18 Mayer, S. E., Maickel, R. P., and Brodie, B. B.: Disappearance of various drugs from the cerebrospinal fluid, J. Pharmacol. Exp. Ther. **128:**41, 1960.

19 Milne, M. D., Scribner, B. H., and Crawford, M. A.: Non-ionic diffusion and excretion of weak acids and bases, Am. J. Med. **24:**709, 1958.

20 Nelson, E.: Kinetics of drug absorption, distribution, metabolism and excretion, J. Pharm. Sci. **50:**181, 1961.

21 Nelson, E.: Physicochemical and pharmaceutic properties of drugs that influence the results of clinical trials, Clin. Pharmacol. Ther. **3:**673, 1962.

22 Odell, G. B.: Studies in kernicterus. I. The protein-binding of bilirubin, J. Clin. Invest. **38:**823, 1959.

23 Orloff, J., and Berliner, R. W.: The mechanism of the excretion of ammonia in the dog, J. Clin. Invest. **35:**223, 1957.

24 Overton, E.: Beiträge zur allgemeinen Muskelund Nervenphysiologie, Pflügers Arch. Ges. Physiol. **92:**115, 1902.

25 Pappenheimer, J. R., Renkin, E. M., and Borrero, L. M.: Filtration, diffusion and molecular sieving through peripheral capillary membrane: contribution to pore theory of capillary permeability, Am. J. Physiol. **167:**13, 1951.

26 Petermann, M. L.: Plasma protein abnormalities in cancer, Med. Clin. North Am. **45:**537, 1961.

27 Peters, L.: Renal tubular excretion of organic bases, Pharmacol. Rev. **12:**1, 1960.

28 Rall, D. P.: Comparative pharmacology and cerebrospinal fluid, Fed. Proc. **26:**1020, 1967.

29 Renkin, E. M., and Pappenheimer, J. R.: Wasserdurchlässigkeit und Permeabilität der Capillarwände, Ergebn. Physiol. **49:**59, 1957.

30 Robertson, J. D.: The ultrastructure of cell membranes and their derivatives, Biochem. Soc. Symp. **16:**3, 1959.

31 Schanker, L. S.: Passage of drugs across body membranes, Pharmacol. Rev. **14:**501, 1962.

32 Solomon, A. K.: The permeability of red cells to water and ions, Ann. N.Y. Acad. Sci. **75:**175, 1958.

33 Varga, F.: Intestinal absorption of chloroquine in rats, Arch. Int. Pharmacodyn. Ther. **163:**38, 1966.

34 Wadell, W. J., and Butler, T. C.: The distribution and excretion of phenobarbital, J. Clin. Invest. **36:**1217, 1957.

35 Walton, R. P.: Sublingual administration of drugs, J.A.M.A. **124:**138, 1944.

36 Weiner, I. M.: Mechanisms of drug absorption and excretion, Annu. Rev. Pharmacol. **7:**39, 1967.

37 Willbrandt, W., and Rosenburg, T.: The concept of carrier transport and its corolarry in pharmacology, Pharmacol Rev. **13:**109, 1961.

38 Wolff, J., Standaert, M. E., and Rall, J. E.: Thyroxine displacement from serum proteins and depressions of serum protein-bound iodine by certain drugs, J. Clin. Invest. **40:**1373, 1961.

REVIEWS

39 Bennett, W. M., Singer, I., and Coggins, C. H.: A practical guide to drug usage in adult patients with impaired renal function, J.A.M.A. **214:**1468, 1970.

40 Dvorchik, B. H., and Vesell, E. S.: Pharmacokinetic interpretation of data gathered during therapeutic drug monitoring, Clin. Chem. **22:**868, 1976.

41 Gibaldi, M., and Levy, G.: Pharmacokinetics in clinical practice, J.A.M.A. **235:**1864 and 1987, 1976.

42 Greenblatt, D. J., and Koch-Weser, J.: Clinical pharmacokinetics, N. Engl. J. Med. 702 and 964, 1975.

43 LaDu, B. N., Mandel, H. G., and Way, E. L.: Fundamentals of drug metabolism and drug disposition, Baltimore, 1971, The Williams & Wilkins Co.

44 Levine, R. R.: Pharmacology: drug actions and reactions, Boston, 1973, Little Brown & Co.

45 Ther, L., and Winne, D.: Drug absorption, Annu. Rev. Pharmacol. **11:**57, 1971.

CHAPTER 4

Drug metabolism and enzyme induction

If the body depended solely on excretory mechanisms for ridding itself of drugs, lipid-soluble compounds would be retained almost indefinitely (p. 25). Drug metabolism generally results in the formation of more water-soluble metabolites that are not well reabsorbed by the renal tubules and are efficiently excreted (Fig. 4-1).

Drug metabolism varies greatly in different species and in individuals of the same species. For example, in humans the effect of a single therapeutic dose of meperidine lasts 3 to 4 hours, but the drug has very transient effects in dogs. This is understandable, since meperidine is metabolized in humans at a rate of 20% per hour, in contrast with 90% per hour in dogs.[55]

DRUG METABOLISM Chemical reactions in drug metabolism

The chemical reactions involved in drug metabolism or *biotransformation* are classified as microsomal oxidations, nonmicrosomal oxidations, reductions, hydrolyses, and conjugations.[24,54,63] The various pathways of drug metabolism will be discussed, with specific examples given. Since microsomal enzymes play a predominant role in biotransformation (Table 4-1), their functions will be summarized first.

Microsomal enzymes

The microsomal enzymes of the liver, which are part of the smooth endoplasmic reticulum, convert many lipid-soluble drugs and foreign compounds into more water-soluble metabolites. Early studies on this system were performed by several investigators.[3,32,63]

The microsomal drug-metabolizing enzymes represent a mixed-function oxidase system. In the presence of nicotinamide adenine dinucleotide phosphate (NADPH) and oxygen the enzyme system transfers one atom of oxygen to the drug while another atom of oxygen is reduced to form water. The general scheme[23] is as follows:

$$NADPH + A + H_2 \rightarrow AH_2 + NADP^+$$

$$AH_2 + O_2 \rightarrow \text{"Active oxygen"}$$

$$\text{"Active oxygen"} + Drug \rightarrow \text{Oxidized drug} + A + H_2O$$

$$NADPH + O_2 + Drug = NADP^+ + H_2O + \text{Oxidized drug}$$

In this general scheme A is cytochrome P_{450}, which is the terminal oxidase for a variety of drug oxidative reactions. Cytochrome P_{450} is so named because this

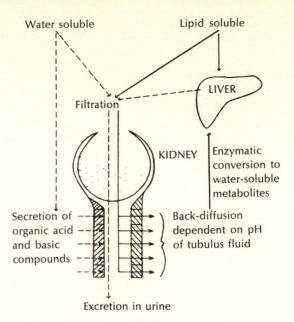

FIG. 4-1. Elimination of drugs. (From Remmer, H.: Am. J. Med. **49:**617, 1970.)

TABLE 4-1. Drug metabolism and enzymes of the endoplasmic reticulum*

Drug metabolism	Enzyme
Oxidations of aliphatic and aromatic groups	Cytochrome P_{450}
Barbiturates	
Diazepoxides	
Phenothiazines	
Meprobamate	
Phenytoin	
Antihistaminics	
Acetophenetidin	
Aminopyrine	
Some synthetic steroids	
Reductions of azo and nitro groups	Flavin enzymes
Hydrolyses of esters and amides	Esterases
Conjugations with glucuronic acid	Transferases
Alcohols	
Phenols	

*Modified from Remmer, H.: Am. J. Med. **49:**617, 1970.

hemoprotein in its reduced form can combine with carbon monoxide, the product having an absorption peak at 450 nm. Other essential enzymes in the reaction include NADPH cytochrome P_{450} reductase, which reduces the oxidized P_{450}.

The reactions catalyzed by the microsomal drug-metabolizing enzymes include hydroxylation of aromatic rings, aliphatic hydroxylations, *N*-dealkylations, *O*-dealkylations, deaminations, sulfoxidations, and *N*-oxidations.

Induction and inhibition of microsomal hydroxylase. Phenobarbital and many other lipid-soluble drugs may cause hypertrophy of the smooth endoplasmic reticulum and an increase in the amount of microsomal hydroxylase.

Premature infants and persons with liver disease may have a deficiency of the microsomal enzymes. Some drugs may also inhibit the drug-metabolizing enzymes.

Hydroxylation of aromatic rings. Acetanilid is changed to p-hydroxyacetanilid, more commonly known as N-acetyl-p-aminophenol. Phenobarbital is changed to the inactive p-hydroxyphenobarbital.

Microsomal oxidations

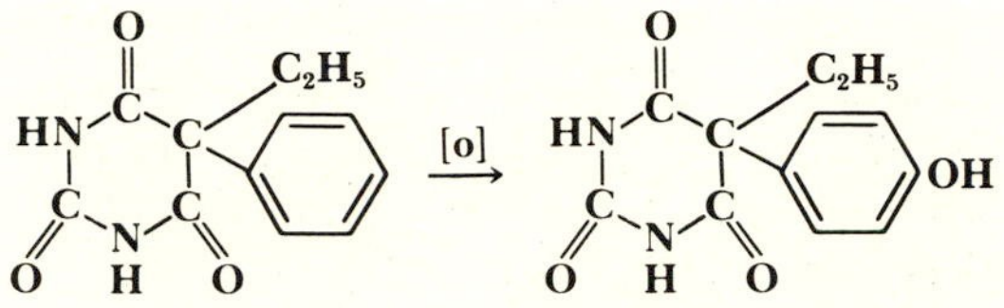

Phenobarbital p-Hydroxyphenobarbital

Side chain oxidation (aliphatic hydroxylation). Pentobarbital is changed to pentobarbital alcohol. Meprobamate is changed to hydroxymeprobamate.

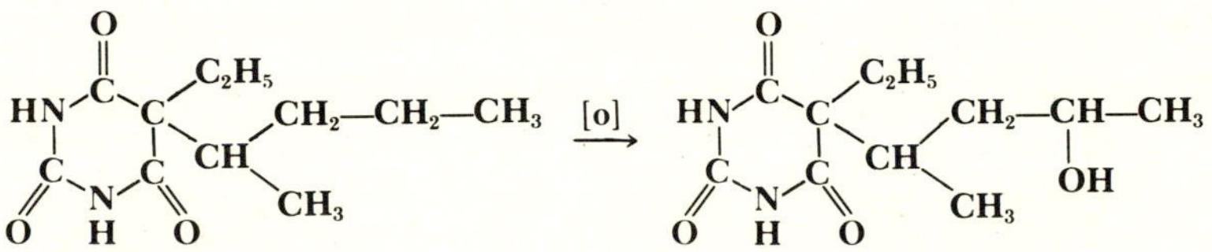

Pentobarbital   Pentobarbital alcohol

N-dealkylation. Mephobarbital is demethylated to phenobarbital.

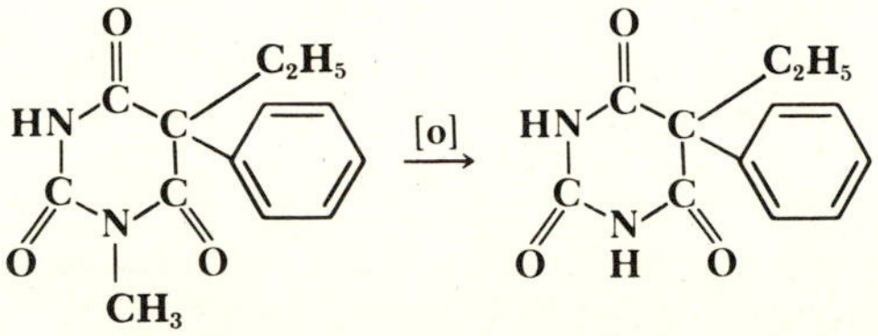

Mephobarbital   Phenobarbital

N-oxidation. Trimethylamine is changed to trimethylamine oxide.

$$(CH_3)_3N \xrightarrow{[o]} (CH_3)_3N = O$$

Trimethylamine   Trimethylamine oxide

Sulfoxidation. Chlorpromazine is changed to chlorpromazine sulfoxide.

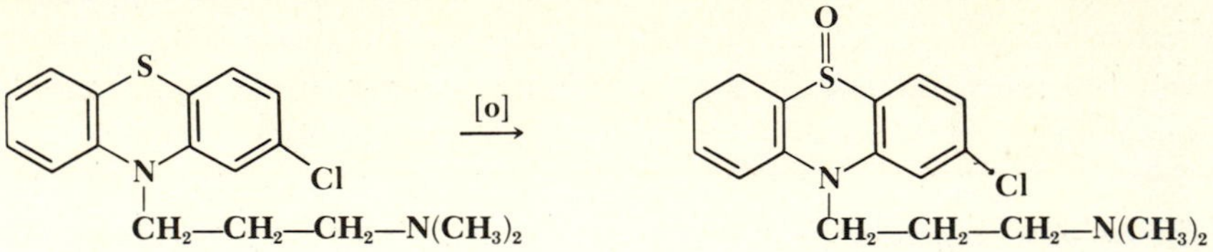

Chlorpromazine $\xrightarrow{[o]}$ Chlorpromazine sulfoxide

O-dealkylation. Acetophenetidin is changed to *N*-acetyl-*p*-aminophenol.

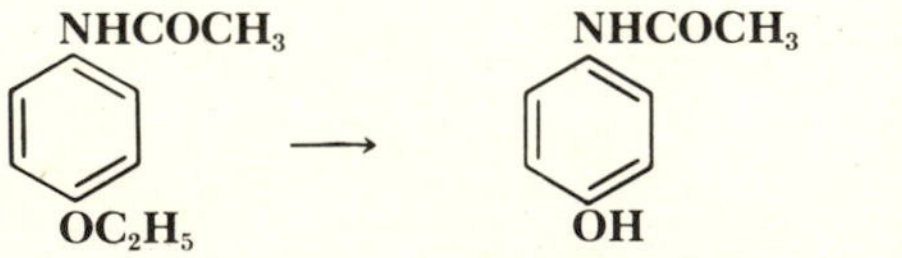

Acetophenetidin → *N*-Acetyl-*p*-aminophenol

S-dealkylation. 6-Methyl thiopurine is changed to 6-mercaptopurine.

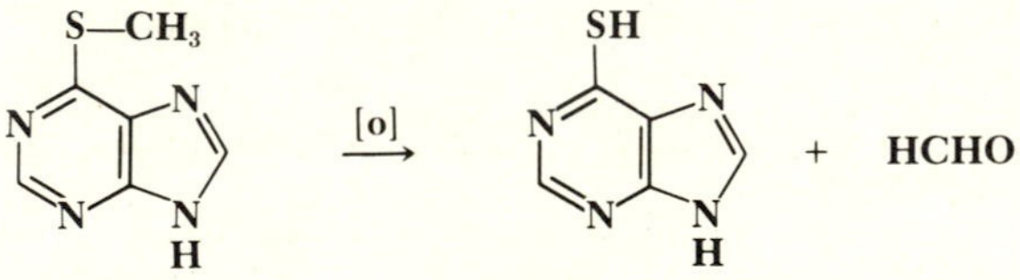

6-Methyl thiopurine $\xrightarrow{[o]}$ 6-Mercaptopurine + HCHO

Deamination. Amphetamine is oxidized to phenylacetone.

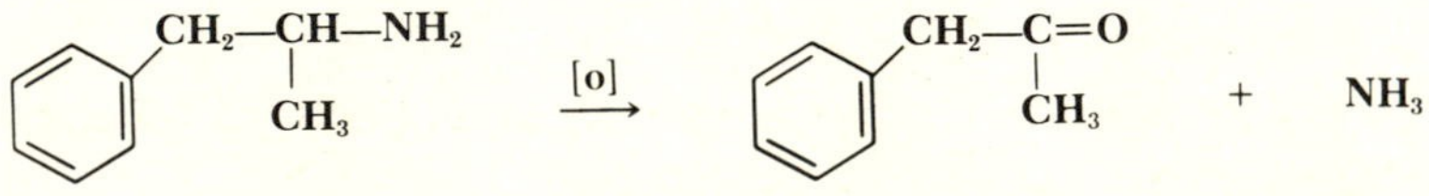

Amphetamine $\xrightarrow{[o]}$ Phenylacetone + NH_3

Desulfuration. Parathion is oxidized to paraoxon.

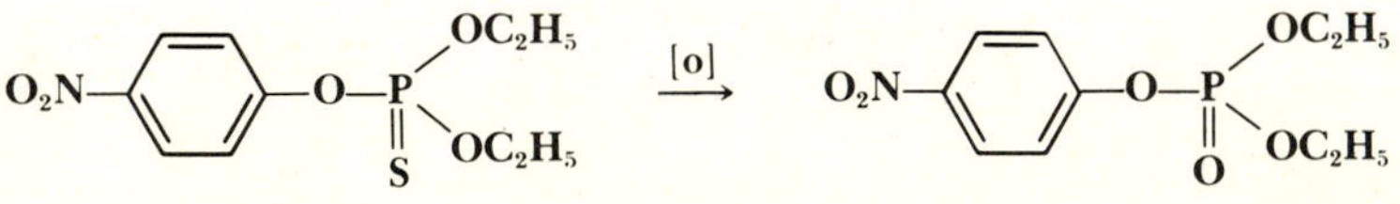

Parathion $\xrightarrow{[o]}$ Paraoxon

Nonmicrosomal (alcohol) oxidation

p-Nitrobenzyl alcohol is changed to *p*-nitrobenzaldehyde.

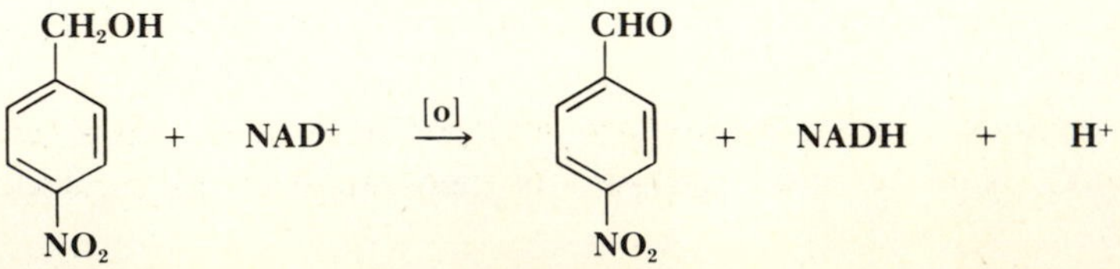

p-Nitrobenzyl alcohol + NAD^+ $\xrightarrow{[o]}$ *p*-Nitrobenzaldehyde + NADH + H^+

Reductions

Nitroreduction. Chloramphenicol is reduced to the arylamine.

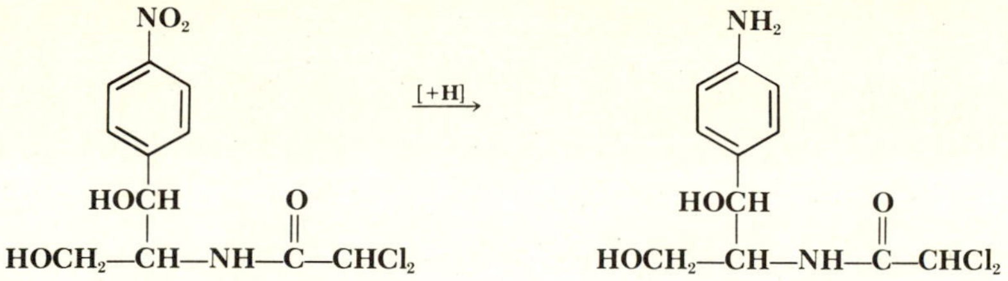
NO2
[+H]
NH2
HOCH
O
HOCH2—CH—NH—C—CHCl2
HOCH
O
HOCH2—CH—NH—C—CHCl2

Chloramphenicol "Arylamine"

Azoreduction. Prontosil is reduced to sulfanilamide.

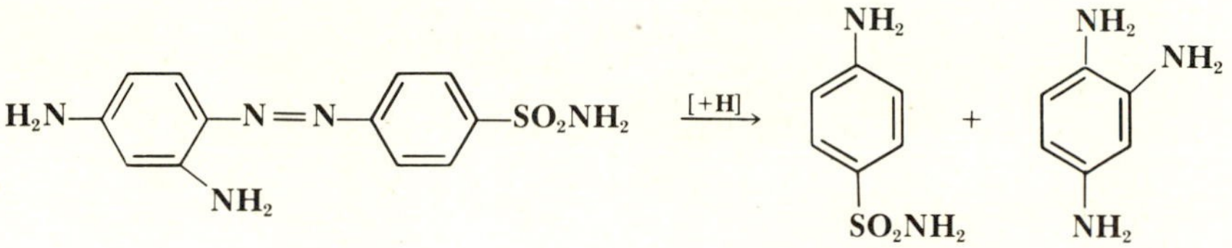
H2N—
—N=N—
—SO2NH2
NH2
[+H]
NH2
SO2NH2
+
NH2
NH2
NH2

Prontosil Sulfanilamide

Alcohol dehydrogenation. Chloral hydrate is changed to trichloroethanol.

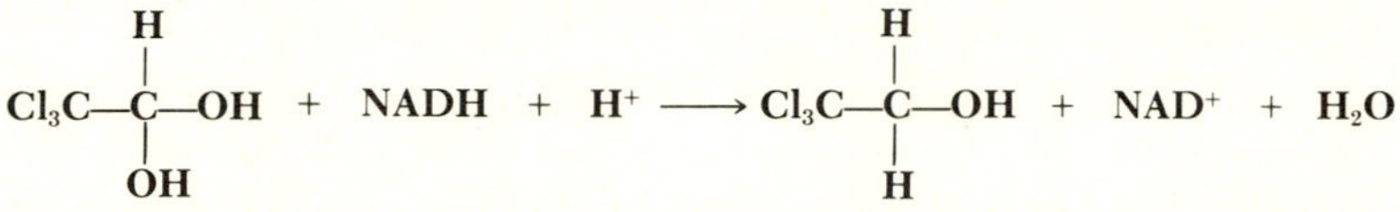
H
Cl3C—C—OH + NADH + H+ → Cl3C—C—OH + NAD+ + H2O
OH
H
H

Chloral hydrate Trichloroethanol

Hydrolyses

Procaine is hydrolyzed to *p*-aminobenzoic acid and diethylaminoethanol.

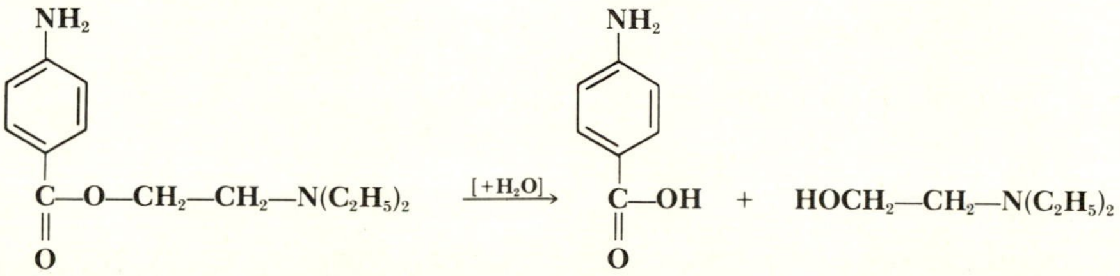
NH2
C—O—CH2—CH2—N(C2H5)2
O
[+H2O]
NH2
C—OH
O
+
HOCH2—CH2—N(C2H5)2

Procaine *p*-Aminobenzoic acid Diethylaminoethanol

Conjugations

The most important conjugation reactions are glucuronide synthesis, glycine conjugation, sulfate conjugation, acetylation, mercapturic acid synthesis, and methylation.

Glucuronide synthesis. Phenols, alcohols, carboxylic acids, and compounds containing amino or sulfhydryl groups may undergo glucuronide conjugation.

Since glucose is generally available in the body, glucuronide formation is a common route of drug metabolism. The mechanism of the reaction is as follows:

$$\text{Uridine diphosphoglucuronate} + \text{ROH} \xrightarrow[\text{transferase}]{\text{Glucuronyl}} \text{RO glucuronide} + \text{Uridine diphosphate}$$

An example of a drug excreted almost entirely as the glucuronide is salicylamide.

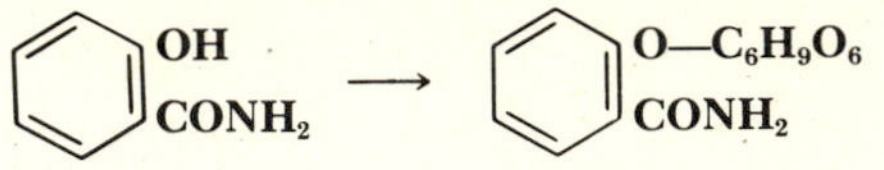

Salicylamide   Salicylamide glucuronide

Glycine conjugation. Glycine conjugation is characteristic for certain aromatic acids. It depends on the availability of coenzyme A, glycine, and glycine-N-acylase. A typical reaction is as follows:

$$\text{Benzoic acid} \xrightarrow{\text{ATP + CoA}} \text{Benzoyl-CoA} \xrightarrow{\text{Glycine}} \text{Hippuric acid}$$

Some of the drugs conjugated with glycine in humans are salicylic acid, isonicotinic acid, and p-aminosalicylic acid. These drugs are metabolized by other pathways also, which may be more important quantitatively than glycine conjugation.

Sulfate conjugation. Phenols, alcohols, or aromatic amines may undergo sulfate conjugation. The sulfate donor is 3'-phospho-adenosine-5-phospho-sulfate (PAPS).

Acetylation. Derivatives of aniline are acetylated in the body. In addition to sulfanilamide and related compounds, such widely used drugs as p-aminosalicylic acid, isoniazid, and aminopyrine are transformed by this mechanism. The general reaction involving an amine, acetyl coenzyme A, and a specific acetylating enzyme may be depicted in the following manner:

$$\text{RNH}_2 + \text{CoASCOCH}_3 \xrightarrow{\text{Acetylase}} \text{RNHCOCH}_3 + \text{CoASH}$$

The acetylating ability of different patients may vary considerably. In the case of isoniazid, a low degree of acetylation shows some correlation with incidence of toxic reactions such as peripheral neuritis.

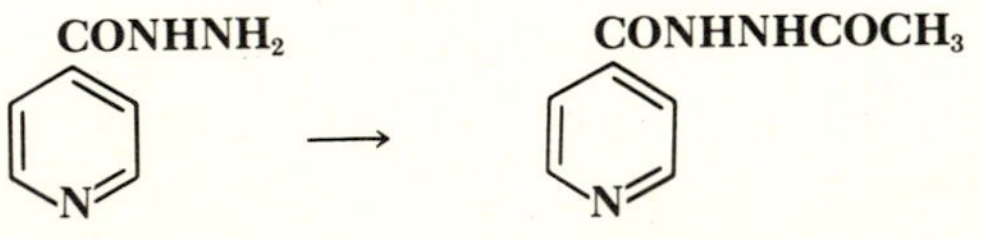

Isoniazid   Acetylated isoniazid

Mercapturic acid synthesis. This is not a common pathway in man, although it may occur. Some drugs containing an active halogen or a nitro group may be changed to mercapturates.

Methylation. Norepinephrine and epinephrine are metabolized in part to normetanephrine and metanephrine by a process of O-methylation, whereas nicotinic acid is metabolized to *N*-methylnicotinic acid, an example of *N*-methylation. The source of methyl groups for drug methylations is *S*-adenosylmethionine.

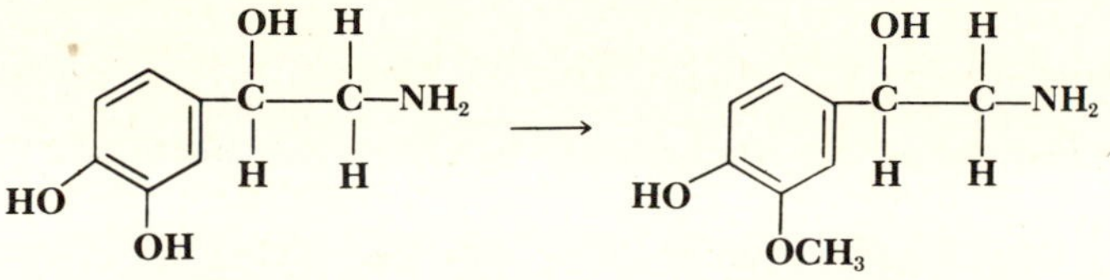

Norepinephrine   Normetanephrine

Drug metabolism generally changes a drug to more water-soluble metabolites. The term *detoxication* is not accurate, since the body can form a toxic metabolite from a less toxic drug. Drug metabolism generally produces inactive metabolites from active drugs. It may, however, produce an active metabolite from an inactive drug or from an initially active drug.

The toxicity of some compounds may be caused by a metabolite. The insecticide parathion is changed in the body to the more toxic paraoxon.

An even more remarkable example of the possible deleterious effects of the so-called detoxication process is given by the example of liver damage caused by carbon tetrachloride and probably some other drugs. Carbon tetrachloride is a well-known hepatotoxic agent. The curious finding that newborn rats are more resistant to the toxic effect of carbon tetrachloride,[37,59] along with the observation that pheno-barbital increases not only the metabolism of the halogenated hydrocarbon but also its toxicity, suggests that drug metabolism is involved in the hepatotoxicity of the compound. It is believed that free radicals are formed as a result of the interaction of some drugs and the drug-metabolizing enzymes. The free radicals may be directly toxic, perhaps through an interaction with membrane phospholipids. They may also make endogenous proteins antigenic, thus accounting for some forms of drug allergy.

Details of metabolism must be considered in connection with the individual drugs, but one very interesting generalization has been made concerning the evolutionary importance of certain detoxication mechanisms.

As we have seen in the previous section, the clearance of weakly acid or basic drugs is hindered by the tubular reabsorption of the undissociated molecule. But for terrestrial animals there is no alternate route of excretion. In contrast, aquatic animals have no difficulty with such foreign compounds because the lipid membranes of the gills offer a ready avenue for their excretion. In the course of evolution, terrestrial organisms seem to have solved this problem by utilizing such mechanisms as side chain oxidation and conjugation, which make these foreign compounds more acid and hence more easily rejected by the renal tubules.

The development of detoxication mechanisms appears to have been an evolutionary necessity, since terrestrial animals ingest many foreign compounds with their food. The mechanisms of detoxication, perhaps developed for the handling of such compounds, serve also at the present time for the biotransformation of a large variety of drugs.

Factors that delay the metabolism of drugs

It has been pointed out that drugs are usually metabolized at rates proportional to their plasma levels because at therapeutic levels their concentration is not high enough to saturate the drug-metabolizing enzymes.[24] Any conditions that lower the concentration of drugs at the level of the metabolizing enzymes or decrease the amount or activity of the enzymes would be expected to prolong the biological half-life of the drug. Several of these factors are of great importance, whereas others may become significant only in particular diseases or in the presence of certain drug combinations. The following are some examples.

1. The reversible protein binding limits drug metabolism. Phenylbutazone, for example, is highly protein bound, up to 98% after therapeutic doses. If the dose is increased so that only 88% of the drug is protein bound, the free portion is metabolized much more rapidly. As a consequence, not much is gained by increasing the dose.
2. Localization of the drug in the adipose tissue (thiopental) or in the liver (quinacrine) protects it against metabolic degradation and prolongs its half-life. Precipitation of the drug in the gastrointestinal tract may similarly prolong its half-life (zoxazolamine).
3. Diseases of the liver and immaturity of drug-metabolizing enzymes during the neonatal period may interfere with the biotransformation of some drugs.
4. A drug may inhibit the metabolism of another drug and thus may prolong and intensify its action. This is why monoamine oxidase (MAO) inhibitors may cause alarming reactions when tyramine-containing food or beverages are ingested. The very interesting experimental drug SKF-525A (β-diethylaminoethyl diphenylpropylacetate) inhibits the microsomal enzymes that metabolize a large variety of drugs. Iproniazid is another inhibitor of drug-metabolizing enzymes.

ENZYME INDUCTION

When several drugs are used simultaneously in a patient, it is difficult enough to keep in mind their various pharmacological interactions. An additional difficulty derives from observations indicating that some drugs can induce the formation of microsomal drug-metabolizing enzymes. Some cases of tolerance to a drug may be caused by microsomal enzyme induction. There are well-authenticated cases in both the experimental and the clinical literature of such drug interactions.

Stimulation of drug-metabolizing enzymes by drugs and foreign compounds

It was first shown in 1954[4] that mice fed the carcinogen 3-methylcholanthrene developed an increased capacity for demethylating 3-methyl-4-dimethylaminoazobenzene by liver microsomal enzymes. Several other examples of increased drug metabolism induced by various preparations followed. The long-acting barbiturate phenobarbital was found to stimulate the metabolism of such short-acting barbiturates as hexobarbital.

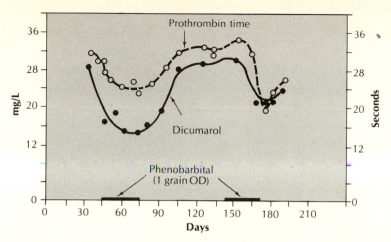

FIG. 4-2. Effect of phenobarbital on plasma levels of dicumarol and on prothrombin time in a human subject treated chronically with 75 mg/day of dicumarol. (From Cucinell, S. A., Conney, A. H., Sansur, M., and Burns, J. J.: Clin. Pharmacol. Ther. **6:**420, 1965.)

The following examples of stimulated drug metabolism have been demonstrated in man.

Phenobarbital stimulates the metabolism of phenytoin (Dilantin),[10] griseofulvin, and dicumarol (Fig. 4-2). Barbiturates stimulate the glucuronide conjugation of bilirubin in mice; this finding suggested the use of phenobarbital in the treatment of congenital nonhemolytic jaundice in infants.[57] The administration of 15 mg of phenobarbital two or three times daily lowered the free serum bilirubin concentration in these infants. Additionally, it improved the conjugation of salicylamide in the same infants, another example of glucuronide formation.

Phenylbutazone speeds the metabolism of aminopyrine.[8] **Meprobamate** and **glutethimide** may induce tolerance to their action by enzyme induction.

Phenytoin interferes with the effect of dexamethasone,[52] probably by promoting microsomal enzyme activity.

The inducers may promote the metabolism of certain hormones as well as that of various drugs and foreign compounds. Oxidative drug-metabolizing enzymes hydroxylate such endogenous compounds as testosterone, estradiol, progesterone, and cortisol.[24]

Although several examples of abnormal drug reactions in inherited diseases are well known, the systematic study of pharmacogenetics is of recent origin.[62] Among the well-known examples of adverse drug reaction occurring in certain inherited diseases are the following: barbiturates may produce severe attacks in congenital porphyria; salicylates are dangerous in individuals in whom glucuronyl transferase is congenitally absent (Crigler-Najjar syndrome); hypersensitivity to atropine occurs in patients suffering from Down's syndrome; and epinephrine or glucagon fail to

Stimulation of drug metabolism in humans

PHARMACO-GENETICS

produce hyperglycemia in individuals who are deficient in the enzyme glucose-6-phosphatase (von Gierke's disease).

A broad classification of pharmacogenetic abnormalities[62] would attribute most genetically conditioned anomalous drug responses to (1) receptor site abnormalities, (2) drug metabolism disorders, (3) tissue metabolism disorders, and (4) anatomical abnormalities.

Although there are not many well-known examples of *receptor site abnormalities*, they must undoubtedly contribute to the variation in drug responses. The resistance of some individuals to the coumarin anticoagulants is probably an example of a receptor site abnormality. The best known examples of pharmacogenetics are provided by *drug metabolism* disorders, in which abnormal blood levels of a drug can be measured after the administration of a normal dose. In *tissue metabolism* disorders an individual may show an adverse reaction to a normal blood level of a drug because of a special vulnerability caused by an abnormality in tissue metabolism. For example, in glucose-6-phosphate dehydrogenase deficiency a usual dose of primaquine may cause hemolytic anemia. Finally, an *anatomical abnormality* may cause adverse drug reactions. For example, in inherited subaortic stenosis, digitalis may cause fatal reactions.[62]

Continuous and discontinuous variation

It is generally recognized that the response to a drug in a population shows *continuous variation*. Drug effects such as the LD_{50} or ED_{50} (p. 47) and rate of destruction of a drug in the body generally show a normal distribution in a population, as shown in Fig. 4-3, *A*. Some of the great discoveries in pharmacogenetics occur when the response to some drug or the metabolism of a drug indicates a *discontinuous variation*, as shown in Fig. 4-3, *B*. Follow-up of such a bimodal distribution often reveals a genetic basis and provides the explanation for unusual responses to drugs, which is more satisfying than simply calling them idiosyncrasies.

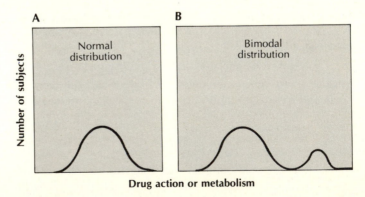

FIG. 4-3. Schematic illustration of *continuous* and *discontinuous* variation. When a standard dose of a drug is given to a large number of persons and a drug effect or metabolism is measured, the usual finding is a normal frequency distribution as in **A.** On the other hand, a discontinuous variation, as exemplified by the bimodal distribution shown in **B,** may indicate a genetically determined abnormality in drug action or metabolism.

Hemolytic anemia caused by the ingestion of the bean *Vicia fava* and reactions to several other drugs have similarly been traced to a deficiency of glucose-6-phosphate dehydrogenase. The following drugs have been suspected: acetophenetidin, acetanilid, probenecid, and others.

As shown in the schema on p. 68, the enzyme glucose-6-phosphate dehydrogenase in the red cell is responsible for the formation of NADPH (reduced form of nicotinamide adenine dinucleotide phosphate, or reduced triphosphopyridine nucleotide). NADPH is a cofactor for glutathione reductase, which converts glutathione to the reduced form. When there is a genetically determined deficiency of glucose-6-phosphate in the red cell, severe hemolytic episodes may be caused by the administration of oxidant drugs.

REFERENCES

1 Beutler, E.: The hemolytic effect of primaquine and related compounds: a review, Blood 14: 103, 1959.

2 Brodie, B. B.: Physiochemical and biochemical aspects of pharmacology, J.A.M.A. 202:600, 1967.

3 Brodie, B. B., Gillette, J. R., and La Du, B. N.: Enzyme metabolism of drugs and other foreign compounds, Annu. Rev. Biochem. 27:427, 1958.

4 Brown, R. R., Miller, J. A., and Miller, E. C.: The metabolism of methylated aminoazo dyes, J. Biol. Chem. 209:211, 1954.

5 Burns, J. J., Evans, C., and Trousof, N.: Stimulatory effect of barbital on urinary excretion of L-ascorbic acid and non-conjugated D-glucuronic acid, J. Biol. Chem. 227:785, 1957.

6 Busfield, D., Child, K. J., Atkinson, R. M., and Tomich, E. G.: An effect of phenobarbitone on blood-levels of griseofulvin in man, Lancet 2:1042, 1963.

7 Bush, M. T., and Sanders, E.: Metabolic fate of drugs: barbiturates and closely related drugs, Annu. Rev. Pharmacol. 7:57, 1967.

8 Chen, W., Vrindten, P. A., Dayton, P. G., and Burns, J. J.: Accelerated aminopyrine metabolism in human subjects pretreated with phenylbutazone, Life Sci. 2:35, 1962.

9 Conney, A. H.: Pharmacological implications of microsomal enzyme induction, Pharmacol. Rev. 19:317, 1967.

10 Conney, A. H.: Drug metabolism and therapeutics, N. Engl. J. Med. 280:653, 1969.

11 Conney, A. H., and Burns, J. J.: Factors influencing drug metabolism, Adv. Pharmacol. 1:31, 1962.

12 Conney, A. H., and Gilman, A. G.: Puromycin inhibition of enzyme induction by 3-methylcholanthrene and phenobarbital, J. Biol. Chem. 238:3682, 1963.

13 Conney, A. H., Miller, E. C., and Miller, J. A.: Substrate-induced synthesis and other properties of benzpyrene hydroxylase in rat liver, J. Biol. Chem. 228:753, 1957.

14 Cooper, J. R., Axelrod, J., and Brodie, B. B.: Inhibitory effects of β-diethylamino-ethyl diphenylpropylacetate on a variety of drug metabolic pathways in vitro, J. Pharmacol. Exp. Ther. 112:55, 1954.

15 Dayton, P. G., Tarcan, Y., Chenkin, T., and Weiner, M.: The influence of barbiturates on coumarin plasma levels and prothrombin response, J. Clin. Invest. 40:1797, 1961.

16 Douglas, J. F., Ludwig, B. J., and Smith, N.: Studies on the metabolism of meprobamate, Proc. Soc. Exp. Biol. Med. 112:436, 1963.

17 Ebert, R. V.: Oral anticoagulants and drug interactions, Arch. Intern. Med. 121:373, 1968.

18 Editorial: Hypertensive reactions to monoamine oxidase inhibitors, Br. Med. J. 1:578, 1964.

19 Evans, D. A. P.: Pharmacogenetics, Am. J. Med. 34:639, 1963.

20 Fouts, J. R., and Brodie, B. B.: On the mechanism of drug potentiation by iproniazid (2-isopropyl-1-isonicotinyl hydrazine), J. Pharmacol. Exp. Ther. 116:480, 1956.

21 Fox, A. L.: The relationship between chemical constitution and taste, Proc. Natl. Acad. Sci. 18:115, 1932.

22 Fox, S. L.: Potentiation of anticoagulants caused by pyrazole compounds, J.A.M.A. 188:320, 1964.

23 Gillette, J. R.: Metabolism of drugs and other foreign compounds by enzymatic mechanisms, Prog. Drug Res. 6:13, 1963.

24 Gillette, J. R.: Biochemistry of drug oxidation

and reduction by enzymes in hepatic endoplasmic reticulum, Adv. Pharmacol. 4:219, 1966.

25 Hertting, G., Axelrod, J., and Whitby, L. G.: Effect of drugs on the uptake and metabolism of H³-norepinephrine, J. Pharmacol. Exp. Ther. 134:146, 1961.

26 Isaac, L., and Goth, A.: The mechanism of the potentiation of norepinephrine by antihistaminics, J. Pharmacol. Exp. Ther. 156:463, 1967.

27 Kalow, W.: Pharmacogenetics: heredity and the response to drugs, Philadelphia, 1962, W. B. Saunders Co.

28 Kuntzman, R.: Drugs and enzyme induction, Annu. Rev. Pharmacol. 9:21, 1969.

29 Landsteiner, K.: The specificity of serological reactions, Cambridge, 1945, Harvard University Press.

30 Loeser, E. W., Jr.: Studies on the metabolism of diphenylhydantoin (Dilantin), Neurology 11:424, 1961.

31 Motulsky, A. G.: Drug reactions, enzymes and biochemical genetics, J.A.M.A. 165:835, 1957.

32 Mueller, G. C., and Miller, J. A.: The reductive cleavage of 4-dimethylaminoazobenzene by rat liver: the intracellular distribution of the enzyme system and its requirement for triphosphopyridine nucleotide, J. Biol. Chem. 180:1125, 1949.

33 Muscholl, E.: Effect of cocaine and related drugs on the uptake of norepinephrine by heart and spleen, Br. J. Pharmacol. 16:352, 1961.

34 Odell, G. B.: Studies in kernicterus. I. The protein-binding of bilirubin, J. Clin. Invest. 38:823, 1959.

35 Parker, C. W., Shapiro, J., Kern, M., and Eisen, H. N.: Hypersensitivity to penicillenic acid derivatives in human beings with penicillin allergy, J. Exp. Med. 115:821, 1962.

36 Ramboer, C., Thompson, R. P. H., and Williams, R.: Controlled trials of phenobarbitone therapy in neonatal jaundice, Lancet 1:966, 1969.

37 Recknagel, R. O.: CCl₄ hepatotoxicity, Pharmacol. Rev. 19:145, 1967.

38 Remmer, H.: The fate of drugs in the organism, Annu. Rev. Pharmacol. 5:405, 1965.

39 Remmer, H., and Merker, H. J.: Drug-induced changes in the liver endoplasmic reticulum: association with drug-metabolizing enzymes, Science 142:1657, 1963.

40 Rubin, E., Gang, H., Misra, P. S., and Lieber, C. S.: Inhibition of drug metabolism by acute ethanol intoxication, Am. J. Med. 49:801, 1970.

41 Shuster, L.: Metabolism of drugs and toxic substances, Annu. Rev. Biochem. 33:571, 1964.

42 Sperber, I.: Secretion of organic anions in the formation of urine and bile, Pharmacol. Rev. 11:109, 1959.

43 Stanbury, J. B., Wyngaarden, J. B., and Fredrickson, D. S.: The metabolic basis of inherited disease, New York, 1960, McGraw-Hill Book Co.

44 Takahara, S.: Progressive oral gangrene probably due to lack of catalase in the blood (acatalasemia), Lancet 2:1101, 1952.

45 Thompson, J. S., and Thompson, M. W.: Genetics in medicine, Philadelphia, 1966, W. B. Saunders Co.

46 Vesell, E. S., and Page, J. G.: Genetic control of drug levels in man: phenylbutazone, Science 159:1479, 1968.

47 Vesell, E. S., Passananti, T., and Greene, F. E.: Impairment of drug metabolism by allopurinol and nortryptyline, N. Engl. J. Med. 283:1484, 1970.

48 Vogel, F.: Moderne probleme der humangenetik, Ergebn. Inn. Med. Kinderheilk. 12:52, 1959.

49 Wadell, W. J., and Butler, T. C.: The distribution and excretion of phenobarbital, J. Clin. Invest. 36:1217, 1957.

50 Walton, R. P.: Sublingual administration of drugs, J.A.M.A. 124:138, 1944.

51 Weiner, I. M., Washington, J. A., II, and Mudge, G. H.: On the mechanism of action of probenecid on renal tubular secretion, Bull. Johns Hopkins Hosp. 106:333, 1960.

52 Werk, E. E., Jr., Choi, Y., Sholiton, L., Olinger, C., and Hague, N.: Interference in the effect of dexamethasone by diphenylhydantoin, N. Engl. J. Med. 281:32, 1969.

53 Willbrandt, W., and Rosenberg, T.: The concept of carrier transport and its corollaries in pharmacology, Pharmacol. Rev. 13:109, 1961.

54 Williams, R. T.: Detoxication mechanisms, New York, 1959, John Wiley & Sons, Inc.

55 Williams, R. T.: Detoxication mechanisms in man, Clin. Pharmacol. Ther. 4:234, 1963.

56 Wolff, J., Standaert, M. E., and Rall, J. E.: Thyroxine displacement from serum proteins and depression of serum protein-bound iodine by certain drugs, J. Clin. Invest. 40:1373, 1961.

57 Yaffe, S. J., Levy, G., Matsuzawa, T., and Baliah, T.: Enhancement of glucuronide-conjugating capacity in a hyperbilirubinemic infant due to apparent enzyme induction by phenobarbital, N. Engl. J. Med. 275:1461, 1966.

58 Yu, T. F., Dayton, P. G., and Gutman, A. B.: Mutual suppression of the uricosuric effects of sulfinpyrazine and salicylate. A study in interactions between drugs, J. Clin. Invest. 42:1330, 1963.

REVIEWS

59 Anders, M. W.: Enhancement and inhibition of drug metabolism, Annu. Rev. Pharmacol. **11:**37, 1971.

60 Conney, A. H., and Burns, J. J.: Metabolic interactions among environmental chemicals and drugs, Science **178:**576, 1972.

61 Gelehrter, T. D.: Enzyme induction, N. Engl. J. Med. **294:**589, 1976.

62 La Du, B. N.: The genetics of drug reactions, Hosp. Pract., p. 97, June, 1971.

63 La Du, B. N., Mandel, H. G., and Way, E. L.: Fundamentals of drug metabolism and drug disposition, Baltimore, 1971, The Williams & Wilkins Co.

64 Remmer, H.: The role of the liver in drug metabolism, Am. J. Med. **49:**617, 1970.

65 Schreiber, E. C.: The metabolic alteration of drugs, Annu. Rev. Pharmacol. **10:**77, 1970.

66 Vesell, E. S.: Pharmacogenetics, N. Engl. J. Med. **287:**904, 1972.

CHAPTER 5

Drug safety and effectiveness

With the expansion of drug therapy and with the introduction of potent agents that have complex effects and even more complex interactions with each other, it is increasingly necessary for the physician to have a scientific attitude and considerable knowledge of drug evaluation.

Since the most extensive studies on drug evaluation are carried out in connection with the development of *new* drugs, this subject will be discussed in some detail along with factors that modify drug safety and effectiveness.

DEVELOPMENT OF A NEW DRUG New drugs originate from many different sources. Accidental observations on natural products, unexpected clinical findings of known compounds, basic physiological or biochemical investigations, and even test tube experiments have provided leads for great therapeutic discoveries. Most new drugs are discovered today by screening. Large numbers of natural products or synthetic compounds are tested for a variety of possible biological activities. A highly effective drug that seems safe enough on preliminary testing is then carried through a series of steps:

1. Animal studies
   a. Acute, subacute, and chronic toxicity
   b. Therapeutic index
   c. Absorption, excretion, distribution, and metabolism
2. Human studies
   a. Phase 1: preliminary pharmacological evaluation
   b. Phase 2: basic controlled clinical evaluation
   c. Phase 3: extended clinical evaluation

Animal studies
Acute, subacute, and chronic toxicity

The most common measure of acute toxicity is the median lethal dose (LD_{50}). The LD_{50} is determined by giving various doses of the drugs to groups of animals. Ordinarily only a single dose is given to each animal. The percentage of animals dying in each group within a selected period, for example, 24 hours, is plotted against the dose. From this curve the dose that kills 50% of the animals is estimated and is referred to as the LD_{50}. This particular dose-mortality figure is chosen because it can be determined more precisely; the curve approaches a straight line at the LD_{50}. It should be emphasized that the LD_{50} of any drug is of interest only to experimental pharmacologists, not to clinicians.

Customarily at least three different species are used for acute toxicity determinations, and observations are made not only on the LD_{50} but also on the type of toxic symptoms that the animals develop.

In subacute toxicity studies the mode of administration and the dosage depend on the proposed clinical trial. Usually the drug is administered orally. Several doses are used, some within the range of the estimated human dose and others that produce toxic manifestations. Careful observations are carried out on these animals, including a variety of laboratory studies such as hematological examinations, renal and hepatic function tests, and many others.

The chronic toxicity studies are of long duration. They may last many months and may be carried through several generations to detect the possible teratogenic effect of a drug. Again several species are necessary because even in prolonged studies some species are much more suitable than others for the demonstration of adverse effects. The animals are killed periodically and thorough pathologic studies are performed.

The LD_{50} of a drug is not nearly as important as its therapeutic index, or thera-   **Therapeutic index** peutic ratio. This concept in *animal experiments* refers to the ratio of the LD_{50} to the median effective dose (ED_{50}), as illustrated in Fig. 5-1.

$$\text{Therapeutic index} = \frac{LD_{50}}{ED_{50}}$$

In clinical medicine the therapeutic index based on median lethal doses has no meaning. Instead, the ratio of a toxic dose over the effective dose is sometimes utilized. Even in animal experiments, the ratio of LD_1/ED_{100} would give a better idea of safety, but it has no particular application. The concept of effectiveness in relation to toxicity is more important than any special ratio.

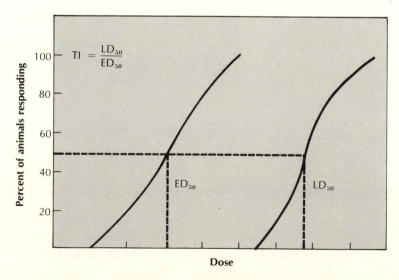

FIG. 5-1. Illustrating concept of therapeutic index (TI).

The concept of toxicity in relation to effectiveness, the basis of the therapeutic index, is of interest to clinicians as well as to experimental pharmacologists. A physician may not be greatly interested in the exact number of milligrams of a drug that will produce toxic effects but is vitally interested in knowing how far the therapeutic dose can be exceeded before adverse effects are likely to be encountered.

Absorption, excretion, distribution, and metabolism

The development of analytic methods for determining the absorption, excretion, distribution, and metabolism of a drug in animals adds much to the proper design of animal experiments on the toxicity and efficacy of the drug. In addition, these methods are desirable for the initiation and pursuit of clinical studies.

Human studies— clinical pharmacology

Animal studies provide a general profile of the toxicity, pharmacological activities, and pharmacokinetics of a new drug. Even with all this information available, the initiation of clinical studies is risky. There are numerous examples of drugs that pass all the preclinical criteria for safety but show serious adverse effects in humans. The clinical pharmacologist should consider not only the data obtained previously in animals but also the chemical nature of the drug and its possible similarity to hazardous drugs.

The lack of correlation between toxicity data in animals and adverse effects in humans is well known. Not only is there great species variation in toxicity, an example of comparative pharmacology, but many adverse effects simply cannot be ascertained in animals. Zbinden[19] claimed that of the 45 most frequent drug-related symptoms observed in 11,000 patients treated with 77 different drugs or drug combinations, at least one half would probably not be recognized in animal experiments. Such symptoms include drowsiness, nausea, dizziness, nervousness, epigastric distress, headache, weakness, insomnia, fatigue, tinnitus, heartburn, skin rash, depression, dermatitis, increased energy, vertigo, lethargy, nocturia, abdominal distention, flatulence, stiffness, and urticaria.

Because of these discrepancies between animal data and human effects, the initial clinical studies on any drug should be undertaken with great care, with the methodology meticulously planned, and with special attention given to *relevance* (pertinence of data), *representativeness* (selection of material to eliminate bias), and *reliability* (repeatability of results).[14] The new drug application must be filed before any clinical evaluation studies are initiated.

Phase 1: preliminary pharmacological evaluation

Very small doses of the drug are administered to human volunteers to obtain a preliminary idea of its safety in humans. With increasing doses, an attempt is made to extend the previously demonstrated effects in animals to humans. The ethical aspects of human experimentation have been the subject of much discussion in recent years and will not be taken up in detail.[17] The important points are, however, that the volunteer must be truly a volunteer (that is, able to give an informed consent) and that the investigator must be competent. In some instances it is essential to have methods for the determination of blood levels of the new drug. Without such determinations the investigator could not tell whether lack of effectiveness in humans is a consequence of lack of absorption or too rapid excretion and metabolism.

Whereas the phase 1 studies are usually performed by one or two clinical investigators, in phase 2 a somewhat larger number of clinical investigators attempt to find out in blind or double-blind studies as much information as possible about the safety and efficacy of the new drug. Adverse effects must be reported promptly to the sponsoring company and to the Food and Drug Administration (FDA), and specific studies are sometimes initiated to ascertain the significance of such unexpected findings.

Phase 2: basic controlled clinical evaluation

As many as 50 to 100 physicians participate in the large-scale clinical trial of a new drug. The investigators must not only be competent clinicians but must also have some experience and training in the field of drug evaluation.

Phase 3: extended clinical evaluation

Assuming that the phase 3 studies demonstrate to the satisfaction of the FDA that the drug is safe and effective, the investigational drug may be approved to be distributed and used when prescribed by a physician.

It would seem that with all these safeguards a drug approved by the FDA would be free of all hazard. Unfortunately there are many unusual side effects, idiosyncrasies, and drug allergies that show up only after extensive use in large numbers of patients.

Experimental studies in animals show that the dose of a drug that will give an all-or-nothing response (such as the death of the animal) varies considerably. Fig. 5-2 illustrates the gaussian distribution of susceptibility, which can be demonstrated easily in animals. The biological variation in drug effect is an important reason why dosages must be individualized and treatment adjusted to the requirements of a given patient.

FACTORS INFLUENCING THE SAFETY AND EFFECTIVENESS OF DRUGS
Biological variation

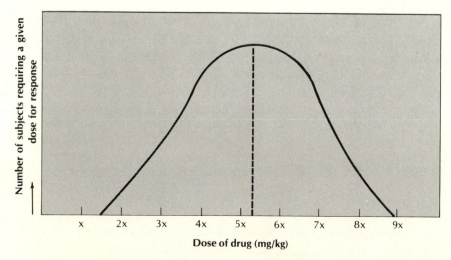

FIG. 5-2. Biological variation in susceptibility to drugs.

Hypersusceptibility

Because of biological variation, disease, or presence of another medication, some persons may show a much greater than normal response to the ordinary dose of a drug. For example, a thyrotoxic patient may respond with exaggerated cardiovascular response to injected epinephrine. A patient with subclinical asthma may evidence symptoms of bronchial constriction from doses of acetyl-β-methylcholine or histamine that would be innocuous in normal persons. In these cases we are dealing with patients who are at the susceptible end of a normal frequency distribution curve and whose responses are quantitatively different. Hypersusceptibility is sometimes referred to as *drug intolerance*.

Drug idiosyncrasy and drug allergy

The term *idiosyncrasy* has been used rather vaguely in medicine to cover drug reactions that are *qualitatively* different from the usual effects obtained in the majority of patients and cannot be attributed to drug allergy. Occasionally extreme susceptibility of an individual to the expected pharmacological effect of a drug has also been included in the drug idiosyncrasies.

With the increasing knowledge of pharmacogenetics, as discussed on p. 54, many drug idiosyncrasies have been found to be genetically conditioned enzymatic deficiencies. Such deficiencies can interfere with the metabolic degradation of a drug, as in prolonged apnea caused by succinylcholine, or they may make certain cells more vulnerable to an adverse effect of a drug, as is the case in hemolytic anemia elicited by primaquine and other drugs in patients whose red cells are deficient in glucose-6-phosphate dehydrogenase.[13]

It is quite likely that all drug idiosyncrasies will turn out to be genetically conditioned abnormalities of enzymes or receptors.

Drug allergy is an altered response to a drug resulting from a previous sensitizing exposure and an immunological mechanism. It differs from drug toxicity in a number of respects. (1) The altered reaction occurs in only a fraction of the population. (2) Its dose-response is unusual in that a minute amount of an otherwise safe drug elicits a severe reaction. (3) The manifestations of the reaction are different from the usual pharmacological effects of the drug. Thus aspirin elicits asthma as a presumably allergic reaction in a few individuals. (4) There is a primary sensitizing period before the individual responds with an unusual reaction to a further exposure. (5) When the sensitizing drug is a protein or a compound that forms covalent bonds with proteins, circulating antibodies may be demonstrated in sensitized individuals and skin tests, although hazardous, may show a positive reaction to the offending drug.

In most drug allergies it is not known what the complete antigen is or in what form the drug acts as a hapten. A patient may react to the ingestion of a sulfonamide by developing a skin rash and still show no positive reaction to the same drug when injected intracutaneously. This is generally true for drugs of small molecular weight and the *immediate* type of allergies elicited by them. In *contact dermatitis*, on the other hand, positive patch tests are regularly obtained.

The terms *immediate* and *delayed reactions* originated from observations of the rapidity with which the positive skin test to allergens becomes manifest. Thus in anaphylactic hypersensitivity, skin test results are immediate, but in delayed states such as tuberculin hypersensitivity, it is many hours before there is a visible change in the skin where the antigen was injected. In addition, there are profound differences in the immunological basis of the two types of hypersensitivities. Circulating antibodies are believed to be important in immediate but not in delayed hypersensitivities. The latter can be transferred to normal individuals only by means of sensitized cells.

Immediate and delayed drug allergies

Among the many types of drug allergies, some are considered immediate, others delayed, and still others are not classifiable at present. *Anaphylaxis, urticaria, angioneurotic edema, drug fever,* and *asthma* clearly belong in the category of immediate reactions. *Serum sickness* reactions are characterized by a delay in the appearance of manifestations following the initial sensitization to a drug; this same delay is observed after the first administration of a foreign serum. Once sensitized, however, an individual often reacts to the same drug rather rapidly. For example, methyldopa (Aldomet) may be taken daily by an individual for 1 to 2 weeks before fever and joint pain develop. The subsequent administration of a small dose of the drug will produce the same reaction in a matter of hours. *Contact dermatitis* is undoubtedly a delayed allergy. Many other cutaneous reactions and *some* severe hematological disturbances elicited by drugs probably also belong in the delayed category.

In experimental investigations, drugs are administered on the basis of a certain number of milligrams per kilogram of body weight, since the volume of distribution of a drug is roughly a function of body mass. For the same reason the weight of the patient should be taken into consideration when a dose is calculated. Certain formulas allow adjustment of dosage according to weight. For example, Clark's rule is as follows:

Age and weight of patient

$$\text{Dose for a child} = \text{Adult dose} \times \frac{\text{Weight of child in pounds}}{150}$$

It is assumed in this formula that a child needs a smaller dose because the weight is less, but this is only an approximation. It has been pointed out that the child is not simply a "small adult" and that reactions to drugs in children may result from problems in growth and development rather than size.[22] Catastrophes have resulted from the routine adaptation of adult dosages for children. The gray syndrome caused by chloramphenicol, kernicterus by vitamin K, and blindness by the use of oxygen in premature infants are examples of the peculiar problems of drug use in pediatrics.

The dose of a drug in children is proportional to weight to the 0.7 power.[21] Since body surface is similarly related to body weight, it has been suggested that pediatric

Dose for children based on surface area

dosages should be calculated on the basis of surface area of the body in square meters. Tables relating the weight of a child in pounds to surface area in square meters and approximate percentage of adult dose are available. According to such tables, a 22-pound child having a surface area of 0.46 sq m should receive 27% of the adult dose. A child weighing 121 pounds with a surface area of 1.58 sq m would receive 91% of the adult dose.

Disease processes influencing susceptibility and detoxication

Pathologic processes influence susceptibility to drugs. In some instances this can be explained by altered detoxication processes induced by the disease, but in other cases the explanation may be obscure.

It is obvious that in severe renal disease one must use with caution those drugs such as phenobarbital that depend on renal clearance for excretion. In severe liver disease, similar care must be exercised in the use of drugs that are normally detoxified by hepatic processes.

Abnormal susceptibility to drugs in disease states may depend on other mechanisms. The asthmatic patient is said to be hypersusceptible to the bronchoconstrictor action of histamine or methacholine, whereas the thyrotoxic patient is hypersusceptible to epinephrine. Patients with subclinical glaucoma may respond with an acute attack to doses of a mydriatic that would be harmless in a normal person.

Presence of other drugs

When more than one drug is used in the same patient, their actions may be completely independent of one another. Often, however, the combined effect may be greater than that which could have been obtained with a single drug, or a drug may have even less effect than if it were given alone.

Additive effect, synergism, and potentiation

When the combined effect of two drugs is the algebraic sum of the individual actions, it is referred to as *summation*, or *additive effect*. Another way of stating the additive effect is in terms of doses rather than effects. If a certain dose of drug A and another dose of drug B produce the same effect quantitatively, the additive effect concept implies that one-half the dose of each drug used simultaneously would elicit the same effect. *Synergism* is defined in various ways. To some it means an additive, or greater than additive, effect. Others reserve the term to cases in which one drug increases the action of another by interfering with its destruction or disposition, thus greatly increasing its action. *Potentiation* generally means a greater than additive effect. The terms synergism and potentiation are commonly abused in pharmaceutical promotion.

Antagonism

Drug antagonism may be of several types: chemical antagonism, physiological antagonism, and pharmacological antagonism.

Chemical antagonism. A drug may actually combine with another in the body. This is the basis of the action of the chemical antidotes. For example, dimercaprol (British anti-lewisite; BAL) can combine with mercury or arsenic in the body. The diuretic effect of a mercurial can be blocked by the injection of BAL.

Physiological antagonism. Two drugs may influence a physiological system in opposite directions, one drug canceling the effect of another. The simultaneous injection of properly adjusted doses of vasodilator and vasoconstrictor drugs may cause no change in blood pressure. Stimulants and depressants of the CNS can antagonize each other by a similar mechanism.

Pharmacological antagonism. Two drugs may compete for the same receptor site, the inactive or weak member of the pair preventing the access of the potent drug. This is the phenomenon of pharmacological antagonism.

Examples of pharmacological antagonism are the histamine-antihistaminic drug relationships and also atropine-acetylcholine antagonism. It is quite likely that many examples of competitive antagonism in pharmacology are not competition for enzymes but rather for receptor surfaces.

The key point in pharmacological antagonism is parallel displacement of the dose-response curve of a drug by a second drug. If the two drugs compete for the same receptor, the curves should remain parallel and the maximal height of the curves should remain the same (p. 12).

A drug may interact with another by many different mechanisms. Some of these are (1) absorption from the gastrointestinal tract, (2) binding to plasma proteins, (3) renal excretion, (4) inhibition of metabolic degradation, (5) promotion of metabolic degradation by enzyme induction, and (6) alteration of electrolyte patterns. These and other drug interactions have acquired such an importance in clinical pharmacology that the problem is discussed in detail in Chapter 63.

Complex drug interactions in clinical pharmacology

Response to dosage can be greatly influenced by certain special features of drug metabolism such as cumulation, tolerance, and tachyphylaxis.

Cumulation, tolerance, and tachyphylaxis

Most drugs are eliminated from the body by a first-order reaction. This means that a constant fraction of the drug present in the body is eliminated per unit time. It also means that it takes four half-lives to eliminate 93% of the drug. If the drug is administered repeatedly and frequently in relation to its half-life, it will accumulate in the body. Eventually, however, a *plateau* will be reached, since elimination is increasing as the amount of drug in the body increases. Digitoxin is a good example of a drug having a long half-life, leading to cumulation when administered daily.

Cumulation

If we plot in a schematic manner the amount of drug in the body against the number of doses, the resulting curve is shown in Fig. 5-3. The plateau in the case of drug *b* (Fig. 5-3) indicates that, in general, the amount of drug metabolized in a day is proportional to the amount in the body.

When we deal with cumulative drugs, the dosage will vary greatly, depending on whether we are administering loading or maintenance doses. The former must be large enough to build up a therapeutically effective level in the body, whereas maintenance doses are adjusted to the daily metabolic and excretory rates.

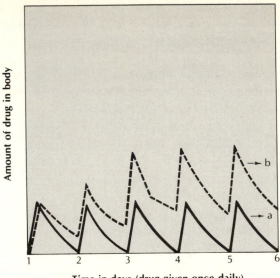

Amount of drug in body

Time in days (drug given once daily)

FIG. 5-3. Illustrating concept of cumulation. Drug *a* is completely destroyed or excreted in less than 24 hours. Thus it does not accumulate when administered once a day. Drug *b* requires more than 24 hours for its metabolic degradation or excretion. It is a cumulative drug when it is administered once a day.

Tolerance   Tolerance is an interesting phenomenon characterized by the need for increasing amounts of a drug to obtain the same therapeutic effect. Drugs vary greatly in their tendency to induce tolerance; perhaps the best-known examples are the opium alkaloids. The adult therapeutic dose of morphine is ordinarily 10 to 15 mg, but if the drug is administered repeatedly to a patient, increasing doses are necessary to obtain the same analgesic effect. Finally, enormous doses are sought by the addict who has gradually developed tolerance. Although it is a well-studied phenomenon, the actual mechanism of tolerance remains mysterious.

Drugs that produce significant tolerance are not numerous. Many are similar to the digitalis glycosides, which can be taken daily for years without tolerance developing.

Tachyphylaxis   Tachyphylaxis is the term reserved for rapidly developing tolerance. This is noted in laboratory experiments with certain drugs—for example, vasopressin or certain adrenergic compounds such as amphetamine. In these experiments the first injection of the drug produces a much greater elevation of blood pressure than subsequent injections given after only a brief interval.

The mechanism of tachyphylaxis is understood only in some cases. For example, indirectly acting sympathomimetic amines such as amphetamine release norepinephrine from adrenergic nerve endings. Tachyphylaxis probably is a consequence of depletion of available norepinephrine. The same mechanism plays a role in tachyphylaxis to histamine releasers. In other instances the action of a drug may persist at the receptor site, but its overt manifestations are concealed by compensatory reflexes or by desensitization of the receptor.

Drug effects are greatly influenced by genetically determined variations in susceptibility. Idiosyncrasies in general are most commonly related to pharmacogenetic abnormalities. This subject is discussed in detail on p. 54.

Pharmacogenetics

REFERENCES

1 Abrams, W. B., Bagdon, R. E., and Zbinden, G.: Drug toxicity and its impact on drug evaluation in man, Clin. Pharmacol. Ther. **5:**273, 1964.

2 Barron, B. A., and Bukantz, S. C.: The evaluation of new drugs. Current Food and Drug Administration regulations and statistical aspects of clinical trials, Arch. Intern. Med. **119:** 547, 1967.

3 Clark, A. J.: General pharmacology. In Heffter, A., editor: Handbuch der experimentellen Pharmakologie, Berlin, 1937, Springer-Verlag.

4 Dearborn, E. H.: Testing drugs for pharmacologic activity and safety, Biomed. Purview 3: 19, 1963.

5 Done, A. K.: Perinatal pharmacology, Annu. Rev. Pharmacol. **6:**189, 1966.

6 Editorial: Therapeutic research and the need for a new look, J.A.M.A. **200:**547, 1967.

7 Karnofsky, D. A.: Drugs as teratogens in animals and man, Annu. Rev. Pharmacol. **5:**447, 1965.

8 Landsteiner, K.: The specificity of serological reactions, Cambridge, 1945, Harvard University Press.

9 Levine, B. B.: Immunochemical mechanisms of drug allergy, Annu. Rev. Med. **17:**23, 1966.

10 Modell, W.: The extraordinary side effects of drugs, Clin. Pharmacol. Ther. **5:**265, 1964.

11 Modell, W.: Drug-induced diseases, Annu. Rev. Pharmacol. **5:**285, 1965.

12 Parker, C. W., Shapiro, J., Kern, M., and Eisen, H. N.: Hypersensitivity to penicillenic acid derivatives in human beings with penicillin allergy, J. Exp. Med. **115:**821, 1962.

13 Prankerd, T. A. J.: Hemolytic effects of drugs and chemical agents, Clin. Pharmacol. Ther. 4:334, 1963.

14 Shaw, D. L.: Clinical evaluation of pharmacologically active compounds, Biomed. Purview 3:30, 1963.

15 Sherlock, S.: Hepatic reactions to therapeutic agents, Annu. Rev. Pharmacol. **5:**429, 1965.

16 Wilson, C. W. M.: The assessment of medical information—a consequence of the drug explosion, J. Irish Med. Assoc. **57:**147, 1965.

17 Wolfensberger, W.: Ethical issues in research with human subjects, Science **155:**47, 1967.

18 Zbinden, G.: Experimental and clinical aspects of drug toxicity, Adv. Pharmacol. **2:**1, 1963.

19 Zbinden, G.: Animal toxicity studies: a critical evaluation, Appl. Ther. **8:**128, 1966.

20 Zbinden, G.: The significance of pharmacologic screening tests in the preclinical safety evaluation of new drugs, J. New Drugs **6:**1, 1966.

REVIEWS

21 Done, A. K.: Drugs for children. In Modell, W., editor: Drugs of choice 1978-1979, St. Louis, 1978, The C. V. Mosby Co.

22 Shirkey, H. C., and Ericson, A. S.: Adverse reactions to drugs—their relation to growth and development. In Shirkey, H. C., editor: Pediatric therapy, ed. 6, St. Louis, 1980, The C. V. Mosby Co.

23 Stewart, G. T.: Allergy to penicillin and related antibiotics: antigenic and immunochemical mechanisms, Annu. Rev. Pharmacol. **13:** 309, 1973.

CHAPTER 6

Pharmacogenetics: the individual response to drugs

VARIATIONS IN DRUG RESPONSE

A perplexing problem for both pharmacologists and physicians concerns the large variations that occur among normal subjects, as well as patients, in response to a particular drug. Such interindividual variations have been demonstrated for many drugs. They signify correspondingly large variations in the dose of these drugs required by different patients. The clinical consequences of such differences among patients in dose requirement cannot be overemphasized.

The magnitude of interindividual variations in rate of elimination of a drug given to a group of subjects, all in the same dose and by the same route, can range from fourfold to fortyfold, depending on both the particular drug and the population. Regardless of this precise value for a particular drug in a defined population, the extent of these variations in pharmacokinetic behavior among normal subjects is larger than that observed for other physiological values, for example, blood pressure, pulse, height, weight, serum electrolytes, blood sugar, blood urea nitrogen, and serum enzymes such as lactate dehydrogenase and the transaminases.

Drug elimination rates and drug toxicity

Every physician learns to take into account large variations among patients in rates of drug elimination by individualizing the dose of certain drugs, particularly drugs with low therapeutic indices. For clinical purposes, the therapeutic index of a drug may be defined as the ratio of the toxic dose of that drug to its effective dose. (For further discussion of this concept and its derivation see p. 45.) If the dose of a drug with a low therapeutic index is not individualized, the same dose administered by the same route can produce toxicity in some patients, the desired pharmacological effect in other patients, and therapeutic ineffectiveness in still others. By contrast, physicians have a greater margin of safety in administering a drug with a high therapeutic index because for such drugs the physician can select from a wider range of nontoxic doses.

In recent years numerous drugs with low therapeutic indices have been introduced, thereby increasing the risk of toxicity when these drugs are administered. Although the frequency of drug toxicity is high, its exact incidence is unknown and probably differs from one hospital to another and from one geographical region to another. On the medical wards of several university hospitals (Cornell and Johns

Hopkins) the incidence of adverse drug reactions was reported to comprise 5% of all admissions.[2] However, this estimate depends on how an adverse drug reaction is defined. Occasionally a patient's symptoms may be incorrectly attributed to a drug when they actually arise from the underlying disease.[20] Once in the hospital, a patient's chances of experiencing an adverse drug reaction rise in direct proportion to the total number of drugs administered.

These epidemiological data on adverse drug reactions emphasize the practical need to understand precise causes for extensive differences among patients in drug response. Understanding these mechanisms could lead to safer ways to use drugs. Probably many adverse drug reactions arise from a failure to tailor the dosage of drugs with low therapeutic indices closely enough to widely different individual needs.

Determining causes of variations in drug elimination rates

Studies designed to identify specific causes of large interindividual variations in drug response are difficult to perform in humans due to the marked heterogeneity of humans with respect to many factors that can influence drug disposition and due to the consequent difficulty of adequately controlling these numerous factors. There-

TABLE 6-1. A partial list of variables affecting drug disposition in experimental animals

Variables in external environment	Variables in internal environment	Pharmacological (drug) variables
Aggregation	Adjuvant arthritis	Short- versus long-term administration
Air exchange and composition	Age	
Barometric pressure	Alloxan diabetes	Bioavailability
Cage design, materials	Cardiovascular function	Dose
Cedar and other softwood bedding	Castration and hormone replacement	Withdrawal
Cleanliness		Presence of other drugs or food
Coprophagia	Circadian and seasonal variations	
Diet (food and water)	Dehydration	Routes of administration
Exercise	Disease—hepatic, renal, malignant, endocrine (thyroid, adrenal, pituitary)	
Gravity		Volume of material injected
Hepatic microsomal enzyme induction or inhibition by insecticides, piperonyl butoxide, heavy metals, detergents, organic solvents, ammonia, vinyl chloride, aerosols containing eucalyptol, etc.	Estrous cycle	Tolerance
	Fever	Vehicle
	Gastrointestinal function, patency, and flora	Other
	Genetic constitution (strain and species differences)	
Handling	Hepatic blood flow	
Humidity	Infection	
Light cycle	Malnutrition, starvation	
Migration	Pregnancy	
Noise level	Sex	
Temperature	Shock (hemorrhagic or endotoxic)	
	Stress	

fore, reliable studies in humans had to await development of safe noninvasive tests for measuring rates of drug elimination in vivo in individual subjects. Problems in developing, using, and interpreting such tests are described later in this chapter, but until such tests appeared, experimental animals served as substitutes for humans in investigations designed to identify and characterize factors capable of affecting rates of drug elimination. The principal advantage of experimental animals is that almost all critical conditions can be carefully controlled, thereby permitting only one factor to be varied independently of the others, which are kept constant. In addition, tissues necessary for measurement of drug-metabolizing enzyme activity, such as liver, are readily accessible in experimental animals, whereas ethical considerations prohibit their use in humans. Despite these advantages, studies in which experimental animals serve as substitutes for humans can yield misleading results because of well-recognized species differences in pathways of hepatic drug metabolism. Table 6-1 shows a partial list of factors that can affect drug disposition, which have been identified over the past 20 years by many studies on experimental animals performed in different laboratories. The term *partial* is used to suggest the existence of several, as yet undiscovered, additional factors.

Pharmacogenetics   As shown in Table 6-1, pharmacogenetics is only one of many causes of large interindividual variations in drug response. Pharmacogenetics deals with genetically caused variations in drug response. Some pharmacogenetic conditions in humans that affect either drug metabolism or the interaction of drugs at different sites, including receptor sites, are listed in Table 6-2. In humans, pharmacogenetic conditions transmitted by genes at a single locus are divided for convenience into those that affect drug absorption, distribution, metabolism, excretion, and receptor action. As yet, no pharmacogenetic condition directly involving either drug absorption or excretion has been described in humans. But the field of pharmacogenetics is new; few systematic searches for such pharmacogenetic entities have been undertaken. One reason is that the necessary analysis of families to establish the mode of inheritance is difficult. Another reason is that few sufficiently simple, sensitive, and safe quantitative tests of individual pharmacokinetic and pharmacodynamic processes are available for family studies or for population screening.

In pharmacogenetics this screening of populations by a simple, rapid, safe test is necessary to ascertain how a particular trait is inherited, what its incidence is in a given group, and how the frequency of the genes controlling the trait varies from one group and geographical area to another. To achieve these aims, the particular test used to measure drug response in families and populations must possess certain characteristics mentioned before. In addition, the test must satisfactorily discriminate among small differences between subjects in gene structure and function and hence must be able to provide information about direct products of that gene. In pharmacogenetics the direct gene product is a protein or enzyme primarily involved in the response of the body to a particular drug.

Whereas in pharmacogenetic studies the plasma half-life or clearance of a drug

TABLE 6-2. Genetic conditions, probably transmitted as single factors, that alter drug response

Condition	Aberrant enzyme and location	Mode of inheritance*	Agent provoking response
Altering the way the body acts on drugs			
Acatalasia	Catalase in erythrocytes	AR	Hydrogen peroxide
Suxamethonium sensitivity or atypical cholinesterase	Cholinesterase in plasma	AR	Suxamethonium or succinylcholine
Slow inactivation of isoniazid	Isoniazid acetylase in liver	AR	Isoniazid, sulfamethazine, sulfamaprine, procainamide, phenelzine, dapsone, and hydralazine
Acetophenetidin-induced methemoglobinemia	? Mixed function oxidase in liver microsomes that deethylates acetophenetidin	AR	Acetophenetidin
Deficient N-glucosidation of amobarbital	? Mixed function oxidase in liver microsomes that N-glucosidates amobarbital	AR	Amobarbital
Polymorphic hydroxylation of debrisoquine in man	? Mixed function oxidase in liver microsomes that 4-hydroxylates debrisoquine	AR	Debrisoquine
Altering the way drugs act on the body			
Warfarin resistance	? Altered receptor or enzyme in liver with increased affinity for vitamin K	AD	Warfarin
Inability to taste phenylthiourea or phenylthiocarbamide	Unknown	AR	Drugs containing $N–C=S$ group such as phenylthiourea methyl and propylthiouracil
Glucose-6-phosphate dehydrogenase deficiency, favism, or drug-induced hemolytic anemia	Glucose-6-phosphate dehydrogenase	XL incomplete codominant	Various analgesics (acetanilid, acetylsalicylic acid, acetophenetidin [phenacetin], antipyrine, aminopyrine [Pyramidon]); sulfonamides and sulfones (sulfanilamide, sulfapyridine, N^2-acetylsulfanilamide, sulfacetamide, sulfisoxazole [Gantrisin], thiazosulfone, sulfoxone, sulfamethoxypyridazine [Kynex]); antimalarials (primaquine, pamaquine, pentaquine, quinacrine [Atabrine]); nonsulfonamide antibacterial agents (furazolidone, nitrofurantoin [Furadantin], chloramphenicol, p-aminosalicylic acid); and miscellaneous drugs (naphthalene, vitamin K, probenecid, trinitrotoluene, methylene blue, dimercaprol [BAL], phenylhydrazine, quinine, and quinidine)

*AR, autosomal recessive; AD, autosomal dominant; XL, X-linked.

has been conveniently employed as the principal test of gene structure and function, such measurements may not be sensitive enough to serve as an index of possible variations among subjects in genes that control proteins, which are directly involved in the disposition of certain drugs. This potential insensitivity of plasma drug half-life and clearance can become serious if the metabolism of the parent drug is mediated by multiple enzymes. Then it is necessary to measure not just the rate of elimination of the parent drug but also the rate of production of each metabolite formed by each enzymatic reaction. Measurement of every one of these enzymatic reactions permits close scrutiny of the direct product of each gene involved in the metabolism of a drug, thereby excluding contributions to the measurement from some of the extraneous factors listed in Table 6-1. In humans, additional factors need to be considered besides those listed in Table 6-1, including cigarette smoking,[7] ethanol ingestion,[34,35] and antifertility pills,[8] all of which can alter the activity of a subject's hepatic drug-metabolizing enzymes.

Distribution curves of drug response

Several curves can be generated when the same dose of a drug is given by the same route to a large population of normal subjects and a specific quantitative response to the drug is measured and plotted. The three most common shapes of this distribution curve are *unimodal*, *bimodal*, and *trimodal*. Pharmacological responses of a normal population generally exhibit large interindividual variations, again indicating that the same dose of drug cannot be administered to all subjects with the expectation of an identical response and that, therefore, the doses of many drugs must be individualized. Although the *shape* of the curve can provide *clues* as to the mechanisms responsible for this large interindividual variation in drug response, the shapes, by themselves, must not be regarded as conclusive evidence. Thus, it must be emphasized that genetic factors, environmental factors, or both may be responsible for producing any shaped curve. For many drugs, when a population is tested, it is customary to obtain a unimodal, normal gaussian distribution curve of drug response. This curve can arise from purely environmental differences among the subjects or, by contrast, from purely genetic differences in which genes at multiple loci contribute to the variation. This latter type of genetic control is called *polygenic*. Polygenic control is generally observed to be at least partially involved in the regulation of such metric traits as blood pressure, intelligence, and intensity of skin color. Similarly, bimodal or trimodal distribution curves of drug response are usually produced by monogenically controlled conditions, such as those listed in Table 6-2, but can also arise from environmental differences among the subjects investigated. Therefore, although the distribution curve cannot itself distinguish among genetic or environmental causes for interindividual variation, the curve can provide a first step toward such a determination.

The second, most critical step is to perform a family study on individuals located at the extremes of the distribution curve. Individuals at the extremes are most likely to exhibit a response to drugs sufficiently distinctive to permit clear-cut identification and tracing through several generations. By determining whether this particular type of drug response is in fact transmitted through several generations in conformity to Mendelian laws for inheritance of dominant and recessive traits, investigators can tell whether a genetic mechanism controls the variation in drug response observed in the population. Furthermore, the specific kind of genetic control (autosomal dominant or recessive; X-linked dominant or recessive) can be discovered. Only pedigree analysis can provide such information, since, as mentioned before, environmental factors can mimic genetic ones in generating each kind of distribution curve as well as in yielding geographical and racial differences in frequency of individuals showing any specific type of response to a drug. Mimicry by environmental factors of genetic effects occurs frequently in human genetics. Such an individual is termed a *phenocopy* because this individual appears to exhibit a genetically determined trait when in fact an environmental factor produced and copied the effect present in another individual solely as a result of the action of a gene.

Before some of the pharmacogenetic conditions listed in Table 6-2 are discussed, the causes of genetic variation in drug response more common than any of those listed in Table 6-2 will be described. Evidence exists that in several populations large interindividual variations in the disposition of numerous drugs are controlled by genetic factors. Twin studies demonstrated that fivefold to tenfold interindividual variations in disposition of antipyrine,[32] phenylbutazone,[31] and bishydroxycoumarin[30] were genetically controlled (Fig. 6-1). For this purpose, twins may be considered to represent partial family units, since monozygotic twins are identical with respect to all their genes, whereas dizygotic twins have approximately 50% of their genes in common, just as do any siblings. Genetic factors controlling interindividual variations in rates of drug elimination proved, unlike most conditions listed in Table 6-2, to occur commonly and to involve many, rather than few, drugs. An appreciable genetic contribution was also discovered over the control of large interindividual variations among normal subjects in the disposition of nortriptyline, phenytoin, ethanol, halothane, salicylate, and amobarbital. The similar results obtained in all these studies suggest that genetic factors might be primarily involved in the regulation of large variations among normal subjects in the disposition of many other untested drugs known to be eliminated primarily by hepatic metabolism.

Although the precise genetic mechanisms responsible for large interindividual variations in the hepatic metabolism of these commonly used drugs have not yet been firmly established, techniques to measure the major metabolites of many of these drugs are now being used in family studies that should soon provide definitive answers to this important question.[11]

Genetic differences that exist among normal subjects in rates of drug elimination from the body help to explain the markedly different dosage requirements of many patients. These results constitute the scientific basis for the long-recognized need to individualize doses of many commonly used drugs.

PHARMACOGENETIC DIFFERENCES IN ELIMINATION RATES OF COMMONLY USED DRUGS

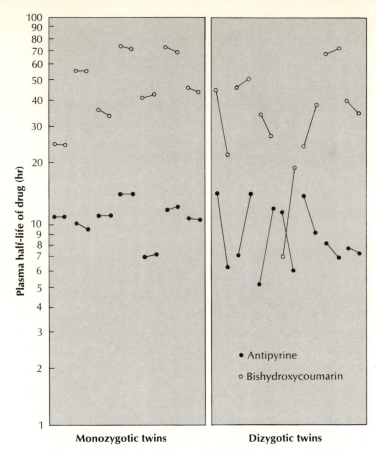

FIG. 6-1. Plasma half-lives of bishydroxycoumarin and antipyrine were measured separately at an interval of more than 6 months in healthy monozygotic (identical) and dizygotic (fraternal) twins. Values for each set of twins for each drug are joined by solid line. Note that intratwin differences in plasma half-life of both bishydroxycoumarin and antipyrine are smaller (as indicated by a shorter line joining the circles) in monozygotic than in dizygotic twins. (Based on data from Vesell, E. S., and Page, J. G.: J. Clin. Invest. **47:**2657, 1968; and Vesell, E. S., and Page, J. G.: Science **161:**72, 1968.)

GENETIC AND ENVIRONMENTAL CAUSES OF VARIATIONS IN DRUG RESPONSE

A rapidly developing area of pharmacogenetics concerns multiple and changing interactions between those genes in a subject that exert control over rates of drug metabolism and numerous factors in the environment of that subject. Despite the underlying genetic control of large interindividual differences in hepatic drug-metabolizing capacity, the enzymes by which the liver biotransforms drugs and the genes controlling them are particularly susceptible to alteration in their activity by many environmental factors. Table 6-1 lists some of these factors, identified from studies in laboratory animals. Quite a few of these factors have been shown to affect drug disposition in humans.

Because so many environmental factors can alter rates of drug elimination in pa-

TABLE 6-3. Applications of the antipyrine test in humans where antipyrine was measured before and after a single environmental change*

Environmental change	Effect of each factor on antipyrine half-life ($t_{1/2}$)
Drugs	
Adrenocorticotropic hormone (ACTH)	Unaltered $t_{1/2}$
Allopurinol	↑ $t_{1/2}$
Aminopyrine (administered simultaneously with antipyrine)	↑ $t_{1/2}$
Amobarbital	↓ $t_{1/2}$
Barbiturate overdose	↓ $t_{1/2}$
Chlorimipramine	↓ $t_{1/2}$
Delta-9-tetrahydrocannabinol	↑ $t_{1/2}$
Dexamethasone	Unaltered $t_{1/2}$
Disulfiram	↑ $t_{1/2}$
Ethanol (for 21 days)	↓ $t_{1/2}$
Ethinyl estradiol plus *dl*-norgestrel	↑ $t_{1/2}$
Fenfluramine	Unaltered $t_{1/2}$
Halofenate	↓ $t_{1/2}$
Hydrocortisone infusion	↓ $t_{1/2}$
	↑ $t_{1/2}$
	Unaltered $t_{1/2}$
Levodopa	↑ $t_{1/2}$
Mandrax^R (diphenhydramine-methaqualone)	↓ $t_{1/2}$
Norethynodrel plus mestranol	↑ $t_{1/2}$
Paracetamol overdose	↑ $t_{1/2}$
Phenobarbital	↓ $t_{1/2}$
Propranolol	↑ $t_{1/2}$
Quinine	↓ $t_{1/2}$
Rifampicin	Unaltered $t_{1/2}$
Spironolactone	↓ $t_{1/2}$
Spironolactone plus butobarbitone	↓ $t_{1/2}$
Tricyclic antidepressants	↓ $t_{1/2}$ or unaltered
Amitriptyline	↑ $t_{1/2}$
Chlorimipramine	
Desmethylimipramine	
Imipramine	
Nortriptyline	
Vitamin C	↓ $t_{1/2}$
Disease states	
Etiocholanolone-induced fever	↑ $t_{1/2}$
Hyperthyroid	↓ $t_{1/2}$
Hypothyroid	↑ $t_{1/2}$
Lead poisoning	↑ $t_{1/2}$

*Based on data from Vesell, E. S.: Clin. Pharmacol. Ther. **26:**675, 1979.

Continued.

TABLE 6-3. Applications of the antipyrine test in humans where antipyrine was measured before and after a single environmental change—cont'd

Environmental change	Effect of each factor on antipyrine half-life ($t_{1/2}$)
Environmental factors and chemicals	
Bed rest (for 3 days)	$\downarrow t_{1/2}$
Brussels sprouts and cabbage diet	Small $\downarrow t_{1/2}$
Charcoal-broiled beef diet	$\downarrow t_{1/2}$
Cigarette smoking	$\downarrow t_{1/2}$
Circadian variations	Circadian variations in antipyrine metabolism occur in some subjects
Cola nut chewing	Unaltered $t_{1/2}$
Obese subjects fasting for 10 days	Unaltered $t_{1/2}$
High carbohydrate–low protein isocaloric diet	$\uparrow t_{1/2}$
Low carbohydrate–high protein isocaloric diet	$\downarrow t_{1/2}$
Menstrual cycle	Small $\downarrow t_{1/2}$ at midcycle (single subject)
Metabolism in the neonate	Antipyrine $t_{1/2}$ 4 days after birth is shorter than at 1 day after birth
Pharmacokinetics of oral and intravenous antipyrine administration	$t_{1/2}$ same after oral or intravenous administration
Piperonyl butoxide	Unaltered $t_{1/2}$
Relationship between D-glucaric acid excretion in urine and antipyrine metabolism	High correlation between antipyrine $t_{1/2}$ and D-glucaric acid excretion in urine
Stress of heat, exercise, and fluid deprivation	Small $\downarrow t_{1/2}$
Miscellaneous factors	
Reproducibility of antipyrine disposition in a subject up to 1 year	$t_{1/2}$ highly reproducible in individual subjects

tients and because the relative role that each of these factors plays in influencing rates of drug metabolism changes even in the same subject with time and with numerous other variables, it is very difficult to identify, even at a particular time, which factors are operating and what contribution each factor actually makes to the total drug-metabolizing capacity of a person. For this reason, the role of each of these factors is generally investigated in normal, nonmedicated volunteer subjects in a near basal state with respect to most of the variables known to alter hepatic drug-metabolizing capacity.[33] Measurements with a test drug, such as antipyrine, are then performed to quantify this basal capacity in each volunteer subject; a single environmental alteration is introduced, during which the subject's drug-metabolizing activity is remeasured; and the change from basal values is taken to quantitate the effect exerted by the single environmental change.[33] This approach, introduced in 1969 and now widely used to explore gene-environment interactions, clearly has limitations, since results cannot always be extrapolated with accuracy to other drugs or will certain environmental factors that alter the disposition of other drugs always alter antipyrine pharmacokinetics. Clearly other test drugs are therefore required.

Furthermore, results obtained in normal volunteer subjects may not apply to patients with a variety of disease states. These drawbacks are often outweighed by the virtues of a carefully controlled approach, with each volunteer subject used as his or her own control. This approach permits investigation of a single factor at a time and elimination of many interfering genetic and environmental variables inherent in the alternative experimental design of comparing a control group with a different experimental group. Thus, in humans the antipyrine test has been successfully utilized to identify the impact of many of the factors listed in Table 6-1 on drug disposition.[29] The results are shown in Table 6-3.[29]

A number of pharmacogenetic conditions result from changes in an enzyme controlling the metabolism of a drug. In these conditions, the mutations result in drug accumulation, which causes toxicity. Drug accumulation and toxicity arise from genetically transmitted defects in metabolism of the drug. These defects cause decreased conversion of pharmacologically active drug to pharmacologically inactive metabolite(s). It is of interest that the genetic abnormality long precedes administration of the drug. Thus, if individuals possessing such genetic abnormalities can be identified *before* they receive the drug, toxicity can be avoided by either not giving the drug or by giving a much reduced dose. For these reasons, familiarity with pharmacogenetic conditions can help physicians administer drugs more safely and can reduce the high incidence of drug toxicity.

PHARMACO-GENETIC CONDITIONS (SINGLE-LOCUS TRANSMISSION) THAT ALTER DRUG METABOLISM

The condition acatalasia was discovered in a patient on application of hydrogen peroxide to the gums to sterilize a wound after surgery. Instead of bubbles of oxygen being evolved due to the action of the enzyme catalase, as occurs in normal individuals, hydrogen peroxide remained unchanged and caused toxicity by denaturing tissue proteins. The patient lacked catalase in her oral mucosa and erythrocytes, as did three of her five siblings. The parents were second cousins—consanguinity is a hallmark of autosomal recessive inheritance, which proved to be the mode of transmission of acatalasia. The incidence of this condition reached 1% in certain regions of Japan and also occurred in slightly lower frequency in certain areas of Switzerland. Only a few sporadic cases have been reported in the United States. An impressive lesson from the discovery of acatalasia is that the clinician (in this case, the Japanese oral surgeon Takahara[24-27]) can make an important contribution if alert to the possibility that genetic differences can cause unusual reactions to drugs. Takahara postulated, after completing oral surgery on his patient who then exhibited a toxic response to the antiseptic hydrogen peroxide, that she responded inappropriately because she lacked the normal form of the enzyme required to eliminate the drug. He proved his theory to be correct by gathering similar cases from 27 Japanese families.

Acatalasia

Another example of how a pharmacogenetic lesion can produce drug toxicity is that of atypical plasma cholinesterase. Individuals possessing a double dose of a

Atypical plasma cholinesterase

mutant gene cannot adequately hydrolyze succinylcholine, a compound administered prior to surgical procedures to produce muscle relaxation. Normally succinylcholine is rapidly metabolized by a plasma esterase. However, in patients with two mutant genes that control the structure of the plasma enzyme cholinesterase, the drug is retained in the body for much longer periods than usual. Succinylcholine can produce respiratory failure for prolonged periods of time and, potentially, death, if appropriate respiratory resuscitation is not available. When succinylcholine was introduced in 1952 and administered widely in England as a preanesthetic agent, several deaths due to paralysis of the respiratory muscles did in fact occur in individuals who had inherited from each parent a mutant gene at the cholinesterase locus. Although 1 in 25 persons carries a single dose of the mutant gene, affected persons with two doses occur only once among 2500 individuals.

Studies on the plasma cholinesterase activity of affected individuals, their families, and normal individuals showed considerable overlap until a refinement in technique was introduced. This refinement consisted of a determination of the "dibucaine number," or percent inhibition of plasma cholinesterase by the drug dibucaine (Nupercaine). The dibucaine numbers of 135 individuals of seven unrelated families gave a trimodal curve with no overlap. It has been postulated that plasma cholinesterase activity is determined by two genes at a single locus (alleles), one responsible for the *usual*, the other for the *atypical* form of the enzyme. Most individuals, having a dibucaine number of around 80, are postulated to have two of the usual alleles, $E_1^u E_1^u$. Individuals of the atypical phenotype, having dibucaine numbers of around 22, have the genotype $E_1^a E_1^a$. Finally, a third or intermediate group, with dibucaine numbers of around 62, may have a genotype of $E_1^u E_1^a$.[10]

Genetic differences in rates of acetylation of isoniazid, hydralazine, procainamide, and some sulfonamides

Isoniazid is used to treat tuberculosis. Individuals with the genetically transmitted trait of fast acetylation of isoniazid may not be adequately treated on a fixed low dose because of rapid biotransformation of the drug. By contrast, slow acetylators, when receiving the higher, normal dose, may develop toxic effects. Isoniazid-induced polyneuritis, that is, pain and tingling and possibly muscular weakness in the upper and lower extremities, occurs more frequently in slow, than in rapid, acetylators of isoniazid.[3,18,19] Fortunately, the neuritis can be effectively treated with vitamin B_6 (pyridoxine).

Isoniazid is metabolized by a liver acetylase. Approximately 50% of the population in this country are acetylators by virtue of possessing a double dose of a recessive form of the gene at this locus. Fast acetylators are either heterozygous or homozygous for the dominant allele. Like several other genetically controlled variations in man, this hereditary variation in acetylation exhibits marked geographical differences in gene frequency. For example, slow inactivation is uncommon in Eskimos, 95% of whom are rapid acetylators, and only slightly more common in Japanese, 90% of whom are rapid acetylators. In Latin America, approximately 67% of the population are rapid acetylators.

Genetically controlled fast and slow acetylation occurs for several other drugs, including certain sulfonamides; the antihypertensive drug hydralazine; procainamide, an antiarrhythmic drug; and phenelzine, an antidepressant drug. However, several drugs metabolized by acetylation, such as the antitubercular drug *p*-aminosalicylic acid, do not show this difference in rate. Therefore, a different enzyme must acetylate these drugs. Continued administration of high doses of hydralazine in slow, but not fast, acetylators can lead to severe toxicity.

Toxicity can develop not only from drug accumulation due to genetically induced retardation in the normal rate of metabolism of a drug but also from the metabolites themselves. For example, rapid acetylators of isoniazid may be more liable than slow acetylators to develop hepatitis after chronic isoniazid administration; presumably a metabolite of the drug is the offending agent. Thus, compared to parent drugs, metabolites cannot all be considered innocuous. An exciting new branch of toxicology is devoted to exploration of how highly reactive, transient drug metabolites covalently bind to tissue components, thereby producing pathologic lesions. In this manner, these metabolites are believed to cause some types of teratogenesis, cancer, drug toxicity, and hypersensitivity. Accordingly, genetically controlled variations in rates of production of these reactive metabolites may determine whether a particular individual is at more or less risk of developing any of these forms of tissue toxicity after exposure to a drug or foreign chemical.

Acetophenetidin-induced methemoglobinemia

Severe methemoglobinemia and hemolysis occurred in a 17-year-old girl after ingestion of the analgesic phenacetin (acetophenetidin).[21] Heritable erythrocytic disorders, including hemoglobinopathies, were excluded as a cause of her hemolysis by multiple laboratory studies. As much as one-half of the patient's hemoglobin was occasionally in the form of methemoglobin. After administration of phenacetin, large amounts of the 2-hydroxyphenetidin metabolite and its conjugates appeared in her urine. In normal persons more than 70% of a single 2 g dose of phenacetin can be accounted for in the urine as *N*-acetyl-*p*-aminophenol (acetaminophen), with only minute amounts of the hydroxylated products that predominated in the patient's urine. One sister, a brother, and both parents of the patient had a normal response to phenacetin, but another sister responded abnormally.

These facts suggested an autosomal recessive mode of inheritance of a defect in which the patient's hepatic drug-metabolizing enzymes were deficient in deethylating capacity. Phenacetin, instead of being deethylated to form acetaminophen, as in normal persons, was hydroxylated in the patient and her 38-year-old sister.

In this patient and her sister, toxicity after phenacetin administration probably arose from these abnormal hydroxylated products, since induction by phenobarbital of hepatic phenacetin-hydroxylating enzymes prior to administration of phenacetin exacerbated the condition, producing severe neurological symptoms, including bilateral positive Babinski responses, and profound methemoglobinemia.[21] By contrast, in a normal volunteer, phenacetin administration after the same pretreatment with phenobarbital failed to give rise to either methemoglobinemia or neurological changes.

Deficient N-glucosidation of amobarbital

A twin study suggested that large interindividual variations in elimination rates of amobarbital were under genetic control.[4] Pursuing their initial observations, Kalow and associates investigated the family of one set of twins with a deficiency in N-hydroxylation, but not C-hydroxylation, of amobarbital.[11] The family study of these twins disclosed that this deficiency probably arose from autosomal recessive transmission of a mutant gene.[11] Later this group reported that the urinary metabolite was mistakenly identified as N-hydroxylamobarbital and that the actual metabolite was instead N-β-D-glucopyranosyl amobarbital.[28] This metabolite showed large variations in the urine of 129 volunteers given a single oral dose of amobarbital—one volunteer completely lacked the metabolite, whereas 14 subjects had it as the primary form.[12] Four of these 14 subjects were of Chinese origin, suggesting possible racial differences in the pattern and pathway of metabolite formation.[12] These studies of amobarbital illustrate several fundamental principles of pharmacogenetics: (1) the utility of searching, whenever possible, for a monogenic origin of pharmacogenetic conditions; (2) the necessity of performing genetic analyses in families; and (3) the need, whenever more than a single metabolite is produced from the parent drug, to measure rates of formation of each metabolite, rather than only the disappearance of the parent drug.

Polymorphic hydroxylation of debrisoquin

The antihypertensive drug debrisoquin is widely used in England, but is not yet employed in the United States. It was observed that patients receiving debrisoquin vary widely in the hypotensive response to the adrenergic-blocking action of the drug and that a close correlation exists between debrisoquin plasma concentrations and the resultant decline in blood pressure.[22] In 94 unrelated volunteers the urinary ratio of the parent drug to the primary metabolite, 4-hydroxydebrisoquin, was measured after a single oral dose of 10 mg debrisoquin.[14] In three of these 94 subjects the ratio was very high, suggesting a possible deficiency of the hepatic cytochrome P-450 dependent monooxygenase that 4-hydroxylates debrisoquin. Furthermore, family studies of these three volunteers with abnormally high ratios of debrisoquin to 4-hydroxydebrisoquin in the 8-hour urinary collection suggested transmission of the metabolic deficiency as an autosomal recessive trait.[14] Most side effects, as well as most pronounced antihypertensive activity, of debrisoquin occurred in the slow metabolizers, those individuals with the highest urinary ratio of parent drug to metabolite. This result, which could have been predicted from the fact that the main metabolite is devoid of antihypertensive action, illustrates both the direct clinical and toxicological consequences of pharmacogenetic conditions and also the need for physicians who observe an unusual drug response in a patient to consider genetic factors as a potential cause.

Another fundamental pharmacogenetic principle is underscored by the work of the British group on the genetic control of debrisoquen metabolism, as well as by the previously described example of genetic differences in isoniazid metabolism. When a genetically controlled variation is discovered in the disposition of a particular drug, a search should be undertaken to determine whether the disposition of structurally related drugs is similarly affected by the same genes. The British group reported that the metabolism of several drugs, in addition to debrisoquen, is regulated by this same genetic locus; these other metabolic reactions include O-deethylation of phenacetin[23] and aromatic hydroxylation of phenytoin.[9]

PHARMACOGENETIC CONDITIONS (SINGLE-LOCUS TRANSMISSION) THAT ALTER DRUG INTERACTIONS

Resistance to warfarin is one of several mutations in humans that modify the pharmacological response to a drug by altering the drug receptor (Table 6-2).[16,17] One might envision the mutation changing the receptor shape so that it is unable to bind the drug as efficiently as the normal receptor does. In subjects bearing the mutant gene, the therapeutic effect is not achieved after normal doses of warfarin. Anticoagulation occurs only after the physician administers many times the normal dose of warfarin.

Warfarin resistance

Warfarin acts by inhibiting the production of several blood components necessary for clotting, probably by competing with vitamin K for the receptor. In cases of warfarin resistance the mutant receptor is an altered molecule that fails to bind warfarin as strongly as the normal one and, therefore, does not produce anticoagulation; this alteration results also in a stronger than normal binding of vitamin K. The first family discovered to exhibit this genetically transmitted resistance to warfarin is shown in Fig. 6-2; the index case was a 71-year-old man who came to the hospital with an acute myocardial infarction, the standard treatment of which includes anticoagulation with warfarin.

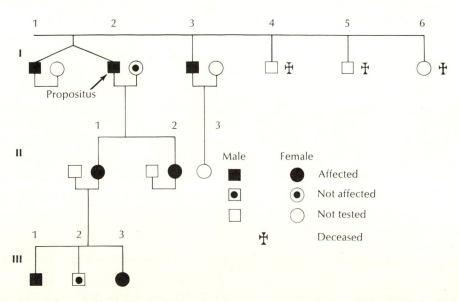

FIG. 6-2. Transmission of warfarin resistance through three generations of a family, indicating autosomal codominant inheritance of resistance to pharmacological effects of this drug. (From O'Reilly, et al. Reprinted by permission. From The New England Journal of Medicine **271:**809, 1964.)

Genetic differences in capacity to taste phenylthiocarbamide

Most persons are able to taste dilute solutions of phenylthiocarbamide (PTC, phenylthiourea) and chemically related compounds containing the thiocyanate group, whereas others, called nontasters, cannot.[1,6,13] These differences in ability to taste PTC, in addition to the fact that metabolism of some thiocyanate compounds appears to be no different in tasters and nontasters, suggest that a receptor mutation exists in nontasters. Enlargement of the thyroid gland, called goiter, can be produced in rats by PTC, and certain of these compounds are utilized as antithyroid drugs in cases of thyroid overactivity. A number of common vegetables including turnips, brussels sprouts, and kale contain a goiter-producing chemical, and nodular goiters are more common among nontasters than among tasters of PTC. These differences in taste threshold may influence food preferences and, thus, consumption of potential goitrogenic compounds.

Genetic control of glucose-6-phosphate dehydrogenase deficiency

A more complicated condition is glucose-6-phosphate dehydrogenase (G-6-PD) deficiency, which affects 100 million people in the world, primarily in areas where malaria is endemic, and 1 in 10 black males in the United States.[5,15,36] Individuals with any one of 80 different mutations that occur at a specific site on the X chromosome develop hemolytic anemia after exposure to a large number of different drugs, some of which are listed in Table 6-2. Some dietary constituents, such as fava beans (beans of the plant *Vicia fava*), can cause hemolysis in susceptible subjects. The mechanism believed responsible for development of hemolysis is complex but probably involves initially a shortage of NADPH, the reduced form of the cofactor nicotinamide adenine dinucleotide phosphate. NADPH is produced by the enzyme G-6-PD. NADPH itself then serves as cofactor for glutathione reductase, an enzyme that converts glutathione to the reduced form. Thus, G-6-PD deficiency ultimately leads to deficiency of reduced glutathione.

In normal individuals, the red cell membrane is maintained in a functional state by having an adequate supply of reduced glutathione available to keep membrane proteins in a reduced and operative condition. Highly reactive drug metabolites oxidize membrane proteins; if these oxidized proteins are not rapidly reduced by glutathione, hemolysis ensues. Thus, a genetically induced enzyme deficiency results in decreased usable glutathione, thereby creating an altered receptor in the cell membrane. Reactive drug metabolites binding to this new receptor produce hemolysis.

It has recently become apparent that there is a high degree of genetically controlled variation among the total complement of enzymes in humans. As many as one-third of all enzymes in humans exist in electrophoretically distinguishable forms that vary markedly within many white populations. These variant forms are determined by genes that, like the previously discussed traits affecting drug disposition, are located at a single genetic locus and transmitted from generation to generation according to Mendelian law. For additional discussion of these and other genetically controlled variations affecting drug response and their relevance to drug administration, the reader is referred to more extensive reviews on pharmacogenetics.[37-43]

PERSPECTIVE

When prescribing drugs with low therapeutic indices, the physician needs to remember that for many different reasons large interindividual variations occur in drug response. Therefore, the dose of such drugs needs to be individualized because the same dose of a drug given to three patients can produce toxicity in one, the desired therapeutic effect in the second, and no pharmacological effect in the third. In this chapter several different monogenically transmitted conditions that cause large interindividual differences in drug response were described. Such conditions involve mainly drug interaction with receptors or drug metabolism, in which, despite usual doses of certain drugs, an inefficient enzyme leads to drug accumulation and consequent toxicity. From a practical point of view physicians need to know that such genetic conditions exist because they can inquire of a patient before administering such drugs whether toxic reactions have been experienced before by that patient or relatives. If so, the drug can be avoided and an appropriate substitute selected. If drug toxicity occurs in a patient due to a genetic condition, the other members of the patient's family should be suspected of being affected and if a simple noninvasive test is available, as in G-6-PD deficiency, they should be studied for this possibility.

Hereditary factors controlling pathways of drug metabolism also cause large interindividual variations in rates of elimination of certain commonly used drugs. In most cases the precise metabolic pathways and mode of transmission of these genetically controlled interindividual differences remain to be established. Superimposed on these genetic factors are many environmental conditions that can alter an individual's inherited capacity to eliminate drugs.

The physician needs to be aware that in a given patient these genetic and environmental factors dynamically interact. Thus, capacity to eliminate drugs involves multiple conditions and factors that themselves can change from day to day in a given patient. For these reasons, the physician must be careful in administering drugs with low therapeutic indices and must be aware that capacity to eliminate such drugs can differ not only from patient to patient, but also in the same patient from day to day.

REFERENCES

1 Blakeslee, A. F.: Genetics of sensory thresholds: taste for phenyl thiocarbamide, Proc. Natl. Acad. Sci. **18:**120, 1932.

2 Cluff, L. E., Thornton, G., Seidl, L., and Smith, J.: Epidemiological study of adverse drug reactions, Trans. Assoc. Am. Physicians **78:**255, 1965.

3 Drayer, D. E., and Reidenberg, M. M.: Clinical consequences of polymorphic acetylation of basic drugs, Clin. Pharmacol. Ther. **22:**251, 1977.

4 Endrenyi, L., Inaba, T., and Kalow, W.: Genetic study of amobarbital elimination based on its kinetics in twins, Clin. Pharmacol. Ther. **20:**701, 1976.

5 Fraser, I. M., Tilton, B. E., and Vesell, E. S.: Alterations in normal and G6PD-deficient human erythrocytes of various ages after exposure to metabolites of hemolytic drugs, Pharmacology **5:**173, 1971.

6 Harris, H., Kalmus, H., and Trotter, W. H.: Taste sensitivity to PTC in goitre and diabetes, Lancet **257:**1038, 1949.

7 Hart, P., Farrel, G. C., Cooksley, W. G. E.,

and Powell, L. W.: Enhanced drug metabolism in cigarette smokers, Br. Med. J. **2:**147, 1976.

8 Homeida, M., Halliwell, M., and Branch, R. A.: Effects of an oral contraceptive on hepatic size and antipyrine metabolism in pre-menopausal women, Clin. Pharmacol. Ther. **24:**228, 1978.

9 Idle, J. R., Sloan, T. P., Smith, R. L., and Wakile, L. A.: Application of the phenotyped panel approach to the detection of polymorphism of drug oxidation in man, Br. J. Pharmacol. **66:**430P, 1979.

10 Kalow, W.: Pharmacogenetics: heredity and the response to drugs, Philadelphia, 1962, W. B. Saunders Co.

11 Kalow, W., Kadar, D., Inaba, T., and Tang, B. K.: A case of deficiency of N-hydroxyla-tion of amobarbital, Clin. Pharmacol. Ther. **21:**530, 1977.

12 Kalow, W., Tang, B. K., Kadar, D., and Inaba, T.: Distinctive patterns of amobarbital metabolites, Clin. Pharmacol. Ther. **24:**576, 1978.

13 Kitchin, F. D., Howel-Evans, W., Clarke, C. A., McDonnell, R. B., and Sheppard, P. M.: PTC taste response and thyroid disease, Br. Med. J. **1:**1069, 1959.

14 Mahgoub, A., Dring, L. G., Idle, J. R., Lancaster, R., and Smith, R. L.: Polymorphic hy-droxylation of debrisoquen in man, Lancet **2:**584, 1977.

15 Motulsky, A. G., Yoshkda, A., and Stamatoyan-nopoulos, G.: Variants of glucose-6-phosphate dehydrogenase, Ann. N.Y. Acad. Sci. **179:**636, 1971.

16 O'Reilly, R. A.: The second reported kindred with hereditary resistance to oral anticoagulant drugs, N. Engl. J. Med. **282:**1448, 1970.

17 O'Reilly, R. A., Aggeler, P. M., Hoag, M. S., Leong, L. S., and Kropatkin, M. L.: Hereditary transmission of exceptional resistance to cou-marin anticoagulant drugs. The first reported kindred, N. Engl. J. Med. **271:**809, 1964.

18 Price Evans, D. A. P.: Individual variations of drug metabolism as a factor in drug toxicity, Ann. N.Y. Acad. Sci. **123:**178, 1965.

19 Price Evans, D. A. P., and White, T. A.: Human acetylation polymorphism, J. Lab. Clin. Med. **63:**394, 1964.

20 Reidenberg, M. M., and Lowenthan, D. T.: Adverse nondrug reactions, N. Engl. J. Med. **279:**678, 1968.

21 Shahidi, N. T.: Acetophenetidin sensitivity, Am. J. Dis. Child **113:**81, 1967.

22 Silas, J. H., Lennard, M. S., Tucker, G. T., Smith, A. J., Malcolm, S. L., and Marten, T. R.: Why hypertensive patients vary in their response to oral debrisoquen, Br. Med. J. **1:**422, 1977.

23 Sloan, T. P., Mahgoub, A., Lancaster, R., Idle, J. R., and Smith, R. L.: Polymorphism of carbon oxidation of drugs and clinical implications, Br. Med. J. **2:**655, 1978.

24 Takahara, S.: Progressive oral gargrene probably due to lack of catalase in the blood (acata-lasemia), Lancet **263:**1101, 1952.

25 Takahara, S., and Doi, K.: Statistical study of acatalasemia (a review of thirty-eight cases appearing in the literature), Acta Med. Okayama **13:**1, 1959.

26 Takahara, S., Hamilton, H. B., Neel, J. V., Kobara, T. Y., Ogura, Y., and Nishimura, E. T.: Hypocatalasemia: a new genetic carrier state, J. Clin. Invest. **39:**610, 1960.

27 Takahara, S., Sato, H., Doi, M., and Mihara, S.: Acatalasemia III. On the hereditary of acata-lasemia, Proc. Japan Acad. **28:**585, 1952.

28 Tang, B. K., Kalow, W., and Grey, A. A.: Amo-barbital metabolism in man: N-glucoside formation, Res. Commun. Chem. Pathol. Pharmacol. **21:**45, 1978.

29 Vesell, E. S.: The antipyrine test in clinical pharmacology: conceptions and misconceptions, Clin. Pharmacol. Ther. **26:**275, 1979.

30 Vesell, E. S., and Page, J. G.: Genetic control of dicumarol levels in man, J. Clin. Invest. **47:**2657, 1968.

31 Vesell, E. S., and Page, J. G.: Genetic control of drug levels in man: antipyrine, Science **161:**72, 1968.

32 Vesell, E. S., and Page, J. G.: Genetic control of drug levels in man: phenylbutazone, Science **159:**1479, 1968.

33 Vesell, E. S., and Page, J. G.: Genetic control of the phenobarbital-induced shortening of plasma antipyrine half-lives in man, J. Clin. Invest. **48:**2202, 1969.

34 Vesell, E. S., Page, J. G., and Passananti, G. T.: Genetic and environmental factors affecting ethanol metabolism in man, Clin. Pharmacol. Ther. **12:**192, 1971.

35 Vesell, E. S., Passananti, G. T., and Lee, C. H.: Impairment of drug metabolism by di-sulfiram in man, Clin. Pharmacol. Ther. **12:**785, 1971.

36 Yoshida, A.: A single amino acid substitution (asparagine to aspartic acid) between normal (B+) and the common negro variant (A+) of human glucose-6-phosphate dehydrogenase, Proc. Nat. Acad. Sci. **57:**835, 1967.

REVIEWS

37 Kalow, W.: Pharmacogenetics: heredity and the response to drugs, Philadelphia, 1962, W. B. Saunders Co.

38 Kalow, W., Tang, B. K., Kadar, D., Endrenyi, L., and Chan, F. -Y.: A method for studying drug metabolism in populations: racial differences in amobarbital metabolism, Clin. Pharmacol. Ther. **26:**766, 1979.

39 LaDu, B. N.: Pharmacogenetics: defective enzymes in relation to reactions to drugs, Annu. Rev. Med. **23:**452, 1972.

40 Motulsky, A. G.: Drugs and genes, Ann. Intern. Med. **70:**1269, 1969.

41 Vesell, E. S.: Pharmacogenetics, N. Engl. J. Med. **287:**904, 1972.

42 Vesell, E. S.: Advances in pharmacogenetics, Progr. Med. Genet. **9:**291, 1973.

43 Vesell, E. S.: Pharmacogenetics: multiple interactions between genes and environment as determinants of drug response, Am. J. Med. **66:**183, 1979.

CHAPTER 7

Effects of age on drug disposition

PROBLEMS OF
INVESTIGATING
In the previous chapter complex, dynamic interactions between environmental factors capable of altering rates of drug elimination and underlying genetic mechanisms that control large interindividual variations in rates of drug metabolism were described. The picture emerges of a very plastic, easily perturbed system. In humans the pharmacokinetic processes of drug absorption, distribution, metabolism, and excretion are indeed subject to change by numerous, continuously impinging environmental factors that can fluctuate greatly in various disease states when hepatic, cardiovascular, and renal status, as well as nutrition, may be changing drastically in short periods of time. By contrast, under stable, near basal conditions, the rate of drug elimination in a given normal subject is generally highly reproducible over long periods of time (Table 7-1). To illustrate how complex the effect of even a single one of the numerous factors in Table 6-1 can be with respect to its influence on drug disposition, the factor of age was selected for consideration in this chapter. Even the subject of age has to be confined for adequate treatment here; space limitations prevent discussion of much recent work on drug disposition during the fetal period and also on effects of age on receptor interactions of drugs.

For many years physicians recognized that patients receiving drugs with low therapeutic indices had to have the usual adult doses reduced to avoid drug toxicity. Precise causes for increased drug sensitivity of geriatric patients have been difficult to identify. Accordingly, only in the last 6 years have some mechanisms responsible for reduced dosage requirements of elderly patients been firmly established. In the last 6 years multiple studies corrected this relative neglect, and the results revealed that, for almost every drug investigated, the values obtained for rates of drug absorption, distribution, metabolism, or excretion differed in geriatric subjects compared to young adults.

Several reasons exist for neglect of geriatric subjects with respect to pharmacological investigations. Until recently elderly subjects have not been recognized as an appropriate group in whom one could and should investigate fundamental pharmacological processes. In 1974 this was changed by creation of the National Institute of Aging, which gave impetus to research on all medical problems of aging. Pharmacological studies in the geriatric population were specially encouraged. In the formation of this institute geriatric patients were identified as a legitimate and worthy group

TABLE 7-1. Reproducibility of plasma half-lives of bishydroxycoumarin and antipyrine in normal volunteers under near basal conditions

Volunteer	Plasma half-life (hour)		
	Initial	Repeat	Percent change
Bishydroxycoumarin			
D. H.	46.0	45.0	2.2
D. W.	44.0	42.5	3.4
Ge. L.	72.0	66.8	7.2
Gu. L.	69.0	70.8	2.6
Ja. T.	74.0	70.8	4.3
Jo. T.	72.0	73.6	2.2
Ja. H.	7.0	7.5	7.1
Je. H.	19.0	18.4	3.2
Antipyrine			
T. Ch.	10.6	11.3	6.6
T. C.	12.5	11.4	8.8
G. Z.	7.7	7.5	2.6
T. L.	12.7	13.2	3.9
R. F.	22.4	20.5	8.5
M. R.	13.1	13.3	1.5
C. H.	9.5	10.0	5.3
P. M.	5.8	6.0	3.5

for fundamental clinical pharmacological studies. Several considerations were particularly compelling. Not only have geriatric subjects constituted an increasingly large proportion of the total population over the past decade, but also this age group experienced more health problems on a per capita basis than any other. Also this group received more prescribed drugs than any other. Consequently, geriatric patients suffered more adverse drug reactions, since the incidence of adverse drug reactions rises in direct proportion to the total number of drugs taken.

Geriatric subjects, compared to middle-aged subjects, present special problems to the pharmacologist and the clinician. To identify how drugs are handled in "normal" geriatric subjects, such subjects must be carefully examined to exclude pathology. However, the very changes that occur in drug disposition in geriatric subjects occur largely because of degenerative alterations in the structure and function of the heart, liver, and kidney. These degenerative changes have as consequences decreased physiological function of each tissue. For example, cardiac output declines approximately 1% per year from age 19 to 86 years, and with age a decreased proportion of the remaining blood goes to the liver and kidneys.[1] Age-induced changes in the structure and function of critical organs probably occur at different rates in different subjects. Accordingly, subjects of the same chronological age can exhibit different degrees of cardiovascular, hepatic, or renal degeneration and hence different degrees of impairment in the physiological function of each organ.

Exogenous environmental factors that can modify drug disposition change with age. These alterations in drug disposition are associated with cigarette smoking, various dietary changes, alcohol ingestion, coffee and tea consumption, and exposure at home or at work to chemicals that can induce or inhibit the hepatic drug-metabolizing enzymes. With age the following changes tend to occur, often concomitantly, thereby complicating analysis of drug disposition and response in the elderly: cigarette smoking decreases or stops; the total caloric intake declines; the amount of exercise is reduced; retirement tends to make life more sedentary; alcohol, tea, and coffee consumption decreases; exposure to chemicals at work and at home decreases. As a result of decreased caloric intake, total body weight tends to decline. Relationships between total body fat, muscle, and extracellular fluid change. For example, body fat increases from 18% to 36% of total body weight in men and from 33% to 48% in women as they increase in age from 18 to 85 years.[19]

Despite these difficulties in defining precisely the causes for age-associated alterations in drug absorption, distribution, metabolism, and excretion and despite the fact that as yet no study has successfully eliminated or adequately assessed all these contributing variables to provide a full description of how aging isolated from all the aforementioned interfering variables affects the individual kinetic processes involved in drug disposition, the following generalizations attempt to present the imperfect state of the art. Hopefully future studies will more rigorously exclude several of the confounding variables enumerated before, thereby permitting a more accurate identification of how and why drug disposition changes with age. Gillette has made suggestions on how to design studies on aging to obtain adequate pharmacokinetic data, claiming that as yet few, if any, of the studies performed in humans have obtained the requisite information.[8]

DRUG ABSORPTION FROM SITES OF ADMINISTRATION

Although complete data concerning effects of age on gastrointestinal absorption of drugs are presently unavailable, certain changes that occur with age should, from a purely theoretical point of view, alter rates of drug absorption from the gastrointestinal tract. For example, with age gastric emptying time decreases, probably secondary to increased stomach pH. Shortened retention of drugs in the stomach would be anticipated to accelerate their absorption, since drug absorption in the gut occurs mainly in the small intestine due to the large absorbing surface available there. However, drug absorption is complex, involving several distinct steps, including disintegration of tablets or capsules and dissolution of active ingredients. Drugs must dissolve in gut fluids before absorption can occur. Rates of these critical processes—gastrointestinal disintegration of tablets and dissolution of drug into gut fluids—may change with age, thereby affecting rates of gastrointestinal drug absorption, which in turn can change the peak plasma drug concentration attained, the time at which this peak is attained, and the duration of both peak and therapeutically effective plasma drug concentrations.

Another critical factor that affects gastrointestinal drug absorption is intestinal blood perfusion, which has been demonstrated to decrease by 40% to 50% from rates measured in young adults.[1] This reduction would be expected to slow drug absorption in the gut due to decreased transfer of some drugs by active transport across the serosal membrane. Reduction with age in the rate of phosphorylation in the intestinal mucosa retards active absorption of galactose, whereas passive absorption of xylose in the gut declines by 40% from ages 18 to 40 years to ages 70 to 80 years.[14]

An additional factor in the elderly that might also tend to slow gastrointestinal drug absorption is increased use of laxatives in the elderly compared to normal young adults. By shortening gastrointestinal transit time laxatives tend to decrease the time available for drug absorption in the gut. Absorption of certain slow-release preparations might not be adequate. Reports have appeared claiming decreased gastrointestinal absorption of xylose, iron, glucose, and calcium in the elderly.

Despite these theoretical considerations suggesting reduced rates of gastrointestinal drug absorption with age, Castleden et al.[4] reported that age exerted no significant effect on either the rate or amount of gastrointestinal absorption of aspirin, an acidic drug, or the β-adrenergic blocker, practolol, a basic drug excreted unchanged by the kidney after absorption from the small intestine. For each drug, the authors measured the lag time (time between dosing and first appearance of drug in plasma), peak hour (time at which maximum plasma concentration of drug occurred), total amount of drug in plasma, and, finally, absorption rate constant (the rate at which the drug crosses the gut mucosa). For aspirin, geriatric and young subjects were not significantly different in any of these measurements. However, geriatric subjects had significantly longer mean practolol lag times, higher plasma practolol concentrations, and higher total amounts of practolol in plasma than did young subjects. These differences between young and geriatric subjects were interpreted as reflecting impairment of renal practolol clearance with age. No change in gastrointestinal absorption of practolol occurred, since young and geriatric subjects showed no difference in absorption rate constant for practolol or in time required to reach maximal plasma practolol concentration.

The paucity of studies quantitating age-associated effects on drug distribution may be due in part to the formidable difficulty of distinguishing between the normal aging process, on the one hand, and physiological dysfunction secondary to degenerative diseases of the heart, liver, and kidney that commonly afflict the elderly, on the other hand. These degenerative diseases can change the composition of fluid compartments of the body, such as total body water, extracellular water, and intracellular water. Therefore, selection of appropriate geriatric subjects for pharmacokinetic investigations influences the results; some conflicting reports can probably be attributed to failure of some studies to employ sufficiently rigorous criteria of "normality" in selecting geriatric subjects.

Albumin concentrations decline with age (Fig. 7-1).[10] Whether this decrease occurs as a consequence of reduced albumin synthesis, increased albumin catabolism, or a combination of these is uncertain. From the theoretical viewpoint of what effect reduced albumin concentration would exert on rates of drug elimination

DRUG DISTRIBUTION

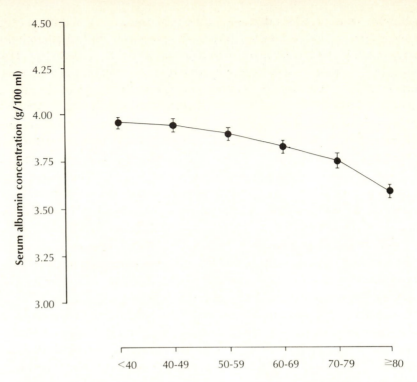

FIG. 7-1. Change in mean (±SE) serum albumin concentrations according to age in 11,090 hospitalized medical patients. (From Greenblatt, D. J.: J. Am. Geriatr. Soc. **27:**20, 1979.)

from the body, one would predict that for drugs not highly bound to albumin, no change in elimination rate would occur. By contrast, one would predict that for highly bound drugs elimination rates would be accelerated. This anticipated acceleration in the elimination rate of highly bound drugs in the elderly would arise from having more of the drug present in its active unbound form, with consequently greater opportunity for metabolism and excretion. In practice, the opposite of this theoretical expectation occurs. In geriatric patients elimination rates of several highly bound drugs either decrease or remain unchanged, but they do not increase. This apparent discrepancy can be explained in several ways: (1) changes in plasma albumin concentrations in elderly subjects may be too small in magnitude to accelerate drug elimination rates appreciably; (2) age-associated alterations in such other pharmacokinetic processes as metabolism and renal excretion exert a quantitatively greater effect on drug disposition; or (3) a combination of these and possibly even additional factors may be responsible.

When the percent binding of specific drugs to albumin is compared in geriatric subjects and normal middle-aged adults, a variety of results are obtained; only a few drugs exhibit reduced binding in older individuals. No changes with age were observed for plasma binding of phenobarbital, penicillin G, or phenytoin, although mean albumin concentrations declined in the subjects investigated from 4.0 g/ml in those under 50 years old to 3.4 g/ml in those over 50 years old.[2] Also in other studies the percent binding of warfarin or diazepam did not change with age. However, another report showed reduced plasma binding of phenylbutazone occurring with age but no change in plasma binding of sulfadiazine or salicylate. In still another study, phenytoin binding declined with age when subjects less than 45 years old, who had a mean serum albumin concentration of 4.1 mg/ml, were compared with subjects over 65 years old whose mean serum albumin concentrations were 2.9 g/ml.[24] In this and a confirmatory paper on phenytoin from a different laboratory,[13,15] the decrease in percent drug binding with age paralleled the decline in plasma albumin concentrations. When groups of young and geriatric subjects were compared in still other studies in which the plasma albumin concentrations declined appreciably in the older subjects, then it could be shown that the percent plasma binding of carbenoxolone,[11] meperidine,[18] and warfarin[12] decreased with age.

Practical consequences of decreased albumin concentrations in geriatric subjects are noteworthy. Wallace et al. showed that the magnitude of interactions affecting displacement from albumin of one drug by another was greater in older than in younger subjects.[24] Binding to plasma proteins of three drugs—phenylbutazone, salicylate, and sulfadiazine—was measured in young and geriatric subjects. In subjects receiving one or more other drugs, geriatric subjects exhibited markedly higher concentrations of the free form of phenylbutazone, salicylate, or sulfadiazine than concentrations found in geriatric subjects not taking other drugs or in younger subjects taking other drugs.[24] The increase in free drug concentration in plasma of geriatric subjects correlated with the number of drugs taken. Wallace et al. suggested that geriatric subjects are more susceptible than younger subjects to displacement of one drug from albumin by another because geriatric subjects have lower plasma albumin concentrations.[24]

With respect to other age-related alterations in drug distribution, it was mentioned before that total body weight declines with age but that the proportion of total body weight occupied by fat increases with age. Thus, it would be expected that, compared to young adults, geriatric subjects should exhibit increased apparent volumes of distribution (aVd) of very lipid-soluble drugs and environmental compounds (such as DDT). Data on this subject are sparse. Klotz et al. reported that with age diazepam aVd increased as a result of elevations in both the initial distribution space and steady state aVd and that this age-associated increase in diazepam aVd was responsible for the four-fold prolongation of plasma diazepam half-life that occurred in the absence of change in diazepam clearance.[17] However, Triggs et al. observed no age-related changes in aVd of acetaminophen, phenylbutazone, or sulfamethizole.[21]

Table 7-2 summarizes studies that show the influence of age on drug disposition in human subjects. Effects of age on drug metabolism had previously been demonstrated in rodents.[9,16] With increasing age rats exhibited reduced activity of several

DRUG METABOLISM

TABLE 7-2. Effects of age on drug disposition

Drug	Elimination rate		aVd	Apparent mechanism for age-related change
	Young adult	Geriatric		
Acetanilid	t½ = 1.45 hr	t½ = 2.07 hr	—	Decreased metabolism
Aminopyrine	t½ = 3.0 hr	t½ = 10.0 hr	—	—
Ampicillin	t½ = 1.0 hr	t½ = 1.2 hr	—	Decreased metabolism
Amylobarbitone (amobarbital)	Urinary metabolite excretion = 14.2%	Urinary metabolite excretion = 4.3%	—	—
Antipyrine	Plasma drug level = 1.3 µg/ml First study: t½ = 12 hr Second study: No change in MCR* of nonsmokers; MCR* decreased with age in smokers	Plasma drug level = 1.0 µg/ml t½ = 17.4 hr	—	—
Chlordiazepoxide	Clearance = 26.6 ml/min	Clearance = 46.3 ml/min	↑ in geriatric subjects	—
Diazepam	t½ = 20 hr	t½ = 80 hr	↑ ×3 in geriatric subjects	—
Digoxin	t½ = 51 hr	t½ = 73 hr	—	Decreased renal function
Dihydrostreptomycin	t½ = 5.2 hr	t½ = 8.4 hr	—	Decreased renal function
Doxycycline	t½ = 11.95 hr	t½ = 17.74 hr	—	Decreased renal function
Flurazepam	Incidence of Flurazepam toxicity increased with age		—	—
Indocyanine green	MCR* decreased with age		—	Decreased liver blood flow
Isoniazid	t½ = 2.5 hr	t½ = 2.9 hr	—	—
Kanamycin	t½ = 107 min	t½ = 282 min	—	Decreased renal function
Lithium	Clearance = 41.5 ml/min	Clearance = 7.7 ml/min	—	—
Lorazepam	Clearance = 0.99 ml/min/kg	Clearance = 0.77 ml/min/kg	↑ ×2.5 in geriatric subjects	—
Nitrazepam	Clearance = 4.1/1 hr	Clearance = 4.7/1 hr	↑ ×2.0 in geriatric subjects	—
Penicillin	t½ = 0.55 hr (penicillin G) t½ = 10 hr (procaine penicillin)	t½ = 1.0 hr (penicillin G) t½ = 18 hr (procaine penicillin)	—	—
Pethidine/meperidine	Plasma levels twice as high in geriatric subjects		—	Decreased metabolism
Phenobarbital	t½ = 71 hr	t½ = 107 hr	—	—
Phenylbutazone	First study: t½ = 81 hr Second study: t½ = 87 hr	t½ = 105 hr t½ = 110 hr	—	—
Phenytoin	Clearance = 26 ml/kg/hr	Clearance = 42 ml/kg/hr	—	Decreased renal function
Practolol	t½ = 7.1 hr	t½ = 8.6 hr	—	Decreased distribution volume
Propicillin	Serum levels are twice as high in geriatric subjects		↓ in geriatric subjects	—
Propranolol	Clearance decreases with age only in smokers		—	
Quinidine	Clearance = 4.04	Clearance = 2.64	No change	Decreased metabolism and renal function
Tetracycline	t½ = 3.5 hr	t½ = 4.5 hr	—	—

*MCR = metabolic clearance rate.

hepatic cytochrome P-450 dependent monooxygenases, the system responsible for biotransformation of most drugs in mammals. Cytochrome P-450 exists in distinct molecular forms, or isozymes, each molecular form probably having different affinity for the same as well as for different drug substrates. These multiple molecular forms have different genetic control and different responses to inducing agents. Heterogeneity of cytochrome P-450 complicates attempts to understand how the drug-metabolizing enzyme system changes under diverse conditions. For example, heterogeneity of cytochrome P-450 may be responsible in part for the complex, age-associated changes observed in both rodents and humans in which, in general, the hepatic drug-metabolizing capacity is very low during the fetal and neonatal periods, reaches a peak in the pediatric age range, and declines thereafter. Possibly different forms of cytochrome P-450 display different developmental patterns.

The main reason for the clarity of the rodent results is that liver could be removed from animals of different ages and the activities of hepatic drug-metabolizing enzymes compared in young and old animals. Ethical reasons prohibit liver biopsies in normal human subjects of different ages. Therefore, less direct methods had to be employed. Innocuous test drugs were administered in the same dose by the same route to subjects of different ages and the pharmacokinetic values obtained in young and geriatric subjects were compared (Figs. 7-2 and 7-3). Differences in pharmacokinetic values suggested that these changes might arise from effects of age on drug disposition. However, major problems arose in interpreting results. For example, changes in drug plasma half-life or clearance could be due to age-associated changes in the independent processes of drug metabolism, distribution, excretion, or a combination of these. Formidable technical difficulties were faced in such studies not only in obtaining the appropriate "normal" subjects and pertinent pharmacokinetic values from them, but also in drawing valid conclusions from these measurements, since frequently concealed environmental factors can contribute to these values.

Studies of two drugs, antipyrine and propranolol, illustrate the complexities of reaching valid interpretations of such pharmacokinetic values obtained in apparently normal subjects of different ages. One of the earliest papers comparing the pharmacokinetics of a drug in young and geriatric subjects revealed that in subjects whose average age was 78 years, antipyrine plasma half-life was 17.4 hours compared to 12.0 hours in subjects of an average age of 26 years.[20] Less marked differences between young and geriatric subjects occurred in antipyrine aVd. Subjects of the same age who differed in sex also had different rates of antipyrine elimination. This paper concluded that older subjects exhibited reduced capacity to eliminate the test drug antipyrine because of age-associated reductions in hepatic drug-metabolizing capacity. Subsequently, an environmental factor, cigarette smoking, was claimed to be mainly responsible for the smaller age-associated reduction in antipyrine elimination observed.[22] In this second study, plasma antipyrine half-life was 16.5% longer and clearance 18.5% less in older subjects than in younger subjects. Cigarette smoking explained 12% of the total variance in antipyrine clearance, whereas age alone explained only 3%.[22] In this study cigarette smoking declined

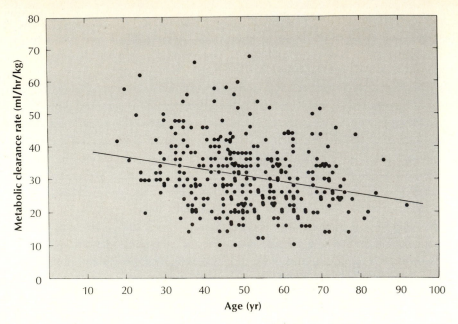

FIG. 7-2. Relationship of age to metabolic clearance rate of antipyrine in 307 normal male subjects. Note wide scatter and low correlation coefficient between age and drug elimination rate (r = −0.25). (From Vestal, R. E., et al.: Clin. Pharmacol. Ther. **18:**425, 1975.)

with age (geriatric subjects smoked fewer cigarettes and the geriatric group contained more nonsmokers than the young group). Thus, geriatric subjects were less exposed to the well-established effects of smoking on enhancing (inducing) the activity of the hepatic drug-metabolizing enzymes. A very recent study suggests that in geriatric subjects the inducing effects of smoking on these hepatic enzymes are reduced compared to those of young subjects.[25] This age difference in inducibility has been documented in rats in which the capacity of phenobarbital to induce declines from fivefold in young rats to less than twofold in old animals.

Not adequately recognized is the complexity of "cigarette smoking" as a habit involving subtle psychological, social, and genetic aspects. Therefore, to consider cigarette smoking as only an environmental factor consisting of exposing the subject to inducing chemicals is to ignore many contributing, but discrete, individual factors associated with the habit. These individual factors ultimately determine whether a subject makes the decision to smoke cigarettes in a sufficiently high dose to alter hepatic drug-metabolizing capacity.

Propranolol illustrates again the complexities inherent in assessing age-associated effects on pharmacokinetics. Two studies published in 1979 reached different conclusions concerning reasons for prolonged propranolol elimination rates and higher plasma concentrations with age.[3,23] The first study claimed that intrinsic total clearance of propranolol decreased with age only in smokers and nonsmokers.[23] No age-related changes occurred in either propranolol, aVd, plasma binding, or sys-

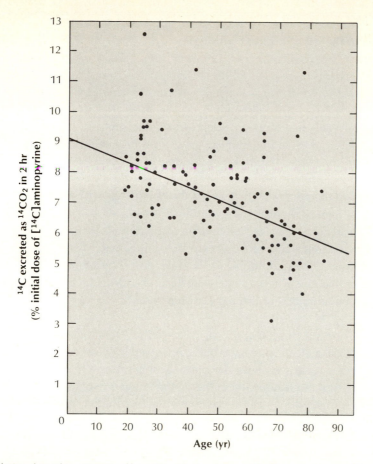

FIG. 7-3. Relationship of age to rate of hepatic aminopyrine metabolism as measured by production of $^{14}[CO_2]$ in breath after a single oral tracer dose of $[^{14}C]$aminopyrine in 112 normal male subjects. Note that scatter is less than for antipyrine, and correlation coefficient is higher (r = −0.44). (See Fig. 7-20.)

temic availability. Thus, smoking was implicated as the main factor responsible for the pharmacokinetic changes observed in propranolol disposition with age and, even more specifically, reduced inducibility by cigarette smoking of hepatic propranolol–metabolizing enzymes with age.[23] The second study, based on similar techniques, but using different doses of propranolol and employing fewer subjects, all but one of whom were nonsmokers, reached different conclusions.[3] This second study observed age-associated effects of propranolol disposition that could not be attributed to cigarette smoking but agreed with the first study in observing higher plasma propranolol concentrations in older subjects, geriatric and young subjects exhibiting similar propranolol aVd.[3] Higher propranolol concentrations in the elderly were attributed both to increased propranolol bioavailability in the elderly, assessed by comparing concentration-time curves after intravenous and oral dosing, and to slowed propranolol distribution to tissues.[3] Increased bioavailability of propranolol after its oral administration in the elderly suggested to the authors that hepatic metabolism of the drug declined with age.

DRUG EXCRETION   Many drugs and their metabolites are eliminated from the body by renal excretion. The extent to which renal mechanisms control drug elimination from the body can vary from 0% to 100%, depending on the drug. For drugs whose elimination depends mainly on renal function, such as barbital, digoxin, gentamicin, and penicillin, impairment of renal function can greatly prolong their sojourn in the body by reducing renal clearance. Estimates of the degree of renal dysfunction as judged by reductions in creatinine clearance form the basis for published nomograms that permit selection of appropriately lowered doses of drugs with relatively small therapeutic indices such as digoxin and gentamicin. Since, on the basis of age-associated reductions in renal perfusion, endogenous creatinine clearance declines in the elderly, even without overt renal disease, to approximately one-half the values observed in normal young adults,[7] these nomograms show, once endogenous creatinine clearance has been measured, what dose of a drug such as digoxin or gentamicin should be administered to a geriatric patient.[5,6]

CONCLUSIONS   Effects of age on drug absorption, distribution, metabolism, elimination, and various combinations of these have been reviewed.[26] The magnitude of such age-related changes depends on both the pharmacological profile of the particular drug and certain critical environmental and genetic characteristics of each geriatric subject. Because so many diverse environmental factors that can influence drug disposition change concomitantly in elderly subjects, it is often difficult to determine what specific factors are responsible for the pharmacokinetic characteristics of a given drug in a particular geriatric patient. Detailed investigations disclosed that the mechanisms involved are more complex than initially suspected and more pharmacokinetic measurements were required for resolution than were actually obtained in the experiments. For these reasons and because of the incompleteness of our present knowledge, physicians need to exercise special care to avoid toxicity when drugs are administered singly or in combination to geriatric patients. Thus, special care is necessary to individualize the dose of many drugs according to the particular requirement of each geriatric patient.

REFERENCES

1 Bender, D. A.: The effect of increasing age on the distribution of peripheral blood flow in man, J. Am. Geriatr. Soc. **13:**192, 1965.
2 Bender, D. A., Post, A., Meier, J. P., Higson, J. E., and Reichard, G.: Plasma protein binding of drugs as a function of age in adult human subjects, J. Pharm. Sci. **64:**1711, 1975.
3 Castleden, C. M., and George, C. F.: The ef-

fect of aging on the hepatic clearance of propranolol, Br. J. Clin. Pharmacol. **7:**49, 1979.
4 Castleden, C. M., Volans, C. N., and Raymond, K.: The effect of aging on drug absorption from the gut, Age Ageing **6:**138, 1977.
5 Christiansen, N. J. B., Kolendorf, K., Siersback-Nielsen, K., and Hansen, J. M.: Serum digoxin values following a dosage regimen

based on body weight, sex, age and renal function, Acta Med. Scand. **194:**257, 1973.

6 Dettli, L. C.: Drug dosage in renal disease, Clin. Pharmacokinet. **1:**126, 1976.

7 Friedman, S. A., Raizner, A. E., Rosen, H., Solomon, N. A., and Sy, W.: Functional defects in the aging kidney, Ann. Intern. Med. **76:**41, 1972.

8 Gillette, J. R.: Biotransformation of drugs during aging, Fed. Proc. **38:**1900, 1979.

9 Gorrod, J. W.: Absorption, metabolism and excretion of drugs in geriatric subjects, Gerontol. Clin. **16:**30, 1974.

10 Greenblatt, D. J.: Reduced serum albumin concentration in the elderly: a report from the Boston Collaborative Drug Surveillance Program, J. Am. Geriatr. Soc. **27:**20, 1979.

11 Hayes, M. J., and Langman, M. J. S.: Analysis of carbenoxolone plasma binding and clearance in young and elderly people. In Symposium Carbenoxolone Proceedings, ed. 4, London, 1974, Butterworth & Co.

12 Hayes, M. J., Langman, M. J. S., and Short, A. H.: Changes in drug metabolism with increasing age. I. Warfarin binding and plasma proteins, Br. J. Clin. Pharmacol. **2:**69, 1975.

13 Hayes, M. J., Langman, M. J. S., and Short, A. H.: Changes in drug metabolism with increasing age. II. Phenytoin clearance and protein binding, Br. J. Clin. Pharmacol. **2:**73, 1975.

14 Holloway, D. A.: Drug problems in the geriatric patient, Drug. Intell. and Clin. Pharmacol. **8:**632, 1974.

15 Hooper, W. D., Bochner, F., Eadie, M. J., and Tyrer, J. H.: Plasma protein binding of diphenylhydantoin; effects of six hormones, renal and hepatic disease, Clin. Pharmacol. Ther. **15:**276, 1974.

16 Kato, R., Vassanelli, P., Frontino, G., and Chiesara, E.: Variation in the activity of liver microsomal drug-metabolizing enzymes in rats in relation to the age, Biochem. Pharmacol. **13:**1037, 1964.

17 Klotz, V., Avant, G. R., Hoyumpa, A., Schenker, S., and Wilkinson, G. R.: The effects of age and liver disease on the disposition and elimination of diazepam in adult man, J. Clin. Invest. **55:**347, 1975.

18 Mather, L. E., Tucker, G. T., Pflug, A. E., Lindop, M. J., and Wilkerson, C.: Meperidine kinetics in man: intravenous injection in surgical patients and volunteers, Clin. Pharmacol. Ther. **17:**21, 1975.

19 Novak, L. P.: Aging, total body potassium, fat free mass, and all mass in males and females between the ages of 18 and 85 years, J. Gerontol. **27:**438, 1972.

20 O'Malley, K., Crooks, J., Duke, E., and Stevenson, I. H.: Effect of age and sex on human drug metabolism, Br. Med. J. **3:**607, 1971.

21 Triggs, E. J., Nation, R. L., Long, A., and Ashley, J. J.: Pharmacokinetics in the elderly, Eur. J. Clin. Pharmacol. **8:**55, 1975.

22 Vestal, R. E., Norris, A. H., Tobin, J. D., Cohen, B. H., Shock, N. W., and Andres, R.: Antipyrine metabolism in man: influence of age, alcohol, caffeine, and smoking, Clin. Pharmacol. Ther. **18:**425, 1975.

23 Vestal, R. E., Wood, A. J. J., Branch, R. A., Shand, D. G., and Wilkinson, G. R.: Effects of age and cigarette smoking on propranolol disposition, Clin. Pharmacol. Ther. **26:**8, 1979.

24 Wallace, S., Whiting, B., and Runcie, J.: Factors affecting drug binding in plasma of elderly patients, Br. J. Clin. Pharmacol. **3:**327, 1976.

25 Wood, A. J. J., Vestal, R. E., Wilkinson, G. R., Branch, R. A., and Shand, D. G.: Effect of aging and cigarette smoking on antipyrine and indocyanine green elimination, Clin. Pharmacol. Ther. **26:**16, 1979.

REVIEW

26 Richey, D. P., and Bender, D. A.: Pharmacokinetic consequences of aging, Annu. Rev. Pharmacol. Toxicol. **17:**49, 1977.

CHAPTER 8

Effects of diet on drug disposition

In addition to age, discussed in Chapter 7, diet can, under certain conditions, markedly alter a subject's rate of drug elimination. Like age, diet is a factor that affects all of us: an old adage states, "You are what you eat." Over the course of a lifetime dietary changes are immense. In certain climates diet changes with season, occupation, or both. Race, culture, religion, and genetic constitution are additional factors that can determine or at least influence diet. Diseases can markedly alter diet. For these reasons, the role of dietary factors on rates of drug elimination merits detailed consideration.

Relationships between diet and drug response in human subjects were not even suspected, much less defined, until recent carefully designed and executed studies not only established a firm foothold on the subject, but also clearly pointed the way for future investigations.[5,7,8,13] At the present time, a few examples exist that show how several dietary factors can alter rates of metabolism of test drugs such as antipyrine and theophylline. More studies are needed with other drugs to establish relationships between dietary factors and the individual processes of drug absorption, distribution, excretion, and receptor interaction.

EFFECTS OF STARVATION ON DRUG DISPOSITION

Of all dietary manipulations, the extreme form, that of starvation, would be expected to produce the most marked pharmacokinetic alteration. When drugs were administered to fasting rodents, greatly reduced rates of hepatic metabolism of some drugs occurred,[4,9] but no major changes in rates of drug metabolism occurred in obese, otherwise healthy, human subjects after 7 to 10 consecutive days on a diet in which the total daily carbohydrate intake was less than 15 g.[16] This diet produced ketoacidosis as well as weight loss that ranged from 3.6 to 15 kg (8 to 33 pounds). When uncorrected for body weight, the apparent volume of distribution (aVd) of both antipyrine and tolbutamide was significantly lower after fasting than before, presumably because during fasting the early loss of body weight is mainly from body water rather than from fat stores or muscle mass. The extent of decrease in aVd was proportional in each subject to the loss of body weight. Therefore, when correction was made for body weight, fasting had no effect on aVd of either antipyrine or tolbutamide. Other hepatic microsomal oxidations were investigated, including those for sulfisoxazole, isoniazid, and procaine.[15] The results disclosed that when allowance was made for body weight, neither half-life nor clearance of these five drugs was changed in obese subjects on a diet containing a total caloric intake of less than 15 g/day of carbohydrates. Although fasting decreased sulfisoxazole excretion, this may be attributed to a decline in rate of urine flow and a fall in urinary pH, both favoring nonionic diffusion of the drug back into the circulation from the renal tubular lumen.

General conclusions regarding the failure of acute fasting to alter rates of hepatic metabolism were further extended by a study of seven female patients with confirmed, classical anorexia nervosa. In these patients, prolonged refusal to eat had produced differing degrees of dehydration, hyponatremia, hypochloremia, hypokalemia, and anemia.[2] Compared with age- and sex-matched normal nurses who served as controls, the patients with anorexia nervosa had normal antipyrine pharmacokinetics when these values were corrected for body weight.

A study performed in India revealed that in 15 men suffering from nutritional edema—a severe manifestation of protein deficiency and resultant hypoalbuminemia—the mean plasma antipyrine half-life of 12.8 hours was not significantly different from that of age- and sex-matched nonsmoking controls (11.2 hours), but higher than that of age- and sex-matched smoking controls (8.9 hours).[10] This same study examined another group of 13 undernourished, hypoalbuminemic men without edema. Their short mean antipyrine half-life of 8.6 hours, similar to that of smoking controls (8.9 hours), could be due to the fact that some of them smoked cigarettes, some drank ethanol, and some were agricultural laborers exposed to pesticides known to induce hepatic drug-metabolizing enzymes. Thus, in this study, severe malnutrition did not by itself markedly alter antipyrine disposition, supporting observations described before for patients with anorexia nervosa and also for obese, but otherwise normal, subjects after a 7- to 10-day fast. Chronic exposure of some subjects in this study to inducing chemicals render the results inconclusive.

A significant contribution to this topic from India measured phenylbutazone pharmacokinetics in four normal male controls (mean age 30) and five undernourished, hypoalbuminemic male subjects (mean age 36), none of whom smoked cigarettes or consumed ethanol chronically. Compared to controls, the malnourished group exhibited shorter mean plasma phenylbutazone half-lives but increased mean phenylbutazone apparent volume of distribution and metabolic clearance rate.[1] These changes in phenylbutazone disposition in undernutrition presumably arose from reduced binding of phenylbutazone to albumin, with a corresponding increase in availability of drug for metabolism and elimination. Because the conclusions could be important therapeutically, these results need to be confirmed in studies on larger groups of undernourished subjects. Nutritionally deprived hypoalbuminemic patients who receive drugs that are highly bound to albumin may require higher doses of these drugs due to their enhanced rates of elimination.

Renal elimination of certain drugs can be altered by fasting or starvation, as mentioned for sulfisoxazole, whose renal excretion decreased during fasting. Also, since plasma free fatty acids (ffa) rise dramatically after 12 hours of fasting[21] and since these ffa bind albumin with an avidity capable of displacing many highly bound drugs, fasting for 24 to 72 hours would be expected to accelerate the rate of elimination of such highly bound drugs as bishydroxycoumarin, diazepam, phenylbutazone, phenytoin, and warfarin. Drug removal from the body would be hastened because displacement of drug from albumin by ffa makes the previously bound, and hence sequestered, drug immediately available for both metabolism and renal elimination, as in the case of undernutrition accompanied by hypoalbuminemia. This hypothesis remains to be established.

MARKED ALTERATIONS IN DRUG METABOLISM CAUSED BY DIETARY MANIPULATION

The most dramatic change in drug metabolism caused by dietary manipulation was described by Kappas and associates,[8] who showed that on an isocaloric diet the rate of antipyrine and theophylline metabolism was prolonged twofold as the percentage of total calories represented by carbohydrate doubled from 35% to 70% and the percentage of protein decreased from 44% to 10%. The percentage of total calories represented by fat remained constant in the two diets at approximately 20%. The pharmacokinetic values indicate that without alteration in total number of calories the switch from high to low protein with a reverse change in carbohydrate content affected only antipyrine and theophylline half-life and clearance, not their aVd (Fig. 8-1). This pattern suggests that this particular type of dietary manipulation affected antipyrine and theophylline metabolism rather than distribution.

Many patients who receive drugs are debilitated and chronically ill; they may have inadequate nutrition and also the proportion of their diet usually occupied by carbohydrate and protein may be reversed due to intravenous therapy. For such patients, due to their dietary alterations, their rate of drug elimination may be significantly changed. Furthermore, a certain percentage of the normal population is involved in various weight-reduction diets; these individuals could also be susceptible to the kinds of changes in drug-metabolizing capacity illustrated in Fig. 8-1. Therefore, drug dosage may also have to be changed according to new requirements in subjects who change their dietary patterns in ways similar to those shown in Fig. 8-1.

The question arises of why starvation produces negligible change in antipyrine metabolism, whereas with an isocaloric diet, simply switching the proportion of carbohydrate to protein exerts profound alterations on antipyrine metabolism. Possibly the body can detect the former dietary manipulation better than the latter type. Through detection of the gross dietary change of starvation, the body can compensate by providing from another source, at least for a limited time, the amino acids required for protein synthesis. By contrast, the body may not be able to detect, and hence compensate for, a much more subtle switch in the proportion of the total number of calories supplied in the diet as either carbohydrate or protein. If this change goes uncompensated, depletion of protein could reduce rates of synthesis of hepatic drug-metabolizing enzymes, which in turn could cause retention in the body of such drugs as antipyrine and theophylline.

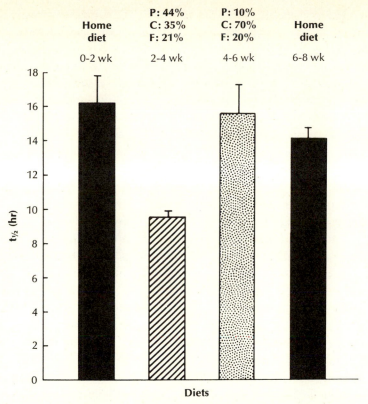

FIG. 8-1. Theophylline half-lives in 6 normal subjects maintained on their usual home diets and on two test-diet periods. Each bar represents mean ± SE for the 6 subjects. *P*, protein; *C*, carbohydrate; *F*, fat. Values for diets *1*, *3*, and *4* are not significantly different from each other. Value for diet *2* is significantly different from that of diet *1* (p = 0.05) and diet *3* (p = 0.01). (From Kappas, S.: Clin. Pharmacol. Ther. **20**:643, 1976.)

Not just the type of food consumed but also the method of its preparation can affect drug concentrations and disposition. In rats, charcoal-broiled beef, compared to beef cooked while covered with foil, thereby preventing formation of polycyclic hydrocarbons on the beef, increased by elevenfold intestinal metabolism of phenacetin in vitro.[11] Similarly designed studies were performed with eight healthy human volunteers in whom plasma antipyrine and theophylline half-lives were measured both before and after 7 days on a charcoal-broiled beef diet.[7] Later these drugs were also measured before and after another 7-day course on a diet containing the same amount of beef, but with the beef cooked while covered with foil. After eating charcoal-broiled beef, the subjects shortened by 22% their plasma antipyrine and theophylline half-lives. No changed occurred in aVd of either drug, but clearance of both drugs increased. Therefore, charcoal broiling appeared to enhance hepatic oxidative metabolism of both drugs.[7] Since, in rats, the consumption of

EFFECTS OF CHARCOAL BROILING ON DRUG DISPOSITION

charcoal-broiled beef greatly stimulated the in vitro oxidative metabolism of both phenacetin and benzo[a]pyrene and since the polycyclic hydrocarbons formed on the surface of beef by charcoal broiling enhance oxidative metabolism of several drugs, it seemed logical to infer that through induction produced by polycyclic hydrocarbons, charcoal broiling stimulated oxidative drug metabolism in the liver and gut. Such induction evidently also occurred in humans by action of polycyclic hydrocarbons in charcoal-broiled beef on gastrointestinal drug-metabolizing enzymes.[13] This study showed markedly decreased plasma phenacetin concentrations in nine normal volunteers after a 4-day diet of charcoal-broiled beef. No change occurred in either plasma phenacetin half-lives or plasma concentrations of the main metabolite of phenacetin, N-acetyl-p-aminophenol. These results suggest that exposure to polycyclic hydrocarbons produced in beef by charcoal broiling induces phenacetin metabolism in the gut. Collectively, these results indicate that, in addition to the relative proportion of carbohydrate and protein in the diet, certain methods by which food is prepared, as exemplified by charcoal broiling, can alter rates of hepatic and gastrointestinal drug metabolism in humans.

STIMULATORY EFFECT OF BRUSSELS SPROUTS AND CABBAGE

In rats a diet containing certain cruciferous vegetables, such as brussels sprouts, cabbage, turnips, broccoli, cauliflower, or spinach, induced intestinal benzo[a]pyrene hydroxylase activity, as well as the intestinal enzymes that metabolize 7-ethoxycoumarin, hexobarbital, and phenacetin.[12,20] Moreover, it was demonstrated that certain indoles present in these cruciferous vegetables were potent inducers of the gut enzymes that metabolize these drugs. Thus, the stage was set for a study in humans to determine whether a dietary regimen rich in these cruciferous vegetables could also exert an inductive effect on drug metabolism. The results obtained in a study on 10 healthy volunteers were positive and showed that on a 7-day diet rich in brussels sprouts and cabbage mean antipyrine half-lives were decreased by 13% and mean plasma phenacetin concentrations were decreased by 34% to 67%.[13] Thus, as in rats, a diet of brussels sprouts or cabbage in humans can accelerate rates of metabolism of certain drugs, presumably due to an inductive effect exerted on the drug-metabolizing enzymes by certain chemicals in these vegetables.

Although statistically significant, very small changes in plasma antipyrine half-life (13%) and in antipyrine clearance (11%) after an intensive and unusual exposure for 1 week to cabbage and brussels sprouts raise the question of how clinically meaningful such dietary manipulations may be. Stated otherwise, could such dietary factors produce a toxic reaction in a patient by changing that patient's dosage requirement of commonly used drugs with low therapeutic indices? Probably they could. While the change in antipyrine clearance produced by a diet high in brussels sprouts and cabbage for 7 days was small, phenacetin plasma concentrations changed much more. For still other drugs, the change produced could be even larger. Thus, more drugs, particularly commonly used drugs with low therapeutic indices, need to be investigated before a firm answer can be given. Finally, it must be emphasized that, in patients, many factors acting simultaneously can influence drug clearance. If, in addition to dietary change, the patient receives drugs with induction potential, then these two factors—dietary change plus inducing compounds—could markedly alter drug clearance and hence the appropriate dosage of a therapeutic agent. Such dosage changes might not be required if each factor had acted alone in the patient without the enhancing effect of the additional factor. On the other hand, both factors could be either nullified or further magnified by impairment of cardiovascular, hepatic, or renal function secondary to numerous diseases.

THEOBROMINE AS A METABOLIC INHIBITOR

Studies described previously established effects on drug disposition of chemically heterogeneous changes in diet. Work on the methylxanthine theobromine, a chemically homogeneous nutritional constituent of such dietary staples as chocolate, coffee, tea, and various cola beverages, revealed that normal subjects, due to daily dietary theobromine intake, are inhibited metabolically with respect to their capacity to eliminate theobromine.[5] After 2 weeks on a methylxanthine-free diet, each of six healthy male subjects increased his capacity to eliminate a test dose of theobromine (Fig. 8-2). Although theobromine is not used as a drug, closely related methylxanthines, such as theophylline are.

In the same patient, during a single course of therapy, theophylline doses may need to be changed abruptly. We hypothesized, on the basis of our studies with theobromine described above, that dietary theobromine intake might influence theophylline dosage requirements. The hypothesis was based on the assumption that theobromine intake in human subjects could inhibit theophylline metabolism. This assumption was recently supported by the demonstration that in human subjects theobromine inhibits rates of theophylline elimination.[3]

COLA NUT INGESTION AND HEPATIC DRUG METABOLISM

All previously mentioned studies on dietary factors utilized a rigorously controlled technique in which carefully selected healthy volunteers, not exposed at home or work to chemicals capable of altering their basal rates of drug elimination, were investigated both before and after imposition of a single dietary change. Thus, each volunteer served as his or her own control. Elimination rates of a test drug such as antipyrine were measured several times in each subject to establish control, basal values. Then after a single environmental change, in this case a change in diet, the test drug was readministered after an appropriate time under the new dietary conditions. This time-consuming method of studying numerous factors affecting drug disposition in humans has proved fruitful since its introduction more than 10 years ago.[17,18] However, certain requirements for screening large numbers of subjects under difficult field conditions led to the introduction of another approach. In this other approach, the subjects differed in age, sex, nutritional status, height, weight, medical condition, smoking habits, and exposure to various inducing agents. Each subject received only a single dose of the test drug so that each subject's pharmacokinetic characteristics could be measured on only one occasion. The statistical device of multiple regression analysis was relied on to help discriminate among the many confounding variables. This statistical method estimated the rela-

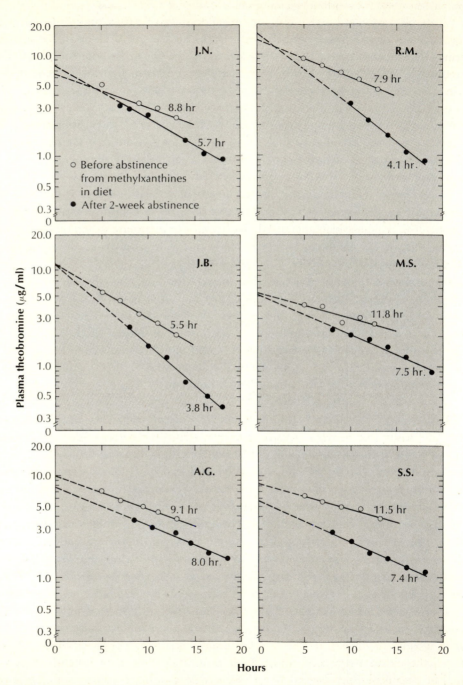

FIG. 8-2. Decay of a single oral dose of theobromine (6 mg/kg) before and after a 2-week dietary abstention from methylxanthines. (From Drouillard, D. D., Vesell, E. S., and Dvorchik, B. H.: Clin. Pharmacol. Ther. **23:**296, 1978.)

tive contribution of each factor that could be identified as a potential source of variation to the total interindividual variability observed.

A study performed in West African villagers identified, through multiple regression analysis, cola nut consumption to be the single best predictor of antipyrine clearance[6]; three other statistically significant predictive factors were sex, hemoglobin in women, and height in men. No attempt was made in these West African villagers to determine effects on antipyrine clearance of cessation of cola nut chewing in chewers or of initiation of chewing in nonchewers. However, a carefully controlled study was performed to determine effects of cola nut chewing on antipyrine clearance in normal male volunteers living in a south central town in Pennsylvania.[19] In these subjects, no alteration in antipyrine clearance occurred after either 2 or 4 weeks of cola nut chewing.

These results do not contradict the earlier ones obtained in West African villagers because the genetic constitutions and environmental conditions of the subjects in each study were so different. Nevertheless, failure of chronic cola nut consumption to alter antipyrine clearance in normal volunteers in this country renders the West African investigation more difficult to interpret. Absence of a controlled study on cola nut chewing in the initial report on the West African villagers is regrettable and prevents firm conclusions from being reached. Consequently, the need to control carefully the conditions of a dietary study so that only one variable is manipulated independently of the others is clear. Such a procedure is required ultimately before firm conclusions can be reached, although multiple regression may provide useful initial clues to potential factors whose actual role needs to be established through testing under the conditions of a controlled experiment.

Multiple, simultaneously acting factors can influence rates of drug elimination in either unselected normal volunteers or patients. Formidable difficulties interfere with accurate assessment of the relative contribution made by each of these simultaneously acting factors to large interindividual variations in rates of drug elimination. The limitations of multiple regression analysis were enumerated, although this statistical device was considered useful as a first step in identifying potential factors that subsequently required testing under carefully controlled conditions before these factors actually could be accepted as affecting rates of drug elimination. Studies performed under carefully controlled conditions revealed that several dietary factors can alter rates of drug elimination. These factors include the relative proportion of protein and carbohydrate in an isocaloric diet, charcoal broiling of beef, and consumption of cruciferous vegetables or theobromine. Although starvation itself without hepatic dysfunction and edema failed to alter clearance of any drug thus far investigated, marked diurnal variations of approximately 35% to 40% in the clearance of some drugs such as aminopyrine were unaffected by 48 hours of sleeplessness,[14] but could be entirely abolished in normal volunteers by 48 hours of starvation. Thus, either alone or operating in concert with still other factors, dietary alterations can appreciably change drug clearance. For this reason,

INTERACTIONS BETWEEN DIET AND OTHER SIMULTANEOUSLY OPERATING CONDITIONS

in considering the appropriate dose of certain drugs for patients whose medical problems necessitate a dietary change, physicians may need to determine whether these dietary changes will cause a change in drug clearance and hence in the appropriate dose of the drug or drugs being adminstered.

REFERENCES

1 Adithan, C., Gandhi, I. S., and Chandrasekar, S.: Pharmacokinetics of phenylbutazone in undernutrition, Indian J. Pharmacol. 10:301, 1978.

2 Bakke, O. M., Aanderud, S., Syversen, G., Bassoe, H. H., and Myking, O.: Antipyrine metabolism in anorexia nervosa, Br. J. Clin. Pharmacol. 5:341, 1978.

3 Caldwell, J., Monks, T. J., Lawrie, S., and Smith, R. L.: Dietary methylxanthines (MXs) as determinants of theophylline (T) metabolism in man, Pharmacologist, 21:1973, 1979.

4 Dixon, R. L., Shultice, R. W., and Fouts, J. R.: Factors affecting drug metabolism by liver microsomes. IV. Starvation, Proc. Soc. Exp. Biol. Med. 103:333, 1960.

5 Drouillard, D. D., Vesell, E. S., and Dvorchik, B. H.: Studies on theobromine disposition in normal subjects, Clin. Pharmacol. Ther. 23:296, 1978.

6 Fraser, H. S., Bulpitt, C. J., Kahn, C., Mould, G., Mucklow, J. C., and Dollery, C. T.: Factors affecting antipyrine metabolism in West African villagers, Clin. Pharmacol. Ther. 20:369, 1976.

7 Kappas, A., Alvares, A. P., Anderson, K. E., Pantuck, E. J., Pantuck, C. B., Chang, R., and Conney, A. H.: Effect of charcoal-broiled beef on antipyrine and theophylline metabolism, Clin. Pharmacol. Ther. 23:445, 1978.

8 Kappas, A., Anderson, K. E., Conney, A. H., and Alvares, A. P.: Influence of dietary protein and carbohydrate on antipyrine and theophylline metabolism in man, Clin. Pharmacol. Ther. 20:643, 1976.

9 Kato, R., and Gillette, J. R.: Sex differences in the effects of abnormal physiological states on the metabolism of drugs by rat liver microsomes, J. Pharmacol. Exp. Ther. 150:285, 1965.

10 Krishnaswamy, K., and Naidu, A. N.: Microsomal enzymes in malnutrition as determined by plasma half-life of antipyrine, Br. Med. J. 1:538, 1977.

11 Pantuck, E. J., Hsiao, K.-C., Kuntzman, R., and Conney, A. H.: Intestinal metabolism of phenacetin in the rat: effect of charcoal-broiled beef and rat chow, Science 187:744, 1975.

12 Pantuck, E. J., Hsiao, K.-C., Loub, W. D., Wattenberg, L. W., Kuntzman, R., and Conney, A. H.: Stimulatory effect of vegetables on intestinal drug metabolism in the rat, J. Pharmacol. Exp. Ther. 198:278, 1976.

13 Pantuck, E. J., Pantuck, C. B., Garland, W. A., Min, B. H., Wattenberg, L. W., Anderson, K. E., Kappas, A., and Conney, A. H.: Stimulatory effect of brussels sprouts and cabbage on human drug metabolism, Clin. Pharmacol. Ther. 25:88, 1979.

14 Poley, G. E., Shively, C. A., and Vesell, E. S.: Failure of sleep deprivation to alter diurnal rhythms of aminopyrine metabolism in normal human volunteers, Clin. Pharmacol. Ther. 24:726, 1978.

15 Reidenberg, M. M.: Obesity and fasting—effects on drug metabolism and drug action in man, Clin. Pharmacol. Ther. 22:729, 1977.

16 Reidenberg, M. M., and Vesell, E. S.: Unaltered metabolism of antipyrine and tolbutamide in fasting man, Clin. Pharmacol. Ther. 17:650, 1975.

17 Vesell, E. S.: Antipyrine test in clinical pharmacology: conceptions and misconceptions, Clin. Pharmacol. Ther. 26:275, 1979.

18 Vesell, E. S., and Page, J. G.: Genetic control of the phenobarbital-induced shortening of plasma antipyrine half-lives in man, J. Clin. Invest. 48:2202, 1969.

19 Vesell, E. S., Shively, C. A., and Passananti, G. T.: Failure of cola-nut chewing to alter antipyrine disposition in normal male subjects from a small town in south central Pennsylvania, Clin. Pharmacol. Ther. 26:287, 1979.

20 Wattenberg, L. W.: Studies of polycyclic hydrocarbon hydroxylases of the intestine possibly related to cancer. Effect of diet on benzpyrene hydroxylase activity, Cancer 28:99, 1971.

21 Wood, F. C., Domenge, L., Bally, P. R., Renold, A. E., and Thorn, G. W.: Studies on the metabolic response to prolonged fasting, Med. Clin. North Am. 44:1371, 1960.

CHAPTER 9

Effects of occupation and disease on drug disposition

In the preceding three chapters host characteristics, specifically genetic constitution, age, and diet, which influence drug response of individual subjects, were described. This chapter considers the additional host factors of occupation and disease that can also affect drug disposition. Emphasis on the critical role played by host factors in drug response reverses the usual textbook approach that incorrectly implies that a given drug in a given dose produces a single, uniform effect in all subjects.

In Chapter 6 it was shown that genetic factors contribute appreciably to large interindividual variations in rates of drug elimination among normal subjects under near basal conditions. However, in unselected subjects chronically exposed to numerous environmental compounds and conditions that can induce or inhibit the activity of hepatic mixed-function oxidases, rates of drug elimination are obviously not basal. In such subjects a dynamic interaction exists between the genes that control hepatic mixed-function oxidases and multiple environmental factors (Table 6-1).

Although for convenience twin studies separate genetic from environmental contributions as though they were discrete unrelated entities, the transcriptional and translational mechanisms by which genetic information is expressed require environmental participation. Conversely, many environmental factors that alter rates of drug disposition in humans do so by affecting genetic mechanisms. Environmental chemicals, such as DDT, polychlorinated biphenyls, and polycyclic hydrocarbons, can alter, through induction, a subject's hepatic drug-metabolizing enzyme activity. As shown later in this chapter, disease states can also markedly change a subject's rate of drug elimination. Assurance of a near basal, relatively uninduced or uninhibited state can never be complete but is partially attainable in a subject through repeated measurements of the rate of elimination of a particular test drug, such as antipyrine as mentioned in Chapter 6, and through a careful history of exposures at work and at home to compounds or conditions capable of altering near basal rates of drug elimination. Simultaneously acting environmental factors (Table 6-1), each with a different capacity in different subjects for changing rates of drug metabolism, make it exceedingly difficult to attribute different portions of the total interindividual variation to

OCCUPATIONAL FACTORS THAT ALTER RESPONSE OF DRUG-METABOLIZING ENZYMES

93

TABLE 9-1. Occupational chemicals that can alter rates of drug elimination, depending on intensity and duration of exposure

Number and sex of subjects	Employed in	Chemical exposure	Test drug	Change in test drug produced by chemical	Reference at end of chapter
26 M 15 M 18 F	Insecticide plant Same insecticide plant as office workers	Lindane and DDT Unexposed (control)	Antipyrine —	Shorter plasma $t_{1/2}$ —	28 —
18 M	DDT plant for more than 5 years	DDT and "DDT-related compounds"	Phenylbutazone and 6β-hydroxy-cortisol excretion in urine	Phenylbutazone $t_{1/2}\downarrow$; urinary excretion of 6β-hydroxy-cortisol↑	41
18 M	Same DDT plant, same time	Unexposed (control)	—	—	—
14 M	Insecticide plant	Spray of solution containing 4% lindane, 0.1% pyrethrum, 2.5% malathion	Phenylbutazone	Phenylbutazone $t_{1/2}\downarrow$	29
9 M	Insecticide plant	Unexposed (control)	—	—	—
26 M	Tree nurseries	Spray of lindane 4%, 2.5% malathion	Antipyrine, phenylbutazone	Antipyrine $t_{1/2}\downarrow$; Phenylbutazone $t_{1/2}\downarrow$	30
23 M 15 M 18 F	Tree nurseries Office	Spray of DDT Unexposed (control)	Oxazepam —	Oxazepam $t_{1/2}$ unchanged —	—

Subjects	Occupation	Exposure	Drug		Effect	Ref
3 M / 2 F	Capacitor manufacturing plant	Polychlorinated biphenyls	Antipyrine	—	Antipyrine $t_{1/2}\downarrow$; clearance$\uparrow$; aVd unchanged	1
3 M / 2 F	Same plant	Unexposed (control)	—	—	—	—
4 MC* / 4 FC*	—	Chronic lead poisoning	Antipyrine, phenylbutazone	—	Antipyrine and phenylbutazone $t_{1/2}\uparrow$; therapy for phenylbutazone poisoning decreased these values toward normal	3
2 ?C* / 1 MC* / 1 FC*	—	Acute lead poisoning / Unexposed (control)	—	—	—	—
8 M	Shipyard	Lead	Antipyrine	—	Antipyrine $t_{1/2}\downarrow$	2
10 M	Unspecified	Chronic lead poisoning	Antipyrine	—	Antipyrine $t_{1/2}\uparrow$; clearance$\downarrow$; these reverted to normal with EDTA therapy	35
23 ?	Anesthesia	OR gases; presumably volatile anesthetic agents (halothane, etc.)	Antipyrine	—	Antipyrine $t_{1/2}\downarrow$ (measured once)	38
23 ?	Anesthesia	Unexposed (control)	—	—	—	—
7 M	Anesthesiology residency	Undefined volatile anesthetic agents	Warfarin	—	Warfarin $t_{1/2}\uparrow$ measured before and after 4 months of exposure to OR	19
5 M	Anesthesiology residency	Unexposed (control)	—	—	—	—

*Children.

specific single environmental factors. In this regard, a major problem in humans is that, even within a single population, most persons are heterogeneous with respect to both the environmental and the genetic factors known to influence drug disposition. The task of partitioning the total interindividual variation in drug elimination of such heterogeneous populations into component parts is further complicated because some seemingly pure "environmental" factors, including diet, smoking, and ethanol consumption, are closely associated with other environmental characteristics as well as with genetic factors.

Physicians should recognize that chronic occupational exposure to the chemicals listed in Table 9-1 can alter a patient's basal rate of drug elimination, mainly by inducing or inhibiting the mixed-function oxidases responsible for hepatic drug metabolism. It should be stressed that choice and pursuit of an occupation, like the factors of diet and cigarette smoking, are not simple, single, isolated events. Rather they represent a complex expression of behavioral choices formed as a result of underlying socioeconomic, psychological, intellectual, and genetic factors. Thus, a given subject's rate of drug elimination may not be attributable *exclusively* to exposure at work to any of the chemicals listed in Table 9-1 that can induce or inhibit hepatic drug-metabolizing enzymes. In addition to occupational exposure, a subject's capacity to metabolize drugs may be markedly affected by several factors listed in Table 6-1 that can change a subject's rate of drug elimination from that expected exclusively from exposure to chemicals encountered at work (Table 9-1). For example, if a woman is exposed at work to chlorinated hydrocarbon insecticides, her rate of elimination of most drugs metabolized by hepatic mixed-function oxidases would be expected to be enhanced due to the inductive effect of insecticides. However, if the woman also took certain steroidal oral contraceptives or if she developed fever, hypothyroidism, or hepatitis, to enumerate a few of the many possibilities, her rate of elimination of a test drug would be retarded relative to that of other women her age or relative to her own, near basal, rate of elimination. The reason is that, by itself, each of these four conditions tends to retard a subject's normal rate of drug elimination. The net inhibitory effect of several of these factors acting simultaneously tends to counterbalance or offset the inductive effect of chronic occupational exposure to an inducing agent such as an insecticide. Thus the simultaneous operation of multiple environmental factors, such as several of those listed in Table 6-1, can change the rate of drug elimination produced solely from occupational exposure to a particular inducing or inhibiting compound.

OCCUPATIONAL CHEMICALS THAT ALTER DRUG-METABOLIZING CAPACITY

A partial list of chemicals encountered in a subject's occupation that are capable of accelerating or retarding rates of hepatic drug metabolism appears in Table 9-1. This list is suggestive rather than complete. Completeness is impossible because of the numerous lipid-soluble organic chemicals to which subjects are chronically exposed in their occupations that can induce their hepatic mixed-function oxidases, thereby accelerating the rates at which these subjects eliminate many drugs and other environmental compounds.

This aspect of occupational medicine (the influence of chemicals encountered at work on a subject's capacity to metabolize drugs) represents only a small portion of the entire subject. In recent years, the field of occupational medicine has expanded greatly due to recognition of the fact that various human diseases develop as a result of chronic exposure to certain chemicals during work. The association between certain diseases and specific conditions at work was documented first in the eighteenth century by Percival Potts. He reported that English chimney sweeps were at high risk of developing cancer of the scrotum. In the twentieth century it was learned that exposure at work to asbestos, benzene, phenol, vinyl chloride, radium, and x rays also increased the risk of developing certain forms of cancer. Chronic intake of large doses of phenacetin by watchmakers in Switzerland to relieve the headaches produced by long hours of eyestrain greatly increased their risk of developing renal disease. Similarly, it was noted that coal miners had a much higher incidence of pulmonary disease than did age-matched controls who were not chronically exposed to the conditions of coal mines.

In this context it would be expected that workers chronically exposed to the lipid-soluble compounds listed in Table 9-1 tend to have accelerated clearance of such test drugs as antipyrine and phenylbutazone. According to this principle, workers chronically exposed to insecticides exhibit accelerated rates of removal of these test drugs, probably due to an inductive response of their hepatic drug-metabolizing enzymes. By contrast, chronic exposure to lead probably inhibits these hepatic drug-metabolizing enzymes, thereby retarding, in both children and adults, clearance of antipyrine and phenylbutazone (Table 9-1). The critical factors of daily dose and total time of exposure influence greatly the extent to which a subject's drug-metabolizing enzymes respond to a chemical encountered at work (see Table 6-1, Pharmacological variables).

Although additional examples could be culled from the literature and fresh examples will undoubtedly be published soon, those enumerated in Table 9-1 illustrate clearly the general principle that many chemicals to which subjects are chronically exposed at work can change their basal rates of drug elimination. This alteration probably results from chronic effects of the chemical on the hepatic mixed-function oxidases. Whether the chemical accelerates or retards the normal rate of drug clearance of the subject depends not only on many environmental and genetic factors affecting the subject (Table 6-1) but also on the properties of the chemical, including its lipid solubility and rate of systemic elimination.

Because this is a pill-oriented society, exposure to potent chemicals that can alter a subject's near basal rate of drug clearance is rarely limited to that subject's occupational exposure. Such chemicals are much more commonly ingested for medicinal, recreational, or nutritional purposes than ingested as a result of occupational exposure only. Persons in certain professions with continuous drug contact have higher drug intake. Thus, complex factors (Table 6-1) and exposure at work and at home through diet, medication, and recreation to numerous chemicals capable of altering rates of drug elimination can render attribution of a particular subject's drug-metabolizing capacity to a simple, single compound difficult, if not impossible.

A controlled experiment is necessary to assess the role of the factors listed in

Table 6-1 and the chemicals listed in Table 9-1 with respect to their role in affecting a subject's capacity to metabolize drugs. In this experiment, only one factor is manipulated independently of the others. Subjects in a near basal state of drug clearance need to be selected for such a study. Then each subject's clearance of a test compound is determined several times before imposition of this factor and again several times after introduction of the factor. By constructing dose-response curves we can assess quantitatively the role exerted by each factor on drug clearance. On the other hand, if only a single measurement of clearance of the test drug is made in unselected subjects of different age, sex, ethnic background, dietary custom, occupation, smoking habit, and medication intake, including birth control pills,[18] no definitive conclusion can be reached concerning the role of occupation, or of any one of these other variables because these variables are all confounded. Moreover, interpretations in this study[18] relied solely on correlation coefficients. In the absence of a controlled experiment, correlation coefficients prove nothing. They may serve as initial clues on which to base a subsequent controlled experiment.

These essential points in experimental design are emphasized here because they may help to explain the discrepant results in Table 9-1 for anesthetists. Table 9-1 shows that anesthetists in one study apparently had accelerated rates of antipyrine elimination,[38] whereas in another study their rates of warfarin elimination were prolonged.[19] In the former study, antipyrine was administered only once and the control group was not concurrent, whereas in the latter study anesthesiology residents served as their own controls with each subject's rate of warfarin elimination being measured on two separate occasions. The initial measurement in each subject represented near basal rates of drug elimination before exposure; the second measurement, taken after 4 months of daily exposure to the conditions of the operating room, represented the effects of occupational exposure to various anesthetic gases. In addition to these critical differences between the two studies in experimental design, other differences between them exist that also could have influenced the results.

For these reasons, results of studies concerning the effects of various chemicals encountered at work on the drug-metabolizing capacity of exposed workers reflect to a large extent the experimental design of the study. They also can be greatly influenced by the multiple individual characteristics of the subjects investigated (Table 6-1), as well as by the dose of the chemical to which the subject is exposed, the route of exposure, and the duration of exposure.

EFFECTS OF DISEASE ON DRUG DISPOSITION   Numerous disease states can, under certain conditions, alter a particular subject's response to some drugs because drug response involves many different physiological processes and tissues. The processes of drug absorption, distribution, metabolism, excretion, and receptor action are complex, located in different tissues, and, most important, are subject to perturbation by multiple factors (Table 6-1). On the other hand, the physician must not be surprised if a particular patient fails to show an expected change in drug response due to a disease, since in that patient the disease process may be insufficiently severe or insufficiently prolonged to have exerted its effect. Thus, both severity and duration of action are critical variables that determine the intensity of effect produced by a disease on the rate of drug elimination in a particular patient. Moreover, an effect on drug disposition due to disease may be compensated for by additional disease-associated changes that balance or offset the initial alteration. For example, early studies on rates of phenylbutazone elimination in patients with alcoholic cirrhosis reported normal values.[12] Later it became clear that patients with alcoholic cirrhosis had reduced hepatic drug-metabolizing capacity but that this reduced capacity was concealed because patients consumed ethanol and other drugs that enhanced their depressed drug metabolism, elevating it to the normal range.[31]

Even by itself, without intervention from factors listed in Table 6-1, a single disease may exert different effects on the separate processes of drug absorption, distribution, metabolism, excretion, and receptor action. When each of these individual effects is measured and all effects summated, the net change in "drug response" may be negligible due to the balancing of one major effect by another acting in an opposite direction. Changes in the patient's condition or treatment may upset this balance and bring to light a major effect that the disease exerts on a single pharmacokinetic or pharmacodynamic process by removing the offsetting effects of the disease on the other processes.

A critical point to remember is that a disease process may affect the disposition of different drugs in different ways. The reason is that each drug has a distinct pharmacological profile and the way a disease process alters the disposition of a particular drug depends on the specific pharmacological characteristics of the drug. For example, in hypoalbuminemia the disposition of drugs such as warfarin and phenylbutazone that are extensively bound to albumin will be changed, whereas the disposition of isoniazid and kanamycin that bind albumin negligibly will not be altered. As another example, hepatocellular disease changes the disposition of drugs biotransformed in the liver much more than it does the disposition of drugs such as barbital and the majority of antibiotics that are not.

Table 9-2 presents a partial list of drugs whose half-lives have been reported to be altered by diseases of the liver or kidney. Since changes in drug half-life can arise from alterations in rates of drug absorption, distribution, metabolism, or excretion, it is useful to consider effects of several prototypical disease states on each of these individual processes. One must also remember that changes in drug half-life do not necessarily indicate a change in rate of drug metabolism, since change in the volume of distribution of a drug can cause changes in drug half-life without a change in drug metabolism. Furthermore, large changes can occur in both the metabolism and volume of distribution of a drug without any change in drug half-life.

Many different disorders and pathological states can alter the normal rates and pathways for drug absorption, distribution, biotransformation, excretion, interaction with receptor sites, or various combinations of these. Since each drug has a distinct profile for these five processes, the extent to which a disease that affects these

TABLE 9-2. A partial list of drugs whose half-lives have been reported to be altered by hepatic or renal dysfunction*

Drug	Change in t½	
	Hepatic dysfunction	Renal dysfunction
Acetaminophen	↑	
Amiloride		↑
Aminopyrine	↑	No change
Ampicillin		↑
Antipyrine	↑↑	No change
Carbenicillin		↑
Cefazolin		↑
Cephacetrile		↑
Cephalexin		↑
Cephaloridine		↑
Cephalothin		↑
Chloramphenicol	↑	No change
Chlorpropamide		↑
Clindamycin	↑	↑
Cloxacillin		↑
Colchicine	↑	↑
Colistimethate		↑
Diazepam	↑	↑
Diazoxide		↑
Dicloxacillin		↓ or no change
Digitoxin		↑
Digoxin	↑	↑
Doxorubicin		
Erythromycin		↑
Ethambutol		↑
Flucytosine		↑
Furosemide		↑
Gentamicin		↑
Hydrocortisone	↑	

Drug	Change in t½	
	Hepatic dysfunction	Renal dysfunction
Indocyanine green	↑	
Isoniazid	↑	
Lidocaine	↑	
Meperidine	↑	No change
Methicillin		↑
Nafcillin	↑	
Niridazole	↑	
Oxacillin		↑
Oxazepam	No change	
Penicillin G		↑
Pentobarbital	No change	No change
Phenacetin		↑
Phenylbutazone	↑ or no change	
Phenytoin		↑
Prednisone		↑
Procainamide		↑
Propranolol	↑	↓ or no change
Rifampicin	↑	
Streptomycin		↑
Sulfadimethoxine		↑
Sulfamethazine		↑ or no change
Sulfamethoxazole		↑
Sulfamethoxy-pyridazine		↑
Tetracycline		↑
Tobramycin		↑
Trimethoprim		↑
Vancomycin		↑
Warfarin	No change	No change

*Data derived from reviews by Creasey,[13] Pagliaro and Benet,[39] Reidenberg,[48] and Vesell.[58]

processes will alter the distribution of a drug depends on the particular drug. There-fore, it is hazardous to extrapolate how pathological processes will affect other drugs on the basis of pathological effects that alter the distribution of one drug.

Clinical consequences of a change in drug distribution produced by disease will be determined also by the therapeutic index of the drug as well as by certain genetic and environmental characteristics of the patient. For example, a change of 200% in the plasma half-life of antipyrine, salicylates, or penicillin will probably have little or no clinical consequence, whereas a change of 20% in the plasma half-life of digoxin, procainamide, or lidocaine may prove critical. By the same token, a change of 1% in the albumin binding of warfarin, which normally is 99% bound, may have profound toxicological results; whereas a change of 1% in the albumin binding of probenecid, which normally is 75% bound, has negligible clinical consequences. Here the crucial factor is the percent change in the free, but not bound, portion of the drug.

Effects of disease states on the rate of absorption of a drug depend on many factors including the site of drug administration. If the drug is administered orally, the influence of disease on rates of drug absorption will depend on the nature of the disease process, whether it affects the areas in the gut where the drug is normally absorbed, and how the disease alters the normal physiological volume, pH, tempera-ture, viscosity, surface tension, and composition of the gastrointestinal secretions and contents.[32] Rates of drug absorption may also be influenced by whether or not food is present, the nature and quantity of bile salts and bacterial flora, the rate of splanchnic blood flow, prior diet, and food intake as well as gastrointestinal motil-ity.[32] Until recently little was known about how disease states altered these factors in man; however, large interindividual differences in rates of absorption of many orally administered drugs occur in hospital patients[6,27,36] as well as in normal volun-teers.[8,45,51] For example, a seven-fold range in the amount of tetracycline absorbed was reported in six fasting, healthy subjects.[44] Variations in gastric emptying may contribute significantly to large interindividual differences in drug absorption rate because numerous physiological conditions, such as posture and autonomic activity as well as the temperature, volume, viscosity, and tonicity of gastric contents, can change gastric emptying time. Grossly impaired absorption of paracetamol occurs in patients with delayed gastric emptying and pyloric stenosis.[20] In patients with slow gastric emptying, L-dopa may be ineffective.[10] Therapeutic failure of orally administered drugs usually accompanies gastric stasis.[20,37,42] In patients with achlorhydria, aspirin was absorbed significantly faster and plasma salicylate concen-trations were higher than those in control subjects.[42] Acetaminophen plasma concentrations were significantly higher after oral administration of the drug to 12 convalescent hospital patients in bed than to 7 healthy ambulant volunteers matched for age and sex.[43]

Since rates of absorption of orally administered pills and capsules are dependent on rates of dissolution and dispersion, some of the factors enumerated above can

Drug absorption

alter such rates, thereby contributing to variations in drug absorption. It is interesting and somewhat surprising that the absorption of p-aminosalicylic acid and isoniazid was unchanged by gastrectomy performed for peptic ulcer, although complete failure of ethionamide absorption occurred in some patients.[34] Furthermore, gastrectomy failed to alter the absorption of sulfisoxazole, quinidine, or ethambutol unless vagotomy had been performed, thereby slowing gastric emptying.[57]

In jejunal disease folic acid absorption is diminished.[21] In ileal disease the transport of bile acids may be impaired, as well as the enterohepatic transport of many lipid-soluble drugs, since bile acids promote the gastrointestinal absorption of fat and certain fat-soluble compounds, including many drugs and vitamins A, D, K, and E. Ileal disease may be associated with impaired vitamin B_{12} absorption, since vitamin B_{12} is absorbed in the ileum after it forms a complex with intrinsic factor produced by the gastric parietal cell. Defective function of the ileum secondary to surgical removal or disease through interference with vitamin B_{12} absorption can lead to pernicious anemia. Vitamin B_{12} absorption can also be impaired in gastric diseases in which parietal cell function is abnormal, producing intrinsic factor deficiency and pernicious anemia. In some patients with pernicious anemia, precipitating or blocking antibodies to intrinsic factor have been identified.[17,50] In addition, regional enteritis as well as tropical sprue, celiac disease, and Whipple's disease, can produce vitamin B_{12} malabsorption. In steatorrhea, fat-soluble drugs and vitamins may be lost in the feces, producing deficiency of the fat-soluble vitamins, a deficiency of vitamin D being by far the most significant chronic problem in gastrointestinal disease.

Some active drugs are produced after metabolism of the inactive form by gut bacteria, the best example being cleavage of salicylazosulfapyridine, the drug of choice in the treatment of chronic ulcerative colitis. Diseases that change the nature of the gastrointestinal flora can affect the disposition of other drugs metabolized by gut bacteria. Possibly the effect of large doses of charcoal on gastrointestinal absorption of phenacetin is mediated by gut bacteria and induction of aryl hydrocarbon hydroxylase activity in these bacteria by charcoal.[40] Absorption of digoxin is reduced by neomycin administration.[33]

Drug distribution   Binding of many drugs to albumin is altered in several disease states, particularly in diseases of the liver and kidney associated with decreased concentrations of serum albumin. For example, phenytoin binding to albumin was decreased in plasma of 15 uremic patients.[46] The size of the unbound fraction correlated well with blood urea nitrogen, serum creatinine, and the clinical state of the patient. In addition to phenytoin, other organic acids including clofibrate, congo red, fluorescein, methyl red, phenytoin, sulfonamides, thyroxine, and tryptophan exhibited decreased protein binding in uremia. By contrast, most organic bases bind normally to plasma from uremic patients. A clinically significant neutral compound, digitoxin, exhibited decreased plasma binding in uremic patients.[52]

Disease states, including cirrhosis and nephritis, that are associated with hypoproteinemia and hypoalbuminemia exhibit elevations in the unbound fraction of most drugs compared with the unbound fraction present under conditions of normal protein and albumin concentrations. These situations illustrate the danger of selecting drug dose solely on the basis of total drug concentrations in plasma rather than on the free concentration, since only the free form is pharmacologically active. In cirrhosis, the plasma binding of the organic bases quinidine, diazepam, and triamterene, as well as of the organic acid fluorescein, are all decreased.

In addition to these disease-associated quantitative changes in drug binding to albumin, qualitative changes can occur in the nature of the binding. Such qualitative changes have been reported in uremia,[49] in which avidity of phenytoin binding to albumin is reduced.

An appropriate answer to the question of how liver disease affects the disposition of a drug normally eliminated primarily by hepatic metabolism requires consideration of several facts. Most drugs metabolized in the liver are converted by multiple reactions, including oxidations, reductions, and conjugations. It is not unusual for such drugs to have 10 to 20 distinctive metabolites, and for some as many as 30 or even 40 metabolites have been identified. Several enzymes responsible for these multiple reactions are cytoplasmic, others are associated with specific subcellular organelles. Under normal conditions the cytochrome P-450 dependent monooxygenases located in the smooth endoplasmic reticulum and responsible for many drug oxidations exist in at least three, and possibly six or more, molecular forms. Diseases of the liver can differentially affect these enzymes and isozymes.

Hepatic drug metabolism

Aside from these physiological considerations, pathophysiological changes in liver disease are relevant to the question at hand. The most common form of liver disease in this country, alcoholic cirrhosis, is a disease characterized by remissions and exacerbations, by a variable progression over a long period of time. During the early part of the disease, rates of metabolism of many drugs in alcoholic subjects may actually be faster than in normal subjects[58] because multiple doses of ethanol induce cytochrome P-450 dependent monooxygenases in hepatic smooth endoplasmic reticulum.[58] However, with time the disease process begins to convert functional hepatocytes into fibrous bands incapable of metabolizing drugs. This insidious process proceeds as follows: first, fatty infiltration of hepatocytes occurs, thereby distending these cells; then septums of connective tissue appear in periportal zones and other areas of active hepatocyte degeneration. The fibrous tissue grows and surrounds small masses of hepatocytes; then these lobular remnants undergo regeneration and form nodules. This entire process proceeds at different rates in different parts of the liver so that drug-metabolizing capacity is not uniform in the liver but varies, depending on the region and the extent of fibrotic tissue.

These facts are presented to show why it is difficult to predict precisely how a particular patient with alcoholic cirrhosis will be able to eliminate a drug whose disposition depends largely on hepatic metabolism. The best course for a physician to take is to give these patients slightly lower than normal doses of such drugs and to watch closely to make sure that the patient does not experience drug toxicity but derives the intended therapeutic benefit from the drugs administered. Such close initial observations after a drug is given may lead to subsequent modifications in the dose.

Fig. 9-1 shows how patients with different forms of liver disease metabolize a relatively safe test, aminopyrine, compared to patients with normal cardiovascular, hepatic, and renal function. This test was developed to measure hepatic capacity to N-demethylate certain drugs.[22,23,24] In humans, aminopyrine is eliminated mainly by N-demethylation accomplished by cytochrome P-450 dependent monooxygenases located in hepatic smooth endoplasmic reticulum. Subsequently, the methyl group removed by these enzymatic reactions is converted to CO_2, excreted in breath, and measurable as $^{14}CO_2$ if a single tracer dose of [dimethylamine-^{14}C]-aminopyrine (2 μCi) is initially administered. Fig. 9-1 shows that patients with certain forms of liver disease, such as fatty liver and cholestasis, do not exhibit marked reduction in their hepatic N-demethylating capacity. On the other hand, patients with hepato-cellular diseases, such as cirrhosis, infectious hepatitis, and certain metastatic cancers or hepatomas, do show reduced N-demethylating capacity.

These observations of reduced rates of aminopyrine elimination in almost all

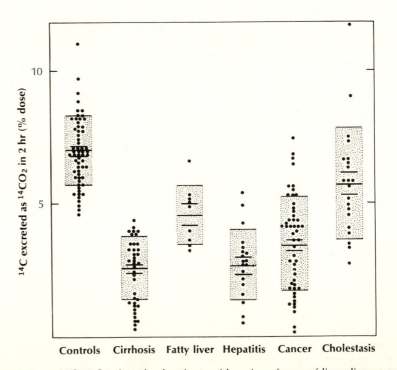

FIG. 9-1. Excretion of $^{14}[CO_2]$ in breath of patients with various forms of liver disease compared to control patients 2 hours after oral administration of a single tracer dose of [^{14}C]aminopyrine. (From Hepner, G. W., and Vesell, E. S.: Ann. Intern. Med. **83**:632, 1975.)

patients with parenchymal liver disease are in agreement with other observations that liver disease is also accompanied by reduced rates of hepatic antipyrine metabolism.[4,5,11] These results can be harmonized with observations that warfarin disposition during acute viral hepatitis is unchanged[60] and that oxazepam disposition is normal during acute viral hepatitis and cirrhosis.[53] Between these extremes, a group of drugs of which clindamycin is an example apparently exhibit intermediate or moderate changes in disposition in liver disease.[7] A wide range, from no change whatever in disposition to significant retardation, has been reported in liver disease, depending on the drug studied and its particular dispositional characteristics. For drugs with high hepatic extraction ratios (greater than 0.8), such as propranolol

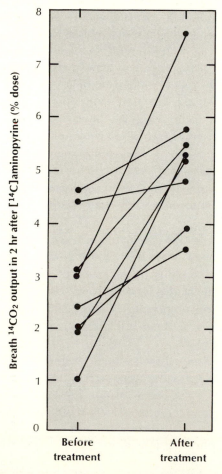

FIG. 9-2. Excretion of $^{14}[CO_2]$ 2 hours after an oral tracer dose of $[^{14}C]$aminopyrine in breath of 8 patients who received $[^{14}C]$aminopyrine before and 7 or 10 days after treatment of congestive heart failure. Note improvement in hepatic capacity to *N*-demethylate aminopyrine with treatment of congestive heart failure as indicated by markedly increased $^{14}[CO_2]$ output in breath after 7 or 10 days of treatment. (From Hepner, G. W., Vesell, E. S., and Tatum, K. R.: Am. J. Med. **65:**271, 1978.)

and lidocaine, alterations in blood flow accompanying liver disease can produce large changes in hepatic clearance of the compound. For drugs with very low hepatic extraction ratios (less than 0.2), such as antipyrine and aminopyrine, large variations in the extent to which hepatocellular disease alters their rates of metabolism cannot be due to abnormal liver blood flow. These variations may be attributed in part to multiple molecular forms of hepatic cytochrome P-450 and to the differential effects that a particular hepatic disorder might exert on these forms.

In addition to the primary diseases of the liver shown in Fig. 9-1 that are associated with reduced aminopyrine N-demethylation, certain disorders of other organs may secondarily involve the liver. For example, in congestive heart failure, liver function may become impaired secondary to pooling of blood in the liver and reduced hepatic perfusion. Reduced blood flow to the liver would be expected to result in decreased hepatic uptake of drugs with a high hepatic extraction, whose clearance by the liver depends on liver blood flow. Therefore, congestive heart failure was demonstrated to result in reduced rates of elimination of such drugs as lidocaine.[54,55] However, for drugs with low hepatic extraction, such as aminopyrine, whose clearance is not dependent on hepatic blood flow, it was not anticipated that reduced hepatic perfusion secondary to congestive heart failure would exert any effect on their rates of elimination. Fig. 9-2 shows that patients admitted to the hospital because of acute congestive heart failure were unable to eliminate aminopyrine as rapidly as they could after 7 to 10 days of treatment for their heart failure. These results with aminopyrine suggest that the hemodynamic changes associated with congestive heart failure impair hepatic drug metabolism, thereby reducing the ability of the body to eliminate drugs through this process.

Renal excretion of drugs   Only relatively few drugs are eliminated primarily by renal excretion. Obviously renal disease impairs the rate of removal of these drugs from the body. Therefore, the dose of these drugs must be reduced, the extent of reduction in dose depending on the severity and duration of the renal disease. Drugs eliminated from the body primarily by renal excretion include colistin, penicillin, procainamide, digoxin, aminoglucoside antibiotics, barbital, cycloserine, ethambutol, methotrexate, and tetracycline.

Since poor renal function is associated with decreased excretion of several drugs, it is important to modify normal drug dosage in uremic patients. Methods for this have been presented.[9,14,15,47] A linear relationship exists between the overall elimination rate constant (k_e) and the endogenous creatinine clearance (V'_{cr}):

$$k_e = k_{nr} + \delta \cdot V'_{cr}$$

In this equation, k_{nr} is the mean extrarenal elimination rate constant in anuric patients and δ is a constant relating V'_{cr} to the renal elimination rate constant (k_r) of the drug. This equation can be used for about 40 drugs; simple nomograms have been devised that allow estimation of rate of drug elimination in a patient with kidney disease from the value of V'_{cr}.[15,59] However, the apparent elimination rates of numerous drugs are unaltered by uremia, including antipyrine, histamine, phenacetin, phenytoin, phenobarbital, propranolol, quinidine, tolbutamide, and vitamin D.[46]

Patients often experience several disorders simultaneously. Moreover, even a single disease process can impair the function of several organs or involve several factors, such as fever,[16,56] that themselves can alter rates of drug elimination. Accordingly, a patient may exhibit a fluctuating course characterized by improvement in function of several tissues but a decline in function of other tissues with corresponding episodic changes in the efficiency of individual pharmacokinetic processes. All these complex, changing conditions render difficult the physician's task of individualizing dosage of drugs with low therapeutic indices. For these reasons, to avoid toxicity, great caution should be exercised in administering such drugs to patients with complex disorders involving multiple organs. Measurement of the concentration of many drugs with low therapeutic indices in the blood of some patients can help physicians adjust dosage of these drugs to fall within therapeutic ranges and out of toxic or ineffective ranges. Although pitfalls occur in this approach and although interpretations of drug blood concentrations must take into account the patient's clinical status and the fact that only the free, unbound form of the drug is available for pharmacological activity, this method has been and is being employed successfully and widely to improve drug safety and efficacy. It is discussed in more detail in Appendix A in which the therapeutic, toxic, and lethal blood concentrations of commonly used drugs are given. Adequate use of drug concentrations in blood requires knowledge of fundamental principles of pharmacokinetics and recognition that drug concentrations in blood change after drug administration, unless a continuous intravenous infusion is maintained. Therefore, the appropriate time to draw blood for drug measurements is before, rather than just after, drug administration.

MONITORING BLOOD CONCENTRATIONS OF CERTAIN DRUGS

PERSPECTIVE

The information provided in chapters 6 to 9 was selected to illustrate the extreme plasticity and sensitivity of human pharmacokinetic processes to perturbation by numerous factors. Five specific host factors were chosen because abundant evidence is available that clearly establishes the influence of each of these factors on rates of drug elimination in man: (1) genetic constitution, (2) age, (3) diet, (4) occupation, and (5) disease. The physician needs to be aware of certain details concerning each of these factors and to question the patient about them. In this way the physician will be more successful in selecting a dosage regimen that is therapeutic rather than toxic or ineffective. Furthermore, several steps are available to help the physician make the right choice: (1) close clinical observation of the patient for therapeutic, as well as toxic, signs of drug action; (2) quantitative endpoints for certain drugs (such as anticoagulants or antihypertensive agents) against which the dose can be titrated; and (3) measurement of drug concentrations in biological fluids of certain drugs whose therapeutic and toxic concentrations have been defined (Appendix A). Thus, despite the fact that dynamic interactions occur among the many factors influencing

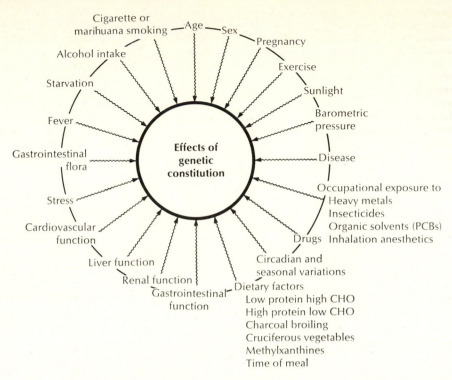

FIG. 9-3. Environmental factors affecting drug disposition in human subjects. Outer circle shows established or suspected environmental factors that can alter genetically controlled rates of drug elimination. A line joins environmental factors to suggest that several are associated and interdependent, rather than independent. Lines from each environmental factor to inner circle are wavy to suggest that modification of genetically controlled rates can occur at multiple levels. Such environmental effects need not occur directly at the genetic level.

rates of drug elimination in individual patients and render dosage selection difficult (Fig. 9-3), the physician can proceed in a rational, deliberate manner to make the correct choice of dose and to derive maximum therapeutic benefit from available drugs, while minimizing risks of toxicity.

REFERENCES

1 Alvares, P., Fischbein, A., Anderson, K. E., and Kappas, A.: Alterations in drug metabolism in workers exposed to polychlorinated biphenyls, Clin. Pharmacol. Ther. 22:140, 1977.

2 Alvares, A. P., Fischbein, A., Sassa, S., Anderson, K. E., and Kappas, A.: Lead intoxication: effects on cytochrome P-450–mediated hepatic oxidations, Clin. Pharmacol. Ther. 19:183, 1976.

3 Alvares, A. P., Kapelner, S., Sassa, S., and Kappas, A.: Drug metabolism in normal children, lead-poisoned children, and normal adults, Clin. Pharmacol. Ther. 17:179, 1975.

4 Andreasen, P. B., Ranek, L., Statland, B. E., and Tygstrup, N.: Clearance of antipyrine-dependence of quantitative liver function, Eur. J. Clin. Invest. 4:129, 1974.

5 Andreasen, P. B., and Vesell, E. S.: Compari-

son of plasma levels of antipyrine, tolbutamide, and warfarin after oral and intravenous administration, Clin. Pharmacol. Ther. **16**:1059, 1974.

6 Armstrong, B. K., Ukich, A. W., and Goatcher, P. M.: Plasma salicylate levels in rheumatoid arthritis produced by four different salicylate preparations, Med. J. Aust. **2**:181, 1970.

7 Avant, G. R., Schenker, S., and Alford, R. H.: The effect of cirrhosis on the disposition and elimination of clindamycin, Am. J. Dig. Dis. **20**:223, 1975.

8 Beermann, B., Hellstrom, K., and Rosen, A.: On the metabolism of propantheline in man, Clin. Pharmacol. Ther. **13**:212, 1972.

9 Bennett, W. M., Singer, I., and Coggins, C. H.: Guide to drug usage in adult patients with impaired renal function, J.A.M.A. **223**:991, 1973.

10 Bianchine, J. R., Calimlim, L. R., Morgan, J. P., Dujvone, C. A., and Lasagna, L.: Metabolism and absorption of L-3, 4-dihydroxyphenylalanine in patients with Parkinson's disease, Ann. N.Y. Acad. Sci. **179**:126, 1971.

11 Branch, R. A., Herbert, C. M., and Read, A. E.: Determinants of serum antipyrine half-lives in patients with liver disease, Gut **14**:569, 1973.

12 Brodie, B. B., Burns, J. J., and Weiner, M.: Metabolism of drugs in subjects with Laennec's cirrhosis, Med. Exp. **1**:290, 1959.

13 Creasey, W. A.: Drug disposition in humans, New York, 1979, Oxford University Press.

14 Dettli, L.: Individualization of drug dosage in patients with renal disease, Med. Clin. North Am. **58**:977, 1974.

15 Dettli, L.: Translation of pharmacokinetics to clinical medicine. In Teorell, T., Dedrick, R., and Condliffe, P., editors: Pharmacology and pharmacokinetics, New York, 1974, Plenum Publishing Corp., pp. 69-86.

16 Elin, R. J., Vesell, E. S., and Wolff, S. M.: Effects of etiocholanolone-induced fever on plasma antipyrine half-lives and metabolic clearance, Clin. Pharmacol. Ther. **17**:447, 1975.

17 Fisher, J. M., Reese, C., and Taylor, K. B.: Intrinsic-factor antibodies in gastric juice of pernicious-anaemia patients, Lancet **2**:88, 1966.

18 Fraser, H. S., Mucklow, J. C., Bulpitt, C. J., Kahn, C., Mould, G., and Dollery, C. T.: Environmental factors affecting antipyrine metabolism in London factory and office workers, Br. J. Clin. Pharmacol. **7**:237, 1979.

19 Ghoneim, M. M., Delle, M., Wilson, W. R., and Ambre, J. J.: Alteration of warfarin kinetics in man associated with exposure to an operating-room environment, Anesthesiology **43**:333, 1975.

20 Hart, P., Farrell, G. C., Cooksley, W. G. E., and Powell, L. W.: Enhanced drug metabolism in cigarette smokers, Br. Med. J. **2**:147, 1976.

21 Hepner, G. W., Booth, C. C., Cowan, J., Hoffbrand, A. V., and Mollin, D. L.: Absorption of crystalline folic acid in man, Lancet **2**:302, 1968.

22 Hepner, G. W., and Vesell, E. S.: Assessment of aminopyrine metabolism in man by breath analysis after oral administration of ^{14}C-aminopyrine, N. Engl. J. Med. **291**:1384, 1974.

23 Hepner, G. W., and Vesell, E. S.: Quantitative assessment of hepatic function by breath analysis after oral administration of [^{14}C]-aminopyrine, Ann. Intern. Med. **83**:632, 1975.

24 Hepner, G. W., Vesell, E. S., Lipton, A., Harvey, H. A., Wilkinson, G. R., and Schenker, S.: Disposition of aminopyrine, antipyrine, diazepam, and indocyanine green in patients with liver disease or on anticonvulsant drug therapy: diazepam breath test and correlations in drug elimination, J. Lab. Clin. Med. **90**:440, 1977.

25 Hepner, G. W., Vesell, E. S., and Tantum, K. R.: Reduced drug elimination in congestive heart failure, Am. J. Med. **65**:271, 1978.

26 Kater, R. M. H., Roggin, G., Tobon, F., Zieve, P., and Iber, F. L.: Increased rate of clearance of drugs from the circulation of alcoholics, Am. J. Med. Sci. **258**:35, 1969.

27 Koch-Weser, J.: Pharmacokinetics of procainamide in man, Ann. N.Y. Acad. Sci. **179**:370, 1971.

28 Kolmodin, B., Azarnoff, D. L., and Sjoquist, F.: Effect of environmental factors on drug metabolism: decreased plasma half-life of antipyrine in workers exposed to chlorinated hydrocarbon insecticides, Clin. Pharmacol. Ther. **10**:638, 1969.

29 Kolmodin-Hedman, B.: Decreased plasma half-life of phenylbutazone in workers exposed to chlorinated pesticides, Eur. J. Clin. Pharmacol. **5**:195, 1973.

30 Kolmodin-Hedman, B.: Decreased plasma half-lives of antipyrine and phenylbutazone in workers occupationally exposed to lindane and DDT. In Morselli, P. L., Cohen, S. N., and Garattini, S.: Drug interactions, New York, 1974, Raven Press.

31 Levi, A. J., Sherlock, S., and Walker, D.: Phenylbutazone and isoniazid metabolism in patients with liver disease in relation to previous drug therapy, Lancet **1**:1275, 1968.

32 Levine, R. R.: Factors affecting gastrointestinal absorption of drugs, Am. J. Dig. Dis. **15**:171, 1970.

33 Lindenbaum, J., Maulitz, R. M., and Butter, V. P., Jr.: Inhibition of digoxin absorption by neomycin, Gastroenterology 71:399, 1976.

34 Mattila, M. J., Friman, A., Larmi, T. K., and Koskinen, R.: Absorption of ethionamid, isoniazid and aminosalicylic acid from the postresection gastrointestinal tract, Ann. Med. Exp. Biol. Fenn. 47:209, 1969.

35 Meredith, P. A., Campbell, B. C., Moore, M. R., and Goldberg, A.: Antipyrine metabolism in lead intoxication, Br. J. Clin. Pharmacol. 3:960P, 1976.

36 Nelson, J. D., Shelton, S., Kusmiesz, H. T., and Haltalin, K. C.: Absorption of ampicillin and nalidixic acid by infants and children with acute shigellosis, Clin. Pharmacol. Ther. 13:879, 1972.

37 Nimmo, J., Heading, R. C., Tothill, P., and Prescott, L. F.: Pharmacological modification of gastric emptying: effects of propantheline and metoclopramide on paracetamol absorption, Br. Med. J. 1:587, 1973.

38 O'Malley, K., Stevenson, I. H., and Wood, M.: Drug metabolizing ability in operating theatre personnel, Br. J. of Anaesth. 45:924, 1973.

39 Pagliaro, L. A., and Benet, L. Z.: Pharmacokinetic data. Critical compilation of terminal half-lives, percent excreted unchanged, and changes of half-life in renal and hepatic dysfunction for studies in humans with references, J. Pharmacokinet. Biopharm. 3:333, 1975.

40 Pantuck, E. J., Hsiao, K. -C., Kuntzman, R., and Conney, A. H.: Intestinal metabolism of phenacetin in the rat: effect of charcoal-broiled beef and rat chow, Science 187:744, 1975.

41 Poland, A., Smith, D., Kuntzman, R., Jacobson, M., and Conney, A. H.: Effect of intensive occupational exposure to DDT on phenylbutazone and cortisol metabolism in human subjects, Clin. Pharmacol. Ther. 11:724, 1970.

42 Prescott, L. F.: Gastrointestinal absorption of drugs, Med. Clin. North Am. 58:907, 1974.

43 Prescott, L. F.: Pathological and physiological factors affecting drug absorption, distribution, elimination and response in man. In Concepts in biochemical pharmacology. III. Berlin-Heidelberg-New York, 1975, Springer-Verlag, p. 241.

44 Prescott, L. F., and Nimmo, J.: Generic inequivalence—clinical observations, Acta Pharmacol. Toxicol. (Kbh) 29(Supp. 3):288, 1971.

45 Prescott, L. F., Steel, R. F., and Ferrier, W. R.: The effects of particle size on the absorption of phenacetin in man, a correlation between plasma concentration of phenacetin and effects on the central nervous system, Clin. Pharmacol. Ther. 11:496, 1970.

46 Reidenberg, M. M.: Kidney disease and drug metabolism, Med. Clin. North Am. 58:1059, 1974.

47 Reidenberg, M. M.: Renal function and drug action, Philadelphia, 1971, W. B. Saunders Co.

48 Reidenberg, M. M., and Drayer, D. E.: Effects of renal disease upon drug disposition, Drug Metab. Rev. 8:293, 1978.

49 Reidenberg, M. M., Odar-Cederlof, I., Von Bahr, C., Borga, O., and Sjoquist, F.: Protein binding of diphenylhydantoin and desmethylimipramine in plasma from patients with poor renal function, N. Engl. J. Med. 285:264, 1971.

50 Schade, S. G., Feick, P., Muckerheider, M., and Schilling, R. F.: Occurrence in gastric juice of antibody to a complex of intrinsic factor and vitamin B_{12}, N. Engl. J. Med. 275:528, 1966.

51 Schroder, H., and Campbell, D. E. S.: Absorption, metabolism, and excretion of salicylazosulfapyridine in man, Clin. Pharmacol. Ther. 13:539, 1972.

52 Shoeman, D. W., and Azarnoff, D. L.: The alteration of plasma proteins in uremia as reflected in their ability to bind digitoxin and diphenylhydantoin, Pharmacology 7:169, 1972.

53 Shull, H. J., Wilkinson, G. R., Johnson, R., and Schenker, S.: Normal disposition of oxazepam in acute viral hepatitis and cirrhosis, Ann. Intern. Med. 84:420, 1976.

54 Thompson, P. D., Melmon, K. L., and Richardson, J. A.: Lidocaine pharmacokinetics in advanced heart failure, Ann. Intern. Med. 78:449, 1973.

55 Thompson, P. D., Rowland, M., and Melmon, M.: The influence of heart failure, liver disease and renal failure on the disposition of lidocaine in man, Am. Heart J. 82:417, 1971.

56 Trenholme, G. M., Williams, R. L., Rieckmann, K. H., Frischer, H., and Carson, P. E.: Quinine disposition during malaria and during induced fever, Clin. Pharmacol. Ther. 19:459, 1976.

57 Venho, V. M. K., Jussila, J., and Aukee, S.: Drug absorption in man after gastric surgery, Fifth International Congress on Pharmacology, San Francisco, 1972, Abstract No. 1445, p. 241.

58 Vesell, E. S., Page, J. G., and Passananti, G. T.: Genetic and environmental factors affecting ethanol metabolism in man, Clin. Pharmacol. Ther. 12:192, 1971.

59 Wagner, J. G.: Biopharmaceutics and relevant pharmacokinetics, Hamilton Ill., 1971, Drug Intelligence Publication.

60 Williams, R. L., Schary, W. L., Blaschke, T. F., Meffin, P. J., Melmon, K. L., and Rowland, M.: Influence of acute viral hepatitis on disposition and pharmacologic effect of warfarin, Clin. Pharmacol. Ther. **20**:90, 1976.

REVIEWS

61 Alvares, A. P.: Interactions between environmental chemicals and drug biotransformation in man, Clin. Pharmacokinet. **3**:462, 1978.
62 Benet, L. Z.: The effect of disease states on drug pharmacokinetics, Washington, D.C., 1976, American Pharmaceutical Association.
63 Vesell, E. S.: The antipyrine test in clinical pharmacology: conceptions and misconceptions, Clin. Pharmacol. Ther. **26**:275, 1979.
64 Vessell, E. S.: Why individuals vary in their response to drugs, Trends in Pharmacological Sciences, pp. 349-351, Aug. 1980.

Drug effects on the nervous system and neuroeffectors

CHAPTER 10

General aspects of neuropharmacology

The more than 10 billion neurons that make up the human nervous system communicate with each other by means of chemical mediators. They exert their effects on peripheral structures by the release of these mediators and not by electric impulses.

In the peripheral portions of the autonomic nervous system acetylcholine and norepinephrine play a predominant role. They act on postjunctional membranes producing excitatory or inhibitory effects as a consequence of depolarization or hyperpolarization of these membranes.

Within the central nervous system (CNS) the neurotransmitters and modulators are biogenic amines, certain amino acids, and numerous peptides. Among the biogenic amines, acetylcholine, norepinephrine, dopamine, serotonin, and probably histamine play a role. Amino acids, such as glutamic and aspartic acid excite the postsynaptic membranes of many neurons. γ-Aminobutyric acid and glycine may be inhibitory transmitters. Among the peptides, about 20 are under consideration as transmitters of nerve signals. Substance P, the endorphins, and the enkephalins are some of the peptides of great current interest.

Numerous drugs mimic or influence the action of the chemical mediators and may be classified as neuropharmacological agents. Others act by unknown mechanisms but may be classified according to their clinical usage as hypnotics, analgesics, anticonvulsants, and general and local anesthetics.

THE CHEMICAL NEUROTRANS-MISSION CONCEPT

The similarity between certain drug effects and those of nerve stimulation was noted prior to this century. Muscarine, from certain mushrooms, was known to slow the heart rate just like vagal stimulation. Adrenal extracts produced effects similar to those following stimulation of sympathetic nerves (Oliver and Shafer, 1895).

Definitive proof of chemical neurotransmission was provided in 1921 by the experiments of Loewi[50] and Cannon and Uridil.[11] In his classic experiment Otto Loewi demonstrated that when the vagus nerve of a perfused frog heart is stimulated, a substance is released that is capable of slowing a second frog heart with no neural connections to the first. Cannon and Uridil[11] found that sympathetic nerve stimulation of the liver causes the release of a substance similar to epinephrine in many respects. This mediator, at first named "sympathin," is now believed to be norepinephrine. Identification of the neurotransmitter in adrenergic axons as norepinephrine was provided by von Euler.[27]

Acetylcholine was first studied systematically by Dale.[19] The "quantum hypothesis" of acetylcholine release and the role of synaptic vesicles in neuromuscular and synaptic transmission is a contribution of Katz and co-workers.[31,48] The discovery by Brodie and Shore[6] of monoamine release by reserpine led to a great expansion of knowledge regarding the metabolism and function of catecholamines in the nervous system. The uptake of catecholamines by sympathetic nerves is mainly a contribution of Axelrod.[2] The importance of these contributions is attested to by the Nobel Prizes that have been awarded to most of the investigators just cited.

After these discoveries it became apparent that drugs need not necessarily act through nerves to influence an effector organ. In fact, it was then clearly seen that nerves could act by releasing chemical compounds, which in turn influenced the effector structures. Instead of classifying drugs as sympathomimetic and parasympathomimetic, it appeared more reasonable to classify nerves on the basis of the mediator released from them. This led to the concept of cholinergic and adrenergic nerve fibers.[18]

SITES OF ACTION OF CHEMICAL MEDIATORS

The role of neurotransmitters at various anatomical sites is well established in some cases and is surmised in others. The generally accepted information on the site of action of these compounds may be summarized as follows:

1. Postganglionic parasympathetic nerve endings on smooth muscle, cardiac muscle, and exocrine glands: acetylcholine
2. Postganglionic sympathetic nerve endings on smooth muscle, cardiac muscle, and exocrine glands: norepinephrine (with the exception of nerve endings on sweat glands)
3. All autonomic ganglionic synapses: acetylcholine (although dopamine may modulate transmission)
4. Motor fiber terminals at skeletal neuromuscular junctions: acetylcholine
5. CNS synapses: acetylcholine, norepinephrine, dopamine, serotonin, histamine, glutamic and aspartic acid, γ-aminobutyric acid (GABA), glycine, and numerous peptides

The site of action of the various mediators in the autonomic nervous system is fairly well established. The situation is much more complex in the CNS where neurophysiological techniques are not sufficient for establishing the role of transmitter at a given site. Immunofluorescence and the biochemical identification of receptors in the brain for the selective localization of active agents are some of the newer approaches for establishing the transmitter role of various compounds.[90]

RECEPTOR CONCEPT IN NEUROPHARMACOLOGY

The neurotransmitters exert their effect on various membranes by interacting with specific receptors. The existence of these receptors may be deduced from structure-activity studies on congeneric series or from parallel shifts of dose-response curves in the presence of specific antagonists. The following receptors may be postulated for some of the neurotransmitters:

1. Acetylcholine has muscarinic and nicotinic receptors. Muscarinic receptors are present in various smooth muscles, cardiac muscle, and exocrine glands. They are termed *muscarinic* because muscarine, a quaternary amine alkaloid, has actions similar to those of acetylcholine at the sites indicated. The muscarinic receptor is competitively blocked by atropine and related drugs.

The nicotinic receptors of acetylcholine are located in autonomic ganglia and at skeletal neuromuscular junctions. They are termed *nicotinic* because nicotine also acts on these receptors. The nicotinic receptors in the autonomic ganglia and in skeletal muscle are not identical. The effects of the acetylcholine in autonomic ganglia are blocked by hexamethonium, whereas the receptors at the skeletal neuromuscular junction are blocked by *d*-tubocurarine and related compounds.

There are muscarinic and nicotinic receptors in the CNS also.[5] Thus the synapse between the collaterals of motor axons and the Renshaw cell is nicotinic, whereas there is good evidence for the presence of muscarinic receptors also within the CNS.

2. Norepinephrine acts on adrenergic receptors that are classified as *alpha* (α) and *beta* (β). Drugs that block these receptors are known as α- and β-*adrenergic blocking agents*. The β-adrenergic receptor may be closely associated with the enzyme adenyl cyclase.

3. Dopamine acts on dopaminergic receptors in the CNS and probably in ganglia. The dopaminergic receptors are blocked specifically by antipsychotic drugs such as phenothiazines and butyrophenones.

4. Serotonin acts on serotoninergic receptors in the CNS and in neuroeffector structures. Its actions are blocked by the antiserotonin compounds, such as methysergide.

5. Histamine acts on histaminergic receptors, which are classified as H_1 and H_2 receptors. The commonly used antihistamines are H_1-receptor antagonists, for example, pyrilamine. H_2-receptor antagonists have only been recently synthesized. A typical example is cimetidine.

Little is known about receptors for the hypothetical amino acid transmitters, but glycine appears to be antagonized by strychnine.[20] Many other receptors are being investigated by radioligand binding techniques.[90]

A partial isolation of the cholinergic receptor has been achieved[80] as a result of studies on some snake venoms that combine irreversibly with such receptors. It was observed that the α toxin of *Bungarus multicinctus*, or bungarotoxin, exerts a postsynaptic blocking action similar to that of *d*-tubocurarine except that it is irreversible. The toxin can be labeled radioactively and serves admirably for the isolation and study of some cholinergic receptors. It has been estimated from such studies that in an end-plate of rat muscle there are about 3×10^7 receptor molecules.

Newer concepts on the cholinergic receptor

Problem 10-1. What accounts for the muscarinic or nicotinic nature of a cholinergic receptor? Crystallographic analysis of acetylcholine and related agonists provides a tentative answer to this question. Acetylcholine is a flexible molecule and rotation is possible at two different bonds.[80]

Muscarinic and nicotinic drugs differ from acetylcholine in the degree of rotation at the sites of torsion. Thus acetylcholine has both muscarinic and nicotinic effects, whereas the purely muscarinic or nicotinic congeners have constraints imposed on them by conformational factors.

SYNAPSES AND NEUROMUSCULAR JUNCTIONS

The synapse is the site of transmission of the nerve impulse between two neurons. The axonal terminal is separated from the postsynaptic membrane by a synaptic cleft of about 200 Å in width. Electron micrographs show that the presynaptic element contains numerous vesicles, which are believed to store the transmitter. They also contain some mitochondria.

Transmission of the nerve impulse across the synapse is quite different from axonal conduction. First, transmission is unidirectional. Second, when the axon is stimulated electrically, there is a delay of about 0.2 second before the postsynaptic element is depolarized.

At somatic motor nerve endings the axon terminal lies within the synaptic gutters. Vesicles containing acetylcholine are present in the axon terminal. Nerve stimulation causes a release of acetylcholine that, diffusing across the gap, causes a change in permeability of the postjunctional membrane to Na^+ and K^+. The release process requires Ca^{++} and is inhibited by Mg^{++}. Botulinus toxin blocks acetylcholine release; hemicholinium, an experimental drug, blocks acetylcholine synthesis, presumably by interfering with the axonal uptake of choline (Fig. 10-1).

At the terminations of autonomic nerve fibers on smooth muscles, cardiac muscle, or exocrine glands, no specialized structures analogous to motor end-plates can be seen. The transmitters apparently are discharged at the terminal plexuses into the extracellular space and reach the receptors by diffusion.

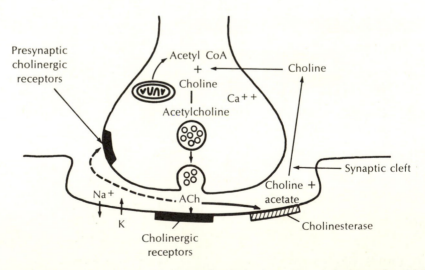

FIG. 10-1. Cholinergic nerve terminal depicting the synthesis, storage, and release of acetylcholine (ACh), its hydrolysis by cholinesterase, and its action on cholinergic receptors on the effector cell and presynaptic receptors.

The role of a mediator in neurotransmission is suggested or established by some or all of the following:

1. The presence of the transmitter in the axon along with the enzyme responsible for its production and destruction
2. Similarity of the mediator's effect to that of nerve stimulation
3. Release of the transmitter by nerve stimulation
4. Blockade of the effect of nerve stimulation by drugs that block the transmitter's action

Most of the criteria can be met in studies of neuromuscular transmission and ganglionic transmission. There are formidable difficulties in proving the transmitter role of a substance in the CNS by these same criteria.

EVIDENCE FOR CHOLINERGIC AND ADRENERGIC NEUROTRANSMISSION

Two apparent exceptions exist to the statement that norepinephrine is the chemical mediator to sympathetically innervated structures. The sweat glands, while receiving sympathetic innervation, are known to be activated by cholinergic drugs and inhibited by anticholinergic drugs, atropine being the great inhibitor of sweating. This apparent anomaly has been explained in a satisfactory manner by demon-

Mediators to sweat glands and adrenal medulla

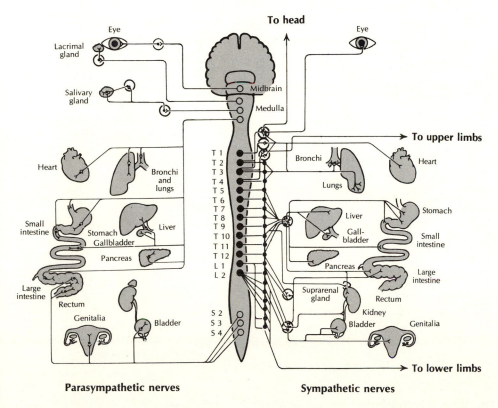

FIG. 10-2. Autonomic innervation of various organs. (Redrawn from a Sandoz Pharmaceuticals publication.)

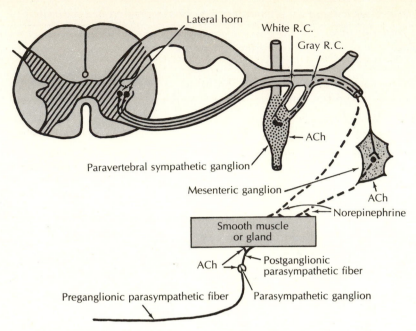

FIG. 10-3. Schematic representation of autonomic innervation of smooth muscle or exocrine gland. *ACh,* Acetylcholine.

strating that the particular fibers innervating the sweat glands are cholinergic. In other words, on stimulation they release acetylcholine rather than norepinephrine.

The adrenal medulla is another apparent exception. This structure secretes epinephrine when cholinergic drugs are injected, but its response may be inhibited by ganglionic blocking agents. The explanation of this apparent anomaly is based on embryological considerations. The adrenal medulla is in reality a modified sympathetic ganglion, and it is therefore not surprising that it should respond to acetylcholine, which is the normal ganglionic mediator for both the sympathetic and parasympathetic nerves.

SEQUENCE OF CHEMICAL EVENTS IN JUNCTIONAL TRANSMISSION   The following steps may be distinguished in junctional transmission: (1) synthesis of the mediator, (2) binding of the mediator in a potentially active form, (3) release of the mediator substance, (4) depolarization of postsynaptic membrane, (5) elimination of the mediator, and (6) repolarization of the postsynaptic membrane. Theoretically, at least, drugs could influence junctional transmission by acting at any of the steps, and, indeed, we have examples of many such interactions, as shown in Table 10-1.

Presynaptic actions of drugs   Although in the foregoing discussion and in Table 10-1 the postjunctional site of action of drugs is emphasized, there is growing evidence of a presynaptic action

TABLE 10-1. Sites of drug action in relation to junctional transmission

Site of drug action	Mediator involved	
	Acetylcholine	Norepinephrine
Synthesis of mediator inhibited by	Hemicholinium*	Methyldopa† α-Methyltyrosine
Binding of mediator in granules inhibited by		Reserpine Guanethidine
Release of mediator enhanced by	Carbachol	Tyramine Amphetamine Reserpine Guanethidine
Release of mediator inhibited by	Botulinus toxin	Bretylium Monoamine oxidase (MAO) inhibitors (?)
Depolarization of postsynaptic membrane promoted by	A. Choline esters Pilocarpine Muscarine B. Nicotine Dimethylphenylpiperazinium (DMPP)* C. Choline esters Nicotine Phenyltrimethylammonium (PTMA)*	Catecholamine and related amines
Depolarization of postsynaptic membrane inhibited by	A. Atropine and related drugs B. Hexamethonium nicotine C. d-Tubocurarine Succinylcholine	α-Receptor blocking agents: phenoxybenzamine β-Receptor blocking agents: propranolol

*Pharmacological tool only.
†Major clinical effect due to norepinephrine release rather than inhibition of synthesis.
A. Cholinergic neuroeffector site.
B. Ganglionic site.
C. Skeletal neuromuscular site.

of many drugs, particularly in relation to catecholamine release and also to neuromuscular transmission.[79,80]

There is good evidence for the presence of α-adrenoreceptors located prejunctionally on postganglionic adrenergic nerve endings, in addition to the α adrenoreceptors that are located postjunctionally. These prejunctional or α_2 receptors tend to reduce norepinephrine output when acted on by an adrenergic agonist.[76,83,84] Blockade of these receptors increases the release of norepinephrine. The physiological significance of these prejunctional receptors is not clear, but the concept has important implications in antihypertensive therapy.

**FACTORS INFLU-
ENCING RESPONSE
OF EFFECTORS TO
CHEMICAL MEDIATORS**

The response of effector cells may be altered remarkably under certain circumstances. The two conditions that have received attention are sensitization following denervation and sensitization in the presence of other drugs.

**Denervation
supersensitivity**

The supersensitivity of denervated structures is based on several mechanisms. Nonspecific supersensitivity may result from chronically reduced activity in a smooth muscle.[35] For example, chronic treatment of a guinea pig with a ganglionic blocking agent leads in a few days to an increased sensitivity of its isolated ileum to acetylcholine, histamine, potassium, and serotonin.[35] On the other hand, organs deprived of their adrenergic innervation become especially sensitive to catecholamines, probably because of absence of the uptake mechanism for the neurotransmitter (p. 127). Preganglionic denervation, also called *deafferentation*, is much less effective in increasing the susceptibility of various effectors to catecholamines. In this case the supersensitivity of smooth muscles may be nonspecific, resulting from chronically reduced activity.[35]

A very interesting mechanism appears to be operating in supersensitive skeletal muscle. A week or two following denervation the whole muscle fiber becomes responsive to externally applied acetylcholine, whereas only the end-plate region was sensitive prior to denervation. It appears as if new acetylcholine receptors had developed as a consequence of denervation.[62]

**Sensitization by
drugs**

In contrast to the supersensitivity induced by denervation and prolonged inactivity, more rapid sensitization to mediators can be produced by certain drugs.

Enzyme inhibitors may be quite effective. The inhibitors of cholinesterase potentiate the actions of acetylcholine. Catechol and pyrogallol may increase the effectiveness of norepinephrine and epinephrine.

Drugs may also interfere with the buffer mechanisms and thereby may allow greater fluctuation in some physiological parameter such as blood pressure when a neuropharmacological agent is administered. It has been suggested that protoveratrine can have this action.[41] The ganglionic blocking agents also increase the effectiveness of injected vasoactive drugs, probably by interfering with buffering responses.

The supersensitivity to catecholamines has been studied mostly on the nictitating membrane where two types of supersensitivity may exist.[68] A "presynaptic" supersensitivity develops after surgical denervation and its correlated with the degeneration of adrenergic nerve terminals. It is specific for catecholamines and related amines and develops within 48 hours after denervation. It is undoubtedly related to the absence of the catecholamine uptake mechanism. Another type of supersensitivity, which is nonspecific in that it applies not only to catecholamines but also to acetylcholine and other agonists, develops slowly after surgical denervation or decentralization. It appears to be postsynaptic and requires weeks for its development. This postsynaptic supersensitivity is a consequence of reduced levels of transmitter.

Cocaine,[52,68] antihistaminics,[47] and tricyclic antidepressants cause presynaptic supersensitivity as a consequence of interference with catecholamine reuptake by the adrenergic terminals. On the other hand, chronic administration of reserpine leads to the postsynaptic type of supersensitivity by chronic depletion of the transmitters. Guanethidine interferes with catecholamine uptake and also produces a long-lasting supersensitivity.[30] It probably exerts both presynaptic and postsynaptic effects.

In general, compounds that have a cocaine-like effect on the uptake of catecholamines sensitize effector cells to their pharmacological effects. The same compounds tend to block the actions of indirectly acting sympathomimetic drugs, such as those of tyramine.

In addition to the mechanisms of sensitization discussed, direct radioligand studies indicate that the *number* of receptors may change under various circumstances. An increase in receptor number is referred to as *up regulation* and a decrease in receptor number as *down regulation*.[85] Thus, high concentrations of adrenergic agents lead to decreased numbers of receptors, whereas a reduction in the tissue or serum levels of catecholamines leads to the opposite effect.[85] These concepts may explain many observations on the changes in sensitivity to mediators in various disease states. They may also explain changes in sensitivity to various mediators induced by hormones and drugs. For example, it is tempting to attribute the propranolol withdrawal syndrome to an increase in receptor number and increased responsiveness to endogenous catecholamines.[85]

AMINE METABOLISM AND THE NERVOUS SYSTEM

The best known neurotransmitters are nitrogenous bases synthesized by the neuron from precursors and stored in vesicles ready to be released. The active amines do not cross the blood-brain barrier efficiently, whereas the precursor amino acids do. The importance of precursor availability and nutritional state in the control of brain neurotransmitter synthesis is receiving increasing attention.[94]

Acetylcholine

The important neurotransmitter acetylcholine is present in certain peripheral nerves and in nerve endings in brain (synaptosomes), where its vesicular localization has been demonstrated.[75]

Acetylcholine is synthesized by the enzyme choline acetyltransferase, previously known as choline acetylase,[56] according to the following schema:

$$\text{Choline} + \text{Acetyl coenzyme A} \rightarrow \text{Acetylcholine} + \text{Coenzyme A}$$

Traditionally acetylcholine has been assayed by biological methods using a skeletal muscle such as the frog rectus abdominis or smooth muscle in the guinea pig ileum as test objects. There are now gas chromatographic techniques available for the same purpose.

During the nerve stimulation, *recently* synthesized acetylcholine may be preferentially released. The experimental compound *hemicholinium* blocks the synthesis of the mediator by interfering with the transport of choline across the neuronal membrane.

Acetylcholine released by a nerve impulse must be destroyed rapidly in order to allow the next impulse to act on a repolarized postsynaptic membrane within a few milliseconds. Hydrolysis of acetylcholine reduces the pharmacological activity of the compound a hundred-thousandfold.

Destruction of acetylcholine is accomplished by the *cholinesterases*, which are of two types. *Acetylcholinesterase*, or specific cholinesterase, hydrolyzes acetyl esters of choline more rapidly than butyryl esters. On the other hand, *pseudocholinesterase*, or nonspecific cholinesterase, is sometimes called butyrylcholinesterase because it hydrolyzes butyryl and other esters of choline more rapidly than the acetyl ester. Acetylcholinesterase is localized in neuronal membranes and surprisingly also in membranes of red cells and the placenta, where its function is unknown. Nonspecific cholinesterase is widely distributed in the body. Plasma cholinesterase is of the nonspecific type. Its presence in plasma is not related to neural activity, although its low titer after exposure to anticholinesterase pesticides is a useful method for diagnosing such poisonings. The titer of plasma cholinesterase is depressed also in advanced liver disease, since the enzyme is manufactured in the liver (p. 144).

Catecholamines   The collective term for norepinephrine, epinephrine, and dopamine is *catecholamine*, since these neurotransmitters are catechols (ortho-dihydroxybenzenes) and contain an amine group in their aliphatic side chain.

Localization   The distribution of catecholamines in the body is well understood, thanks to the availability of suitable methods for their determination, such as the fluorometric assay. In addition, the histochemical fluorescence microscopy techniques developed by Swedish investigators[45] allow an actual visualization of the catecholamine-containing structures (Fig. 15-1), their precise localization, and their susceptibility to drug effects.

Norepinephrine is present in adrenergic fibers and in certain pathways within the CNS. *Epinephrine* constitutes most of the catecholamine present in the human adrenal medulla, although adrenal medullary tumors may contain largely norepinephrine. Small amounts of epinephrine may occur also in various organs and in the CNS, but its main function recognized so far has to do with the adrenal medulla. *Dopamine* is present in relatively high concentration in the brain and is particularly concentrated in the caudate nucleus and the putamen (Table 10-2).

The distribution of norepinephrine in various organs corresponds well with their adrenergic innervation. Although there is considerable species variation, the heart, arteries, and veins of most mammals contain norepinephrine of the order of 1 μg/g of tissue.[27] The liver, lungs, and skeletal muscle contain considerably less, whereas the vas deferens has about five to ten times as much.

TABLE 10-2. Distribution of norepinephrine and dopamine in the human brain (micrograms/gram)*

	Norepinephrine	Dopamine
Frontal lobe	0.00-0.02	0.00
Caudate nucleus	0.04	3.12
Putamen	0.02	5.27
Hypothalamus (anterior part)	0.96	0.18
Substantia nigra	0.04	0.40
Pons	0.04	0.00
Medulla oblongata (dorsal part)	0.13	0.00
Cerebellar cortex	0.02	0.02

*Based on data from Bertler, A.: Acta Physiol. Scand. **51**:97, 1961.

Biosynthesis

The biosynthesis of catecholamines represents a small but very important portion of the metabolism of tyrosine. Other pathways lead to the formation of thyroxine, *p*-hydroxyphenylpyruvate, and melanin and to protein synthesis. Tyrosine itself may arise from hydroxylation of phenylalanine or may be taken up directly by the neurons for catecholamine synthesis.

The various steps in the biosynthesis of catecholamines are shown below (for structural formulas see Fig. 10-4):

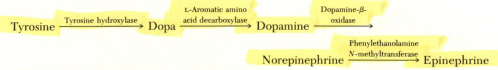

Tyrosine hydroxylase,[69] a cytoplasmic enzyme, catalyzes the rate-limiting step in catecholamine biosynthesis. Thus inhibition of this enzyme by amino acid analogues such as α-methyltyrosine leads to a depletion of catecholamines in brain and various sympathetic nerves, with important functional consequences.

L-*Aromatic amino acid decarboxylase* is a cytoplasmic enzyme that decarboxylates a number of substrates in addition to dopa, for example, 5-hydroxytryptophan to serotonin.

Dopamine-β-oxidase, a copper-containing enzyme bound to the membranes of the exoplasmic granules, catalyzes the conversion of dopamine to norepinephrine. The enzyme is inhibited by copper reagents such as disulfiram and diethyldithiocarbamate. Because the enzyme is associated with the catecholamine vesicles, sympathetic stimulation leads to the appearance of dopamine-β-oxidase activity in the circulation.[74]

Phenylethanolamine-N-methyltransferase is a cytoplasmic enzyme present largely in the adrenal medulla where it catalyzes the transfer of a methyl group from S-adenosylmethionine to norepinephrine for the formation of epinephrine.

Negative feedback of catecholamine biosynthesis. Sympathetic nerve stimulation does not cause catecholamine depletion in the axon, suggesting that increased synthesis can keep up with loss. With the discovery of tyrosine hydroxylase as the rate-

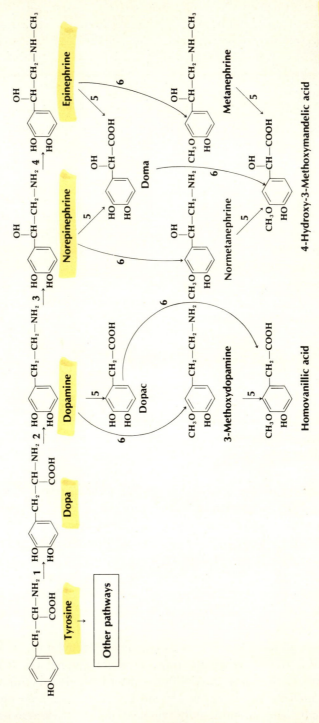

FIG. 10-4. Pathways of synthesis and metabolism of catecholamines. Enzymes catalyzing various reactions are as follows: *1,* tyrosine hydroxylase; *2,* aromatic amino acid decarboxylase; *3,* dopamine-β-hydroxylase; *4,* phenylethanolamine-*N*-methyltransferase; *5,* MAO plus aldehyde dehydrogenase; *6,* catechol-*O*-methyltransferase. *Dopa,* 3,4-Dihydroxyphenylalanine; *Dopac,* 3,4-dihydroxyphenylacetic acid; *Doma,* 3,4-dihydroxymandelic acid. (From Crout, J. R.: Catecholamine metabolism. In Manger, C. W., editor: Hormones and hypertension, Springfield, Ill., 1966, Charles C Thomas, Publisher.)

limiting enzyme in catecholamine biosynthesis, the relative constancy of catechol-amine stores can be explained. Norepinephrine and dopamine inhibit tyrosine hydroxylase. It becomes understandable, then, that increased catecholamine release through sympathetic activity will lead to accelerated synthesis of catecholamines at nerve terminals. On the other hand, monoamine oxidase (MAO) inhibitors, which elevate catecholamine levels in adrenergic neurons, also lead to a slowdown in cate-cholamine biosynthesis.

The release and synthesis of catecholamines are influenced in an important way by a neuronal feedback, most clearly shown for dopamine in the brain.[7,14] It has been shown that dopamine receptor blockade by phenothiazines or haloperidol leads to a compensatory increase in the activity of dopaminergic cells by a neuronal feed-back mechanism.[14]

Catecholamines are stored in vesicles in association with adenosine triphosphate and a soluble protein *chromogranin*. The vesicles are formed originally in the nerve cell body and are transported to the endings by axoplasmic flow. Constriction of an adrenergic nerve causes the accumulation of vesicles proximal to the ligature.[17]

Storage and release

Release of catecholamines is believed to take place by a specialized form of exocy-tosis. During the release process adenosine triphosphate, chromogranin, and dopa-mine-β-oxidase appear in the perfusate of adrenal medullary tissue[22] in addition to catecholamines. Although these findings suggest that the vesicles empty their con-tent, other evidence indicates that recently synthesized catecholamine is released preferentially.

In contrast with release by exocytosis, reserpine causes the release of the granu-lar catecholamines into the axoplasm, where they are deaminated by the enzyme monoamine oxidase (MAO) present in the axonal mitochondria.

Catecholamine release requires calcium[22] and is in this respect similar to acetyl-choline release from cholinergic nerves and to histamine release from mast cells.

The relative constancy of catecholamine stores in adrenergic neurons is not only a consequence of feedback regulation of its biosynthesis. It is also an expression of a remarkable ability of these neurons to take up the amines after their release. More than half the released catecholamine may be conserved by this mechanism, which will be discussed in greater detail (p. 184).

Disposition of the released catecholamine

The portion of the released catecholamine that escapes the amine pump reuptake is attacked by two enzymes: *catechol-O-methyl transferase* and *MAO*. The latter is widely distributed in the body, not only in adrenergic axonal mitochondria but also in nonneural structures. Catechol-*O*-methyltransferase is also widely distributed and is particularly concentrated in the liver and kidneys. Although the precise rela-tionship of these enzymes to sympathetic function is not understood, it is clearly not as crucial as the acetylcholine-cholinesterase interdependence. For example, inhibition of catechol-*O*-methyltransferase by catechol or pyrogallol does not cause a significant increase in sympathetic activity or potentiation of the action of injected catecholamines. Similarly, drugs that inhibit MAO fail to potentiate the action of catecholamines and do not increase sympathetic functions in the periphery.

The detailed metabolic pathways of catecholamines are shown in Fig. 10-4. The role of many of these pathways may be appreciated from data on the urinary excretion of catecholamine metabolites in normal humans; the percentages of endogenous catecholamines and metabolites are as follows:

Norepinephrine + Epinephrine	1.1%
Normetanephrine + Metanephrine	7.6%
Vanillylmandelic acid (VMA)	91.0%

The 24-hour VMA excretion in normal individuals is 10 mg. Much larger amounts may be excreted by patients with adrenal medullary tumors (p. 188).

Interaction of drugs with catecholamine storage and release mechanisms

Numerous clinically useful drugs interact with the storage and release of catecholamines. They are listed in Table 10-3 and will be discussed in some detail in the appropriate chapters.

Chemical sympathectomy: 6-hydroxydopamine

The administration of 6-hydroxydopamine, an interesting experimental tool, causes an extremely long-lasting depletion of catecholamines in organs innervated by the sympathetic division. Electron microscopic studies indicate that the drug causes a selective destruction of peripheral adrenergic nerve terminals. In newborn animals the whole neuron is destroyed irreversibly, whereas in adults only the terminals are affected so that regeneration of the fibers is possible.[92] To destroy adren-

TABLE 10-3. Drugs interacting with catecholamine storage and release mechanisms*

Drug	Clinical use	Site of action
Norepinephrine depletors Reserpine Guanethidine	Antihypertensive	Blockade of intraneuronal storage
False transmitters α-Methyldopa	Antihypertensive	Substitution of norepinephrine by false transmitter in storage granules
MAO inhibitors Pargyline	Antihypertensive	Inhibition of norepinephrine release by free norepinephrine or false transmitter
Neuron blockers Bretylium Debrisoquin	Antihypertensive	Prevention of norepinephrine release; also MAO inhibition
Amphetamine Ephedrine	Sympathomimetic	Norepinephrine release from granules
Tricyclic drugs Imipramine Amitriptyline	Antidepressant	Inhibition of adrenergic neuronal membrane amine carrier system

*Modified from Shore, P. A. In Jones, R. J., editor: Proceedings of the Second International Symposium, New York, 1970, Springer-Verlag New York, Inc., p. 528.

ergic terminals in the CNS, 6-hydroxydopamine must be injected into the ventricles because it does not cross the blood-brain barrier.

Serotonin, or 5-hydroxytryptamine, is present in high concentrations in the enterochromaffin cells of the intestinal tract and in the pineal gland. It is also present in the brain, in platelets, and in mast cells of rats and mice. Serotonin occurs also in some fruits such as bananas.

The steps in the biosynthesis of serotonin are as follows:

$$\text{Tryptophan} \xrightarrow[\text{hydroxylase}]{\text{Tryptophan}} \text{5-Hydroxytryptophan} \xrightarrow[\text{decarboxylase}]{\text{L-Aromatic amino acid}} \text{5-Hydroxytryptamine}$$

Serotonin is degraded to 5-hydroxyindolacetic acid by the enzyme MAO. The daily excretion of 5-hydroxyindolacetic acid in humans is about 3 mg. It may increase greatly in patients with carcinoid tumor or after the administration of reserpine. The ingestion of bananas also results in elevated concentrations of 5-hydroxyindolacetic acid in the urine.

In the pineal gland there is not only a high concentration of serotonin but also a biosynthetic product of the amine, 5-methoxy-N-acetyltryptamine, also known as melatonin. This unique product lightens skin color by affecting melanocytes. It also exerts an effect on gonadal functions in female rats. Interestingly melatonin synthesis is greatly influenced by light.[78]

In addition to the previously discussed neurotransmitters, several endogenous compounds may play a role in neural function, although the available evidence is hardly sufficient for characterizing them as mediators of neurotransmission.

Histamine is present in the hypothalamus along with serotonin and catecholamines. Its presence in adrenergic nerves is interesting but may be related to the presence of mast cells close to these nerves. The brain can form histamine from histidine and is rich in the methylating enzyme that inactivates this biogenic amine. Unfortunately no powerful inhibitors of the methylating enzyme are available.

Glutamic and *aspartic acids* are remarkably potent in causing depolarization of nerve cells when applied by iontophoresis. Since these amino acids are normally present in the brain, they could conceivably have some neurotransmitter function. Nevertheless, most criteria for proving the neurotransmitter role of a compound cannot be met by these amino acids.

Glycine is recognized increasingly as a probable inhibitory transmitter in the spinal cord. This simple amino acid is present in high concentration in the spinal cord and causes hyperpolarization of motoneurons.[93] Since strychnine is known to antagonize the effects of the naturally occurring inhibitory transmitter released from Renshaw cells to motoneurons, it was of great interest to examine the possible relationship between the alkaloid and glycine.[20] Antagonism of the hyperpolarizing effect of glycine by strychnine applied by microelectrophoresis has been clearly demonstrated. Interestingly tetanus toxin in the same system does not antagonize the actions of glycine, implying a presynaptic site of action for the toxin.

γ-*Aminobutyric acid* (*GABA*) has also received some attention as a naturally occurring amine that may have a role in brain function. This compound is made by brain tissue through decarboxylation of glutamic acid.

$$\underset{\textbf{Glutamic acid}}{HOOC-\overset{\overset{\displaystyle NH_2}{|}}{CH}-CH_2-CH_2-COOH} \qquad \underset{\textbf{γ-Aminobutyric acid}}{H_2N-CH_2-CH_2-CH_2-COOH}$$

Brain tissue contains significant quantities of GABA. Its destruction is accomplished through transamination. The study of the effects of GABA on brain function has been greatly handicapped by the fact that it does not cross the blood-brain barrier effectively when injected.

Crustacean stretch receptors are inhibited by GABA, and studies of Purpura and co-workers[59] suggest that GABA and related omega amino acids may have inhibitory properties on central synaptic transmission when applied directly to the brain surface.

Polypeptides are candidates for a neurotransmitter or neuromodulator role. Substance P, for example, is found not only in parts of the brain and spinal cord, but also in sensory nerves. Substance P contains II amino acids and may have great importance in pain pathways. The *prostaglandins*, which are acidic lipids, probably play a role in neural function. They are discussed in Chapter 22.

CLASSIFICATION OF NEUROPHAR-MACOLOGICAL AGENTS

The rational classification of neuropharmacological agents should be based on their site of action and mode of action, reflecting drug-receptor interactions. This can be done very satisfactorily for drugs acting on autonomic end organs, autonomic nerve endings, autonomic ganglia, and skeletal neuromuscular junctions. At each site we have agonists and antagonists or drugs that promote or inhibit the release of neurotransmitters.

AUTONOMIC AND RELATED DRUGS
Classification by *site of action* **and** *mode of action*

I. Drugs acting on autonomic receptors in end organs
   A. Agonists mimicking postganglionic transmitters
      1. Cholinergic drugs (parasympathomimetics)
         a. Direct action on effector cell (effective after denervation)—acetylcholine, pilocarpine
         b. Indirect action (potentiate endogenous ACh; ineffective after denervation)
            (1) Competitive cholinesterase inhibitors—physostigmine
            (2) Noncompetitive cholinesterase inhibitors—isoflurophate (DFP) (enzyme reactivated by pralidoxime)
      2. Adrenergic drugs (sympathomimetics)
         a. Direct action on effector cell (effective after denervation)—norepinephrine, epinephrine, isoproterenol
         b. Indirect action (release norepinephrine from adrenergic nerve endings; ineffective peripherally after denervation)—tyramine, amphetamine
         c. Mixed action (direct and indirect)—ephedrine, metaraminol

B. Antagonists acting on end-organ receptors
  1. Cholinergic receptor antagonists (cholinergic blocking drugs)
    a. Competitive antagonists of "muscarinic" receptors—atropine
  2. Adrenergic receptor antagonists (adrenergic blocking drugs)
    a. Antagonize α-adrenergic receptors
      (1) Competitive—phentolamine
      (2) Noncompetitive—phenoxybenzamine
    b. Antagonize β-adrenergic receptors
      (1) Competitive—propranolol

II. Drugs acting on autonomic nerve endings
  A. Agonists that cause the release of transmitters
    1. Cholinergic neurons—none
    2. Adrenergic neurons—indirect and mixed acting sympathomimetics
  B. Drugs that inhibit the release of transmitters
    1. Cholinergic neurons—botulinum toxin
    2. Adrenergic neurons—bretylium, guanethidine
  C. Drugs that inhibit the synthesis of transmitters
    1. Cholinergic neurons (inhibits synthesis of ACh)—hemicholinium
    2. Adrenergic neurons (inhibits synthesis of norepinephrine)—α-methyl-p-tyrosine
  D. Drugs that inhibit the storage of transmitters in neurons
    1. Cholinergic neurons—none
    2. Adrenergic neurons (deplete norepinephrine)—reserpine, guanethidine
  E. Drugs that cause the formation of false transmitters in neurons
    1. Cholinergic neurons—none
    2. Adrenergic neurons—methyldopa, metaraminol, MAO inhibitors
  F. Drugs that inhibit the uptake of transmitters into neurons
    1. Cholinergic neurons—none
    2. Adrenergic neurons—cocaine, desmethylimipramine and congeners

III. Drugs acting on autonomic ganglia
  A. Agonists that stimulate postganglionic neurons ("nicotinic" stimulants)
    1. Both cholinergic and adrenergic neurons—nicotine
  B. Antagonists that inhibit "nicotinic" receptors or postganglionic neurons
    1. Both cholinergic and adrenergic neurons (competitive antagonists)—hexamethonium, mecamylamine

NONAUTONOMIC DRUGS

I. Drugs acting on the skeletal muscle neuromuscular junction
  A. Agonists mimicking the motor nerve transmitter, acetylcholine
    1. Direct action on muscle cell—neostigmine
    2. Indirect action (cholinesterase inhibitors)
      a. Competitive—neostigmine, physostigmine
      b. Noncompetitive—isoflurophate
  B. Antagonists that block skeletal muscle receptors
    1. Depolarizing—succinylcholine
    2. Nondepolarizing (competitive)—d-tubocurarine

II. Drugs acting on sensory nerve endings
  A. "Sensitize" stretch receptors monitoring blood pressure—Veratrum alkaloids

III. Drugs acting on all nerves to block conduction of action potentials
  A. Local anesthetics

IV. Drugs acting on vascular smooth muscle
  A. Vasoconstrictors—angiotensin, vasopressin
  B. Vasodilators—nitrites, papaverine
  C. Antihypertensive drugs—hydralazine, diazoxide

V. Other endogenous biologically active compounds
  A. Serotonin, histamine, bradykinin, prostaglandins, etc.

For the sake of simplicity, autonomic drugs will be classified in the succeeding chapter as cholinergic drugs, anticholinergic drugs (various types), adrenergic drugs, and adrenergic blocking drugs (alpha [α]and beta [β]).

REFERENCES

1 Ahlquist, R. P.: A study of the adrenotropic receptors, Am. J. Physiol. **153**:586, 1948.

2 Axelrod, J.: The metabolism of catecholamines in vivo and in vitro, Pharmacol. Rev. **11**:402, 1959.

3 Bertler, A.: Occurrence and localization of catechol amines in the human brain, Acta Physiol. Scand. **51**:97, 1961.

4 Boura, A. L. A., and Green, A. F.: Adrenergic neuron blocking agents, Annu. Rev. Pharmacol. **5**:183, 1965.

5 Brimblecombe, R. W.: Drug actions on cholinergic systems. In Bradley, P. B., editor: Pharmacology monographs, Baltimore, 1974, University Park Press.

6 Brodie, B. B., Spector, S., and Shore, P. A.: Interaction of drugs with norepinephrine in the brain, Pharmacol. Rev. **11**:548, 1959.

7 Bunney, B. J., Walters, J. R., Roth, R. H., and Aghajanian, G. K.: Dopaminergic neurons: effect of antipsychotic drugs and amphetamine on single cell activity, J. Pharmacol. Exp. Ther. **185**:560, 1973.

8 Burgen, A., and MacIntosh, F.: The physiological significance of acetylcholine. In Elliott, K. A. C., editors: Neurochemistry, Springfield, Ill., 1955, Charles C Thomas, Publisher.

9 Burn, J. H.: Release of noradrenaline from the sympathetic postganglionic fibre, Br. Med. J. **2**:196, 1967.

10 Burn, J. H., and Rand, M. J.: A new interpretation of the adrenergic nerve fiber, Adv. Pharmacol. **1**:1, 1962.

11 Cannon, W. B., and Uridil, J. E.: Studies on conditions of activity in endocrine glands: some effects on the denervated heart of stimulating nerves of the liver, Am. J. Physiol. **58**:353, 1921.

12 Carlsson, A.: The occurrence, distribution and physiological role of catecholamines in the nervous system, Pharmacol. Rev. **11**:490, 1959.

13 Carlsson, A., and Hillarp, N. A.: On the state of catechol amines of the adrenal medullary granules, Acta Physiol. Scand. **44**:163, 1958.

14 Carlsson, A., and Lindquist, M.: Effect of chlorpromazine and haloperidol on formation of 3-methoxytyramine and normetanephrine in mouse brain, Acta Pharmacol. Toxicol. **20**:140, 1963.

15 Curtis, D., Phillips, J., and Watkins, J.: The depression of spinal neurones by γ-amino-n-butyric acid and β-alanine, J. Physiol. **146**: 185, 1959.

16 Dahlström, A., and Fuxe, K.: Evidence for the existence of monoamine-containing neurons in the central nervous system. I. Demonstration of monoamines in the cell bodies of brain stem neurons, Acta Physiol. Scand. **62**(Supp. 232): 1, 1965.

17 Dahlström, A., and Häggendal, J.: Studies on the transport and life-span of amine storage granules in a peripheral adrenergic neuron system, Acta Physiol. Scand. **67**:278, 1966.

18 Dale, H. H.: On some physiological actions of ergot, J. Physiol. **34**:163, 1906.

19 Dale, H. H.: The action of certain esters and ethers of choline and their relation to muscarine, J. Pharmacol. Exp. Ther. **6**:147, 1914.

20 Davidoff, R. A., Aprison, M. H., and Werman, R.: The effects of strychnine on the inhibition of interneurons by glycine and γ-aminobutyric acid, Int. J. Neuropharmacol. **8**:191, 1969.

21 Dengler, H. J., Spiegel, H. E., and Titus, E. O.: Effect of drugs on uptake of isotopic norepinephrine by cat tissues, Nature **19**:816, 1961.

22 Douglas, W. W.: Stimulus-secretion coupling: the concept and clues from chromaffin and other cells, Br. J. Pharmacol. **34**:451, 1968.

23 Eccles, J. C.: The physiology of nerve cells, Baltimore, 1957, The Johns Hopkins University Press.

24 Elliott, T. R.: The action of adrenalin, J. Physiol. **32**:401, 1905.

25 Engleman, K., Lovenberg, W., and Sjoerdsma, A.: Inhibition of serotonin synthesis by parachlorophenylalanine in patients with the carcinoid syndrome, N. Engl. J. Med. **277**:1103, 1967.

26 Eränkö, O.: Histochemistry of nervous tissues: catecholamines and cholinesterases, Annu. Rev. Pharmacol. **7**:203, 1967.

27 von Euler, U. S.: Noradrenaline: chemistry, physiology, pharmacology and clinical aspects, Springfield, Ill., 1956, Charles C Thomas, Publisher.

28 von Euler, U. S.: Pieces in the puzzle, Annu. Rev. Pharmacol. **11**:1, 1971.

29 von Euler, U. S., and Pernow, B.: Nuerotropic

effects of substance P, Acta Physiol. Scand. 36: 265, 1956.

30 Evans, B., Iwayama, T., and Burnstock, G.: Long-lasting supersensitivity of the rat vas deferens to norepinephrine after chronic guanethidine administration, J. Pharmacol. Exp. Ther. 185:60, 1973.

31 Fatt, P., and Katz, B.: Spontaneous subthreshold activity at motor nerve endings, J. Physiol. 117:109, 1952.

32 Ferguson, J., Henriksen, S., Cohen, H., Mitchell, G., Barchas, J., and Dement, W.: "Hypersexuality" and behavioral changes in cats caused by the administration of p-chlorophenylalanine, Science 168:499, 1970.

33 Ferry, C. B.: Cholinergic link hypothesis in adrenergic neuroeffector transmission, Physiol. Rev. 46:420, 1966.

34 Ferry, C. B.: The autonomic nervous system, Annu. Rev. Pharmacol. 7:185, 1967.

35 Fleming, W. W.: Nonspecific supersensitivity of the guinea-pig ileum produced by chronic ganglion blockade, J. Pharmacol. Exp. Ther. 162:277, 1968.

36 Fleming, W. W., and Trendelenburg, U.: Development of supersensitivity to norepinephrine after pretreatment with reserpine, J. Pharmacol. Exp. Ther. 133:41, 1961.

37 Galindo, A.: Curare and pancuronium compared: effects on previously undepressed mammalian myoneuronal junctions, Science 178: 753, 1972.

38 Gewirtz, G. P., and Kopin, I. J.: Effect of intermittent nerve stimulation on norepinephrine synthesis and mobilization in the perfused cat spleen, J. Pharmacol. Exp. Ther. 175:514, 1970.

39 Giachetti, A., and Shore, P. A.: Studies in vitro of amine uptake mechanisms in heart, Biochem. Pharmacol. 15:607, 1966.

40 Ginsborg, B. L.: Ion movements in junctional transmission, Pharmacol. Rev. 19:289, 1967.

41 Goth, A., and Harrison, F.: Influence of protoveratrine on effect of vasoactive drugs, Proc. Soc. Exp. Biol. Med. 87:437, 1954.

42 Govier, W. C., Sugrue, M. F., and Shore, P. A.: On the inability to produce supersensitivity to catecholamines in intestinal smooth muscle, J. Pharmacol. Exp. Ther. 165:71, 1969.

43 Harrison, F., and Goth, A.: Effect of reserpine on the hypothalamic pressor response, J. Pharmacol. Exp. Ther. 116:262, 1956.

44 Hertting, G., Axelrod, J., and Whitby, L. G.: Effect of drugs on the uptake and metabolism of H^3-norepinephrine, J. Pharmacol. Exp. Ther. 134:146, 1961.

45 Hillarp, N. A., Fuxe, K., and Dahlström, A.: Demonstration and mapping of central neurons containing dopamine, noradrenaline, and 5-hydroxytryptamine and their reactions to psychopharmaca, Pharmacol. Rev. 18:727, 1966.

46 Holzbauer, M., and Vogt, M.: Depression by reserpine of the noradrenaline of the hypothalamus of the cat, J. Neurochem. 1:8, 1956.

47 Isaac, L., and Goth, A.: The mechanism of the potentiation of norepinephrine by antihistaminics, J. Pharmacol. Exp. Ther. 156:463, 1967.

48 Katz, B., and Miledi, R.: Propagation of electric activity in motor nerve terminals, Proc. R. Soc. Biol. 161:483, 1965.

49 Koelle, G. B.: The elimination of enzymatic diffusion artifacts in the histochemical localization of cholinesterases and a survey of their cellular distributions, J. Pharmacol. Exp. Ther. 103: 152, 1951.

50 Loewi, O.: Über humorale Übertragbarkeit der Herznervenwirkung, Arch. Ges. Physiol. 189: 239, 1921.

51 Longenecker, H. E., Hurlbut, W. P., Mauro, A., and Clark, A. W.: Effect of black widow spider venom on the frog neuromuscular junction, Nature 225:701, 1970.

52 MacMillan, W. H.: A hypothesis concerning the effect of cocaine on the action of sympathomimetic amines, Br. J. Pharmacol. 14:385, 1969.

53 Maxwell, R. A., Plummer, A. J., Povalski, H., and Schneider, F.: Concerning a possible action of guanethidine (SU-5864) in smooth muscle, J. Pharmacol. Exp. Ther. 129:24, 1960.

54 McLennan, H.: Synaptic transmission, Philadelphia, 1963, W. B. Saunders Co.

55 Miledi, R.: The acetylcholine sensitivity of frog muscle fibers after complete or partial denervation, J. Physiol. 151:1, 1960.

56 Nachmansohn, D., and Machado, A. L.: The formation of acetylcholine. A new enzyme: "choline acetylase," J. Neurophysiol. 6:397, 1943.

57 Okamoto, M., Longenecker, H. E., and Riker, W. F.: Destruction of mammalian motor nerve terminals by black widow spider venom, Science 172:733, 1971.

58 Palade, G. E., and Palay, S. L.: Electron microscope observations of interneuronal and neuromuscular synapses, Anat. Rec. 118:335, 1954.

59 Purpura, D. P., Girado, M., Smith, T. G., Callan, D. A., and Grundfest, H.: Structure-activity determinants of pharmacological effects of

amino acids and related compounds on central synapses, J. Neurochem. **3:**238, 1959.

60 Riker, W. F.: Pharmacologic considerations in a reevaluation of the neuromuscular synapse, Arch. Neurol. **3:**488, 1960.

61 Salmoiraghi, G. C., Costa, E., and Bloom, F. E.: Pharmacology of central synapses, Annu. Rev. Pharmacol. **5:**213, 1965.

62 Shore, P. A.: Release of serotonin and catecholamines by drugs, Pharmacol. Rev. **14:**531, 1962.

63 Shore, P. A., and Olin, J.: Identification and chemical assay of norepinephrine in brain and other tissues, J. Pharmacol. Exp. Ther. **122:**295, 1958.

64 Snyder, S. H., Young, A. B., Bennett, J. P., and Mulder, A. H.: Synaptic biochemistry of amino acids, Fed. Proc. **32:**2039, 1973.

65 Symposium: Adrenergic mechanisms, Ciba Foundation and Committee for Symposium on Drug Action, Boston, 1960, Little, Brown & Co.

66 Thesleff, S., and Quastel, D. M. J.: Neuromuscular pharmacology, Annu. Rev. Pharmacol. **5:**263, 1965.

67 Trendelenburg, U.: The supersensitivity caused by cocaine, J. Pharmacol. Exp. Ther. **125:**55, 1959.

68 Trendelenburg, U.: Mechanisms of supersensitivity and subsensitivity to sympathomimetic amines, Pharmacol. Rev. **18:**629, 1966.

69 Udenfriend, S.: Tyrosine hydroxylase, Pharmacol. Rev. **18:**43, 1966.

70 Varma, D. R., and McCullough, H. N.: Dissociation of the supersensitivity to norepinephrine caused by cocaine from inhibition of H^3-norepinephrine uptake in cold stored smooth muscle, J. Pharmacol. Exp. Ther. **166:**26, 1969.

71 Vogt, M.: Catecholamines in brain, Pharmacol. Rev. **11:**483, 1959.

72 Volle, R. L.: Pharmacology of the autonomic nervous system, Annu. Rev. Pharmacol. **3:**129, 1963.

73 Weiner, N., and Trendelenburg, U.: The effect of cocaine and of pretreatment with reserpine on the uptake of tyramine-2-C^{14} and DL-epinephrine-2-C^{14} into heart and spleen, J. Pharmacol. Exp. Ther. **137:**56, 1962.

74 Weinshilboum, R. M., Thoa, N. B., Johnson, D. G., Kopin, I. J., and Axelrod, J.: Proportional release of norepinephrine and dopamine-β-hydroxylase from sympathetic nerves, Science **174:**1349, 1971.

75 Whittaker, V.: Identification of acetylcholine and related esters of biological origin. In Heffter, A., and Heubner, W., editors: Handbuch der experimentellen Pharmakologie, vol. 15, Berlin, 1963, Springer-Verlag.

REVIEWS

76 Berthelsen, S., and Pettinger, W. A.: A functional basis for classification of α-adrenergic receptors, Life Sci. **21:**595, 1977.

77 Bhagat, B. D.: Recent advances in adrenergic mechanisms, Springfield, Ill., 1971, Charles C Thomas, Publisher.

78 Cooper, J. R., Bloom, F. E., and Roth, R. H.: The biochemical basis of neuropharmacology, New York, 1970, Oxford University Press, Inc.

79 Galindo, A.: The role of prejunctional effects in myoneural transmission, Anesthesiology **36:**598, 1972.

79a Hoffman, B. B., and Lefkowitz, R. J.: Radioligand binding studies of adrenergic receptors: new insights into molecular and physiological regulation, Annu. Rev. Pharmacol. Toxicol. **20:**581, 1980.

80 Hubbard, J. I., and Quastel, D. M. J.: Micropharmacology of vertebrate neuro-muscular transmission, Annu. Rev. Pharmacol. **13:**199, 1973.

81 Izquierdo, I., and Izquierdo, J. A.: Effects of drugs on deep brain centers, Annu. Rev. Pharmacol. **11:**189, 1971.

82 Kirshner, N., and Viveros, O. H.: In Schümann, H. J., and Kroneberg, G., editors: New aspects of storage and release of catecholamines, Berlin, 1970, Springer-Verlag.

83 Langer, S. Z.: Presynaptic regulation of catecholamine release, Biochem. Pharmacol. **23:**1793, 1974.

84 Langer, S. Z.: Presynaptic receptors and their role in the regulation of transmitter release, Br. J. Pharmacol. **60:**481, 1977.

85 Lefkowitz, R. J.: Direct binding studies of adrenergic receptors: biochemical, physiologic and clinical implications, Ann. Intern. Med. **91:**450, 1979.

86 Pohorecky, L. A., and Wurtman, R. J.: Adrenocortical control of epinephrine synthesis, Pharmacol. Rev. **23:**1, 1971.

87 Rubin, R. P.: The role of calcium in the release of neurotransmitter substances and hormones, Pharmacol. Rev. **22:**389, 1970.

88 Shore, P. A.: Drugs affecting catecholamine metabolism and storage in the adrenergic neurone. In Jones, R., editor: Atherosclerosis, Proceedings of the Second International Symposium, New York, 1970, Springer-Verlag New York Inc.

89 Shore, P. A.: Transport and storage of biogenic amines, Annu. Rev. Pharmacol. **12:**209, 1972.

90 Snyder, S. H., and Bennett, J. P., Jr.: Neurotransmitter receptors in the brain: biochemical identification, Annu. Rev. Physiol. **38:**153, 1976.

91 Sulser, F., and Sanders-Bush, E.: Effect of drugs on amines in the CNS, Annu. Rev. Pharmacol. **11:**209, 1971.

92 Thoenen, H., and Tranzer, J. P.: The pharmacology of 6-hydroxydopamine, Annu. Rev. Pharmacol. **13:**169, 1973.

93 Willis, W. D.: The case for the Renshaw Cell. In Riss, W., editor: Brain, behavior and evolution, vol. 5, Basel, 1971, S. Karger AG.

94 Wurtman, R. J., and Fernstrom, J. D.: Control of brain neurotransmitter synthesis by precursor availability and nutritional state, Biochem. Pharmacol. **25:**1691, 1976.

CHAPTER 11

Cholinergic (cholinomimetic) drugs

The various cholinergic drugs can be divided into two major groups: directly acting cholinergic drugs and cholinesterase inhibitors.

DIRECTLY ACTING CHOLINERGIC DRUGS
Choline esters

Although acetylcholine is an essential compound from the standpoint of its role in body physiology, two important considerations render it useless as a drug. First, even when it is injected intravenously, its actions are very brief because of its rapid destruction by the ubiquitous cholinesterases. Second, it has so many diverse effects that no selective therapeutic purpose can be achieved through its use. The various derivatives of acetylcholine, however, differ from the parent compound by being more resistant to the action of the cholinesterases and by having a certain amount of selectivity in their sites of action.

If we depict the acetylcholine-receptor combination in a manner similar to that postulated for acetylcholine-cholinesterase, as shown in Fig. 11-1, it can be seen that slight changes in the structure should alter the union of the drug with the receptor. Some of these changes can prevent an enzymatic attack on the molecule while still allowing an interaction of the drug with some of the receptors. Drugs in this group that have some importance are the following:

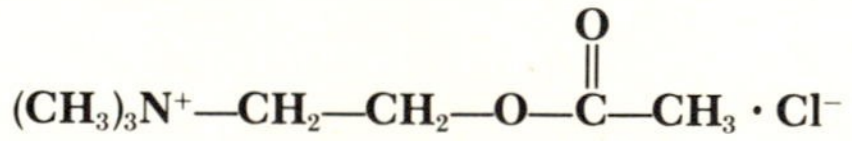

$$(CH_3)_3N^+ \!-\! CH_2 \!-\! CH_2 \!-\! O \!-\! \overset{\overset{\displaystyle O}{\|}}{C} \!-\! CH_3 \cdot Cl^-$$

Acetylcholine chloride

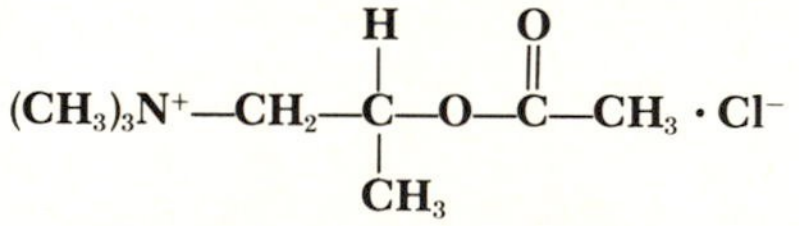

$$(CH_3)_3N^+ \!-\! CH_2 \!-\! \underset{\underset{\displaystyle CH_3}{|}}{\overset{\overset{\displaystyle H}{|}}{C}} \!-\! O \!-\! \overset{\overset{\displaystyle O}{\|}}{C} \!-\! CH_3 \cdot Cl^-$$

Methacholine chloride

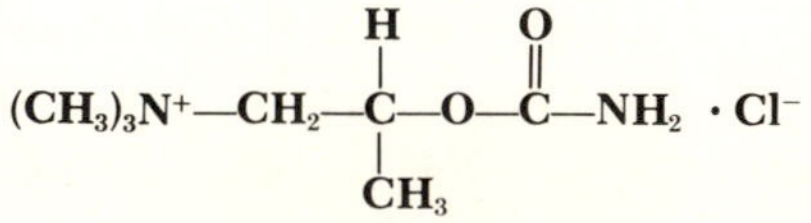

$$(CH_3)_3N^+ \!-\! CH_2 \!-\! \underset{\underset{\displaystyle CH_3}{|}}{\overset{\overset{\displaystyle H}{|}}{C}} \!-\! O \!-\! \overset{\overset{\displaystyle O}{\|}}{C} \!-\! NH_2 \cdot Cl^-$$

Bethanechol chloride

$$(CH_3)_3N^+ \!-\! CH_2 \!-\! CH_2 \!-\! O \!-\! \overset{\overset{\displaystyle O}{\|}}{C} \!-\! NH_2 \cdot Cl^-$$

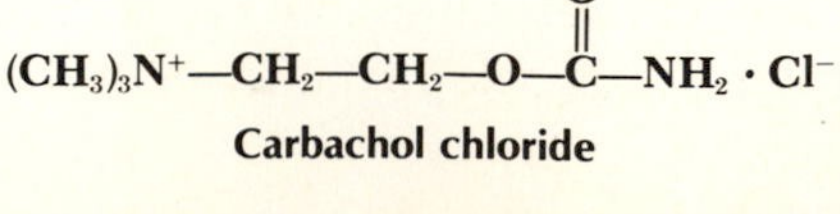

Carbachol chloride

136

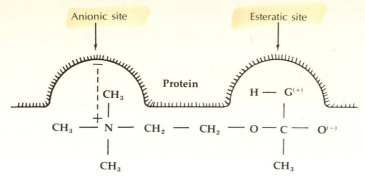

FIG. 11-1. Interaction of acetylcholine and acetylcholinesterase. (From Wilson, I. B.: Neurology **8**[Supp. 1]:41, 1958.)

All drugs in this group are quaternary amines. Replacement of the acetyl group by carbamate protects the drug against cholinesterases and thus prolongs its half-life in the body. Substitution in the β carbon, as in acetyl-β-methylcholine, protects against the action of the nonspecific cholinesterase.

Bethanechol and methacholine have many of the actions of acetylcholine on smooth muscles and glands without significantly affecting ganglia and skeletal neuro-muscular transmission.

Bethanechol (Urecholine) has selective effects on the gastrointestinal and urinary tracts and is the parasympathomimetic drug of choice for the treatment of postoperative abdominal distention and postoperative urinary retention. Bethanechol is not destroyed by cholinesterases and thus has prolonged effects. The usual cholinergic side effects are sweating, flushing, salivation, and aggravation of bronchial asthma. Hypotension may be caused by the drug but is not common. Contraindications to its use include bronchial asthma, severe cardiac disease, hyperthyroidism (atrial fibrillation may occur), and mechanical obstruction of the gastrointestinal and urinary tracts. Preparations include tablets of 5, 10, and 25 mg and solutions for subcutaneous injection, 5 mg/ml. The dosage for adults is 5 to 30 mg three or four times daily by mouth or 2.5 to 5 mg three or four times daily by subcutaneous injection.

Methacholine (Mecholyl) has few uses in medicine. It possesses mostly muscarinic activity, especially on the cardiovascular system. Because it is an acetyl ester, it is hydrolyzed by acetylcholinesterase, although more slowly than acetylcholine. Methacholine has been used in the treatment of paroxysmal atrial tachycardia because it abolishes the ectopic focus in the atrium, probably as a consequence of hyperpolarization. It is seldom used for this purpose because it can cause alarming syncopal attacks when injected by the subcutaneous route. Patients with adrenal medullary tumors respond to methacholine with a rise of blood pressure, since it stimulates the output of catecholamines from the tumor. The methacholine test for pheochromocytoma has had some popularity but is seldom used at present. Preparations include tablets containing 200 mg and powder for injectable solution, 25 mg. For adults the oral dosage is 50 to 600 mg three or four times daily; the subcutaneous dosage, 10 to 25 mg.

Carbachol is a very potent choline ester having both muscarinic and nicotinic effects. Its only use at present is in the treatment of glaucoma. Solutions of 0.5% to 1%, applied to the conjunctiva, cause miosis and reduction of intraocular pressure. The antidote to carbachol is atropine.

The muscarinic and nicotinic actions of the choline esters can be illustrated by a simple experiment. Fig. 11-2 shows the effect of injected choline esters on blood pressure responses of a dog before and after atropine administration.

In summary, the essential actions of the choline esters following subcutaneous injection are cutaneous vasodilatation with flushing, sweating, salivation, and increased tone of the smooth muscle of the gastrointestinal tract and urinary bladder. There are variable effects on heart rate and blood pressure. There is a precipitous fall in the blood pressure of some individuals, whereas in others the changes in blood pressure and heart rate are slight because compensatory reflexes remain active. It should always be kept in mind that asthmatic patients are particularly susceptible to the bronchoconstrictor action of these compounds. The antidote, atropine, should always be on hand before a choline ester is administered.

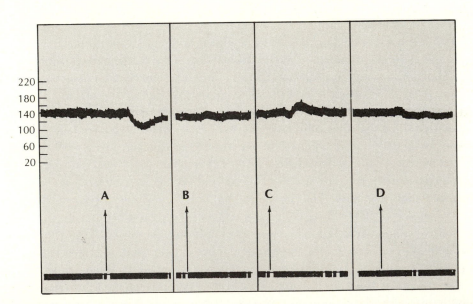

FIG. 11-2. Effect of acetylcholine on blood pressure before and after atropine. The following drugs were administered intravenously to a dog anesthetized with pentobarbital: *A,* acetylcholine, 10 μg/kg; between *A* and *B,* atropine, 1 mg/kg; *B,* acetylcholine, 10 μg/kg; *C,* acetylcholine, 100 μg/kg; between *C* and *D,* phentolamine, 5 mg/kg; *D,* acetylcholine, 100 μg/kg. Note that atropine prevented blood pressure lowering induced by small dose of acetylcholine. Large dose of acetylcholine actually caused elevation of blood pressure, the so-called nicotinic effect of acetylcholine. This response is blocked by phentolamine, an adrenergic blocking agent.

The two alkaloids pilocarpine and muscarine have the curious property of acting like acetylcholine on receptors of smooth muscles and glandular cells. Muscarine is present in the mushroom *Amanita muscaria*, along with toxic peptides,[23] whereas pilocarpine is found in the leaves of the plant *Pilocarpus jaborandi*.

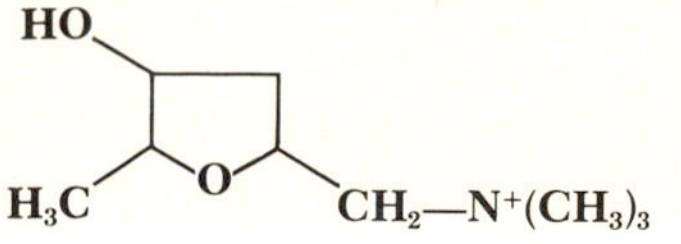

Pilocarpine and muscarine

Muscarine 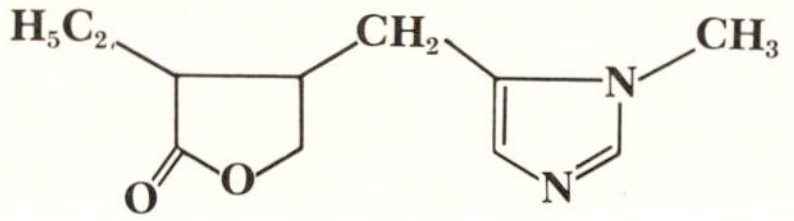   Pilocarpine

Both alkaloids show the so-called muscarinic effects of acetylcholine without having significant nicotinic action. Atropine blocks these muscarinic effects. Muscarine, being a quaternary ammonium compound, shows some similarity to acetylcholine, but it is puzzling why pilocarpine, which is a tertiary amine, should also mimic the muscarinic effects of acetylcholine. It is well established, however, that this is not the result of cholinesterase inhibition.

Of these two drugs, muscarine has only academic interest. Pilocarpine, however, is employed in ophthalmology as a miotic and is occasionally used for stimulating the flow of saliva in patients who complain of dryness of the mouth during therapy with ganglionic blocking agents. For ophthalmological applications, pilocarpine is employed in a 1% solution. The usual dose for stimulating the secretion of saliva is 5 mg, given either orally or by subcutaneous injection. In addition to stimulating the flow of saliva, the drug greatly increases sweating. Its antidote is atropine.

Problem 11-1. The fixed dilated pupil may be an ominous sign caused by an involvement of the third nerve by an intracranial disease. How can this be distinguished from the accidental application to the eye of an anticholinergic (mydriatic) drug? In an interesting article,[21] topical application of pilocarpine is used to establish the diagnosis. The pupil responds well to pilocarpine in the case of nerve damage, whereas it is unresponsive if the dilated pupil is caused by the application of a mydriatic drug. Could an anticholinesterase such as physostigmine be substituted for pilocarpine in this diagnostic test?

Some drugs inhibit the destruction of acetylcholine and thereby produce a higher concentration of the agent at those sites where it is released. They can also potentiate the action of some of the exogenous choline esters when these are administered.

ANTICHOLIN-ESTERASES

The cholinesterase inhibitors are of great interest in medicine. They have been found very useful in the treatment of myasthenia gravis and in the management of glaucoma. The group has also yielded some of our most potent insecticides, which are of great toxicological importance because of their widespread use. Cholinesterase inhibitors are valuable investigative tools. They are also potential chemical warfare agents. Physostigmine is also becoming useful in the treatment of atropine poisoning.

<table>
<tr><td>

Physostigmine, neostigmine, and related drugs

</td><td>

Physostigmine and neostigmine are reversible anticholinesterases. Physostigmine is a tertiary amine used in the treatment of glaucoma and as an antidote in poisoning caused by atropine-like drugs. Neostigmine is a quaternary ammonium compound used in myasthenia gravis, in glaucoma, and as a gastrointestinal and urinary tract stimulant.

Physostigmine (eserine), an alkaloid obtained from the seeds of *Physostigma venenosum*, also known as calabar or ordeal bean, has been familiary to pharmacologists since the latter part of the nineteenth century. Synthesis of compounds related to physostigmine led to the development of neostigmine in 1931.[1]

</td></tr>
</table>

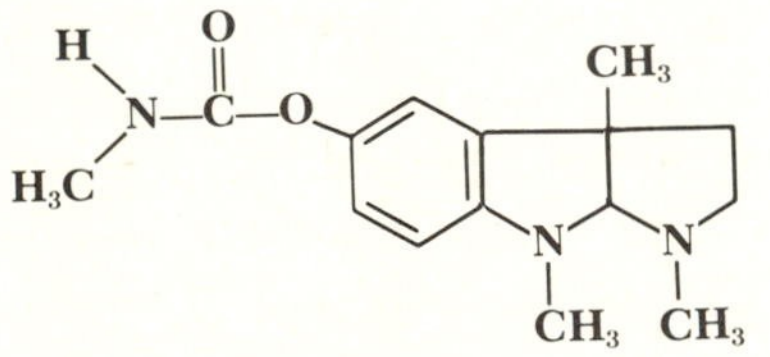

Physostigmine 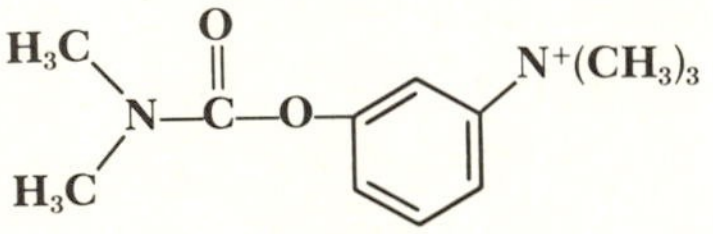   Neostigmine

Pharmacological investigations have shown that physostigmine is an antagonist of curare. In 1934 the British physician Mary Walker[22] tried physostigmine in the treatment of myasthenia gravis because of the clinical similarity of this disease to a curarized state. The results were impressive, and when neostigmine became available, it was tried also.

Action and uses of physostigmine

The actions of physostigmine may be attributed entirely to cholinesterase inhibition on the basis of the following considerations. The drug inhibits cholinesterase in vitro. Its affinity for the enzyme may be 10,000 times greater than that of acetylcholine. After combination with the enzyme, it seems to be gradually dissociated and inactivated in the body. Consequently, the drug is a reversible inhibitor of the cholinesterases.

Physostigmine exerts no effect on the denervated pupil or on the denervated skeletal muscle, even when given by close intra-arterial injection. It has potent effects on structures with normal innervation because of its ability to protect the endogenously released acetylcholine.

Physostigmine salicylate is the specific antidote for anticholinergic intoxication. Given intravenously or intramuscularly in doses of 1 mg, it counteracts the abnormal mental state caused by atropine or scopolamine. Physostigmine salicylate has also been used topically in the treatment of primary open-angle glaucoma, although pilocarpine is preferred. For open-angle glaucoma the drug is applied as a drop of 0.25% to 1% solution. Effects of physostigmine on long-term memory processes are interesting but still investigational.[3]

Neostigmine and related compounds

Some of the actions of neostigmine are caused by cholinesterase inhibition, whereas others are the result of a combination of enzyme inhibition plus a direct acetylcholine-like effect. On the denervated eye, for example, neostigmine acts like physostigmine, producing no pupillary constriction. On the other hand, intra-arterially injected neostigmine will elicit an effect at the neuromuscular junction even when the nerves are degenerated and all cholinesterase has been previously destroyed by diisopropyl fluorophosphate. This evidence suggests that the muscarinic actions of neostigmine are produced by cholinesterase inhibition, whereas the nicotinic actions, at least at the neuromuscular site, are in part a result of a direct effect.

The intramuscular injection of 0.5 to 1 mg of neostigmine methylsulfate (Prostigmin methylsulfate) into a normal human being will produce the usual cholinergic effects: elevation of skin temperature, sweating, salivation, intestinal contractions with a desire to defecate, contraction of smooth muscles of the urinary tract with an urgency to micturate, some slowing of the heart rate with possible hypotension, and muscle fasciculations. Atropine will antagonize the muscarinic effects but not the neuromuscular nicotinic actions of neostigmine. This antidote should be available whenever neostigmine is employed.

In addition to the injectable methylsulfate, neostigmine can be given by mouth as the bromide salt. Much larger doses are given orally, 15 to 30 mg, because much of the drug is inactivated in the gastrointestinal tract. Absorption may be variable, and untoward reactions may occur if too much of the drug is suddenly absorbed.

Drugs related to neostigmine. Edrophonium (Tensilon) has a structure that is similar to that of neostigmine. This drug has been introduced as an anticurare agent. It also has diagnostic and investigative uses in myasthenia.

$$OH-\underset{\text{Edrophonium chloride}}{\bigcirc}-N^{+}{\overset{\displaystyle CH_3}{\underset{\displaystyle CH_3}{-C_2H_5}}} \cdot Cl^{-}$$

The essential feature of edrophonium is its short duration of action. From a practical standpoint it may be considered an extremely short-acting neostigmine. In the myasthenic patient the intravenous injection of 2 to 5 mg of edrophonium will cause rapid and transient improvement of muscular strength. This may be used for diagnostic purposes and also for "titrating" the degree of effectiveness of other treatment. The physician may be in doubt as to whether to increase or decrease the dosage of neostigmine for a myasthenic patient. If intravenous edrophonium causes further improvement in the patient, it is likely that previous therapy has been inadequate. On the other hand, if the reaction to this edrophonium test is unfavorable, indicating overtreatment, increasing the neostigmine dosage would be undesirable. The action of edrophonium in this test lasts only a few minutes.

The drug is a potent antidote to curare. It acts more rapidly than neostigmine, and its action is more transient. Although the drug has some cholinesterase inhibitory properties, its neuromuscular effect is probably a direct one.

Neostigmine substitutes. Pyridostigmine (Mestinon) is used in the treatment of myasthenia gravis, in single doses of 60 mg orally. Its duration of action is 4 hours.

Ambenonium (Mytelase) is also used in the treatment of myasthenia gravis in single doses of 10 mg orally. Its duration of action is 8 hours.

Organophosphorus anticholinesterases

Diisopropyl fluorophosphate (DFP; isofluorophate) and a variety of other alkyl phosphates are highly toxic compounds that produce irreversible inactivation of the cholinesterases. They were developed as potential chemical warfare agents and have had some therapeutic applications, but their principal interest is toxicological because of their widespread use as insecticides.

The structural formulas of some of the organophosphorus compounds are shown below:

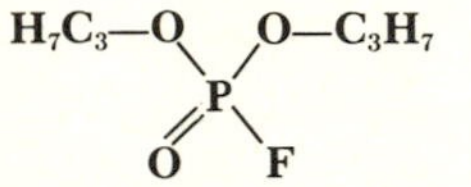

Diisopropyl fluorophosphate

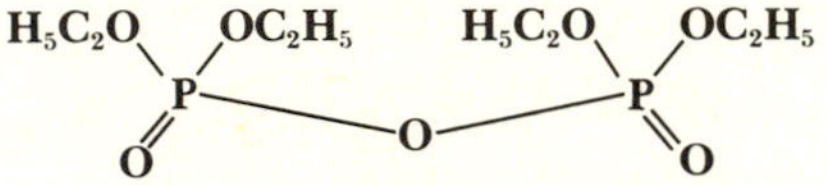

Tetraethyl pyrophosphate

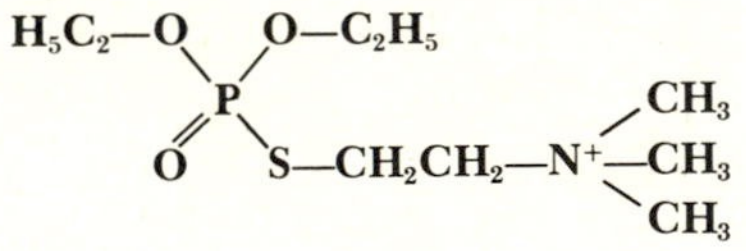

Echothiophate

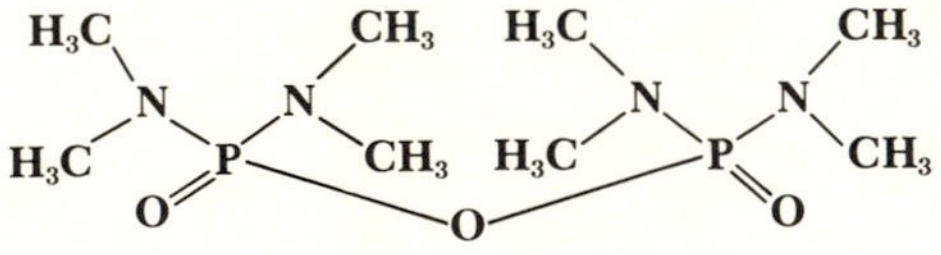

Octamethyl pyrophosphoramide

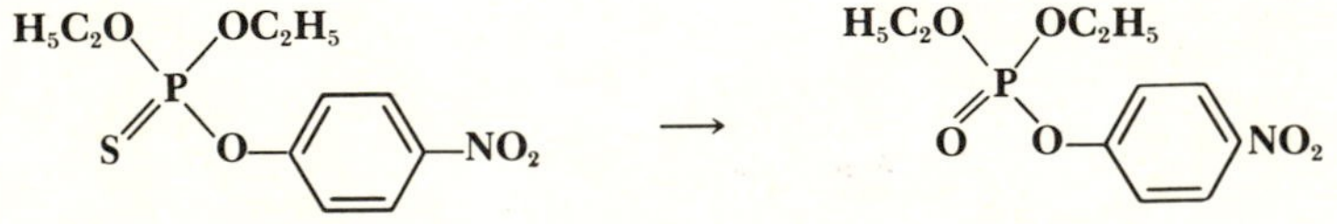

Parathion

Paraoxon

Whereas the reversible anticholinesterases depress enzymatic activity for a few hours following a single administration, the organophosphorus compounds produce an effect that may persist for weeks or months. The difference may be attributed to the fact that the organophosphorus compounds combine with the cholinesterases, which then become phosphorylated. The phosphorylated enzyme is stable, does not hydrolyze, and is inactive against acetylcholine. As a consequence, enzymatic activity will remain reduced until new enzyme material is synthesized, unless some reactivator of cholinesterase is employed as an antidote.

The nonspecific cholinesterase of plasma is affected preferentially and primarily by the alkyl phosphates. With sufficient doses, however, there is increasing destruction of acetylcholinesterase in red cells and in neural tissue. Nonspecific cholinesterase of plasma is regenerated by the liver in about 2 weeks. It may take 3 months to regenerate acetylcholinesterase activity at synapses and neuromuscular junctions.

When DFP or other alkyl phosphate anticholinesterases are injected or inhaled, the clinical picture that develops is a combination of peripheral cholinergic effects and involvement of the CNS (Table 11-1). Muscle fasciculations, constricted pupils, salivation, sweating, abdominal cramps, and respiratory distress are consequences of cholinesterase inactivation in the periphery. Anxiety, restlessness, electroencephalographic changes, and perhaps even terminal convulsions may be related to the actions of the inhibitor on the CNS. Atropine protects against the peripheral muscarinic effects and the involvement of the CNS. It exerts no protective effect against muscle fasciculations and skeletal muscle weakness.[10] The cause of death in organophosphate poisoning is respiratory paralysis.

Pharmacological effects

Pralidoxime (pyridine-2-aldoxime-methiodide; PAM) is a tailor-made molecule developed on the basis of a mechanism postulated by Wilson[24] to explain the action of the alkyl phosphate anticholinesterases. Experimental studies have shown that hydroxylamine and oximes are capable of regenerating the enzyme when it is presumably phosphorylated by the alkyl phosphates. With this knowledge, a molecule was designed in which the distance between the quaternary nitrogen and the oxime is the same as that postulated for acetylcholine. It was predicted that such a compound would fit into the cholinesterase enzyme and would act as a more efficient regenerator than would an ordinary oxime. This work led to the synthesis of pralidoxime.

Antidotal action of pralidoxime

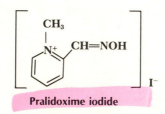

Pralidoxime iodide

TABLE 11-1. Signs and symptoms of organophosphate poisoning*

Muscarinic manifestations	Nicotinic manifestations	CNS manifestations
Bronchoconstriction	Muscular fasciculation	Restlessness
Increased bronchial secretions	Tachycardia	Insomnia
Sweating	Hypertension	Tremors
Salivation		Confusion
Lacrimation		Ataxia
Bradycardia		Convulsions
Hypotension		Respiratory depression
Miosis		Circulatory collapse
Blurring of vision		
Urinary incontinence		

*Modified from Namba, T., Nolte, C. T., Jackrel, J., and Grob, D.: Am. J. Med. **50:**475, 1971.

The interactions of organophosphates, cholinesterases, and reactivators such as pralidoxime may be visualized in the following manner:

$$\underset{\text{Organophosphate}}{\underset{\textstyle R_2 \quad \text{Acyl}}{R_1 \diagdown \overset{\textstyle O}{\underset{\textstyle P}{\diagup}} }} + \underset{\text{Cholinesterase}}{H \cdot \text{Esterase}} \longrightarrow \underset{\text{Phosphorylated esterase}}{\underset{\textstyle R_2 \quad \text{Esterase}}{R_1 \diagdown \overset{\textstyle O}{\underset{\textstyle P}{\diagup}}}} \xrightarrow{\text{Pralidoxime}} \underset{\text{Reactivated esterase}}{H \cdot \text{Esterase}}$$

Pralidoxime must be administered parenterally. It is usually given by intravenous infusion, 50 mg/kg of body weight dissolved in 1000 ml of saline solution. The drug has some depolarizing effect of its own in addition to reactivation of the phosphorylated cholinesterases.

Other reactivator oximes such as diacetylmonoxime (DAM) and bisquaternary oximes have been studied.

Medical uses of organophosphates

Although the organophosphates are used most widely as insecticides (Malathion, Diazinon) and are potential chemical warfare agents, some have medical uses.

Isoflurophate, echothiophate, and demecarium are used in the treatment of glaucoma. When applied locally, the action of the drugs remains localized. They may produce a prolonged decrease of intraocular pressure over a period of weeks. The effect of the organophosphorus compounds may be partially blocked in glaucoma by the prior application of physostigmine or neostigmine.

A very high percentage of presently available insecticides contain organophosphorus anticholinesterases. Acute and chronic poisoning resulting from these pesticides is not uncommon.

The *treatment of organophosphorus poisoning* is as follows. Atropine sulfate, 1 to 2 mg, should be administered as symptoms appear. This antidote may be given every hour up to 25 to 50 mg in a day. The skin, stomach, and eyes should be decontaminated. Pralidoxime is administered by slow intravenous infusion in a dose of 1 g for adults if the patient fails to respond to atropine. Certain drugs are contraindicated in organophosphorus poisoning. These include morphine, theophylline, or aminophylline. If the patient is cyanotic, artificial respiration should be administered even before atropine.

General features of cholinesterase inhibition

Much has been learned about the importance of the cholinesterases from studies on the action of anticholinesterases. It appears from these studies that serum cholinesterase is probably of no great physiological importance but may have a significant effect when exogenous labile choline esters are administered. Serum cholinesterase can be reduced to very low levels with DFP treatment without important consequences. Measurements of serum cholinesterase activity may be altered by disease of the liver or by the previous administration of anticholinesterases. Such measurements are of importance in industrial medicine to evaluate the extent of exposure to anticholinesterases, thus preventing inadvertent poisoning.

The specific acetylcholinesterase appears to exist in excess at the various junctions at which acetylcholine functions as a mediator of neural transmission. Moderate decreases of acetylcholinesterase have little physiological consequence. On the other hand, a severe reduction of brain cholinesterase, down to 10% of normal, has been observed in animals when death occurs from the administration of an anticholinesterase.

The presence of acetylcholinesterase in the red cell is puzzling since no obvious physiological reason for it seems to exist. It has been suggested that the acetylcholine-cholinesterase system has a much broader significance than that expected from its neuroeffector function.

Cholinesterase activity of the red cell mass can reflect hematopoietic activity. The regeneration of acetylcholinesterase activity of red blood cells following the administration of irreversible anticholinesterases is directly proportional to the production of new cells.

Myasthenia gravis is a neuromuscular disease characterized by muscle fatigability. The density of the acetylcholine receptor at the neuromuscular junction is reduced by humoral and possibly cell-mediated immune factors, resulting in impairment of neuromuscular transmission.[28]

Repetitive stimulation of a motor nerve in a myasthenic patient rapidly leads to fatigue of the muscles innervated by that particular nerve. Intra-arterial injection of acetylcholine, neostigmine, or edrophonium increases the strength of the fatigued

PHARMACO-LOGICAL ASPECTS OF MYASTHENIA GRAVIS

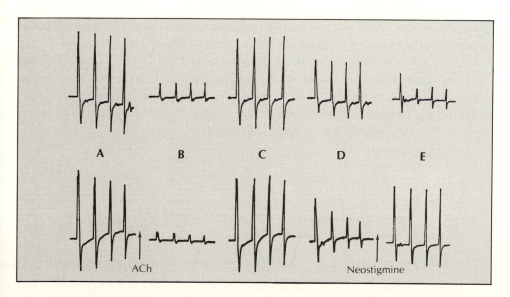

FIG. 11-3. Effect of acetylcholine and neostigmine on the muscle action potential response to nerve stimulation in a normal subject (upper row) and a patient with myasthenia gravis (lower row). *A*, Control response to four supramaximal nerve stimuli at 40 msec intervals; *B*, prompt depression 7 seconds after intra-arterial injection of 5 mg of acetylcholine; *C*, recovery 15 seconds after injection; *D*, late depression 1 hour after injection; *E*, effect of 0.5 mg neostigmine. (From Grob, D.: J. Chron. Dis. **8:**536, 1958.)

TABLE 11-2. Anticholinesterase preparations

Drug	Preparations	Usual route of administration
Physostigmine (eserine)	0.1% to 1% solution	Topical (eye)
Neostigmine bromide (Prostigmin bromide)	Tablets, 15 mg	Oral
Neostigmine methylsulfate (Prostigmin methylsulfate)	Injectable solutions, 0.25, 0.5, and 1 mg/ml	Subcutaneous or intramuscular
Pyridostigmine (Mestinon)	Tablets, 60 mg	Oral
Ambenonium (Mytelase)	Tablets, 10 and 25 mg	Oral
Demecarium (Humorsol)	0.25% solution	Topical (eye)
Edrophonium (Tensilon)	Injectable solution, 10 mg/ml	Intravenous
Echothiophate (Phospholine)	0.25% solution	Topical (eye)

muscles. In normal persons the intra-arterial injection of these drugs produces fasciculation and weakness, probably as a result of persistent depolarization of the neuromuscular end-plates (Fig. 11-3). Also, myasthenic patients are susceptible to doses of *d*-tubocurarine or quinine that scarcely affect normal persons.

It is currently believed that the defect in myasthenic neuromuscular transmission is both prejunctional[5] and postjunctional.[6] Thus the amount of acetylcholine in each synaptic vesicle is low, and the junctional acetylcholine receptors are reduced in number by an immunological mechanism.

Various anticholinesterases are useful for the diagnosis and management of myasthenia. For diagnostic purposes, neostigmine in a dose of 1 to 2 mg may be injected by the intramuscular route with atropine, 0.6 mg. Smaller doses (0.5 mg) of neostigmine may be used by the intravenous route. Edrophonium may be given for diagnosis in a dose of 2 to 8 mg intravenously.

For the management of weakness, neostigmine and related drugs are most useful. Neostigmine bromide is administered orally in doses of 15 to 30 mg, sometimes as often as every 3 hours (Table 11-2). Much smaller doses of neostigmine as the methylsulfate suffice when given by the intramuscular route.

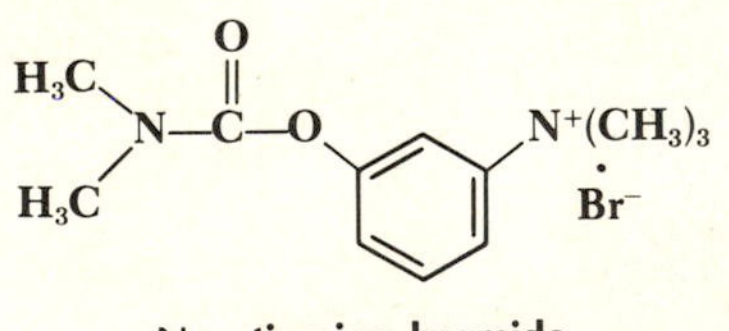

Neostigmine bromide

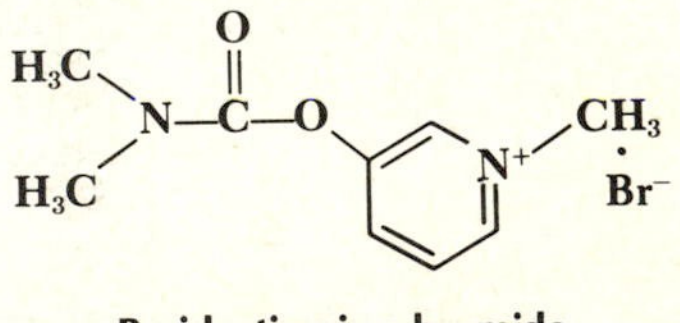

Pyridostigmine bromide

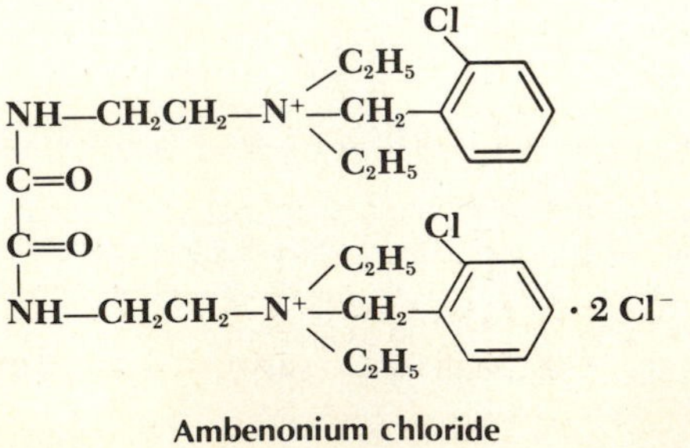

Ambenonium chloride

Excessive doses of anticholinesterases produce what is often called a cholinergic **Cholinergic crisis** crisis. Its muscarinic signs are miosis, sweating, salivation, lacrimation, and a hyperactive bowel. Its nicotinic signs are revealed by muscle fasciculations and paralysis. The diagnosis of anticholinesterase poisoning can be made on the basis of these symptoms and signs, since there are essentially no other diagnostic possibilities.[8]

An intravenous injection of 2 mg of edrophonium may be useful in distinguishing between cholinergic crisis and myasthenic crisis. If the injection is followed by increased strength, it is an indication of undertreatment rather than overtreatment.[16]

Quinine, *d*-tubocurarine, and decamethonium aggravate the symptoms of the myasthenic patient. Provocation of these symptoms for diagnostic purposes should be done only under careful supervision with adequate facilities for artificial respiration.

REFERENCES

1 Aeschlimann, J. A., and Reinert, M.: Pharmacological action of some analogues of physostigmine, J. Pharmacol. Exp. Ther. **43**:413, 1931.

2 Becker, B., and Ballin, N.: Glaucoma, Annu. Rev. Med. **17**:235, 1966.

3 Davis, K. L., Mohs, R. C., Tinklenberg, J. R., Pfefferbaum, A., Hollister, L. E., and Kopell, B. S.: Physostigmine: improvement of long-term memory processes in normal humans, Science **201**:272, 1978.

4 Duvoison, R. C., and Katz, R.: Reversal of central anticholinergic syndrome in man by physostigmine, J.A.M.A. **206**:1963, 1968.

5 Elmquist, D. M., Hoffmann, W. W., Kugelberg, J., and Quastel, D. M. J.: An electrophysiological investigation of neuromuscular transmission in myasthenia gravis, J. Physiol. **174**:417, 1964.

6 Fambrough, D. M., Drachman, D. B., and Satyamurti, S.: Neuromuscular junction in myasthenia gravis: decreased acetylcholine receptors, Science **182**:293, 1973.

7 Glaser, G. H.: Pharmacological considerations in the treatment of myasthenia gravis, Adv. Pharmacol. **2**:113, 1963.

8 Hallett, M., and Cullen, R. F.: Intoxication with echothiophate iodide, J.A.M.A. **222**:1414, 1972.

9 Hanin, I., Jenden, D. J., and Cho, A. K.: The influence of pH on the muscarinic action of oxotremorine, arecoline, pilocarpine, and their quaternary ammonium analogs, Mol. Pharmacol. **2**:269, 1966.

10 Kanagaratnam, K., Boon, W. H., and Hoh, T. K.: Parathion poisoning from contaminated barley, Lancet **1**:538, 1960.

11 Leopold, I. H., and Keates, E.: Drugs used in the treatment of glaucoma. I. Clin. Pharmacol. Ther. **6**:130, 1965.

12 Leopold, I. H., and Keates, E.: Drugs used in the treatment of glaucoma. II. Clin. Pharmacol. Ther. **6**:262, 1965.

13 Levy, B., and Ahlquist, R. P.: A study of sympathetic ganglionic stimulants, J. Pharmacol. Exp. Ther. **137**:219, 1962.

14 Moore, H.: Advantages of pyridostigmine bromide (Mestinon) and edrophonium chloride (Tensilon) in the treatment of transitory myasthenia gravis in the neonatal period, N. Engl. J. Med. **253**:1075, 1955.

15 Namba, T., Nolte, C. T., Jackrel, J., and Grob, D.: Poisoning due to organophosphate insecticides, Am. J. Med. **50**:475, 1971.

16 Osserman, K. E., and Kaplan, L. I.: Studies in myasthenia gravis: use of edrophonium chloride (Tensilon) in differentiating myasthenic from cholinergic weakness, Arch. Neurol. Psychiatr. **70**:385, 1953.

17 Quinby, G. E., Loomis, T. A., and Brown, H. W.: Oral occupational parathion poisoning treated with 2-PAM iodide, N. Engl. J. Med. **268**:639, 1963.

18 Richter, J. A., and Goldstein, A.: Effects of morphine and levorphanol on brain acetylcholine content in mice, J. Pharmacol. Exp. Ther. **175**:685, 1970.

19 Strauss, A. J. L., Seegal, B. C., Hsu, K. S., Burkholder, P. M., Nastuk, W. L., and Osserman, K. E.: Preliminary observations by immunofluorescence technique of a muscle-binding complement-fixing globulin in the serum of patients with myasthenia gravis, Proc. Soc. Exp. Biol. Med. **105**:184, 1960.

20 Thesleff, S., and Quastel, D. M. J.: Neuromuscular pharmacology, Annu. Rev. Pharmacol. **5:**263, 1965.

21 Thompson, H. S., Newsome, D. A., and Loewenkfeld, I. E.: The fixed dilated pupil, Arch. Ophthalmol. **86:**21, 1971.

22 Walker, M. B.: Case showing effect of prostigmine on myasthenia gravis, Proc. R. Soc. Med. **28:**759, 1935.

23 Wieland, T.: Poisonous principles of mushrooms of the genus Amanita, Science **159:**946, 1968.

24 Wilson, I. B.: A specific antidote for nerve gas and insecticide (alkylphosphate) intoxication, Neurology 8(Supp. 1):41, 1958.

REVIEWS

25 Brimblecombe, R. W.: Drug actions on cholinergic systems. In Bradley, P. B., editor: Pharmacology monographs, Baltimore, 1974, University Park Press.

26 Cohen, J. B., and Changeux, J-P.: The cholinergic receptor protein in its membrane environment, Annu. Rev. Pharmacol. **15:**83, 1974.

27 Drachman, D. B.: Myasthenia gravis, I and II. N. Engl. J. Med. **298:**136, 186, 1978.

28 Elias, S. B., and Appel, S. H.: Recent advances in myasthenia gravis, Life Sci. **18:**1031, 1976.

29 Hofmann, W. W.: The treatment of myasthenia gravis, Ration. Drug Ther. **13:** No. 2, Feb. 1979.

30 Koelle, G. B.: Acetylcholine—current status in physiology, pharmacology and medicine, N. Engl. J. Med. **286:**1086, 1972.

31 Lindstrom, J., and Dau, P.: Biology of myasthenia gravis, Annu. Rev. Pharmacol. Toxicol. **20:**337, 1980.

CHAPTER 12

Atropine group of cholinergic blocking drugs

GENERAL CONCEPT

Atropine and related drugs are important therapeutic agents and have widespread uses as pharmacological tools. They are competitive antagonists of acetylcholine on organs innervated by postganglionic cholinergic nerves. Atropine, scopolamine, and related drugs find important applications in ophthalmology, anesthesia, and cardiac and gastrointestinal diseases. In addition to their peripheral anticholinergic effects, most of these drugs act on the CNS and are used in the treatment of Parkinson's disease and vestibular disorders, as proprietary hypnotics, and as antidotes for the anticholinesterases. In this last instance both peripheral and central actions of the drugs are of great benefit.

GENERAL CONCEPT

Atropine and scopolamine are among the oldest drugs in medicine. Many solanaceous plants have been used for centuries because of their active principles of *l*-hyoscyamine and *l*-hyoscine. The name *hyoscyamine* is derived from *Hyoscyamus niger* (henbane). It is of some toxicological interest to know that the common jimsonweed, *Datura stramonium*, also contains these alkaloids. These drugs also are often called the belladonna alkaloids because they are found in the deadly nightshade, *Atropa belladonna*.

ATROPINE AND SCOPOLAMINE

The alkaloids as they occur in the plants are *l*-hyoscyamine and *l*-hyoscine (scopolamine). Atropine is *dl*-hyoscyamine, with racemization occurring during the extraction process. Just as acetylcholine is an ester of an amino alcohol, the blocking drugs of the belladonna group are esters of complex organic bases with tropic acid. Atropine and scopolamine differ only slightly in the structure of the organic base part of the molecule, as is evident from comparison of their structural formulas.

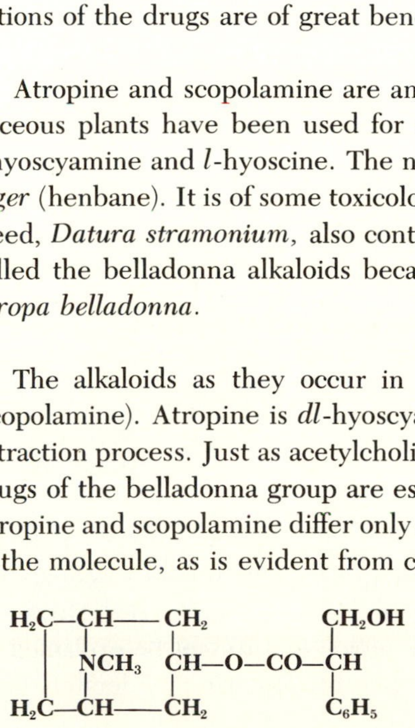

Chemistry

$$
\begin{array}{cc}
\text{H}_2\text{C}-\text{CH}-\!\!-\text{CH}_2 \qquad \text{CH}_2\text{OH} & \text{HC}-\text{CH}-\!\!-\text{CH}_2 \qquad \text{CH}_2\text{OH} \\
\quad\; |\quad\; \text{NCH}_3 \; \text{CH}-\text{O}-\text{CO}-\text{CH} & \text{O} \triangleleft \quad | \quad \text{NCH}_3 \; \text{CH}-\text{O}-\text{CO}-\text{CH} \\
\text{H}_2\text{C}-\text{CH}-\!\!-\text{CH}_2 \qquad\quad \text{C}_6\text{H}_5 & \text{HC}-\text{CH}-\!\!-\text{CH}_2 \qquad\quad \text{C}_6\text{H}_5
\end{array}
$$

Atropine 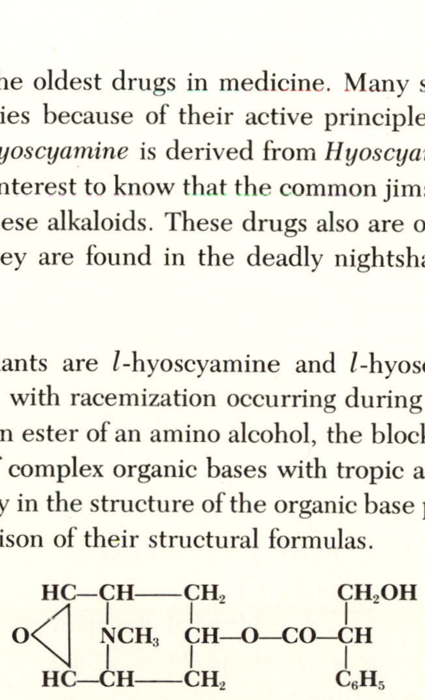   **Scopolamine**

Atropine and scopolamine are competitive antagonists of acetylcholine at receptor sites in smooth muscles, cardiac muscle, and various glandular cells. (See Fig.

Mode of action

2-2, p. 12.) The effectiveness of this competition is greatest against the muscarinic effects of injected cholinergic drugs and against the tonic effect of the vagus nerve on the heart. These drugs are less effective in blocking the actions of parasympathetic nerves on the gastrointestinal tract and urinary bladder.

The actions of atropine and scopolamine on the cardiovascular system and on the eye are very similar. The two drugs differ mainly in their CNS effects. In therapeutic doses, given parenterally, scopolamine tends to produce considerable sleepiness, whereas atropine is not likely to produce this evidence of CNS depression. While it is generally believed that scopolamine is a CNS depressant and atropine is a stimulant, in reality the effect depends on the dose. In low doses both drugs tend to cause sedation. In larger doses both cause stimulation, which may progress to delirium. Finally, after very high doses of either drug, coma may supervene.

There is definite gradation in the sensitivity of various functions mediated by acetylcholine to inhibition by atropine and scopolamine. Therapeutic doses of 0.6 mg of atropine or 0.3 mg of scopolamine may cause dryness of the mouth and inhibit sweating. Blockade of the cardiac vagus requires somewhat larger doses. Gastrointestinal and urinary tract smooth muscle is even more resistant to the action of atropine and scopolamine. Finally, the inhibition of gastric secretion requires such large doses in humans that side effects on the more susceptible sites would make that therapeutic objective completely impractical.

Pharmacological effects

Cardiovascular system effects. The effects of atropine and scopolamine on blood pressure are not impressive. Most vascular areas in the body do not receive parasympathetic innervation. It is common experience in the laboratory to inject atropine intravenously into a dog, 1 mg/kg of body weight, without observing a significant change in the mean pressure.

The effect of atropine on the heart rate in humans is complex. With large enough doses, tachycardia develops, as expected, from blockade of vagal influences on the heart. With smaller doses, paradoxical as it may seem, the heart rate may be slowed. Ablation experiments have shown that atropine stimulates vagal nuclei in the medulla, an action that results in bradycardia unless large enough doses are used to prevent such an action at the muscarinic receptors. In one study the final effect of scopolamine on heart rate was found to be the result of two separate actions, one tending to produce tachycardia, the other bradycardia.[20]

A distinctly anomalous vascular effect of atropine is its production of cutaneous dilatation. In warm environments, atropine may promote cutaneous vasodilatation because it tends to block sweating, thus causing body temperature to rise. However, atropine has an additional cutaneous vasodilator action that cannot be explained on this basis. Flushing of the skin may be very noticeable following moderately large doses of atropine.

Gastrointestinal effects. In large enough doses the belladonna alkaloids will reduce motility and tone of the gastrointestinal tract and may even reduce the volume of its various secretions. Motility is more easily reduced by therapeutic doses than is gastric secretion, particularly if a peptic ulcer is present.

Effect on urinary tract. Atropine has little effect on the ureters. It relaxes the fundus of the bladder but promotes contraction of the sphincter, thus favoring urinary retention.

Effect on eye. The actions of atropine on the eye are straightforward. When it is applied directly to the conjunctiva (0.5% to 1% solutions), the drug will produce mydriasis and paralysis of accommodation (cycloplegia). In addition, in patients subject to glaucoma it may precipitate an acute attack with catastrophic increases in intraocular pressure.

The circular muscle of the iris receives cholinergic innervation through fibers traveling in the third nerve. Atropine blocks the actions of acetylcholine on this sphincter muscle, and the resulting predominance of the radial fibers produces mydriasis. The atropinized pupil does not react to light. Cycloplegia is caused by paralysis of the ciliary muscles, which are normally innervated by cholinergic fibers. Increased intraocular pressure is generally attributed to impeded drainage of aqueous humor through the canals of Schlemm.

It should be recalled that the adrenergic drugs also can produce mydriasis. They act, however, by contracting the radial muscle of the iris. Accommodation is not paralyzed by the adrenergic drugs, in contrast to the atropine-like compounds.

CNS effects. In atropine poisoning the CNS effects are very striking; patients become excited and maniacal. Large therapeutic doses stimulate respiration and may prevent death from respiratory depression in poisoning caused by the alkyl phosphate cholinesterase inhibitors.

There are additional reasons for believing that the belladonna alkaloids affect the CNS. Scopolamine in particular is valuable in the management of Parkinson's

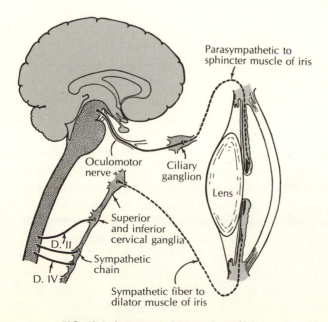

FIG. 12-1. Autonomic innervation of iris.

disease and in the prevention of motion sickness.[4] When it is given by injection, the drug promotes a state of sedation and twilight sleep and may cause amnesia.[16]

Absorption, excretion, and metabolism

Atropine and scopolamine are well absorbed from the gastrointestinal tract and following subcutaneous injection. They may even be absorbed following topical application. Accidents may occur in ophthalmologic use, particularly in children, if the drug is allowed to reach the nasal mucosa through the nasolacrimal duct after its application to the conjunctival sac.

Atropine is rapidly excreted from the body and about 50% of an injected dose appears in the urine within 4 hours. The remainder is excreted within 24 hours in the form of metabolites and the unchanged drug.[35] The duration of the pharmacological effects reflects the rapidity of excretion except for the dilatation of the pupils and paralysis of accommodation, which may persist for a long time, particularly when atropine is applied topically to the conjunctiva.

Preparations and clinical uses

The belladonna alkaloids are used either in galenic preparations* or in a pure form. Belladonna tincture is given orally in a dose of 0.6 ml, which is equivalent to 0.2 mg of atropine. Atropine sulfate tablets are available in several different sizes. The usual dose is 0.6 mg. Scopolamine hydrobromide tablets are available in sizes of 0.3 and 0.6 mg. The usual dose is 0.6 mg. Solutions of atropine sulfate are available for instillation into the conjunctival sac. The usual strength of these solutions is 0.5% to 1%.

Ophthalmologic use. The anticholinergic drugs are applied topically for producing mydriasis and cycloplegia. Atropine itself has such a long duration of action that its use in ophthalmology is impractical. Homatropine and cyclopentolate are much more commonly employed and have a much shorter duration of action.

Preoperative uses. It is customary to administer atropine or scopolamine before operative procedures and general anesthesia. The drug protects the patient from excessive salivation and bradycardia. Scopolamine is often used in obstetrics because it produces sedation and amnesia. The anticholinergics were particularly important when ether was widely employed. With the newer anesthetics, excessive tracheobronchial secretions are not produced and the need for routine preanesthetic anticholinergics is questioned by some.[35]

Cardiac uses. Atropine is being used increasingly after myocardial infarction for reversing bradycardia caused by excessive vagal activity. The drug is also useful in digitalis-induced heart block. Although many physicians will use atropine after myocardial infarction if the heart rate falls below 60,[35] there is no certainty about the need or safety of this procedure unless hypotension or arrhythmias justify it. Large intravenous doses of atropine may cause dangerous tachycardia and ventricular arrhythmias in cardiac patients.

---

*Galenic preparations contain one or several organic ingredients as contrasted with pure chemical substances.

Uses in gastrointestinal disease. Anticholinergic drugs are used widely in the treatment of peptic ulcer. The drugs may diminish vagally mediated secretion, relieve spasm, and prolong the time during which antacids remain in the stomach by slowing down gastric emptying. To be effective, the anticholinergics must often be administered in large enough doses to cause discomfort, such as difficulty of vision and urination. Although there is no evidence for a favorable effect of anticholinergics on the long-term progress of ulcer disease, these drugs are unquestionably of considerable symptomatic benefit. The quaternary anticholinergics are preferred by many gastroenterologists. In large doses they may cause postural hypotension in addition to other predictable atropine-like effects. In addition to the usual contraindications, atropine should not be used in the presence of obstructive lesions, since it promotes retention.

Antiparkinsonism drugs. These drugs are discussed on p. 158. *Atropine-like drugs for vestibular disorders* are discussed along with the antihistaminic drugs on p. 250. The use of scopolamine as a hypnotic in combination with antihistaminics is unimportant except from a commercial standpoint. The presence of scopolamine in such over-the-counter preparations should be kept in mind in relation to possible drug interactions and in cases in which atropine-like drugs are contraindicated.

Toxicity and antidotes

The belladonna alkaloids and atropine-like drugs are generally safe medications. Large doses in a normal individual may cause unpleasant effects but are not life-threatening. Blurred vision, tachycardia, dry mouth, constipation, and urinary retention are among these unpleasant effects. Patients with glaucoma and prostatic hypertrophy may have disastrous reactions even to therapeutic doses of these drugs. Normal individuals have survived doses as high as 1 g taken by mouth.[1]

Full-blown atropine poisoning is characterized by excitement and maniacal tendencies, hot and dry skin, dilated pupils, and tachycardia. The subcutaneous injection of 25 mg of methacholine will not elicit cholinergic effects in such patients.

Patients with atropine poisoning should be managed with supportive care. Sedatives such as chlordiazepoxide or diazepam may be helpful in controlling violent excitement.

Physostigmine has been found remarkably effective as an antidote in atropine poisoning. The drug may be injected subcutaneously in doses of 1 to 4 mg.[23] The injection may be repeated in 1 hour if necessary. Although the effectiveness of physostigmine in atropine poisoning has been known for years on the basis of animal experiments, its clinical usefulness became obvious more recently as a consequence of clinical observations made on patients with Parkinson's disease who received excessive amounts of atropine-like drugs.[23]

Problem 12-1. Why is physostigmine preferable to neostigmine in reversing the CNS effects of atropine? The answer undoubtedly has some connection with the relative rates of penetration of the two drugs across the blood-brain barrier. Physostigmine is not a quaternary compound, but neostigmine is.

Numerous drugs, such as antihistamines and tricyclic antidepressants, have atropine-like effects and may contribute to atropine poisoning. Atropine-like drugs counteract the extrapyramidal side effects of the phenothiazines.

ATROPINE SUBSTITUTES

The atropine substitutes will be classified on the basis of their primary usefulness, which to a certain extent reflects their selectivity. On this basis they fall into three groups: the atropine-like mydriatics, the antispasmodics, and the antiparkinsonism drugs.

Atropine-like mydriatics

Atropine itself is a powerful mydriatic and cycloplegic, but its long duration of action is generally a disadvantage except in the treatment of iritis. For examination of the fundus and measurement of refractive errors, a number of shorter-acting agents are preferred. Some of these are homatropine, eucatropine, cyclopentolate, and tropicamide. In addition, adrenergic drugs such as phenylephrine (Neo-Synephrine) produce mydriasis without cycloplegia when applied topically to the eye.

Homatropine is the oldest of the atropine-like mydriatic drugs. It differs from atropine only in the fact that it is an ester of mandelic rather than of tropic acid. Homatropine is applied to the eye in 2% solutions. It produces mydriasis fairly rapidly, but its action lasts only 1 or 2 days. It is a less potent cycloplegic than atropine and is commonly used in ophthalmology.

$$H_2C-CH{-\!\!-\!\!-}CH_2 \qquad OH$$
$$\Big| \qquad\quad NCH_3 \quad CH-O-CO-CH$$
$$H_2C-CH{-\!\!-\!\!-}CH_2 \qquad C_6H_5$$

Homatropine

Eucatropine (Euphthalmine) is a weaker drug than homatropine. It produces mydriasis in 30 minutes, which lasts only about 12 hours. The drug has little cycloplegic action. It is used in 2% to 5% solutions.

Cyclopentolate hydrochloride (Cyclogyl) produces mydriasis in 30 to 60 minutes, with return of normal vision in less than 24 hours. It is used in 0.5% and 1% solutions, although for deeply pigmented eyes a 2% solution may be necessary.

Tropicamide (Mydriacyl) is a very rapidly acting mydriatic and cycloplegic. It produces mydriasis in less than 30 minutes, and its action lasts only 15 to 20 minutes. It is used in 0.5% and 1% solutions.

Anticholinergic smooth muscle relaxants

A large group of atropine substitutes have been synthesized for the purpose of obtaining some selective action on the gastrointestinal tract. The great incentives for this search are the prevalence of peptic ulcer and the belief that desirable objectives in its management are relief of smooth muscle spasm and hypersecretion.

Conversion of the usual tertiary atropine-like drugs to quaternary amines introduces a number of important changes into their pharmacology. (1) Quaternary amines are less lipid soluble and do not penetrate the CNS. (2) The quaternary atropine-like drugs exert some ganglionic blocking effect that may reinforce their actions on the gastrointestinal tract. Thus the quaternary atropine methylbromide

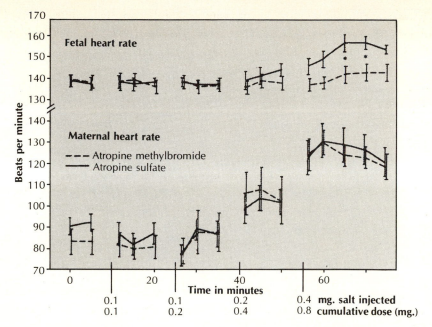

FIG. 12-2. Effect of atropine sulfate and atropine methylbromide on maternal and fetal heart rates. The lesser effect of the quaternary anticholinergic drug on fetal heart rate illustrates a basic difference between the two types of drugs as regards their passage across biological membranes. (From dePadua, C. B., and Gravenstein, J. S.: J.A.M.A. **208:**1022, 1969.)

would not be expected to penetrate into the CNS as efficiently as atropine sulfate. The difference between the two in regard to penetration across biological membranes is shown in Fig. 12-2.

Quaternary anticholinergic drugs used in 2 to 15 mg doses include methscopolamine (Pamine), homatropine methylbromide (Novatran), propantheline (Pro-Banthine), oxyphenonium (Antrenyl), penthienate (Monodral), valethamate (Murel), pipenzolate (Piptal), and poldine (Nacton). Quaternary anticholinergics used in doses of 50 to 100 mg or more include methantheline (Banthine), tridihexethyl (Pathilon), mepiperphenidol (Darstine), tricyclamol (Elorine), diphemanil (Prantal), amolanone (Amethone), and hexocyclium (Tral).

Quaternary anticholinergic drugs

Propantheline bromide

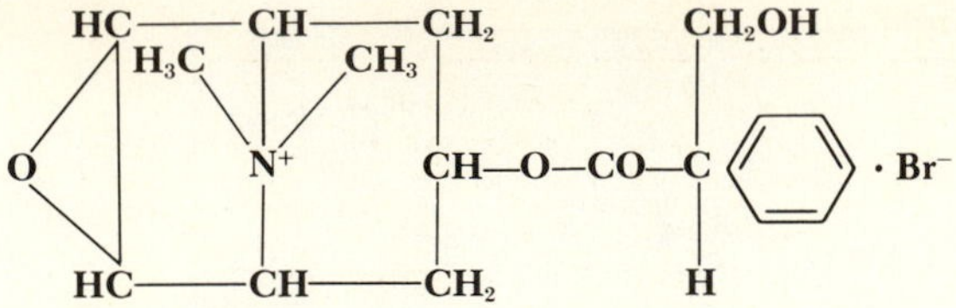

Methscopolamine bromide 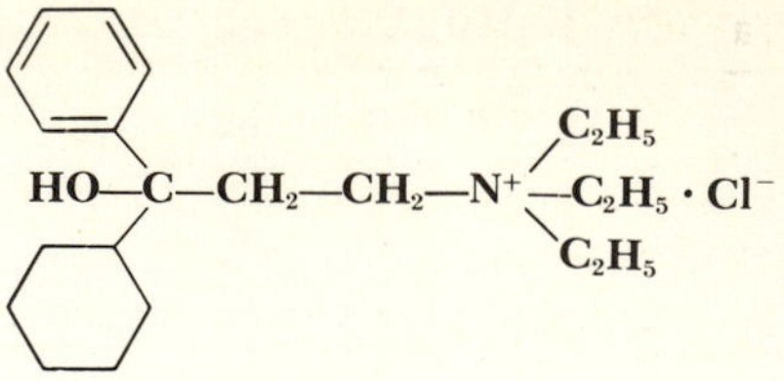   Tridihexethyl chloride

Tertiary anticholinergic drugs   Among these synthetic atropine substitutes the most potent, used in doses of 10 mg, are dicyclomine (Bentyl) and oxyphencyclimine (Daricon). Drugs of this group used in doses of 50 mg or more are piperidolate (Dactil), aminocarbofluorene (Pavatrine), and amprotropine (Syntropan). Adiphenine (Trasentine), largely obsolete, also belongs to this group.

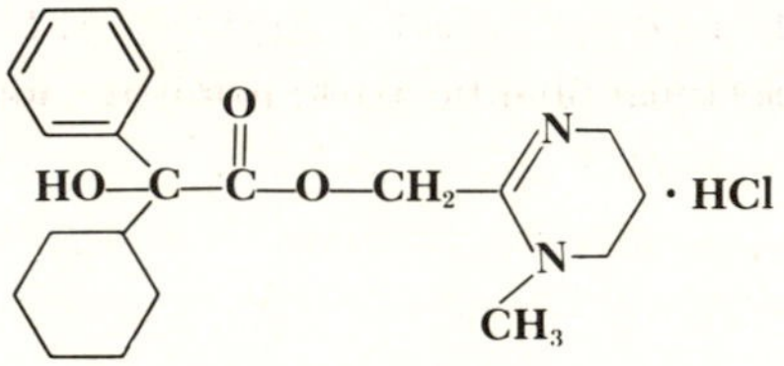

Oxyphencyclimine hydrochloride

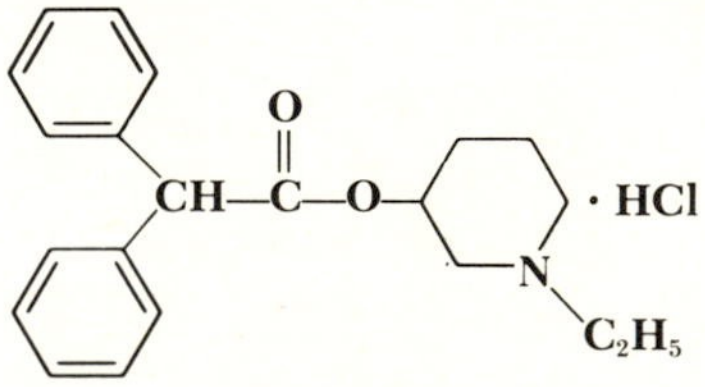

Piperidolate hydrochloride 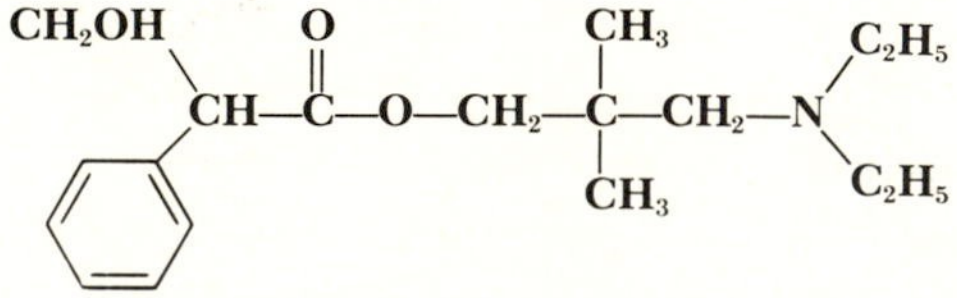   Amprotropine

Dual antispasmodic action   Some anticholinergics, such as dicyclomine hydrochloride (Bentyl), are not only parasympatholytic but possess a direct depressant action on the intestinal smooth muscle. The evidence for this statement is based on the ability of dicyclomine to counteract not only the effects of acetylcholine but also those of bradykinin on the intestinal smooth muscle. The clinical significance of this *musculotropic* antispasmodic action is difficult to evaluate.

Antiparkinsonism drugs   The pharmacology of parkinsonism has been revolutionized during the last few years by the discovery of the effectiveness of L-dopa in its treatment and the role of dopamine in extrapyramidal function. Until recently the treatment of this common and disabling condition was based on the empiric use of (1) belladonna alkaloids and their synthetic congeners, (2) antihistamines, (3) drugs with both anticholinergic and antihistaminic properties (benztropine), and (4) dextroamphetamine for some

Table 12-1. Drug effects in parkinsonism

Drugs that aggravate or cause parkinsonism	Drugs that relieve parkinsonism
Reserpine	Belladonna alkaloids
Chlorpromazine (phenothiazines)	Synthetic anticholinergic drugs
Haloperidol	Antihistamines
α-Methyldopa	Drugs having both anticholinergic and antihistaminic properties
	Levodopa
	Amantadine
	Dextroamphetamine
	Apomorphine

manifestations of postencephalitic parkinsonism, such as oculogyric crisis and rigidity.

Parkinsonism, characterized by tremor, rigidity, and akinesia, includes idiopathic paralysis agitans, postencephalitic parkinsonism, and other disturbances of the extrapyramidal system. It may also be caused by drugs. It was suggested more than 100 years ago that the belladonna alkaloids might be useful in the management of the syndrome, and drug studies have contributed greatly to current concepts of its pathophysiology (Table 12-1).

The effectiveness of belladonna alkaloids in the treatment of parkinsonism called attention to the possible role of cholinergic mechanisms in its causation. It seemed reasonable to theorize that some brain centers must have become supersensitive to acetylcholine in the parkinsonian patient, perhaps as a form of denervation supersensitivity or as a consequence of removal of an inhibitory influence.

Cholinergic and dopaminergic mechanisms in parkinsonism

The role of cholinergic mechanisms in parkinsonism was supported by experiments that showed that *tremorine*, a cholinomimetic drug, produces a syndrome in animals resembling parkinsonism.[27] The injection of acetylcholine into the globus pallidus of patients undergoing stereotaxic surgery resulted in increased tremor contralaterally.[31] Furthermore, the anticholinesterase physostigmine was found to exacerbate the symptoms of parkinsonian patients.[13] In this last study the suggestion was made that the role of the cholinergic system may be secondary to the involvement of a dopaminergic mechanism.[13]

Histochemical fluorescence techniques have shown[2] that the characteristic green fluorescence of catecholamines is present in the nerve cell bodies of the *substantia nigra* and in the nerve terminals of the *striatum*, both areas being rich in dopamine. Furthermore, lesions placed in the substantia nigra of rats resulted in a decrease in dopamine in the ipsilateral striatum.[2]

The nigro-striatal dopaminergic system probably plays an important pathogenetic role in parkinsonism. In idiopathic parkinsonism the most conspicuous lesions are found in the substantia nigra, and the level of dopamine is found to be decreased in the striatum where the axonal terminations of the striatal neurons are located. The effectiveness of L-dopa in the treatment of parkinsonism suggests also that this precursor of dopamine, when administered in large doses, may overcome the deficiency of dopamine that is known to exist in the nigro-striatal dopaminergic pathway.

The proposal of antagonistic roles of cholinergic and dopaminergic pathways and loss of dopaminergic inhibitory functions at the level of the striatum serves admirably for explaining the mode of action of drugs that aggravate or relieve parkinsonism.

Drugs that aggravate parkinsonism. Both reserpine and chlorpromazine aggravate the symptoms of parkinsonism. Reserpine causes a depletion of dopamine in the striatum and thus, according to the theory, would remove an inhibitory influence on a cholinergic system. L-Dopa reverses the effect of reserpine, since it is converted to dopamine.

Chlorpromazine and haloperidol have some adrenergic and dopaminergic receptor-blocking effects and antagonize dopamine at central receptor sites.

Drugs that relieve parkinsonism. The anticholinergic drugs would be expected to be effective if the cholinergic system is hyperactive as a consequence of removal of dopaminergic inhibitory influences. Most of the antihistaminics also have anticholinergic actions, which may account for their effectiveness.

Dextroamphetamine may be useful in the treatment of certain manifestations of postencephalitic parkinsonism, such as rigidity and oculogyric crisis. Dextroamphetamine promotes presynaptic dopamine release and blocks its reuptake.[18]

Amantadine, an antiviral drug, has been reported to be beneficial in parkinsonism. Although the mode of action of this drug is uncertain, dopamine release from neuronal storage sites following its injection has been claimed on the basis of animal experiments.[22]

Apomorphine, a dopaminergic amine, and related aporphines appear promising in the treatment of parkinsonism.[8]

Major antiparkinsonism agents

The available antiparkinsonism drugs fall into the following groups on the basis of their pharmacological properties:
1. Belladonna alkaloids, including atropine and scopolamine
2. Synthetic anticholinergics, such as trihexyphenidyl hydrochloride (Artane), biperiden hydrochloride (Akineton), cycrimine hydrochloride (Pagitane), and procyclidine hydrochloride (Kemadrin)
3. Antihistamines such as diphenhydramine hydrochloride (Benadryl) and orphenadrine citrate (Norflex) or orphenadrine hydrochloride (Disipal)
4. Drugs with both anticholinergic and antihistaminic properties, such as benztropine mesylate (Cogentin mesylate)
5. Phenothiazines with anticholinergic and antihistaminic actions, such as ethopropazine (Parsidol)
6. Levodopa (L-dopa), acting on dopaminergic mechanisms

7. Miscellaneous drugs probably acting on dopaminergic mechanisms, such as amantadine and dextroamphetamine

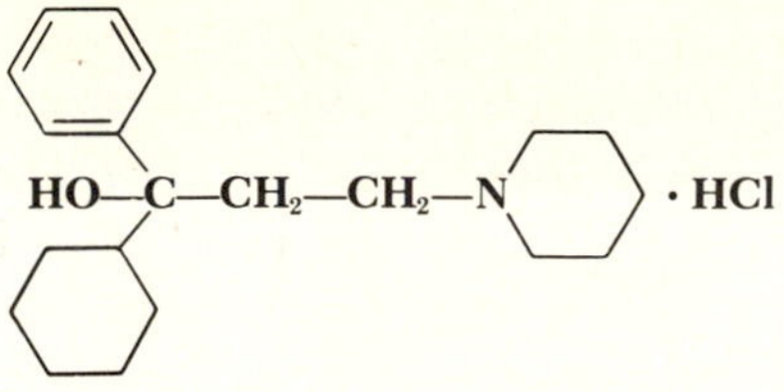

Trihexyphenidyl hydrochloride

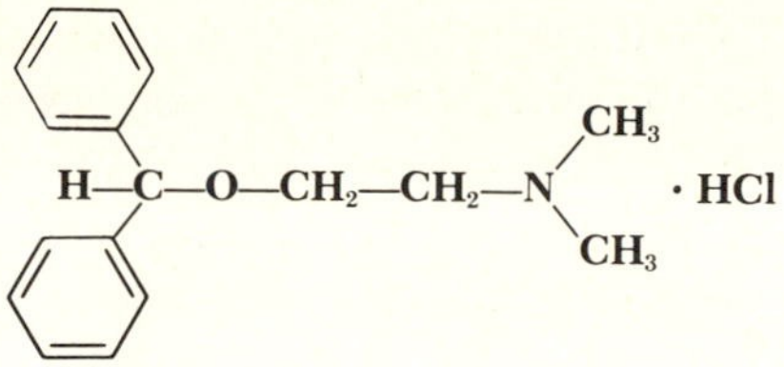

Diphenhydramine hydrochloride

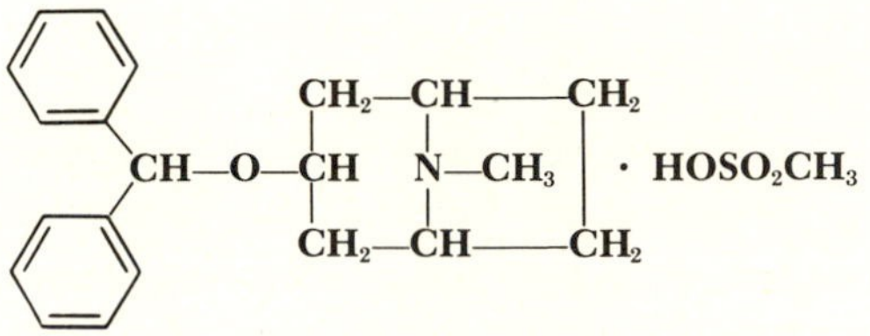

Benztropine mesylate

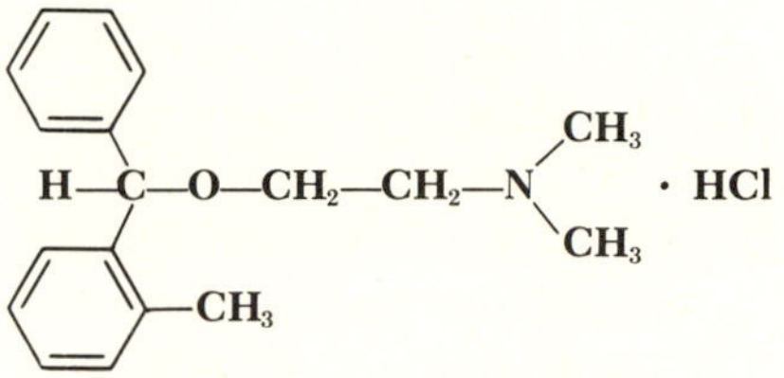

Orphenadrine hydrochloride

Belladonna alkaloids and synthetic anticholinergics. The naturally occurring belladonna alkaloids atropine and scopolamine have been used for years in treatment of parkinsonism. They have been replaced by the newer synthetics because the latter do not produce as powerful peripheral anticholinergic symptoms for a given amount of relief of parkinsonian disability.

The action and uses of the synthetic anticholinergics are similar. All are chemically related to trihexyphenidyl, and all produce atropine-like untoward effects such as dryness of the mouth, blurred vision, dizziness, and dysuria.

Trihexyphenidyl hydrochloride (Artane) is available in tablets of 2 and 5 mg, timed-release capsules of 5 mg, and elixir, 2 mg/5 ml. Dosage ranges from 1 mg initially to a maximum of 20 mg daily.

Biperiden hydrochloride (Akineton hydrochloride) is available in 2 mg tablets for oral administration; **biperiden lactate** (Akineton lactate) is available as a solution, 5 mg/ml, for injection.

Cycrimine hydrochloride (Pagitane hydrochloride) is available in tablets of 1.25 and 2.5 mg.

Procyclidine hydrochloride (Kemadrin) is available in tablets of 2 and 5 mg.

Antihistamines. Diphenhydramine and the closely related orphenadrine have some usefulness in the treatment of parkinsonism including that induced by drugs such as the phenothiazines. They are not as effective as the anticholinergics but produce fewer atropine-like untoward effects. On the other hand, they produce considerable drowsiness.

Diphenhydramine hydrochloride (Benadryl) is available in 25 and 50 mg cap sules, elixirs of 12.5 mg/5 ml, and solutions for intravenous and intramuscular injections containing 10 or 50 mg/ml.

Orphenadrine citrate (Norflex) is available in tablets, 100 mg, and solutions for injection, 30 mg/ml.

Orphenadrine hydrochloride (Disipal) is available in tablets, 50 mg.

Drugs with both anticholinergic and antihistaminic properties. The major representative of this class is benztropine mesylate. An examination of its chemical structure reveals similarities to atropine and a typical antihistaminic. Its pharmacological properties resemble those of atropine not only with regard to untoward effects but also from the standpoint of duration of action, which is long.

Benztropine mesylate (Cogentin mesylate) is available in tablets of 0.5, 1, and 2 mg and in solution for intramuscular or intravenous injection, 1 mg/ml.

Ethopropazine hydrochloride (Parsidol), a phenothiazine with both anticholinergic and antihistaminic actions, may be useful as an adjunct to the anticholinergic drugs. It causes considerable drowsiness, muscle cramps, and paresthesia and may cause agranulocytosis and hypotension. Its preparations include tablets of 10, 50, and 100 mg.

Levodopa. Levodopa is considered the most effective medication for parkinsonism. When administered orally in increasing doses, it is likely to benefit at least 50% of the patients, although it may take several weeks for the improvement to become manifest. Fortunately it is not necessary to discontinue the usual anticholinergic medications while the dosage is being built up. The initial daily dose is 300 mg to 1 g. Dosage is built up gradually until marked improvement occurs or adverse reactions make further increases impractical.

MAO inhibitors, when used concomitantly with levodopa, may cause hypertensive crises. Pyridoxine in large doses (more than 5 mg) reverses the effects of levodopa by promoting its peripheral decarboxylation. Sympathomimetic amines may have exaggerated effects in patients treated with levodopa. Anticholinergics should be used cautiously and in reduced dosages. Antihypertensive drugs should also be used with caution because postural hypotension may occur as a reaction to levodopa. Phenothiazines may cause parkinsonian-like symptoms that are usually resistant to levodopa. Many antihistamines have anticholinergic effects and should be used with caution in association with levodopa.

Levodopa (Dopar, Larodopa) is available in capsules containing 100, 250, and 500 mg.

Levodopa has been combined with an inhibitor of aromatic amino acid decarboxylase, carbidopa, and introduced under the trade name of **Sinemet.** Carbidopa is the hydrazino derivative of methyldopa. Carbidopa inhibits the decarboxylation of peripheral levodopa, but it does not enter the CNS. As a consequence more levodopa is available for transport to the brain and the amount of levodopa required is reduced by about 75%. Sinemet is available in tablets of two strengths: Sinemet 10/100 contains 10 mg of carbidopa and 100 mg of levodopa; Sinemet 25/250 contains 25 mg of carbidopa and 250 mg of levodopa.

Patients receiving levodopa must discontinue their medication at least 8 hours before taking the levodopa-carbidopa combination. Common serious adverse effects of the combination are choreiform and other involuntary movements, mental changes, nausea, arrhythmias, postural hypotension, and many others. Dosage must be determined by careful titration for each patient.

Amantadine. This antiviral agent produces clinical improvement in some patients having parkinsonian symptoms and does so more rapidly than levodopa. The mode of action of amantadine is not understood, although there is a highly suggestive experimental finding of an amantadine-dopamine interaction.[22]

Adverse effects of amantadine include hyperexcitability, slurred speech, ataxia, insomnia, and gastrointestinal disturbances. Convulsions have occurred after the administration of excessive doses.

Amantadine hydrochloride (Symmetrel) is available in capsules of 100 mg and as a syrup containing 50 mg/ml. Initial dose for adults is 100 mg once daily for 5 to 7 days.

REFERENCES

1 Alexander, E., Jr., Morris, D. P., and Eslick, R. L.: Atropine poisoning: report of a case, with recovery after the ingestion of one gram, N. Engl. J. Med. **234**:258, 1946.

2 Anden, N. E., Carlsson, A., Dahlstrom, A., Fuxe, K., Hillarp, N. A., and Larsson, K.: Demonstration and mapping out of nigro-neostriatal dopamine neurons, Life Sci. **3**:523, 1964.

3 Barbeau, A.: The pathogenesis of Parkinson's disease: a new hypothesis, Can. Med. Assoc. J. **87**:802, 1962.

4 Brand, J. J., and Perry, W. L. M.: Drugs used in motion sickness. A critical review of methods available for the study of drugs of potential value in its treatment and of the information which has been derived by these methods, Pharmacol. Rev. **18**:895, 1966.

5 Calne, D. B., Laurence, D. R., and Stern, G. M.: L-Dopa in postencephalitic parkinsonism, Lancet **1**:744, 1969.

6 Cotzias, G. C., and Papavasiliou, P. S.: Blocking the negative effects of pyridoxine on patients receiving levodopa, J.A.M.A. **215**:1504, 1971.

7 Cotzias, G. C., Papavasiliou, P. S., and Gellene, R.: Modification of parkinsonism—chronic treatment with L-dopa, N. Engl. J. Med. **280**:337, 1969.

8 Cotzias, G. C., Papavasiliou, P. S., Tolosa, E. S., Mendez, J. S., and Bell-Midura, M.: Treatment of Parkinson's disease with aporphines, N. Engl. J. Med. **294**:567, 1976.

9 Cotzias, G. C., Van Woert, M. H., and Schiffer, L. M.: Aromatic amino acids and modification of parkinsonism, N. Engl. J. Med. **276**:374, 1967.

10 DePadua, C. B., and Gravenstein, J. S.: Atropine sulfate vs atropine methyl bromide: effect on maternal and fetal heart rate, J.A.M.A. **208**:1022, 1969.

11 Doshay, L. J., and Constable, K.: Treatment of paralysis agitans with orphenadrine (Disipal): results in one hundred seventy-six cases, J.A.M.A. **163**:1352, 1957.

12 Doshay, L. J., Constable, K., and Zier, A.: Five-year follow-up of treatment with trihexyphenidyl (Artane), J.A.M.A. **154**:1334, 1954.

13 Duvoisin, R. C.: Cholinergic-anticholinergic antagonism in parkinsonism, Arch. Neurol. **17**:124, 1967.

14 Eger, E. I.: Atropine, scopolamine, and related compounds, Anesthesiology **23**:365, 1962.

15 Friend, D. G.: Anti-parkinsonism drug therapy, Clin. Pharmacol. Ther. **4**:815, 1963.

16 Frumin, M. J., et al.: Amnesic actions of diazepam and scopolamine in man, Anesthesiology **45**:406, 1976.

17 Gershon, S., Neubauer, H., and Sundland, D. M.: Interaction between some anticholinergic agents and phenothiazines, Clin. Pharmacol. Ther. **6**:749, 1965.

18 Glowinski, J., Axelrod, J., and Iversen, L. I.: Regional studies of catecholamines in the rat brain. IV. Effects of drugs on the disposition and metabolism of H³-norepinephrine and H³-

dopamine, J. Pharmacol. Exp. Ther. **153**:30, 1966.

19 Gosselin, R. E., Gabourel, J. D., and Wills, J. H.: The fate of atropine in man, Clin. Pharmacol. Ther. **1**:597, 1960.

20 Gravenstein, J. S., Ariet, M., and Thornby, J. I.: Atropine on the electrocardiogram, Clin. Pharmacol. Ther. **10**:660, 1969.

21 Gravenstein, J. S., and Thornby, J. I.: Scopolamine in heart rates in man, Clin. Pharmacol. Ther. **10**:395, 1969.

22 Grelak, R. P., Clark, R., Stump, J. M., and Vernier, V. G.: Amantadine-dopamine interaction: possible mode of action in parkinsonism, Science **169**:203, 1970.

23 Heiser, J. F., and Gillin, J. C.: The reversal of anticholinergic drug-induced delirium and coma with physostigmine, Am. J. Psychiatry **127**:1050, 1971.

24 Hornykiewicz, O.: Die topische Lokalisation und das Verhalten von Noradrenalin and Dopamin (3-Hydroxytyramin) in der Substantia nigra der normalen und Parkinsonkranken Menschen, Wien, Klim. Wochenschr. **75**:309, 1963.

25 Hornykiewicz, O.: Dopamine (3-hydroxytyramine) and brain function, Pharmacol. Rev. **18**: 925, 1966.

26 Ingelfinger, F. J.: In Symposium on clinical drug evaluation and human pharmacology. XIX. Clinical judgment in clinical research, Clin. Pharmacol. Ther. **3**:685, 1962.

27 Ingelfinger, F. J.: Anticholinergic therapy of gastrointestinal disorders, N. Engl. J. Med. **268**:1454, 1963.

28 Klawans, H. L., Jr.: The pharmacology of parkinsonism (a review), Dis. Nerv. Sys. **29**: 805, 1968.

29 Levine, R. M., Blair, M. R., and Clark, B. B.: Factors influencing the intestinal absorption of certain monoquaternary anticholinergic compounds with special reference to benzomethamine [N-diethylaminoethyl-N'-methylbenzilamide methobromide (MC-3199)], J. Pharmacol. Exp. Ther. **114**:78, 1955.

30 McGreer, P. L., Boulding, J. E., Gibson, W. C., and Foulkes, R. G.: Drug-induced extrapyramidal reactions. Treatment with diphenhydramine hydrochloride and dihydroxyphenylalanine, J.A.M.A. **177**:665, 1961.

31 Nashold, B. S.: Cholinergic stimulation of globus pallidus in man, Proc. Soc. Exp. Biol. Med. **101**:68, 1959.

32 Schwab, R. S., England, A. C., Jr., Poskanzer, D. C., and Young, R. R.: Amantadine in the treatment of Parkinson's disease, J.A.M.A. **208**: 1168, 1969.

33 Stern, J., and Ward, A.: Inhibition of the muscle spindle discharge by ventrolateral thalamic stimulation, Arch. Neurol. Psychiatry **3**:193, 1960.

34 Toman, J. E. P.: Some aspects of central nervous pharmacology, Annu. Rev. Pharmacol. **3**: 153, 1963.

REVIEWS

35 Greenblatt, D. J., and Shader, R. I.: Anticholinergics, N. Engl. J. Med. **288**:1215, 1973.

36 Lieberman, A., Estey, E., Kupersmith, M., Gopinathan, G., and Goldstein, M.: Treatment of Parkinson's disease with lergotrile mesylate, J.A.M.A. **238**:2380, 1977.

37 Schwartz, B.: The glaucomas, N. Engl. J. Med. **299**:182, 1978.

38 Yahr, M. D., editor: The basal ganglia. In Research publications: Association for Research in Nervous and Mental Disease, vol. 55, New York, 1976, Raven Press.

39 Yahr, M. D., and Duvoisin, R. C.: Drug therapy of parkinsonism, N. Engl. J. Med. **287**: 20, 1972.

CHAPTER 13

Ganglionic blocking agents

GENERAL CONCEPT

Ganglionic transmission can be blocked either by compounds that prevent the depolarizing actions of acetylcholine or by drugs that produce persistent depolarization. In concentrations that have little effect at other sites, the clinically useful ganglionic blocking agents prevent the actions of acetylcholine on ganglionic neurons.

In addition to the important nicotinic receptors, ganglionic neurons have muscarinic and α-adrenergic receptors. Blockade of these receptors has little effect on ganglionic transmission, since all useful ganglionic blocking agents act on the nicotinic receptors.

There are few uses for ganglionic blocking agents. **Trimethaphan** (Arfonad) is of value in producing controlled hypotensive states for surgery, and **mecamylamine hydrochloride** (Inversine) is used occasionally in hypertension.

GANGLIONIC STIMULANTS

Certain ganglionic stimulants such as tetramethylammonium, small doses of nicotine, and the experimental drug dimethylphenylpiperazinium (DMPP) will cause vasoconstriction and blood pressure elevations as a consequence of their stimulant action on ganglia. This type of drug effect has not yet found therapeutic applications. It should be remembered, however, that some of the drugs used in the diagnosis of pheochromocytoma (for example, methacholine) cause catecholamine release. This is analogous to ganglionic or adrenomedullary stimulation.

GANGLIONIC BLOCKING AGENTS

Development

The curious ability of nicotine to block ganglionic transmission following initial stimulation has been known for many years. During the latter part of the nineteenth century Langley made extensive use of the local application of nicotine for charting sympathetic ganglia in the cat and the distribution of the fibers emanating from them.

The ability of tetraethylammonium to block the effect of ganglionic stimulants was also known for many years. Such blocking agents received little attention, however, until 1946, when the mode of action of tetraethylammonium on the mammalian circulation was thoroughly investigated.[1] These studies suggested the possibility of blocking ganglionic transmission in a fairly selective manner.

A variety of ganglionic blocking agents were developed for practical use, particularly in treating hypertension and in producing controlled hypotension. Some of the most widely used compounds are hexamethonium, pentolinium, chlorisondamine, and trimethaphan camphorsulfonate. More recently, mecamylamine and pempidine have received clinical applications.

Chemistry   The chemical formulas of some of the ganglionic blocking agents are as follows:

$$(C_2H_5)_3N^+ —CH_2—CH_3 \cdot Cl^-$$

Tetraethylammonium chloride

$$N^+(CH_3)_3—CH_2—(CH_2)_4—CH_2—N^+(CH_3)_3 \cdot 2Cl^-$$

Hexamethonium chloride

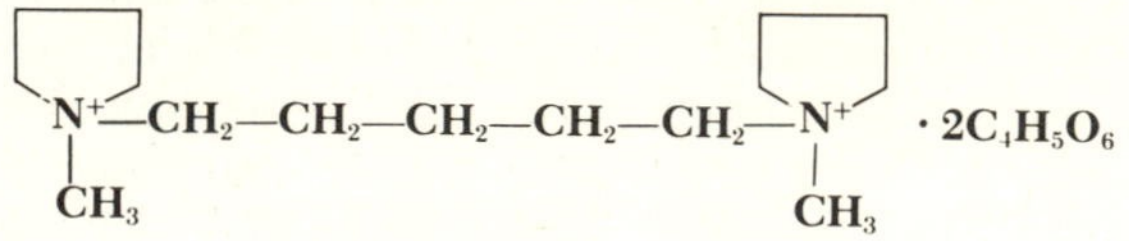

$$\overset{|}{\underset{CH_3}{N^+}}—CH_2—CH_2—CH_2—CH_2—CH_2—\overset{|}{\underset{CH_3}{N^+}} \cdot 2C_4H_5O_6$$

Pentolinium tartrate

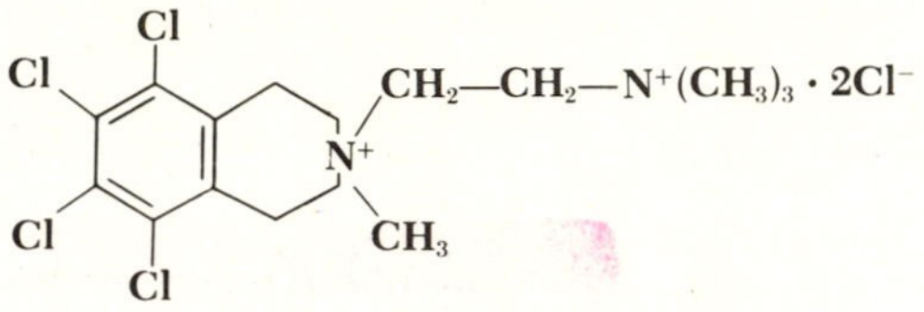

$$CH_2—CH_2—N^+(CH_3)_3 \cdot 2Cl^-$$

Chlorisondamine chloride

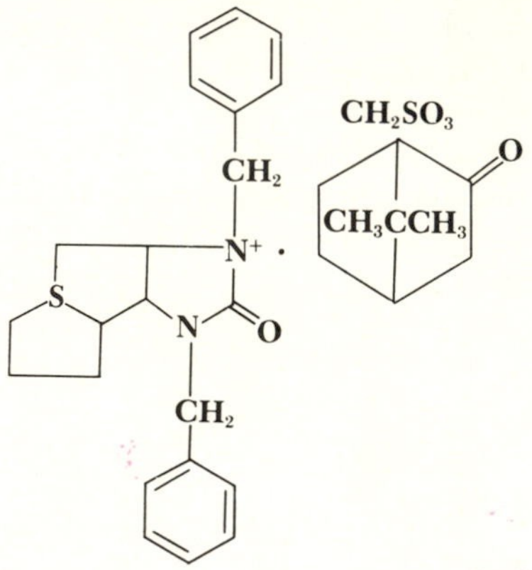

Trimethaphan camphorsulfonate

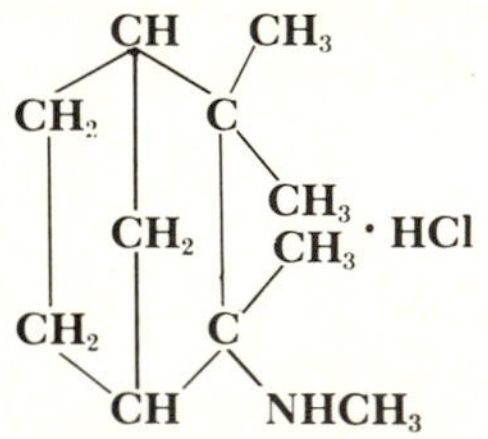

Mecamylamine hydrochloride 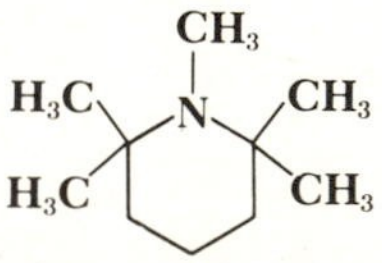   **Pempidine** 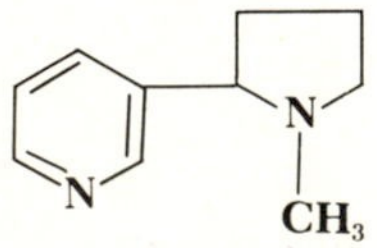   **Nicotine**

The majority of the ganglionic blocking drugs are quaternary ammonium compounds, just as acetylcholine has a quaternary nitrogen. Mecamylamine and pempidine, however, are not quaternary amines.

Clinical pharmacology

The pharmacological effects of the ganglionic blocking agents depend on the prevailing autonomic tone to an organ, since they block both sympathetic and parasympathetic ganglia.

The ganglionic blocking agents are used principally for decreasing the influence of the sympathetic division of the autonomic nervous system on the circulation. These compounds will also affect transmission across parasympathetic ganglia and can produce numerous side effects.

A very picturesque description of the actions of a typical ganglionic drug was given by Paton in his account of the "hexamethonium man."

(kiu) — wait in a line
vasodilitation

He is a pink complexioned person, except when he has stood in a queue for a long time,— when he may get pale and faint. His handshake is warm and dry. He is a placid and relaxed companion; for instance he may laugh, but he can't cry because the tears cannot come. Your rudest story will not make him blush, and the most unpleasant circumstances will fail to make him turn pale. His collars and socks stay very clean and sweet. He wears corsets and may, if — *anhidrosis* you meet him out, be rather fidgety (corsets to compress his splanchnic vascular pool, fidgety — *xerostomia* to keep the venous return going from his legs). He dislikes speaking much unless helped *mydriasis, cycloplegia* with something to moisten his dry mouth and throat. He is long-sighted and easily blinded by bright light. The redness of his eyeballs may suggest irregular habits and in fact his head is rather weak. But he always behaves like a gentleman and never belches nor hiccups. He *frostbite* tends to get cold and keeps well wrapped up. But his health is good; he does not have chil- blains and those diseases of modern civilization, hypertension and peptic ulcer, pass him by. He is thin because his appetite is modest; he never feels hunger pains and his stomach never— *↓ tone & motility* rumbles. He gets rather constipated so that his intake of liquid paraffin is high. As old age — *constipation* comes on, he will suffer from retention of urine and impotence, but frequency, precipitancy, — *urinary retention* and strangury will not worry him. One is uncertain how he will end, but perhaps if he is not careful, by eating less and less and getting colder and colder, he will sink into a symptomless, hypoglycemic coma and die, as was proposed for the universe, a sort of entropy death.*

difficulty in micturition

Circulatory effects. The ganglionic blocking drugs tend to lower blood pressure by decreasing sympathetic tone to various vascular areas. The intensity of this hypo- tensive action depends on a number of factors. First, the position of the patient has a great influence. There may be only slight lowering of the pressure while the patient is in the recumbent position. When the patient stands, however, the mean pressure may fall precipitously to the point of faintness. This is known as postural hypoten- sion and undoubtedly results from pooling of blood in the extremities in the absence of compensatory vasoconstriction there.

Side effects and complications. In addition to the unavoidable postural hypo- tension reflecting decreased sympathetic outflow, the ganglionic blocking drugs may produce side effects from blockade of parasympathetic ganglia.

The smooth muscle tone of the gastrointestinal and urinary tracts may be re- laxed by the ganglionic blocking agents, resulting in constipation or difficulty in voiding. As one might expect, the pupils may dilate and there can be interference with accommodation for near vision. Salivary secretion may be inhibited, and the resulting dry mouth may be sufficiently uncomfortable to require administration of pilocarpine. Sweating is also reduced, not by an atropine-like effect, but because of decreased sympathetic activity as a consequence of the ganglionic block.

Metabolism

The quaternary ammonium ganglionic blocking agents are poorly absorbed from the gastrointestinal tract. Drugs such as tetraethylammonium or trimethaphan cam- phorsulfonate cannot be used by mouth because of poor absorption. Although chlorisondamine and pentolinium are given by oral administration, their absorption is far from complete. The oral-intravenous LD_{50} ratio of these drugs in mice is about

---

*From Paton, W. D. M.: The principles of ganglionic block. In Scientific basis of medicine, vol. 2, London, 1954, Athlone Press.

20:1. On the other hand, the secondary amine, mecamylamine, is much better absorbed, giving an oral-intravenous LD_{50} ratio of about 4:1.[4]

The ganglionic blocking agents of the quaternary ammonium group are eliminated through renal excretion. Their distribution in the body is largely extracellular.

Differences among various ganglionic blocking agents

The various ganglionic blocking drugs differ with respect to potency, oral absorption, and duration of action.

Mecamylamine hydrochloride (Inversine) is a potent drug that is well absorbed from the gastrointestinal tract and has a duration of action of 4 to 12 hours. The initial oral dose is 2.5 mg twice daily. This dose is gradually increased until a satisfactory effect is obtained, usually at a dose level of 30 mg/day.

The drug may cause CNS stimulation and neuromuscular blockade in large doses.

Pempidine (Perolysen) is similar in action to mecamylamine. It is well absorbed from the gastrointestinal tract and is used in doses of 2.5 mg twice daily by mouth. In large doses it may cause CNS stimulation and neuromuscular blockade.

Hexamethonium (Methium), at the other end of the spectrum, is poorly and irregularly absorbed and is now obsolete.

Pentolinium (Ansolysen) is about five times as potent as hexamethonium in lowering blood pressure. The subcutaneous injection of 3 mg of pentolinium has about the same effect as 15 mg of hexamethonium by the same route.

Chlorisondamine (Ecolid) appears to be a potent ganglionic blocking agent that has a long duration of action. The recommended daily dose is about 100 to 200 mg, usually given in two doses (only by intravenous infusion).

Trimethaphan camphorsulfonate (Arfonad) is a very short-acting ganglionic blocking agent. It is chiefly used for producing controlled hypotension during special surgical operations. Although it is a potent histamine-releasing agent in dogs, no adverse effects that could be attributed to histamine release have occurred in human beings. Intravenous infusion of a solution containing 1 mg/ml will significantly lower blood pressure. When the infusion is stopped, blood pressure returns to its normal levels in about 5 minutes. Trimethaphan camsylate (Arfonad) is available as a 50 mg/ml solution that is diluted to 1 mg/ml for intravenous infusion.

REFERENCES

1 Acheson, G. H., and Moe, G. K.: The action of tetraethylammonium ion on the mammalian circulation, J. Pharmacol. Exp. Ther. **87:**220, 1946.
2 Aviado, D. M.: Hemodynamic effects of ganglion blocking drugs, Circ. Res. **8:**304, 1960.
2a Eränkö, O.: Small intensely fluorescent (SIF) cells and nervous transmission in sympathetic ganglia, Annu. Rev. Pharmacol. Toxicol. **18:**417, 1978.
3 Paton, W. D. M.: The principles of ganglionic block. In Scientific basis of medicine, vol. 2, London, 1954, Athlone Press.

4 Stone, C. A., Torchiana, M. L., Navarro, A., and Beyer, K. H.: Ganglionic blocking properties of 3-methylaminoisocamphane hydrochloride (mecamylamine): a secondary amine, J. Pharmacol. Exp. Ther. **117:**169, 1956.
5 Volle, R. L.: Modification by drugs of synaptic mechanisms in autonomic ganglia, Pharmacol. Rev. **18:**839, 1966.
6 Winbury, M. M.: Comparison of the vascular actions of 1-1-dimethyl-4-piperazinium (DMPP), a potent ganglionic stimulant, J. Physiol. **147:**1, 1959.

CHAPTER 14

Neuromuscular blocking agents and muscle relaxants

The clinically useful neuromuscular blocking drugs act postsynaptically by one of two major mechanisms: (1) competition with acetylcholine for the end-plate receptor (nondepolarizing blocking agents) and (2) initial depolarization followed by densensitization to the transmitter despite repolarization. An example of a nondepolarizing blocking agent is *d*-tubocurarine; succinylcholine acts by the second mechanism.

Skeletal muscle relaxation may be achieved by other mechanisms also. The centrally acting agents, such as mephenesin, meprobamate, and other antianxiety agents including diazepam, produce muscle relaxation by a primary action on the CNS. Finally, drugs such as dantrolene act on the skeletal muscle itself to cause relaxation.

In addition to the therapeutically useful muscle relaxants, many drugs cause disorders of neuromuscular transmission as an unwanted side effect. For example, antibiotics such as the aminoglycosides and polymyxins, local anesthetics, and others may cause postoperative respiratory depression or may aggravate myasthenia gravis.

Experimentation with the South American arrow poison, *curare*, was one of the earliest examples of scientific work in pharmacology. In the nineteenth century Magendie and his pupil Claude Bernard studied the effects of curare on nerve-muscle preparations. Claude Bernard was able to show that the drug prevented the response of the muscle to nerve stimulation. Surprisingly, it did not prevent the muscle from responding to direct stimulation, and it failed to block conduction in the nerve. It therefore seemed to exert its effect at the junction of nerve and muscle.

The active principle of *Chondodendron tomentosum* roots is *d*-tubocurarine, which has been isolated and its structure established.[5] It is a fairly large molecule in which two quaternary ammonium structures appear to be separated by an estimated distance of 14 Å, compared with the critical distance of 7 Å in acetylcholine.

The neuromuscular blocking agents are of two types: *nondepolarizing* and *depolarizing*. The nondepolarizing agents are *d*-tubocurarine, gallamine, benzoquinonium, and pancuronium. Depolarizing drugs are succinylcholine and decamethonium. This second category of drugs produces initial depolarization followed by desensitization of the receptors to acetylcholine.

GENERAL CONCEPT

NEUROMUSCULAR BLOCKING AGENTS
Development

The intravenous injection of 5 to 10 mg of *d*-tubocurarine produces flaccid paralysis of the extremities. Doubling these doses may produce apnea. The effects last for 10 minutes, with muscle strength returning in 40 minutes. There is a characteristic progression of effects, with the extrinsic muscles of the eye being affected first and then those of the face, the extremities, and finally the diaphragm.

The usual therapeutic doses of *d*-tubocurarine are unlikely to produce significant CNS action, since the blood-brain barrier represents a considerable defense against quaternary ammonium compounds. The beneficial effect on pain in certain clinical conditions is ascribed to the relaxation of contracted muscles and not to primary analgesic or hypnotic effect.

Drug interactions with nondepolarizing muscle relaxants such as *d*-tubocurarine are of great importance. General anesthetics such as ether, halothane, cyclopropane, and methoxyflurane intensify the action of nondepolarizing agents, making a reduction of their dosage necessary. Antibiotics such as neomycin, streptomycin, polymyxin B, colistin, kanamycin, and viomycin potentiate neuromuscular blockade. Quinine and quinidine also potentiate the action of neuromuscular blocking drugs. Anticholinesterase insecticides such as parathion, malathion, and tetraethyl pyrophosphate have some properties similar to those of the depolarizing blocking agents, and prolonged apnea may result when the patient exposed to such insecticides is treated with neuromuscular blocking drugs. Finally, patients with myasthenia gravis, acidosis, or severe renal disease react excessively to the usual doses of *d*-tubocurarine.

Adverse reactions to the nondepolarizing neuromuscular blocking drugs include prolonged apnea, bronchospasm, and hypotension, the last two being partly a consequence of histamine release.[18,22]Ganglionic blockade may contribute to the hypotension. Neostigmine and edrophonium (Tensilon) are antagonists of the early nondepolarizing actions of *d*-tubocurarine. Nevertheless, the most important antidotal measure is artificial respiration.

Mode of action   It is generally believed that acetylcholine is released from synaptic vesicles with passage of the nerve impulse.[6] The mediator produces a small electric charge known as the *end-plate potential*. Under normal circumstances this produces in turn the propagated *action potential*. In a partially curarized preparation the small end-plate potential is clearly visible, since it is not followed by the larger action potential. The effect of curare on the end-plate potential and the anticurare action of physostigmine are shown in Fig. 14-1.

The administration of the depolarizing agents results in muscle fasciculations as the initial response, whereas the competitive blocking agents do not have this effect.

Mixed block. Initial depolarization followed by block is referred to as mixed block.

When a depolarizing drug is applied to a muscle, the depolarization is not sustained but tends to fade.[30] It appears as if the acetylcholine receptors become in-

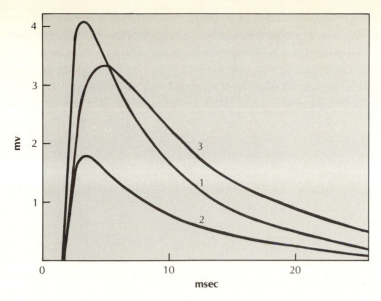

FIG. 14-1. Effect of curarine on the end-plate potential of the frog sartorius and the antagonistic action of physostigmine. *1*, After 6 μM of curarine; *2*, after 9 μM of curarine; *3*, after 9 μM of cu- plus physostigmine 10^{-5}. (From Eccles, J. C., et al.: J. Neurophysiol. **5:**211, 1942.)

active. The term "receptor inactivation" has been introduced to describe this phenomenon, which is probably of great importance in the second phase of the action of succinylcholine.

The various neuromuscular blocking agents differ with respect to potency, mode of action, and the nature of their side effects.

d-**Tubocurarine** is injected intravenously in the form of solutions containing 3 or 15 mg/ml. *d*-Tubocurarine chloride (Tubarine) is available for injection in a solution, 3 mg/ml. Its action is transient. About one-third of the amount administered is excreted unchanged in the urine, whereas the rest is metabolically altered. It is probably still the most important competitive neuromuscular blocking agent, although the newer **dimethyltubocurarine chloride** (Mecostrin) has a potency about three times as great. A solution of dimethyltubocurarine iodide (Metubine iodide), 2 mg/ml, is available for injection.

Differences among more common neuromuscular blocking agents

d-**Tubocurarine chloride**

Pancuronium dimethobromide is a recently introduced nondepolarizing neuro-muscular blocking agent that differs from *d*-tubocurarine in its greater potency and lack of histamine-releasing or ganglionic blocking actions. As indicated in its structural formula, the drug has a steroid nucleus with two quarternary amines attached. Its potency is such that, administered intravenously, 2 mg of pancuronium dimethobromide produces about the same effect as 10 to 15 mg of *d*-tubocurarine.[17]

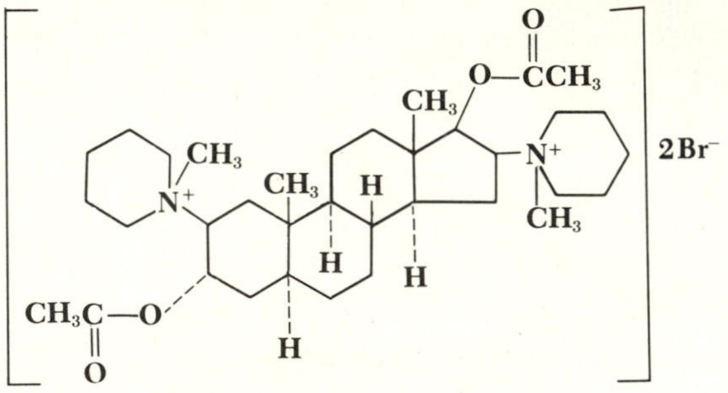

Pancuronium dimethobromide

Gallamine triethiodide (Flaxedil triethiodide) and **benzoquinonium** (Mytolon) are also neuromuscular blocking drugs of the competitive type. They have certain side effects that are not observed following the use of *d*-tubocurarine. Gallamine has an atropine-like effect on the cardiac branch of the vagus nerve and can produce considerable tachycardia.[23] Gallamine triethiodide is available in solutions for injection of 20 and 100 mg/ml. The actions of gallamine triethiodide are very similar to those of tubocurarine. It may have a slightly shorter duration of action, and it does not cause histamine release. This may be an advantage in asthmatic persons. On the other hand, its tendency to cause tachycardia by its vagolytic and perhaps catecholamine-releasing action may be a disadvantage in patients in whom tachycardia may represent a hazard.

Decamethonium bromide (Syncurine; C-10), one of the methonium compounds, is a depolarizing blocking agent that has been largely replaced by succinylcholine. Decamethonium bromide solution, 1 mg/ml, is available for injection.

$$Br^- \cdot N(CH_3)_3-(CH_2)_{10}-N^+(CH_3)_3 \cdot Br^-$$

Decamethonium bromide

It is interesting to note that the difference between this drug and hexamethonium consists of four additional methylene groups in decamethonium. This change in the distance between the two quaternary ammonium groups is sufficient to change the drug from a primary ganglionic blocking agent to one that is principally active on the neuromuscular junction.

Succinylcholine (Anectine) has the following structural formula:

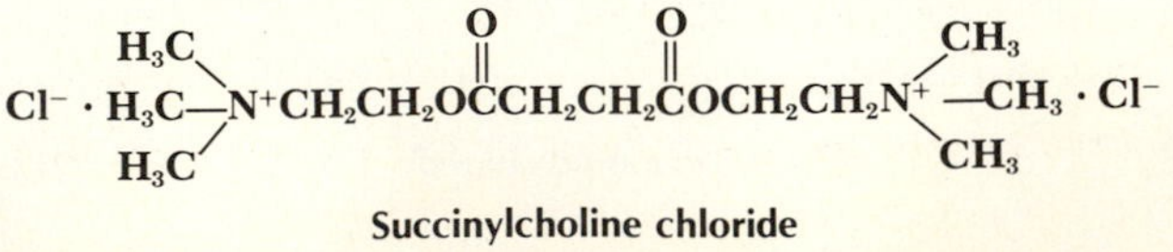

Succinylcholine chloride

When succinylcholine chloride, 0.5 to 1 mg/kg of body weight, is injected intravenously, there may be considerable muscular contraction for several seconds before paralysis develops. The muscles remain paralyzed for about 5 minutes and resume their function in another 5 minutes.

The drug has a selective action on the neuromuscular receptor sites, although in large doses it may cause some effects similar to those of acetylcholine on the heart and circulation.

The actions of succinylcholine are prevented by *d*-tubocurarine, whereas neostigmine is definitely not an antidote and may even aggravate the muscle paralysis caused by succinylcholine.

The short duration of action of succinylcholine may be attributed to its rapid metabolic degradation. The compound is hydrolyzed by plasma cholinesterase to succinylmonocholine and choline. In a second step, succinylmonocholine is hydrolyzed to succinic acid and choline by the cholinesterases.[11]

In some patients, succinylcholine has produced prolonged apnea caused by quantitative or qualitative differences in cholinesterase, a genetic abnormality (p. 64).

Succinylcholine is a valuable agent for producing short periods of muscular relaxation. It may be given in single intravenous doses or by intravenous infusion. Preparations of succinylcholine chloride (Anectine chloride) for injection include powder, 500 mg and 1 g, and solutions of 20, 50, and 100 mg/ml. Facilities for artificial respiration are essential, since this appears to be the only effective antidotal measure to apnea.

Usefulness

The greatest usefulness of the neuromuscular blocking agents is in anesthesia, in which they contribute to muscular relaxation. They also are employed for facilitating endotracheal intubation.

Succinylcholine is employed for protecting patients against severe convulsions in electroconvulsive therapy. Curare-like drugs have also been used in the treatment of tetanus, but they are not the drugs of choice for this condition.

SKELETAL MUSCLE DEPRESSANTS THAT ACT ON THE SPINAL CORD
Centrally acting skeletal muscle relaxants

In addition to those acting at the neuromuscular junction, other drugs can cause muscle relaxation by acting on internuncial spinal neurons to depress polysynaptic pathways (Fig. 14-2). These centrally acting muscle relaxants also act on higher centers and are commonly used as antianxiety agents. Although experimentally these drugs can depress the spinal cord at dose levels that do not cause sleep or anesthesia, in clinical practice it is difficult to say how much of their muscle-relaxing power is simply a consequence of the antianxiety effects. Although some drugs in this series are promoted as centrally acting muscle relaxants, others almost identical in structure are widely used for thier antianxiety properties.

Indications for these drugs include the treatment of muscle spasm resulting from sprains, arthritis, myositis, and fibrositis. Drugs in this group can cause adverse effects such as drowsiness, lethargy and ataxia, allergic manifestations, and psychic dependence, particularly to the meprobamate and chlordiazepoxide group of compounds.

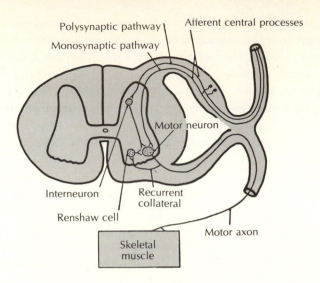

FIG. 14-2. Innervation of skeletal muscle.

Mephenesin

Mephenesin carbamate

Methocarbamol

Meprobamate

Carisoprodol

Zoxazolamine

Chlormezanone

Chlorzoxazone

Mephenesin and mephenesin carbamate. These propanediol derivatives were the first drugs introduced as centrally acting muscle relaxants. Their selective action on spinal neurons was shown by abolition of strychnine convulsions in animals at dose levels that, in contrast to general anesthetics, did not cause sleep. These drugs are rather weak and must be given in large doses to obtain an effect. Preparations for mephenesin (Tolserol) include tablets, 500 mg, and elixir, 500 mg/5 ml. Mephenesin carbamate (Tolseram) is available in tablets, 500 mg, and elixir, 1 g/5 ml.

Methocarbamol. Closely related to mephenesin carbamate, the drug has the same indication, uses, and limitations. Methocarbamol (Robaxin) is available in tablets, 500 and 750 mg, and, for injection, in solution of 100 mg/ml in 50% polyethylene glycol.

Chlorphenesin carbamate. This drug is closely related to mephenesin and has the same moderate effectiveness as a centrally acting muscle relaxant. Chlorphenesin carbamate (Maolate) is available in tablets, 400 mg.

Meprobamate. Another drug closely related to mephenesin, this propanediol has become extremely popular as a so-called minor tranquilizer. Its use and abuse are discussed on p. 290. Preparations of meprobamate (Miltown; Equanil) include capsules and tablets containing 200 and 400 mg.

Carisoprodol. Closely related to meprobamate, this drug has some limited usefulness in the treatment of muscle spasms. Preparations of carisoprodol (Soma) include tablets, 350 mg, and capsules, 250 mg.

Benzoxazole derivatives. The centrally acting muscle relaxants zoxazolamine (Flexin) and chlorzoxazone (Paraflex) were developed on the basis of the observation that benzimidazole had depressant effects on polysynaptic pathways of the spinal cord. Zoxazolamine turned out to be hepatotoxic and was removed from the market. The closely related chlorzoxazone has some usefulness in muscle spasms caused by neurological diseases. It also may cause jaundice in an occasional patient. It is available in tablets, 500 mg.

Chlormezanone. Chlormezanone (Trancopal) is used more as an antianxiety agent and has no specific effects on muscle rigidity. It is available in tablets, 100 and 200 mg.

Metaxalone. Chemically unrelated to the propanediols, this drug is 5-[3,5,(-dimethylphenoxyl)methyl]-2-oxazolidinone. Its usefulness in spastic conditions is probably related to its sedative effect. Metaxalone (Skelaxin) is available in tablets, 400 mg.

The diazepoxides. Chlordiazepoxide (Librium) and diazepam (Valium) are generally viewed as antianxiety agents and are discussed in Chapter 24. These drugs may be useful for reducing spasm in musculoskeletal disorders and may be considered as centrally acting skeletal muscle relaxants. They are available in tablet form and also as injectable solutions.

Baclofen. Baclofen (Lioresal) is a new skeletal muscle relaxant related to GABA (γ-aminobutyric acid). It appears to be useful in muscle spasm associated with multiple sclerosis and may be of value in conditions related to spinal cord injuries. Baclofen is 4-amino-3 (p-chlorophenyl) butyric acid. It is supplied in tablets, 10 mg.

Cyclobenzaprine. Cyclobenzaprine hydrochloride (Flexeril) is chemically and pharmacologically related to the tricyclic antidepressants. It is indicated for the short-term treatment of acute, painful musculoskeletal conditions. The drug has numerous side effects just as the tricyclic antidepressants. It should not be used in patients receiving MAO inhibitors. Cyclobenzaprine hydrochloride is available in tablets, 10 mg.

Dantrolene: a new approach to spasticity. Dantrolene sodium (Dantrium) is a new hydantoin derivative that acts on the skeletal muscle beyond the neuromuscular junction. The drug may act by interfering with the release of calcium.[8,9] Although quite new, dantrolene has produced some improvement in patients with strokes, multiple sclerosis,[13] and postencephalitic athetosis and dystonia.

The drug is useful in the treatment of anesthetic-induced malignant hyperthermia probably because it uncouples excitation and contraction in skeletal muscle by interfering with calcium release from the sarcoplasmic reticulum.

Dantrolene may cause numerous serious reactions and side effects. When used chronically, hepatic damage, seizures, pleural effusion with pericarditis, and skin reactions suggesting hypersensitivity have been noted. Gastrointestinal, neurological, psychiatric, and cardiovascular adverse effects have also been reported.

The starting dose in adults is 25 mg twice a day orally. This dosage may have to be increased gradually to a maximum of 400 mg daily. Beneficial effects may require treatment for a week. Dantrolene sodium (Dantrium Intravenous) is available in vials containing 20 mg of the drug. It is indicated, along with other supportive measures, for the management of malignant hyperthermia crisis.

REFERENCES

1 Beecher, H. K., and Todd, D. P.: A study of the deaths associated with anesthesia and surgery, based on a study of 599,548 anesthesias in ten institutions, Ann. Surg. **140**:2, 1954.

2 Berger, F. M.: Spinal cord depressant drugs, Pharmacol. Rev. **1**:243, 1949.

3 Bridenbaugh, P. O., and Churchill-Davidson, H. C.: Response to tubocurarine chloride and its reversal by neostigmine methylsulfate in man, J.A.M.A. **203**:541, 1968.

4 Comroe, J. H., Jr., and Dripps, R. D.: The histamine-like action of curare and tubocurarine injected intracutaneously and intaarterially in man, Anesthesiology **7**:260, 1946.

5 Dutcher, J. D.: The isolation and identification of additional physiologically active alkaloids in extracts of Chondodendron tomentosum ruiz and pavon, Ann. N.Y. Acad. Sci. **54**:326, 1951.

6 Eccles, J. C.: The physiology of nerve cells, Baltimore, 1957, The Johns Hopkins University Press.

7 Ehrenpreis, S.: The interaction of quaternary ammonium ions with various macromolecules, Georgetown Med Bull. **16**:148, 1963.

8 Ellis, K. O., and Bryant, S. H.: Excitation-contraction uncoupling in skeletal muscle by dantrolene sodium, Naunym-Schmiedebergs Arch. Pharmacol. **274**:107, 1972.

9 Ellis, K. O., and Carpenter, J. F.: Studies on the mechanism of action of dantrolene sodium, a skeletal muscle relaxant, Naunyn-Schmiedebergs Arch. Pharmacol. **275**:83, 1972.

10 Foldes, F. F.: The mode of action of quaternary ammonium type neuromuscular blocking agents, Br. J. Anesth. **26**:394, 1954.

11 Foldes, F. F., Vandervort, R. S., and Shanor, S. P.: The fate of succinylcholine in man, Anesthesiology **16**:11, 1955.

12 Friend, D. G.: Pharmacology of muscle relaxants, Clin. Pharmacol. Ther. **5**:871, 1964.

13 Gelenberg, A. J., and Poskanzer, D. C.: The effect of dantrolene sodium on spasticity in multiple sclerosis, Neurology **23**:1313, 1973.

14 Griffith, H. R., and Johnson, G. E.: The use of curare in general anesthesia, Anesthesiology **3**:418, 1942.

15 Henneman, E., Kaplan, A., and Unna, K.: A neuropharmacological study on the effect of

myanesin (Tolserol) on motor systems, J. Pharmacol. Exp. Ther. **97:**331, 1949.

16 Karczmar, A. G.: Neuromuscular pharmacology, Annu. Rev. Pharmacol. **7:**241, 1967.

17 Kariss, J. H., and Gissen, A. J.: Evaluation of new neuromuscular blocking agents, Anesthesiology **35:**149, 1971.

18 Mongar, J. L., and Whelan, R. F.: Histamine release by adrenaline and *d*-tubocurarine in the human subject, J. Physiol. **120:**146, 1953.

19 Paton, W. D. M.: A theory of drug action based on the rate of drug-receptor combination, Proc. R. Soc. Biol. **154:**21, 1961.

20 Riker, W. F.: Pharmacologic considerations in a reevaluation of the neuromuscular synapse, Arch. Neurol. **3:**488, 1960.

21 Riker, W. F., and Okamoto, M.: Pharmacology of motor nerve terminals, Annu. Rev. Pharmacol. **9:**173, 1969.

22 Riker, W. F., and Wescoe, W. C.: The pharmacology of Flaxedil, with observations on certain analogs, Ann. N.Y. Acad. Sci. **54:**373, 1951.

23 Salem, M. R., Kim, Y., and El Etr, A. A.: Histamine release following the intravenous injection of *d*-tubocurarine, Anesthesiology **29:**380, 1968.

24 Thesleff, S.: The mode of neuromuscular block caused by acetylcholine, nicotine, decamethonium, and succinylcholine, Acta Physiol. Scand. **34:**218, 1955.

25 Thesleff, S., and Quastel, D. M. J.: Neuromuscular pharmacology, Annu. Rev. Pharmacol. **5:**263, 1965.

26 Van Winkle, W. B.: Calcium release from skeletal muscle sarcoplasmic reticulum: site of action of dantrolene sodium? Science **193:**1130, 1976.

REVIEWS

27 Argov, Z., and Mastaglia, F. L.: Disorders of neuromuscular transmission caused by drugs, N. Engl. J. Med. **301:**409, 1979.

27a Baclofen (Lioresal): new muscle relaxant for multiple sclerosis, Med. Lett. **20:**43, 1978.

28 Galindo, A.: The role of prejunctional effects in myoneural transmission, Anesthesiology **36:**598, 1972.

29 Herman, R., Mayer, N., and Mecomber, S. A.: Clinical pharmaco-physiology of dantrolene sodium, Am. J. Phys. Med. **51:**296, 1972.

30 Hubbard, J. I., and Quastel, D. M. J.: Micropharmacology of vertebrate neuromuscular transmission, Annu. Rev. Pharmacol. **13:**199, 1973.

CHAPTER 15

Adrenergic (sympathomimetic) drugs

The adrenergic or sympathomimetic drugs comprise a large group of compounds that act *directly* on adrenergic receptors or that release catecholamines from nerve endings and thus act *indirectly*. Some of these drugs have a *mixed effect*, acting directly on receptors and also releasing the catecholamines.

The adrenergic group includes the endogenous biogenic amines norepinephrine, epinephrine, dopamine, and the related synthetic catecholamines, such as isoproterenol. It also includes ephedrine and miscellaneous adrenergic vasoconstrictors, bronchodilators, CNS stimulants, and anorexiants.

The effect of these drugs can be predicted from a knowledge of (1) the type of adrenergic receptor with which they interact, (2) the direct, indirect, or mixed nature of their action, and (3) their penetration or lack of penetration into the CNS.

CATECHOLAMINES

Norepinephrine, epinephrine, and dopamine are the endogenous catecholamines, whereas isoproterenol is a synthetic, chemically related analog. These substances are termed *catecholamines* because their structure consists of catechol (*o*-dihydroxybenzene) and an amino group on the side chain.

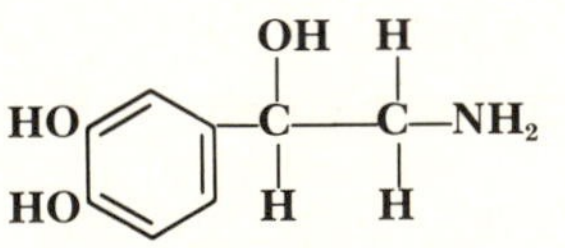

Norepinephrine

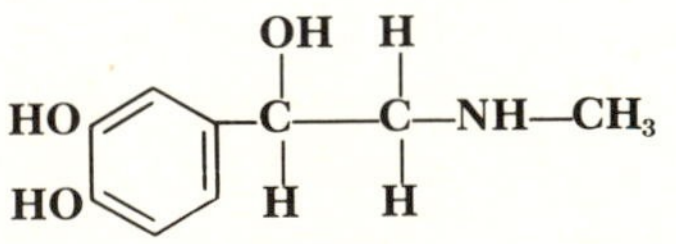

Epinephrine

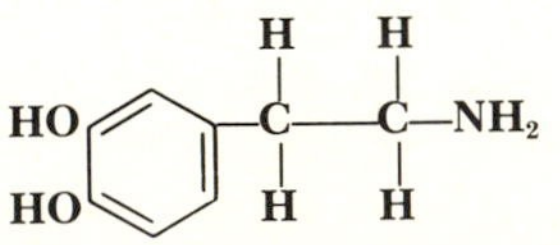

Dopamine

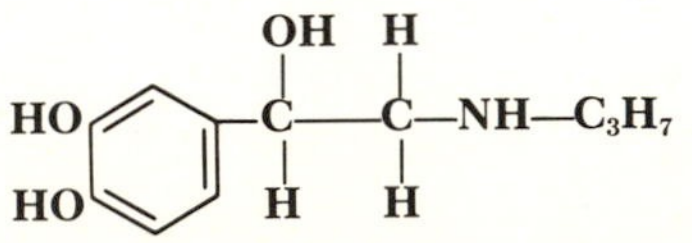

Isoproterenol

As shown in their structural formulas, epinephrine differs from norepinephrine in having a methyl group on the nitrogen, isoproterenol has an isopropyl group on the nitrogen, and dopamine lacks the β-hydroxyl on the side chain. The prefix *nor-* in norepinephrine is derived from German chemical terminology. It is the abbreviation of *Nitrogen ohne Radikal,* which means nitrogen without radical.

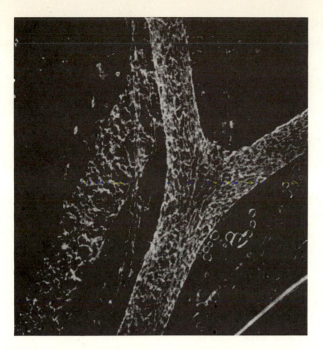

FIG. 15-1. Fluorescent adrenergic terminals around small arteries and a vein in the rat mesentery. (From Falck, B.: Acta Physiol. Scand. **56**[Supp. 197]:19, 1962.)

The presence of norepinephrine in adrenergic nerve fibers was demonstrated by von Euler in 1946.[22] It had been suspected that the "sympathin" released following adrenergic nerve stimulation was norepinephrine.

The relationship between adrenergic nerves and blood vessels and the presence of catecholamines in the nerves is strikingly demonstrated by the fluorescence technique of the Swedish investigators Falck, Hillarp, and Carlsson, as shown in Fig. 15-1.

Epinephrine is highly concentrated in the granules of the adrenal medulla. It is also present in many other organs, probably in chromaffin cells. Sympathetic denervation affects the norepinephrine content of an organ without a significant decrease in epinephrine concentration. From this observation it is suspected that epinephrine is present in chromaffin cells, which have nothing to do with adrenergic innervation.[22]

The adrenal medullary granules and probably the adrenergic axonal vesicles contain catecholamines along with adenosine triphosphate in the proportion of 4:1. They also contain a special soluble protein, *chromogranin*, and the enzyme dopamine-β-oxidase.

In the human adrenal medulla, norepinephrine may represent as much as 20% of the total catecholamine content. It may constitute a much higher percentage in the adrenal medulla of the newborn infant and in tumors of the adrenal medulla.

Occurrence and physiological functions

The main functions of norepinephrine appear to be the maintenance of normal sympathetic tone and adjustment of circulatory dynamics. Epinephrine appears to be the great emergency hormone that stimulates metabolism and promotes blood flow to skeletal muscles, preparing the individual for "fight or flight."

Dopamine is localized in certain areas of the CNS where it serves as an important transmitter. Dopamine is also the precursor of norepinephrine and epinephrine at other sites. The role of dopamine in Parkinson's disease and in the actions of psychoactive drugs is discussed on pp. 157 and 277.

Pharmacological actions

The catecholamines act directly on adrenergic and dopaminergic receptors. An understanding of their effects requires knowledge of present concepts of the adrenergic and dopaminergic receptors.

Adrenergic and dopaminergic receptors. The classification of adrenergic receptors as *alpha* (α) and *beta* (β), originally proposed by Ahlquist[3] in 1948, is now generally accepted. The concept was based on the order of activity of a series of sympathomimetic drugs at various effector sites and was greatly strengthened when specific blocking agents were developed for each receptor. As shown in Table 15-1, the functions associated with α receptors are vasoconstriction, mydriasis, and intestinal relaxation. β receptors mediate adrenergic influences for vasodilatation, cardioacceleration, bronchial relaxation, positive inotropic effect, and intestinal relaxation.

TABLE 15-1. Receptors mediating various adrenergic drug effects*

Effector organ	Receptor	Response
Heart		
Sinoatrial node	β	Tachycardia
Atrioventricular node	β	Increase in conduction rate and shortening of functional refractory period
Atrial and ventricles	β	Increased contractility
Blood vessels		
To skeletal muscle	α and β	Contraction or relaxation
To skin	α	Contraction
Bronchial muscle	β	Relaxation
Gastrointestinal smooth muscle		
To stomach	β	Decreased motility
To intestine	α and β	Decreased motility
Gastrointestinal sphincters		
To stomach	α	Contraction
To intestine	α	Contraction
Urinary bladder		
Detrusor	β	Relaxation
Trigone and sphincter	α	Contraction
Eye		
Radial muscle, iris	α	Contraction (mydriasis)
Ciliary muscle	β	Relaxation

*Based on data from Epstein, S. E., and Braunwald, E.: N. Engl. J. Med. **275:**1106, 1966.

These adrenergic receptors are on postsynaptic elements. In recent years there has developed evidence for the presence of adrenergic receptors on adrenergic neuron terminals, their function being to modulate norepinephrine release from the neurons.[46,69] The evidence for the presence of presynaptic α receptors is especially strong. The modulation system may be a further control in regulating the amount of transmitter at an effector cell.

Metabolic effects of the catecholamines, such as glycogenolysis and fatty acid release, are largely β functions. Insulin release is promoted by drugs acting on β receptors, whereas release tends to be inhibited by α-receptor agonists.[64]

Norepinephrine acts on both α and β receptors. Epinephrine also acts on both receptors, but its β effects predominate. Isoproterenol is a pure β agonist and its actions are blocked by propranolol, a β-adrenergic blocking agent. Other drugs such as methoxamine and phenylephrine act on α receptors, and their effects are blocked by phenoxybenzamine or by phentolamine, both α-adrenergic blocking agents. Thus we have a graduation from pure α agonists to pure β agonists.

β Receptors are of two types: β_1 and β_2. Lands[45] termed β_1 the receptors responsible for cardiac stimulation and also lipolysis. The β_2 receptors mediate adrenergic bronchodilatation and vasodepression. The β_2 agonists are especially useful in the treatment of asthma (p. 191) because they produce bronchodilatation without much cardiac stimulation.

The nomenclature, α_1, and α_2, is sometimes used, but in this case the differentiation refers to the localization of the α receptor, α_1 referring to postsynaptic and α_2 referring to presynaptic localization.

Although dopamine acts on cardiac β receptors and also on vascular α receptors (in larger doses), some of its vasodilator effects suggest the existence of specific dopamine receptors.[80] Dopamine produces vasodilatation in the renal, mesenteric, coronary, and intracerebral arteries. This action is not antagonized by propranolol but is selectively attenuated by haloperidol and the phenothiazines. The dopaminergic receptors are probably present not only in certain vascular beds but also in the basal ganglia and some other parts of the CNS (p. 117).

In recent years the development of adrenergic radioligand binding techniques has permitted direct studies of the molecular properties of α and β receptors as well as the mechanisms of physiological and pathological receptor alterations.[83a] The techniques also permit the quantitation of receptors in isolated tissues.

Norepinephrine and epinephrine

The various aspects of the pharmacology of norepinephrine (levarterenol; Levophed) and epinephrine (adrenaline) will be discussed first, followed by those of dopamine, ephedrine, and other adrenergic, sympathomimetic drugs.

The differences between the pharmacological effects of norepinephrine and epinephrine are a consequence of the generally greater influence of norepinephrine on α receptors, whereas epinephrine has a stronger action on β receptors. Nevertheless, both drugs have effects on both receptors.

Cardiovascular effects   The actions of norepinephrine and epinephrine on the cardiovascular system may be quite different when both drugs are administered in small doses. They are not very different if large unphysiological doses are used.

Net effects of small doses in humans. When norepinephrine is infused intravenously into a normal person, it is generally given in a solution containing 4 mg of the drug in 1 L of isotonic fluid. If this solution containing 4 μg/ml is infused at such a rate that the patient receives about 10 μg/min, the hemodynamic changes listed in Table 15-2 will be observed. If a similar infusion of epinephrine were to be given to an individual, the changes listed in Table 15-3 would generally be observed. The differences in heart rate elicited by the two drugs are illustrated in Fig. 15-2.

The difference between the circulatory effects of epinephrine and norepinephrine reflects their different potency at various sites within the cardiovascular system. Norepinephrine has widespread vasoconstrictor properties, whereas epinephrine constricts some vascular areas and dilates others. The blood pressure elevation produced by norepinephrine brings into play reflexes that will cause bradycardia, which can be eliminated by the administration of atropine.

Epinephrine, on the other hand, stimulates the heart, and since there is no elevation of mean pressure, no reflex mechanisms come into play to slow the heart. The differences observed in humans following the infusion of dilute solutions of the two drugs may be attributed to their different peripheral actions, which affect the heart through reflex mechanisms.

Response of heart and various vascular areas. The actions of epinephrine on the heart consist of increased rate,* increased force of contraction, increased irritability, and increased coronary blood flow.

---

*Heart rate may be decreased by epinephrine as a consequence of reflex vagal activity, which can be blocked by atropine.

TABLE 15-2. Cardiovascular effects of small dose of norepinephrine in humans

Systolic pressure	Increased
Diastolic pressure	Increased
Mean pressure	Increased
Heart rate	Slightly decreased
Cardiac output	Slightly decreased
Peripheral resistance	Increased

TABLE 15-3. Cardiovascular effects of small dose of epinephrine in humans

Systolic pressure	Increased
Diastolic pressure	Decreased (increased by large dose)
Heart rate	Increased
Mean pressure	Unchanged
Cardiac output	Increased
Peripheral resistance	Decreased

Norepinephrine has cardiac accelerator action also, but this inherent chronotropic effect is opposed by reflex slowing secondary to vasoconstriction and elevated blood pressure.

The increased coronary blood flow following the injection of epinephrine is largely a result of the increased cardiac work and metabolism. It has no usefulness in relieving precordial pain and may even precipitate anginal attacks in patients with coronary atherosclerosis.

The differences between epinephrine and norepinephrine tend to disappear when they are injected in large doses. Under these circumstances both will elevate

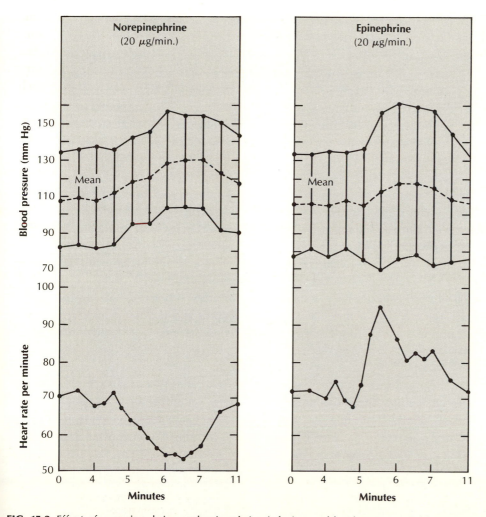

FIG. 15-2. Effect of norepinephrine and epinephrine infusion on blood pressure and heart rate in humans. Note increased mean pressure and decreased heart rate following infusion of norepinephrine and also essentially unchanged mean pressure, increase in pulse pressure, and elevated heart rate following infusion of epinephrine. (From Barcroft, H., and Konzett, H.: Lancet **1:**147, 1949.)

diastolic pressure, increase peripheral resistance, and reduce blood flow through skeletal muscles.[28]

The effects of epinephrine on renal hemodynamics have received considerable attention. It is generally accepted that the drug decreases renal plasma flow but does not influence glomerular filtration, the net effect being an increased filtration fraction.[58] Large doses of epinephrine, however, may decrease the filtration fraction by stopping blood flow through some nephrons.

Cerebral blood flow is affected in a complex manner by norepinephrine and epinephrine. Through their direct action these drugs cause constriction of the cerebral vessels. The elevation of systemic pressure, however, can oppose this direct action to such an extent that no significant change in cerebral blood flow may occur.

Bronchodilator effect

Epinephrine is a dilator of the bronchial smooth muscle; norepinephrine is a much weaker dilator on this particular effector, whereas isoproterenol is a more active bronchodilator than epinephrine. The bronchodilator effect is not important when these drugs are administered to a normal individual. It becomes prominent when the bronchi are constricted by some pharmacological agent such as histamine or methacholine or in disease states such as bronchial asthma. Epinephrine is a time-honored remedy in the latter condition.

Other smooth muscle effects

Under special circumstances epinephrine causes mydriasis by contracting the radial muscle of the iris. This effect does not usually occur with direct application of the drug, but cocaine sensitizes the radial muscle to topically applied epinephrine. Norepinephrine has less effect on the eye.

The capsule of the spleen is contracted by epinephrine in some animals such as the dog. It is questionable that this effect occurs in humans.

The catecholamines have some slight inhibitory actions on the gastrointestinal smooth muscle. This action has little physiological and no therapeutic importance. The same may be said for the complex and variable effects of epinephrine on the uterus.

Neural actions

It is believed at present that injected catecholamines do not cross the blood-brain barrier efficiently. Alterations in norepinephrine content in the CNS may be associated with altered brain function and behavior, but injected catecholamines do not exert prominent effects. Nevertheless, the injection of epinephrine into normal humans produces anxiety and weakness.

Certain adrenergic drugs such as amphetamine have a marked stimulant action on the CNS.

Metabolic actions

Oxygen consumption may be increased by 25% following the injection of a therapeutic dose of epinephrine. Norepinephrine has considerably weaker effects on both oxygen consumption and lactic acid production in man.

Epinephrine and isoproterenol, and to a lesser degree norepinephrine, exert complex effects on carbohydrate metabolism. They elevate blood sugar by glycogenolysis and also inhibit glucose utilization.[19] By stimulating glycogenolysis, glucose is released from the liver and lactic acid from muscle. The influence on phosphorylase has been studied extensively by Sutherland and Rall.[71-73] It appears that epinephrine in many tissues promotes the formation of a cyclic adenylic acid, adenosine-3',5'-monophosphate.

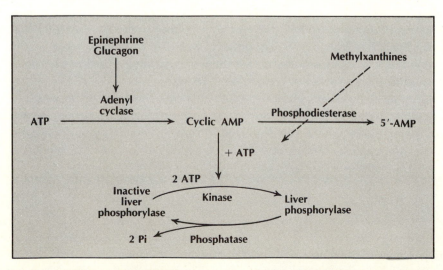

Adenosine-3',5'-monophosphate
(cyclic adenylic acid)

The formation of cyclic adenylate and some of its functions are shown in Fig. 15-3.

Catecholamines promote the release of fatty acids from adipose tissue and elevate the level of unesterified fatty acids in the blood. Thus the sympathetic nervous system, through catecholamine release, provides not only glucose but also free fatty acids as energy sources. The important effect on fatty acid release can be blocked by adrenergic blocking agents.

Marked elevations of plasma potassium may occur following the injection of epinephrine. It is believed that the source of this potassium is the liver.

FIG. 15-3. Cyclic AMP and phosphorylase activation. Site of action of epinephrine, glucagon, and methylxanthines. (From Butcher, R. W.: N. Engl. J. Med. **279:**1378, 1968.)

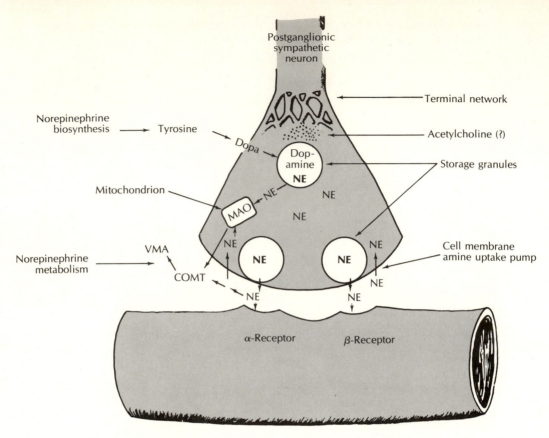

FIG. 15-4. Norepinephrine metabolism in the postganglionic sympathetic neuron. (From Abrams, W. B.: Dis. Chest **55**:148, 1969.)

Biosynthesis   Catecholamines are made in the body from tyrosine through a series of steps involving dopa (3,4-dihydroxyphenylalanine), dopamine, norepinephrine, and finally epinephrine (p. 125). It is believed that these catecholamines are synthesized at the sites at which they are stored prior to their release.

The steps in the synthesis of norepinephrine by sympathetic nerves are shown in Fig. 15-4. Norepinephrine synthesis varies directly in relation to nerve stimulation. Catecholamine synthesis is regulated by *tyrosine hydroxylase*, the rate-limiting enzyme. An inhibitor of tyrosine hydroxylase, α-methyltyrosine, blocks the increased catecholamine synthesis that results from nerve stimulation.

There is much evidence to indicate that norepinephrine inhibits tyrosine hydroxylase.[76] Thus the regulation of norepinephrine synthesis in adrenergic nerves is achieved by end-product inhibition.

Termination of action   The termination of action of norepinephrine and epinephrine is largely a consequence of reuptake by adrenergic nerves. This reuptake is achieved by an amine

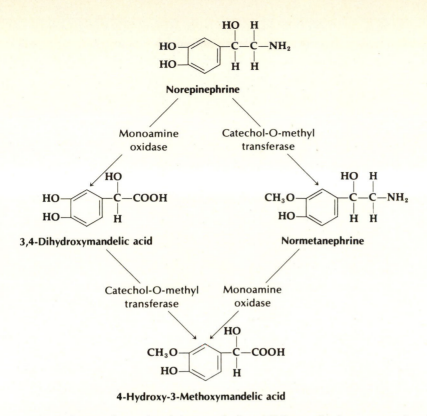

FIG. 15-5. Major pathways of norepinephrine metabolism. MAO actually changes norepinephrine and normetanephrine to the corresponding mandelic aldehydes. These products are then transformed to mandelic acids by aldehyde dehydrogenase. (For other details see text.)

pump in the nerve membrane that requires sodium and is inhibited by cocaine, the tricyclic antidepressants (such as desipramine), and also ouabain. That portion of norepinephrine and epinephrine that escapes the reuptake is attacked by the enzymes catechol-O-methyltransferase (COMT) and MAO (Fig. 15-5).

The normal urinary excretion of catecholamines and metabolites in man is as follows:

Norepinephrine + Epinephrine	1.1%
Normetanephrine + Metanephrine	7.6%
4-Hydroxy-3-methoxymandelic acid (VMA)	91%

The 24-hour VMA excretion in normal individuals is 10 mg. Much larger amounts may be excreted by patients with adrenal medullary tumors (p. 188).

A number of experimental facts suggest that uptake of catecholamines by nerves is the most important mechanism for the termination of the action of catecholamines. First, the injection of small physiological doses of tritiated norepinephrine results in its rapid clearance from the blood by the heart and other organs innervated by adrenergic fibers.[31] That this uptake is in adrenergic fibers has been demonstrated by histochemical techniques in vitro.[4] Furthermore, sympathetic nerve stimulation or reserpine treatment causes release of tritiated catecholamine.

Denervated structures take up only very small quantities of tritiated norepinephrine. Such structures, of course, are supersensitive to the action of catecholamines. Cocaine, imipramine, and certain antihistaminics[37] block the uptake of norepinephrine and potentiate the action of catecholamines. These relationships may become clear by an examination of Fig. 15-6 (see also p. 127).

The neuronal uptake of norepinephrine is often referred to as uptake$_1$.[81] In addition, there is a second uptake system in various smooth muscles and glandular tissues, called *uptake$_2$*. The significance of uptake$_2$ is not at all clear. It is not blocked by cocaine or desipramine.

The amine pump and false transmitters

The relatively nonspecific amine pump of the adrenergic neuron transports not only catecholamines but also tyramine, metaraminol,[68] α-methylnorepinephrine, and even serotonin. Some of these, such as metaraminol, may be held by the axon terminal and released on nerve stimulation, thereby acting as *false transmitters*.[15] The antihypertensive drug α-methyldopa is taken up by the neuron and transformed to α-methylnorepinephrine, which also acts as a false transmitter when released. A hypotensive action may result in part from the lower potency of the false transmitters compared with norepinephrine, which they displace.

Despite the low specificity of the amine pump, the adrenergic neuron is protected against the accumulation of all sorts of amines by the much greater specificity of the granular storage mechanism. Thus when tyramine is taken up, it is not only deaminated by MAO but the amine is also rejected by the granules, since only

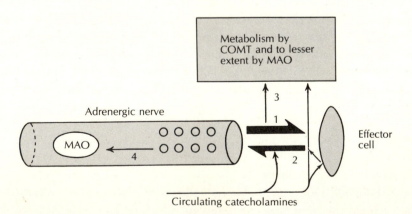

FIG. 15-6. Fate of norepinephrine released from adrenergic nerve. *1*, Release and interaction with receptor on effector cell; *2*, reuptake into the nerve of a portion of released norepinephrine; *3*, metabolism by COMT and to a lesser extent by MAO; *4*, metabolic degradation within the nerve by MAO of norepinephrine released within the axoplasm (such as following ingestion of reserpine).

β-hydroxylated amines are held there. After the use of MAO inhibitors, however, tyramine, which is protected against deamination, is transformed by the fairly non-specific dopamine-β-oxidase into the β-hydroxy derivative *octopamine*, which can be stored in the granules and acts as a false transmitter. The hypotensive action of MAO inhibitors has been attributed to this mechanism,[82] although the explanation is not entirely satisfying.

Adrenergic nerve terminals can take up compounds that may be injurious to them. The experimental drug *6-hydroxydopamine* causes degenerative changes in adrenergic nerve terminals,[74] leading to *chemical sympathectomy*. Desipramine, a known blocker of the amine pump, prevents these effects.[52]

The therapeutic uses of epinephrine and norepinephrine are based on the vasoconstrictor, cardiac stimulant and bronchodilator properties of these compounds.

Therapeutic applications

Vasoconstrictor uses. Epinephrine is commonly added to local anesthetic solutions because its vasoconstrictor action delays the absorption of the local anesthetic and thereby restricts its effect to a given area. Because of its vasoconstrictor ability, epinephrine is widely used in the treatment of urticaria and angioneurotic edema.

Norepinephrine (Levophed) infusions have been widely used in the management of hypotension and shock. The initial enthusiasm decreased considerably once it was realized that in shock there is already a greatly increased sympathetic activity and that correction of underlying abnormalities such as decreased blood volume or fluid balance disturbances is more important.

Cardiac uses. Either epinephrine or the newer drug isoproterenol is indicated in the management of heart block or Adams-Stokes syndrome. These drugs act partly to improve atrioventricular conduction but mostly by stimulating ventricular automaticity, thus producing an increased ventricular rate. Caution should be exercised in the so-called states of prefibrillation, since the drug may precipitate ventricular arrhythmias. It is permissible to inject epinephrine directly into the heart in asystole in an attempt to achieve resuscitation. Cardiac massage is gaining much favor over the simple epinephrine resuscitation.

Bronchodilator action. Epinephrine is a time-honored remedy in the treatment of bronchial asthma. For this purpose it may be given subcutaneously in the amount of 0.2 to 0.5 ml of a 1:1000 solution. It may also be given by inhalation. For this purpose a stronger solution (up to 1:100) is employed in a nebulizer. Isoproterenol has been replacing epinephrine in this type of treatment.

Overdoses of norepinephrine or epinephrine may cause severe hypertension, pulmonary edema, and arrhythmias (particularly following the use of certain general anesthetics). In addition, extravasation ischemia may result at the site of intravenous infusions of levarterenol. This can be treated by the local infiltration of phentolamine (Regitine), an α-adrenergic blocking agent.

Patients receiving tricyclic antidepressants or guanethidine, which block the amine uptake mechanism in adrenergic nerves, may show exaggerated responses to norepinephrine and epinephrine.

Catecholamines and
disease states

Hypertension. Hypertension is clearly not caused solely by an increase in sympathetic activity. No significant increase in catecholamine excretion has been found in persons with essential hypertension. On the other hand, plasma catecholamines may be elevated in this condition.[49]

Pheochromocytoma. A rare form of hypertension is caused by tumors of adrenomedullary tissue that secrete norepinephrine with variable amounts of epinephrine. Although pheochromocytoma is a rare tumor, its diagnosis is most important because it represents one of the few forms of completely curable hypertension.

Several tumors have been examined by chemical methods. It appears that most of them contain very high concentrations of norepinephrine and smaller amounts of epinephrine. There may be as much as 10 to 15 mg/g of tissue, and the total catecholamine content of a large tumor may be more than 1 g.

Several methods have been introduced during the last few years for the diagnosis of pheochromocytoma. Some of these are based on neuropharmacological principles and others on the determination of catecholamines in the urine. Although pharmacological tests are inaccurate and hazardous as compared with chemical tests, they illustrate interesting principles.

Pharmacological tests. Drug tests for pheochromocytoma are of two types: those that can promote the secretion of catecholamines from the tumor and cause blood pressure elevation, and those that inhibit the actions of norepinephrine and thereby cause lowering of the elevated blood pressure.

Among those drugs that elevate blood pressure in patients with pheochromocytoma are histamine, methacholine, and tetraethylammonium. Drugs that lower blood pressure in patients with pheochromocytoma are phenoxybenzamine, and phentolamine.

The most widely used drug in diagnosis of pheochromocytoma is phentolamine (Regitine). A dose of 5 mg is injected intravenously or intramuscularly. If systolic blood pressure falls more than 35 mm Hg and diastolic pressure more than 25 mm Hg, the test is considered positive.

Chemical tests. The diagnosis of pheochromocytoma may be established by the determination of normetanephrine plus epinephrine or norepinephrine plus epinephrine or VMA in a 24-hour urine specimen. There is a rapid screening procedure for VMA in many laboratories, but its diagnostic accuracy is not as great as that of other procedures. Methyldopa, tetracycline, and quinidine may falsely increase norepinephrine plus epinephrine values. MAO inhibitors will increase normetanephrine plus metanephrine. Anxiety and excitement do not elevate the excretion of catecholamines sufficiently to cause diagnostic errors. On the other hand, acute myocardial infarction, surgical trauma, and shock may cause abnormally high urinary output of the catecholamines and their metabolites.[14]

Preparations

Levarterenol bitartrate (Levophed bitartrate) is available for injection in a 0.2% solution equivalent to 1 mg of base per milliliter in 2 and 4 ml ampules. For intravenous infusion in adults 4 to 8 ml of the 0.2% solution is added to 500 ml of 5% dextrose injection. The injection rate is regulated to keep the systolic blood pressure somewhat below normal.

Epinephrine hydrochloride (Adrenalin chloride) is a solution containing for injection, 1 mg/ml, and for inhalation, 10 mg/ml.

Epinephrine bitartrate is available in special devices (Medihaler-epi) for inhalation, deliver 0.3 mg per dose.

Epinephrine suspension, aqueous or in oil, for injection contains 2.5 or 2 mg/ml.

Epinephrine bitartrate and epinephrine hydrochloride are also available for ophthalmic uses in 1% and 2% solutions.

Dopamine

This catecholamine has important functions as a chemical mediator in some parts of the CNS. In addition it has been introduced as a therapeutic agent under the trade name Intropin.

Dopamine acts on β receptors in the heart, causing increased contractility and heart rate. In large enough doses it acts on α receptors in blood vessels, causing vasoconstriction. Dopamine exerts some unusual vasodilator effects on the renal, mesenteric, coronary, and intracerebral vessels, which suggest the existence of specific dopaminergic receptors. These are not blocked by propranolol but are inhibited by haloperidol and the phenothiazines.[80] These dopamine vascular receptors may be similar to the dopaminergic receptors in the basal ganglia (p. 157).

The hemodynamic effects of dopamine depend on the dose with some individual variations. Intravenous infusion of 1 to 10 μg^2/kg/min leads to increased cardiac contractility, cardiac output, and renal blood flow. Heart rate and mean blood pressure do not change significantly. With higher infusion rates arterial pressure rises and heart rate decreases.

Dopamine infusions are used in some cases of shock and in chronic refractory congestive failure. In shock, dopamine should not be administered until blood volume becomes adequate as reflected by a central venous pressure of 10 to 15 cm H_2O.

Ventricular arrhythmia is the most serious adverse effect. Nausea, vomiting, and hypotension may also occur. If the blood pressure becomes elevated, it is comforting to know that the action of the drug is dissipated in a few minutes.

The cardiac actions of dopamine are antagonized by propranolol, its hypertensive effects are inhibited by phentolamine, and dopaminergic vasodilation is blocked by haloperidol or the phenothiazines. Furthermore, MAO inhibitors cause exaggerated responses to dopamine.

Dopamine hydrochloride (Intropin) is available in 5 ml ampules that contain 200 mg of dopamine. The drug should be diluted in a 250 or 500 ml sterile intravenous solution. Infusion rates should be adjusted so that 2 to 5 μg/kg/min of the drug are given.

MISCELLANEOUS ADRENERGIC DRUGS

The various sympathomimetic drugs may act *directly* on α and β receptors, or they may act *indirectly* by releasing endogenous catecholamines. Some also have a *mixed* action, both direct and indirect. Some important examples are as follows.

	α agonists	β agonists
Direct acting drugs	Methoxamine	Isoproterenol
Mixed acting drugs	Metaraminol	Ephedrine (indirect
		on α receptors)
Indirect acting drugs	Tyramine	
	Amphetamine	

The evidence for this classification is based on various considerations. It has been demonstrated that tyramine, ephedrine, amphetamine, and phenylethylamine, now considered to be indirectly acting agents, had less effect in animals in whose tissue the norepinephrine content had been depleted by reserpine[9] (Fig. 15-7).

The infusion of norepinephrine restored the capacity of the animals to react to these drugs. In a reserpinized animal the *responses* to some adrenergic drugs are normal or augmented. Other adrenergic drugs are suppressed, and still others are partly antagonized by reserpine.[55] Drugs of the first type include norepinephrine, epinephrine, and phenylephrine. They are direct acting. Among those suppressed by norepinephrine depletion are tyramine, amphetamine, phenylethylamine, and hydroxyamphetamine. Partially suppressed and having presumably a mixed effect are ephedrine and phenylpropanolamine.

Another line of evidence that suggests norepinephrine release as the mode of action of many sympathomimetic drugs is the observation that indirectly acting amines are ineffective on chronically denervated structures.

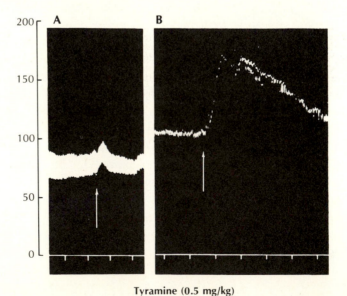

FIG. 15-7. Blood pressure response to tyramine. **A,** Reserpinized cat. **B,** Control cat. Dose of reserpine: 7 mg/kg subcutaneously. Dose of tyramine: 0.5 mg/kg intravenously. Arrow indicates times of injection. (From Carlsson, A., Rosengren, E., Bertler, Å., and Nilsson, J.: Psychotropic drugs, Amsterdam, 1957, Elsevier Publishing Co.)

A discussion of the sympathomimetic amines may be simplified by placing them into categories based on their clinical usage. There are three such categories: the vasoconstrictors, the bronchodilators, and the CNS stimulants. Despite some overlap in these activities, it is possible to select sympathomimetics for therapeutic purposes on the basis of predominant action. Ephedrine, a prototype of the sympathomimetic amines, belongs to a special category. It is used for its cardiovascular, bronchodilator, and stimulant properties.

Classification based on clinical usage

Adrenergic vasoconstrictors are phenylephrine, methoxamine, mephentermine, metaraminol, and the nasal vasoconstrictors phenylephrine hydrochloride, hydroxyamphetamine, phenylpropranolamine, propylhexedrine, cyclopentamine, tuaminoheptane, methylhexaneamine, naphazoline, and tetrahydrozoline. Dopamine is also being advocated in the treatment of hypotension.[51]

Adrenergic bronchodilators are isoproterenol, protokylol, isoetharine, and methoxyphenamine. Related vasodilators are nylidrin and isoxsuprine. The newer β_2 bronchodilators such as terbutaline and metaproterenol will be discussed in Chapter 40.

Adrenergic vasodilators include nylidrin, isoxsuprine, and isoproterenol.

Adrenergic CNS stimulants and anorexiants are amphetamine sulfate, dextroamphetamine, methamphetamine, and the related appetite suppressants phenmetrazine and diethylpropion.

Used in China for centuries and introduced into the United States in 1923, ephedrine is a naturally occurring sympathomimetic drug. Its action is similar to that of epinephrine and norepinephrine except for a much longer duration of action, effectiveness after oral administration, CNS stimulation, and occurrence of tachyphylaxis on frequent administration. On a weight basis it is about 100 times weaker; thus it is administered in doses of about 25 mg. Its action lasts for hours, and it is well absorbed from the gastrointestinal tract. From the standpoint of intestinal absorption of sympathomimetic drugs, the generalization may be made that the *phenyl* amines are much better absorbed than are the catechol derivatives.

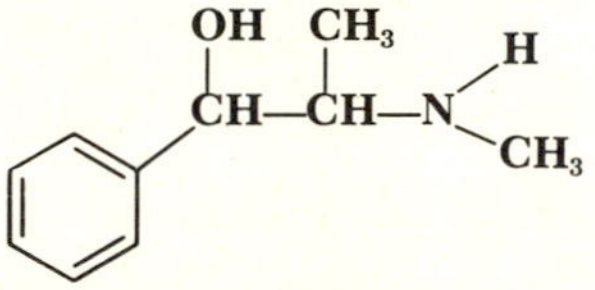

Ephedrine

Ephedrine

Ephedrine is an indirectly acting phenylisopropylamine. Its peripheral actions are reduced by intensive pretreatment with reserpine or by sympathetic denervation.

In addition to its vasopressor effects, ephedrine acts on the heart, with the heart rate usually increasing. Ephedrine dilates the bronchi and is useful in the treatment of asthma. It causes mydriasis when applied to the eye, produces CNS stimulation with anxiety and wakefulness, and has some slight anticurare action on the skeletal muscles. It is occasionally useful in myasthenia gravis.

Ephedrine sulfate USP is available for oral administration in the form of capsules containing 25 and 50 mg and also as an elixir containing 5 and 10 mg/5 ml. For injection, solutions containing 20, 25, or 50 mg/ml are available.

Adrenergic vaso-constrictors related to epinephrine or ephedrine

Phenylephrine (Neo-Synephrine) is a direct-acting α-receptor agonist. Subcutaneous injection of 5 mg has been used for the prevention of hypotension during spinal anesthesia and for the treatment of orthostatic hypotension. It is also a nasal decongestant.

Methoxamine (Vasoxyl) is a direct-acting α receptor agonist lacking cardiac stimulant properties. It is available for injection as a solution containing 10 and 20 mg/ml.

Mephentermine (Wyamine) is both a direct and indirect vasoactive drug acting on both α and β receptors. The duration of its vasoconstrictor and myocardial stimulant action is 60 minutes following subcutaneous injection of 10 to 30 mg.

Metaraminol (Aramine) resembles phenylephrine in its properties, but it acts both directly and indirectly. It is taken up by sympathetic fibers and released as a false transmitter.[68] The drug is administered subcutaneously or intramuscularly in doses of 2 to 10 mg. It is available as metaraminol bitartrate in injectable solutions containing 10 mg/ml.

Hydroxyamphetamine (Paredrine) resembles ephedrine in its action except for having little CNS effect. The drug is available in tablet form, 20 mg, for oral administration and as an ophthalmic preparation in a 1% solution.

Phenylpropanolamine is used almost entirely as an oronasal decongestant.

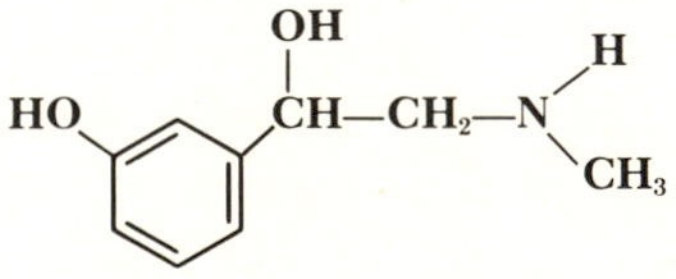

Phenylephrine

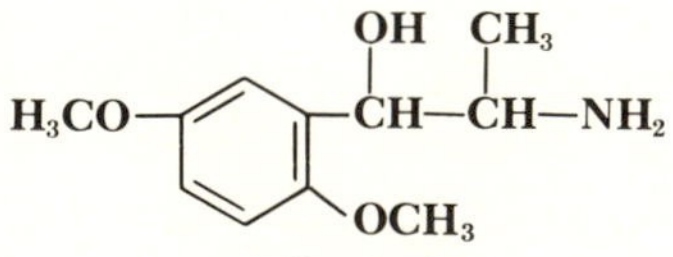

Methoxamine

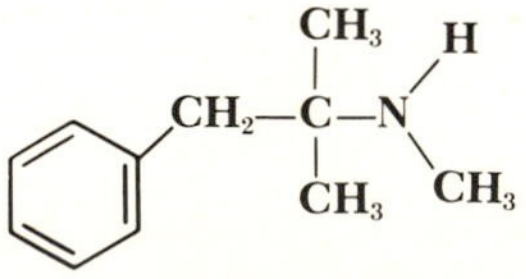

Mephentermine

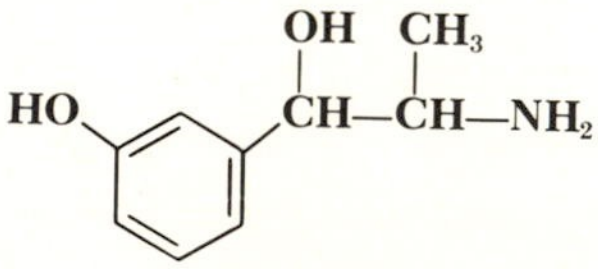

Metaraminol

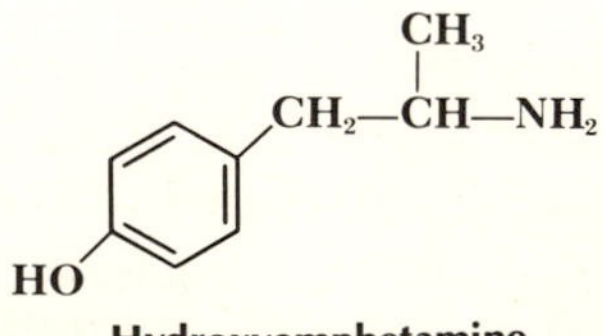

Hydroxyamphetamine

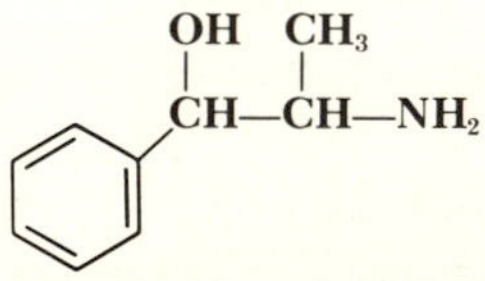

Phenylpropanolamine

Some of the commonly used nasal decongestants are the following.

Phenylephrine hydrochloride (Neo-Synephrine hydrochloride) is available in solutions of 0.125% for topical application; it may cause rebound swelling of the nasal mucosa. Oral administration of the drug in capsules of 10 and 25 mg is somewhat unpredictable in its effect.

Phenylpropanolamine hydrochloride (Propadrine hydrochloride) is available in capsules of 25 mg; it has also been used as an anorexiant but is ineffective.

Propylhexedrine (Benzedrex) is commonly administered by inhalation. It has many of the properties of amphetamine but with lesser pressor effect and much less CNS stimulation.

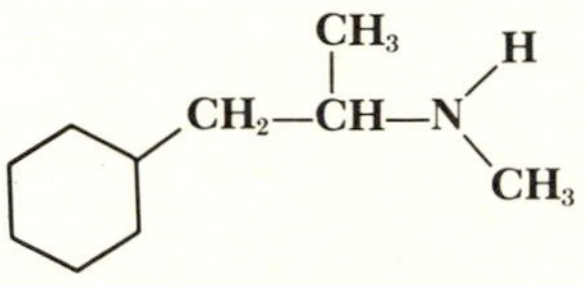

Propylhexedrine

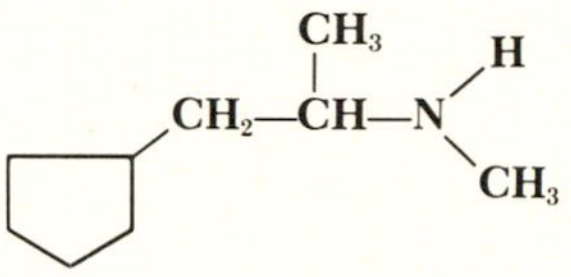

Cyclopentamine

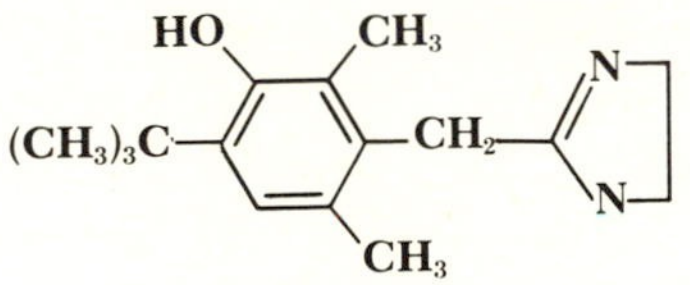

Oxymetazoline

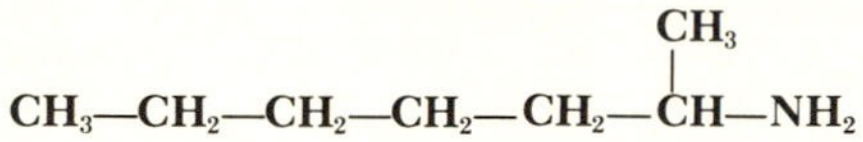

Tuaminoheptane

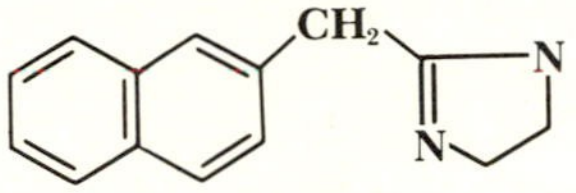

Naphazoline

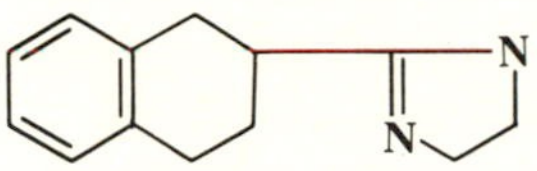

Tetrahydrozoline

Cyclopentamine hydrochloride (Clopane hydrochloride) is applied topically as a 0.5% solution.

Oxymetazoline hydrochloride (Afrin) is available in 0.05% solution as nose drops and spray.

Tuaminoheptane (Tuamine) is available as a 1% solution and also as an inhalant.

Naphazoline hydrochloride (Privine hydrochloride), an imidazoline derivative, is available in 0.05% solutions as nose drops and a spray. It may cause profound drowsiness and coma in children and also rebound swelling of the mucosa and cardiac irregularities when used excessively.

Tetrahydrozoline hydrochloride (Tyzine) is similar to naphazoline chemically and in its adverse effects.

Current concept of nasal vasoconstrictors. The nasal vasoconstrictors or decongestants are sympatomatic medications that have some usefulness but are not harmless. Continued use of these medications may actually induce chronic congestion of the nasal mucosa, probably because ischemia leads to rebound swelling. In excessive doses the nasal decongestants produce the usual adrenergic effects such as increased blood pressure, dizziness, palpitation, and in some cases CNS stimulation.

In addition, the imidazoline derivatives naphazoline and tetrahydrozoline have produced drowsiness and coma in children.

The nasal decongestants are frequently combined with antihistamines. Thus preparations containing phenylephrine and an antihistamine have become very popular as nasal decongestants that are taken orally.

Adrenergic bronchodilators
Isoproterenol

Isoproterenol (isopropylnorepinephrine) is a potent activator of β receptors. It dilates the bronchial smooth muscle and has powerful effects on the heart. It also dilates blood vessels, particularly in skeletal muscle. When used in the treatment of bronchial asthma, it may cause tachycardia, arrhythmias, and hypotension. Some instances of sudden death in asthmatic persons have been attributed to excessive use of isoproterenol.[85]

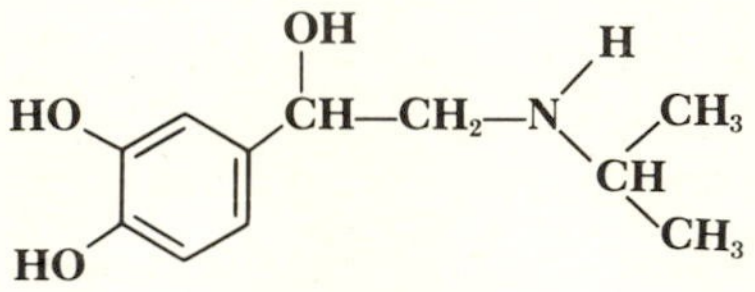

Isoproterenol

Isoproterenol is used primarily in the treatment of bronchial asthma, atrioventricular block, and cardiac arrest.

Palpitations, arrhythmias, anginal pain, and headache may occur following the use of isoproterenol. The drug may intensify arrhythmias caused by digitalis. Cyclopropane, halogenated anesthetics, and propellants may sensitize the myocardium to isoproterenol. The effects of the drug are blocked by propranolol.

Isoproterenol hydrochloride (Isuprel hydrochloride) is available in solutions of 1:100 (10 mg/ml), 1:200 (5 mg/ml), and 1:400 (2.5 mg/ml) for oral inhalation; solutions containing 0.2 mg/ml for injection; and sublingual tablets of 10 and 15 mg. The effects of the tablets are somewhat unpredictable because of erratic absorption.

Other bronchodilators

In addition to isoproterenol, several adrenergic drugs and theophylline derivatives are used as bronchodilators. Epinephrine and ephedrine are widely used and have already been discussed (pp. 179 and 182). Protokylol, isoetharine, and methoxyphenamine are additional adrenergic bronchodilators. Among the theophylline derivatives, aminophylline (theophylline ethylenediamine), oxtriphylline, theophylline in 20% alcohol, and theophylline sodium glycinate are commonly used in asthmatic individuals. The corticosteroids, although not primarily bronchodilators, are also of great importance in the treatment of severe asthma.

In addition to these bronchodilators, certain β-receptor agonists, such as metaproterenol sulfate (Alupent), terbutaline (Brethine), and salbutamol, are being employed in the treatment of asthma because they have fewer cardiac side effects.

The bronchodilators are discussed in Chapter 40 in connection with drug effects on the respiratory tract.

Isoproterenol is a β-adrenergic stimulant that dilates blood vessels while it stimulates the heart. Certain vasodilators have been developed that probably act through a similar mechanism. These are **nylidrin** (Arlidin) and **isoxsuprine** (Vasodilan). Although these drugs can dilate peripheral blood vessels experimentally, their effectiveness in the management of peripheral vascular disease is not universally accepted among clinical investigators. Nylidrin is used orally in doses of 6 mg and isoxsuprine is also used orally in doses of 10 to 20 mg. Although the action of these drugs resembles that of isoproterenol, they probably act indirectly by releasing catecholamines.

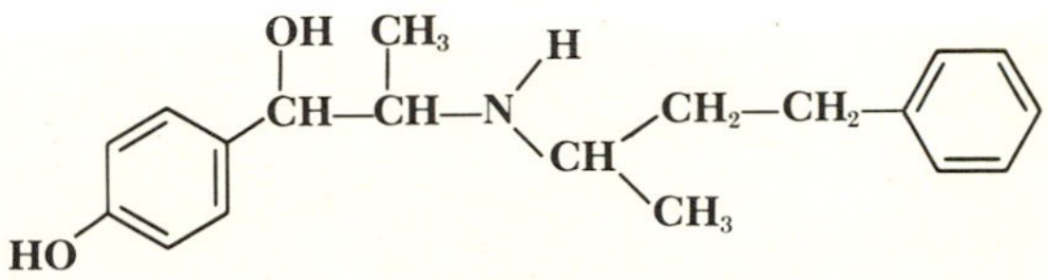

Adrenergic vasodilators

Nylidrin

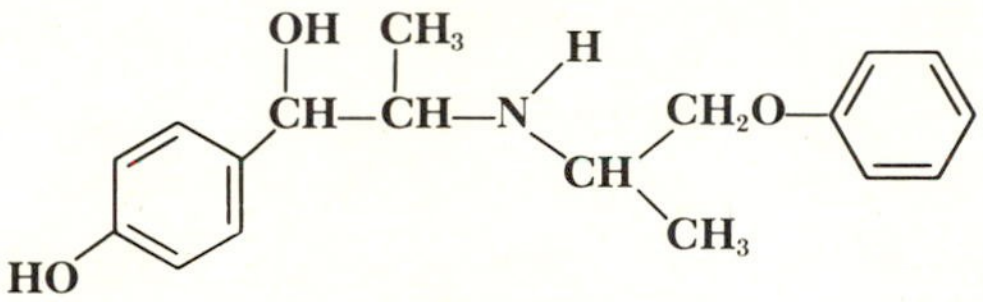

Isoxsuprine

The amphetamines are powerful stimulants of the CNS. *Dextro*amphetamine has relatively greater central, and less cardiovascular, effects than the *levo* isomer. The drug is used and also abused mainly in relation to its anorexiant effect, and even this use is questioned by many authorities. In addition to being an anorexiant, dextroamphetamine finds some application as an analeptic in the treatment of narcolepsy, as an antidepressant, in the management of hyperkinetic children, and in postencephalitic reactions.

Adrenergic CNS stimulants and anorexiants
Amphetamines

Numerous anorexiants have been developed and are used by the medical profession, often without the realization that these drugs are essentially relatives of dextroamphetamine without significant advantages over the anorexiant prototype. Some of the drugs are methamphetamine (Desoxyn), phenmetrazine (Preludin), diethylpropion (Tenuate; Tepanil), phenylpropanolamine (Propadrine), phentermine (Ionamin; Wilpo), chlorphentermine (Pre-Sate), benzphetamine (Didrex), and phendimetrazine (Plegine). In addition, numerous mixtures of adrenergic stimulants with barbiturates and other depressants have been prepared and are used widely anorexiants. Despite their popularity, such mixtures are generally not recommended.

The disadvantages in the use of anorexiants are related to the development of psychic dependence and to untoward effects resulting from adrenergic actions. Toxic psychosis may result from large doses of many of these drugs.

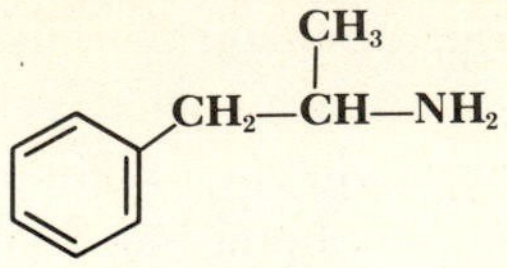

$$CH_2-CH-NH_2$$

with CH₃ above the CH, attached to a benzene ring.

Amphetamine

The vascular effects of the amphetamines may be attributed to endogenous catecholamine release, since they do not elevate blood pressure in a reserpinized animal.

The central stimulant effects of amphetamine are not inhibited by catecholamine depletion by reserpine, but blockade of catecholamine synthesis quickly inhibits the behavioral actions of amphetamine. These findings suggest that although the drug's cardiovascular effects stem from the release of preformed peripheral norepinephrine, the drug's behavioral actions are mediated through a newly synthesized fraction of brain catecholamines.

Certain central stimulants, such as methylphenidate, while mimicking amphetamine's central effects, clearly act by a different mechanism, since the central effects of such drugs are blocked by reserpine but not by catecholamine synthesis blockade, unless synthesis inhibition is prolonged until catecholamine depletion occurs.

Habituation and tolerance develop to the central effects of amphetamine. Large and repeated doses may produce a psychosis that has many of the characteristics of paranoid schizophrenia.

Amphetamine is well absorbed from the gastrointestinal tract. The main metabolite of amphetamine is phenylacetone, a product of microsomal deamination. A minor metabolite, p-hydroxyamphetamine, is taken up by adrenergic nerves and transformed to p-hydroxynorephedrine, which is stored in vesicles, thus forming a false transmitter.[63]

Amphetamine (Benzedrine) is available in tablets, 5, 10, and 15 mg; sustained action capsules; and injectable solutions containing 20 mg/ml.

Dextroamphetamine (Dexedrine) is available in tablets 5, 10, and 15 mg; sustained action capsules; elixir, 5 mg/5 ml; and injectable solutions containing 20 mg/ml.

Methylphenidate (Ritalin) is available in tablets, 5, 10, and 20 mg, and in injectable solutions containing 10 mg/ml.

Methamphetamine (d-deoxyephedrine) is closely related from a structural standpoint to both ephedrine and amphetamine. It is a potent CNS stimulant and has a considerable pressor effect on blood vessels. It is used for the same purposes as amphetamine in approximately the same dosage.

Phenmetrazine (Preludin) is used as an appetite suppressant, a questionable approach to the treatment of obesity. It has considerable CNS effects.

Diethylpropion (Tenuate; Tepanil) is employed as an anorexigenic agent. It is basically an amphetamine-like drug, although it is claimed that it causes less jitteriness and insomnia and also fewer cardiovascular effects than does amphetamine. The drug is considerably weaker than dextroamphetamine and is used in doses of 25 mg orally.

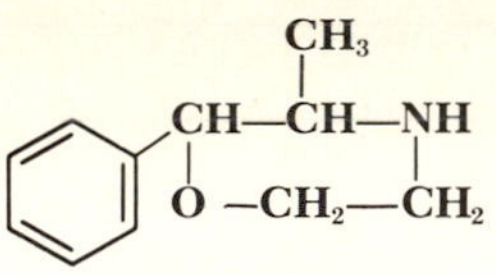

Phenmetrazine 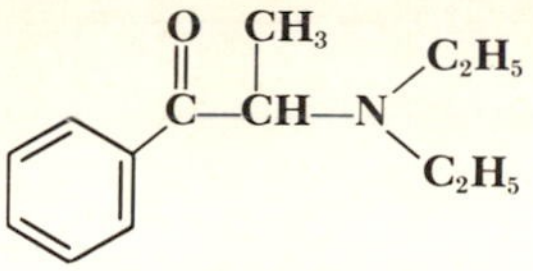   **Diethylpropion**

Clortermine hydrochloride (Voranil), **fenfluramine hydrochloride** (Pondimin), and **mazindol** (Sanorex) are additional anorexiants that have been recently evaluated.[78] They are comparable to other anorexiants in suppressing appetite. They may be used as short-term adjuncts to other measures that include caloric restriction, exercise, and psychotherapy. Of these drugs, mazindol (Sanorex) is not a phenethylamine and is claimed to have a different mode of action from the others. Fenfluramine (Pondimin) is unusual in causing CNS depression along with appetite suppression.

Miscellaneous anorexiants

Clortermine and fenfluramine are said to affect the appetite control centers in the hypothalamus. This is also true for all phenethylamines. Mazindol reportedly facilitates the electric activity in the septal region of the brain.

All the CNS stimulants and anorexiants may cause hypertensive crises in patients taking MAO inhibitors. All, except fenfluramine, antagonize the antihypertensive action of guanethidine (Ismelin). Fenfluramine may potentiate the antihypertensive action of guanethidine and methyldopa (Aldomet). Fenfluramine, being a sedative, may increase the effects of alcohol and other CNS depressants. Mazindol potentiates the vasopressor effect of levarterenol in dogs and probably should not be combined with vasopressor medications.

Drug interactions

A great deal is known about the relationships between structure and activity in adrenergic drugs. Such knowledge in general is important to the pharmaceutical chemist as a guide in synthetic work on new drugs. Structure-activity relationships are also of fundamental importance in that they should reflect basic characteristics of receptor mechanisms. In the case of adrenergic drugs the problem is complicated by the fact that many sympathomimetic drugs act indirectly through the release of endogenous catecholamines. The differences in action of these drugs may be related to the predominant site of catecholamine release.

Structure-activity relationships in adrenergic series

A few generalities may serve to illustrate the concept of structure-activity relationships.

The basic adrenergic structure is phenylethylamine.

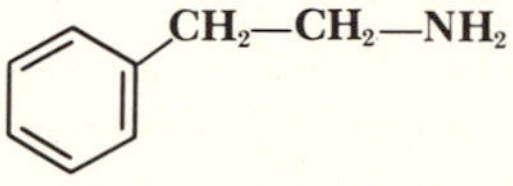

Phenylethylamine

Hydroxyl groups on the benzene ring or on the side chain influence the metabolic rate and absorption of the drugs as well as their actions on receptors. Sympathomimetics that are not catechols are generally absorbed better and are, of course, not attacked by O-methylation.

Substitutions on the nitrogen have a great influence on the type of receptor with which the drug will interact. Thus norepinephrine, lacking substitutions, acts on α receptors, epinephrine with one methyl group acts on both receptors, and isoproterenol acts almost entirely on β receptors.

Substitutions on the α carbon tend to prolong the action of the drug, probably because of protection against enzymatic destruction. The OH group on the β carbon is necessary for granular storage in adrenergic neurons.

REFERENCES

1 Abboud, F. M.: Clinical importance of adrenergic receptors, Arch. Intern. Med. **118:**418, 1966.

2 Abboud, F. M., Eckstein, J. W., Zimmerman, B. G., and Graham, M. H.: Sensitization of arteries, veins and small vessels to norepinephrine after cocaine, Circ. Res. **15:**247, 1964.

3 Ahlquist, R. P.: A study of the adrenotropic receptors, Am. J. Physiol. **153:**586, 1948.

4 Angelakos, E. T.: Histochemical demonstration of uptake of exogenous norepinephrine by adrenergic fibers in vitro, Science **145:**503, 1964.

5 Armstrong, M. D., McMillan, A., and Shaw, K. N.: 3-Methoxy-4-hydroxy-D-mandelic acid, a urinary metabolite of norepinephrine, Biochim. Biophys. Acta **25:**422, 1957.

6 Axelrod, J., Inscoe, J. K., Senoh, S., and Witkop, B.: O-methylation, the principal pathway for the metabolism of epinephrine and norepinephrine in the rat, Biochim. Biophys. Acta **27:**210, 1958.

7 Axelrod, J., and Laroche, M. J.: Inhibitor of O-methylation of epinephrine and norepinephrine in vitro and in vivo, Science **130:**800, 1959.

8 Boura, A. L. A., and Green, A. F.: Adrenergic neuron blocking agents, Annu. Rev. Pharmacol. **5:**183, 1965.

9 Burn, J. H., and Rand, M. J.: The action of sympathomimetic amines in animals treated with reserpine, J. Physiol. **144:**314, 1958.

10 Burn, J. H., and Rand, M. J.: Acetylcholine in adrenergic transmission, Annu. Rev. Pharmacol. **5:**163, 1965.

11 Butcher, R. W.: Role of cyclic AMP in hormone action, N. Engl. J. Med. **279:**1378, 1968.

12 Carlsson, A., and Hillarp, N. A.: On the state of the catecholamines of the adrenal medullary granules, Acta Physiol. Scand. **44:**163, 1958.

13 Costa, E., and Garattini, S., editors: International Symposium on amphetamines, New York, 1970, Raven Press.

14 Crout, J. R.: Sampling and analysis of catecholamines and metabolites, Anesthesiology **29:**661, 1968.

15 Crout, J. R., Alpers, H. S., Tatum, E. L., and Shore, P. A.: Release of metaraminol (Armine) from the heart by sympathetic nerve stimulation, Science **145:**828, 1964.

16 Crout, J. R., Pisano, J. J., and Sjoerdsma, A.: Urinary excretion of catecholamines and their metabolites in pheochromocytoma, Am. Heart J. **61:**375, 1961.

17 Dale, H. H.: On some physiological actions of ergot, J. Physiol. **34:**163, 1906.

18 Dengler, H. J., Michaelson, I. A., Spiegel, H. E., and Titus, E. O.: The uptake of labeled norepinephrine by isolated brain and other tissues of the cat, Int. J. Neuropharmacol. **1:**23, 1962.

19 Drury, D. R., and Wick, A. N.: Epinephrine and carbohydrate metabolism, Am. J. Physiol. **194:**465, 1958.

20 Engelman, K., and Sjoerdsma, A.: A new test for pheochromocytoma, J.A.M.A. **189:**81, 1964.

21 Espelin, D. E., and Done, A. K.: Amphetamine poisoning: effectiveness of chlorpromazine, N. Engl. J. Med. **278:**1361, 1968.

22 von Euler, U. S.: A specific sympathomimetic ergone in adrenergic nerve fibers (sympathin) and its relation to adrenaline and noradrenaline, Acta Physiol. Scand. **12:**73, 1946.

23 von Euler, U. S.: Noradrenaline: chemistry, physiology, pharmacology, and clinic, Springfield, Ill., 1956, Charles C Thomas, Publisher.

24 Frederickson, D. S., and Gordon, R. S.: Transport of fatty acids, Physiol. Rev. **38:**585, 1958.

25 Friend, D. G.: Drugs for peripheral vascular disease, Clin. Pharmacol. Ther. **5:**666, 1964.

26 Furchgott, R. F.: The receptors for epinephrine and norepinephrine (adrenergic receptors), Pharmacol. Rev. **11:**429, 1959.

27 Goldberg, L. I., McDonald, R. H., and Zimmerman, A. M.: Sodium diuresis produced by dopamine in patients with congestive heart failure, N. Engl. J. Med. 269:1060, 1963.

28 Goldenberg, M., Pines, K. L., Baldwin, E. deF., Greene, D. G., and Roh, C. E.: The hemodynamic response of man to norepinephrine and epinephrine and its relation to the problem of hypertension, Am. J. Med. 5:792, 1948.

29 Govier, W. C.: A positive inotropic effect of phenylephrine mediated through alpha adrenergic receptors, Life Sci. 6:1361, 1967.

30 Haddy, F. J., and Scott, J. B.: Cardiovascular pharmacology, Annu. Rev. Pharmacol. 6:49, 1966.

31 Hertting, G., Axelrod, J., and Whitby, L. G.: Effect of drugs on the uptake and metabolism of H^3-norepinephrine, J. Pharmacol. Exp. Ther. 134:146, 1961.

32 Hertting, G., Kopin, I. J., and Gordon, E.: The uptake, release, and metabolism of norepinephrine-7-H^3 in the isolated perfused rat heart, Fed. Proc. 21:331, 1962.

33 Hertting, G., Potter, L. T., and Axelrod, J.: Effect of decentralization and ganglionic blocking agents on the spontaneous and reserpine-induced release of H^3-norepinephrine, J. Pharmacol. Exp. Ther. 136:289, 1962.

34 Hess, M. E., and Haugaard, N.: Actions of autonomic drugs on phosphorylase activity and functions, Pharmacol. Rev. 17:27, 1965.

35 Hillarp, N. A., Hökfelt, B., and Nilson, B.: The cytology of the adrenal medullary cells with special reference to the storage and secretion of the sympathomimetic amines, Acta Anat. 21:155, 1954.

36 Himms-Hagen, J.: Sympathetic regulation of metabolism, Pharmacol. Rev. 19:367, 1967.

37 Isaac, L., and Goth, A.: Interaction of antihistaminics with norepinephrine uptake: a cocaine-like effect, Life Sci. 4:1899, 1965.

38 Iversen, L. L.: The uptake of adrenaline by the rat isolated heart, Br. J. Pharmacol. Chemother. 24:387, 1965.

39 Iversen, L. L.: The uptake of catecholamines at high perfusion concentrations in the rat isolated heart: a novel catecholamine uptake process, Br. J. Pharmacol. Chemother. 25:18, 1965.

40 Iversen, L. L.: The uptake and storage of noradrenaline in sympathetic nerves, New York, 1967, Cambridge University Press.

41 James, T. N., Bear, E. S., Lang, K. F., and Green, E. W.: Evidence for adrenergic alpha receptor depressant activity in the heart, Am. J. Physiol. 215:1366, 1958.

42 Kasuya, Y., and Goto, K.: The mechanism of supersensitivity to norepinephrine induced by cocaine in rat isolated vas deferens, Eur. J. Pharmacol. 4:355, 1958.

43 Koch-Weser, J.: Beta adrenergic blockade and circulating eosinophils, Arch. Intern. Med. 121:255, 1968.

44 Kopin, I. J.: Storage and metabolism of catecholamines: the role of monamine oxidase, Pharmacol. Rev. 16:179, 1964.

45 Lands, A. M., Arnold, A., and McAnliff, J. P.: Differentiation of receptor systems activated by sympathomimetic amines, Nature 214:597, 1967.

46 Langer, S. Z.: Presynaptic regulation of catecholamine release, Biochem. Pharmacol. 23:1793, 1974.

47 Lasagna, L., and McCann, W.: Effect of tranquilizing drugs on amphetamine toxicity in aggregated mice, Science 125:1241, 1957.

48 Lewis, C. M., and Weil, M. H.: Hemodynamic spectrum of vasopressor and vasodilator drugs, J.A.M.A. 208:1391, 1969.

49 Louis, W. J., Doyle, A. E., Anavekar, S. N., Johnston, C. I., Geffen, L. B., and Rush, R.: Plasma catecholamine, dopamine-beta-hydroxylase, and renin levels in essential hypertension, Circ. Res. 34-35(Supp. 1):1-57, 1974.

50 Lundholm, L., Mohme-Lundholm, E., and Svedmyr, N.: Metabolic effects of catecholamines. In Bittar, E. E., and Bittar, N., editors: The biological basis of medicine, vol. 2, New York, 1968, Academic Press, Inc.

51 MacCannell, K. L., McNay, J. L., Meyer, M. B., and Goldberg, L. I.: Dopamine in the treatment of hypotension and shock, N. Engl. J. Med. 275:1389, 1966.

52 Malmfors, T.: Histochemical studies of adrenergic neurotransmission. In Adrenergic neurotransmission, Ciba Foundation Study Group No. 33, Boston, 1968, Little, Brown & Co.

53 Marley, E.: The adrenergic system and sympathomimetic amines, Adv. Pharmacol. 3:168, 1964.

54 Maxwell, R. A., Plummer, A. J., Povalski, H., and Schneider, F.: Concerning a possible action of guanethidine (SU-5864) in smooth muscle, J. Pharmacol. Exp. Ther. 129:24, 1960.

55 Maxwell, R. A., Povalski, H., and Plummer, A. J.: A differential effect of reserpine on pressor amine activity and its relationship to other agents producing this effect, J. Pharmacol. Exp. Ther. 125:178, 1959.

56 Meyer, M. B., McNay, J. L., and Goldberg, L. I.: Effects of dopamine on renal function and hemodynamics in the dog, J. Pharmacol. Exp. Ther. 156:186, 1967.

57 Modell, W., and Hussar, A. E.: Failure of dextroamphetamine sulfate to influence eating and sleeping patterns in obese schizophrenic patients, J.A.M.A. **193:**275, 1965.

58 Moyer, J. H., and Handley, C. A.: Norepinephrine and epinephrine effect on renal hemodynamics, Circulation **5:**91, 1952.

59 Moyer, J. H., Morris, G., and Snyder, H.: A comparison of the cerebral hemodynamic response to Aramine and norepinephrine in the normotensive-hypotensive subject, Circulation **10:**265, 1954.

60 Nickerson, M.: Vasoconstriction and vasodilation in shock. In Hershey, S. G., editor: Shock, Boston, 1964, Little, Brown & Co.

61 Norberg, K. A., and Hamberger, B.: The sympathetic adrenergic neuron, Acta Physiol. Scand. **63**(Supp. 238):1, 1964.

62 Patel, N., Mock, D. C., and Hagans, J. A.: Comparison of benzphetamine, phenmetrazine, d-amphetamine, and placebo, Clin. Pharmacol. Ther. **4:**330, 1963.

63 Rangno, R. E., Kaufmann, J. S., Cavanaugh, J. H., Island, D., Watson, J. T., and Oates, J.: Effects of a false neurotransmitter, *p*-hydroxynorephedrine, on the function of adrenergic neurons in hypertensive patients, J. Clin. Invest. **52:**952, 1973.

64 Renold, A. E.: Insulin biosynthesis and secretion—a still unsettled topic, N. Engl. J. Med. **282:**173, 1970.

65 Schmid, P. G., Eckstein, J. W., and Abboud, F. M.: Comparison of effects of deoxycorticosterone and dexamethasone on cardiovascular responses to norepinephrine, J. Clin. Invest. **46:**590, 1967.

66 Scroop, G. C., Walsh, J. A., and Whelan, R. F.: A comparison of the effects of intra-arterial and intravenous infusions of angiotensin and noradrenaline on the circulation in man, Clin. Sci. **29:**315, 1965.

67 Second symposium on catecholamines, Pharmacol. Rev. **18:**1, 1966.

68 Shore, P. A., Busfield, D., and Alpers, H. S.: Binding and release of metaraminol: mechanism of norepinephrine depletion by alpha-methyl-M-tyrosine and related agents, J. Pharmacol. Exp. Ther. **146:**194, 1964.

69 Starke, K., and Montel, H.: Alpha-receptor mediated modulation of transmitter release from central noradrenergic neurones, Naunyn-Schmiedebergs Arch. Pharmacol. **279:**53, 1973.

70 Steer, M. L., Atlas, D., and Levitzki, A.: Interrelations between β-adrenergic receptors, adenylate cyclase and calcium, N. Engl. J. Med. **292:**409, 1975.

71 Sutherland, E. W.: The effect of the hyperglycemic factor and epinephrine on enzyme systems of liver and muscle, Ann. N. Y. Acad. Sci. **54:**693, 1951.

72 Sutherland, E. W., and Rall, T. W.: The relationship of adenosine-3′,5′-phosphate to the action of catechol amines. In Adrenergic mechanisms, Ciba Foundation and Committee for Symposium on Drug Action, Boston, 1960, Little, Brown & Co.

73 Sutherland, E. W., and Rall, T. W.: The relation of adenosine-3′,5′-phosphate and phosphorylase to the actions of catecholamines and other hormones, Pharmacol. Rev. **12:**265, 1960.

74 Thoenen, H., and Tranzer, J. P.: Chemical sympathectomy by selective destruction of adrenergic nerve endings with 6-hydroxydopamine, Naunyn-Schmiedebergs Arch. Exp. Pathol. **261:**271, 1968.

75 Trendelenburg, U.: Supersensitivity and subsensitivity to sympathomimetic amines, Pharmacol. Rev. **15:**225, 1963.

76 Udenfriend, S.: Physiological regulation of noradrenaline biosynthesis. In Adrenergic neurotransmission, Ciba Foundation Study Group No. 33, Boston, 1968, Little, Brown & Co.

77 Wurtman, R. J.: Catecholamines, N. Engl. J. Med. **273:**637 and 693, 1965.

REVIEWS

78 Dykes, M. H.: Evaluation of three anorexiants, J.A.M.A. **230:**270, 1974.

79 Geffen, L. B., and Livett, B. G.: Synaptic vesicles in sympathetic neurons, Physiol. Rev. **51:**98, 1971.

80 Goldberg, L. I.: Dopamine—clinical uses of an endogeneous catecholamine, N. Engl. J. Med. **291:**707, 1974.

81 Iversen, L. L.: Uptake mechanisms for neurotransmitter amines, Biochem. Pharmacol. **23:**1927, 1974.

82 Kopin, I. J., et al.: False neurochemical transmitters and the mechanism of sympathetic blockade by monoamine oxidase inhibitors, J. Pharmacol. Exp. Ther. **147:**186, 1965.

83 Lefkowitz, R. J.: β-Adrenergic receptors: recognition and regulation, N. Engl. J. Med. **295:**323, 1976.

83a Lefkowitz, R. J.: Direct binding studies of adrenergic receptors: biochemical, physiologic, and clinical implications, Ann. Intern. Med. **91:**450, 1979.

84 Shore, P. A.: Transport and storage of biogenic amines, Annu. Rev. Pharmacol. **12:**209, 1972.

85 Stolley, P. D.: Asthma mortality, Am. Rev. Respir. Dis. **105:**883, 1972.

86 Weil, M. H., Shubin, H., and Carlson, R.: Treatment of circulatory shock, J.A.M.A. **231:**1280, 1975.

CHAPTER 16

Adrenergic blocking agents

Adrenergic blocking agents are drugs that competitively inhibit the actions of catecholamines and other adrenergic agonists on their specific receptors. They are effective against catecholamines released from sympathetic nerve endings.

Adrenergic blocking drugs are classified as *alpha* (α) and *beta* (β) adrenergic blocking agents, reflecting the existence of two types of receptors. In tissues that possess both types of receptors, such as most blood vessels, α stimulation causes contraction and β stimulation causes relaxation. The α-adrenergic blocking drugs in such a tissue cause vasodilation. In organs whose receptors are almost entirely β, such as the heart, the β blockers oppose the excitatory effects of norepinephrine released from sympathetic nerve endings.

Drugs that deplete catecholamines or prevent their release in adrenergic nerves should be called *catecholamine depleters* and *adrenergic neuronal blocking drugs*, respectively, and should not be confused with the *adrenergic blocking agents* that act on α and β receptors. Certain imprecise older terms such as *adrenolytic*, *sympatholytic*, and *sympathoplegic* should be abandoned.

The single most characteristic feature of the α-adrenergic blocking drugs is their ability to transform the pressor effect of injected epinephrine into a depressor response. This "epinephrine reversal" was first observed by Dale in 1905 following the injection of certain ergot preparations.

The epinephrine reversal caused by phentolamine is shown in Fig. 16-1.

The facts fit the hypothesis that arteriolar smooth muscle has both α and β receptors, the former mediating vasoconstriction and the latter mediating vasodilatation by adrenergic drugs. Epinephrine acts on both receptors. An α blocker such as phentolamine prevents access of the drug to α receptors and thus unmasks its action on β receptors, the result being vasodilatation instead of the usual vasoconstriction.

Norepinephrine, on the other hand, has no effect on vascular β receptors. Thus the α blockers prevent blood pressure rise by the drug without causing a norepinephrine reversal.

The α-adrenergic blocking drugs inhibit the effect of various agonists on the α receptor. They reverse the actions of epinephrine on the blood pressure, oppose the actions of norepinephrine, but do not prevent β-receptor–mediated effects of adrenergic drugs, such as cardiac effects and vasodilatation.

GENERAL CONCEPT

CONCEPT OF EPINEPHRINE REVERSAL

α-ADRENERGIC BLOCKING AGENTS
General features

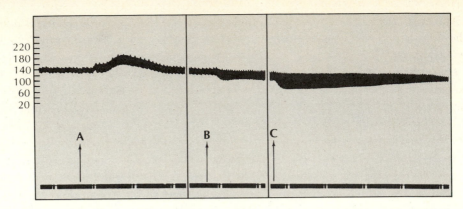

FIG. 16-1. Epinephrine reversal by phentolamine. Effect of epinephrine on blood pressure before and after injection of phentolamine. Dog was anesthetized with pentobarbital sodium. At *A*, epinephrine was injected intravenously, 1 μg/kg. At *B*, phentolamine was injected, 5 mg/kg. At *C*, epinephrine injection was repeated. Time is given in seconds. Note lowering of mean pressure by epinephrine following adrenergic blocking agent. Increased pulse pressure under these circumstances is an indication that adrenergic blocking agent does not prevent the cardiac stimulant effect of epinephrine.

Differences among various α-adrenergic blocking agents

The various drugs in this group differ from each other in potency and duration of action. They may also possess pharmacological properties entirely unrelated to adrenergic blockade.

Phenoxybenzamine hydrochloride

Phenoxybenzamine. Phenoxybenzamine (Dibenzyline), when administered in doses of 20 to 100 mg, produces lowering of blood pressure and orthostatic hypotension. The effects of the drug last more than 24 hours. It is available in capsules of 10 mg.

The long duration of action of phenoxybenzamine is probably a consequence of a stable combination between the drug and the α receptor. In this case, although competition exists between the drug and catecholamines for the receptor during the early stages of blockade, such competition becomes ineffective as the blockade develops fully. The term *nonequilibrium blockade*[23] has been applied to such an interaction between agonist and antagonist.

Occasional indications for the use of phenoxybenzamine include peripheral vascular diseases in which vasospasm is an important feature, such as Raynaud's disease, and the management of pheochromocytoma both prior to and during the operation.

Among the many adverse effects that may be caused by phenoxybenzamine, orthostatic hypotension, tachycardia, nasal congestion, and miosis are common and predictable.

Tolazoline hydrochloride. Tolazoline hydrochloride (Priscoline), a weak α blocker, causes peripheral vasodilatation largely by a direct relaxant effect on vascular smooth muscle. In addition, the drug is a direct cardiac stimulant and its use is often accompanied by tachycardia.

Tolazoline is used in the treatment of peripheral vascular diseases for the relief of vasospasm. It is available in tablets of 25 mg, timed-release tablets of 80 mg, and solution for injection, 25 mg/ml.

Adverse effects to the drug include pilomotor stimulation (gooseflesh), tachycardia, and increased gastrointestinal motility and hydrochloric acid secretion. Tolazoline is related structurally to histamine.

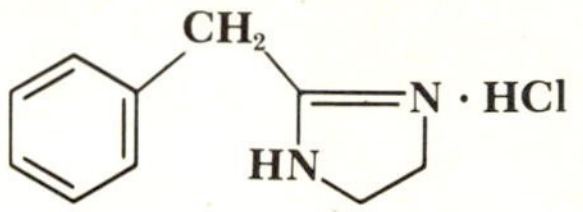

Tolazoline hydrochloride 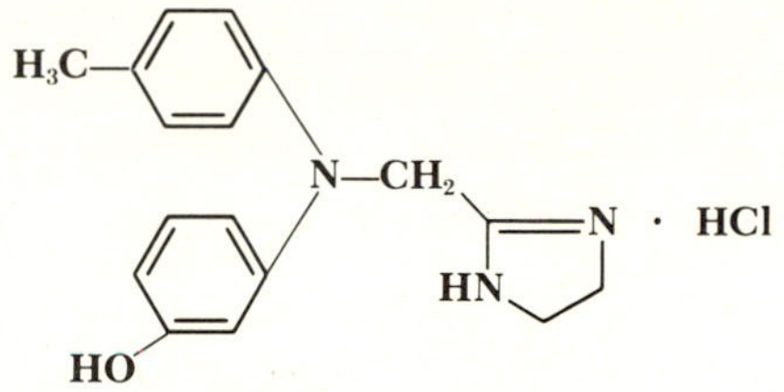   Phentolamine hydrochloride

Phentolamine. Phentolamine is an α blocker used almost exclusively for the diagnosis of pheochromocytoma and for the prevention of hypertension during operative removal of the tumor. Preparations include phentolamine hydrochloride (Regitine hydrochloride) in tablets, 50 mg, and phentolamine mesylate (Regitine mesylate) in powder for injection, 5 mg. In addition to its blocking action on receptors, the drug has other pharmacological actions similar to those of tolazoline, to which it is chemically related.

Adverse effects include orthostatic hypotension, tachycardia, nasal stuffiness, and gastrointestinal disturbances such as nausea, vomiting, and diarrhea.

In patients having an adrenal medullary tumor, the intravenous injection of 5 mg of phentolamine generally causes a rapid fall of blood pressure, 25 mm Hg diastolic and 33 mm Hg systolic. False positive and false negative reactions may occur, however, and the pharmacological tests for pheochromocytoma are being replaced by the more reliable chemical tests (p. 188).

Azapetine phosphate. Azapetine phosphate (Ilidar), an α-adrenergic blocking drug with additional smooth muscle–relaxing actions on the peripheral vasculature, is used in vasospastic diseases. It is available in tablets, 25 mg.

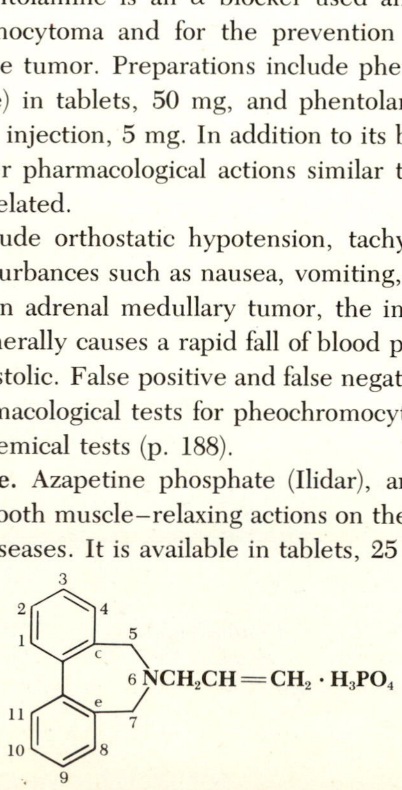

Azapetine phosphate

Prazosin. Prazosin is a recently introduced antihypertensive drug, which initially was thought to act by a direct relaxant effect on vascular smooth muscle. It was later found, however, that prazosin is a powerful but unusual α-blocking agent.[39] It is a useful antihypertensive, which has fewer side effects than the other available α blockers, probably due to its selective action on postsynaptic α receptors. The drug does not cause the marked tachycardia as seen, for example, with phenoxybenzamine. The reason for the difference may lie in the action of phenoxybenzamine in blocking both presynaptic and postsynaptic α receptors. Blockade of the presynaptic receptor prevents released norepinephrine from acting on this receptor to inhibit further transmitter release. Consequently, enhanced norepinephrine release occurs with phenoxybenzamine and can then stimulate unprotected cardiac β receptors. The weak action of prazosin on presynaptic receptors would result in less cardiac stimulation.

Prazosin hydrochloride (Minipress) is available in 1, 2, and 5 mg capsules. Adverse effects include a marked postural hypotension following the first dose. Fortunately, this effect does not generally persist with continued drug usage.

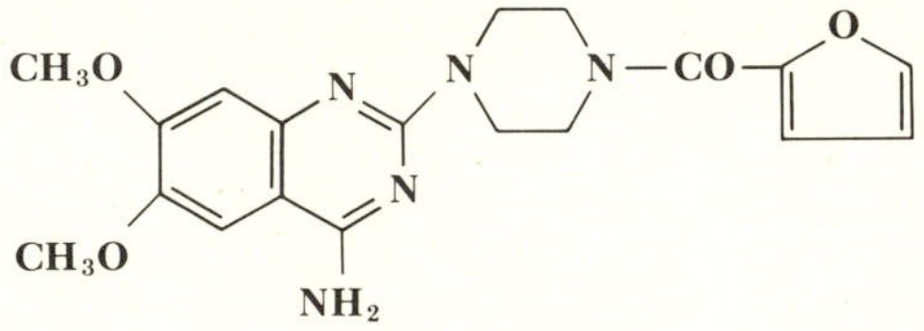

Prazosin

Ergot alkaloids. Certain alkaloids of ergot, such as ergotamine, have some α-adrenergic blocking action. They are not used as adrenergic blocking agents. Their pharmacology is discussed in Chapter 21.

β-ADRENERGIC BLOCKING AGENTS

The β-adrenergic blocking agents competitively inhibit the actions of adrenergic agonists on β receptors.

Development

The first β-adrenergic blocking agent, dichlorisoproterenol, was discovered in 1957.[28] As it had some intrinsic β-receptor stimulant activity, it was not clinically useful. Later, pronethalol, a fairly pure β blocker was synthesized.[1] Subsequently,

TABLE 16-1. Effects of β-adrenergic receptor blockade

Heart rate	Decreased
Myocardial contractility	Decreased
Cardiac output	Decreased
Arterial blood pressure	Unaffected or decreased
Effect of exercise on heart rate and cardiac output	Decreased
Effects of isoproterenol	Blocked
β-adrenergic drug effects (myocardial, arterial, bronchial, metabolic)	Blocked

propranolol (Inderal) was introduced and approved by the Food and Drug Administration, initially for the treatment of cardiac arrhythmias (1968), then for the treatment of angina pectoris (1973), and finally as an antihypertensive agent (1976). Numerous β blockers have been developed in addition to propranolol. They differ from propranolol in their relative effects on cardiac and bronchial β receptors, intrinsic agonist activity on β receptors, and membrane depressant properties. Recently metoprolol has been approved as an antihypertensive, and nadolol as an antihypertensive and antianginal agent.

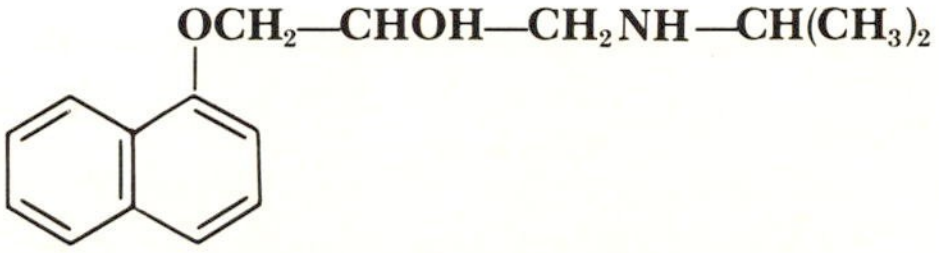

Propranolol

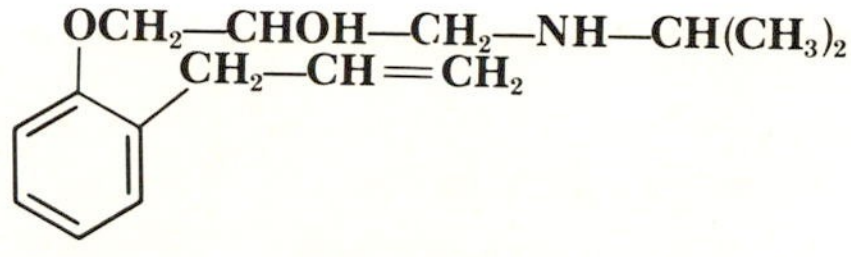

Alprenolol

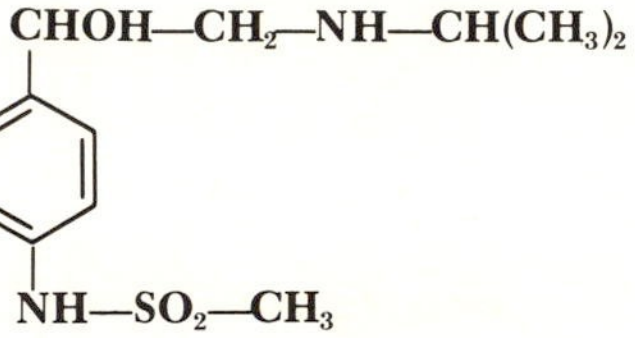

Sotalol

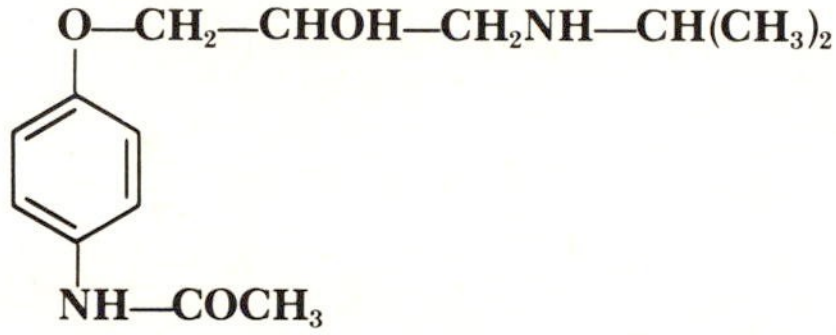

Practolol

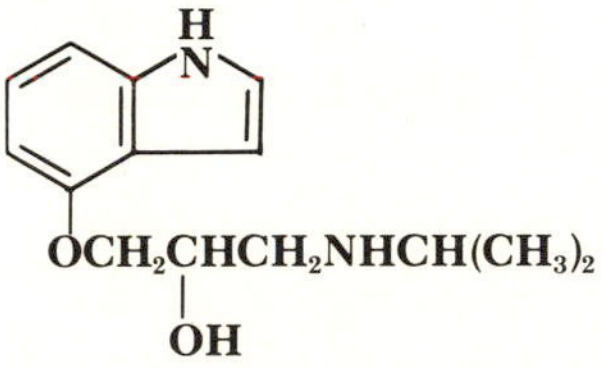

Pindolol

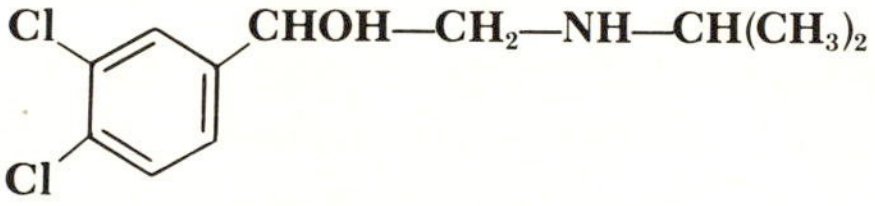

Dichloroisoproterenol

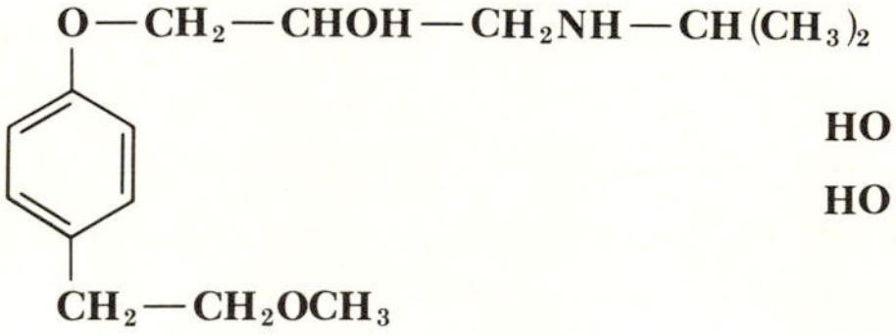

Metoprolol

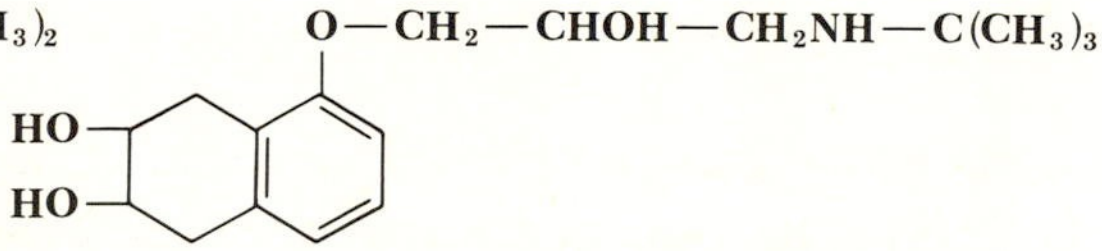

Nadolol

Pharmacological effects. Propranolol antagonizes competitively the effects of catecholamines released from adrenergic nerves or from the adrenal medulla on all β receptors. As a consequence the drug exerts negative chronotropic and inotropic effects on the heart, slows atrioventricular conduction, promotes bronchoconstriction, lowers plasma renin activity, and may cause hypoglycemia. It also exerts some quinidine-like actions on the heart.

The effects of propranolol may be overcome by sufficiently large doses of iso-

Propranolol

proterenol, which is a β agonist, or by glucagon, which acts on a different receptor but also activates adenyl cyclase.

Pharmacokinetics. Propranolol is absorbed completely from the gastrointestinal tract. About 50% is extracted by the liver as the drug is being absorbed, the so-called first pass effect. Plasma concentrations are low and variable. The half-life of the drug is 3 hours. The major metabolite, 4-hydroxypropranolol, is active as a β blocker but has a short half-life.[10,15]

Despite its short half-life, propranolol may be administered at 6- to 8-hour intervals in order to achieve therapeutic effects. Altered renal function has little effect on the dosage regimens. On the other hand, phenobarbital decreases the half-life of the drug.[5]

Clinical uses. The generally accepted uses of propranolol are in the treatment of arrhythmias, angina pectoris, hypertension, hypertrophic subaortic stenosis, thyrotoxicosis, and pheochromocytoma. Investigational uses include action tremors and migraine.

The *antiarrhythmic effect* of propranolol results largely from β blockade. Its quinidine-like effect may contribute to its effectiveness in digitalis-induced arrhythmias. Propranolol is a racemic mixture. The *levo* form is the β blocker, but the *dextro* form has a greater membrane effect. Propranolol is used in supraventricular tachyarrhythmias, such as in thyrotoxicosis. Ventricular tachycardias caused by catecholamines or digitalis are also important indications, but in other types of ventricular tachycardias propranolol is not the first choice.

Angina pectoris is benefited by propranolol in selected patients who do not respond to conventional measures, such as sublingual nitroglycerin. The drug should not be used in patients in whom angina is precipitated only by great effort because of the adverse effects of the drug on some properties of the myocardium.

The *antihypertensive effect* of propranolol has not been explained in a completely satisfactory manner.[15] Reduction of cardiac output, inhibition of renin release, and some CNS effect have all been suggested as possible mechanisms of the antihypertensive action of propranolol, but there are arguments against each one of these suggestions.[15] When propranolol is used in combination with a peripheral vasodilator, such as hydralazine, its beneficial effect is more easily understandable. Peripheral vasodilation leads to reflex cardiac stimulation, which is blocked by propranolol.

Hypertrophic subaortic stenosis is accompanied by symptoms such as angina, which are made worse by increased cardiac contractility. The usefulness of propranolol then becomes obvious.

Hyperkinetic cardiocirculatory states are benefited by propranolol as a consequence of the ability of the drug to depress cardiac function.

Propranolol is used both before and during surgical intervention for *pheochromocytoma*. By itself, propranolol may cause a rise in arterial pressure in these patients. Thus α-receptor blocking agents must be used simultaneously.

The investigational uses of propranolol in *action tremors*[37] and in *migraine* appear promising, but further studies are required.

Adverse effects and drug interactions. The major adverse effects of propranolol result from depression of cardiac contractility, heart block, and bronchial constriction. Sudden withdrawal of propranolol in patients with coronary disease may precipitate angina or even myocardial infarction.[1]

Propranolol may cause hypoglycemia and may interfere with the recovery from hypoglycemia following insulin administration. Propranolol may increase the hypotensive actions of the phenothiazines, and it inhibits the β-adrenergic effects of dopamine administered or formed from levodopa. Propranolol may aggravate the negative inotropic effects of quinidine. The β blocker is used in the treatment of digitalis-induced arrhythmias but may exaggerate bradycardia caused by digitalis. Bradycardia induced by propranolol responds to atropine.

Preparations. Propranolol (Inderal) is available in tablets, 10 and 40 mg, and injectable solutions containing 1 mg/ml in 1 ml containers.

Newer β-blocking drugs

Recently approved for use in the United States are **metoprolol** (Lopressor) and **nadolol** (Corgard). Metoprolol has been approved for use as an antihypertensive agent. It has a preferential effect on β_1 receptors and thus is relatively cardioselective in its β-blocking actions. Because of this it may be somewhat less hazardous in patients with bronchospastic disease, but cannot be considered without effect on bronchial smooth muscle. The drug has no intrinsic sympathomimetic activity and weak membrane effects. Nadolol has been approved as an antihypertensive and antianginal agent. It is not a selective β blocker, but lacks membrane actions or intrinsic agonist activity. Its potency and duration of action appear to be greater than those of propranolol.

A drug recently introduced for the treatment of glaucoma is timolol maleate (Timoptic). This drug is a β blocker, but it is unclear at the present time as to whether this action is involved in the drug's ability to lower intraocular pressure.

Certain other β blockers have been developed but are not yet approved for use in the United States. The various actions of these drugs are given in Table 16-2.

TABLE 16-2. Actions of newer β-blocking drugs in comparison with propranolol*

Generic name	Trade name	Potency (blocker)	Cardiac action	Arteriolar action	Bronchial action	β-Stimulation	Membrane activity
Propranolol	Inderal	1.0	++	+++	+++	0	+
Alprenolol	Aptine	1.0	++	+	+	++	+
Oxprenolol	Trasicor	2.0	++	+	+	++	+
Pindolol	INPEA	0.04	++	+	++	+	0
Sotalol	—	0.1	++	+	+	0	0
Practolol	—	0.5	++	0	0	0	0

*From Miller, R. R., Amsterdam, E. A., and Mason, D. T.: Ration. Drug Ther. **8:**1, 1974.

REFERENCES

1 Alderman, E. L., Coltart, D. J., Wettach, G. E., and Harrison, D. C.: Coronary artery syndromes after sudden propranolol withdrawal, Ann. Intern. Med. **81**:625, 1974.

2 Antonis, A., Clark, M. L., Hodge, R. L., Molony, M., and Pilkington, T. R.: Receptor mechanisms in the hyperglycaemic response to adrenaline in man, Lancet **1**:1135, 1967.

3 Belleau, B.: Relationships between antagonists and receptor sites. In Adrenergic mechanisms, Ciba Foundation and Committee on Drug Action, Boston, 1960, Little, Brown & Co.

4 Bloch, J. H., Pierce, C. H., and Lillehei, R. C.: Adrenergic blocking agents in the treatment of shock, Annu. Rev. Med. **17**:483, 1966.

5 Branch, R. A., Shand, D. G., Wilkinson, G. R., et al.: Increased clearance of antipyrine and *d*-propranolol after phenobarbital treatment in the monkey: relative contributions of enzyme induction and increased hepatic blood flow, J. Clin. Invest. **53**:1101, 1974.

6 Cohen, L. S., and Braunwald, E.: Amelioration of angina pectoris in idiopathic hypertrophic subaortic stenosis with beta-adrenergic blockade, Circulation **35**:847, 1967.

7 Dollery, C. T., Paterson, J. W., and Conolly, M. E.: Clinical pharmacology of beta-receptor-blocking drugs, Clin. Pharmacol. Ther. **10**:765, 1969.

8 Dornhorst, A. C., and Robinson, B. F.: Clinical pharmacology of a beta-adrenergic blocking agent (nethalide), Lancet **2**:413, 1962.

9 Epstein, S. E., and Braunwald, E.: Beta-adrenergic receptor blocking drugs, N. Engl. J. Med. **275**:1106, 1175, 1966.

10 Evans, G. H., and Shand, D. G.: Disposition of propranolol. V. Drug accumulation and steady-state concentrations during chronic oral administration in man, Clin. Pharmacol. Ther. **14**:487, 1973.

11 Fitzgerald, J. D.: Perspectives in adrenergic beta-receptor blockade, Clin. Pharmacol. Ther. **10**:292, 1969.

12 Fourneau, E., and Bovet, D.: Récherches sur l'action sympathicolytique d'un nouveau dérivé du dioxane, Arch. Int. Pharmacodyn. **46**:178, 1933.

13 Frohlich, E. D., and Page, I. H.: The clinical meaning of cardiovascular beta-adrenergic receptors, Physiol. Pharmacol. Physicians **1**(11):1, 1966.

14 Hamer, J., Grandjean, T., Melendez, L., and Sowton, G. E.: Effect of propranolol (Inderal) in angina pectoris: preliminary report, Br. Med. J. **2**:720, 1964.

15 Holland, O. B., and Kaplan, N. M.: Propranolol in the treatment of hypertension, N. Engl. J. Med. **294**:930, 1976.

16 Irons, G. V., Ginn, W. N., and Orgain, E. S.: Use of a beta adrenergic receptor blocking agent (propranolol) in the treatment of cardiac arrhythmias, Am. J. Med. **43**:161, 1967.

17 Kelliher, G. J., and Roberts, J.: The effect of d (+) and l (−) practolol on ouabain-induced arrhythmia, Eur. J. Pharmacol. **20**:243, 1972.

18 Kosinski, E. J., and Malindzak, G. S.: Glucagon and isoproterenol in reversing propranolol toxicity, Arch. Intern. Med. **132**:840, 1973.

19 Lands, A. M., Arnold, A., and McAnliff, J. P.: Differentiation of receptor systems activated by sympathomimetic amines, Nature **214**:597, 1967.

20 Levy, B.: Adrenergic blocking activity of N-tertiary-butylmethoxamine (butoxamine), J. Pharmacol. Exp. Ther. **151**:413, 1966.

21 Miller, R. R., Amsterdam, E. A., and Mason, D. T.: The pharmacologic basis for clinical use of beta adrenergic blocking drugs, Ration. Drug Ther. **8**:1, 1974.

22 Nickerson, M.: The pharmacology of adrenergic blockade, Pharmacol. Rev. **1**:27, 1949.

23 Nickerson, M.: Nonequilibrium drug antagonism, Pharmacol. Rev. **9**:246, 1957.

24 Nickerson, M.: Vasoconstriction and vasodilation in shock. In Hershey, S. G., editor: Shock, Boston, 1964, Little, Brown & Co.

25 Nickerson, M., and Goodman, L. S.: Pharmacological properties of a new adrenergic blocking agent; N,N-dibenzyl-β-chlorethylamine (Dibenamine), J. Pharmacol. Exp. Ther. **89**:167, 1947.

26 Pettinger, W. A., Campbell, W. B., and Keeton, K.: The adrenergic component of renin release induced by vasodilating antihypertensive drugs in the rat, Circ. Res. **33**:82, 1973.

27 Pettinger, W. A., and Mitchell, H. C.: Minoxidil: a possible alternative to nephrectomy for hypertension, N. Engl. J. Med. **289**:167, 1973.

28 Powell, C. E., and Slater, I. H.: Blocking of inhibitory adrenergic receptors by a dichloro analog of isoproterenol, J. Pharmacol. Exp. Ther. **122**:480, 1958.

29 Prichard, B. N. C., and Gillam, P. M. S.: Use of propranolol (Inderal) in treatment of hypertension, Br. Med. J. **2**:725, 1964.

30 Sandler, G., and Clayton, G. A.: Clinical eval-

uation of practolol, a new cardioselective beta-blocking agent in angina pectoris, Br. Med. J. 1:399, 1970.

31 Schelling, J. L., Scazziga, B., Dufour, R. J., Milinkovic, N., and Weber, A. A.: Effect of pindolol, a beta receptor antagonist, in hyperthyroidism, Clin. Pharmacol. Ther. 14:158, 1973.

32 Srivastava, S. C., Dewar, H. A., and Newell, D. J.: Double-blind trial of propranolol (Inderal) in angina of effort, Br. Med. J. 2:724, 1964.

33 Stallworth, J. M., and Jeffords, J. V.: Clinical effects of azapetine (Ilidar) on peripheral vascular disease, J.A.M.A. 161:840, 1956.

34 Taylor, R. R., Johnston, C. I., and José, A. D.: Reversal of digitalis intoxication by beta adrenergic blockade with pronethalol, N. Engl. J. Med. 271:877, 1964.

35 Traub, Y., Shaver, J. A., McDonald, R. H., and Shapiro, A. P.: Effects of practolol on pressor responses to noxious stimuli in hypertensive patients, Clin. Pharmacol. Ther. 14:165, 1973.

36 Westfall, T. C., Cipolloni, P. B., and Edmundowicz, A. C.: Influence of propranolol on hemodynamic changes and plasma catecholamine levels following cigarette smoking and nicotine, Proc. Soc. Exp. Biol. Med. 123:174, 1966.

37 Winkler, G. F., and Young, R. R.: Efficacy of chronic propranolol therapy in action tremors of the familial, senile or essential varieties, N. Engl. J. Med. 290:984, 1974.

REVIEWS

38 Prichard, B. N. C.: β-Adrenergic receptor blockade in hypertension, past, present, and future, Br. J. Clin. Pharmacol. 5:379, 1978.

39 Stokes, G. S., and Oates, H. F.: Prazosin—new alpha adrenergic blocking agent in treatment of hypertension, Cardiovasc. Med. 3:41, 1978.

CHAPTER 17

Drugs acting on the adrenergic neuron

GENERAL CONCEPT   Drugs can influence sympathetic functions by affecting the storage and release of catecholamines, thus providing tools for an entirely new pharmacological approach to the nervous system. Such drugs have found wide application as *antihypertensive agents* and in the field of *psychopharmacology.*

This field was opened up by the discovery that reserpine, a *Rauwolfia* alkaloid, caused a release of serotonin (5-hydroxytryptamine) from its binding sites in various tissues.[33] Subsequently it was shown that reserpine also releases norepinephrine and dopamine. Decreased sympathetic functions induced by reserpine, such as hypotension and bradycardia, are now generally attributed to the catecholamine depletion at the adrenergic nerve endings.

Other drugs can influence catecholamine stores also. Guanethidine causes depletion of peripheral amine stores. On the other hand, bretylium blocks adrenergic fibers without depleting their catecholamine content.

The MAO inhibitors raise the catecholamine content of neural tissues in several species. This finding suggests that the enzyme may have a regulatory function on the concentration of bound catecholamines. Hypotension that follows the use of MAO inhibitors may be related to the accumulation of norepinephrine or some other amine in ganglia and adrenergic fibers.[24]

Studies on the catecholamine-depleting agents led to the concept that tyramine and many other sympathomimetic amines act indirectly by releasing catecholamines in the body. These studies led to the discovery that certain amines such as metaraminol are taken up by adrenergic nerves, where they may function as false transmitters.[31]

MECHANISMS OF CATECHOLAMINE RELEASE   Drugs may release catecholamines by one of two mechanisms, and these mechanisms may be further influenced by at least four additional pharmacological actions.

The *two basic* mechanisms of release and the drugs that illustrate them are as follows:

Interference with granular storage mechanism
    Reserpine
    Guanethidine

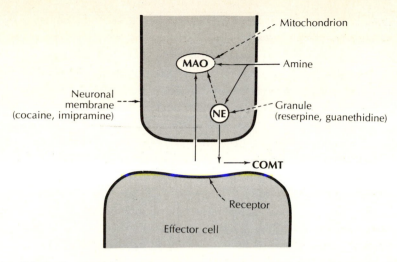

FIG. 17-1. Schematic representation of nerve ending and effector cell. (For details see text.)

Displacement of catecholamines
    Tyramine
    Amphetamine
    Metaraminol
    Methyldopa (through its metabolite α-methylnorepinephrine)

1. *Interference with granular storage mechanism.* As shown in Fig. 17-1, when catecholamines are released physiologically, a small granule is extruded and its amine acts on the receptor. On the other hand, when the amine is released by drugs such as reserpine or guanethidine, it is freed from the granule within the axoplasm, making it subject to attack by MAO. Instead of the active amine, mostly its inactivated products appear outside the nerve. This is likely the reason why the injection of reserpine, although causing massive depletion of catecholamines, does not result in an elevation of blood pressure.

2. *Displacement of catecholamines.* The indirectly acting sympathomimetic drugs such as tyramine and amphetamine can cause release of catecholamines. Other amines not only displace catecholamines but also are incorporated into the granule. These include metaraminol[3] and α-methylnorepinephrine. The latter is a metabolite of methyldopa, which undoubtedly causes amine depletion by this indirect mechanism.

The basic mechanisms of catecholamine release can be modified by at least four pharmacological influences.

The *MAO inhibitors* protect the intraneuronally released catecholamines from inactivation.

Certain drugs, the *adrenergic neuronal blocking agents*, prevent catecholamine release induced by nerve stimulation or by the indirectly acting amines such as tyramine. The best known example of such drugs is bretylium. Conceptually, these drugs behave as if they anesthetized the adrenergic fibers. Indeed, they have local anesthetic properties and they concentrate in adrenergic fibers.

Drugs that act at the neuronal membrane (Fig. 17-1) such as cocaine and imipramine have several important actions on catecholamine release. They block the action of tyramine and other indirectly acting amines. They do not block the action of reserpine, a point in favor of a difference in the site of action of tyramine and reserpine. Cocaine and other drugs that inhibit the membrane pump for amines cause an apparent "sensitization" of the receptor by allowing the local accumulation of catecholamine.

Drugs may act on presynaptic α or β receptors that modulate catecholamine release.[25]

Although the physiological significance of this modulation in the normal functioning of the adrenergic neuron is not clear at present, it appears that some of the side effects of certain α-blocking drugs might arise in part from blockade of presynaptic α receptors. The resulting excessive norepinephrine release may contribute via actions on β receptors to the tachycardia and the high renin secretion seen, for example, after administration of phenoxybenzamine.

Basic differences between the actions of reserpine and guanethidine

Although both reserpine and guanethidine deplete nerves of their catecholamine by acting on the granular storage mechanism, guanethidine has additional effects. Its intravenous injection regularly leads to a transient elevation of blood pressure, caused by a *tyramine-like* effect that can be blocked by cocaine. To make matters more complex, guanethidine has an early *bretylium-like* effect that somehow interferes with norepinephrine release after nerve stimulation.

An additional difference between reserpine and guanethidine is of great importance. Reserpine depletes catecholamines and serotonin from many sites, including the brain. Guanethidine apparently fails to cross the blood-brain barrier and thus has no effect on brain amines.

Mechanism of decreased sympathetic activity induced by catecholamine depletion

When the catecholamine content of a nerve is decreased to below 50%, stimulation of the nerve results in a lessened response. The rate of depletion varies in different organs. Cardiac catecholamine declines rapidly, and adrenal stores are more resistant. The rate of depletion is a function not only of the dose of reserpine but also of the rate of turnover of the amine at the various sites.[11,26] It has been estimated that the half-time of catecholamines in the heart is 4 to 8 hours, in contrast with their half-time of 7 days in the adrenal medulla.[8] Depletion must be rapid in arterioles and venules. This is why reserpine is useful as an antihypertensive drug.

Catecholamine uptake

Several experiments suggest that catecholamines are taken up by adrenergic nerves.[2] It has been shown that in a reserpinized animal neither sympathetic stimulation nor injected tyramine will cause a pressor response.[9] After an infusion of norepinephrine, the pressor response to nerve stimulation and tyramine is restored, although only a small fraction of the catecholamine stores is replenished.

It appears, then, that there must be a pool of available norepinephrine[30] that is essential for function of the sympathetic endings. It has been shown that the H^3-norepinephrine taken up by the pool is actually released by sympathetic nerve stimulation and appears in the venous effluent blood.[2]

Alkaloids of *Rauwolfia serpentina* have antihypertensive and tranquilizing properties. Reserpine and some other *Rauwolfia* alkaloids produce depletion of norepinephrine, dopamine, and also serotonin from various binding sites in the brain and peripheral nerves. The drug not only causes a release of amines but also blocks their granular uptake. It does not, however, block the action of catecholamines. It may have some blocking effect on norepinephrine synthesis by preventing the uptake of dopamine into storage granules that contain dopamine-β-oxidase. **RESERPINE**

The antihypertensive drug guanethidine (Ismelin)[16,27] causes decreased sympathetic activity by a dual mechanism, depleting norepinephrine at peripheral nerve endings in the manner of reserpine and also causing early sympathetic neuronal blockade at a time when catecholamines are not yet depleted in the nerve. It is not a ganglionic blocking agent and does not prevent the action of catecholamines (p. 225). **GUANETHIDINE**

Debrisoquin (Declinax) is structurally related to guanethidine, but it produces adrenergic neuronal blockade by the same mechanisms as bretylium. It is a potent antihypertensive agent when used in the same dosage as guanethidine.[28] **DEBRISOQUIN**

The studies showing that debrisoquin as well as bretylium inhibits MAO and is apparently concentrated in the adrenergic neurons throw new light on the mode of action of these drugs.[21]

Bretylium (Darenthin)[4] produces a selective block on the peripheral sympathetic nervous system without opposing the action of injected or released catecholamines. **BRETYLIUM**

Bretylium tosylate

Bretylium blocks the adrenergic fiber without depleting its catecholamine content and may act as a local anesthetic that concentrates in adrenergic fibers.[4]

Bretylium blocks the enzyme MAO[21]; perhaps this action in the adrenergic nerves explains its action.

Although bretylium is basically a very interesting drug, its clinical use has been attended by so many toxic effects, including muscular weakness and mental confusion, that it is no longer available. There is some interest in its experimental use as an antiarrhythmic drug.

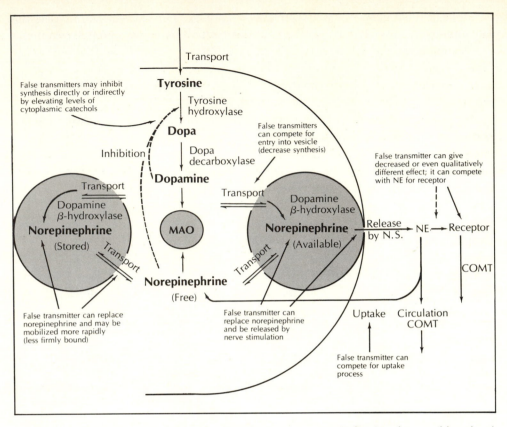

FIG. 17-2. Catecholamine metabolism in the adrenergic neuron, indicating the possible role of false transmitters. (From Kopin, I. J.: In Adrenergic neurotransmission, Ciba Foundation Study Group No. 33, Boston, 1968, Little, Brown & Co.)

METHYLDOPA   Methyldopa (Aldomet), an analog of dihydroxyphenylalanine, competes with this precursor of norepinephrine for the enzyme that decarboxylates aromatic L-amino acids. Although it inhibits the synthesis of both norepinephrine and serotonin, norepinephrine levels in the brain remain low for a much longer time than serotonin levels.[3] This and other evidence suggests that much of the catecholamine depletion induced by methyldopa is caused by the drug's being metabolized to form α-methyl-norepinephrine that replaces norepinephrine and acts as a "false transmitter."[29] The various consequences of the presence of false transmitters are summarized in Fig. 17-2.

MAO INHIBITORS   MAO inhibitors were introduced as antidepressants. One of their surprising side effects was orthostatic hypotension, which suggested interference with sympathetic functions.

Experimentally, the MAO inhibitors elevate the levels of norepinephrine and serotonin in the brain, ganglia, and other peripheral tissues.[15] In addition, they prevent many of the actions of reserpine, including its ability to lower amine levels.

Although it has been suggested that the MAO inhibitors block the amine release phenomenon directly, it is more likely that they prevent the metabolic degradation of endogenous amines released from subcellular structures, thus causing elevation of their levels in the axoplasm of adrenergic neurons. MAO inhibitors may also promote the formation of false transmitters such as octopamine.[22] False transmitters, in turn, may block norepinephrine release (Fig. 17-2).

One of the serious disadvantages of the MAO inhibitors is the increased likelihood of adverse reactions to ingested foods and to drugs that may release monoamines in the body.[19,35] The ingestion of aged cheese, beer, or certain wines has caused hypertensive emergencies in patients who were being treated with MAO inhibitors. These serious reactions have been traced to the presence of tyramine in these foods and beverages. Tyramine would normally be deaminated by MAO. When its deamination is inhibited by drugs, it releases catecholamines in the body. Adverse reactions to indirectly acting sympathomimetic drugs have also occurred under similar circumstances.

Although most MAO inhibitors are used as antidepressants, one of these, pargyline (Eutonyl), was introduced as an antihypertensive agent.[7]

REFERENCES

1 Aviado, D. M., and Dil, A. H.: The effects of a new sympathetic blocking drug (bretylium) on cardiovascular control, J. Pharmacol. Exp. Ther. **129:**328, 1960.

2 Axelrod, J., Whitby, L. G., and Hertting, G.: Effect of psychotropic drugs on the uptake of H³-norepinephrine by tissues, Science **133:** 383, 1961.

3 Boura, A. L., and Green, A. F.: Adrenergic neurone blocking agents, Annu. Rev. Pharmacol. **5:**183, 1965.

4 Boura, A. L., Green, A. F., McCoubrey, A., Laurence, D. R., Moulton, R., and Rosenheim, M. L.: Darenthin: hypotensive agent of new type, Lancet **2:**17, 1959.

5 Brodie, B. B., Olin, J. S., Kuntzman, R. G., and Shore, P. A.: Possible interrelationships between release of brain norepinephrine and serotonin by reserpine, Science **125:**1293, 1957.

6 Brooks, V. B.: The action of botulinum toxin on motor-nerve filaments, J. Physiol. **123:**501, 1954.

7 Bryant, J. M., Torosdag, S., Schvartz, N., Fletcher, L., Fertig, H., Schwartz, S., and Quan, R. B. F.: Antihypertensive properties of pargyline hydrochloride, J.A.M.A. **178:**406, 1961.

8 Burack, W. R., and Draskoczy, P. R.: The turnover of endogenously labeled catecholamines in several regions of the sympathetic nervous system, J. Pharmacol. Exp. Ther. **144:**66, 1964.

9 Burn, J. H., and Rand, M. J.: A new interpretation of the adrenergic nerve fiber, Adv. Pharmacol. **1:**1, 1962.

10 Butterfield, J. L., and Richardson, J. A.: Acute effects of guanethidine on myocardial contractility and catecholamine levels, Proc. Soc. Exp. Biol. Med. **106:**259, 1961.

11 Carlsson, A.: Physiological and pharmacological release of monoamines in the central nervous system. In von Euler, U. S., Rosell, S., and Ulvnas, B., editors: Mechanisms of release of biogenic amines, New York, 1966, Pergamon Press, Inc.

12 Carlsson, A., and Lindquist, M.: In vivo decarboxylation of α-methylDOPA and α-methyl metatyrosine, Acta Physiol. Scand. **54:**87, 1962.

13 Carlsson, A., Lindquist, M., Magnusson, T., and Waldeck, B.: On the presence of 3-hydroxytyramine in brain, Science **127:**471, 1958.

14 Cass, R., and Spriggs, T. L. B.: Tissue amine levels and sympathetic blockade after guanethidine and bretylium, Br. J. Pharmacol. **17:**442, 1961.

15 Chessin, M., Kramer, E. R., and Scott, C. C.: Modifications of the pharmacology of reserpine and serotonin by iproniazid, J. Pharmacol. **119:** 453, 1957.

16 Cohn, J. N., Liptak, T. E., and Freis, E. D.:

Hemodynamic effects of guanethidine in man, Circ. Res. **12:**298, 1963.

17 Costa, E., and Brodie, B. B.: A role for norepinephrine in ganglionic transmission, J. Am. Geriatr. Soc. **9:**119, 1961.

18 Eccles, J. C.: The physiology of nerve cells, Baltimore, 1957, The Johns Hopkins University Press.

19 Editorial: Hypertensive reactions to monoamine oxidase inhibitors, Br. Med. J. **1:**578, 1964.

20 Fleming, W. W., and Trendelenburg, U.: Development of supersensitivity to norepinephrine after pretreatment with reserpine, J. Pharmacol. Exp. Ther. **133:**41, 1961.

21 Giachetti, A., and Shore, P. A.: Monoamine oxidase inhibition in the adrenergic neuron by bretylium, debrisoquin, and other adrenergic neuronal blocking agents, Biochem. Pharmacol. **16:**237, 1967.

22 Kopin, I. J.: False adrenergic transmitters, Annu. Rev. Pharmacol. **8:**377, 1968.

23 Kopin, I. J.: The influence of false adrenergic transmitters on adrenergic neurotransmission. In Adrenergic neurotransmission, Ciba Foundation Study Group No. 33, Boston, 1968, Little, Brown & Co.

24 Kopin, I. J., Fischer, J. E., Musacchio, J. M., Horst, W. D., and Weise, V. K.: False neurochemical transmitters and the mechanism of sympathetic blockade by monamine oxidase inhibitors, J. Pharmacol. Exp. Ther. **147:**186, 1965.

25 Langer, S. Z.: Presynaptic regulation of catecholamine release, Biochem. Pharmacol. **23:**1793, 1974.

26 Lee, F. L.: The relation between norepinephrine content and response to sympathetic nerve stimulation of various organs of cats pretreated with reserpine, J. Pharmacol. Exp. Ther. **156:**137, 1967.

27 Maxwell, R. A., Plummer, A. J., Schneider, F., Povalski, H., and Daniel, A. I.: Pharmacology of [2-(octahydro-1-axocinyl)ethyl] guanethidine sulfate (SU-5864), J. Pharmacol. Exp. Ther. **128:**22, 1960.

28 Moe, R. A., et al.: Cardiovascular effects of 3,4,-dihydro-2(1H) isoquinoline carboxamidine (Declinax), Curr. Ther. Res. **6:**299, 1964.

29 Muscholl, E.: Effect of drugs on smooth muscle: newer mechanisms of adrenergic blockade, Annu. Rev. Pharmacol. **6:**107, 1966.

30 Shore, P. A.: Release of serotonin and catecholamines by drugs, Pharmacol. Rev. **14:**531, 1962.

31 Shore, P. A., Busfield, D., and Alpers, H. S.: Binding and release of metaraminol: mechanism of norepinephrine depletion by α-methyl-M-tyrosine and related agents, J. Pharmacol. Exp. Ther. **146:**194, 1964.

32 Shore, P. A., and Giachetti, A.: Dual actions of guanethidine on amine uptake mechanisms in adrenergic neurons, Biochem. Pharmacol. **15:**899, 1966.

33 Shore, P. A., Silver, S. L., and Brodie, B. B.: Interaction of reserpine, serotonin, and lysergic acid diethylamide in brain, Science **122:**284, 1955.

34 Starke, K., and Montel, H.: Alpha-receptor mediated modulation of transmitter release from central noradrenergic neurones, Naunyn-Schniedebergs Arch. Pharmacol. **279:**53, 1973.

35 Thomas, J. C. S.: Monoamine oxidase inhibitors and cheese, Br. Med. J. **2:**1406, 1963.

36 Udenfriend, S., Connamacher, R., and Hess, S. M.: On the mechanism of release of norepinephrine by alpha-methyl-M-tyrosine and alpha-methyl-M-tyramine, Biochem. Pharmacol. **8:**419, 1962.

REVIEWS

37 Maxwell, R. A., and Wastila, W. B.: Adrenergic neuron blocking drugs, Handbook Exp. Pharmacol. **39:**161, 1977.

38 Shore, P. A.: Transport and storage of biogenic amines, Annu. Rev. Pharmacol. **12:**209, 1972.

CHAPTER 18

Antihypertensive drugs

GENERAL CONCEPT

Effective treatment of hypertension is one of the major developments in medicine. Beginning in 1949 when ganglionic blocking agents were introduced, a series of important discoveries occurred, which led to the present availability of numerous antihypertensive drugs that are capable of exerting a favorable effect on life expectancy and the complications of hypertension.[92,98,99]

Some of the most significant developments that led to the present state of antihypertensive treatment were the introduction of hydralazine in 1952, reserpine in 1953, the thiazide diuretics in 1959, guanethidine in 1960, followed by methyldopa and clonidine in 1967, β-adrenergic blocking drugs in 1968, and, recently, prazosin, an α-adrenergic blocking drug. It appears at present that the introductions of the thiazide diuretics and the β-adrenergic blocking drugs have had the greatest impact on the management of hypertension.

The antihypertensive drugs act by many different mechanisms, as summarized in Table 18-1. An understanding of these mechanisms is essential for tailoring antihypertensive therapy to the individual patient's requirement. A diagrammatic representation of blood pressure–regulating mechanisms is shown in Fig. 18-1.

RELATION OF ANGIOTENSIN AND ALDOSTERONE TO HYPERTENSION

The demonstration that renal ischemia leads to hypertension[27] resulted in the discovery of a kidney enzyme, renin, which is in the granules of the juxtaglomerular apparatus.[28] When this enzyme is released by ischemia or perhaps by a decreased caliber of the afferent arteriole, it acts on a substrate in blood and eventually yields angiotensin, a potent vasopressor polypeptide. This sequence of events is shown in Table 18-2.

The amino acid composition of angiotensin I is as follows:

Asp-Arg-Val-Tyr-Ileu-His-Pro-Phe-His-Leu

The converting enzyme removes the terminal histidyl-leucine to form angiotensin II. Angiotensin I has little or no biological activity, although it may have some effect on aldosterone release, as does angiotensin III. Oral contraceptives increase the renin substrate concentrations and promote angiotensin formation.[56]

Saralasin (I-sarcosyl-8-alanyl-angiotensin II) is a specific angiotensin antagonist with essentially no other pharmacological action.[66] Given intravenously it serves as an investigational tool for determining the contribution of angiotensin to the blood pressure elevation.

TABLE 18-1. Site of action of antihypertensive drugs

Site of action	Mode of action	Drug	Trade name
Arteriolar smooth muscle	Direct vasodilatation	Hydralazine Diazoxide Minoxidil Nitroprusside	Apresoline Hyperstat Nipride
α-Adrenergic receptors	Receptor blockade	Phentolamine Phenoxybenzamine Prazosin	Regitine Dibenzyline Minipress
β-Adrenergic receptors	CNS effect Myocardial depression Renin release inhibition	Propranolol Metoprolol	Inderal Lopressor
Sympathetic fibers	Blockade of norepinephrine release (also depletion) Inhibition of MAO	Guanethidine Pargyline	Ismelin Eutonyl
Paravertebral ganglia	Ganglionic blockade	Chlorisondamine Hexamethonium Mecamylamine Pentolinium Trimethaphan	Ecolid Inversine Ansolysen Arfonad
CNS	Depression of cardiovascular control center False neurotransmitter Norepinephrine depletion	Clonidine Methyldopa Reserpine	Catapres Aldomet Many
Carotid sinus	Reflex sympathetic depression	Veratrum Electric stimulation	
Kidney	Sodium excretion Volume depletion	Many diuretics	

TABLE 18-2. Metabolism of angiotensin

Sequence	Inhibitors
Renin in kidney ↓ Renin released	β Blockers
+ Angiotensinogen ↓ Angiotensin I (decapeptide) +	
Converting enzyme ↓	Inhibitors (captopril)
Angiotensin II (octapeptide) +	Antagonists (saralasin)
Angiotensinases A, B, C ↓ ↘	
Angiotensin III Split product (heptapeptide)	

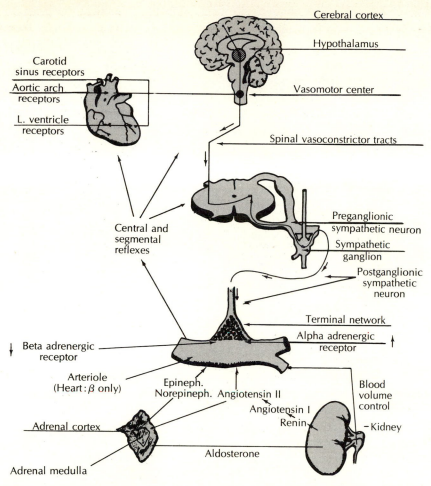

FIG. 18-1. Diagrammatic representation of blood pressure–regulating mechanisms. (From Abrams, W. B.: Dis. Chest **55:**148, 1969.)

Renin release

The release of renin from the juxtaglomerular apparatus of the kidney is under intensive investigation. Lowering of blood pressure and renal perfusion pressure promotes the release of the enzyme.[76] Some of the effect of lowered blood pressure on renin release may be mediated through sympathetic fibers. In fact, catecholamines can cause renin release. They do this apparently by acting on β receptors, since propranolol blocks catecholamine-induced renin release.[83]

Pharmacological effects

The pharmacological effects of angiotensin II (hereafter referred to as angiotensin) are as follows: (1) elevation of blood pressure, (2) contraction of isolated smooth muscle preparations, (3) release of aldosterone, and (4) release of catecholamines from adrenal medulla and adrenergic nerves.[20,64] Not only does angiotensin release catecholamines but it also prevents their reuptake by adrenergic nerves.[87]

The vasopressor effects of angiotensin are exerted primarily on peripheral resistance vessels in the skin, splanchnic area, and kidney. It has little cardiac stimulant action. The capacitance vessels are not greatly affected by it, differing in this respect from the response to catecholamines.

Several features of the action of angiotensin are of great interest in research on hypertension. This polypeptide has an effect on the vasomotor centers, resulting in increased sympathetic activity. It also potentiates the actions of catecholamines. It causes sodium retention by promoting the release of aldosterone from the adrenal cortex. Angiotensin is also a potent central dipsogenic agent in experimental animals.

The renin-angiotensin system along with the sympathetic nervous system plays a role in many hypertensive states. Since both plasma renin activity and catecholamine concentrations can be measured, the selection of antihypertensive medications is increasingly influenced by these measurements.

CLASSIFICATION OF ANTIHYPERTENSIVE DRUGS   The various antihypertensive drugs may be classified according to their mode of action as shown in Table 18-1. They will be discussed under the headings of direct vasodilators, α-adrenergic blocking drugs, β-adrenergic blocking drugs, MAO inhibitors, ganglionic blocking agents, central depressants of sympathetic functions, reflex inhibitors of central sympathetic function, and antihypertensive drugs that promote salt excretion.

DIRECT VASODILATORS   Direct vasodilators act on the vascular smooth muscle. They include hydralazine (Apresoline) and minoxidil (Loniten) for chronic use. Diazoxide (Hyperstat) and sodium nitroprusside (Nipride) are reserved for acute hypertensive emergencies.

Hydralazine   Hydralazine hydrochloride (1-hydrazinophthalazine hydrochloride) (Apresoline) is a direct relaxant of the vascular smooth muscle that is used commonly in chronic hypertension. Although the drug relaxes the vascular smooth muscle, it often produces considerable cardiac stimulation through reflex mechanisms. The cardiac effects may be prevented by β-adrenergic blocking agents.[13]

Adverse effects   Headache, palpitations, and gastrointestinal disturbances are not uncommon after taking the drug. A unique and more serious adverse effect is seen frequently when doses larger than 200 mg daily are administered. Many such patients develop a syndrome resembling systemic lupus erythematosus. This syndrome is reversible in most cases.

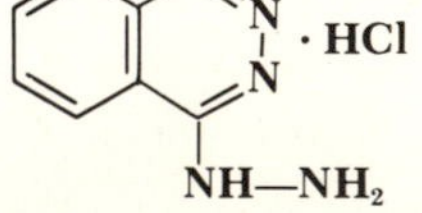

Hydralazine hydrochloride

The combined use of hydralazine and propranolol is becoming widely accepted in the management of hypertension. With the addition of a diuretic, the combination is quite effective.

Hydralazine hydrochloride (Apresoline) is obtainable in tablets of 10, 25, 50, **Preparations** and 100 mg and in a solution for injection, 20 mg/ml.

Minoxidil (Loniten) is a recently introduced powerful vasodilator, which is **Minoxidil** administered orally. It is indicated only for patients with severe hypertension who do not respond to other drugs. Minoxidil causes considerable sodium retention and edema, tachycardia, and hirsutism. The sodium retention may be controlled by the use of potent diuretics, and the tachycardia responds to β blockers. In addition, minoxidil has produced hemorrhagic right atrial lesions in dogs, an effect that apparently does not occur in humans.[95]

Minoxidil is available in tablet form. The initial dose should be 5 mg, and dosage is increased gradually to 40 mg a day in single or divided doses. The antihypertensive effect of the drug lasts at least 12 hours.

Diazoxide (Hyperstat) is a nondiuretic congener of the thiazide drugs. Admin- **Diazoxide** istered intravenously, it can be used for the rapid lowering of blood pressure in hypertensive emergencies. The effect lasts about 12 hours. Injection of diazoxide causes hyperglycemia as a consequence of inhibition of insulin release.

Diazoxide (Hyperstat) is supplied in a 20 ml ampule containing 300 mg of the **Preparation and** drug. The preparation is injected intravenously and rapidly. Blood pressure de- **dosage** creases within 2 minutes to its lowest level. Then it increases fairly rapidly for 30 minutes and more slowly for the next 2 to 12 hours.

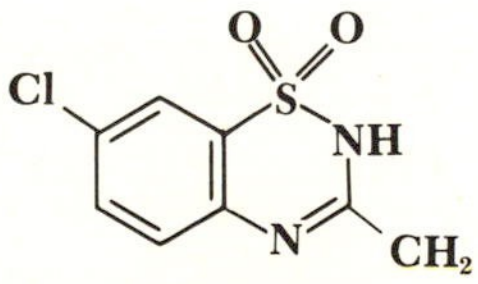

Diazoxide

Sodium nitroprusside (Nipride) is a direct vasodilator that has been approved **Sodium** for use in hypertensive crises. A dose of 1 μg/kg/min administered by intravenous **nitroprusside** infusion produces a rapid lowering of the blood pressure. The infusion rate must be adjusted by monitoring the blood pressure. The drug is very sensitive to light, and the infusion system should be protected against light.

Adverse effects of nitroprusside include nausea, disorientation, and muscle spasms. The metabolic product of nitroprusside, thiocyanate, is excreted by the kidney. Toxic effects may develop in patients who have renal impairment. Also, patients with hepatic impairment will detoxify the drug more slowly. When infused for prolonged periods to create a bloodless field in surgical procedures, thiocyanate and cyanide concentrations in the blood may become elevated, and delayed metabolic acidosis may supervene. The dosage of sodium nitroprusside should probably not exceed 500 μg/kg in order to avoid these toxic effects.

Sodium nitroprusside (Nipride) is available in 5 ml amber-colored vials containing the equivalent of 50 mg sodium nitroprusside dihydrate for reconstitution with dextrose in water for intravenous infusion.

α-ADRENERGIC BLOCKING DRUGS

The α-adrenergic blocking drugs, such as phenoxybenzamine and phentolamine (Chapter 16), have not been useful in the management of hypertension because of their tendency to produce postural hypotension and marked reflex tachycardia. A relatively new α-adrenergic blocking drug, prazosin (Minipress) does not cause as much tachycardia as the other drugs of the same class or as hydralazine.

Prazosin

Prazosin (Minipress) exerts its antihypertensive action by blocking postsynaptic α_1- adrenergic receptors in blood vessels. Its superiority over other α-blocking drugs is attributed to its greater affinity for postsynaptic receptors than for presynaptic α_2-adrenergic receptors. Blockade of presynaptic receptors by phenoxybenzamine or phentolamine results in increased release of norepinephrine. Prazosin has little effect on presynaptic receptors.[89]

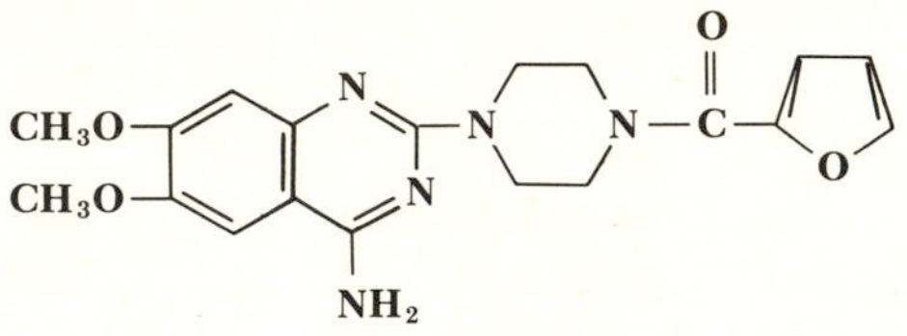

Prazosin

Following oral administration, plasma concentrations of prazosin peak between 1 and 3 hours, the drug having a half-life of about 4 hours. Prazosin is excreted mainly through biliary excretion in the form of inactive metabolites.

Prazosin is an effective antihypertensive drug, particularly when combined with a diuretic. It may be especially useful in patients who do not respond well to a β blocker–diuretic combination. Prazosin dilates both the systemic arterial and venous beds and has been found useful in the treatment of heart failure, since it reduces preload and afterload without causing cardiac acceleration.

Untoward effects

A commonly encountered effect of prazosin is often called the *first dose phenomenon*,[89] characterized by weakness often progressing to syncope, which occurs within 1 hour after the first dose is taken. It is probably caused by postural hypotension and is aggravated by exercise and sodium depletion. The drug may aggravate angina. Prazosin hydrochloride (Minipress) is available in 1 and 5 mg tablets. The initial dose should be 1 mg two or three times a day.

Problem 18-1. Why is it necessary to use an α blocker during the operation for pheochromocytoma when a β blocker is being administered? Manipulation of the tumor results in the release of norepinephrine and epinephrine from the tumor. These catecholamines would produce excessive hypertension in the presence of a β blocker. Thus an α blocker must be added.

β-ADRENERGIC BLOCKING DRUGS

The β-adrenergic blocking drugs are widely used in the treatment of hypertension. In combination with a diuretic they are quite effective and produce fewer adverse effects than most antihypertensive drugs. For several years propranolol (Inderal) was the only β blocker available in this country. The antihypertensive effect of this drug was quite unexpected and was discovered accidentally when patients with hypertension and angina were treated with β blockers in England.[96] With the recognition of the existence of β_1, or cardiac receptors,[46] efforts were made to develop specific blocking drugs for these receptors, which would not affect the β_2 receptors mediating catecholamine effects on the bronchial tree and vasodilator influences. Such a cardioselective β_1-receptor blocker is now available in the form of metoprolol (Lopressor). Nadolol (Corgard) is a longer acting nonselective β blocker.

Despite extensive investigations, the mechanism of the antihypertensive action of the β-blocking drugs is not known.[90] Various theories invoke (1) inhibition of renin release, (2) CNS effects, (3) decrease in cardiac output, and (4) increased sensitivity of baroreceptors.[90] None of these theories is sufficient to explain all the effects of the β blockers in hypertension, although they may partly explain the lowering of blood pressure observed.

Mechanism of action

Propranolol (Inderal) is the most widely used β blocker in hypertension. Its mechanism of action is still poorly understood. Although the drug blocks renin release and reduces cardiac output,[91] these effects cannot explain the usefulness of the drug as an antihypertensive agent. Propranolol may exert its effect by actions on the CNS as well as on the renin-angiotensin system.[91]

Propranolol

Propranolol is well absorbed from the intestine, but 50% to 70% of an oral dose is extracted and metabolized by the liver during the first pass. The major metabolite, 4-hydroxypropranolol is active but has a shorter half-life. Propranolol has a half-life of 4 to 6 hours. Despite its short half-life, twice-daily dosage may be sufficient in most patients.

Pharmacokinetics

It has been shown in a cooperative study[99] that blood pressure was well controlled only in 52% of patients when propranolol was taken alone. In combination with a diuretic this percentage increased to 81%, and the addition of hydralazine to the propranolol-diuretic combination produced good results in 92% of the patients. Propranolol then has a major role in combination therapy, particularly because it can counteract some of the adverse hemodynamic effects of other antihypertensive agents. Propranolol is very useful in patients who have anginal pain.

Effectiveness

Propranolol does not cause orthostatic hypotension. It may produce congestive failure and asthmatic attacks in susceptible individuals. Bradycardia is common but is not a contraindication to continued therapy. Gastrointestinal side effects, Raynaud's phenomenon, and worsening of claudication are rare. The drug has a disadvantage in insulin-dependent diabetics, since it may mask the symptoms of hypoglycemia. The majority of patients taking propranolol show no adverse effects of any kind.

Adverse effects

Dosage and administration   Propranolol (Inderal) is available in 10, 40, and 80 mg tablets. Dosage for the treatment of hypertension must be individualized. Initial dose is 80 mg daily in divided doses. The usual effective dose range is 160 to 480 mg daily.

Metoprolol   Metoprolol (Lopressor) is a cardioselective agent, since it blocks β receptors in the heart preferentially.[93] The drug can be used in patients with asthma and in those having intermittent claudication. The plasma half-life of metoprolol is 3 to 6 hours, but the antihypertensive effect is longer, and the drug may be given twice daily in a total daily dose of 50 to 200 mg. The drug is available in 50 and 100 mg tablets.

Nadolol   Nadolol (Corgard) is a β blocker characterized by slow elimination, having a plasma half-life of 12 hours. Thus, it may be used once a day in the chronic management of hypertension. The drug is excreted unchanged in the urine and stool.

ADRENERGIC NEURONAL BLOCKING DRUGS   A number of drugs, such as guanethidine, other guanidine compounds, and bretylium, can block the release of catecholamines from adrenergic nerve fibers. Among these drugs, guanethidine (Ismelin) has become the most widely used antihypertensive drug.

Guanethidine   Guanethidine sulfate (Ismelin) is an adrenergic neuronal blocking agent, which is a highly effective antihypertensive drug. In addition to blocking adrenergic neurons, guanethidine causes catecholamine release and depletion. In this respect it resembles reserpine with the important difference that it does not cross the blood-brain barrier.

Mode of action   Guanethidine blocks adrenergic neurons selectively because it is concentrated within the neurons by the same membrane transport system that pumps norepinephrine into the nerves following its release.[54] The tricyclic antidepressants oppose the antihypertensive actions of guanethidine because they block its uptake into the adrenergic neurons.

In addition to its adrenergic neuronal blocking actions, guanethidine causes some catecholamine depletion, which may be termed a *reserpine-like effect*. Other less important actions consist of a *tyramine-like effect*, meaning that the drug can cause release of catecholamines, and a *cocaine-like effect*, which refers to blockade of the membrane amine pump. The adrenergic neuronal blocking action is sometimes referred to as a *bretylium-like effect*.

Clinical pharmacology   The onset of action of guanethidine is slow. Maximal effects may not develop for 2 or 3 days after initiation of treatment. For this reason patients are started on small doses such as 10 mg once daily, which are maintained for 5 to 7 days before the amount of drug administered is increased. Guanethidine is a drug with long duration of action. Its effect may persist for 7 days after its administration has been discontinued.

Guanethidine sulfate

The absorption of guanethidine is only about 50% of the orally administered dose. The drug is largely excreted by the kidney.

In contrast to reserpine, guanethidine causes postural hypotension with some frequency. The reason for this difference is probably related to the adrenergic neuronal blocking properties of guanethidine. In addition to postural hypotension, guanethidine causes the usual consequences of reduced sympathetic activity, such as diarrhea, bradycardia, weakness, and nasal stuffiness.

Guanethidine has a great advantage over reserpine in that it does not cross the blood-brain barrier and thus does not cause sedation and depression. It has replaced the ganglionic blocking agents because it does not inhibit parasympathetic ganglia. It has a strange effect on male sexual function, preventing ejaculation without affecting erection.

Guanethidine and related adrenergic neuronal blocking guanidiniums are accumulated in the adrenergic neurons by the same transport system that carries norepi-

Drug interactions

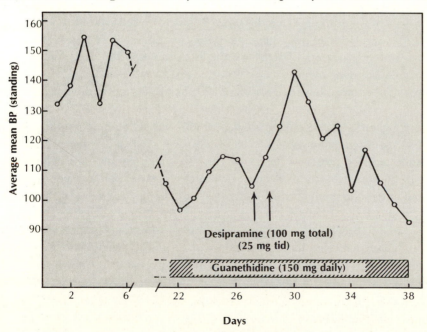

FIG. 18-2. Antagonism of guanethidine by desipramine. Guanethidine was given in increasing doses between days 6 and 21 until blood pressure was controlled (150 mg daily). Dose was maintained during experimental period. Desipramine was administered between arrows. (From Mitchell, J. R., Arias, L., and Oates, J. A.: J.A.M.A. **202**:973, 1967.)

nephrine to its storage site.[54] Desipramine and related tricyclic antidepressants block the membrane transport system and prevent the accumulation of guanethidine in the adrenergic neuron. As a consequence the tricyclic antidepressants block the antihypertensive effect of the drug, as shown in Fig. 18-2.

Preparations   Guanethidine sulfate (Ismelin) is available in tablets containing 10 and 20 mg. No parenteral forms are available because the drug is not useful for the treatment of hypertensive emergencies. In fact, it could aggravate them.

MAO INHIBITORS

One of the common side effects of MAO inhibitors is postural hypotension (p. 293). Although the mechanism of this is not well understood, at least one member of the series has been introduced as an antihypertensive agent.

Pargyline (Eutonyl) is administered orally in doses of 25 to 50 mg once daily. Side effects consist of orthostatic hypotension, gastrointestinal disturbances, insomnia, and headaches.

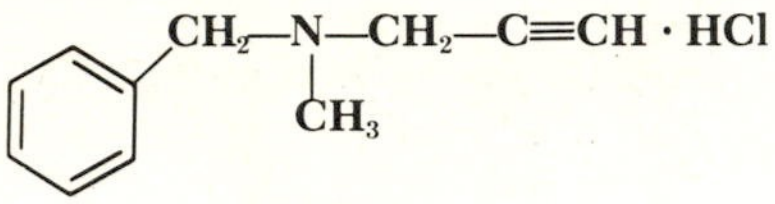

$$CH_2-N-CH_2-C\equiv CH \cdot HCl$$
$$CH_3$$

Pargyline hydrochloride

Probably the greatest disadvantage of the MAO inhibitors is their incompatibility with a large variety of drugs. Thus in patients receiving pargyline the indirect sympathomimetics would be contraindicated, as shown by the violent reaction to tyramine-containing foods in such patients. Also, combinations of antidepressants are strictly contraindicated (p. 294). It is difficult to see why the drug should be used in the face of so many dangers.

Pargyline comes in tablets containing 10, 25, and 50 mg of the drug.

GANGLIONIC BLOCKING AGENTS

The ganglionic blocking agents (Chapter 13) such as hexamethonium, pentolinium, and mecamylamine have received extensive trial in hypertensive diseases. Reductions of blood pressure, particularly in the standing position, can be achieved, but again the inevitable side effects of orthostatic hypotension and parasympathetic ganglionic blockade complicate this approach to the management of hypertension.

CENTRAL DEPRESSANTS OF SYMPATHETIC FUNCTIONS
Clonidine

Clonidine hydrochloride (Catapres) acts by α_2-receptor stimulation in the CNS to lower blood pressure. In combination with a diuretic, clonidine is suitable for long-term therapy. A rebound increase in blood pressure has been reported following rapid withdrawal of clonidine.[44,94]

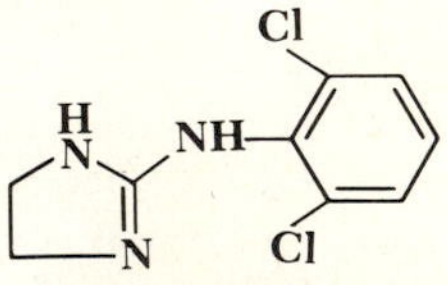

Clonidine

The intravenous administration of clonidine is followed by a transient pressor response and a more sustained depressor effect accompanied by bradycardia. It is believed that the initial pressor response is exerted on peripheral α receptors. The antihypertensive action is probably the result of an action of the drug on α receptors within the CNS and on cardiovascular centers in the medulla.

Mode of action

It is believed that there is a noradrenergic component in the central baroreceptor reflex pathway.[44] Norepinephrine lowers the blood pressure when injected into the cisterna magna. Clonidine may act on the same receptors as norepinephrine, thus mimicking the actions of baroreceptor stimulation.

Drowsiness and dryness of the mouth are common adverse effects. Constipation occurs in some patients. Postural hypotension is rare. Withdrawal symptoms on discontinuation of clonidine therapy include restlessness, tachycardia, and a rebound increase in blood pressure. Desipramine and other tricyclic antidepressants may interfere with the antihypertensive effects of clonidine.

Adverse reactions and drug interactions

Clonidine is absorbed well after oral administration. Plasma levels reach their peak within 3 to 5 hours and the half-life is 12 to 16 hours. Following oral administration, 60% of the drug is excreted by the kidney, mostly in the form of metabolites.

Metabolism

Clonidine hydrochloride (Catapres) is available in the form of tablets, 0.1 and 0.2 mg. The initial dose for adults is 0.1 mg two or three times daily. The usual maintenance dose is 0.2 to 0.8 mg daily. Dosage must be adjusted to the patient's requirement. The drug is more effective if it is given in association with a diuretic. It is also more potent for reducing the blood pressure in the upright position. Withdrawal symptoms are more likely to occur if larger doses, more than 1.2 mg daily, are employed.

Preparations and dosages

Methyldopa (Aldomet) was introduced as an antihypertensive drug on the theory that, being an inhibitor of aromatic amino acid decarboxylase, it would lower catecholamine concentrations in the body by that mechanism. It was found, however, that the drug is taken up and metabolized to α-methylnorepinephrine.[10,39,58]

Methyldopa

The mode of antihypertensive action of methyldopa is not completely understood. It appears to act on central adrenergic mechanisms through its metabolite α-methylnorepinephrine.

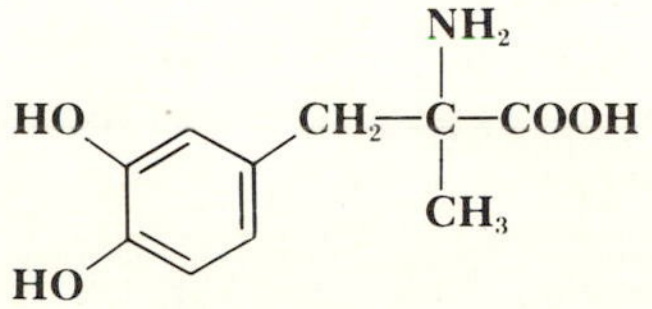

Methyldopa

Methyldopa is recommended for the treatment of most types of hypertension. It is preferred by some for patients with chronic renal disease and in hypertensive emergencies. For the latter, the drug may be injected intravenously—in contrast with guanethidine, which is only used orally. Methyldopa causes much less orthostatic hypotension than guanethidine, ganglionic blocking drugs, or MAO inhibitors.

Adverse reactions   Adverse reactions to methyldopa include marked drowsiness in many patients, depression, and nightmares. In some individuals the administration of methyldopa is followed in about a week by an influenza-like reaction that may be caused by sensitization to the drug. In some of these individuals, subsequent administration of small doses of methyldopa will elicit the same reaction. This syndrome is accompanied rarely by alterations in serum glutamic oxaloacetic transaminase levels and mild hepatitis.

Pharmacokinetics   Methyldopa is absorbed well from the gastrointestinal tract. Its elimination is largely renal, with a half-life of 2 hours. Some of the drug is eliminated much more slowly, however, and cumulation may occur when renal function is inadequate. The drug and its metabolites may give false positive tests in the diagnosis of pheochromocytoma.

Preparations   Methyldopa (Aldomet) is available in 250 mg tablets. Methyldopa hydrochloride (Aldomet ester hydrochloride) is available as a solution for intravenous injection, 250 mg/5 ml.

Reserpine   Reserpine is the prototype of several alkaloids present in *Rauwolfia serpentina*, or Indian snakeroot. Used in India for centuries, it was introduced into Western medicine in the 1950s.[4] At first reserpine seemed as important for its tranquilizing properties as for its usefulness in the treatment of hypertension. It was gradually replaced as an antipsychotic drug by the phenothiazines. It is still important as an antihypertensive drug and as a fascinating pharmacological tool.

Basic action and effects   Reserpine has one basic action responsible for most, if not all, of its pharmacological effects. The drug causes a depletion of catecholamines and serotonin in the central and peripheral nervous system and some other sites. Depletion is a consequence of amine release. Not only are the amines released from their binding sites, but their reaccumulation is also prevented. Some interference by reserpine with catecholamine synthesis has been reported.[70]

What is the mechanism of amine release induced by reserpine? It was thought at first that reserpine must destroy the binding sites for the amines, since its depleting action lasted for a long time, although its half-life in the body was only about 2 hours.[36] Most recent studies indicate, however, that a small fraction of the administered reserpine clings tenaciously to tissue elements. It is quite likely that reserpine is not a "hit-and-run" drug. Rather, a small fraction of the administered dose interferes with granular uptake of catecholamines in neural structures.[1]

Parasympathetic effects of reserpine are in part a result of decreased sympathetic activity. Bradycardia, aggravation of peptic ulcer, increased gastrointestinal motility, and miosis may all be explained as results of parasympathetic predominance.

The *CNS effects* of the drug are among its greatest disadvantages in the treatment of hypertension. An unpleasant type of drowsiness and lethargy is particularly disliked by individuals who must be intellectually alert and creative. Depression and suicides have occurred during chronic reserpine administration. Reserpine increases the CNS depressant actions of other drugs such as barbiturates and alcohol. It predisposes patients to severe hypotension during surgery and anesthesia.

Various derivatives of reserpine are very similar in action to the parent compound. Syrosingopine produces fewer central effects in relation to its antihypertensive action. This selectivity has been attributed to the fact that its norepinephrine-depleting action is largely limited to the peripheral nervous system. It is also much less potent.

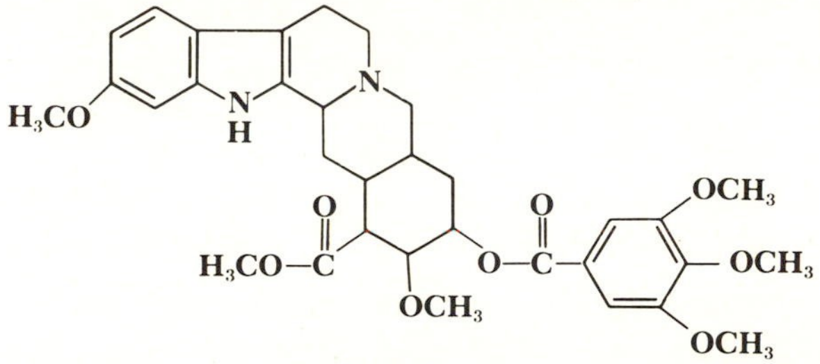

Reserpine

The dried root of *Rauwolfia serpentina* Benth (Raudixin) is available in tablets containing 50 and 100 mg. Preparations of *reserpine* include tablets of 0.1, 0.25, and 1 mg; an elixir containing 0.25 mg/4 ml; and solution for injection, 2.5 mg/ml.

Syrosingopine (Singoserp) is available in tablets of 1 mg.

Preparations

The veratrum alkaloids, protoveratrines A and B, act through the remarkable mechanism of promoting the activity of afferent nerves from the carotid sinus and aortic arch and thereby causing a reflex inhibition of central sympathetic activity with subsequent parasympathetic predominance. Unfortunately, the protoveratrines cause considerable nausea in many patients, and their dosage must be carefully adjusted to obtain a good hypotensive effect. These disadvantages have limited the usefulness of these compounds, but their pharmacology illustrates some unique mechanisms of drug action.

A number of alkaloids occur in plants of the species *Veratrum viride* and *Veratrum album*. They are classified as (1) tertiary amine esters and (2) secondary amines and their glycosides. The various alkaloids are polycyclic ring structures showing some resemblance to the cardiac glycosides.

If a small dose, less than 2 mg, of a mixture of protoveratrines A and B (Veralba) is injected intravenously into a human being, the characteristic effect consists of

REFLEX INHIBITORS OF CENTRAL SYMPATHETIC FUNCTION

Effects of protoveratrines A and B

bradycardia and fall of blood pressure. When proportionately larger doses are given to animals, temporary apnea is produced in addition to the circulatory effects.

The mechanism of these circulatory actions is quite unusual and is related to what is known as the Bezold-Jarisch effect. It was suggested many years ago on the basis of investigations of the effect of veratrine in rabbits[5] that the cardiovascular actions of the preparation were caused by stimulation of afferent nerve fibers within the thorax and probably within the heart itself. Later investigations indicate that the conclusions of Bezold were essentially correct.[40,67]

It has been suggested that these veratrum alkaloids may sensitize the afferent endings in the baroreceptors of the carotid sinus and other areas so that they have greater response to the normally effective stretch stimulus.[67]

ANTIHYPERTEN-SIVE DRUGS THAT PROMOTE SALT EXCRETION

Drugs that promote salt secretion, such as the thiazides, are important in the treatment of hypertension because sodium is involved in some way in the pathogenesis of the disease.

Rats on a high salt intake develop hypertension.[53] Also, the hypertensive effect of deoxycorticosterone and aldosterone[47,65] is probably attributable to salt retention. Conversely, the antihypertensive action of a low salt diet is generally accepted at present. The mechanism whereby an excess of salt in the body contributes to hypertension is not definitely known. Expansion of extracellular fluid volume and alterations in the salt concentration in arteriolar walls have been suggested as important factors.

Chlorothiazide and related drugs

Most investigators believe that thiazide diuretics exert their antihypertensive action through salt depletion. Isolated observations suggest that these drugs may also have extrarenal effects. In any case, they have been a welcome addition to antihypertensive therapy because it is much easier to accomplish salt depletion through this means than by strict limitation of salt intake.

The most useful oral diuretics, discussed in greater detail in Chapter 38, are the thiazides and the related drugs chlorthalidone (Hygroton) and quinethazone (Hydromox). They are widely used in the treatment of hypertension because of their safety and effectiveness and their ability to increase the antihypertensive action of other unrelated drugs.

Another potent diuretic, metolazone (Zaroxolyn) has also been introduced recently as an antihypertensive agent administered once daily.

The aldosterone antagonist spironolactone is sometimes combined with the thiazide diuretics, mainly to reduce potassium loss. The same is true for triamterene (Dyrenium).

The adverse effects of the thiazide diuretics, such as hypokalemia, hyperuricemia, and aggravation of diabetes, are discussed in Chapter 38. On the whole, these drugs are very useful in the treatment of hypertension.

REFERENCES

1 Alpers, H. S., and Shore, P. A.: Specific binding of reserpine—association with norepinephrine depletion, Biochem. Pharmacol. **18**:1363, 1969.

2 Baker, D. R., Schrader, W. H., and Hitchcock, C. R.: Small bowel ulceration apparently associated with thiazide and potassium therapy, J.A.M.A. **190**:586, 1964.

3 Baum, T., Shropshire, A. T., and Varner, L. L.: Contribution of the central nervous system to the action of several antihypertensive agents (methyldopa, hydralazine and guanethidine), J. Pharmacol. Exp. Ther. **182**:135, 1972.

4 Bein, H. J.: The pharmacology of Rauwolfia, Pharmacol. Rev. **8**:435, 1956.

5 von Bezold, A., and Hirt, L.: Ueber die physiologischen Wirkungen des essigsauren Veratrins, Untersuchungen Physiol. Lab. Würzburg **1**:73, 1867.

6 Biron, P., Kolw, E., Nowaczynski, W., Brouillet, J., and Genest, J.: The effects of intravenous infusions of valine-5 angiotensin II and other pressor agents on urinary electrolytes and corticosteroids, including aldosterone, J. Clin. Invest. **40**:338, 1960.

7 Borison, H. L., and Wang, S. C.: Physiology and pharmacology of vomiting, Pharmacol. Rev. **5**:193, 1953.

8 Bowlus, W. E., and Langford, H. G.: A comparison of the antihypertensive effect of chlorthalidone and hydrochlorothiazide, Clin. Pharmacol. Ther. **5**:708, 1964.

9 Buhler, F. R., Laragh, J. H., Baer, L., Vaughan, E. D., and Brunner, H. R.: Propranolol inhibition of renin secretion, N. Engl. J. Med. **287**:1209, 1972.

10 Colwill, J. M., Dutton, A. M., Morrissey, J., and Yu, P. N.: Alpha-methyldopa and hydrochlorothiazide. A controlled study of their comparative effectiveness as antihypertensive agents, N. Engl. J. Med. **71**:696, 1964.

11 Conn, J. W.: Aldosteronism and hypertension, Arch. Intern. Med. **107**:813, 1961.

12 Dahlström, A., Fuxe, K., and Hillarp, N-A.: Site of action of reserpine, Acta Pharmacol. **22**:277, 1965.

13 Dahr, A. S., George, C. F., and Dollery, C. T.: The effect of selective adrenergic β-blockade on the hypotensive effect of hydralazine, Experientia **27**:545, 1971.

14 Davis, J. O.: Aldosterone and angiotensin, J.A.M.A. **188**:1062, 1964.

15 Dawes, G. S., and Comroe, J. H., Jr.: Chemoreflexes from the heart and lungs, Physiol. Rev. **34**:167, 1954.

16 DeCharme, D. W., Freyburger, W. A., Graham, B. E., and Carlson, R. G.: Pharmacologic properties of minoxidil: a new hypotensive agent, J. Pharmacol. Exp. Ther. **184**:662, 1973.

17 Dickinson, C. J., and Lawrence, J. R.: A slowly developing pressor response to small concentrations of angiotensin. Its bearing on the pathogenesis of chronic renal hypertension, Lancet **1**:1354, 1963.

18 Ehrlich, E. N.: Aldosterone, the adrenal cortex, and hypertension, Annu. Rev. Med. **19**:373, 1968.

19 Erdös, E. G.: Angiotensin I converting enzyme, Circ. Res. **36**:247, 1975.

20 Feldberg, W., and Lewis, G. P.: The action of peptides on the adrenal medulla. Release of adrenalin by bradykinin and angiotensin, J. Physiol. (London) **171**:98, 1964.

21 Flacke, W., Caviness, V. S., Jr., and Samaha, F. G.: Treatment of myasthenia gravis with germine diacetate, N. Engl. J. Med. **275**:1207, 1966.

22 Freis, E. D., Wanko, A., Wilson, I. M., and Parrish, A. E.: Chlorothiazide in hypertensive and normotensive patients, Ann. N.Y. Acad. Sci. **7**:450, 1958.

23 Friend, D. G.: Antihypertensive drugs, Clin. Pharmacol. Ther. **3**:269, 1962.

24 Frolich, E. D., et al.: The paradox of beta-adrenergic blockade in hypertension, Circulation **37**:417, 1968.

25 Gifford, R. W., Jr.: Bethanidine sulfate: a new antihypertensive agent, J.A.M.A. **193**:901, 1965.

26 Gilmore, E., Weil, J., and Chidsey, C.: Treatment of essential hypertension with a new vasodilator in combination with beta-adrenergic blockade, N. Engl. J. Med. **282**:521, 1970.

27 Goldblatt, H.: The renal origin of hypertension, Springfield, Ill., 1948, Charles C Thomas, Publisher.

28 Goormaghtigh, N.: Existence of an endocrine gland in the media of the renal arterioles, Proc. Soc. Exp. Biol. Med. **42**:688, 1939.

29 Gordon, R. D., Küchel, O., Liddle, G. W., and Island, D. P.: Role of the sympathetic nervous system in regulating renin and aldosterone production in man, J. Clin. Invest. **46**:599, 1967.

30 Goth, A., and Harrison, F. L.: Influence of

protoveratrine on effect of vasoactive drugs, Proc. Soc. Exp. Biol. Med. **87**:437, 1954.

31 Gottlieb, T. B., Katz, F. H., and Chidsey, C. A.: Combined therapy with vasodilator drugs and beta-adrenergic blockade in hypertension: a comparative study of hydralazine and minoxidil, Circulation **45**:571, 1972.

32 Green, A. F.: Antihypertensive drugs, Adv. Pharmacol. **1**:162, 1962.

33 Gross, F., editor: Antihypertensive therapy, an international symposium, Berlin, 1966, Springer-Verlag.

34 Gross, F., Druey, J., and Meier, R.: Eine neue Gruppe Blutdrucksenkender Substanzen von Besonderem Wirkungscharacter, Experientia **6**:19, 1950.

35 Heath, W. C., and Freis, E. D.: Triamterene with hydrochlorothiazide in the treatment of hypertension, J.A.M.A. **186**:119, 1963.

36 Hess, S. M., Shore, P. A., and Brodie, B. B.: Persistence of reserpine action after the disappearance of drug from brain: effect on serotonin, J. Pharmacol. Exp. Ther. **118**:84, 1956.

37 Hoobler, S. W.: Treatment of hypertension, Am. J. Med. **17**:259, 1954.

38 Hoobler, S. W., and Dontas, A. S.: Drug treatment of hypertension, Pharmacol. Rev. **5**:135, 1953.

39 Igloe, M. C.: Effects of methyldopa in hypertension, J.A.M.A. **189**:188, 1964.

40 Jarisch, A., and Richter, H.: Die afferenten Bahnen des Veratrineffektes in den Herznerven, Arch. Exp. Pathol. Pharmakol. **193**:355, 1939.

41 Johnsson, G., Henning, M., and Ablad, B.: Studies on the mechanism of the vasoconstrictor effect of angiotensin II in man, Life Sci. **4**:1549, 1965.

42 Johnston, L. C., and Grieble, H. G.: Treatment of arterial hypertensive disease with diuretics, Arch. Intern. Med. **119**:225, 1967.

43 Kopin, I. J., Fischer, J. E., Musacchio, J. M., Horst, W. D., and Weise, V. K.: "False neurochemical transmitters" and the mechanism of sympathomimetic blockade by monoamine oxidase inhibitors, J. Pharmacol. Exp. Ther. **147**:186, 1965.

44 Kosman, M. E.: Evaluation of clonidine hydrochloride (Catapres), J.A.M.A. **233**:174, 1975.

45 Krayer, O.: Antiaccelerator cardiac agents, J. Mt. Sinai Hosp., N.Y. **19**:53, 1952.

46 Lands, A. M., Arnold, A., and McAnliff, J. P.: Differentiation of receptor systems activated by sympathomimetic amines, Nature **214**:597, 1967.

47 Laragh, J. H.: Aldosterone in fluid and elec-

trolyte disorders: hyper- and hypoalderosteronism, J. Chron. Dis. **11**:292, 1960.

48 Laragh, J. H., Ulick, S., Januszewicz, V., Deming, Q. B., Kelly, W. G., and Lieberman, S.: Aldosterone secretion and primary and malignant hypertension, J. Clin. Invest. **39**:1091, 1960.

49 Lindmar, R., and Muscholl, E.: Die Wirkung von Bharmaka auf die Elimination von Noradrenalin aus der Perfusionsflüssigkeit und die Noradrenalinaufnahme in das isolierte Herz, Arch. Exp. Pathol. Pharmakol. **247**:469, 1964.

50 Luria, M. H., and Freis, E. D.: Treatment of hypertension with debrisoquin sulfate (Declinax), Curr. Ther. Res. **7**:289, 1965.

51 Mason, D. T., and Braunwald, E.: Effects of guanethidine, reserpine, and methyldopa on reflex venous and arterial constriction in man, J. Clin. Invest. **43**:1449, 1964.

52 Maxwell, R. A., Povalski, H., and Plummer, A. J.: A differential effect of reserpine on pressor amine activity and its relationship to other agents producing this effect. J. Pharmacol. Exp. Ther. **125**:178, 1959.

53 Meneely, G. R., Tucker, R. G., Darby, J., and Auerbach, S. H.: Chronic sodium chloride toxicity: hypertension, renal and vascular lesions, Ann. Intern. Med. **39**:991, 1953.

54 Mitchell, J. R., and Oates, J. A.: Guanethidine and related agents. I. Mechanism of the selective blockade of adrenergic neurons and its antagonism by drugs, J. Pharmacol. Exp. Ther. **172**:100, 1970.

55 Muelheims, G. H., Entrup, R. W., Paiewonsky, D., and Mierzwiak, D. S.: Increased sensitivity of the heart to catecholamine-induced arrhythmias following guanethidine, Clin. Pharmacol. Ther. **6**:757, 1965.

56 Newton, M. A., Sealy, J. E., Ledingham, J. G., and Laragh, J. H.: High blood pressure and oral contraceptives, Am. J. Obstet. Gynecol. **101**:1037, 1968.

57 Oates, J. A.: Antihypertensive drugs that impair adrenergic neuron function, Pharmacol. Phys. **1**(6):1, 1967.

58 Oates, J. A., Seligmann, A. W., Clark, M. A., Rousseau, P., and Lee, R. E.: The relative efficacy of guanethidine, methyldopa and pargyline as antihypertensive agents, N. Engl. J. Med. **273**:729, 1965.

59 Onesti, G., Schiazza, D., Brest, A. N., and Moyer, J. H.: Cardiac and renal hemodynamic effects of debrisoquin sulfate in hypertensive patients, Clin. Pharmacol. Ther. **7**:17, 1966.

60 Page, I. H.: A new hormone, angiotensin, Clin. Pharmacol. Ther. **3**:758, 1962.

61 Page, I. H., Corcoran, A. C., Dustan, H. P., and Koppanyi, T.: Cardiovascular actions of sodium nitroprusside in animals and hypertensive patients, Circulation 11:188, 1955.

62 Page, I. H., and Dustan, H. P.: A new potent, antihypertensive drug: preliminary study of [2-(octahydro-1-azocinyl)-ethyl] guanidine sulfate (guanethidine), J.A.M.A. 170:1265, 1959.

63 Panisset, J. C., and Bourdois, P.: Effect of angiotensin on the response to noradrenaline and sympathetic nerve stimulation, and on the 3H-noradrenaline uptake in cat mesenteric blood vessels, Can. J. Physiol. Pharmacol. 46:125, 1968.

64 Pardo, E. G., Vargas, R., and Virdrio, H.: Antihypertensive drug action, Annu. Rev. Pharmacol. 5:77, 1965.

65 Perera, G. A., and Blood, D. W.: Pressor activity of deoxycorticosterone acetate in normotensive and hypertensive subjects, Ann. Intern. Med. 27:401, 1947.

66 Pettinger, W. A., and Mitchell, H. C.: Renin release, saralasin and vasodilator-beta-blocker drug interaction in man, N. Engl. J. Med. 292:1214, 1975.

67 Richardson, A. P., Walker, H. A., Farrar, C. B., Griffith, W., Pound, E., and Davidson, J. R.: The mechanism of the hypotensive action of veratrum alkaloids, Proc. Soc. Exp. Biol. Med. 79:79, 1952.

68 Rubin, A. A., Roth, F. E., Taylor, R. M., and Rosenkilde, H.: Pharmacology of diazoxide, an antihypertensive, nondiuretic benzothiadiazine, J. Pharmacol. Exp. Ther. 136:344, 1962.

69 Ruedy, J.: A comparative clinical trial of guanoxan and guanethidine in essential hypertension, Clin. Pharmacol. Ther. 8:38, 1967.

70 Rutledge, C. O., and Weiner, N.: The effect of reserpine upon the synthesis of norepinephrine in the isolated rabbit heart, J. Pharmacol. Exp. Ther. 157:290, 1967.

71 Schirger, A., and Sheps, S. G.: Prazosin—new antihypertensive agent, J.A.M.A. 237:989, 1977.

72 Sellers, E. M., and Koch-Weser, J.: Protein binding and vascular activity of diazoxide, N. Engl. J. Med. 281:1141, 1969.

73 Tobian, L.: Why do thiazide diuretics lower blood pressure in essential hypertension? Annu. Rev. Pharmacol. 7:399, 1967.

74 Trendelenburg, U.: Supersensitivity and subsensitivity to sympathomimetic amines, Pharmacol. Rev. 15:225, 1963.

75 Udhoji, V. N., and Weil, M. H.: Circulatory effects of angiotensin, levarterenol and metaraminol in the treatment of shock, N. Engl. J. Med. 270:501, 1964.

76 Vander, A. J.: Control of renin release, Physiol. Rev. 47:359, 1967.

77 Vane, J. R.: The release and fate of vaso-active hormones in the circulation, Br. J. Pharmacol. 35:209, 1969.

78 Veterans Administration Cooperative Study on Antihypertensive Agents: A double-blind control study of antihypertensive agents: comparative effectiveness of reserpine, reserpine and hydralazine, and three ganglionic blocking agents, chlorisondamine, mecamylamine, and pentolinium tartrate, Arch. Intern. Med. 106:81, 1960.

79 Veterans Administration Cooperative Study on Antihypertensive Agents: Chlorothiazide alone and in combination with other agents: preliminary results, Arch. Intern. Med. 110:134, 1962.

80 Weidmann, P., Maxwell, M. H., Lupu, A. N., Lewin, A. J., and Massry, S. G.: Plasma renin activity and blood pressure in terminal renal failure, N. Engl. J. Med. 285:757, 1971.

81 Wilkins, R. W.: Studies on antihypertensive action of chlorothiazide (abstract), Clin. Res. 6:831, 1958.

82 Wilkins, R. W., Hollander, W., and Chobanian, A. V.: Chlorothirazide in hypertension: studies on its mode of action, Ann. N.Y. Acad. Sci. 71:465, 1958.

83 Winer, N., Chokshi, D. S., and Freedman, A. D.: Adrenergic receptor mediation of renin secretion, J. Clin. Endocrinol. 29:1168, 1969.

84 Yeh, B. K., Nantel, A., and Goldberg, L. I.: Antihypertensive effect of clonidine, Arch. Intern. Med. 127:233, 1971.

85 Zacest, R., Gilmore, E., and Koch-Weser, J.: Treatment of essential hypertension with combined vasodilation and beta-adrenergic blockade, N. Engl. J. Med. 286:617, 1972.

86 Zbinden, G.: The antihypertensive effect of the monoamine oxidase inhibitors—mechanism of action. In Brest, A. N., and Moyer, J. H., editors: Hypertension: recent advances, Philadelphia, 1961, Lea & Febiger.

87 Zimmerman, B. G., and Gisslen, J.: Pattern of renal vasoconstriction and transmitter release during sympathetic stimulation in presence of angiotensin and cocaine, J. Pharmacol. Exp. Ther. 163:320, 1968.

REVIEWS

88 Davis, J. O.: What signals the kidney to release renin? Circ. Res. 28:301, 1971.

88a Freis, E. D.: Salt in hypertension and the effects of diuretics, Annu. Rev. Pharmacol. Toxicol. 18:13, 1979.

89 Graham, R. M., and Pettinger, W. A.: Prazosin, N. Engl. J. Med. 300:232, 1979.

90 Hammond, J. J., and Kirkendall, W. M.: Beta blocking drugs and the treatment of hypertension, Tex. Med. **74**:43, 1978.

91 Holland, O. B., and Kaplan, N. M.: Propranolol in the treatment of hypertension, N. Engl. J. Med. **294**:930, 1976.

92 Hypertension Detection and Follow-up Program Cooperative Group: Five-year findings of the hypertension detection and follow-up program. I. Reduction in mortality of persons with high blood pressure, including mild hypertension, J.A.M.A. **242**:2562, 1979.

93 Koch-Weser, J.: Metoprolol, N. Engl. J. Med. **301**:698, 1979.

94 Pettinger, W. A.: Recent advances in the treatment of hypertension, Arch. Intern. Med. **137**:679, 1977.

95 Pettinger, W. A., and Mitchell, H. C.: Minoxidil—an alternative to nephrectomy for refractory hypertension, N. Engl. J. Med. **289**:167, 1973.

96 Prichard, B. N. C., and Gillam, P. M. S.: Treatment of hypertension with propranolol, Br. Med. J. **1**:7, 1969.

97 Proger, S.: Antihypertensive drugs: praise and restraint (editorial), N. Engl. J. Med. **286**:155, 1972.

97a Scriabine, A.: β-adrenoceptor blocking drugs in hypertension, Annu. Rev. Pharmacol. Toxicol. **19**:269, 1979.

98 Veterans Administration Cooperative Study Group on Antihypertensive Agents: Effects of treatment on morbidity in hypertension. II. Results in patients with diastolic blood pressure averaging 90 through 114 mm. Hg, J.A.M.A. **213**:1143, 1970.

99 Veterans Administration Cooperative Study Group on Antihypertensive Agents: Propranolol in the treatment of essential hypertension, J.A.M.A. **237**:2303, 1977.

CHAPTER 19

Histamine

Histamine is of interest in pharmacology and medicine because of its potent pharmacological activity and its wide distribution in tissues. When released from its binding sites, histamine can elicit reactions that range in intensity from mild itching to shock and death.

It would seem that such a potent and easily released endogenous compound would have important functions in the body. There is indeed evidence for a local role of histamine in inflammation. It is also quite certain that the amine plays a role in anaphylaxis, allergies, and drug reactions.

The role of histamine in normal physiology is not clearly established. It is probably one of the neurotransmitters, and it undoubtedly functions in the process of gastric secretion. Many other "local hormonal functions" have been attributed to it.

HISTAMINE RECEPTORS

Histamine acts on two separate and distinct receptors, termed H_1 and H_2 *receptors*. Contraction of the smooth muscle of the bronchi and intestine is mediated by H_1 receptors and is antagonized by a typical antihistamine. On the other hand, H_2 receptors mediate the actions of histamine or gastric secretion, cardiac acceleration, and inhibition of the contractions of the rat uterus. These actions are antagonized by a new type of antihistamine exemplified by burimamide[67] and the related drugs metiamide and cimetidine.

Both H_1 and H_2 receptors mediate the vasodilator effects of histamine.[41] The H_1 receptors are generally more important, except for certain areas. For example, vasodilatation along the distribution of the temporal artery in humans is more strongly influenced by H_2 receptors.

TABLE 19-1. Distribution of histamine receptors in the body

Histamine receptor	Tissue	Antagonist
H_1	Smooth muscle of intestine, bronchi, blood vessels	Classical antihistamines (diphenhydramine)
H_2	Gastric parietal cell Smooth muscle of some blood vessels Guinea pig atria Rat uterus	Cimetidine Metiamide Burimamide

DEVELOPMENT OF CONCEPTS

Histamine was first synthesized in 1906 by Windaus. It was also found to occur naturally in ergot as the product of bacterial contamination. The pharmacological properties of histamine were extensively studied by Sir Henry Dale, who was impressed with the similarities in the actions of histamine and the manifestations of anaphylaxis in several species such as the guinea pig, rabbit, and dog. Once histamine was found widely distributed in mammalian tissues, numerous roles were assigned to it, often uncritically. Studies by Thomas Lewis on the release of "H substance" from the skin in response to injury had a great influence.

When the antihistaminic drugs were developed in the 1940s, many of the histaminic theories of various physiological functions and pathological processes were abandoned because of the inability of these drugs to modify them.

The demonstration in the 1950s of a close association between mast cells and histamine created much interest, and research concerning histamine focused on mechanisms of its release from mast cells. It was soon realized, however, that there is also an important non–mast cell pool of histamine, the function of which is still being investigated.

In addition to the interest in preformed histamine in the tissues and its release, there has also been a great interest in newly formed histamine as a consequence of activation of histidine decarboxylase.[49] The role of this nascent histamine is uncertain.

TISSUE DISTRIBUTION AND FORMATION

Histamine is widely distributed in the body. Its concentration varies in different species; in humans the highest concentrations are found in the lungs, skin, and stomach. Details of its distribution are given in Table 19-2.

TABLE 19-2. Histamine content of human tissues*

Tissue	Histamine content
Lung	33 ± 10 μg/g†
Mucous membrane (nasal)	15.6 μg/g
Stomach	14 ± 4.0 μg/g†
Duodenum	14 ± 0.9 μg/g†
Skin	6.6 μg/g (abdomen)
	30.4 μg/g (face)
Spleen	3.4 ± 0.97 μg/g†
Kidney	2.5 ± 1.2 μg/g†
Liver	2.2 ± 0.76 μg/g†
Heart	1.6 ± 0.07 μg/g†
Thyroid	1.0 ± 0.13 μg/g†
Skeletal muscle	0.97 ± 0.13 μg/g†
Central nervous tissue	0-0.2 μg/g
Plasma	2.6 μg/L
Basophils	1,080 μg/10^9 cells
Eosinophils	160 μg/10^9 cells
Neutrophils	3.0 μg/10^9 cells
Lymphocytes	0.6 μg/10^9 cells
Platelets	0.009 μg/10^9 platelets
Whole blood	16-89 μg/L

*Based on data from Van Arsdel, P. P., Jr., and Beall, G. N.: Arch. Intern. Med. **106**:192, 1960.
†Mean ± Standard error.

It is generally believed that most of the histamine present in tissues arises locally as a consequence of decarboxylation of histidine. Various foods may contain histamine and intestinal bacteria may form large amounts, but whatever histamine is absorbed is rapidly altered and does not contribute to the body's stores of this amine.

With the availability of experimental drugs that destroy mast cells, such as compound 48/80, it has become possible to identify two pools of histamine in the body. The mast cell pool is widely distributed in the connective tissue and is depleted experimentally by the mast cell–destroying agents.

The circulating basophils behave like the mast cells and contain very high concentrations of histamine. The non–mast cell pool includes the gastric mucosa and the small amounts present in the brain, heart, and other organs. It is not known with certainty what the cellular localization of non–mast cell histamine is, but it is suspected that with the exception of the gastric mucosa, it is present in neural elements.[28] It differs from mast cell histamine in its more rapid turnover rate and its resistance to the usual histamine releasers such as compound 48/80.

Chemically, histamine is 2(4-imidazolyl) ethylamine. Its structure is as follows:

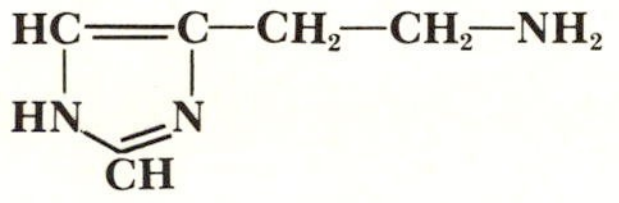

HISTIDINE DECARBOXYLASES

$$HC = C - CH_2 - CH_2 - NH_2$$
$$HN \diagdown N$$
$$CH$$

Histamine

Histamine is derived from the decarboxylation of histidine. It represents another example of a powerful pharmacological agent resulting from the decarboxylation of an amino acid.

Mammalian tissues contain two different histidine decarboxylases. The one known as specific histidine decarboxylase, present in mast cells, is inhibited by methylhistidine and the hydrazine analog of histidine, but not by methyldopa. The other enzyme, also known as aromatic L-amino acid decarboxylase, decarboxylates several aromatic L-amino acids (dopa, for example). It is inhibited by methyldopa. There is every reason to believe that specific histidine decarboxylase is more important physiologically.

DEGRADATION OF HISTAMINE IN THE BODY

The degradation of histamine in the body takes place through two main pathways, with considerable species variation in their relative importance. In humans, histamine is primarily methylated to 1-methylhistamine.[48] This product is converted to 1-methyl-imidazole-4-acetic acid by the enzyme MAO. In the other pathway, which also occurs in humans, histamine is oxidized by diamine oxidase to imidazole-4-acetic acid, much of which is conjugated with ribose and is excreted as the riboside. The known pathways are shown in Fig. 19-1.

In addition to these compounds, some N-acetylhistamine also appears in the urine. The acetyl compound appears to reflect orally ingested histamine and amine formed by intestinal bacteria. The exact site of acetylation is still in doubt. There are suggestions that intestinal bacteria can acetylate histamine,[60] and some investigators believe that no acetylation occurs outside the gastrointestinal tract.

It has been estimated that about 1% of histamine slowly injected intravenously appears in the urine in the free form, whereas most orally ingested histamine is found in the conjugated form in the urine. It has been estimated that in a normal person 2 to 3 mg of histamine may be released daily from the tissues. Urticaria in humans or

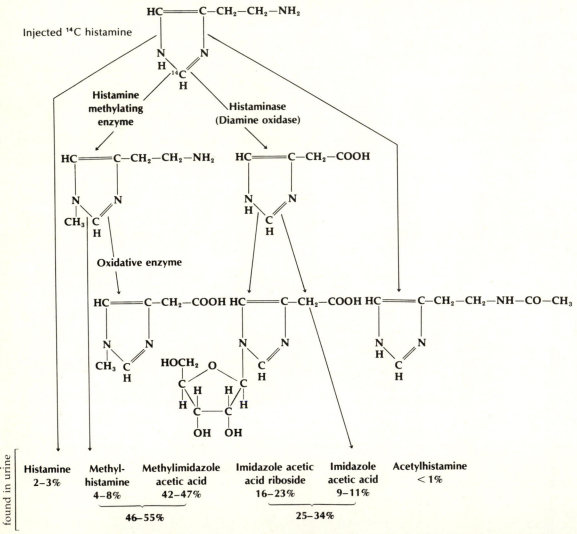

FIG. 19-1. Known pathways of histamine metabolism. Relative importance of the different pathways in human males is indicated by figures at bottom, which are expressed as percent of the total ^{14}C excreted in the urine during 12 hours after intradermal injection of ^{14}C histamine. Of the injected ^{14}C, 74% to 93% was excreted in 12 hours. (From Nilsson, K., Lindell, S.-E., Schayer, R. W., and Westling, H.: Clin. Sci. **13:**313, 1959.)

the injection of histamine-releasing agents into animals causes an increase in the urinary excretion of histamine.

BINDING AND RELEASE OF MAST CELL HISTAMINE

Histamine is highly concentrated in the granules of the mast cell. These granules also contain large amount of heparin, proteolytic enzymes, and, in some species (rats and mice), serotonin. Histamine release is visualized as a two-step process. In the first step the granules are suddenly extruded; in the second, as the granules are exposed to the cations in the extracellular environment, histamine is released by ion exchange. The amine is held within the granule by electrostatic forces.

Although granule release generally accompanies histamine release, it is possible that release of the amine could occur within the cell also. The appearance of granules within the mast cell is shown in Fig. 19-2.

Histamine is released from mast cells by physical and chemical agents, antigen-antibody reactions, and a variety of drugs.

Release by chemicals and drugs

Many early isolated observations suggested that simple chemicals can cause release of histamine in the body. Intracutaneous morphine injection in humans produces the "triple response of Lewis" consisting of localized redness, localized edema, and a diffuse redness. This was suspected of being an example of a chemical causing

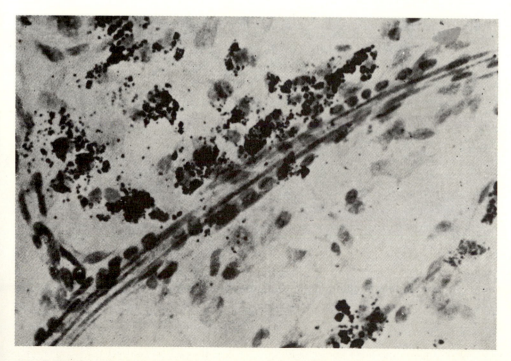

FIG. 19-2. Mast cells of rat mesentery 3 hours after intraperitoneal injection of compound 48/80. (From Riley, J. F., and West, A. B.: J. Pathol. Bacteriol. **69**:269, 1955.)

release of H substance.[29] It has also been shown that curare alkaloids can liberate histamine, and this was thought to explain the episodes of bronchial constriction accompanying intravenous curare injections. With the discovery of adverse reactions to certain diamidines and polypeptide antibiotics (licheniformin, polymyxin), interest in this problem increased greatly.

The chemical histamine-releasing agents may be divided into two classes: small-molecule amines and certain large-molecule compounds such as dextran, polyvinylpyrrolidone, and ovomucoid, which are active only in some species.

A variety of organic bases can cause release of histamine from mast cells. The most active compound known is compound 48/80, a condensation product of *p*-methoxyphenylethylmethylamine with formaldehyde (Fig. 19-2).

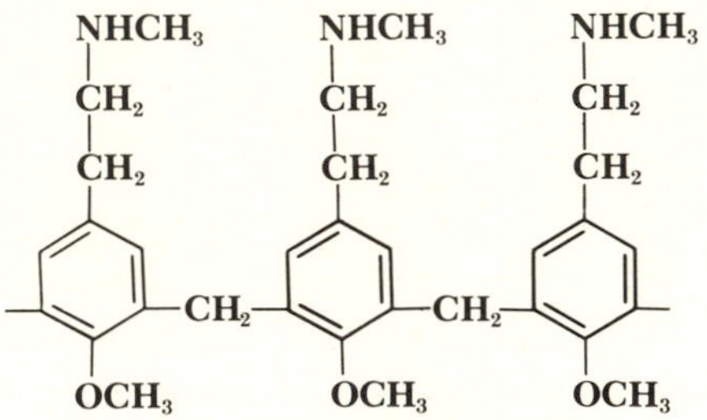

$$\text{NHCH}_3 \quad \text{NHCH}_3 \quad \text{NHCH}_3$$

Compound 48/80

It has been suggested that histamine release may be caused not only by the curare alkaloids but also by such commonly used drugs as morphine, codeine, papaverine, meperidine, atropine, hydralazine, and even sympathomimetic amines.[39] Histamine release by these drugs may not be significant unless they are administered intravenously in fairly large doses.

The histamine-releasing agents of small molecular size exert their effect in most species. On the other hand, there are a number of large-molecule compounds whose action appears to be limited to one species or family of animals. Dextran and ovomucoid (from egg white) produce a condition resembling angioneurotic edema in rats[52] and release histamine in this species[12] but do not have this effect in dogs or in humans. Large-molecule dextran can cause reactions in humans also. Curiously, polyvinylpyrrolidone and polysorbate 80 (Tween 80) exert similar effects in the dog but not in the rat.[16,26] The reason for this species-specific action of certain polymers has not been elucidated.[67]

A characteristic feature of histamine release by chemical compounds is the development of tachyphylaxis to subsequent injections. When one obtains a marked fall in blood pressure following intravenous injection of 100 to 200 μg/kg of compound 48/80 in a dog, a second injection of the drug may have no effect whatever for several hours. Tachyphylaxis to Tween 20 or polyvinylpyrrolidone may last 14 to 20 hours.

Release in anaphylaxis and allergy   Histamine release plays an important role in the symptomatology of experimental anaphylactic shock in several species. In 1910 Dale and Laidlaw[2] observed that the symptoms elicited by histamine in guinea pigs, dogs, and rabbits were very similar to the manifestations of anaphylactic shock in these species. In guinea pigs the dominant symptom is bronchial constriction and asphyxial death from intravenous doses as small as 0.4 mg/kg. In dogs profound hypotension and acute enlargement of the liver are caused by both histamine and anaphylaxis. In the rabbit the pulmonary arterioles are constricted and acute dilatation of the right side of the heart ensues when either histamine is injected or antigen is administered to the previously sensitized animal.

In addition, in the dog the blood may become incoagulable in anaphylaxis but not after histamine injection. Much was made of this difference until it was demonstrated that anaphylaxis in the dog also releases heparin, presumably from the mast cells, which are abundant in the dog's liver.

The release of histamine by injecting antigens into the sensitized animal has been demonstrated also by perfusion expiments of the skin[6] and on addition of the antigen in vitro to sensitized minced tissues.[34]

In acute anaphylactic reactions in humans, histamine probably plays an important role. In anaphylaxis the human being reacts like the dog and the guinea pig, exhibiting profound hypotension, bronchial constriction, or laryngeal edema.[22]

Important new observations have been made on histamine release from human leukocytes by specific antigens such as ragweed extract.[31,32] These studies suggest that the cyclic AMP and drugs that activate adenyl cyclase have an inhibitory action on histamine release. There is a possibility that drugs widely used in allergic diseases, such as the catecholamines and theophylline, may exert an inhibitory effect on histamine release in addition to their well-known antagonism to many of its pharmacological actions. Anaphylactically induced histamine release is inhibited by the drug disodium cromoglycate (Intal) in vitro (p. 718).[27] It is enhanced by phosphatidylserine in rat mast cells.[11]

PHARMACO-LOGICAL EFFECTS

Histamine taken by mouth has essentially no effect because it is altered by the intestinal bacteria, the gastrointestinal wall, and also the liver.

If injected intravenously, however, as little as 0.1 mg of histamine phosphate causes a sharp decline in the blood pressure, acceleration of the heart rate, elevation of the cerebrospinal fluid pressure, flushing of the face, and headache. There is also stimulation of gastric hydrochloric acid secretion. All these effects last only a few minutes. If a similar injection is given to an asthmatic individual, even while he or she is free of demonstrable breathing difficulty, there will be a marked decrease in vital capacity, and a severe attack of asthma may be precipitated.

When larger doses of histamine are administered intravenously, which can be done only in animals, the blood pressure remains low for a considerable length of time, and there is marked elevation of the hematocrit reading. Histamine shock may ensue, with possibly fatal termination. The lethal dose in species such as the dog, in which the circulatory action of histamine predominates, may be as high as several milligrams per kilogram of body weight.

Circulatory effects   The two factors involved in the circulatory actions of histamine are arteriolar dilatation and increased capillary permeability. These cause loss of plasma from the circulation.

A striking demonstration of the histamine effect on capillaries is seen when very low concentrations are injected intracutaneously in humans. The injection of as little as 10 μg of the drug produces the "triple response of Lewis."[30] The sequence of events consists of localized redness, localized edema or wheal, and diffused redness or flare.

The localized redness and wheal are the consequences of vasodilatation and increased capillary permeability. The diffuse flare involves neural mechanisms, perhaps axon reflexes, since it can be abolished by previous sectioning of sensory nerves.

The triple response is interesting because human skin seems to respond to a variety of injuries in the same manner as it does to histamine injections. This similarity led Sir Thomas Lewis to suggest that perhaps various injuries may cause release of a histamine-like substance, or H substance, from the skin; this substance then mediates the manifestations of evanescent skin inflammations.

Histamine increases the rate and force of contraction of the heart in several species.[71] Both H_1 and H_2 receptors are present in the heart, and species variations in their distribution are great. Histamine stimulates adenylate cyclase in the human heart. This is not blocked by propranolol. The significance of cardiac histamine receptors is not entirely clear. Large doses of histamine cause norepinephrine release from the heart.[9]

Other smooth muscle effects   Human beings and guinea pigs are very susceptible to the bronchoconstrictor action of histamine. Persons with a previous history of asthma are particularly vulnerable and may respond with an acute asthmatic attack to a dose of histamine that would only cause minor decreases in vital capacity in a normal person. This is generally interpreted as increased susceptibility to histamine of the bronchial smooth muscle in asthmatic persons. Asthmatic individuals are highly susceptible not only to histamine but also to methacholine.

Effect on secretions   Histamine is a potent stimulant of gastric hydrochloric acid secretion. As little as 0.025 mg of the drug injected subcutaneously in humans will cause marked increase in hydrochloric acid secretion but few other effects in the body. This response to histamine is utilized in tests for complete achlorhydria. Histamine-resistant achlorhydria has diagnostic importance in such conditions as addisonian pernicious anemia.

The polypeptide gastrin is an extremely potent stimulant of gastric acid secretion, being 500 times as potent as histamine.[54] Its actions are also antagonized by the H_2 antihistamines, which brings up interesting speculations on the relationship between gastrin and histamine.

Histamine stimulates to a slight extent the secretory activities of many other glandular cells. Effects on salivary and bronchial secretions can be demonstrated, but these actions are not important in a normal person. Its effect on catecholamine secretion has been mentioned before.

Very little is known about the possible physiological roles of histamine. The presence of this potent capillary and arteriolar dilator in mast cells, which are in intimate contact with blood vessels, suggests some role more significant than causation of hives. Just what this role may be cannot be stated at present.

In one interesting experiment,[7] normal rats exposed to ultraviolet light, after having been injected previously with hematoporphyrin, reacted in about a day with edema of the skin. When these rats were pretreated for a week with the histamine-releasing agent compound 48/80 in order to deplete the histamine content of their skin, they did not react to the ultraviolet light.

Histamine undoubtedly plays a role in gastric secretion. It acts on H_2 receptors and may have a "permissive" enhancing effect on the actions of gastrin and acetylcholine. This will be discussed further in relation to cimetidine (p. 253).

Histamine probably plays an important role in neural function. The brain has receptors for this amine, and the enzymes for its synthesis and inactivation by methylation are also present. A ganglionic stimulant effect of histamine has been demonstrated.[59] Histamine releases catecholamines in pheochromocytoma and in animal experiments. Drugs used in parkinsonism and the tricyclic antidepressants have potent antihistaminic effects.

It has also been suggested that certain types of vascular headaches may be caused by histamine.[21] The evidence for the histaminic etiology in this instance is largely indirect. It is based on the facts that injected histamine can reproduce the symptoms and that repeated administration produces "desensitization" and symptomatic improvement.

Histamine is useful as a diagnostic adjunct for differentiating pernicious anemia from other diseases of the stomach on the basis of achlorhydria. It is also used occasionally in the diagnosis of pheochromocytoma, since it stimulates the output of catecholamines from the adrenal medullary tumor. Intracutaneous injections of histamine may be used for revealing the integrity of blood supply and innervation to an area. Other medical uses based on its vasodilator action are obsolete.

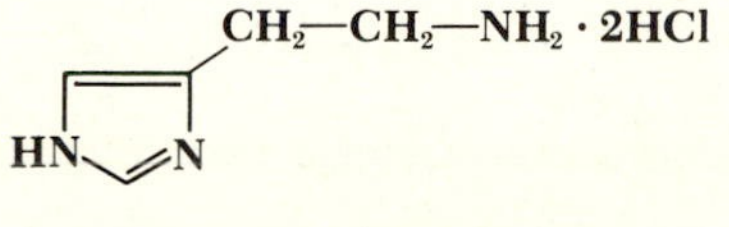

Histamine dihydrochloride 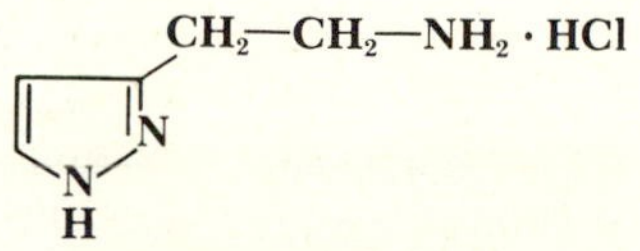   Betazole hydrochloride

Betazole is an isomer of histamine that stimulates gastric secretion but has only one-fiftieth the potency of histamine. Furthermore, it has relatively less effect than histamine on the cardiovascular system and may be safer for determination of gastric acidity. However, the drug may be dangerous in asthmatic persons.

Histamine preparations include histamine phosphate solutions for injection, containing 0.275, 0.55, and 2.75 mg/ml. Betazole hydrochloride (Histalog) is available as a solution for injection, 50 mg/ml.

REFERENCES

1 Copenhaver, J. H., Jr., Nagler, M. E., and Goth, A.: The intracellular distribution of histamine, J. Pharmacol. Exp. Ther. **109**:401, 1953.

2 Dale, H. H., and Laidlaw, P. P.: The physiological action of β-iminozolethylamine, J. Physiol. **41**:318, 1910.

3 Diana, J. N., and Kaiser, R. S.: Pre- and postcapillary resistance during histamine infusion in isolated dog hindlimb, Am. J. Physiol. **218**:132, 1970.

4 Dragstedt, C. A.: The role of histamine and other metabolites in anaphylaxis, Ann. N.Y. Acad. Sci. **50**:1039, 1950.

5 Feldberg, W., and Loeser, A. A.: Histamine content of human skin in different clinical disorders, J. Physiol. **126**:286, 1954.

6 Feldberg, W., and Schachter, M.: Histamine release by horse serum from skin of the sensitized dog and the nonsensitized cat, J. Physiol. **188**:124, 1952.

7 Feldberg, W., and Talesnik, J.: Reduction of tissue histamine by compound 48/80, J. Physiol. **120**:550, 1953.

8 Flacke, W., Atamackovic, D., Gillis, R. A., and Alper, M. H.: The actions of histamine on the mammalian heart, J. Pharmacol. Exp. Ther. **155**:271, 1967.

9 Fredholm, B. B., and Frisk-Holmberg, M.: Lipolysis in canine subcutaneous tissue following release of endogenous histamine, Eur. J. Pharmacol. **13**:254, 1971.

10 Goth, A.: Inhibition of anaphylactoid edema in the rat by 2-deoxyglucose, Am. J. Physiol. **197**:1056, 1959.

11 Goth, A., Adams, H. R., and Knoohuizen, M.: Phosphatidylserine: selective enhancer of histamine release, Science **173**:1034, 1971.

12 Goth, A., Nash, W. L., Nagler, M., and Holman, J.: Inhibition of histamine release in experimental diabetes, Am. J. Physiol. **199**:25, 1957.

13 Green, J. P.: Binding of some biogenic amines in tissues, Adv. Pharmacol. **1**:349, 1962.

14 Haddy, F.: Effect of histamine on small and large vessel pressures in the dog foreleg, Am. J. Physiol. **198**:161, 1960.

15 Halpern, B. N.: Histamine release by long chain molecules. In Ciba Foundation Symposium on Histamine, Boston, 1956, Little, Brown & Co.

16 Halpern, B. N., and Briot, M.: Mecanisme histaminique de l'action de la polyvinylpyrrolidone chez le chien, C. R. Soc. Biol. **147**:643, 1953.

17 Haverback, B. J., Tecimer, L. B., Tyce, B. J., Cohen, M., Stubrin, M. L., and Santa Ana, A. D.: The effect of gastrin on stomach histamine in the rat, Life Sci. **3**:637, 1964.

18 Haverback, B. J., and Wirtschafter, S. K.: The gastrointestinal tract and naturally occurring pharmacologically active amines, Adv. Pharmacol. **1**:309, 1962.

19 Högberg, B., and Uvnas, B.: The mechanism of the disruption of mast cells produced by compound 48/80, Acta Physiol. Scand. **41**:344, 1957.

20 Högberg, B., and Uvnas, B.: Further observations on the disruption of rat mesentery mast cells caused by compound 48/80, antigen-antibody reaction, lecithinase A and decylamine, Acta Physiol. Scand. **48**:133, 1960.

21 Horton, B. T.: Management of vascular headache, Angiology **10**:43, 1959.

22 James, L. P., and Austen, K. F.: Fatal systemic anaphylaxis in man, N. Engl. J. Med. **270**:597, 1964.

23 Kahlson, G.: A place for histamine in normal physiology, Lancet **1**:67, 1960.

24 Kahlson, G., and Rosengren, E.: Histamine, Annu. Rev. Pharmacol. **5**:305, 1965.

25 Kim, K. S., and Shore, P. A.: Mechanism of action of reserpine and insulin on gastric amines and gastric acid secretion, and the effect of monoamine oxidase inhibition, J. Pharmacol. Exp. Ther. **141**:321, 1963.

26 Krantz, J. C., Jr., Carr, C. J., Bird, J. G., and Cook, S.: Sugar alcohols: pharmacodynamic studies of polyoxyalkylene derivatives of hexitol anhydride partial fatty acid esters, J. Pharmacol. Exp. Ther. **93**:188, 1948.

27 Kusner, E. J., Dunnick, B., and Herzog, D. J.: The inhibition by disodium cromoglycate in

vitro of anaphylactically induced histamine release from rat peritoneal mast cells, J. Pharmacol. Exp. Ther. **184**:41, 1973.

28 Levine, R. J., Sato, T. L., and Sjoerdsma, A.: Inhibition of histamine synthesis in the rat by hydrazino analog of histidine and 4-bromo-3-hydroxy benzyloxyamine, Biochem. Pharmacol. **14**:139, 1965.

29 Lewis, T.: The blood vessels of the human skin and their responses, London, 1927, Shaw & Sons, Ltd.

30 Lewis, T., and Grant, R. T.: Vascular reactions of the skin to injury: the liberation of histamine-like substance in injured skin; the underlying cause of factitious urticaria and of wheals produced by burning; and observations upon the nervous control of certain skin reactions, Heart **11**:209, 1924.

31 Lichtenstein, L. M., Henney, C. S., Bourne, H. R., and Greenough, W. B.: Effects of cholera toxin on in vitro models of immediate and delayed hypersensitivity, J. Clin. Invest. **52**:691, 1973.

32 Lichtenstein, L. M., and Margolis, S.: Histamine release in vitro: inhibition by catecholamines and methylxanthines, Science **161**:902, 1968.

33 MacMillan, W. H., and Vane, J. R.: The effects of histamine on the plasma potassium levels of cats, J. Pharmacol. Exp. Ther. **118**:182, 1956.

34 Mongar, J. L., and Schild, H. O.: A comparison of the effects of anaphylactic shock and of chemical histamine releasers, J. Physiol. **118**:461, 1952.

35 Mongar, J. L., and Schild, H. O.: Effect of antigen and organic bases on intracellular histamine in guinea-pig lung, J. Physiol. **131**:207, 1956.

36 Mongar, J. L., and Schild, H. O.: Cellular mechanisms in anaphylaxis, Physiol. Rev. **42**:226, 1962.

37 Norton, S., and de Beer, E. J.: Effect of some antibiotics on rat mast cells in vitro, Arch. Int. Pharmacodyn. **102**:352, 1955.

38 Orange, R. P., Valentine, M. D., and Austen, K. F.: Release of slow reacting substance of anaphylaxis in the rat: polymorphonuclear leukocyte, Science **157**:318, 1967.

39 Paton, W. D. M.: Histamine release by compounds of simple chemical structure, Pharmacol. Rev. **9**:269, 1957.

40 Piper, P. J., and Vane, J. R.: Release of additional factors in anaphylaxis and its antagonism by anti-inflammatory drugs, Nature **223**:29, 1969.

41 Powell, J. R., and Brody, M. J.: Participation of H_1 and H_2 histamine receptors in physiolog-

ical vasodilator responses, Am. J. Physiol. **231**:1002, 1976.

42 Riley, J. F.: The effects of histamine-liberators on the mast cells of the rat, J. Pathol. Bact. **65**:471, 1953.

43 Rocha e Silva, M., subeditor: Histamine and antihistaminics. Encyclopedia of experimental pharmacology, vol. 18, Berlin, 1966, Springer-Verlag.

44 Rowley, D. A., and Benditt, E. P.: 5-Hydroxy-tryptamine and histamine as mediators of the vascular injury produced by agents which damage mast cells in rats, J. Exp. Med. **103**:399, 1956.

45 Schayer, R. W.: Biogenesis of histamine, J. Biol. Chem. **199**:245, 1952.

46 Schayer, R. W.: Studies on histamine-metabolizing enzymes in intact animals, J. Biol. Chem. **203**:787, 1953.

47 Schayer, R. W.: Catabolism of physiological quantities of histamine in vivo, Physiol. Rev. **39**:116, 1959.

48 Schayer, R. W., and Cooper, J. A. D.: Metabolism of C^{14} histamine in man, J. Appl. Physiol. **9**:481, 1956.

49 Schayer, R. W., and Ganley, O. H.: Adaptive increase in mammalian histidine decarboxylase activity in response to nonspecific stress, Am. J. Physiol. **197**:721, 1959.

50 Schayer, R. W., and Karjala, S. A.: Ring N methylation: a major route of histamine metabolism, J. Biol. Chem. **221**:307, 1956.

51 Schayer, R. W., and Smiley, R. L.: Binding and release of radioactive histamine in intact rats, Am. J. Physiol. **177**:401, 1954.

52 Selye, H.: Effect of ACTH and cortisone upon an "anaphylactoid reaction," Can. Med. Assoc. J. **61**:553, 1949.

53 Shore, P. A., Burkhalter, A., and Cohn, V. H., Jr.: A method for the fluometric assay of histamine in tissues, J. Pharmacol. Exp. Ther. **127**:182, 1959.

54 Silen, W. B.: Advances in gastric physiology, N. Engl. J. Med. **277**:864, 1968.

55 Smith, D. E.: Nature of the secretory activity of the mast cell, Am. J. Physiol. **193**:573, 1958.

56 Snyder, S. H., and Epps, L.: Regulation of histidine decarboxylase in rat stomach by gastrin: the effect of inhibitors of protein synthesis, Mol. Pharmacol. **4**:187, 1968.

57 Tabor, H.: Metabolic studies on histidine, histamine, and related imidazoles, Pharmacol. Rev. **6**:299, 1954.

58 Thompson, J. C.: Gastrin and gastric secretion, Annu. Rev. Med. **20**:291, 1969.

59 Trendelenburg, U.: Non-nicotinic ganglion-

stimulating substances, Fed. Proc. **18**:1001, 1959.

60 Urbach, K. F.: Nature and probable origin of conjugated histamine excreted after ingestion of histamine, Proc. Soc. Exp. Biol. Med. **70**:146, 1949.

61 Uvnas, B.: The mechanism of histamine liberation, J. Pharm. Pharmacol. **10**:1, 1958.

62 Van Arsdel, P. P., Jr., and Beall, G. N.: The metabolism and functions of histamine, Arch. Intern. Med. **106**:192, 1960.

63 Vick, J. A.: Bioassay of the prominent humoral agents involved in endotoxin shock, Am. J. Physiol. **209**:75, 1965.

64 Walton, R. P., Richardson, J. A., and Thompson, W. L.: Hypotension and histamine release following intravenous injection of plasma substitutes, J. Pharmacol. Exp. Ther. **127**:39, 1959.

65 West, G. B.: Studies on the mechanism of anaphylaxis: a possible basis for the pharmacologic approach to allergy, Clin. Pharmacol. Ther. **4**:749, 1963.

REVIEWS

66 Beaven, M. A.: Histamine, N. Engl. J. Med. **294**:30, 1976.

67 Black, J. W., Duncan, W. A. M., Durant, C. J., Ganellin, C. R., and Parsons, E. M.: Definition and antagonism of histamine H_2-receptors, Nature **236**:385, 1972.

67a Ginsburg, R., Bristow, M. R., Stinson, E. B., and Harrison, D. C.: Histamine receptors in the human heart, Life Sci. **26**:2245, 1980.

68 Goth, A.: Histamine release by drugs and chemicals. In Schachter, M., editor: International encyclopedia of pharmacology and therapy: histamine and antihistamines, vol. 1, New York, 1973, Pergamon Press Inc.

69 Goth, A.: On the general problem of the release of histamine. In Rocha e Silva, M., editor: Handbook of experimental pharmacology, 18/2:57, Berlin, 1978, Springer-Verlag.

70 Goth, A., and Johnson, A. R.: Current concepts on the secretory function of mast cells, Life Sci. **16**:1201, 1975.

71 Verma, S. C., and McNeill, J. H.: Cardiac histamine receptors and cyclic AMP, Life Sci. **19**:1797, 1976.

CHAPTER 20

Antihistaminic drugs

Drugs that block the effects of histamine competitively at various receptor sites are referred to as antihistaminic drugs. The actions of histamine on bronchial and intestinal smooth muscles can be blocked by the conventional antihistamines, as exemplified by mepyramine. On the other hand, the effects of histamine on gastric secretion are not blocked by the usual antihistamines but are prevented by the newer type of competitor, as exemplified by cimetidine.

The antihistaminics are classified as H_1-and H_2-receptor antagonists. Diphenhydramine and tripelennamine were the first H_1 antihistaminics introduced in this country many years ago. Cimetidine, a congener of burimamide and metiamide,[20] was introduced fairly recently and is an H_2-receptor antagonist.

The H_1 antihistaminic drugs are useful not only in allergic diseases but also for the prevention of motion sickness and in the treatment of parkinsonism. Also, their sedative effect may be of some benefit. The H_2 antihistamines, such as cimetidine, are useful in the treatment of peptic ulcer disease.[2]

The field of antihistaminics was opened up by the discovery that certain phenolic ethers could protect guinea pigs against anaphylactic shock and histamine. The response of the guinea pig to the inhalation of histamine aerosol has been used widely in subsequent development of new antihistaminics. With the recognition of the structural requirements for antihistaminic action, compounds of considerable potency and low toxicity were synthesized. Such compounds as N-benzyl-N',N'-dimethyl-N-phenylethylenediamine (Antergan), diphenhydramine, and tripelennamine were found to protect guinea pigs against as many as 50 lethal doses of histamine. These were introduced into therapeutics and were followed by an enormous number of other antihistaminics.

ANTIHISTAMINES: H_1-RECEPTOR ANTAGONISTS Development

The basic structure of the antihistaminics may be represented as a substituted ethylamine:

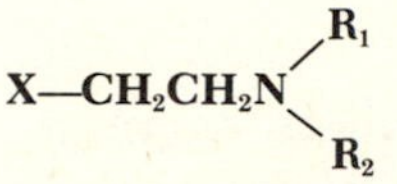

Chemistry

$$X-CH_2CH_2N\begin{array}{c} R_1 \\ \\ R_2 \end{array}$$

If it is recalled that histamine is 2-(4-imidazolyl)ethylamine, it is apparent that some relationship may exist between the ethylamine portion of the histamine molecule and the fact that the antihistamines are substituted ethylamines. Perhaps this portion of the histamine molecule is essential for its attachment to some of the receptor structures.

The R groups in the ethylamine structure are in most cases CH_3. If the X in the basic structure is nitrogen, the compound may be looked on as a substituted ethylenediamine. Examples of this type of antihistaminic drugs are tripelennamine (Pyribenzamine; PBZ), methapyrilene (Thenylene; Histadyl), thonzylamine (Neohetramine), pyrilamine (Neo-Antergan), and many others. The structural formulas of tripelennamine and methapyrilene are shown on p. 248.

Diphenhydramine (Benadryl), being a dimethylaminoethoxy compound, is an example of an antihistaminic in which the X of the basic structure is represented by oxygen. Its structural formula is shown on p. 248.

Dimenhydrinate (Dramamine) is a combination of diphenhydramine and 8-chlorotheophylline.

An example of an antihistaminic in which the X is carbon is chlorpheniramine (Chlor-Trimeton) (p. 249).

Promethazine (Phenergan) contains the phenothiazine structure (p. 249).

In some antihistaminics the ethylamine structure is within a heterocyclic ring. For example, cyclizine (Marezine) is 1-diphenylmethyl-4-methylpiperazine (p. 249).

Cyclizine and another piperazine derivative, meclizine (Bonamine), have been recommended particularly for the prevention of motion sickness.

Clinical pharmacology   If a recommended dose of one of the antihistaminics is taken orally by a normal person, the only noticeable effects will be on the CNS. Drowsiness is quite common, and barbiturates taken simultaneously appear to be synergistic in causing sleepiness. There is no relationship between the antihistaminic potency of these drugs and their central depressant action. Chlorpheniramine produces less sedation for an equivalent antihistaminic action than diphenhydramine. An unusual histaminic, phenindamine (Thephorin), may even have CNS stimulant properties.

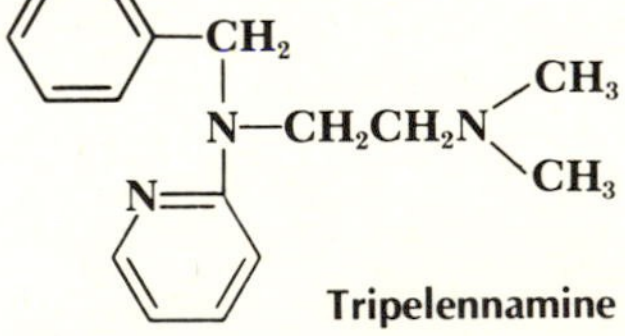

Tripelennamine

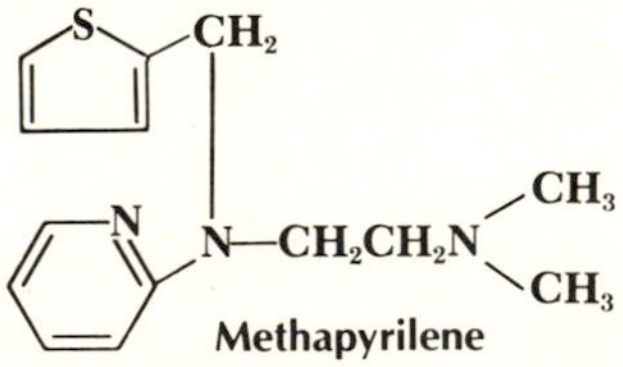

Methapyrilene

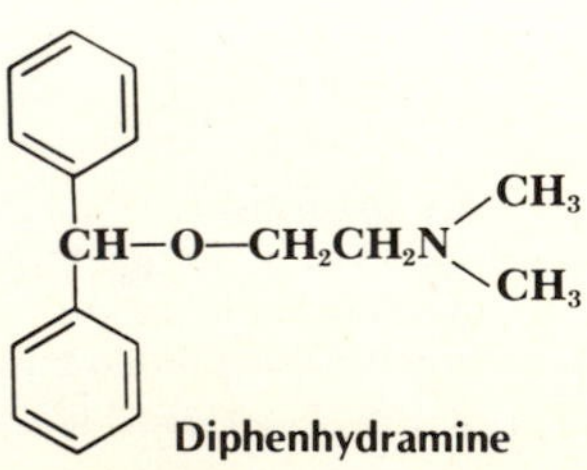

Diphenhydramine

Dimenhydrinate

Chlorpheniramine   **Promethazine**   **Cyclizine**

If the patient suffers from urticaria or hay fever, the various antihistaminics will produce considerable relief with variable sedation. Surprisingly, these drugs have very little benefit in the treatment of asthma, and this ineffectiveness has led to some doubt concerning the role of histamine in asthma.

It is important to recall that even in animal experiments the antihistaminics are more effective against exogenously administered histamine, particularly when the antihistaminic precedes the administration of histamine.

With the recognition of two separate receptors for histamine and the discovery of H_2-receptor antagonists, many puzzling aspects of the pharmacology of antihistamines can be clarified. Gastric secretion is mediated by H_2 receptors and is not blocked by the commonly available antihistamines, which are H_1-receptor antag-

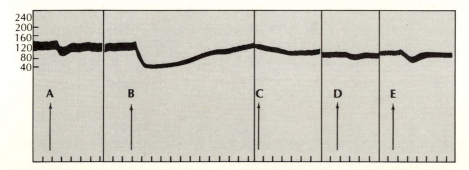

FIG. 20-1. Effect of histamine on blood pressure and its antagonism by an antihistaminic drug. *A*, Histamine, μg/kg IV. *B*, Histamine, 5 μg/kg IV. *C*, Diphenhydramine, 5 mg/kg IV. *D*, Histamine, 1 μg/kg IV. *E*, Histamine, 5 μg/kg IV. Blood pressure recording of dog anesthetized with pentobarbital sodium. Time in 15 seconds. Note that the antihistaminic drug, although exerting considerable protection against vasodepressor action of histamine, failed to eliminate it completely.

onists.[20] It appears also that vasodilatation and increased capillary permeability are mediated by both types of receptors and that such actions of histamine can be blocked completely only by a combination of H_1- and H_2-receptor antagonists[20] (Fig. 20-1).

Antihistaminics are often applied topically to obtain symptomatic improvement in itching skin conditions, but in several cases contact dermatitis developed as a consequence of sensitization of the patient to the topically applied antihistaminics.

Miscellaneous actions

Besides being competitive antagonists of histamine, the antihistaminics have a number of additional actions. These are (1) CNS effect, (2) anticholinergic effect, (3) local anesthetic properties, and (4) antiserotonin action.

Antihistaminics produce a *sedative CNS effect* different from the actions of barbiturates and other sedative-hypnotics. The sedative effect of the antihistaminics is not pleasant. Furthermore, if the dose of the antihistamine is increased, sedation is replaced by marked irritability, leading to convulsions, hyperpyrexia, and even death. Toxic doses are likely to produce excitation in children. Additional CNS effects are probably related to anticholinergic properties.

The *anticholinergic effect* manifests itself as a drying of salivary and bronchial secretions, similar to the effect of atropine. For the same reason these drugs may have adverse effects in the treatment of bronchial asthma by increasing the viscosity of secretions in the respiratory tract.

The anticholinergic effect of the antihistaminics may be related to their usefulness in the prevention of motion sickness.[8,9] Dimenhydrinate is widely used for this. There is good indication from clinical studies that the drug owes its antimotion sickness properties to diphenhydramine, one of its components. Certain antihistaminics such as cyclizine and meclizine are especially recommended for the prevention of motion sickness. The effectiveness of diphenhydramine in Parkinson's disease may also result from its anticholinergic properties.

The *local anesthetic properties* of antihistaminics make them suitable as antipruritic agents in topical applications. Unfortunately they may cause sensitization, and their use as topical agents is best avoided.

Antiserotonin properties are quite common in antihistaminic drugs. At least one, cyproheptadine (Periactin), is generally viewed as a combined antihistamine-antiserotonin. There is no reason to believe, however, that antagonism to serotonin confers any special advantages in an antihistaminic.

Therapeutic uses

There are many conditions in which antihistaminics are helpful. There are others in which they are used but perhaps should not be.[10]

Conditions in which the antihistaminics are helpful include allergic rhinitis, urticaria, some types of asthma, and motion sickness. Conditions in which antihistaminics are not the drugs of choice include acute anaphylactic emergencies (epinephrine is much more useful), most cases of asthma, diseases of the skin, eyes, and nose, and the common cold.

TABLE 20-1. Doses and sedative properties of various antihistamines*

Generic name	Trade name	Usual adult dose (mg)	Degree of sedation
Carbinoxamine	Clistin	4	+
Chlorothen	Tagathen	25	+
Phenindamine	Thephorin	25	+†
Chlorpheniramine	Chlor-Trimeton	4	++
Brompheniramine	Dimetane	4	++
Triprolidine	Actidil	2.5	++
Doxylamine	Decapryn	12.5	++
Chlorcyclizine	Di-Paralene	50	++
Methapyrilene	Histadyl	25	++
Dimethindene	Forhistal	1	++
Pyrilamine	Neo-Antergan	25	++
Cyproheptadine	Periactin	4	++
Tripelennamine	Pyribenzamine	50	++
Diphenhydramine	Benadryl	50	+++
Promethazine	Phenergan	12.5	+++

*Based on data from Feinberg, S. M.: Pharmacol. Phys. **1**(12):1, 1967.
†Stimulation possible.

In the selection of antihistaminics, their sedative action is a major consideration. Potency is not so important, since it only influences the size of the tablets used. The duration of action of most antihistamines when given in a therapeutic dose is about 4 hours and is greatly influenced by the dose. The usual adult doses and sedative potencies of a number of antihistamines are shown in Table 20-1.

Absorption and metabolism

The H_1 antagonists are absorbed rapidly and completely from the gastrointestinal tract. They cause systemic effects in less than 30 minutes, and absorption is complete in 4 hours. In the case of diphenhydramine, peak blood levels occur in 1 hour, declining to essentially zero in 6 hours.[11] The H_1 antagonists are metabolized in the liver by hydroxylation, and these drugs may stimulate the hepatic microsomal enzymes.[25]

Toxicity

On the whole the antihistaminics are remarkably nontoxic compounds when used in the recommended doses. It is possible that the widespread use of these drugs may contribute to automobile accidents because of their sedative properties. It is also likely that the simultaneous use of antihistaminics and other depressant drugs such as barbiturates or alcohol may exert synergistic depressant actions.[12] A few cases of skin sensitization have been reported following topical use of antihistaminics.

Acute poisoning has occurred following ingestion of very large doses of the antihistaminics, particularly in children. Surprisingly, the symptoms consisted of CNS excitation and convulsive phenomena. The management of acute poisoning is purely symptomatic. The anticonvulsant barbiturates must be tried very cautiously because there is experimental evidence that their toxicity may be additive to that of the antihistaminics.

Some of the antihistaminics commonly used for the prevention of motion sickness have been found to be teratogenic in rats. As a consequence, meclizine, cyclizine, and chlorcyclizine should not be used in pregnant women and preparations offered for self-medication must bear a warning to that effect.[15] The teratogenic effect is not related to an antihistaminic effect but seems related to a structural feature, all of these drugs being piperazines.

Antihistaminics with antiserotonin action

Among the antihistaminic drugs, promethazine has considerable antiserotonin action on smooth muscles, approaching LSD in this activity. Chlorpromazine, a tranquilizer, is about half as active. A relatively new antihistaminic, cyproheptadine hydrochloride, is a potent antiserotonin drug as well.

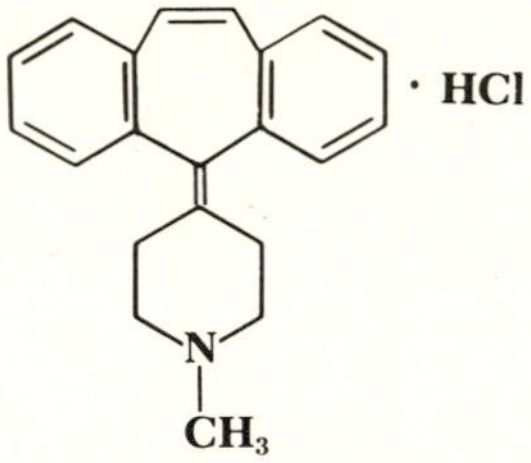

Cyproheptadine hydrochloride

Administered in doses of 4 to 20 mg daily, cyproheptadine is available for the same indications as other antihistaminics. In addition, there are claims for its effectiveness in the postgastrectomy dumping syndrome and other conditions, but further experience is needed for evaluating these claims.

H₂-RECEPTOR ANTAGONISTS

The H_1-receptor antagonists or classical antihistamines do not block the gastric secretory effect of histamine. To explain this anomaly it was proposed in 1966[1] that there were two histamine receptors. In 1972 Black and co-workers described the first antagonist, burimamide, which competitively antagonized the effects of histamine on gastric parietal cells, guinea pig atria, and rat. These histamine receptors were called H_2-receptor antagonists. Further studies led to the synthesis of metiamide, which had effects similar to those of burimamide, but which was better absorbed from the gastrointestinal tract.[25] Following extensive clinical use, several patients developed agranulocytosis while on metiamide. Because of this a newer H_2 antagonist, cimetidine, was introduced,[7] which so far has not caused serious hematological toxicity. In cimetidine, the thiourea in the side chain is changed to cyanoguanidine.

Differences between H₁ and H₂ antihistamines

These two groups of drugs differ in their chemistry, pharmacokinetics, and clinical uses, in addition to acting on different receptors.

In the H_1 antihistamines the imidazole ring structure is extensively modified or replaced by other substituents. In the H_2 antagonists the imidazole part of histamine is preserved and the side chain is extensively modified. More than 700 compounds had to be synthesized before burimamide was obtained.

In contrast with the H_1 antagonists, the H_2 antihistamines are generally less lipid-soluble compounds, do not cross the blood-brain barrier, and do not cause sedation.

Cimetidine

Cimetidine causes a significant reduction in diurnal gastric acid secretion.[2] After 6 weeks of treatment most ulcer patients were cured as compared with members of the placebo group. When the drug was administered in doses of 200 mg three times a day, even stimulated gastric secretion was inhibited. The drug was found to be effective even in the Zollinger-Ellison syndrome.[21]

Mechanism of inhibition of gastric secretion

The H_2-receptor antagonists, such as cimetidine, inhibit gastric secretion caused by histamine, gastrin, acetylcholine, and food.[27] There are several possible explanations for this apparent lack of specificity of the inhibitory action. Histamine could be the final common pathway for the various stimuli. Or there could be separate receptors on the parietal cell for histamine, gastrin, and acetylcholine, but occupation of the histamine receptor interferes in some way with the others. Finally, histamine could have a "permissive" effect on the actions of the other stimuli.

Clinical pharmacology, indications, and toxicity

A 300 mg dose of cimetidine at bedtime causes a significant reduction of gastric acidity for at least 8 hours. The drug is well absorbed when given orally, has a plasma half-life of 2 hours, and is excreted in the urine, 70% unchanged.

Approved indication for cimetidine are active duodenal ulcer disease and hypersecretory states in Zollinger-Ellison syndrome and mastocytosis. Investigational uses include reflux esophagitis, pancreatic insufficiency, stress ulcers, and upper gastrointestinal hemorrhage.

Adverse effects of cimetidine are rare. The drug is not very lipophilic and does not cause drowsiness because of poor penetration into the CNS. In very large doses, the drug has caused renal and hepatic damage in dogs, but the doses required were of the order of 500 mg/kg. Rare instances of elevations of creatinine and transient elevations of transaminase, gynecomastia and galactorrhea, and mental confusion and neutropenia have been reported.

Cimetidine (Tagamet) is available in 300 mg tablets and in vials containing 300 mg/2 ml.

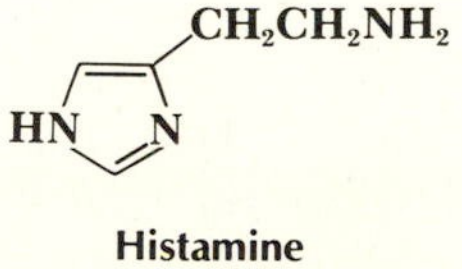

Histamine

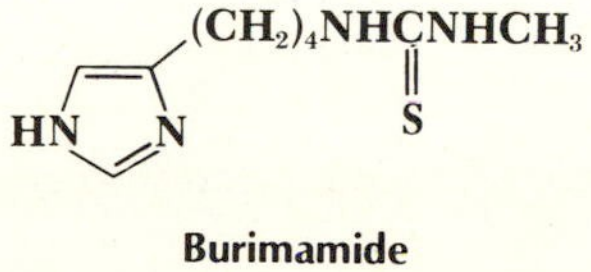

Burimamide

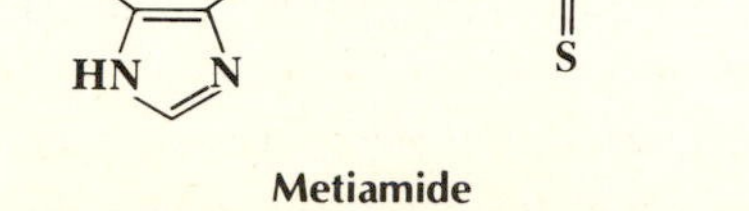

Metiamide

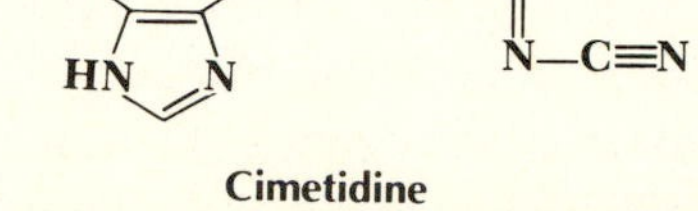

Cimetidine

REFERENCES

1 Ash, A. S. F., and Schild, H. O.: Receptors mediating some actions of histamine, Br. J. Pharmacol. **27**:427, 1966.

2 Bodemar, G., and Walan, A.: Cimetidine in treatment of active duodenal and prepyloric ulcers, Lancet **2**:161, 1976.

3 Bodemar, G., and Walan, A.: A double blind trial of cimetidine on patients with active duodenal or prepyloric ulcers, Scand. J. Gastroenterol. **11**(Supp. 38):108, 1976.

4 Bovet, D., and Staub, A.: Action protrectrice des éthers phénoliques au cours de l'intoxication histaminique, C. R. Soc. Biol. **124**:547, 1937.

5 Brand, J. J.: The pharmacologic basis for the control of motion sickness by drugs, Pharmacol. Phys. **2**(3):1, 1968.

6 Brand, J. J., and Perry, W. L. M.: Drugs used in motion sickness, Pharmacol. Rev. **18**:895, 1966.

7 Brimblecombe, R. W., Duncan, W. A. M., Durant, G. J., et al.: Cimetidine: a non–thiourea H_2-receptor antagonist, J. Int. Med. Res. **3**:86, 1975.

8 Chinn, H. I., and Milch, L. J.: Comparison of airsickness preventives, J. Appl. Physiol. **5**:162, 1952.

9 Chinn, H. I., and Oberst, F. W.: Effectiveness of various drugs in prevention of airsickness, Proc. Soc. Exp. Biol. Med. **73**:218, 1950.

10 Feinberg, S. M.: The antihistamines: pharmacologic principles in their use, Pharmacol. Phys. **1**(12):1, 1967.

11 Glazko, A. J., and Dill, W. A.: Biochemical studies on diphenhydramine (Benadryl): distribution in tissues and urinary excretion, J. Biol. Chem. **179**:403, 1949.

12 Hughes, F. W., and Forney, R. B.: Comparative effects of three antihistaminics and ethanol on mental and motor performance, Clin. Pharmacol. Ther. **5**:414, 1964.

13 Isaac, L., and Goth, A.: Interaction of antihistaminics with norepinephrine uptake: a cocaine-like effect, Life Sci. **4**:1899, 1965.

14 Isaac, L., and Goth, A.: The mechanism of the potentiation of norepinephrine by antihistaminics, J. Pharmacol. Exp. Ther. **156**:463, 1967.

15 Sadusk, J. F., and Palmisano, P. A.: Teratogenic effect of meclizine, cyclizine and chlorcyclizine, J.A.M.A. **194**:139, 1965.

16 Stavorski, J. M., and Ross, C. A.: Antiserotonin-antihistaminic properties of cyproheptadine, J. Pharmacol. Exp. Ther. **131**:73, 1961.

17 Weinman, E. O., and Geissman, T. A.: The distribution, excretion, and metabolism of C^{14}-labeled tripelennamine (Pyribenzamine) by pigs, J. Pharmacol. Exp. Ther. **125**:1, 1959.

18 Winbury, M. M., and Alworth, B. L.: Suppression of experimental atrial arrhythmias by several antihistamines, Arch. Int. Pharmacodyn. **122**:318, 1959.

19 Zeppa, R., and Hemingway, G. C.: Inhibition of histamine release from mast cells, Surg. Forum **14**:56, 1963.

REVIEWS

20 Black, J. W., Duncan, W. A. M., Durant, C. J., Ganellin, C. R., and Parsons, E. M.: Definition and antagonism of histamine receptors, Nature **236**:385, 1972.

21 Danilevicius, Z.: A new star: how brightly will it shine? J.A.M.A. **237**:2224, 1977.

22 Finkelstein, W., and Isselbacher, K. J.: Cimetidine, N. Engl. J. Med. **299**:992, 1978.

23 Fleischer, D., and Samloff, I. M.: Cimetidine therapy in a patient with a metiamide-induced agranulocytosis, N. Engl. J. Med. **296**:342, 1977.

24 Goth, A.: Antihistamines. In Middleton, E., Jr., Reed, C. E., and Ellis, E. F.: Allergy: principles and practice, St. Louis, 1978, The C. V. Mosby Co., pp. 454-463.

25 Kuntzman, R.: Drugs and enzyme induction, Annu. Rev. Pharmacol. **9**:21, 1969.

26 Melville, K. I.: Antihistamine drugs. In Schacter, M., editor: Histamine and antihistamines, vol. 1, International Encyclopaedia of Pharmacology and Therapeutics, Oxford, 1973, Pergamon Press, pp. 3-24.

27 Schlippert, W.: Cimetidine. H_2-receptor blockade in gastrointestinal disease, Arch. Intern. Med. **138**:1257, 1978.

28 Wood, C. J., and Simkins, M. A., editors: International Symposium on histamine H_2-receptor antagonists, London, 1973, Research and Development Division, Smith, Kline & French Laboratories, Ltd.

CHAPTER 21

Serotonin and antiserotonins

Serotonin, or 5-hydroxytryptamine, occupies a surprisingly prominent position in the medical literature, considering the ignorance that surrounds its functions in the body. The reasons for this paradox are many. This endogenously produced amine is almost certainly one of the central neurotransmitters. It is also present in large quantities in the enterochromaffin system of the intestine and in platelets, where its functions are unknown. Moreover, studies on serotonin have contributed greatly to theories on biochemical mechanisms in disease states ranging from mental disease to migraine. The relationships between lysergic acid diethylamide (LSD) and serotonin and the release of the amine by reserpine provided potent stimuli for psychopharmacological research. The same can be said of the hallucinogenic properties of many serotonin derivatives.

In addition to serotonin, some of its therapeutically useful antagonists will be discussed in this chapter. Furthermore, the pharmacology of ergot alkaloids, lysergic acid derivatives that are generally serotonin antagonists, will also be considered at this point.

SEROTONIN

The discovery of serotonin (5-hydroxytryptamine; 5-HT) as a normally occurring amine resulted from independent studies on the vasoconstrictor substance in serum[13] at the Cleveland Clinic and the active substance in intestinal enterochromaffin cells,[7] named *enteramine* by investigators in Italy. The compound investigated by both groups was eventually shown to be 5-HT.

Occurrence and distribution

Serotonin is widely distributed in the animal and plant kingdom. Some fruits such as bananas contain a high concentration but represent no threat of causing serotonin poisoning because the amine is not well absorbed from the gastrointestinal tract and is rapidly metabolized. Ingestion of such fruits, however, may increase the urinary excretion of serotonin metabolites, giving false positive tests in the diagnosis of carcinoid tumor.

In mammals about 90% of the total serotonin is in the enterochromaffin cells of the intestine, about 8% in platelets, and 2% in the CNS, particularly in the pineal gland and the hypothalamus. In rats and mice serotonin is also present in mast cells along with histamine. Human mast cells probably do not contain serotonin, since in mastocytosis the excretion of the serotonin metabolite 5-hydroxyindoleacetic acid in the urine is not increased.

At the various sites mentioned except the platelets, which actively concentrate the amine but do not make it, serotonin is synthesized from tryptophan.

Biosynthesis and metabolic degradation

Serotonin is made from tryptophan. Normally only a small fraction of the dietary tryptophan is utilized for serotonin synthesis. In patients with carcinoid tumors this fraction may increase so greatly that pellagra may result.

The various steps in the biosynthesis and biodegradation of serotonin are as follows:

Tryptophan → 5-Hydroxytryptophan → 5-Hydroxytryptamine → 5-Hydroxyindoleacetic acid

Tryptophan

5-Hydroxytryptophan

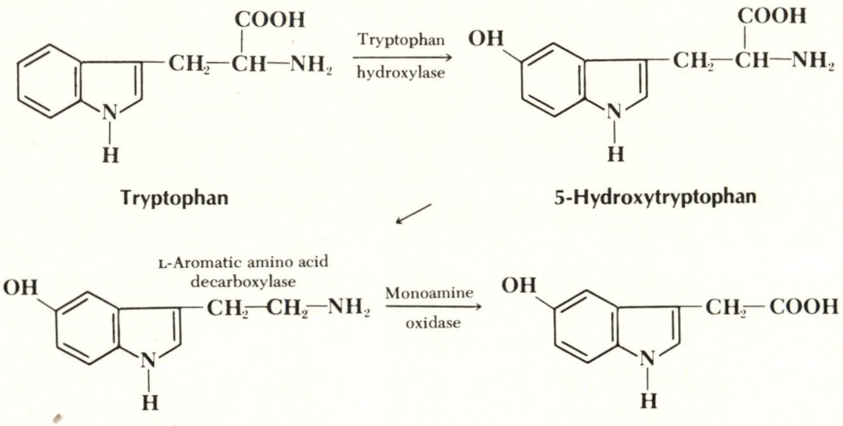

5-Hydroxytryptamine (serotonin)

5-Hydroxyindoleacetic acid

In addition, serotonin is converted in the pineal gland to *N*-acetyl serotonin and its *O*-methyl derivative, *melatonin*.

The biosynthesis of serotonin is blocked by *p-chlorophenylalanine*, which inhibits tryptophan hydroxylase, the rate-limiting enzyme. Degradation of serotonin is blocked by the MAO inhibitors. Turnover of serotonin is quite rapid in the CNS and also in the intestine. MAO inhibitors can double the serotonin content of brain in less than 1 hour.

The daily excretion of 5-hydroxyindoleacetic acid in the urine is 3 to 10 mg in a normal adult. It increases greatly in the presence of a carcinoid tumor and also with the ingestion of bananas and the administration of reserpine, which releases serotonin from its binding sites. Excretion of 5-hydroxyindoleacetic acid is decreased by MAO inhibitors.[7]

Pharmacological effects

The actions of serotonin are exerted on smooth muscles and on nerve elements including afferent nerve endings. The smooth muscle effects are prominent in the cardiovascular system and the gastrointestinal tract.

Intravenous injection of a few micrograms of serotonin as the creatinine sulfate complex produces a *triphasic* response: (1) a transient fall of blood pressure, (2) a brief period of hypertension, and (3) a more prolonged period of pressure lowering. The early depressor phase is probably caused by a reflex elicited by stimulation of chemoreceptors (Bezold-Jarisch effect). The blood pressure elevation is a consequence of constriction of blood vessels in many areas. Finally, the late depressor phase is attributed to the vasodilator action of serotonin in areas such as the skeletal muscle. Continuous intravenous infusion of serotonin produces only the prolonged lowering of peripheral resistance, with lowering of mean blood pressure.

In addition to its effect on the cardiovascular system, serotonin stimulates the gastrointestinal and bronchial smooth muscles. The gastrointestinal effects are both direct and also a consequence of excitation of ganglion cells. The direct effects are blocked by serotonin antagonists such as LSD; the ganglionic action is, interestingly, blocked by morphine. The bronchial stimulant action of the drug is probably unimportant in humans, although asthmatic individuals may be unduly responsive to it.

Serotonin can stimulate afferent nerve endings, ganglion cells, and adrenal medullary cells. It does not cross the blood-brain barrier but exerts striking effects when injected into the lateral ventricles of cats.[8] Sleep, catatonia, and fever have been elicited by such injections.

The possible role of serotonin in mood and behavior and in mental disease comes from speculations based on several lines of evidence. First, the powerful psychotomimetic drug LSD was early found to inhibit the actions of serotonin on smooth muscles. The simple hypothesis based on these facts found little support, however, when it was shown that other antiserotonins, even the closely related D-2-bromolysergic acid diethylamide, were not psychotomimetic.

Role in health and disease

The final remaining speculation in regard to a link between serotonin and mental disease is the demonstrated hallucinogenic effect of a variety of compounds structurally related to the amine. For example, bufotenine is 5-hydroxy-dimethyltryptamine, and psilocin is 4-hydroxy-dimethyltryptamine. Bufotenine is present in some plants and in toads. Psilocin and its phosphoryl ester psilocybin are very potent LSD-like hallucinogens. Many other tryptamine derivatives have psychotomimetic effects, and it is intriguing to speculate on biochemical explanations of schizophrenia. A critical review of this problem[10] concluded that all such speculations are interesting but up to then, at least, not convincing.

Serotonin probably plays a role in intestinal motility, since there is an abundance of this amine in the enterochromaffin cells that can be released by distention and other mechanical stimuli. Morphine blocks the effects of serotonin on intramural ganglion cells.

Serotonin probably plays a role in the causation of symptoms in the *carcinoid syndrome*. Flushing and increased intestinal motility have been attributed to serotonin release. However, the flush that occurs in carcinoid patients cannot be elicited by the injection of serotonin but will occur, on the other hand, after the administration of epinephrine or bradykinin.[12] It has been shown that kinin-producing enzymes are released from the carcinoid tumor. In addition, in the gastric carcinoid syndrome histamine plays an important role. The ameliorating effects of *p*-chlorophenylalanine on intestinal motility of carcinoid patients suggests a role for serotonin in its causation.[5]

The role of serotonin in platelets is completely unknown, although for years it was believed to play a role in hemostasis as the vasoconstrictor of serum. This hypothesis was put to a test when reserpine became available as a serotonin depletor.[9] Reserpine was administered to patients in sufficient dosage to reduce serotonin levels to negligible amounts. This procedure had no effect on bleeding time or clotting time, a result that casts doubt on the role of serotonin in hemostasis.

Because of the effectiveness of several serotonin antagonists in the prevention of *migraine*, a role for the amine in the causation of vascular headaches has been suggested. The evidence for this is poor.

SEROTONIN ANTAGONISTS, OR ANTISEROTONINS

Serotonin antagonists include numerous *lysergic acid derivatives*, many of which are naturally occurring ergot alkaloids. Methysergide (Sansert) is a potent antiserotonin of clinical usefulness in the prevention of vascular headaches. Other lysergic acid derivatives that are potent antiserotonins include LSD and D-2-bromolysergic acid diethylamide. Many *antihistamines* have antiserotonin effects also. Among these *cyproheptadine* (Periactin) is potent and has been discussed among the antihistamines (p. 252). *Chlorpromazine*, other *phenothiazines*, and *α-adrenergic blocking agents* such as *phenoxybenzamine* also block the effects of serotonin.

For practical purposes methysergide (Sansert) and cyproheptadine (Periactin) are the only two drugs available for antagonizing symptoms that might be attributed to serotonin clinically.

Methysergide maleate

Methysergide is closely related to the ergot alkaloid methyl-ergonovine, which is used as an oxytocic drug. It is 1-methyl-*d*-lysergic acid butanolamide and was introduced specifically as a prophylactic agent for migraine headaches. It is a potent serotonin antagonist, even more potent than ergotamine or LSD. The drug is useful only for the prevention and not for the treatment of migraine. Its mode of action is not well understood, since connections between migraine and serotonin are in the realm of speculation.

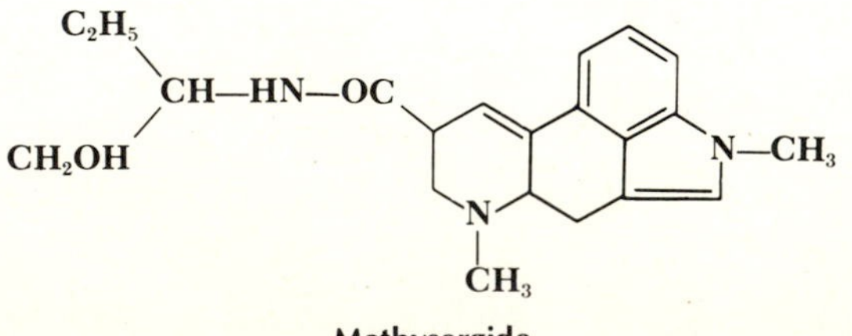

Methysergide

Adverse reactions to methysergide are many and include nausea, dizziness, insomnia, behavioral changes (reminiscent of mild LSD reactions), gastrointestinal disturbances, and others. A serious complication seen in several patients after long-term use of methysergide was retroperitoneal fibrosis and pleural pulmonary fibrosis. Retroperitoneal fibrosis may lead to urinary tract obstruction.

Contraindications to the use of methysergide are peripheral vascular disease, hypertension, peptic ulcer, coronary artery disease, and pregnancy.

Methysergide maleate (Sansert) is available in tablets containing 2 mg.

Cyproheptadine hydrochloride

Cyproheptadine hydrochloride is an antihistaminic drug that also has potent antiserotonin properties. It has been proposed for some indications that are different from those requiring the usual antihistamines. The drug is effective in the treatment of allergic rhinitis and for the relief of pruritus in a variety of skin disorders. In addition, it is claimed to be effective in promoting weight gain in children by mechanisms that are not understood.

The main untoward effect seen after the administration of cyproheptadine is drowsiness. Preparations of cyproheptadine hydrochloride (Periactin hydrochloride) include tablets, 4 mg, and syrup, 2 mg/5 ml.

Ergot alkaloids

Some of the ergot alkaloids are quite useful in treating vascular headaches, some are employed for stimulating the uterine smooth muscle, and still others have been tried as hypotensive agents. The work on LSD is an outgrowth of pharmacological studies on ergot alkaloids.

There is increasing interest in new semisynthetic ergot alkaloids such as bromocriptine, which act as dopaminergic agonists. Such drugs inhibit the release of prolactin from the pituitary gland and have been used successfully to suppress postpartum lactation and to treat galactorrhea and amenorrhea in patients with increased prolactin levels.

Historical aspects of pharmacology

It has been known for centuries that ingestion of diseased rye can cause poisoning characterized by gangrene, abortion, and sometimes convulsions. The fungus that causes this disease of rye is *Claviceps purpurea*, often called *ergot*. It contains a large variety of potent pharmacological agents referred to as the ergot alkaloids, many of which are derivatives of lysergic acid. The structural formulas of lysergic acid and ergonovine, one of the ergot alkaloids, are shown below.

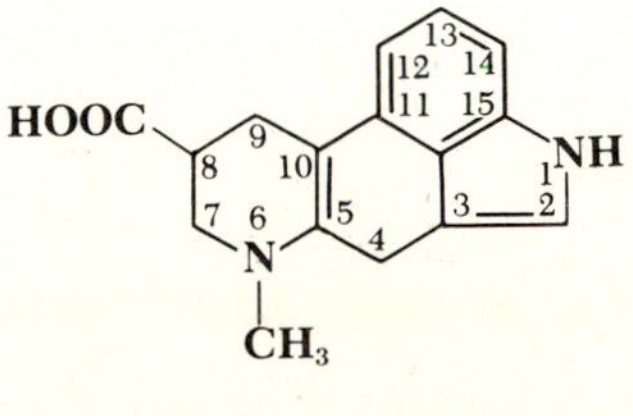

Lysergic acid 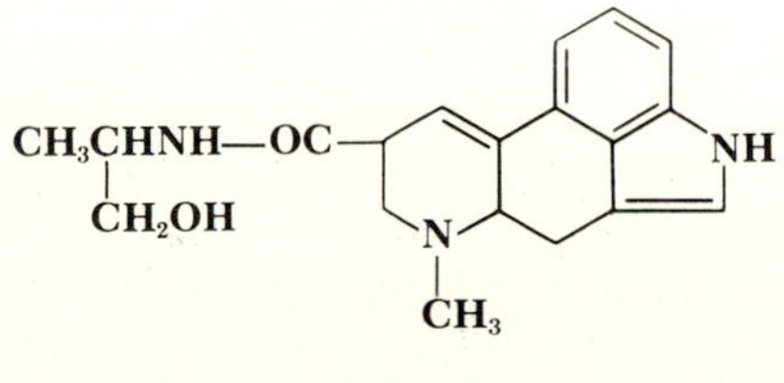   Ergonovine

The isolation of ergotamine and ergotoxine, a mixture of ergot alkaloids, led to the belief that most of the pharmacological properties of ergot resulted from these compounds. It was later shown, however, that crude ergot extracts had a greater effect on the uterus than did ergotamine or ergotoxine.[4] Soon the alkaloid ergonovine was also isolated, and this unsuspected new compound served to explain the greater activity of the crude extracts.

Chemistry   The important alkaloids of ergot are ergotamine, ergotoxine, and ergonovine. In addition, ergotoxine has been shown to be a mixture of three compounds: ergocristine, ergocryptine, and ergocornine.

From a chemical standpoint, ergonovine is the simplest compound. Its structural formula indicates that it is a combination of lysergic acid with *d*-2-aminopropranol.

In contrast to ergonovine, ergotamine and the ergotoxine group yield amino acids on hydrolysis and have a considerably higher molecular weight than ergonovine, although they also are lysergic acid derivatives.

Pharmacological effects   The ergot alkaloids have three major actions in the body: smooth muscle contraction, particularly evident on blood vessels and the uterus, adrenergic blocking effect, and CNS effects leading to hypotension. These actions are present to a varying extent in the different alkaloids. Ergonovine has powerful smooth muscle effects without the other properties characteristic of many of the other alkaloids. Ergotamine and the ergotoxine group have smooth muscle actions and can also block norepinephrine and epinephrine.

The two most commonly used ergot alkaloids in therapeutics are ergotamine (Gynergen) and ergonovine (Ergotrate). Ergotamine is extensively employed in the treatment of vascular headaches such as migraine, whereas ergonovine finds its greatest usefulness in obstetrics for its stimulant effect on the uterine smooth muscle.

Ergotamine tartrate   Ergotamine tartrate is used almost exclusively in the treatment of migraine and other vascular headaches, and its effects can be best illustrated by describing its actions when administered to a patient suffering from such headaches.

It is believed that during the early stages of the attack there is constriction of blood vessels, followed by their marked dilatation.[19] The early visual disturbances are attributed to constriction of retinal vessels, whereas the headache itself may be related to dilatation and edema of the extracranial vessels.

Ergotamine tartrate is the drug of choice in the treatment of migraine and is believed to act by vasoconstriction. The drug may be given orally or injected subcutaneously or intramuscularly. Its effectiveness in relieving a headache is considered to be of diagnostic value.

Although the drug is very effective, it is not suitable for long-continued or prophylactic use because of serious adverse effects such as severe vasoconstriction and gangrene of the extremities. For prophylaxis of migraine, methysergide (discussed previously) is commonly used, but it also has many untoward effects and contraindications.

Adverse effects. Ergotamine tartrate may cause nausea, vomiting, diarrhea, vasoconstriction, and gangrene of the extremities. Because of its adverse effects the drug is contraindicated in pregnancy and all vascular diseases.

Preparations. Ergotamine tartrate (Gynergen) is available in 1 mg tablets and solution for injection, 0.5 mg/ml. Ergotamine tartrate is also available in sublingual tablets, 2 mg, and for inhalation in Medihalers, which dispense 0.36 mg of the drug in each inhalation.

Ergonovine maleate (Ergotrate maleate) and its derivative, methylergonovine (Methergine), are used exclusively in obstetrics. They are less effective than ergotamine in migraine.

Ergonovine maleate

Ergonovine and methylergonovine are powerful oxytocics and have significant vasoconstrictor effects, but they lack the adrenergic blocking action of ergotamine. They are well absorbed from the gastrointestinal tract, whereas the larger amino acid alkaloids are only partially absorbed. They may produce hypertension.

Ergonovine and methylergonovine are used in obstetrics in the third stage of labor, principally to decrease postpartum bleeding through their powerful effect on direct contraction of the uterine smooth muscle.

Although ergonovine and methylergonovine have powerful effects on the uterus, they do not promote normal uterine contractions as does oxytocin. For this reason they should not be employed for initiation of labor.

Adverse effects. Adverse effects of ergonovine and methylergonovine include nausea, vomiting, and elevations of blood pressure.

Preparations. Ergonovine maleate (Ergotrate maleate) is available in tablets containing 0.2 mg and in solution for injection, 0.2 mg/ml. Methylergonovine maleate (Methergine) is available in tablets, 0.2 mg, and solution for injection, 0.2 mg/ml.

The dihydrogenated alkaloids of the ergotoxine group are available in sublingual tablets containing 0.167 mg each of dihydroergocornine, dihydroergocristine, and dihydroergokryptine as the mesylates. Hydergine is used in elderly patients in whom it may produce modest improvements in self-care and various symptoms commonly attributed to cerebral atherosclerosis, although without definitive evidence regarding etiology. Hydergine does not have vasoconstrictor properties and the sublingual tablets do not produce serious side effects.

Dihydroergotoxine mesylate (Hydergine)

From a pharmacological standpoint the dihydrogenated ergotoxine alkaloids are expected to produce some adrenergic blockade and an inhibitory effect on central sympathetic functions. Nevertheless, the effects of Hydergine sublingual tablets in elderly patients cannot be definitely attributed to a specific pharmacological action.

Poisoning with ergot alkaloids occasionally follows ingestion of bread prepared from ergot-contaminated rye. There were large epidemics in the past, and occasional outbreaks still occur in some parts of the world. Poisoning may also be pro-

Ergot poisoning

duced when patients take ergot alkaloids in fairly large doses over a long period of time for migraine or for the purpose of inducing abortion.

The symptoms and signs of ergot poisoning depend on whether the poisoning is acute or chronic. In chronic poisoning the clinical picture is dominated by gangrene. In acute poisoning there may be vomiting, diarrhea, headache, vertigo, paresthesia, convulsions, and gangrene of the fingers, toes, nose, or ears. The skin may be cold and cyanotic. The pulse rate may slow, but more frequently it is rapid and weak. Treatment with vasodilators such as papaverine and sympathetic nerve block has been tried, but there is no consensus on its effectiveness. The most important preventive measure is avoidance of long-continued use of ergotamine tartrate for vascular headaches.

REFERENCES

1 Aghajanian, G. K., and Wang, R. Y.: Physiology and pharmacology of central serotonergic neurons. In Lipton, M. A., Di Mascio, A., and Killam, K. F., editors: Psychopharmacology: a generation of progress, New York, 1978, Raven Press, pp. 171-183.

1a Brodie, B. B., Olin, J. S., Kuntzman, R. G., and Shore, P. A.: Possible interrelationship between release of brain norepinephrine and serotonin by reserpine, Science 125:1293, 1957.

2 Brodie, B. B., Spector, S., Kuntzman, R. G., and Shore, P. A.: Rapid biosynthesis of brain serotonin before and after reserpine administration, Naturwissenschaften 45:343, 1958.

3 Dahlstrom, A., and Fuxe, K.: Evidence for the existence of monoamine-containing neurons in the central nervous system. I. Demonstration of monoamines in the cell bodies of brain stem neurons, Acta Physiol. Scand. 62(Supp. 232): 1, 1965.

4 Dudley, H. W., and Moir, C.: Substance responsible for traditional clinical effect of ergot, Br. Med. J. 1:520, 1935.

5 Engleman, K., Lovenberg, W., and Sjoerdsma, A.: Inhibition of serotonin synthesis by parachlorophenylalanine in patients with the carcinoid syndrome, N. Engl. J. Med. 277:1103, 1967.

6 Erspamer, V.: Pharmacology of indolealkylamines, Pharmacol. Rev. 6:425, 1954.

7 Erspamer, V., subeditor: Handbook of experimental pharmacology. 5-Hydroxytryptamine and related indolealkylamines, vol. 19, New York, 1966, Springer-Verlag New York Inc.

8 Feldberg, W., and Sherwood, S. L.: Injections of drugs into the lateral ventricles of the cat, J. Physiol. (London) 123:148, 1954.

9 Haverback, B. J., Dutcher, T. F., Shore, P. A.,

Tomich, E. G., Terry, L. L., and Brodie, B. B.: Serotonin changes in platelets and brain induced by small daily doses of reserpine, N. Engl. J. Med. 256:343, 1957.

10 Kety, S. S.: Biochemical theories of schizophrenia, Science 129:1528, 1590, 1959.

11 Lauer, J. W., Inskip, W. M., Bernsohn, J., and Zeller, E. A.: Observations on schizophrenic patients after iproniazid and tryptophan, Arch. Neurol. Psychiatry 80:122, 1958.

12 Oates, J. A., Melmon, K., Sjoerdsma, A., Gillespie, L., and Mason, D.: Release of a kinin peptide in the carcinoid syndrome, Lancet 1: 514, 1964.

13 Page, I. H.: Serotonin (5-hydroxytryptamine), Physiol. Rev. 34:563, 1954.

14 Purpura, D. P., Girado, M., Smith, T. G., Callan, D. A., and Grundfest, H.: Structure-activity determinants of pharmacological effects of amino acids and related compounds on central synapses, J. Neurochem. 3:238, 1959.

15 Rapport, M. M., Green, A. A., and Page, I. H.: Serum vasoconstrictor (serotonin): isolation and characterization, J. Biol. Chem. 176:1243, 1948.

16 Salmoiraghi, G. C., Costa, E., and Bloom, F. E.: Pharmacology of central synapses, Annu. Rev. Pharmacol. 5:213, 1965.

17 Sandler, M.: The role of 5-hydroxyindoles in the carcinoid syndrome, Adv. Pharmacol. 6B: 127, 1968.

18 Toman, J. E. P.: Some aspects of central nervous pharmacology, Annu. Rev. Pharmacol. 3: 153, 1963.

19 de Whurst, W. G.: New theory of cerebral amine function and its clinical application, Nature 218:1130, 1968.

20 Wolff, H. G.: Headache and other pains, London, 1948, Oxford University Press.

CHAPTER 22

Kinins and prostaglandins

In addition to various amines that act as neurotransmitters, there are numerous polypeptides and acidic lipids that exert powerful effects on various smooth muscles and glands. Since these compounds occur normally in the body, they probably perform important regulatory functions. The *kinins* are vasodilator polypeptides; among them the plasma kinins *bradykinin* and *kallidin* are of greatest interest. The *prostaglandins* are acidic lipids widely distributed in the body and having great pharmacological activity.

A variety of polypeptides have effects somewhat similar to those of histamine on vascular smooth muscle, capillary permeability, and bronchial and intestinal smooth muscle.

KININS
General concept

Bradykinin is a biologically active nonapeptide, a product of the enzyme *kallikrein* on its α_2-globulin substrate. It is a potent agent to which many functions have been attributed, such as the regulation of the microcirculation of exocrine glands, circulatory changes occurring after birth, and mediation of inflammatory processes.

Numerous related kinins occur widely distributed in nature, such as in wasp venom and in the skin of amphibia. What makes bradykinin of special interest, however, is the ease with which it may be made and destroyed in the body. It could have great importance in physiological and pathological processes, but its exact role is not likely to be defined until specific antagonists become available.

The early studies on the kinins were carried out by two groups of investigators, one in Germany (Werle and co-workers[16]) and the other in Brazil (Rocha e Silva and co-workers[23]). Until recently the nomenclature on kinins was quite confusing because of the conflicting terms used by the various groups. The German group named their polypeptide *kallidin* and its plasma precursor *kallidinogen;* the enzyme that acted on kalidinogen was named *kallikrein.* The hypotensive substance was found in the urine and also in the pancreas, whose Greek name is *kallikreas* (although some Greeks disagree).

History and
nomenclature

Independently the Brazilian group found that when snake venoms or trypsin acted on plasma globulin, a substance was produced that caused a slow contraction of the guinea pig ileum. The term *bradykinin* (from the Greek word *bradys*, meaning "slow") was coined to designate this substance.

Bradykinin is a polypeptide composed of a chain of nine amino acids (arginine-proline-proline-glycine-phenylalanine-serine-proline-phenylalanine-arginine). Kallidin is a decapeptide that contains an additional *N*-terminal lysine residue. The precursor of the kinins is called *kininogen*, sometimes referred to as bradykininogen or kallidinogen. The precursor of active *kallikrein* is *prekallikrein*. Enzymes that release kinins in general should be called *kininogenases*. Thus kallikrein and trypsin are kininogenases. The relationships between these factors are shown below:

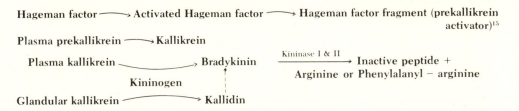

Bradykinin is split by at least two enzymes. Kininase I[7] is also known as carboxypeptidase N. Kininase II appears to be identical with the angiotensin I converting enzyme.[40] Kininase I inactivates other biologically active peptides,[32] for example, an anaphylatoxin derived from the activation of the complement system.[2] Kininase I acts mostly in blood, whereas kininase II acts in various organs such as the lung.

The actual events are much more complex than indicated in the schema. Some of the kallidin released by glandular kallikrein may be converted to bradykinin.[7,32] Kininogen may be acted on by trypsinlike proteases. There are activators in tissues that are not well characterized. Glandular tissues, such as salivary glands or pancreas and also urine, are among the richest sources of kallikrein. There are also numerous kallikrein inhibitors in tissues and in blood.

Kininogen has a role in blood clotting, and liberated plasma kallikrein activates factor XII (Hageman factor) by a positive feedback.

Kallikrein inhibitor. Aprotinin (Trasylol) is a peptide extracted from bovine lung. It inhibits kallikrein and many other proteases. It has been used clinically, particularly in Germany, in various types of shock, acute pancreatitis, and fibrinolytic states. It has not been approved for use by the Food and Drug Administration.

Roles of bradykinin. Some interesting relationships may exist between bradykinin and angiotensin (p. 217). Both are polypeptides split from plasma proteins. Angiotensin is a potent vasoconstrictor, whereas bradykinin has the opposite effect on vascular smooth muscle. The converting enzyme in the angiotensin system is a powerful inactivator of bradykinin.

Converting enzyme inhibitors are being tested at present both in treatment of hypertension and for their effect on the destruction of bradykinin. A nonapeptide (Pyr-Trp-Pro-Arg-Pro-Gln-Ile-Pro-Pro) blocks the conversion of angiotensin I to angiotensin II. It was found effective in the early phases of experimental renal hypertension if given intravenously. A newer inhibitor, captopril, is active orally.

The plasma kinins very likely play a role in inflammatory processes. They can reproduce the cardinal signs of inflammation such as vasodilatation, increased capillary permeability, and pain. Furthermore, they can be produced rather easily in the tissues following injury.

It is attractive to think of some types of inflammation as having two phases. In an early phase histamine and other mediators are released rather explosively. In a secondary phase kinins may be constantly produced and destroyed to perpetuate the inflammatory process. Interestingly, many of the kinins in fairly high concentration can cause histamine release from mast cells,[14] although their primary action in the body is probably not a consequence of histamine release.

On a molar basis the plasma kinins are the most potent vasodilators known. They also cause increased capillary permeability and pain when applied to a denuded surface such as the base of a blister or after intraperitoneal injection. Pain produced by bradykinin is increased by prostaglandins.

Pharmacological effects

Bradykinin also constricts the bronchial smooth muscle. Aspirin antagonizes the action of the peptide on guinea pig bronchi.[4] This may be a result of an interaction between aspirin and prostaglandins released by the kinin.

Other smooth muscle effects. Bradykinin constricts the uterine smooth muscle and most gastrointestinal smooth muscles. The anomalous relaxing effect on the rat duodenum may be a consequence of catecholamine release. Bradykinin can cause the release of catecholamines from the adrenal medulla,[10] histamine from mast cells,[14] and prostaglandin from the kidney.

In view of the ease with which plasma and tissue prekallikreins are activated and the availability of kininogen in the plasma, it is not surprising that numerous roles are being attributed to the kinins in health and disease. Plasma prekallikrein may be activated by the prior activation of the Hageman factor, antigen-antibody reactions, inflammation, trauma, trypsin, snake venoms, acid milieu, endotoxins, and heat. Similarly, tissue kallikreins may be activated and released by trauma, inflammation, toxins, and heat.

Clinical significance of plasma kinins

Some of the clinical conditions in which the kinins are believed to play a pathogenetic role are endotoxin shock, carcinoid syndrome (p. 257), hereditary angioneurotic edema[5] with its deficiency of a kallikrein inhibitor, anaphylaxis, arthritis (particularly gout where urate crystals activate the Hageman factor), and acute pancreatitis. In addition, bradykinin may play a role in constricting the umbilical artery and the ductus arteriosus and in the transformation of the fetal to the neonatal circulation.[18] An orthostatic syndrome, hyperbradykinemia, has recently been described.[27]

The significance of the kallikrein-bradykinin system may increase as a consequence of the observation indicating that some hypertensive patients excrete less kallikrein than normal controls.[34] This is an old observation that has been confirmed recently.

In addition to bradykinin and kallidin, there are other peptides with somewhat similar properties. *Substance P* is present in the brain and in larger amounts in the

Other hypotensive peptides

intestine.[7] *Eledoisin* is a powerful hypotensive peptide obtained from the salivary gland of the octopus.[7]

PROSTAGLANDINS

The prostaglandins, so named because they were first isolated from seminal fluid, represent a series of acidic lipids having powerful pharmacological activity. Their widespread occurrence in tissues (including those of the nervous system) suggests for these acidic compounds a regulatory function that may be exerted as a very basic control system related to adenyl cyclase. Great efforts are being made to develop this new class of agents into medically useful drugs. Preliminary indications are that they may find applications in the induction of labor, as abortifacients, and as nasal vasoconstrictors. All these uses and the many others that are being investigated must be considered as strictly experimental at present.

History and nomenclature

In 1930 two New York gynecologists reported that fresh human semen could cause contraction or relaxation of strips of human uterus. A few years later, Goldblatt in England[12] and von Euler in Sweden[8] studied the pharmacological effects of lipid extracts of seminal fluid. The name *prostaglandin* was coined by von Euler in 1935, and the structures of two were established by Sune Bergström at the Karolinska Institute. Work on the pharmacology of prostaglandins has accelerated greatly since synthetic compounds have become available.

Prostaglandins are present in greatest amounts in human and sheep seminal plasma. In various species they occur also in the uterus, lung, brain, iris, thymus, pancreas, and kidney, and they are found in human menstrual blood. It is quite likely that the numerous acidic lipids with pharmacological activity isolated over the years from various tissues are actually prostaglandins.

As shown in the schema on p. 267, the prostaglandins are analogs of *prostanoic acid*, a C_{20} acid that contains a five-membered ring. Biosynthetically they originate from arachidonic acid or dihomo-γ-linolenic acid. The four major groups of prostaglandins are designed as E, F, A, and B on the basis of their ring structure. The numeral in the subscript position indicates the degree of unsaturation in the side chains.

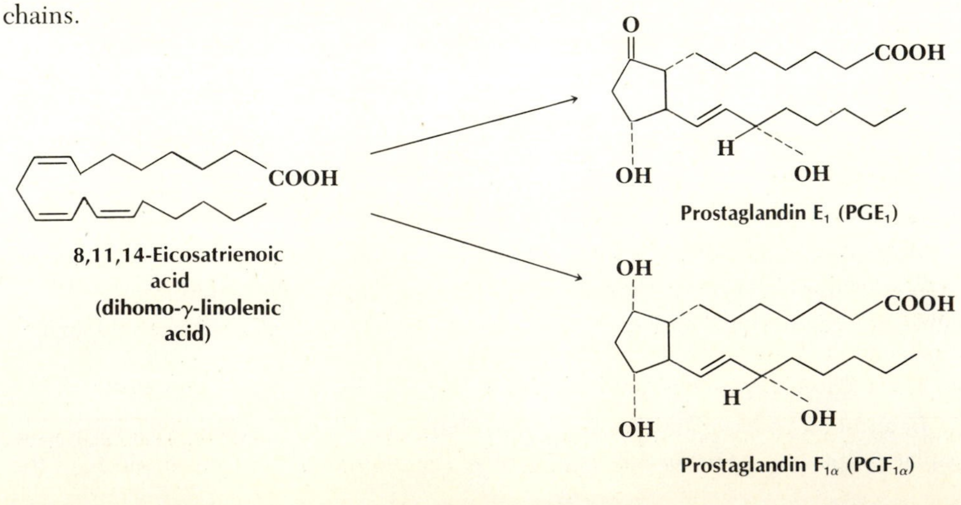

8,11,14-Eicosatrienoic acid
(dihomo-γ-linolenic acid)

Prostaglandin E_1 (PGE$_1$)

Prostaglandin $F_{1\alpha}$ (PGF$_{1\alpha}$)

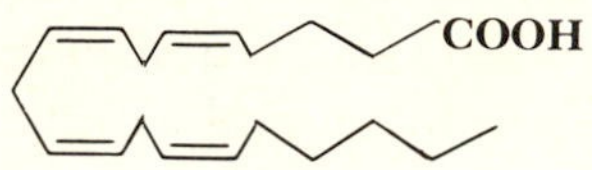

5,8,11,14-Eicosatetraenoic
acid
(arachidonic acid)

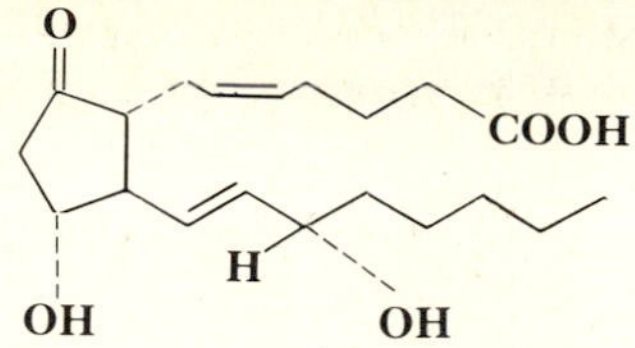

Prostaglandin E_2 (PGE$_2$)

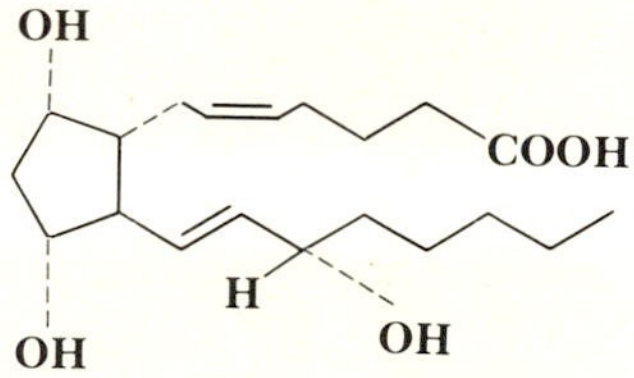

Prostaglandin $F_{2\alpha}$ (PGF$_{2\alpha}$)

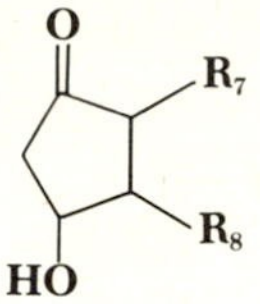

E 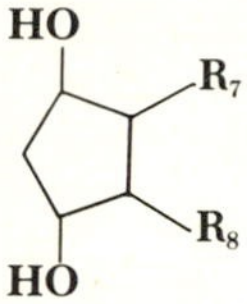   F 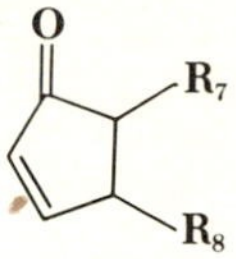   A 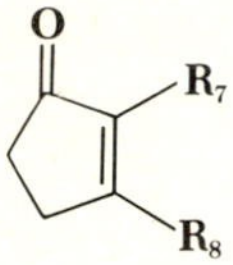   B

Biosynthesis

As shown in the formulas on p. 266 and above, prostaglandins are made from dihomo-γ-linolenic acid and arachidonic acid. These fatty acids are probably released from phospholipids by phospholipases. According to current views, arachidonic acid is first converted by the enzyme prostaglandin synthetase to the cyclic endoperoxides, of very short half-life, also known as prostaglandin G_2 or H_2. This reaction is blocked by aspirin and indomethacin:

$$\text{Arachidonic acid} \xrightarrow[\quad]{\text{Aspirin, indomethacin}} \begin{array}{l}\text{Prostaglandins } G_2, H_2 \\ \text{(cyclic endoperoxides)}\end{array}$$

From the cyclic endoperoxides, the synthetic process may follow three different paths, forming several prostaglandins, thromboxanes, and prostacyclin.

$$\text{Cyclic endoperoxides} \begin{array}{l} \longrightarrow \text{PGE}_2, \text{PGF}_{2\alpha}, \text{PGD}_2 \\ \longrightarrow \text{Thromboxane A}_2 \rightarrow \text{thromboxane B}_2 \\ \longrightarrow \text{Prostacyclin} \end{array}$$

In addition to the cyclooxygenase pathway, which yields the endoperoxides, arachidonic acid may follow a lipoxygenase pathway, which produces hydroxy acids (HETE) and leukotrienes. One of these in combination with cysteine is SRS-A, slow reacting substance of anaphylaxis, which may play an important role in bronchial asthma.

The metabolic pathways of arachidonic acid are shown on pp. 268 and 269.*

---

*From Moncada, S., and Vane, J. R.: Pharmacology of endogenous roles of prostaglandin endoperoxides, thromboxane A_2 and prostacyclin, Pharmacol. Rev. **30**:293, 1979.

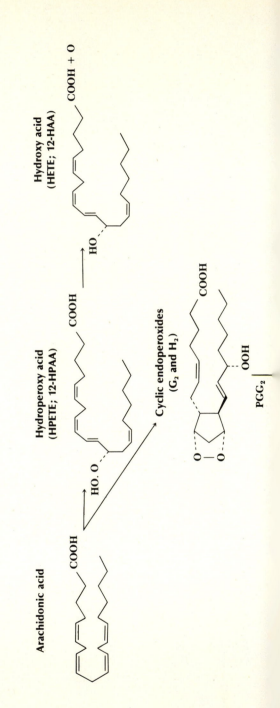

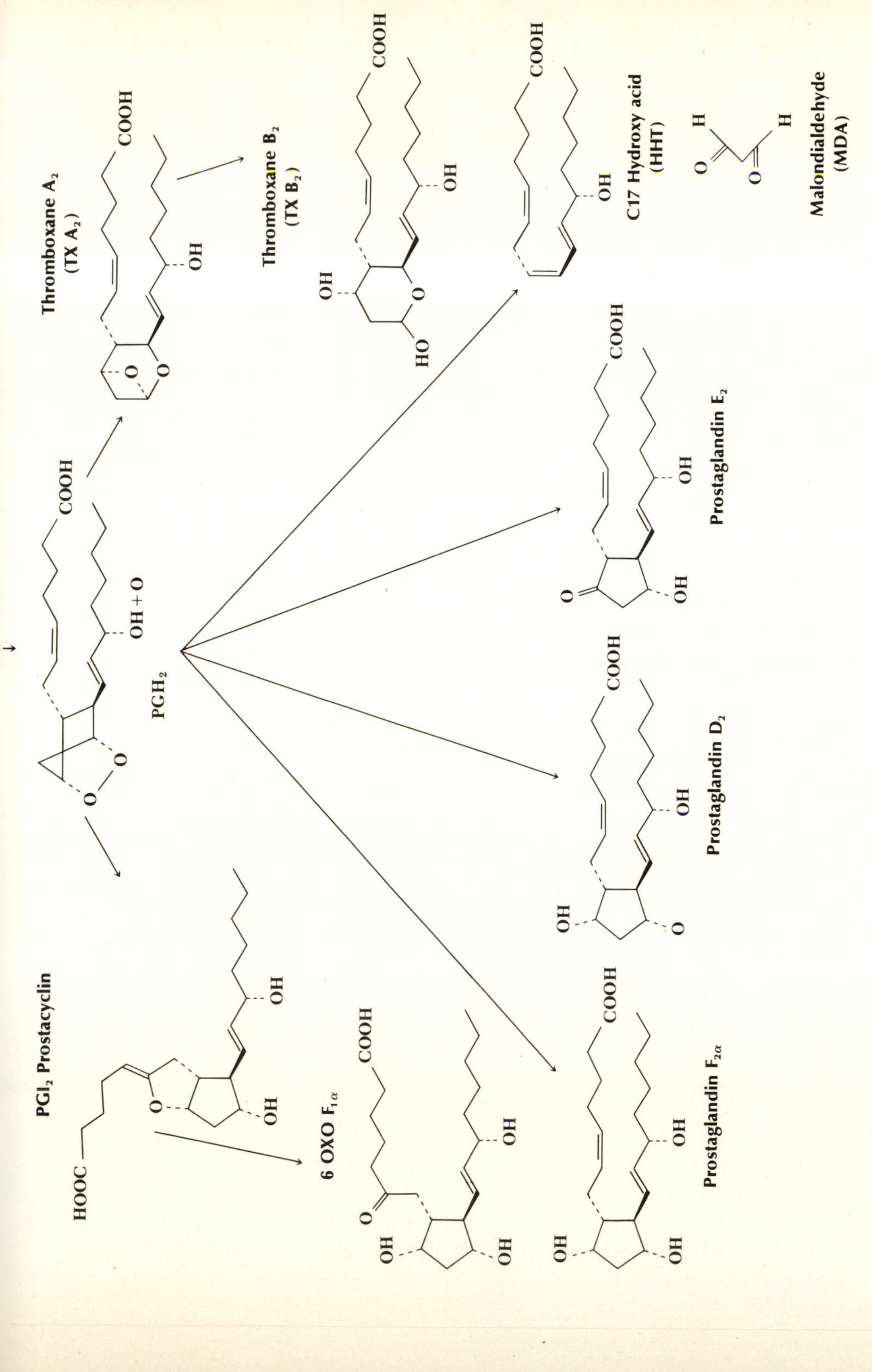
Thromboxane A₂
(TX A₂)
Thromboxane B₂
(TX B₂)
C17 Hydroxy acid
(HHT)
Malondialdehyde
(MDA)
PGH₂
OH + O
Prostaglandin E₂
Prostaglandin D₂
Prostaglandin F₂α
PGI₂ Prostacyclin
6 OXO F₁α
COOH
HOOC
OH
HO
O
H

Pharmacological effects

The mechanism of action of the prostaglandins may involve the stimulation of cyclic AMP production and calcium utilization by various cells. The synthesis of these compounds is inhibited by aspirin, indomethacin, and other nonsteroidal anti-inflammatory agents. Antagonists include the arachidonic acid analog eicosatetraynoic acid (ETYA) and polyphloretin phosphate.

The complex effects of the various prostaglandins may be summarized as follows: *cardiovascular*—PGE causes a decrease in blood pressure, PGF produces an increase in blood pressure; *kidney*—PGE but not PGF causes vasodilatation, natriuresis, diuresis, and renin release; *respiratory*—PGE is a bronchodilator, PGF is a bronchoconstrictor; *gastrointestinal*—PGE and PGF contract the smooth muscle and cause diarrhea, whereas PGE inhibits gastric secretion; *eye*—PGE and PGF cause miosis; and *reproductive system*—PGE relaxes the nonpregnant but contracts the pregnant uterus, whereas PGF contracts both the pregnant and nonpregnant uterus.

The possible role of the prostaglandins in inflammation and immune phenomena is of great interest. The intracutaneous injection of various prostaglandins has histamine-like effects.[28] In addition, it has been shown[25] that aspirin blocks the synthesis of prostaglandins by human platelets, guinea pig lungs, and some other tissues. On the basis of these findings it has been suggested[28] that the action of aspirin and perhaps other nonsteroidal anti-inflammatory drugs may be attributed to inhibition of prostaglandin synthesis.[28] The antithrombotic actions of aspirin are probably caused by this enzymatic effect.[39]

Although the prostaglandins do not produce much pain, there are reasons to believe that they may reinforce the pain-producing actions of bradykinin.

Precursors of prostaglandins, such as arachidonic acid, may have effects similar to the final product when injected. On the other hand the *endoperoxide* intermediates in the synthesis of the prostaglandins may have pharmacological effects of their own.

The thromboxanes are powerful but short-lived platelet aggregating agents. The newly discovered prostacyclin, or PGX, prevents platelet aggregation. It is postulated that the balance of these compounds, elaborated by the vascular endothelium, may play an important role in thrombosis and its prevention.

Diseases associated with excess production of prostaglandins

Various diseases may be associated with excessive prostaglandin production. The main evidence for such an association is based on the improvement that can be achieved by prostaglandin synthesis inhibitors. Some of these conditions are primary dysmenorrhea, Bartter's syndrome, threatened abortion, patent ductus arteriosus, pancreatic cholera, hypercalcemia of cancer, idiopathic orthostatic hypotension, and inflammation. The nonsteroidal anti-inflammatory drugs, such as aspirin, indomethacin, ibuprofen, and others may owe their effectiveness to prostaglandin synthesis inhibition.

Possible therapeutic applications

Dinoprost tromethamine (Prostin F_2 Alpha) was introduced as an abortifacient in the second trimester of pregnancy. Synthetic analogs are being used investigationally in the treatment of peptic ulcer, hypertension, asthma, and hypercalcemia.[31] As an abortifacient, dinoprost tromethamine is administered intraamniotically. Adverse effects caused by the drug include nausea, vomiting, hypertension, allergic reactions, bronchospasm, hypotension, syncope, and uterine lacerations.

REFERENCES

1 Bergström, S., and Samuelsson, B.: Prostaglandins, Annu. Rev. Biochem. **34:**101, 1965.
2 Bokisch, V. A., and Muller-Eberhard, H. J.: Anaphylatoxin inactivator of human plasma: its isolation and characterization as a carboxypeptidase, J. Clin. Invest. **49:**2427, 1970.
3 Coffman, J. D.: The effect of aspirin on pain and hand blood flow responses to intraarterial injection of bradykinin in man, Clin. Pharmacol. Ther. **7:**26, 1966.
4 Collier, H. O. J.: The action and antagonism of kinins on bronchioles, Ann. N.Y. Acad. Sci. **104:**290, 1963.
5 Donaldson, V. H.: Serum inhibitor of C'1-esterase in health and disease, J. Lab. Clin. Med. **68:**369, 1966.
6 Ellis, E. F., Oelz, O., Roberts, L. J., Payne, N. A., Sweetman, B. J., Nies, A. S., and Oates, J. A.: Coronary arterial smooth muscle contraction by a substance released from platelets: evidence that it is thromboxane A_2, Science **193:**1135, 1976.
7 Erdös, E. G., editor: Structure and function of biologically active peptides: bradykinin, kallidin, and congeners, Ann. N.Y. Acad. Sci. **104:**1, 1963.
8 von Euler, U. S.: Zur Kenntnis der pharmakologischen Wirkungen von Nativsekreten und Extrakten männlicher accessorischer Geschlechtdrüsen, Arch. Exp. Pathol. Pharmakol. **175:**78, 1934.
9 von Euler, U. S.: Prostaglandins, Clin. Pharmacol. Ther. **9:**228, 1968.
10 Feldberg, W., and Lewis, G. P.: The action of peptides on the adrenal medulla release of adrenaline by bradykinin and angiotensin, J. Physiol. (London) **171:**98, 1964.
11 Frey, E. K., Kraut, H., and Werle, E.: Das Kallikrein-kinin Systemund seine Inhibitoren, Stuttgart, 1968, Ferdinand Enke Verlag.
12 Goldblatt, M. W.: A depressor substance in seminal fluid, J. Soc. Chem. Ind. **52:**1056, 1933.
13 Horton, E. W.: Hypotheses on physiological roles of prostaglandins, Physiol. Rev. **49:**122, 1969.
14 Johnson, A. R., and Erdös, E. G.: Release of histamine from mast cells by vasoactive peptides, Proc. Soc. Exp. Biol. Med. **142:**1252, 1973.
15 Kaplan, A. P., and Austen, K. F.: A prealbumin activator of prekallikrein, J. Immunol. **105:**802, 1970.
16 Kraut, F., Frey, E. K., and Werle, E.: Der Nach weis eines Kreislaufhormons in der Pankreasdrüse, Z. Physiol. Chem. **189:**97, 1930.
17 Lim, R. K. S., Guzman, F., Rodgers, D. W., Goto, K., Braun, C., Dickerson, G. D., and Engle, R. J.: Site of action of narcotic and nonnarcotic analgesics determined by blocking bradykinin-evoked visceral pain, Arch. Int. Pharmacodyn. **152:**28, 1964.
18 Melmon, K. L., Cline, M. J., Hughes, T., and Nies, A. S.: Kinins: possible mediators of neonatal circulatory changes in man, J. Clin. Invest. **47:**1295, 1968.
19 Milton, A. S., and Wendlandt, S.: Effects on body temperature of prostaglandins of the A, E and F series on injection into the third ventricle of unanaesthetized cats and rabbits, J. Physiol. **218:**325, 1971.
20 Oates, J. A., Pettinger, W. A., and Doctor, R. B.: Evidence for the release of bradykinin in carcinoid syndrome, J. Clin. Invest. **45:**173, 1966.
21 Orloff, J., Handler, J. S., and Bergström, S.: Effect of prostaglandin (PGE_1) on the permeability response of toad bladder to vasopressin, theophylline and adenosine 3',5'-monophosphate, Nature **205:**397, 1965.
22 Ramwell, P. W., Shaw, J. E., Corey, E. J., and Andersen, N.: Biological activity of synthetic prostaglandins, Nature **221:**1251, 1969.
23 Rocha e Silva, M., Beraldo, W. T., and Rosenfeld, G.: Bradykinin, a hypotensive and smooth muscle stimulating factor released from plasma globulin by snake venoms and by trypsin, Am. J. Physiol. **156:**261, 1949.
24 Rowley, D. A.: Venous constriction as the cause of increased vascular permeability produced by 5-hydroxytryptamine, histamine, bradykinin, and compound 48/80 in the rat, Br. J. Exp. Pathol. **45:**56, 1964.
25 Smith, J. B., and Willis, A. L.: Aspirin selectively inhibits prostaglandin production in human platelets, Nature **231:**235, 1971.

26 Steinberg, D., Vaughan, M., Nestel, P. J., and Bergstrom, S.: Effects of prostaglandin E opposing those of catecholamines on blood pressure and on triglyceride breakdown in adipose tissue, Biochem. Pharmacol. 12:764, 1963.

27 Streeten, D. H. P., Kerr, C. B., Kerr, L. P., Prior, J. C., and Dalakos, T. G.: Hyperbradykinism: a new orthostatic syndrome, Lancet 2:1048, 1972.

28 Vane, J. R.: Inhibition of prostaglandin synthesis as a mechanism of action for aspirin-like drugs, Nature 231:232, 1971.

REVIEWS

29 Andersen, N. H., and Ramwell, P. W.: Biological aspects of prostaglandins, Arch. Intern. Med. 133:30, 1974.

30 Bonta, I. L., and Parnham, M. J.: Prostaglandins and chronic inflammation, Biochem. Pharmacol. 27:1611, 1978.

31 Clayman, C. B.: The prostaglandins, J.A.M.A. 233:904, 1975.

32 Erdös, E. G., editor: Handbook of experimental pharmacology: bradykinin, kallidin, and kallikrein, Berlin, 1970, Springer-Verlag.

33 Erdös, E. G.: Conversion of angiotensin I to angiotensin II, Am. J. Med. 60:749, 1976.

34 Karim, S. M. M.: Prostaglandins as abortifacients, N. Engl. J. Med. 285:1534, 1971.

35 Margolius, H. S., Geller, R. G., deJong, W., Pisano, J. J., and Sjoerdsma, A.: Urinary kallikrein excretion in hypertension, Circ. Res. 30:11, 1972.

36 Moncada, S., and Vane, J. R.: Pharmacology of endogenous roles of prostaglandin endoperoxides, thromboxane A_2 and prostacyclin, Pharmacol. Rev. 30:293, 1979.

37 Ramwell, P. W., and Shaw, J. E., editors: Prostaglandins, Ann. N.Y. Acad. Sci. 180:1971.

38 Schachter, M.: Kallikreins (kininogenases)—a group of serine proteases with bioregulatory actions, Pharmacol. Rev. 31:1, 1979.

39 Vane, J. K.: The mode of action of aspirin and similar compounds, J. Allergy Clin. Immunol. 58:691, 1976.

40 Yang, H. Y. T., Erdös, E. G., and Levin, Y.: A dipeptidyl carboxypeptidase that converts angiotensin I and inactivates bradykinin, Biochim. Biophys. Acta 214:374, 1970.

Psychopharmacology

CHAPTER 23

General concepts of psychopharmacology

Before the 1950s there were no effective pharmacotherapeutic agents available for the treatment of the major mental diseases. Large doses of barbiturates were used to calm agitated psychotic patients, and amphetamine was sometimes used in an attempt to combat acute depression. In the early 1950s two drugs were introduced for the management of psychotic patients. These drugs, reserpine and chlorpromazine, proved to be agents that allowed a vast improvement in the medical management of psychotic persons and also provided the investigational tools for a major breakthrough in understanding the central transmitters and neuronal circuits involved in the antipsychotic actions of the drugs, as well as, possibly, in the etiology of the disease processes. At hand now are a large number of agents useful in the specific management of schizophrenia, depression, manic-depressive psychoses, and anxiety states.

MONOAMINE BASIS OF PSYCHOPHARMACOLOGY
Antischizophrenic drugs

Reserpine, the major active substance of *Rauwolfia serpentina* and related plants, provided the earliest insights into specific brain amines associated with mental disease. It was initially found that the drug depletes stores of serotonin (5-hydroxytryptamine) in the brain as well as peripheral organs and that only psychoactive alkaloids of *Rauwolfia* shared this action. It was later discovered that the drug also depletes stores of norepinephrine and epinephrine in the brain and periphery in a similar manner. Still later, after the identification of dopamine stores in the brain, it was found that reserpine and other psychoactive analogs also depleted the brain stores of this amine. Coupled with the observation that monoamine oxidase (MAO) inhibitors interfere with the metabolism of all of these brain amines and that the MAO inhibitors also altered the behavioral effects of reserpine in animals, it seemed apparent that one or more of the amines was involved in the central actions of reserpine.[9]

The inability of the phenothiazine antipsychotic, chlorpromazine, to affect brain amine concentrations was at first an obstacle to further advances, but it was this drug that later allowed an important additional breakthrough when it was demonstrated that chlorpromazine and related drugs are blockers of dopamine receptors in various brain areas.[1] With the further elucidation of central dopaminer-

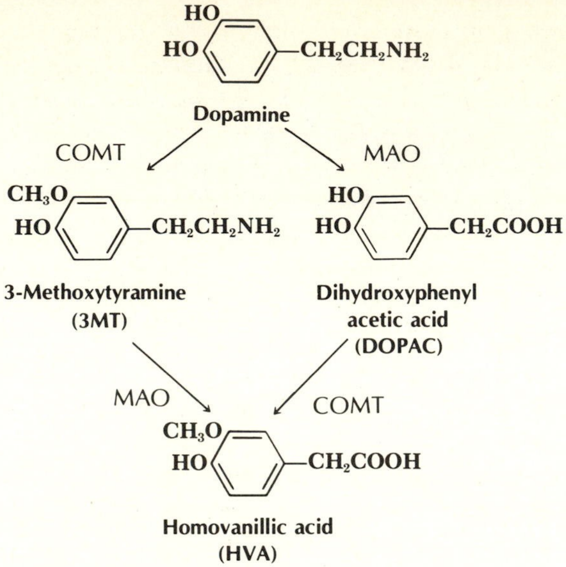

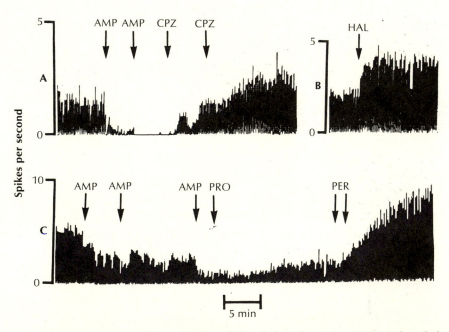

FIG. 23-1. Metabolism of dopamine in the brain.

FIG. 23-2. A, Antagonism by chlorpromazine (CPZ) of *d*-amphetamine (AMP)-induced slowing of dopaminergic cell activity in a nonanesthetized animal. AMP significantly decreased firing rate. After CPZ, cell firing resumed and increased. **B,** Effect of haloperidol on a dopaminergic cell in the nonanesthetized animal. Haloperidol increased basal activity. **C,** Effect of promethazine (PRO) on cell firing rate subsequent to *d*-amphetamine depression in an anesthetized animal. AMP markedly decreased unit activity. Promethazine failed to increase the rate usually seen with the antipsychotic phenothiazines. Perphenazine produced a rapid increase in rate to above baseline levels. (From Bunney, B. S., et al.: J. Pharmacol. Exp. Ther. **185:**560, 1973. Copyright 1973, The Williams & Wilkins Co., Baltimore.)

gic neuronal pathways, increasingly it appears that the major antipsychotic action of the phenothiazine and related drugs is by blockade of dopamine receptors in mesolimbic or mesocortical brain areas, whereas the blockade of dopamine receptors in the corpus striatum is responsible for the major central side effects of these drugs.[11]

Some of the major evidence for a role of dopamine in the therapeutic action of antischizophrenic drugs may be summarized as follows:

1. The potencies of antipsychotic drugs to stimulate dopamine turnover in general correlate well with their clinical potencies. This effect is seen in the elevation of the concentration of the dopamine metabolites, homovanillic acid (HVA) and dihydroxyphenylacetic acid in dopamine neuronal brain areas. Blockade of dopamine receptors causes a compensatory increase in the firing rate of dopamine neurons and in dopamine synthesis. The metabolic fate of dopamine in the brain is shown in Fig. 23-1.

2. Electrophysiological studies on dopamine neurons demonstrate again that there is a correlation between clinical antipsychotic potency and the ability of the drugs to alter dopamine neuronal firing rate. Some examples are given in Fig. 23-2.

3. Inhibition of tyrosine hydroxylase, the rate-limiting enzyme in the biosynthesis of catecholamines, in schizophrenic patients allows a major reduction in the dose of antipsychotic drug required to control their symptoms (Fig. 23-3).

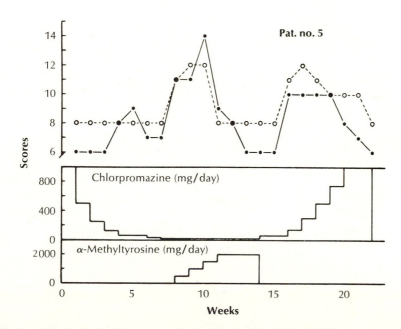

FIG. 23-3. Social behavior (solid lines) and mental symptoms (dashed lines) in a patient with chronic schizophrenia. Patient had been receiving 1000 mg of chlorpromazine daily. The patient's condition worsened when this dose was reduced but improved when α-methyltyrosine was given with a small dose of chlorpromazine. (From Carlsson, A., Persson, T., Roos, B.-E., and Walinder, J.: J. Neural Transm. **33:**83, 1972.)

4. Ligand-binding studies have shown a generally close association between clinical potency and affinity of binding of antipsychotic drugs to an apparent dopamine receptor on brain membrane fractions (Fig. 23-4).[2]

It is known that in certain neural tissues including dopaminergic brain areas there exists a dopamine-activated adenylate cyclase, which may be involved in dopamine receptor activation and coupling. This cyclase is inhibited by many antipsychotics in proportion to clinical potency. An excellent correlation appears in the case of phenothiazines, but haloperidol and other butyrophenones are relatively inactive.[3]

Recently it has been observed that antipsychotic drugs also bind to the calcium-dependent regulatory protein, calmodulin.[15] As this protein appears to be involved in adenylate cyclase activation and in phosphodiesterase activation, it may represent an appropriate target site for the action of antipsychotics. However, the correlation of binding affinity and clinical antipsychotic potency is limited.

It presently appears that there may be multiple receptors for dopamine, some linked to the adenylate cyclase and others not.[4] Such a dichotomy of receptor types may help clarify the overall interpretation of dopamine receptor–ligand-binding studies.

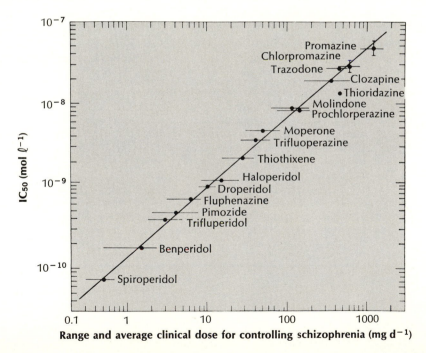

FIG. 23-4. Concentration of various antipsychotic drugs required to produce a 50% inhibition of binding of haloperidol to a preparation of caudate nucleus are plotted against the average clinical dose in humans to control schizophrenic symptoms. (From Seeman, P., Lee, T., Chau-Wong, M., and Wong, K. Reprinted by permission from *Nature* **261**:717. Copyright 1976, Macmillan Journals Ltd.)

5. Administration of drugs such as amphetamines, known to release dopamine in the brain, can exacerbate schizophrenic symptoms or, in large, repeated doses, can initiate symptoms of paranoid schizophrenia. These effects are blocked by dopamine-blocking agents such as chlorpromazine.[10]

Although this brief summary for a role of dopamine is not a complete citation, it is an impressive array of evidence. It must be pointed out, however, that these findings do not, in themselves, constitute evidence for a role of dopamine neuronal abnormality in the *etiology* of schizophrenia. Furthermore, certain newer, experimental drugs thought to be useful in schizophrenia, appear to have only subtle effects on dopamine receptors.

Of current interest are observations that certain dopamine agonists may act preferentially on dopamine neuronal presynaptic receptors to inhibit neuronal activity. It has been reported that low doses of the dopamine receptor agonist, apomorphine, lessen the symptoms of schizophrenia.[12] The possible development of more specific presynaptic dopamine agonists will be awaited with interest.

Endogenous psychotogenic substances

Based on the fact that ingestion of certain chemicals can result in abnormal mental function, for a number of years there have been suggestions that there might exist an endogenous substance capable of causing psychosis. The evidence for most such suggestions has proven inconclusive. A recent candidate for such a substance is phenylethylamine.[8] Small quantities have been reported in the brain, and injection can lead to amphetamine-like effects. It has been reported that higher than normal amounts are excreted in the urine of paranoid schizophrenics.[7] Interestingly, there is evidence that injected phenylethylamine may act through a dopaminergic mechanism.[13]

Antidepressant drugs

Basic and clinical investigations have led to the development of drugs useful in the treatment of depression and to increased understanding of their basic actions. The first of these drugs, MAO inhibitors, were tried because they altered the unusual central depressant effects seen in animals given reserpine and because of an unusual stimulant effect seen in humans. The MAO inhibitors are thought to act through enhancement of free monoamines in central neuronal systems. These drugs have largely been replaced in clinical practice by the safer and more effective tricyclic antidepressants such as imipramine. Although the latter drugs are not MAO inhibitors, they inhibit the norepinephrine reuptake mechanism in adrenergic neurons. Serotonin uptake is also inhibited. Interestingly, the tricyclics have little effect on the dopamine uptake system in dopamine neurons.

It is currently thought that although uptake inhibition may be involved in the action of tricyclic antidepressants, this alone cannot explain their effects, since uptake inhibition occurs rapidly yet there is a delay of about 2 weeks for a clinical antidepressant effect. Recently it has been shown that with chronic administration of these drugs there occurs slowly developing changes in the sensitivity of central adrenergic receptors, presynaptic[5] and postsynaptic[14] or of serotonin receptors.[6]

Chronic, but not acute, administration as well as electroconvulsive treatment, causes a decrease in the sensitivity of norepinephrine-stimulated adenylate cyclase in the brain.[14]

The actions and current view of the mechanisms of action of lithium and the antianxiety drugs are discussed in subsequent chapters.

REFERENCES

1 Carlsson, A., and Lindqvist, M.: Effects of chlorpromazine or haloperidol on formation of 3-methoxytyramine and normetanephrine in mouse brain, Acta Pharmacol. Toxicol. **20**:140, 1963.

2 Creese, I., Burt, D. R., and Snyder, S. H.: Dopamine receptor binding predicts clinical and pharmacological potencies of antischizophrenic drugs, Science **192**:481, 1976.

3 Iversen, L. L.: Dopamine receptors in the brain, Science **188**:1084, 1975.

4 Kehabian, J. M., and Calne, D. B.: Multiple receptors for dopamine, Nature **277**:93, 1979.

5 McMillen, B. A., Warnack, W., German, D. C., and Shore, P. A.: Effects of chronic desipramine treatment on rat brain noradrenergic responses to α-adrenergic drugs, Eur. J. Pharmacol. **61**:239, 1980.

6 Montigny, C. de, and Aghajanian, G. K.: Tricyclic antidepressants: long-term treatment increases responsivity of rat forebrain neurons to serotonin, Science **202**:1303, 1978.

7 Potkin, S. G., Karoum, F., Chuang, L.-W., Cannon-Spoor, H. E., Phillips, I., and Wyatt, R. J.: Phenylethylamine in paranoid chronic schizophrenia, Science **206**:471, 1979.

8 Sabelli, H. C., Borison, R. L., Diamond, B. I., Havdala, H. S., and Narasimhachari, N.: Phenylethylamine and brain function, Biochem. Pharmacol. **27**:1707, 1978.

9 Shore, P. A.: Release of serotonin and catecholamines by drugs, Pharmacol. Rev. **14**:531, 1962.

10 Snyder, S. H., Banerjee, S. P., Yamamura, H. I., and Greenberg, D.: Drugs, transmitters, and schizophrenia, Science **184**:1243, 1974.

11 Stevens, J. R.: An anatomy of schizophrenia, Arch. Gen. Psychiatry **29**:177, 1973.

12 Tamminga, C. A., Schaeffer, M. H., Smith, R. C., and Davis, J. M.: Schizophrenic symptoms improve with apomorphine, Science **200**:567, 1978.

13 Tinklenberg, J. R., Gillen, J. C., Murphy, G. M., Staub, R., and Wyatt, R. J.: Phenylethylamine in rhesus monkeys: interactions with α-methyl-p-tyrosine and L-dopa, Am. J. Psychiatry **136**:311, 1979.

14 Vetulani, J., and Sulser, F.: Action of various antidepressant treatments reduces reactivity of noradrenergic cyclic AMP generating system in limbic forebrain, Nature **257**:495, 1975.

15 Weiss, B., and Levin, R. M.: Mechanism for selectively inhibiting the activation of cyclic nucleotide phosphodiesterase and adenylate cyclase by antipsychotic agents, Adv. Cyclic Nucleotide Res. **9**:285, 1978.

REVIEW

16 Carlsson, A.: Does dopamine have a role in schizophrenia? Biol. Psychiatry **13**:3, 1978.

CHAPTER 24

Antipsychotic and antianxiety drugs

Antipsychotic and antianxiety drugs are the newer terms for major and minor tranquilizers, respectively. The antipsychotic drugs, represented by the *phenothiazines*, *thioxanthenes*, and *butyrophenones*, produce a specific improvement in the mood and behavior of psychotic patients without excessive sedation and without causing addiction.

The antianxiety drugs include the *benzodiazepines*, *meprobamate*, and related drugs. The antianxiety drugs may not be basically different from the sedative-hypnotics except for some characteristics of the benzodiazepines that probably account for their great popularity and overuse. They are less likely to produce tolerance and physical dependence, and they are much safer than the sedative-hypnotics when taken in suicidal overdoses.

DEVELOPMENT

The field of tranquilizing agents was opened up by the almost simultaneous introduction of two powerful drugs, chlorpromazine and reserpine. Chlorpromazine originated in France as a result of studies on those antihistaminics having a phenothiazine structure, such as promethazine. Preparations of *Rauwolfia serpentina* have been used in India for centuries for the treatment of various illnesses. Reserpine, one of its alkaloids, was isolated in 1952.

A key feature of the central effects of reserpine is depletion of the stores of the brain monoamines—serotonin, norepinephrine, and dopamine—whereas the phenothiazines and similarly acting drugs are blockers of dopamine receptors.

It was soon found that even at subhypnotic levels these drugs exert striking calming effects on the behavior of wild animals and disturbed patients. The knowledge that these drugs could influence spontaneous and learned behavior in animals led to the development of extensive screening procedures for new drugs of a tranquilizing type. This activity produced not only a variety of phenothiazine derivatives and reserpine-like compounds but also many antianxiety drugs such as meprobamate, chlordiazepoxide, and diazepam. The list of these drugs is still growing.

ANTIPSYCHOTIC DRUGS

The development of the current antipsychotic drugs is an outgrowth of research on antihistamines. The prototype of the phenothiazine drugs, chlorpromazine, was developed as an antihistamine related to promethazine (Phenergan). Once the unusually beneficial effect of the drug in psychotic patients was recognized, a large number of related compounds were introduced. As a group, these drugs are characterized by their calming effect on psychotic persons without excessive sedation, by their extrapyramidal effects, and by their unusual property of not inducing dependence. Most of these drugs have indications also as antiemetics, and some are used as antipruritics.

From a chemical standpoint the antipsychotic drugs comprise the *phenothiazines*, *thioxanthenes*, and *butyrophenones*. The properties of these drugs are so similar that emphasis in this discussion will be placed primarily on the phenothiazines. Reserpine was at one time used as a "major tranquilizer" but has been essentially abandoned in psychiatric practice. Its use as an antihypertensive is discussed in Chapter 18.

The term *neuroleptic* is often used as a synonym for antipsychotic. A neuroleptic is a drug that causes psychomotor slowing, emotional quieting, and, in higher doses, psychic indifference to the environment. It may or may not have a sedative effect and is not a hypnotic. The term is currently synonymous with antipsychotic because all antischizophrenic drugs used at the present time are neuroleptics. It is conceivable that at some time drugs will be developed that control the symptoms of schizophrenia but that are not frank neuroleptics.

Phenothiazine derivatives   Numerous phenothiazine derivatives are in current use. They resemble chlorpromazine in action but differ from it in potency, clinical indications, and toxicity.

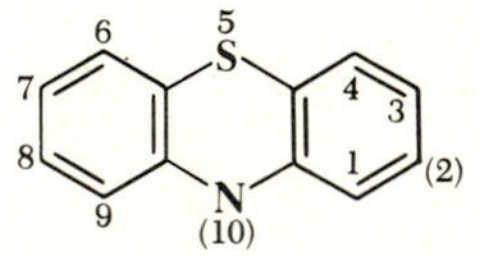

Phenothiazine nucleus

The pharmacological effects of the phenothiazine tranquilizers are quite complex. In addition to their behavioral effects, these drugs are potent antiemetics and have important actions on the autonomic nervous system at various levels. In large doses they also produce significant toxic side effects such as parkinsonism.

The phenothiazines are classified on the basis of their chemistry and pharmacology into three groups (p. 283). The differences result mainly from substitutions on the nitrogen in the phenothiazine ring. Among the numerous *piperazines* some of the most widely used are prochlorperazine (Compazine), trifluoperazine (Stelazine), perphenazine (Trilafon), fluphenazine (Prolixin; Permitil), and thiopropazate (Dartal). The *aliphatic* compounds include chlorpromazine (Thorazine), promazine (Sparine), and triflupromazine (Vesprin). The *piperidines* are represented by mesoridazine (Serentil) and thioridazine (Mellaril).

The *thioxanthene* group of antipsychotic drugs resembles in all respects the phenothiazines. The thioxanthenes include chlorprothixene (Taractan) and thio-

	Substitution in (2)	Substitution in (10)	Average oral dose (mg)
		Piperazine	
Prochlorperazine (Compazine)	Cl	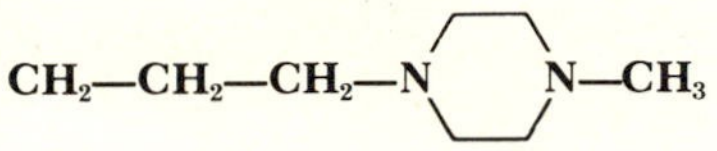 CH_2—CH_2—CH_2—N⟨ ⟩N—CH_3	5-10
Trifluoperazine (Stelazine)	CF_3	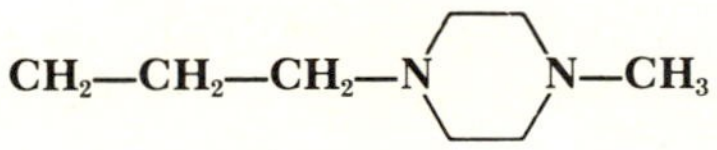 CH_2—CH_2—CH_2—N⟨ ⟩N—CH_3	2-10
Perphenazine (Trilafon)	Cl	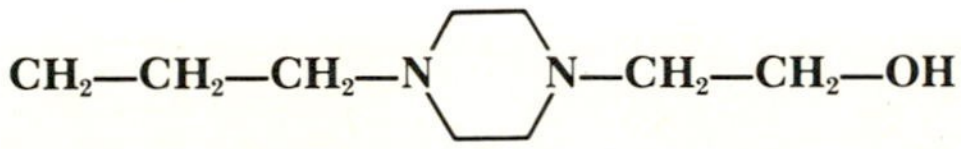 CH_2—CH_2—CH_2—N⟨ ⟩N—CH_2—CH_2—OH	4-8
Fluphenazine (Prolixin; Permitil)	CF_3	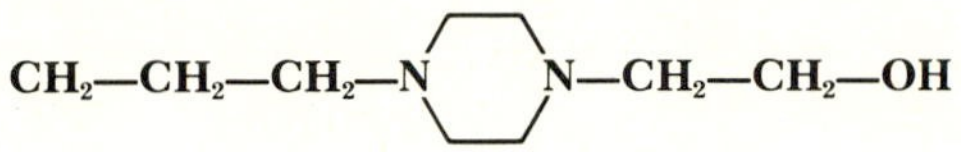 CH_2—CH_2—CH_2—N⟨ ⟩N—CH_2—CH_2—OH	0.25-0.5
Thiopropazate (Dartal)	Cl	CH_2—CH_2—CH_2—N⟨ ⟩N—CH_2—CH_2—O$\overset{\displaystyle O}{\overset{\|}{C}}$—$CH_3$	10
		Aliphatic	
Chlorpromazine (Thorazine)	Cl	CH_2—CH_2—CH_2—N—$(CH_3)_2$	25-50
Promazine (Sparine)	—	CH_2—CH_2—CH_2—N—$(CH_3)_2$	25-50
Triflupromazine (Vesprin)	CF_3	CH_2—CH_2—CH_2—N—$(CH_3)_2$	10-25
		Piperidine	
Mesoridazine (Serentil)	$\overset{\displaystyle SCH_3}{\underset{O}{\|}}$	CH_2—CH_2—⟨N—CH_3⟩	50-200
Thioridazine (Mellaril)	SCH_3	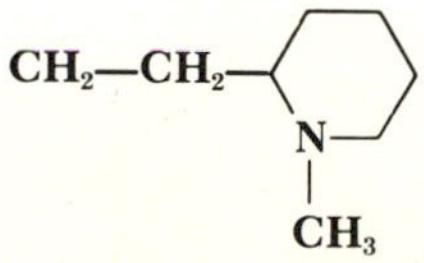 CH_2—CH_2—⟨N—CH_3⟩	25-100

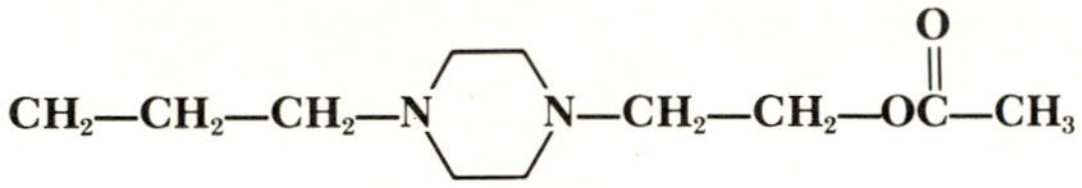

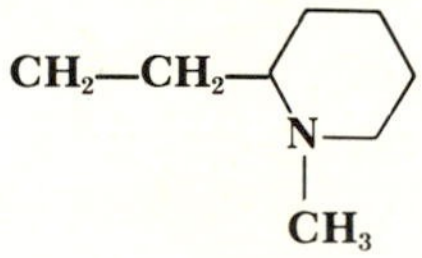

thixene (Navane). The *butyrophenone* haloperidol (Haldol) is also very similar pharmacologically to the phenothiazines.

Major differences among derivatives. The various phenothiazines differ from the standpoint of their potency, extrapyramidal effects, and sedative effects. The piperazines are more potent than other phenothiazines, cause significant extrapyramidal effects, and are not very sedative. The piperidines are least potent, cause fewer extrapyramidal effects, and produce sedation. The aliphatic compounds are between the piperazines and the piperidines as regards these properties.

Since the extrapyramidal effects may be antagonized by the anticholinergic drugs, it is possible that differences in causing extrapyramidal side effects reflect intrinsic anticholinergic potency of some of the phenothiazines.

Chlorpromazine will be discussed as the prototype of the phenothiazine drugs.

Chlorpromazine

Chlorpromazine (Thorazine), an aliphatic or dimethylaminopropyl phenothiazine, is a sedative antipsychotic drug. In addition to its usefulness in agitated psychotic persons, the drug has other medical applications such as prevention of nausea and vomiting. It is used also for its ability to potentiate the actions of other drugs such as anesthetics.

The structural formulas of chlorpromazine (Thorazine) and the antihistaminic drug promethazine (Phenergan) are as follows:

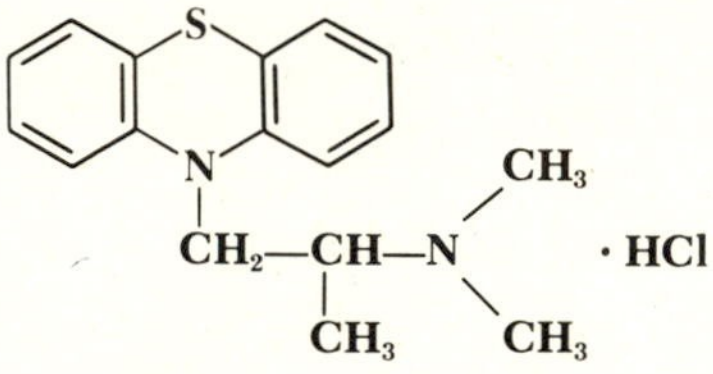

Promethazine hydrochloride

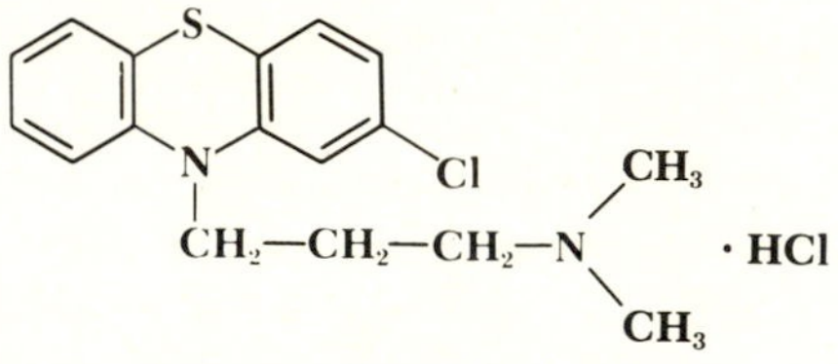

Chlorpromazine hydrochloride

Pharmacological effects. The pharmacological effects of chlorpromazine and other phenothiazines are antipsychotic, abnormal movements, anticholinergic and antiadrenergic, interference with temperature regulation, antiemetic,and endocrine.

Antipsychotic effects. The phenothiazines produce emotional quieting, psychomotor slowing, and affective indifference. They tend to decrease paranoid ideation, anxiety, delusions, and agitation, thus being very useful in the treatment of schizophrenia.[37] In normal subjects the phenothiazines produce dysphoria and impairment of intellectual functions.

Abnormal involuntary movements. The phenothiazines can produce tremors, dystonias, dyskinesias, parkinsonism, akathisias, and tardive dyskinesias. These disorders are reversible except for tardive dyskinesia. The extrapyramidal symptoms are generally related to dopamine receptor blockade and increased cholinergic predominance. Many of these side effects may be controlled by anticholinergic medications, such as benztropine (Cogentin) or diphenhydramine (Benadryl).

Tardive dyskinesia is increasingly recognized as a major medical problem in long-term use of antipsychotics. It has been estimated that up to 50% of the patients receiving such drugs for 1 year or more develop some form of this syndrome, which is most often seen as grossly abnormal orofacial movements, although other body areas may be involved. Unfortunately, there is no generally effective treatment of this syndrome at the present time, and it may be irreversible.

Unlike the situation with other neuroleptic-induced extrapyramidal symptoms, the anticholinergic drugs are of no benefit in tardive dyskinesia. It is of interest that the neuroleptics, which cause the syndrome, also tend to suppress its clinical signs.

Anticholinergic and antiadrenergic effects. Chlorpromazine has some atropine-like effects that manifest themselves by such symptoms as dry mouth, constipation, urinary retention, and paralysis of accommodation. On the other hand dilatation of the pupil and tachycardia are not usually caused by the phenothiazines.

Chlorpromazine can produce postural hypotension that has generally been attributed to an α-adrenergic blocking action of the drug. It appears, however, that the mechanism of this hypotensive action may be explained by an exaggeration of β-adrenergic vasodilatation, since chlorpromazine does not block the pressor action of norepinephrine. Marked hypotension may occur following the parenteral administration of the phenothiazines.

Temperature regulation. Although chlorpromazine is not an effective antipyretic, it does cause some lowering of body temperature and it prevents shivering. It is used sometimes when it is desirable to produce hypothermia, such as in hypothermic anesthesia.

Antiemetic effects. Chlorpromazine blocks the emetic effect of apomorphine, which is exerted primarily on the chemoreceptor trigger zone. The phenothiazines in general are more effective in preventing vomiting caused by chemical agents than against motion sickness. In the latter condition the atropine-like drugs and the antihistaminics are more commonly used.

Endocrine effects. Chlorpromazine may cause galactorrhea, delayed menstruation, amenorrhea, and weight gain. It is generally believed that these actions of the phenothiazine are exerted on the hypothalamus.

Adverse effects and drug interactions. In addition to the extrapyramidal effects, chlorpromazine may cause numerous adverse reactions such as blood dyscrasias, cholestatic jaundice, increased responsiveness to barbiturates and other hypnotics, postural hypotension, electrocardiographic changes, skin reactions and photosensitivity, skin pigmentation, deposition of pigments in the cornea and lens, and the toxic consequences of its anticholinergic effect.

Drug interactions include aggravation of the effects of alcohol, hypnotics, morphine-like analgesics, anesthetics, and antihypertensive and anticholinergic drugs.

Pharmacokinetics. Chlorpromazine, the prototype phenothiazine, is absorbed somewhat erratically when given by mouth. Peak plasma levels occur in 2 to 4 hours, a plateau is maintained for several hours, and predose levels occur in 12 hours. Plasma half-lives are extremely variable, averaging 9 hours.

The distribution of chlorpromazine in various tissues is quite uneven.[37] The brain contains about four times as much as the plasma. Elimination takes place through the kidney and bile. The drug is excreted also in the milk. Chlorpromazine has numerous metabolites. The glucuronides and sulfoxides are excreted in the urine, and the demethylated, nonpolar metabolites enter the bile and may undergo reabsorption, excretion in the feces, or storage in the tissues.

Clinical uses. Chlorpromazine is used for many purposes, but the most common uses are based on the tranquilizing and antiemetic properties.

Chlorpromazine and other antipsychotics are effective in controlling the fundamental symptoms of schizophrenia, such as disturbances of affective responses and autism, as well as the secondary symptoms such as delusions and hallucinations. Agitated patients may be calmed and made more receptive to psychotherapy. The drugs also find use in the treatment of toxic psychosis.

Chlorpromazine and other phenothiazines are also useful as antiemetics, particularly in controlling nausea and vomiting by agents acting on the chemoreceptor trigger zone. The drugs are effective against emesis caused by narcotics and anesthetics, radiation sickness, and uremia. The drugs are not effective against nausea produced by digitalis, veratrum alkaloids, or motion sickness. In this case, the antihistaminic and anticholinergic drugs are more effective. The non-antipsychotic phenothiazine, promethazine, is also effective in treatment of motion sickness.

Antihistaminic activity   Some of the phenothiazines with powerful antihistaminic activity are widely used and are effective in the relief of itching of various skin diseases. **Promethazine hydrochloride** is a powerful antihistaminic having a phenothiazine structure. **Trimeprazine tartrate** (Temaril) is related structurally to promazine. **Methdilazine** (Tacaryl) is another antihistaminic phenothiazine commonly used as an antipruritic. In general, these antihistaminic phenothiazines can cause drowsiness and all the toxic effects described previously. All precautions applicable to the other phenothiazines should be observed in their use.

Preparations   The phenothiazines, as well as the thioxanthenes and butyrophenones, are available in a variety of dosage forms such as tablets, capsules, syrups, elixirs, injectables, and rectal suppositories. Fluphenazine, as the decanoate or enanthate ester, may be used for extended duration of action after intramuscular or subcutaneous injection.

Thioxanthene derivatives   The thioxanthene derivatives **chlorprothixene** (Taractan) and **thiothixene** (Navane) are similar chemically and pharmacologically to the phenothiazine derivatives. In the thioxanthene drugs a carbon is substituted for the nitrogen that is present in the central ring of the phenothiazines.

Thiothixene is considerably more potent than chlorprothixene. It may be noted that the side chain on the carbon atom, which replaces the nitrogen of the phenothiazines, influences the activity in a similar way. Thiothixene has a piperazine side chain, whereas chlorprothixene is an alkylamine thioxanthene.

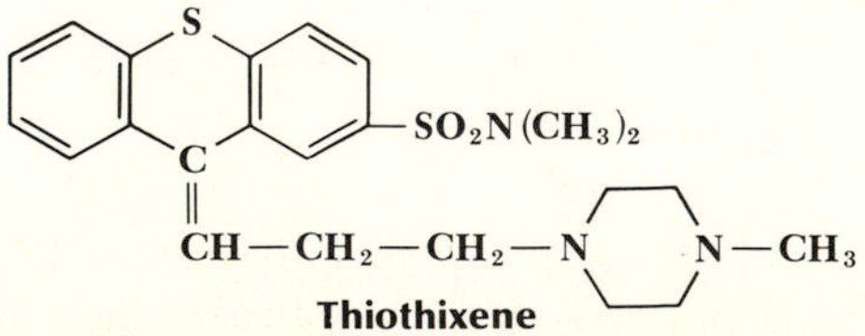

Thiothixene

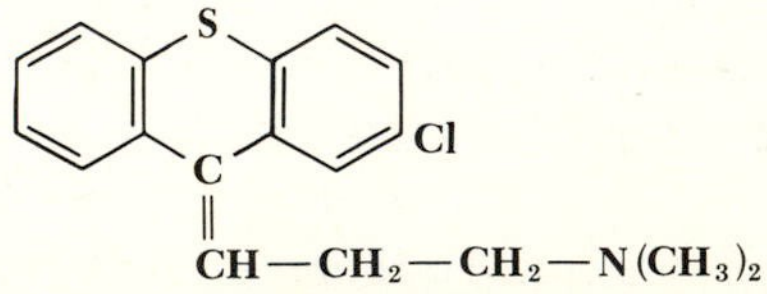

Chlorprothixene

Chlorprothixene (Taractan) is effective in psychotic conditions in which agitation and anxiety are prominent symptoms. The drug is available in tablets of 10, 25, 50, and 100 mg and in solutions for injection containing 12.5 mg/ml.

Thiothixene (Navane) is useful in the treatment of chronic schizophrenic patients who are apathetic. The drug is available in capsules containing 1, 2, 5, and 10 mg.

Butyrophenones

A series of substituted butyrophenones synthesized in Belgium since 1956 have been used increasingly as major tranquilizers, particularly in psychiatry and anesthesiology. **Haloperidol** (Haldol), the prototype of this series, has the following structure:

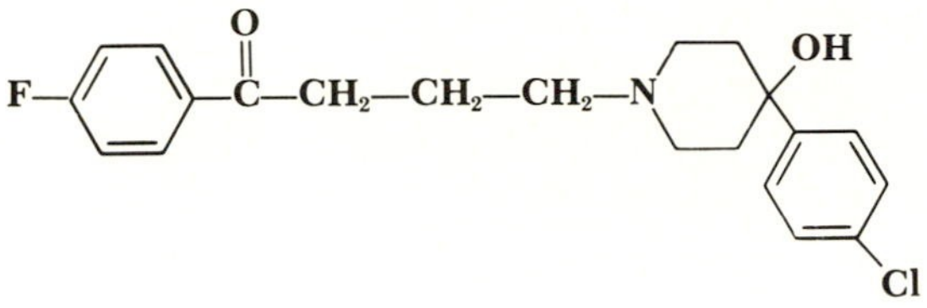

Haloperidol

Haloperidol is a potent antipsychotic and antiemetic. Although there is no obvious chemical resemblance, pharmacologically the drug resembles the piperazine phenothiazines, thus causing frequent extrapyramidal reactions.

Many other butyrophenone-type drugs are currently being tested or are in use in other countries. It is likely that some of these will be introduced in the United States.

The tranquilizing butyrophenones are also used in anesthesiology in combination with some potent narcotic analgesic. The substituted butyrophenone droperidol, in combination with a meperidine-like analgesic (fentanyl), has been introduced recently for so-called neuroleptanalgesia. The combination is available under the trade name Innovar.

Other antipsychotic drugs

Two recently introduced drugs are **loxapine** (Loxitane) and **molindone** (Lidone). In general, the pharmacology of these drugs resembles that of the other antipsychotic drugs. Thus, they have antischizophrenic and antiemetic actions and cause extrapyramidal effects. At present it is difficult to define their role in therapeutics.

Choosing antipsychotic drugs

In a number of clinical trials it has been concluded that although the many antipsychotic drugs differ greatly in their potencies, side effects, and duration of action, there is little or no difference in efficacy when the drugs are used at optimal dosage regimens. Thus it is generally accepted that the best medical practice is to become familiar with a few of the drugs representative of the various types rather than to use a great number of drugs.

Lithium carbonate in manic psychosis

Lithium carbonate, a simple inorganic compound, shows effectiveness in the treatment of the manic phases of manic-depressive psychosis. In 1949 Cade[3] of

Australia instituted the study of its effect on pyschotic behavior following the observation that lithium carbonate caused lethargy in guinea pigs.

Patients in acute manic phases usually require doses as high as 600 mg three times a day, which should produce a serum lithium level of 0.5 to 1.5 mEq/L. As soon as a good response is achieved, the dosage should be reduced to 300 mg three times a day. Serum lithium levels should be monitored and should not be allowed to exceed 2 mEq/L. Diarrhea, vomiting, drowsiness, and ataxia are among the early signs of lithium intoxication. Thyroid involvement may occur. Lithium is distributed in the total body water. Its renal clearance is proportional to its concentration in plasma. By interfering with sodium reabsorption, lithium may promote sodium depletion.[24,25]

The dose-related adverse effects of lithium carbonate administration may progress from *mild* symptoms such as nausea, vomiting, diarrhea, and muscle fasciculations to *moderately severe* symptoms that include hyperactive reflexes, epileptiform convulsions, and somnolence, leading finally to peripheral circulatory collapse, generalized convulsions, coma, and death. The very severe reactions are associated with serum lithium levels of 2.5 mEq/L or more.

The mechanism of action of lithium carbonate in manic psychosis is not understood. Since there are many similarities in the biological actions of sodium and lithium and since sodium is required for catecholamine uptake by the amine pump, current research is focusing on the possible effect of lithium on catecholamine uptake. Lithium appears to accelerate the uptake of norepinephrine by isolated nerve-ending particles (synaptosomes).[30]

Lithium carbonate is available in capsules (Eskalith; Lithonate) and in tablets (Lithane), all containing 300 mg of the drug.

ANTIANXIETY DRUGS   In contrast with the antipsychotic drugs, a group of compounds termed *antianxiety agents* are commonly prescribed, sometimes unnecessarily, for nervousness and tension in normal or neurotic individuals. These drugs are sometimes referred to as "minor tranquilizers," a term that should be abandoned because it implies a similarity to the antipsychotic drugs, or "major tranquilizers." The majority of the antianxiety drugs have sedative and even hypnotic effects and are centrally acting skeletal muscle relaxants; they do not produce extrapyramidal side effects or interfere with autonomic nervous system functions. On the other hand, and in contrast to the phenothiazines, they produce physical dependence.

The major group of antianxiety drugs, benzodiazepines and drugs related to meprobamate, includes chlordiazepoxide hydrochloride (Librium), diazepam (Valium), oxazepam (Serax), meprobamate (Equanil; Miltown), oxanamide (Quiactin), phenaglycodol (Ultran), mephenoxalone (Trepidone), hydroxyphenamate (Listica), and tybamate (Solacen; Tybatran).

A miscellaneous group of drugs includes certain antihistaminic and anticholinergic drugs and others that are difficult to classify. Hydroxyzine (Atarax; Vistaril) and buclizine (Softran) are antihistaminic and anticholinergic agents, and benactyzine (Suavitil) is an anticholinergic drug.

The benzodiazepines, **chlordiazepoxide hydrochloride** (Librium), **diazepam** (Valium), and **oxazepam** (Serax), are widely used antianxiety drugs having central skeletal muscle–relaxing properties. The related drug **flurazepam** (Dalmane) is used as a hypnotic. Their pharmacology is basically similar to that of the barbiturate hypnotics except that in some tests they can achieve effects without excessive sedation or ataxia. Thus they have a taming effect on monkeys and other animals in doses that are not incapacitating, and behavioral studies in animals indicate that these drugs have a greater margin between the dosage needed for altering behavior and the one that is generally depressant. The benzodiazepines prevent convulsions caused by strychnine or pentylenetetrazole. In this respect they are similar to the barbiturates and are quite different from the phenothiazines or reserpine, which are not anticonvulsants. They have no significant extrapyramidal or autonomic side effects.

Recently introduced benzodiazepines include **lorazepam** (Ativan) and **clonazepam** (Clonopin). The latter drug is promoted for its anticonvulsant actions.

The great popularity of the benzodiazepines is probably dependent on two differences between them and the barbiturates.[27] They are not as likely to produce tolerance and physical dependence, and they are remarkably safe when taken in large suicidal doses.[32]

Adverse effects produced by the benzodiazepines include drowsiness, ataxia, syncope, paradoxic excitement, rash, nausea, and altered libido.[13] Benzodiazepines such as diazepam should be used with caution in patients who are taking concomitantly such drugs as barbiturates, alcohol, antihypertensive drugs, anticonvulsants, opiates, or other drugs that depress the central nervous system.[8]

The drugs are psychologically addictive, leading to overuse. This can lead to a definite physical dependence, which may be manifested by convulsions following abrupt withdrawal from chronic usage at the higher doses.

The half-life of chlordiazepoxide in the body is of the order of 24 hours. Diazepam is also a long-acting drug, and one of its major metabolic products is oxazepam.

Preparations. Chlordiazepoxide (Libritabs) is available in tablets containing 5, 10, and 25 mg. Preparations of chlordiazepoxide hydrochloride (Librium) include capsules of 5, 10, and 25 mg and power for injection, 100 mg. Preparations of diazepam (Valium) include tablets containing 2, 5, and 10 mg and solution for injection, 5 mg/ml. Oxazepam (Serax) is available in capsules containing 10, 15, and 30 mg and in tablets containing 15 mg.

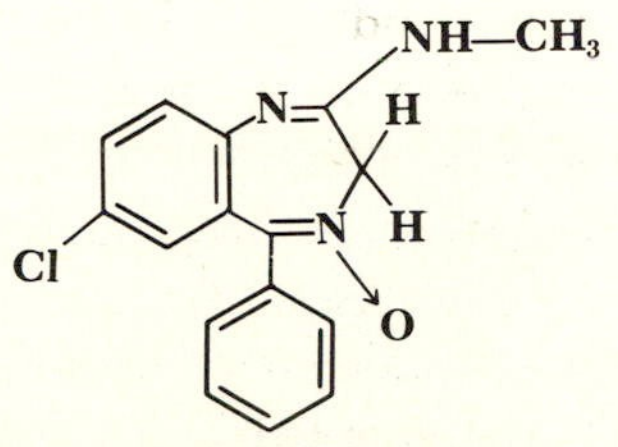

Benzodiazepine drugs

Chlordiazepoxide 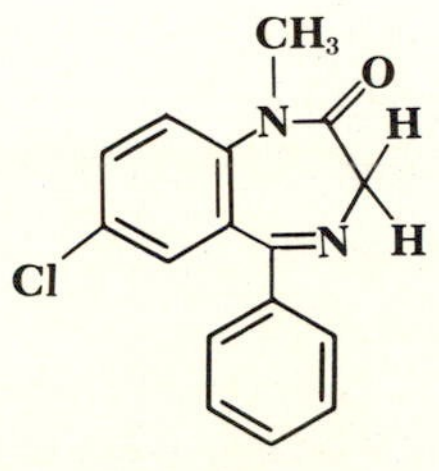   Diazepam 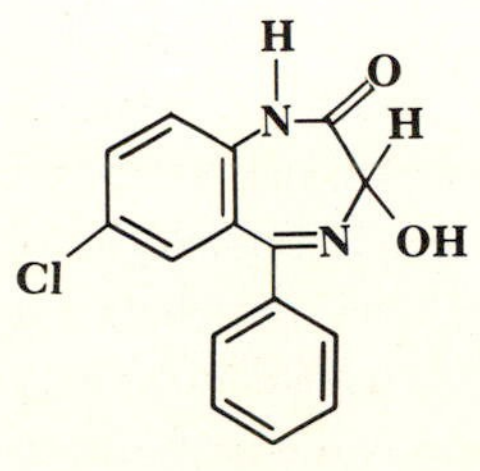   Oxazepam

Mechanism of action. Although the exact mechanism of action is unknown at the present time, very interesting interactions of the benzodiazepines with the inhibitory neurotransmitter,[33] γ-aminobutyric acid (GABA) have been observed at widespread receptors in the brain. It has been demonstrated that the electrophysiological effects of GABA are enhanced in the presence of the drugs. Furthermore, high affinity binding sites for both GABA and benzodiazepines have been demonstrated, and an interaction can be seen in that GABA enhances the binding of the drugs, whereas GABA antagonists inhibit benzodiazepine binding. The drug-binding sites appear to be involved in the pharmacological actions of the drugs, since the ability of various benzodiazepines to displaced labeled, bound diazepam parallels their clinical potency. At the present time efforts are being made to identify a possible endogenous ligand for the drug-binding sites.

Meprobamate   Meprobamate (Miltown; Equanil) was developed as a result of studies on mephenesin-like drugs. Clinical trials of this central muscle relaxant indicated that the drug has sedative and tranquilizing properties.

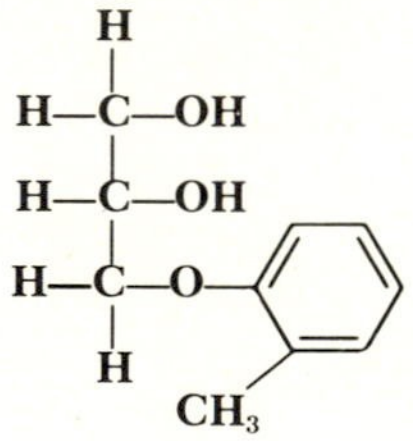

Mephenesin 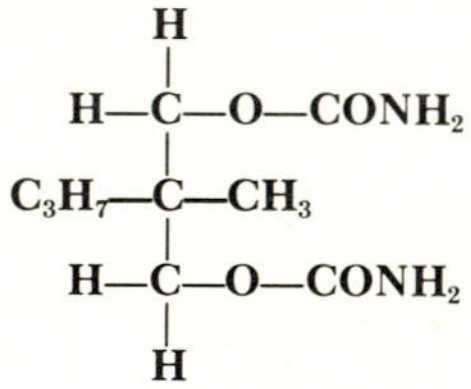   Meprobamate

Meprobamate is available in 400 mg tablets. The oral administration of one of these tablets has very slight effects, causing only very mild sedation. Larger doses tend to produce some drowsiness and reduction of muscle spasm without interference with normal proprioceptive tone. In sufficiently large doses the drug causes ataxia.

The central muscle relaxant effect of meprobamate is illustrated by its reduction of experimental tremors induced by strychnine. The drug is also a fairly potent anticonvulsant and can protect mice against convulsions and death produced by pentylenetetrazol.

Mode of action. It is believed that meprobamate has a blocking action on interneurons, since it has been shown that the drug has no effects on knee jerk, whereas flexor and crossed extensor reflexes are diminished by it. There are no interneurons interposed between the afferent and efferent reflex arcs in knee jerk. Thus the drug produces muscle relaxation without directly influencing transmission from motor nerve to skeletal muscle.

It is the opinion of many clinical pharmacologists that the muscle relaxant sedatives, although offered as tranquilizers, should be regarded simply as nonspecific sedatives similar in action to the barbiturates.[10] Not only do they cause somnolence and ataxia when used in large enough doses but also addiction, generally similar to barbiturate addiction, develops in patients who take large doses for a long time. Serious withdrawal symptoms characterized by muscle twitching and even convulsions may result when these drugs are discontinued abruptly.

Despite their lack of specificity, the muscle relaxants are used widely, perhaps too widely. Their mild sedative effect and lack of autonomic and extrapyramidal actions make them very attractive to physicians and patients alike.

Metabolism. Studies so far indicate that meprobamate is largely metabolized in the body. Only about 10% of the drug is excreted unchanged in the urine. Conjugation with glucuronic acid appears to be important in the metabolism of meprobamate, although it is first changed to hydroxymeprobamate.

Side effects and toxicity. Drowsiness occurs when fairly large doses of meprobamate are used. Skin rash, gastrointestinal disturbances, and purpura may rarely be caused by the drug. Severe hypotension associated with acute cardiac failure has been observed following the ingestion of large doses of meprobamate.[2]

Habituation and addiction to the drug may occur when large doses of meprobamate are taken for long periods of time. Sudden withdrawal may result in muscular twitching and even convulsions. It is very unlikely for these withdrawal symptoms to occur if the patient takes only two or three tablets a day. The drug should be withdrawn slowly and gradually.

REFERENCES

1 Berger, F. M.: The similarities and differences between meprobamate and barbiturates, Clin. Pharmacol. Ther. 4:209, 1963.
2 Blumberg, A. G., Rosett, H. L., and Dobrow, A.: Severe hypotensive reactions following meprobamate overdosage, Ann. Intern. Med. 51:607, 1959.
3 Cade, J. F. J.: Lithium salts in the treatment of psychotic excitement, Med. J. Aust. 36:349, 1949.
4 Cerletti, A., and Bove, F. J.: The present status of psychotropic drugs, Amsterdam, 1969, Excerpta Medica Foundation.
5 Cook, L., and Kelleher, R. T.: Effects of drugs on behavior, Clin. Pharmacol. Ther. 3:599, 1962.
6 Creese, I., Burt, D. R., and Snyder, S. H.: Dopamine receptor binding predicts clinical and pharmacological potencies of antischizophrenic drugs, Science 192:481, 1976.
7 Dasgupta, S. R., and Werner, G.: Inhibition of hypothalamic, medullary and reflex vasomotor responses by chlorpromazine, Br. J. Pharmacol. 9:389, 1954.
8 Diazepam as a muscle relaxant, Med. Letter 15:1, 1973.
9 Domino, E. F.: Human pharmacology of tranquilizing drugs, Clin. Pharmacol. Ther. 3: 599, 1962.
10 Domino, E. F.: Sites of action of some central nervous system depressants, Annu. Rev. Pharmacol. 2:215, 1962.
11 Essig, C. F.: Newer sedative drugs that can cause states of intoxication and dependence of barbiturate type, J.A.M.A. 196:714, 1966.
12 Friend, D. G.: Current concepts of therapy, tranquilizers. III. Meprobamate, phenaglycodol and chlordiazepoxide, N. Engl. J. Med. 264:870, 1961.
13 Friend, D. G., and Cummins, J. F.: Use of chlorpromazine in the treatment of nausea and vomiting of uremia, N. Engl. J. Med. 250: 997, 1954.
14 Glaviano, V. V., and Wang, S. C.: Dual mechanism of the antiemetic action of chlorpromazine, Fed. Proc. 13:358, 1954.
15 Hollister, L. E.: Complications from psychotherapeutic drugs—1964, Clin. Pharmacol. Ther. 5:322, 1964.
16 Itil, T. M.: Electroencephalography and pharmacopsychiatry. In Freyhan, F. A., Petrilowitsch, N., and Pichot, P., editors: Modern problems of pharmacopsychiatry, vol. 1, Clinical psychopharmacology, Basel, 1968, S. Karger, A. G.

17 Jansen, P. A. J.: The pharmacology of halo-peridol, Int. J. Neuropsychiatry 3(Supp.):10, 1967.

18 Lasagna, L., and McCann, W.: Effect of tranquilizing drugs on amphetamine toxicity in aggregated mice, Science 125:1241, 1957.

19 Levis, S., Preat, S., Beersaerts, J., Dauby, J., Beelen, L., and Baugniet, V.: Pharmacological study on hydroxyzine, U.C.B. 492, a disubstituted piperazine derivative, Arch. Int. Pharmacodyn. 109:127, 1957.

20 Moyer, J. H., Kinross-Wright, V., and Finney, R. M.: Chlorpromazine as a therapeutic agent in clinical medicine, Arch. Intern. Med. 95: 202, 1955.

21 National Institute of Mental Health Psychopharmacology Service Center (collaborative study group): Phenothiazine treatment in acute schizophrenia, Arch. Gen. Psychiatry 10:246, 1964.

22 Prensky, A. L., Raff, M. C., Moore, M. J., and Schwab, R. S.: Intravenous diazepam in the treatment of prolonged seizure activity, N. Engl. J. Med. 276:779, 1967.

23 Scheckel, C. L.: Pharmacology and chemistry of thioxanthenes with special reference to chlorprothixene. In Freyhan, F. A., Petrilowitsch, N., and Pichot, P., editors: Modern problems of pharmacopsychiatry, vol. 2, The thixanthenes, Basel, 1969, S. Karger, A. G.

24 Schildkraut, J. J.: Neuropsychopharmacology and the affective disorders, N. Engl. J. Med. 281:197, 248, 302, 1969.

25 Schou, M.: Lithium in psychiatric therapy and prophylaxis, J. Psychiatry Res. 6:67, 1968.

26 Shepherd, M., and Wing, L.: Pharmacological aspects of psychiatry, Adv. Pharmacol. 1:229, 1962.

27 Symposium on anxiety and a decade of tranquilizer therapy, J. Neuropsychiatry 5:1, 1964.

28 Zbinden, G., and Randall. L. O.: Pharmacology of benzodiazepines: laboratory and clinical correlations, Adv. Pharmacol. 5:213, 1967.

REVIEWS

29 Blackwell, B.: Rational drug use in the management of anxiety, Ration. Drug Ther. 9:1, 1975.

30 Davis, J. M., and Fann, W. E.: Lithium Annu. Rev. Pharmacol. 11:285, 1971.

31 Greenblatt, D. J., and Shader, R. I.: Benzodiazepines, N. Engl. J. Med. 291:1011, 1974.

32 Hollister, L. E.: Mental disorders—antianxiety and antidepressant drugs, N. Engl. J. Med. 286:1195, 1972.

33 Iversen, L. L.: GABA and benzodiazepine receptors, Nature 275:477, 1978.

34 Kobayashi, R. M.: Drug therapy of tardive dyskinesia, N. Engl. J. Med. 296:257, 1977.

35 Murphy, D. L., Goodwin, F. K., and Bunney, W. E.: A reevaluation of biogenic amines in manic and depressive states, Hosp. Practice, p. 85, Dec. 1972.

36 Randall, L. O., Scheckel, C. L., and Pool, W.: Pharmacology of medazepam and metabolites, Arch. Int. Pharmacodyn. Ther. 185:135, 1970.

37 Rivera-Calimlim, L.: The pharmacology and therapeutic application of the phenothiazines, Ration. Drug Ther. 11(4):1, 1977.

38 Singer, I., and Rotenberg, D.: Mechanisms of lithium action, N. Engl. J. Med. 289:254, 1973.

CHAPTER 25

Antidepressant and psychotomimetic drugs

The *monoamine oxidase (MAO) inhibitors* were introduced as the first antidepressants. *Iproniazid* was soon replaced by somewhat less toxic MAO inhibitors such as phenelzine (Nardil), isocarboxazid (Marplan), and tranylcypromine (Parnate).

The *tricyclic antidepressant* imipramine (Tofranil) was discovered accidentally during clinical testing for antipsychotic drugs. It was followed soon by related drugs such as amitriptyline (Elavil) and protriptyline (Vivactil) and their demethylated metabolites, such as desipramine (Pertofrane) and nortriptyline (Aventyl).

In addition to these groups of antidepressants, *central stimulants* such as dextroamphetamine (Dexedrine) and methylphenidate (Ritalin) are still used occasionally for depressed patients.

On the basis of chemical structure, the MAO inhibitors may be placed into two categories: hydrazine and nonhydrazine drugs. Most MAO inhibitors are of the hydrazine type; the major ones in current, but limited, use are **phenelzine** (Nardil) and **isocarboxazid** (Marplan). Tranylcypromine (Parnate) is the only nonhydrazine in current use. Although both types cause a long-lasting inhibition of the enzyme, tranylcypromine also causes a rapid central stimulation, probably related to its amphetamine-like structure.

Hydrazine-type inhibitors cause a variety of side effects including hepatotoxicity, overstimulation, postural hypotension, and hypertensive crises. The latter effect, which may be fatal, is generally associated with the ingestion of foods and drinks containing a high content of monoamines such as tyramine. Such foods and drinks include aged cheeses, some wines and beer, and others. For this reason, the hypertensive crisis is often referred to as a "cheese reaction." The monoamines are normally broken down by MAO in the intestine and the liver. If this enzyme is blocked, the amines may enter the circulation in sufficient concentration to release norepinephrine from adrenergic neurons.

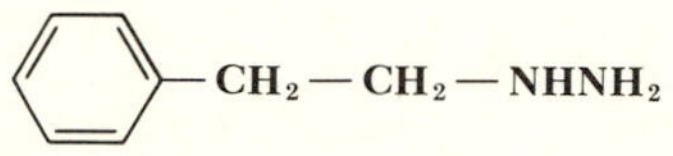

MAO INHIBITORS
Types and actions

Phenelzine

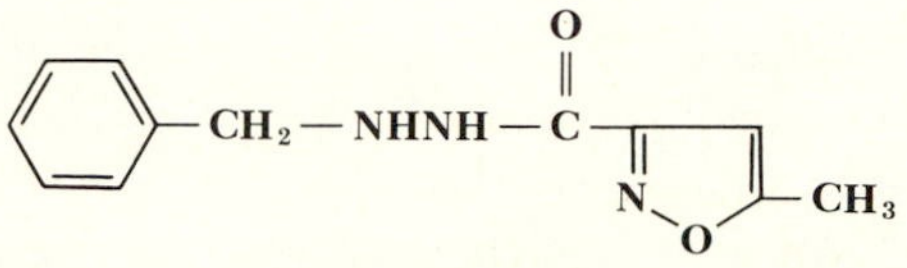

Isocarboxazid

293

Tranylcypromine

Tranylcypromine (Parnate) is a potent *nonhydrazine MAO inhibitor* that also has a direct amphetamine-like stimulant action. Thus it is a *bimodal antidepressant.* The drug is closely related to amphetamine.

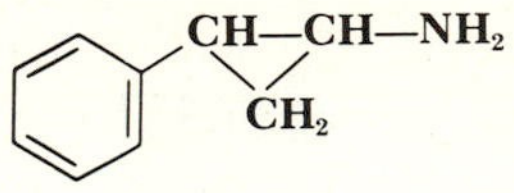

$$CH-CH-NH_2$$
$$CH_2$$

Tranylcypromine

Tranylcypromine provides fast, direct stimulation similar to that of amphetamine, but its action is sustained, probably as a consequence of its MAO inhibitory action. Its fast action is an advantage over the hydrazine drugs, but it shares with the latter the ability to cause postural hypotension. It is a remarkable fact that all MAO inhibitors cause postural hypotension. Tranylcypromine may cause overstimulation, and its use may be combined with a phenothiazine to combat the overstimulation.

Tranylcypromine is an extremely potent MAO inhibitor. It, too, can cause hypertensive crises following ingestion of certain foods. This drug's use is restricted to hospitalized or closely supervised patients.

Drug interactions

The MAO inhibitors are generally reserved for depressed patients not responding to other antidepressant therapy. Combined use of these drugs with the tricyclic antidepressants may cause a dangerous interaction resulting in hypertensive crisis, fever, and convulsions. At least a 1-week withdrawal period should be allowed for either the MAO inhibitor or the tricyclics before therapy with the other drug is initiated.

•   •   •

Pargyline is discussed with the antihypertensive drugs on p. 226.

TRICYCLIC ANTIDEPRESSANTS

The tricyclic antidepressants have become the most widely used medications in the treatment of depression. These drugs include imipramine (Tofranil), amitriptyline (Elavil), their desmethyl derivatives desipramine (Pertofrane; Norpramin), nortriptyline (Aventyl), protriptyline (Vivactil), and **doxepin** (Sinequan; Adapin).

Pharmacological effects

The major effects of the tricyclic antidepressants are their antidepressant and anticholinergic actions. Minor effects are related to sedation, antihistaminic action, and potentiation of the action of adrenergic drugs. They also have some quinidine-like effect on the heart.

Antidepressant effect. After a delay of several days, the tricyclic compounds elevate mood, increase alertness, and improve appetite in about 80% of patients suffering from depression.

Current ideas of the mechanisms of action of the antidepressants may be found in Chapter 23.

Other than their antidepressant action, the pharmacological effects of the tricyclic antidepressants are seen as adverse effects and drug interactions.

Adverse effects and drug interactions

The anticholinergic action of the tricyclic compounds causes symptoms such as dryness of the mouth, blurred vision, constipation, and urinary retention. Disorientation and mental confusion may also be related to central anticholinergic (atropine-like) effects, since they can be effectively treated with physostigmine.[19]

Sedation may be considerable, and there is an increasing tendency for prescribing the tricyclic drugs in a single dose at bedtime. The antihistaminic action of these drugs is of no practical importance.

Cardiovascular side effects of the tricyclic antidepressants include tachycardia, arrhythmias, and prolongation of atrioventricular conduction time.[28]

The tricyclic antidepressants prevent and reverse the antihypertensive actions of guanethidine by blocking the membrane amine pump, which transports guanethidine into the adrenergic fiber. Anticholinergic drugs and barbiturates should be used cautiously in patients who are taking one of the tricyclic antidepressants because of additive effects. MAO inhibitors are strictly contraindicated in these same patients.

Imipramine (Tofranil; Presamine) is available as oral tablets of 10, 25, and 50 mg and injectable solution containing 12.5 mg/ml.

Preparations

Amitriptyline hydrochloride (Elavil hydrochloride) is available in oral tablets of 10, 25, and 50 mg and injectable solution containing 10 mg/ml.

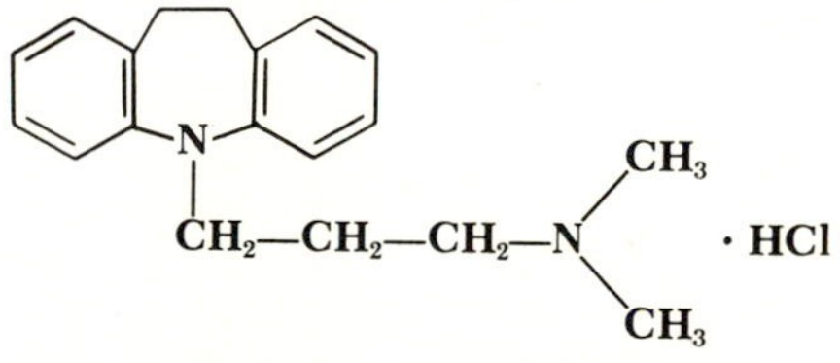

Imipramine hydrochloride

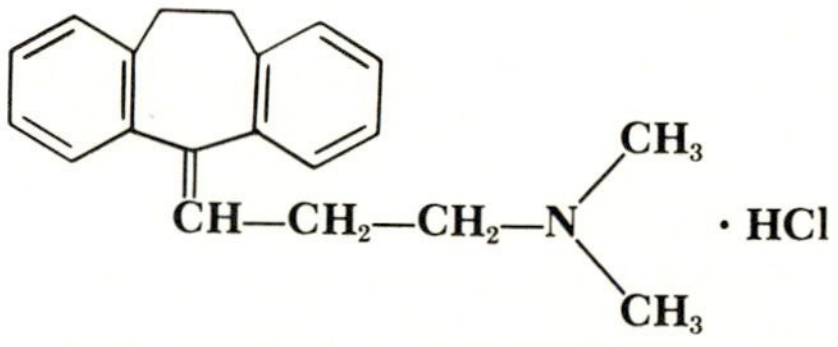

Amitriptyline hydrochloride

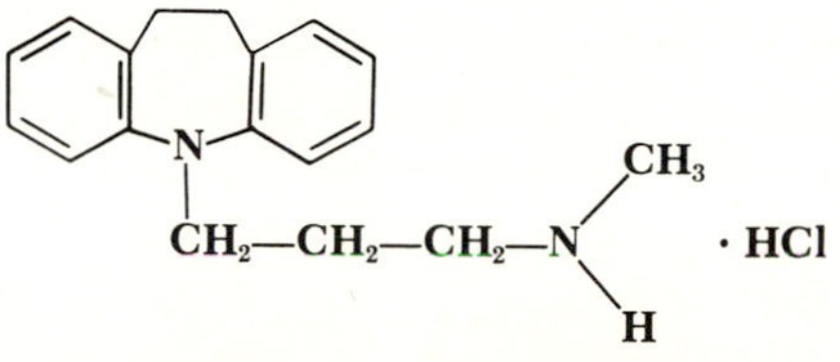

Desipramine hydrochloride

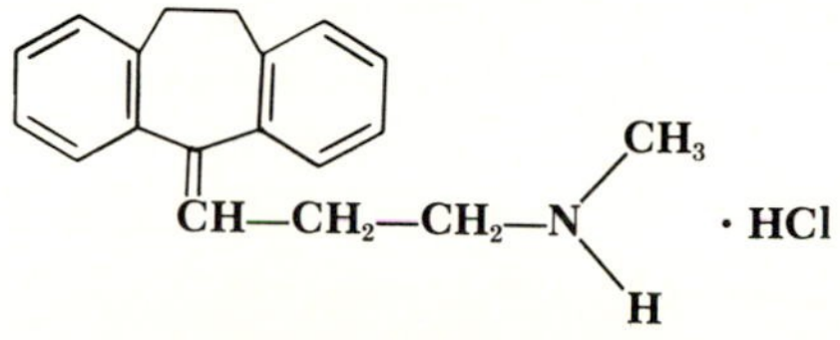

Nortriptyline hydrochloride

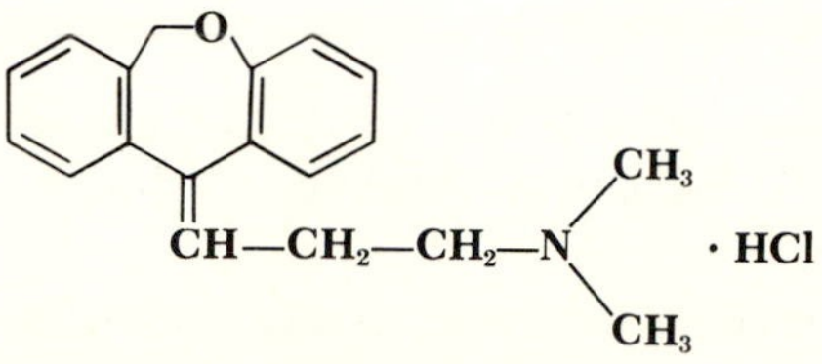

Doxepin hydrochloride

Desipramine hydrochloride (Norpramin; Pertofrane) is available in oral tablets of 25 to 50 mg and capsules of 25 and 50 mg.

Nortriptyline hydrochloride (Aventyl hydrochloride) is available in capsules of 10 and 25 mg and liquid containing 10 mg/5 ml.

Protriptyline hydrochloride (Vivactil hydrochloride) is available in oral tablets, 5 and 10 mg.

Doxepin hydrochloride (Sinequan; Adapin) is available in capsules, 10, 25, and 50 mg.

**PSYCHOTO-MIMETIC DRUGS
Psychomotor
stimulants**

Amphetamine, particularly the more potent *dextro* form, has been used for years as a mood elevator in depressed patients. Its disadvantages are its cardiovascular effects and the letdown that follows the short period of stimulation. Other stimulants are also sometimes used in depressive states. These are pipradrol (Meratran) and methylphenidate (Ritalin).

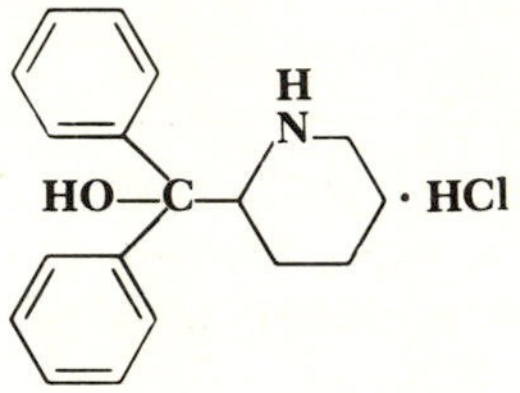

Pipradrol hydrochloride 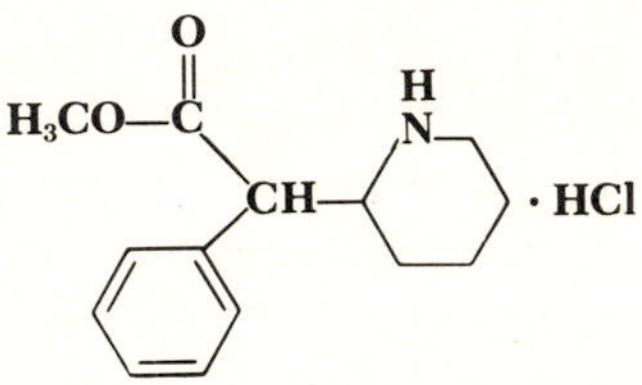   Methylphenidate hydrochloride

Pipradrol has been used as an antidepressant in depressive states, but its effectiveness is questionable. The related drug, methylphenidate hydrochloride, is more widely used and abused.

Methylphenidate resembles dextroamphetamine in its pharmacology except for its lower potency. The drug is used widely as a mild stimulant in depressive states but is not basically superior to dextroamphetamine. Its use in hyperkinetic children may be justified and is quite effective. It is often used in the treatment of narcolepsy and is one of the favorites of medical students just before examinations.

Although methylphenidate in the usual adult dose of 10 mg taken orally does not elevate the blood pressure, it should not be used in hypertensive persons or in any patients in whom sympathetic stimulation may be hazardous.

Preparations of methylphenidate hydrochloride (Ritalin hydrochloride) include tablets containing 5, 10, and 20 mg and powder for injection, 100 mg.

Types and actions

Psychomotor stimulants may be divided into two general types: amphetamine and nonamphetamine. Examples of the first are amphetamine and methamphetamine and, of the latter type, methylphenidate, cocaine, and certain newer agents such as nomifensine and amfonelic acid.

This differentiation is not only on the basis of chemical structure, but also on mechanism of action. The central stimulant effect of amphetamine is dependent on a small, rapidly turning over pool of catecholamine. Thus its central actions are blocked by α-methyltyrosine, a catecholamine synthesis inhibitor. Its action is not blocked by amine depletion by reserpine. The nonamphetamines, on the other hand, act by the release of stored catecholamines. Their central actions are inhibited by reserpine but not by α-methyltyrosine.

Both types of stimulants can exacerbate, or in high chronic doses, induce schizophrenic symptoms. This, and other central actions of the drugs, can be blocked by dopamine receptor blocking agents such as chlorpromazine or haloperidol.

Although the nonamphetamines do not directly release dopamine, as does amphetamine, it is interesting to note that a common property of the nonamphetamine stimulants is blockade of the dopamine neuronal uptake mechanism. The stimulant activity of the drugs parallels their potencies as dopamine uptake inhibitors, and it has been proposed that such inhibition results in an intraneuronal translocation of stored dopamine so as to make more transmitter available for impulse-induced release.[24]

One of the nonamphetamines, nomifensine, is used as an antidepressant in certain countries but not in the United States.

Hallucinogens

Certain drugs can produce toxic psychosis in small doses. Interest in these compounds has been great, partly because they have some usefulness in experimental psychiatry and partly because their actions suggest that perhaps there may be a chemical basis for mental illness.

A significant difference between the central effects of the hallucinogens and the mental effects of high doses of the psychomotor stimulants such as amphetamine is that in the case of the hallucinogens, human subjects generally retain insight into their experience, realizing that their reaction is drug induced. Thus their hallucinations might better be termed *pseudohallucinations*. In the case of amphetamine and related drugs, they are more truly psychotomimetic and may cause symptoms of paranoid schizophrenia indistinguishable from the actual disease.

Some of the most interesting psychotomimetic agents are lysergic acid diethylamide, mescaline, and psilocybin.

Lysergic acid diethylamide (LSD; Delysid) is closely related to the ergot alkaloids. Discovery of its hallucinogenic properties was made by the chemist who synthesized the drug and noted these reactions on himself. Subjects who take a few micrograms of LSD develop auditory and visual hallucinations. The body may feel distorted, the arms, for example, appearing to be at a great distance. The subject may become fearful and irrational.

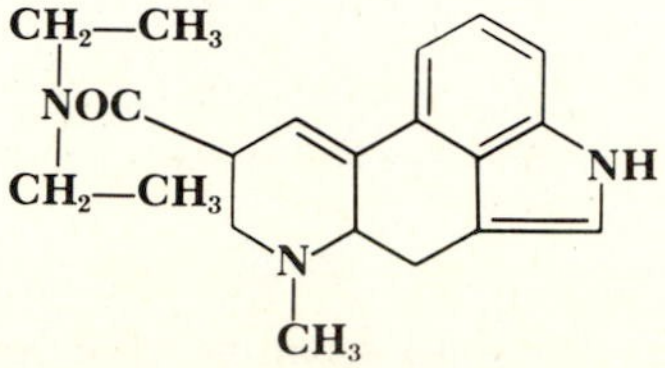

Lysergic acid diethylamide

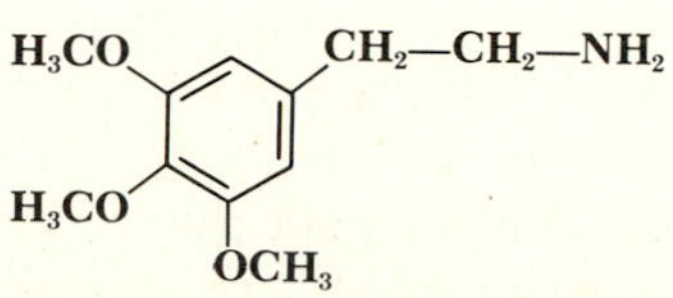

Mescaline

In animal experiments, LSD may cause excitement and hyperthermia. With repeated administration, considerable tolerance to the drug develops.

LSD is a potent antagonist of the action of serotonin on smooth muscles. The association of this antiserotonin activity and the psychic effects suggested many interesting speculations concerning the role of serotonin in behavior. It should be remembered, however, that there is no evidence to indicate that the central actions of LSD result from its antagonistic effect on serotonin. Brom-lysergic acid diethylamide has antiserotonin effects on smooth muscles similar to those of LSD, but the drug has no hallucinogenic properties. There is also no evidence for the normal occurrence of an LSD-like substance in mammals.

Mescaline is obtained from the cactus known as peyote or mescal (*Lophophora williamsii*) found in the southwestern region of the United States. This cactus is used by some Indians in religious ceremonies. Persons who have ingested dried peyote buttons report that they cause a stuporous state with unusual visual hallucinations. Colored lights, reported to be extremely beautiful, are the most striking feature of these hallucinations. Interestingly, some volunteers report that they have seen colors they did not know existed.

Mescaline, the active principle of peyote, is 3,4,5-trimethoxyphenethylamine, a structure resembling the sympathomimetic amines. The compound has some interest in experimental psychiatry. It is used experimentally in doses of 300 to 500 mg.

Psilocybin (*O*-phosphoryl-4-hydroxy-*N*,*N*-dimethyltryptamine) has been isolated from Mexican mushrooms that have hallucinogenic effects. Chemically it is closely related to serotonin.

It is of great interest that compounds related to the endogenously occurring amines have hallucinogenic properties. Further research is needed to explain why this should be so.

The abuse of psychotomimetic drugs is discussed in detail in Chapter 30.

REFERENCES

1 Carlsson, A., Corrodi, H., Fuxe, K., and Hokfelt, T.: Effect of antidepressant drugs on the depletion of intraneuronal brain 5-hydroxytryptamine stores caused by 4-methyl-α-ethyl-meta-tyramine, Eur. J. Pharmacol. **5**:357, 1969.

2 Cohen, S.: Psychotomimetic agents, Annu. Rev. Pharmacol. **7**:301, 1967.

3 Davies, E. B.: Tranylcypromine and cheese, Lancet **2**:691, 1963.

4 De Ritter, E., Drekter, L., Scheiner, J., and Rubin, S. H.: Urinary excretion of hydrazine derivatives of isonicotinic acid in normal humans, Proc. Soc. Exp. Biol. Med. **79**:654, 1952.

5 Dengler, H. J., Michaelson, I. A., Spiegel, H. E., and Titus, E. O.: The uptake of labeled norepinephrine by isolated brain and other tissues of the cat, Int. J. Neuropharmacol. **1**:23, 1962.

6 Friend, D.: Antidepressant drug therapy, Clin. Pharmacol. Ther. **6**:805, 1965.

7 Glowinski, J., and Axelrod, J.: Inhibition of uptake of tritiated-noradrenaline in the intact rat brain by imipramine and structurally related compounds, Nature **204**:1318, 1964.

8 Himwich, W. A., and Petersen, J. C.: Effect of combined administration of imipramine and monoamine oxidase inhibitor, Am. J. Psychiatry **117**:928, 1961.

9 Hollister, L. E.: Chemical psychoses, Annu. Rev. Med. **15**:203, 1964.

10 Hollister, L. E.: Overdoses of psychotherapeutic drugs, Clin. Pharmacol. Ther. **7:**142, 1966.
11 Iversen, L. L.: Inhibition of norepinephrine uptake by drugs, J. Pharm. Pharmacol. **17:**62, 1965.
12 Jacobsen, E.: The clinical pharmacology of the hallucinogens, Clin. Pharmacol. Ther. **4:**480, 1963.
13 Kety, S. S.: Biochemical theories of schizophrenia, Science **129:**1528, 1590, 1959.
14 Luby, E. D., and Domino, E. F.: Toxicity from large doses of imipramine and MAO inhibitor in suicidal intent, J.A.M.A. **177:**68, 1961.
15 Rickels, K., Raab, E., DeSilverio, R., and Etemad, B.: Drug treatment of depression, J.A.M.A. **201:**675, 1967.
16 Rowe, G. G., Afonso, S., Castillo, C. A., Kyle, J. C., Leicht, T. R., and Crumpton, C. W.: Systemic and coronary hemodynamic effects of an amine oxidase inhibitor and of serotonin, Clin. Pharmacol. Ther. **4:**467, 1963.
17 Schuckit, M., Robins, E., and Feighner, J.: Tricyclic antidepressants and monoamine oxidase inhibitors, Arch. Gen. Psychiatry **24:**509, 1971.

REVIEWS

18 Axelrod, J.: Biogenic amines and their impact in psychiatry, Sem. Psychiatry **4:**199, 1972.
19 Burks, J. S., Walker, J. E., Rumack, B. H., and Ott, J. E.: Tricyclic antidepressant poisoning, J.A.M.A. **230:**1405, 1974.
20 Himwich, H. E., and Alpers, H.: Psychopharmacology, Annu. Rev. Pharmacol. **10:**313, 1970.
21 Hollister, L. E.: Mental disorders—antianxiety and antidepressant drugs, N. Engl. J. Med. **286:**1195, 1972.
22 Kety, S. S.: Toward hypotheses for a biochemical component in the vulnerability to schizophrenia, Sem. Psychiatry **4:**223, 1972.
23 Lennard, H. L., Epsteinn, L. J., Bernstein, A., and Ransom, D. C.: Hazards implicit in prescribing psychoactive drugs, Science **169:**438, 1970.
24 Shore, P. A., McMillen, B. A., Miller, H. H., Sanghera, M. K., Kiser, R. S., and German, D. C.: The dopamine neuronal storage system and nonamphetamine stimulants: a model for psychosis. In Catecholamines: basic and clinical frontiers, New York, 1979, Pergamon Press, Inc., p. 722.
25 Snyder, S. H., Banerjee, S. P., Yamamura, H. I., and Greenberg, D.: Drugs, transmitters and schizophrenia, Science **184:**1243, 1974.
26 Sulser, F., and Sanders-Bush, E.: Effect of drugs on amines in the CNS, Annu. Rev. Pharmacol. **11:**209, 1971.
27 Sulser, F., Vetulani, J., and Mobley, P. L.: On the mode of action of antidepressant drugs, Biochem. Pharmacol. **27:**257, 1978.
28 Vohra, J., Burrows, G. D., and Sloman, G.: Assessment of cardiovascular side effects of therapeutic doses of tricyclic antidepressant drugs, Aust. N. Z. J. Med. **5:**7, 1975.

SECTION FOUR

Depressants and stimulants of the central nervous system

CHAPTER 26

Hypnotic drugs

A variety of drugs can produce a state of depression of the central nervous system (CNS) resembling normal sleep. These drugs are referred to as *hypnotics*. In smaller doses many of these drugs can produce a state of drowsiness, and when used in this manner, they are referred to as *sedatives*. When used in larger doses, hypnotics may produce anesthesia, poisoning, and death. These progressive dose-related effects may be indicated as follows:

$$\text{Sedation} \rightleftarrows \text{Hypnosis} \rightleftarrows \text{Anesthesia} \rightleftarrows \text{Coma} \rightarrow \text{Death}$$

Hypnotics have many important uses in medicine. Sleeping pills are used properly and improperly by many people. In addition, hypnotics are helpful in combination with analgesics in painful states, are antidotes for stimulant and convulsant drugs, and are useful in convulsive disorders and as adjuncts to anesthesia.

The most important hypnotics are the barbiturates, which were introduced as early as 1903 by Fischer and von Mering. When properly used, they are highly effective and safe medications. Whereas the barbiturates are habit-forming and may even lead to addiction, the newer sedative-hypnotics, offered with the implication of being safer, are not truly superior. The piperidinediones such as glutethimide and methyprylon, introduced as "nonbarbiturate hypnotics," are actually chemically related to the barbiturates and offer no special advantages.

In addition to the barbiturates and the piperidinediones, there are many other classes of drugs that properly belong to the sedative-hypnotic group. Carbamates such as urethan and related drugs, bromides, alcohols, and paraldehyde are also classified as sedative-hypnotics.

A new benzodiazepine, flurazepam (Dalmane), has been introduced as a hypnotic agent for all types of insomnia. The excessive use of flurazepam and other hypnotics is being increasingly condemned.

The combination of urea with organic acids results in monoureides and diureides that have hypnotic properties. The combination of urea and malonic acid is malonylurea, or barbituric acid, the parent compound of the barbiturate series.

The majority of the clinically useful barbiturates are obtained by making appropriate substitutions in position 5 of the molecule. Thus phenobarbital is ethylphenylbarbituric acid. In some cases an additional substitute is made by replacing a hydro-

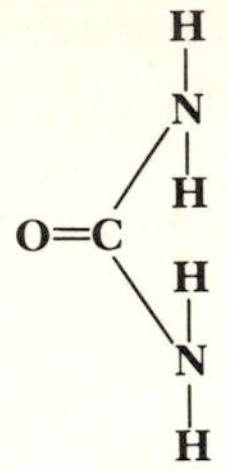

H
|
N
|
H
|
O=C
|
N
|
H

Urea

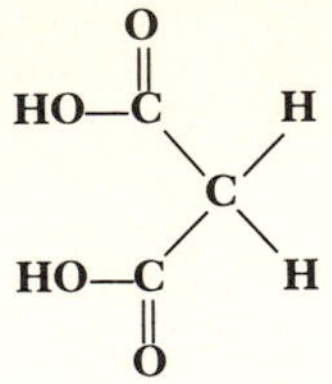

O
‖
HO—C   H
\   \
              C
/   /
HO—C   H
‖
O

Malonic acid

H   O
| ‖
N—C   H
1   6   \
O=C 2   5 C
| 3   4 /
N—C   H
| ‖
H   O

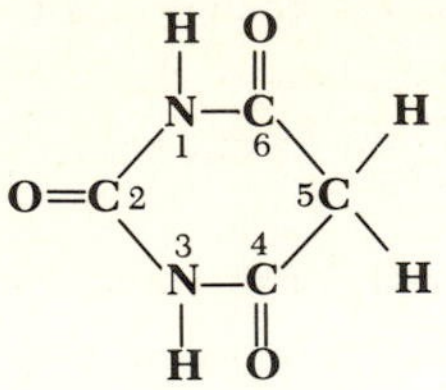

Barbituric acid

gen in the ring. Thus mephobarbital (Mebaral) differs from phenobarbital in having a CH_3 group attached to a nitrogen atom. Finally, if thiourea instead of urea is combined with malonic acid, the resulting thiobarbituric acid is the parent compound of the ultrashort-acting barbiturate intravenous anesthetics such as thiopental (Pentothal).

Classification   The therapeutically useful barbiturates have traditionally been classified according to their duration of action, based on animal experiments.[42] Thus the pharmacological literature describes ultrashort-, short-, intermediate-, and long-acting barbiturates, as indicated in Table 26-1.

Clinical experience indicates, however, that this classification is misleading.[41,42] In particular, the distinction between short- and long-acting barbiturates is not borne out by controlled clinical trials. Thus 100 mg doses of secobarbital, pentobarbital, and phenobarbital were equally effective in inducing sleep in patients with chronic diseases. In the same study, hangover was not greater with the long-acting phenobarbital than with secobarbital or pentobarbital.

It is a reasonable suggestion that barbiturates be simply classified according to their therapeutic indications as "sedative-hypnotic barbiturates" and "anesthetic bar-

TABLE 26-1. Classification, structure, and dosage of commonly used barbiturates

Names	Substituents in position 5	Hypnotic dose	Duration of action
Thiopental* (Pentothal) Thiamylal* (Surital) Hexobarbital† (Evipal)	Ethyl, 1-methylbutyl Allyl, 1-methylbutyl Methyl, cyclohexenyl		Ultrashort (intravenous anesthetics)
Secobarbital (Seconal) Pentobarbital (Nembutal)	Allyl, 1-methylbutyl Ethyl, 1-methylbutyl	0.1-0.2 g 0.1 g	Short
Butabarbital (Butisol) Amobarbital (Amytal) Vinbarbital (Delvinal)	Ethyl, sec-butyl Ethyl, isoamyl Ethyl, 1-methyl-1-butenyl	0.1-0.2 g 0.05-0.2 g 0.1-0.2 g	Intermediate
Phenobarbital (Luminal) Mephobarbital† (Mebaral) Barbital (Veronal)	Ethyl, phenyl Ethyl, phenyl Ethyl, ethyl	0.1-0.2 g 0.1-0.2 g 0.3-0.5 g	Long

*Thiobarbiturate.
†A CH_3 group is attached to the nitrogen atom.

biturates."[42] Within the former group the physician may find that phenobarbital may be more slowly absorbed and metabolized and is thus more suitable for maintained sedation than secobarbital or pentobarbital. Nevertheless, for their most common usage, the promotion of sleep, duration of action has been overemphasized.

Barbiturates are weak acids that cross biological membranes in their undissociated form as a function of their *lipid solubility*. The variations in absorption, distribution, protein binding, speed of metabolic degradation, tissue localization, duration of action, and renal excretion are well correlated with the lipid solubility of the undissociated barbituric acid derivative.

The relationship between lipid solubility of a series of barbiturates and their therapeutic classification is shown in Table 26-2. Clearly, the ultrashort-acting intravenous anesthetics are highly lipid soluble, the short- and intermediate-acting sedative-hypnotics are much less so, and the long-acting drugs such as phenobarbital and barbital are even less lipid soluble.

Table 26-3 shows the pharmacokinetic characteristics of three representative bar-

Physicochemical factors and pharmacokinetic behavior

TABLE 26-2. Lipid solubility of a series of barbiturates as determined by their partition coefficients between methylene chloride and water*

Drug	Partition coefficient†	Classification
Methohexital	1000	Intravenous anesthetic
Thiopental	580	Intravenous anesthetic
Secobarbital	52	Sedative-hypnotic, short acting
Amobarbital	42	Sedative-hypnotic, short or intermediate acting
Pentobarbital	39	Sedative-hypnotic, short or intermediate acting
Phenobarbital	3	Sedative-hypnotic, long acting
Barbital	1	Sedative-hypnotic, long acting

*Based on data from Bush, M. T. In Root, W. S., and Hofmann, F. G., editors: Physiological pharmacology, vol. 1, New York, 1963, Academic Press, Inc.
†Partition coefficient between methylene chloride and water at approximately 25° C of the unionized form. The partition coefficient is defined as the ratio : (concentration in organic solvent)/(concentration in aqueous phase) at equilibrium. Methylene chloride is a typical lipid solvent.

TABLE 26-3. Pharmacokinetic behavior of three representative barbiturates in relation to their lipid solubility

Characteristics	Phenobarbital	Secobarbital	Thiopental
Partition coefficient*	3	52	580
Absorption from stomach †	Slow	Rapid	Rapid (not used orally)
Plasma protein binding †	2%	44%	65%
Rate of entry into CNS	Slow	Rapid	Very rapid
Renal excretion of unchanged drug	30%	Negligible	Negligible

*Between methylene chloride and water.
†Data from Bush, M. T. In Root, W. S., and Hofmann, F. G., editors: Physiological pharmacology, vol. 1, New York, 1963, Academic Press, Inc.

biturates in relation to their lipid solubilities. Phenobarbital, having a low lipid solubility compared with secobarbital or thiopental, is generally classified as a "long-acting" sedative-hypnotic. This is a consequence of its slow absorption from the gastrointestinal tract and its slower rate of metabolism. The renal excretion of 30% of the administered phenobarbital is a consequence of several factors—slower rate of metabolism, less protein binding, and less tubular reabsorption. In the case of barbital, which is even less lipid soluble, as much as 65% to 90% of the administered dose is excreted unchanged.

The rate of entry into the CNS is strongly influenced by lipid solubility. When thiopental is injected intravenously, it produces anesthesia almost instantaneously. On the other hand, when sodium phenobarbital was injected intravenously into mice, there was a delay of 12 minutes before anesthesia occurred.[7]

In addition to lipid solubility, ionization of barbiturates plays a role in their distribution and excretion. For practical purposes this is important only when the pK_a of the drug is about the same as the physiological pH. The pK_a of phenobarbital is 7.3. As a consequence, relatively slight changes in the pH of the body fluids will exert a significant effect on the degree of ionization of phenobarbital. It has been demonstrated that alkalinization with sodium bicarbonate infusions or hyperventilation will favor a movement of phenobarbital from the tissues to the plasma. For the same reasons administration of sodium bicarbonate, with its alkalinizing effect on the urine, will favor the excretion of the phenobarbital.

Pharmacological effects   The primary action of the barbiturates is on nervous tissue. The consequences of this primary action are manifested as (1) hypnosis and anesthesia, (2) anticonvulsant effects, and (3) miscellaneous effects such as analgesia, autonomic nervous system actions, respiratory effects, and others.

Hypnosis and anesthesia. Following the administration of a hypnotic dose of a barbiturate, the only significant effect consists of sleep from which the individual can be awakened by various stimuli. When larger amounts are administered, a state of anesthesia ensues from which the person or animal cannot be awakened until the drug is metabolized or, in the case of the ultra short-acting compounds, until the blood level of the drug falls as a consequence of its distribution in the body. The same barbiturate may be a sedative, a hypnotic, or an anesthetic or may be lethal as increasing doses are administered. This relationship between dosage and effect is illustrated in Fig. 26-1.

It may be seen from the data that the therapeutic index, expressed as LD_{50}/hypnotic $dose_{50}$, is quite favorable. On the other hand, the anesthetic dose is dangerously close to the lethal dose. This is an important reason why the ordinary sedative-hypnotic barbiturates are not suitable for general anesthesia in patients, although they are commonly used in experimental animals. The ultrashort-acting barbiturates are used in anesthesia for induction and supplementation of inhalation agents because their rapid redistribution in the body allows a minute-to-minute adjustment of the intensity of their effect. The cause of death following administra-

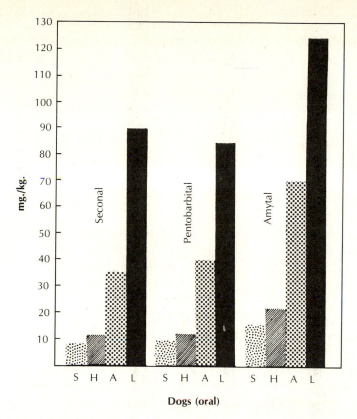

FIG. 26-1. Activity of three barbiturates in dogs. A comparison of three barbiturates with regard to sedative, hypnotic, anesthetic, and lethal doses. *S,* Sedative dose$_{50}$; *H,* hypnotic dose$_{50}$; *A,* anesthetic dose$_{50}$; *L,* lethal dose$_{50}$. Note that SD$_{50}$ is approximately one-fourth of AD$_{50}$, HD$_{50}$ is about one-third of AD$_{50}$, and AD$_{50}$ is about one-half of LD$_{50}$. (From Chen, K. K.: In Symposium on sedative and hypnotic drugs, Baltimore, 1954, The Williams & Wilkins Co.)

tion of large doses is respiratory failure as a consequence of depression of the respiratory center.

Of great current interest is the effect of barbiturates and other drugs on the various sleep states. It is now recognized that sleep consists of two main functional states. One is called "slow wave," nondreaming, or non–rapid eye movement (NREM) sleep. The other is referred to as "paradoxic," dreaming, or rapid eye movement (REM) sleep. Dream deprivation or suppression of REM sleep causes adverse effects in normal persons. Since sedative-hypnotic drugs tend to suppress REM sleep, evaluation of the long-range consequences of their chronic use is an important research problem.[47] Certain newer sedative-hypnotics that are being promoted are claimed to have less effect on REM sleep, but any such conclusion would seem premature. The recently introduced drug flurazepam hydrochloride (Dalmane), for example, is said not to decrease dream time as reflected by REM.

The studies of Magoun[37] indicate that barbiturates have a selective effect on the reticular activating system and are capable of blocking ascending conduction in this area. It has also been shown that the barbiturates increase the recovery time and raise the threshold for neurons in general. The selective effect on the ascending reticular formation may be related to the extensive chain of synaptic connections in this area or to a lower factor of safety at the individual synapses.

Anticonvulsant effects. The barbiturates are potent antidotes of the convulsant drugs, and they can also abolish convulsions that arise in disease states such as tetanus and eclampsia. Some of the barbiturates are effective also as antiepileptic drugs, but not all are useful in this respect.

The antidotal action of the barbiturates against convulsant drugs is of great practical importance. It is possible to protect experimental animals against as many as 10 lethal doses of strychnine and pentylenetetrazol and also against the convulsant and lethal action of local anesthetics such as procaine and cocaine. It is important to point out, however, that whereas the barbiturates are potent antidotes against the convulsant drugs, the mutual antagonism works much better in this sequence than in the reverse direction; that is, convulsant drugs are only moderately effective against barbiturate depression and can protect experimental animals against only *very few* lethal doses of barbiturates.

The barbiturates are often employed for preventing or abolishing convulsions in disease states. For this purpose the drugs are usually injected intravenously or intramuscularly.

When a barbiturate is used as an anticonvulsant, it is important to realize that if the duration of action of the barbiturate outlasts the duration of action of the convulsant, serious depression of respiration may result. For this reason the ultrashort-acting or short-acting barbiturates are much preferred in the management of convulsive emergencies.

In addition to this general usefulness of the barbiturates as anticonvulsants, some members of the series are also antiepileptic drugs. Phenobarbital, mephobarbital, and metharbital have special anticonvulsant and antiepileptic properties. Clinically these drugs are potent in the management of grand mal epilepsy, and experimental studies indicate also that these three barbiturates have anticonvulsant actions in situations in which other members of the series are ineffective.

Miscellaneous effects. Miscellaneous effects include analgesia, autonomic nervous system actions, respiratory effects, and others.

Analgesia. It is generally believed that barbiturates are not primarily analgesic, or at least they do not elevate the pain threshold significantly. A patient still perceives painful stimuli when subanesthetic doses of barbiturates are given. Also, a patient experiencing severe pain may become agitated and delirious if barbiturates are administered without analgesics. On the other hand, barbiturates may modify the reaction to pain. It has been shown that intravenous hypnotic doses of pentobarbital produce relief from postoperative pain in 50% of the patients in one series, whereas a placebo relieved only 20%. Morphine produced relief in 80% of these patients.

Autonomic nervous system actions. Ordinary hypnotic doses of the barbiturates have no important actions on the autonomic nervous system. On the other hand, anesthetic doses can produce many effects on autonomic function.

Central autonomic regulations are influenced by these drugs. The body temperature tends to fall in barbiturate anesthesia, partly as a result of central interference with temperature regulation. Direct hypothalamic stimulation produces a lessened blood pressure rise in barbiturate-anesthetized animals.

The influence of various autonomic blocking agents is altered considerably by pentobarbital anesthesia.[75] For example, the intravenous administration of hexamethonium produces tachycardia in the unanesthetized dog but causes bradycardia following administration of pentobarbital.

Respiratory effects. Although hypnotic doses of barbiturates cause only minor depression of respiration, larger doses depress the respiratory center and diminish its responsiveness to carbon dioxide. The cause of death in acute barbiturate poisoning is respiratory depression.

It is generally believed that in severe barbiturate depression the respiratory center is still responsive to anoxia through the carotid chemoreceptor mechanism. There is experimental evidence to indicate that oxygen may further depress respiration in profound barbiturate anesthesia by eliminating the anoxic drive.[2]

Other effects. Hypnotic doses of the barbiturates exert no effects on the heart. In heart-lung preparations, large experimental doses of the barbiturates can produce failure, which responds to digitalis glycosides. However, concentrations used in these experiments are much higher than those that can be obtained in patients. The low blood pressure in barbiturate poisoning is probably a consequence of both impaired gaseous exchange secondary to respiratory depression and actions on central and peripheral components of the autonomic nervous system.

Metabolism

The barbiturates are absorbed rapidly from the stomach, intestine, rectum, subcutaneous tissue, and muscle. Their sodium salts are employed when given by injection.

Following absorption, the barbiturates are bound to a varying extent to plasma proteins. Thiopental is bound up to 60% or 70%, pentobarbital about 50%, and the long-acting phenobarbital only to a very slight extent.

Just as plasma binding varies with the different barbiturates, their binding by tissue also shows important differences. The concentration of thiopental or pentobarbital in the brain is not very different from their concentration in plasma. On the other hand, thiopental slowly becomes six times more concentrated in body fat than in plasma, whereas pentobarbital is not concentrated in fatty tissue.[3]

Some of the barbiturates penetrate into the brain more slowly than others, even following intravenous injection. Barbital shows an "anesthetic lag," which has been correlated with its slow equilibration with brain tissue. This in turn correlates well with the low fat solubility of the nonionized barbital, as contrasted with that of pentobarbital.

The metabolic degradation of the various barbiturates follows four general paths:

(1) oxidation of radicals in the 5 position, (2) removal of *N*-alkyl radicals, (3) conversion of thiobarbiturates to their oxygen analogs, and (4) cleavage of the ring. The first mechanism is important for pentobarbital, phenobarbital, and many others, including the thiobarbiturates. The second mechanism has been demonstrated for mephobarbital,[8] whereas the importance of mechanisms 3 and 4 in humans is not known.

The long-acting barbiturate phenobarbital is metabolized quite slowly to *p*-hydroxyphenobarbital. As a consequence, as much as 30% of a dose of phenobarbital in humans may be recovered in the urine. Renal handling of the various barbiturates appears to be glomerular filtration with partial tubular reabsorption. In the case of phenobarbital, excretion of the drug is markedly influenced by the urinary pH. Excretion of the drug is promoted by an alkaline pH.

Factors that influence Many factors have been described that either oppose or potentiate the action of
action the barbiturates, but only a few of these have practical significance.

The various CNS stimulants such as caffeine, strychnine, picrotoxin, pentylenetetrazol, and bemegride (β,β-methylethylglutarimide; Megimide) tend to oppose the action of the barbiturates, particularly when they are administered at about the same time. This antagonism does not have the same specificity as the well-known antagonism of nalorphine and morphine. In severe, prolonged barbiturate anesthesia the antidotal action of the CNS stimulants is weak.

With the exception of the stimulants, the only procedures that may shorten the action of the barbiturates are those that promote the removal of the drug from the body. Alkalinization of the urine promotes excretion of phenobarbital but cannot be expected to be effective in the case of the short-acting and intermediate-acting compounds, since their pK′ is higher.

The action of the barbiturates is intensified by several factors. These can be divided into two categories: factors that interfere with the metabolism or excretion of the barbiturates and drugs that exert synergistic effects with the barbiturates on the CNS.

Factors that interfere with metabolism or excretion of barbiturates. Liver and kidney diseases may intensify the action of the barbiturates by interfering with their metabolism or excretion. The side chain oxidation of the barbiturates is carried out in the liver microsomes. The factor of safety must be great, however, since degradation of the barbiturates proceeds quite adequately even in patients with cirrhosis. Kidney disease is expected to prolong the half-life of those barbiturates normally excreted in the urine. In uremia the toxicity of the barbiturates is increased out of proportion to the deficient clearance of the drugs by the kidney; the mechanisms are not clear.

Drugs that inhibit the hepatic microsomal enzymes interfere with the metabolism of barbiturates. An experimental preparation, SKF-525 A, the propyl derivative of adiphenine (Trasentine), is a powerful inhibitor of microsomal enzymes. Some MAO inhibitors have an additional effect on microsomal enzymes and prolong the action of barbiturates.

Drugs that intensify the action of barbiturates. Alcohol, reserpine, the phenothiazine tranquilizers, other sedative-hypnotics, and many other drugs may intensify the actions of the barbiturates. For this reason it is inadvisable to administer drugs in combination with barbiturates without considering possible drug interactions. Another reason is the capacity of some barbiturates (phenobarbital, for example) to accelerate the metabolism of a variety of drugs by enzyme induction in the hepatic microsomes (p. 38).

Toxicity

The barbiturates are safe and effective drugs when administered in hypnotic doses to normal persons. Untoward effects may arise in an occasional person as unexplained idiosyncrasies or in all persons as a result of acute or chronic overdosage. Barbiturates are strictly contraindicated in porphyria, since they may produce severe toxic effects, even paralysis.[61]

A few persons, particularly elderly persons, may exhibit idiosyncratic excitement instead of depression following the use of the barbiturates. A few may also show skin reactions, vague pains and aches, and gastrointestinal symptoms. The incidence of these unusual responses is extraordinarily low.

Acute barbiturate poisoning

Barbiturate poisoning is one of the most common problems in toxicology. The intake of large doses of barbiturates may be intentional in suicide or it may be accidental.

The cause of death in acute, overwhelming barbiturate poisoning is undoubtedly cessation of respiration as a consequence of depression of the respiratory center. If the ingested dose is not quite lethal or absorption from the gastrointestinal tract is delayed, the individual may survive for many hours or days. Under these conditions he will often be comatose, with respiration slow, skin and mucous membranes cyanotic, and various reflexes diminished or absent. Body temperature will be low, blood pressure may be diminished, and pupils may be somewhat constricted and may or may not respond to light.

Although respiratory depression is the primary cause of death in acute, overwhelming barbiturate poisoning, other factors may contribute to lethality if the patient does not succumb in the first few hours. Impairment of circulation, hypostatic pneumonia, and perhaps unknown mechanisms may still cause death even if adequate oxygenation is ensured.

Treatment. Maintenance of adequate respiration and circulation should be the most important objectives in the treatment of acute poisoning. In addition, efforts at eliminating the drug may contribute to recovery. Such efforts include the administration of osmotic diuretics such as mannitol or hemodialysis and in phenobarbital poisoning the administration of sodium bicarbonate to produce an alkaline urine.

Alkalinization of the urine in the case of phenobarbital is based on a sound principle that has been confirmed by animal experiments. The pK_a of phenobarbital is 7.3. At a urinary pH of 8, achievable with bicarbonate administration, 86% of the phenobarbital in the renal tubular fluid becomes ionized and 14% nonionized. It will be recalled (p. 25) that it is the ionized fraction that escapes tubular reabsorption. The reason for the ineffectiveness of alkalinization in promoting the urinary excretion of other commonly used barbiturates becomes obvious by examining their acid dissociation constants. The pK_a of pentobarbital is 8.1. Even if the urinary pH is brought to 8 with bicarbonate, as much as 44% of the drug would still be un-ionized and thus reabsorbable by the tubules.

The experimental administration of CNS stimulants in the early stages of poisoning can protect animals against an otherwise lethal dose of barbiturates. Artificial respiration will do the same by reversing the adverse effects of hypoxia and hypercapnia. Although CNS stimulants were widely used at one time in the treatment of barbiturate poisoning, they have fallen into disfavor as compared with the physiological approach first promoted by a Danish group of investigators.[46] Excessive use of CNS stimulants can lead to secondary depression of respiration and aggravation of the clinical state of the poisoned individual. There are no specific pharmacological antagonists for sedative-hypnotic drugs.

According to the best current evidence, supportive therapy with early gastric aspiration and efforts at elimination of the drug from the body are more rewarding than "desperate efforts at arousal."[43]

Psychic and physiological dependence

The barbiturates are unquestionably habit-forming. Some individuals who perhaps unnecessarily become accustomed to taking one of these drugs at bedtime may find it difficult to give up the habit and may develop some craving for the drug. For many years it was assumed that chronic habituation to the barbiturates was an unimportant problem when compared with the chronic use of the morphine type of narcotics. It is now generally accepted that chronic administration of large doses of barbiturates results in serious withdrawal symptoms in both humans and animals.[25] The manifestations of withdrawal consist of anxiety, tremors, occasional convulsive phenomena, and craving for the barbiturate.

The most important principle in the medical management of the barbiturate addict is gradual withdrawal of the drug. Sudden withdrawal can produce marked excitement and even convulsions.

The tolerance to barbiturates that develops with their chronic use is not nearly so great as the tolerance to morphine and similar narcotics. Most barbiturate addicts ingest about 10 to 15 hypnotic doses, or 1 to 1.5 g of the drug in 24 hours, whereas the morphine addict may take a hundred times the usual therapeutic dose of morphine. Tolerance to the lethal effect of the barbiturates is probably not very great in the addict, whereas the morphine addict is resistant to many lethal doses of the narcotic.

NONBARBITURATE SEDATIVE-HYPNOTICS

Although the barbiturates are quite satisfactory as sedative-hypnotics, a large variety of other drugs are available for essentially the same indications. Some (chloral hydrate, for example) are old but still quite useful medications. Others, introduced more recently for competitive reasons, have few, if any, advantages over the barbiturates.

Bromides and ethanol also belong to the sedative-hypnotic group of drugs. Both are obsolete as therapeutic agents but are of interest because of their toxicology, basic mechanisms of action, and (at least in the case of ethanol) widespread abuse. A classification of sedative-hypnotic drugs follows:

Alcohols
   Tertiary alcohols
      Ethchlorvynol (Placidyl)
      Methylparafynol (Dormison)
   Other alcohols
      Ethanol
      Trichloroethanol
      Phenaglycodol (Ultran)
   Piperidinediones
      Methyprylon (Noludar)
      Glutethimide (Doriden)
      Thalidomide

Carbamates
   Urethan
   Ethinamate (Valmid)
Chloral hydrate and related drugs
   Chloral hydrate
   Petrichloral (Perichlor)
   Chloral betaine (Beta-Chlor)
Cylic ether
   Paraldehyde
Bromides
Miscellaneous sedative-hypnotics
   Methaqualone (Quaalude)
   Flurazepam (Dalmane)

Alcohols
Tertiary alcohols

The structural formulas of **ethchlorvynol** (Placidyl) and **methylparafynol** (Dormison) follow.

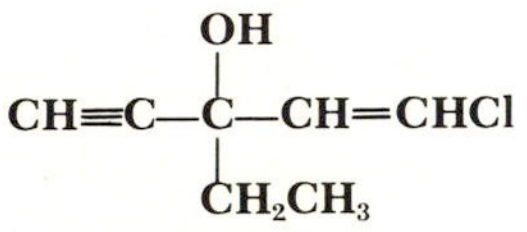

Ethchlorvynol 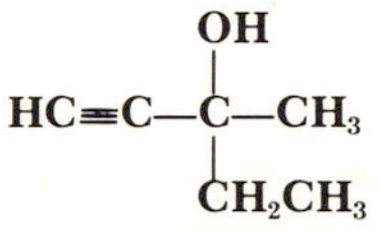   Methylparafynol

Ethchlorvynol induces sleep rapidly when administered in doses of 0.3 to 0.5 g. Its duration of action is similar to that of secobarbital, although it has considerably less potency. In insomnia as much as 1 g may have to be administered for a satisfactory result.

Methylparafynol is so weak that it seldom deserves consideration as a hypnotic.

Other alcohols

Ethanol is undoubtedly the most widely used sedative, although it is not commonly prescribed by physicians. Its pharmacology will be discussed at the end of this chapter.

Trichloroethanol is a metabolic product of chloral hydrate and will be discussed in relation to the action of that hypnotic (p. 315).

Phenaglycodol (Ultran) is a sedative related structurally and in its pharmacology to meprobamate. Phenaglycodol is a derivative of butanediol, whereas meprobamate and its congeners are derivatives of propanediol. The drug is used as a sedative in the form of capsules (300 mg) and tablets (200 mg), which may be administered to an adult three times a day.

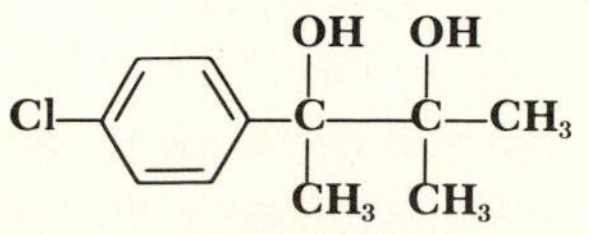

Phenaglycodol

Piperidinediones   The two widely used piperidinedione hypnotics, **methyprylon** (Noludar) and **glutethimide** (Doriden), are structurally related to the barbiturates, with few if any advantages over the older drugs. Methyprylon is used much the same way as pentobarbital or secobarbital. The usual adult dose is one capsule (300 mg) or one to two tablets (200 mg per tablet).

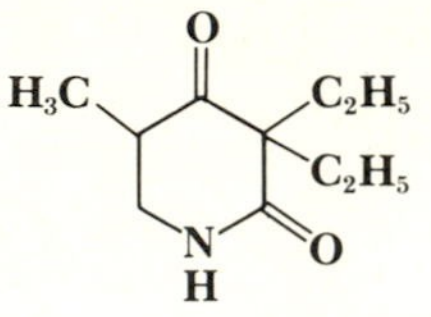

Methyprylon 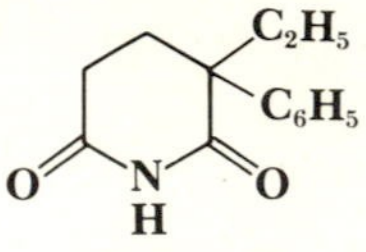   Glutethimide

Glutethimide is similar in its clinical uses to a moderately long-acting barbiturate. In its toxicology it has some unusual features. In glutethimide intoxication the pupils may be widely dilated; the patient may go into coma many hours after return to consciousness and may die unexpectedly. It has been suggested that very slow absorption from the intestine may be responsible for the irregular course of glutethimide intoxication. Laryngospasm and convulsions are other unusual features. In addition to these disadvantages, hemodialysis is of only limited usefulness in the treatment of glutethimide poisoning. Glutethimide is just as addictive as the barbiturates, and sudden withdrawal may lead to convulsions. It is difficult to see what advantages this nonbarbiturate hypnotic could have over the barbiturates. Glutethimide is available in the form of tablets and capsules, and the usual adult dose for insomnia is 0.5 g.

The piperidinedione hypnotic **thalidomide** was responsible for the birth of thousands of children with disastrous defects such as absence of limbs. This occurred especially in Germany. Pregnant women ingesting a single hypnotic dose of the drug between the twenty-fourth and thirty-sixth day of their pregnancy have delivered severely deformed babies. Although the potent teratogenic action of the drug precludes its clinical use, its pharmacology is quite remarkable. Despite its hypnotic potency, which is similar to that of the barbiturates, its acute toxicity is so low that it would be almost impossible to commit suicide by taking the drug. Except for its teratogenic action, thalidomide is almost an ideal hypnotic. Elucidation of its basic mechanism of action would probably contribute to the understanding of the chemical basis of sleep.

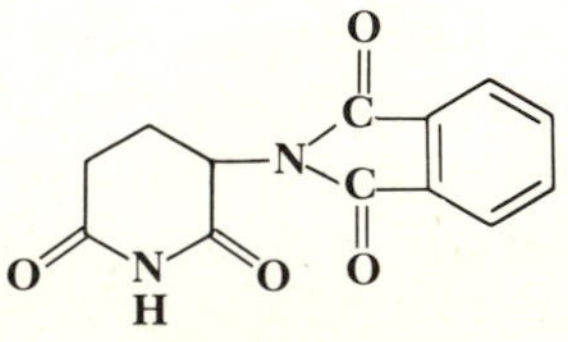

Thalidomide

It is believed that the teratogenic action of thalidomide is mediated by some of its metabolites, among which phthalyglutamic acid and its decarboxylated derivative may play an important role. Interference with glutamic acid metabolism is an interesting possibility.

The thalidomide disaster stimulated the adoption of strict regulations in the testing of new drugs in the United States. It also called attention to the teratogenic potential of other drugs when used during pregnancy. The common antiemetic antihistaminic drugs such as cyclizine must now carry a warning of their possible teratogenicity as demonstrated in rat experiments. Also, physicians are becoming cautious in the use of almost any drug during the first trimester of pregnancy.

Carbamates

Carbamic acid esters of various alcohols have sedative and hypnotic properties. Ethyl carbamate, or **urethan,** is a weak hypnotic used as an injectable anesthetic in animals only. Although it is obsolete as a hypnotic in medicine, it exerts some antineoplastic effect (p. 588 in the fifth edition).

Several of the carbamates are used as mild sedatives, hypnotics, and muscle relaxants. **Ethinamate** (Valmid) is a short-acting sedative hypnotic. Available in 0.5 g tablets, the drug is administered in doses of one to two tablets.

A number of dicarbamates such as meprobamate (Miltown; Equanil) and related drugs are viewed by the medical profession as "minor tranquilizers" or antianxiety drugs rather than ordinary mild sedatives. These drugs are discussed in Chapter 24.

Chloral hydrate and related drugs

Chloral hydrate is an old but still useful hypnotic. It is often prescribed for elderly patients who may show idiosyncratic reactions to the barbiturates. It is metabolically altered in the tissues to trichloroethanol.[6] Since this compound is also effective as a hypnotic, it is quite likely that much of the hypnotic action of chloral hydrate may be mediated by this metabolic product.[6] Some of the drug is oxidized also to trichloroacetic acid. Trichloroethanol is excreted as the glucuronide. It gives a false positive reaction for glucose in the urine by reducing Fehling's solution or similar alkaline copper reagents.

$$Cl_3C-\underset{\underset{\textstyle OH}{|}}{C}HOH$$

Chloral hydrate

Chloral hydrate is administered to adults in the usual dosage of 1 g. It causes some gastric irritation in the concentrated form. When diluted in some flavored solution, it is less irritating but still not as convenient to take as the barbiturates. The drug produces refreshing sleep, usually for 4 to 8 hours.

The toxicity of chloral hydrate is low but is increased by the simultaneous administration of alcohol. This is the basis of "knockout drops." The lethal dose of the drug is quite variable but probably lies between 3 and 30 g. It is likely that heart disease or impaired detoxication may account for the wide variation in the lethal dose of chloral hydrate. Although ordinary hypnotic doses have no demonstrable adverse effect on the heart, overdosage may affect the cardiac muscle and should be avoided in patients suffering from heart disease.

The main disadvantage of chloral hydrate as compared with the barbiturates is gastric irritation and its characteristic odor. To avoid these disadvantages, preparations have been created that can be administered in tablet form, chloral hydrate being released from these tablets in the gastric juice.

Perichloral (Perichlor) is a combination of chloral and pentaerythritol, from which the hypnotic is released slowly in the stomach. It is claimed that the combination causes less gastric irritation than does chloral hydrate. The hypnotic dose of petrichloral is 0.3 to 0.6 g for adults.

Chloral betaine (Beta-Chlor) is a combination of chloral and betaine. It is available in stable, tasteless tablets. In the tablet form, 870 mg of the complex is equivalent to 500 mg of chloral hydrate. The complex is absorbed as such from the gastrointestinal tract and is hydrolyzed in the tissues. The hypnotic dose of chloral betaine is one of two tablets for adults, which is equivalent to 0.5 to 1 g of chloral hydrate. It is claimed that the betaine complex causes less gastric irritation than chloral hydrate alone.

Cyclic ether   **Paraldehyde,** a cyclic ether obtained through the polymerization of acetaldehyde, is an effective hypnotic with limited usefulness because of its offensive odor. It is unique among the hypnotics in that a significant fraction of the administered dose is excreted through the lungs. The remainder is metabolized through the stage of acetaldehyde. Drugs that block the oxidation of acetaldehyde, such as disulfiram, elicit severe reactions when paraldehyde is ingested.

Paraldehyde is administered orally, usually in a cold beverage to disguise its taste. A dose of 4 to 8 ml is sufficient to facilitate sleep. Its use is restricted almost entirely to the management of hospitalized patients undergoing alcohol withdrawal and convulsive states such as eclampsia or tetanus. It is sometimes employed in patients with renal shutdown, since as much as 28% of the drug administered may be eliminated through the pulmonary route and the remainder is metabolized to carbon dioxide and water.

Paraldehyde may be injected by the intramuscular route, although it is quite damaging to tissues at the site of injection. Intravenous use of the drug has resulted in fatalities and should be avoided. Paraldehyde is well absorbed following rectal administration. When administered rectally, the drug is often dissolved in 2 or 3 parts of olive oil.

The lethal dose of paraldehyde is quite variable, depending on the route of administration and other factors. As little as 12 to 24 ml of the drug administered rectally has caused death, whereas doses as high as 100 ml have been given to some patients with ultimate recovery. Liver damage increases the toxicity of paraldehyde, probably because of delayed metabolic transformation. For the same reason the drug should not be prescribed for any patient who is taking disulfiram.

The bromide ion exerts a sedative and antiepileptic effect. Until recently it has been widely utilized in medicine and by the laity. With recognition of the dangers of chronic bromide intoxication and the cumulative action of the drug and with the development of much more effective sedatives and antiepileptic drugs, the modern physician finds few uses for bromides.

Bromides

The administration of 2 to 5 g of sodium bromide or other bromide salt produces sedation, drowsiness, and sleep. The mechanism whereby this halide influences the CNS is mysterious. Since the body does not easily distinguish the bromide from the chloride ion, it is suspected that the replacement of brain chloride by bromide may alter the functions of nerve cells. Chronic administration of several grams of bromide tends to produce mental depression, confusion, and lethargy.

Pharmacological effects

Bromide is the oldest antiepileptic drug, having been introduced for this purpose in 1857 by Charles Locock.

When a bromide is ingested, it becomes distributed in the body in a manner very similar to that of chloride. Bromide remains largely extracellular, with the exception of the red cell, which normally contains a high concentration of chloride.

Metabolism

If administration of bromide is stopped, considerable time is required to rid the body of the drug. Large amounts of chloride given to such a patient will accelerate the elimination of bromide because the total daily halide excretion will be increased.

Mental and neurological symptoms are most prominent, and it is important for the physician to consider the possibility of chronic bromide intoxication in the differential diagnosis of confused and lethargic patients.

Toxicity

In addition, various skin lesions, gastrointestinal disturbances, and involvement of the mucous membranes of the eyes and respiratory passages are not uncommon in bromide intoxication.

Many of the "minor tranquilizers" and "antianxiety agents" are difficult to distinguish from the sedative-hypnotic class of drugs from the standpoint of clinical pharmacology, although sophisticated neurophysiological and behavioral experiments performed in animals do reveal some differences.

Miscellaneous sedative-hypnotics

Some of the antihistaminic drugs exert considerable sedative-hypnotic effects, and they are promoted as sleep-inducing medications in over-the-counter products. One such antihistaminic, doxylamine, has proved effective as a hypnotic in a controlled clinical trial.[56] In doses of 25 and 50 mg the drug performed better than a 100 mg dose of secobarbital but was somewhat inferior to a dose of 200 mg secobarbital. The pharmacology of the antihistaminics is discussed in Chapter 20.

Methaqualone (Quaalude), a relatively new hypnotic, is similar in action to the barbiturates. It has no proved advantages except in patients who show idiosyncratic reactions to the barbiturates. Chemically, methaqualone is 2-methyl-3-*o*-tolyl-4(3H) quinazolone. It is available in 150 mg tablets, and the dose for adults is 150 to 300 mg given at bedtime.

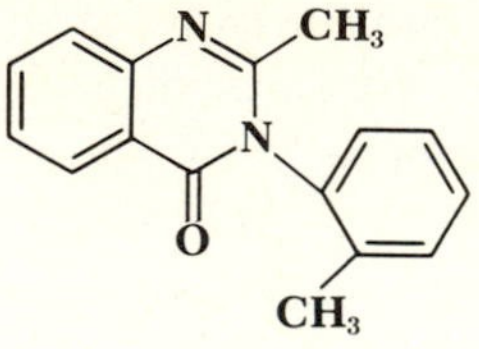

Methaqualone

Flurazepam is structurally related to the benzodiazepines, such as chlordiazepoxide (Librium). It has certain definite advantages, so much so that some clinical pharmacologists are beginning to refer to the barbiturates as "archaic . . . hypnotics."[74] Although this conclusion may be premature, flurazepam has some impressive properties as a hypnotic.

Flurazepam is an effective hypnotic. It has the following advantages over the barbiturates:

1. It leaves the REM sleep relatively intact.
2. Hepatic microsomal enzymes are not induced by the drug.
3. Flurazepam has a low addiction potential.
4. The drug has a high therapeutic index, and fatal poisoning is unlikely.

Although psychic and physical dependence can develop to flurazepam and several minor adverse effects have been reported following its use, the drug is a remarkably safe and effective hypnotic. The adult dose is 15 to 30 mg.

Flurazepam hydrochloride (Dalmane) is available in capsules, 15 and 30 mg.

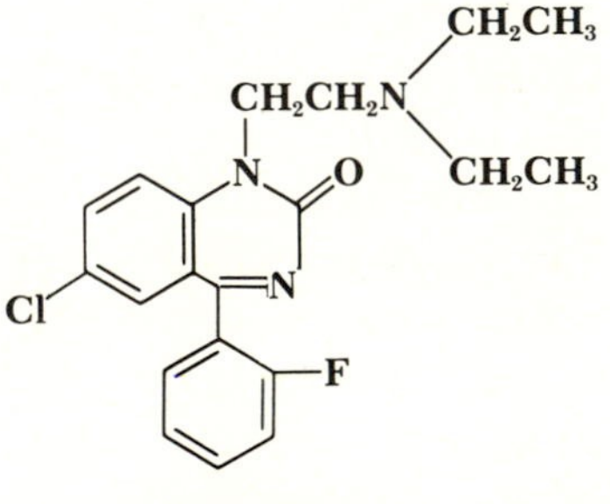

Flurazepam

CLINICAL PHARMACOLOGY OF HYPNOTICS   The safe and effective use of hypnotics requires the application of certain simple pharmacological principles.[34]

1. Hypnotics should be used only if obvious causes of insomnia such as painful conditions or too much coffee have been eliminated. The drugs should be used only when necessary and in doses as low as possible.

2. Inability to go to sleep is somewhat different from difficulty in staying asleep, the latter being the more common problem. A few minutes' delay in going to sleep should not require sleep medications, all of which are habit-forming.

3. Although there are differences in the onset of action of the various hypnotics, these differences are of little practical significance. Liquid preparations of chloral hydrate, paraldehyde, or elixirs of the barbiturates act rapidly but are inconvenient to use. Capsules of secobarbital, pentobarbital, and chloral hydrate act quite rapidly, whereas phenobarbital may have a somewhat delayed effect.

4. The duration of action of the various hypnotics has received much attention in pharmacology and in drug promotion, but the rigid classifications of "short acting," "medium acting," and "long acting" are not very important in actual practice (p. 304). It should be remembered that duration of action is greatly influenced by dose. Nevertheless, it is traditional to look on secobarbital, pentobarbital, chloral hydrate, paraldehyde, and methyprylon as short-acting hypnotics; amobarbital and glutethimide as intermediate-acting hypnotics; and phenobarbital as long-acting hypnotics. The antianxiety agents are also employed as hypnotics, with the meprobamate-type drugs being intermediate-acting and the benzodiazepines such as flurazepam behaving as long-acting sedative-hypnotics.

5. The hypnotic dose of a drug varies greatly in different individuals and should be adjusted carefully. On the other hand, liver disease and moderate impairment of renal function do not greatly influence the duration of action of hypnotics. Other sedative-hypnotics, tranquilizers, or alcohol do modify the dose and duration of action of sleep-producing medications. Sudden withdrawal of all such drugs is dangerous.

6. Habituation, addiction, and the dangers of sudden withdrawal are greater hazards than direct toxic effects when sedative-hypnotics are properly used in therapeutics.

ALCOHOL

As a therapeutic agent, alcohol is only of moderate importance. Alcohol has great toxicological interest, however, and chronic alcoholism is one of the great social problems of mankind.

Pharmacological effects

The main action of alcohol is exerted on the CNS. It may be looked on as an unusual hypnotic and anesthetic. There is general agreement that the apparent stimulant action of the drug is a consequence of primary depression of the higher centers, resulting in uninhibited behavior.

In addition to its action on behavior and consciousness, alcohol influences cardiovascular, gastrointestinal, and renal functions.

Cutaneous vasodilation and a feeling of warmth are generally observed following the ingestion of an alcoholic beverage. This vasodilation is not a direct effect of the drug on blood vessels but is a consequence of its CNS actions. There is a popular impression that alcohol dilates the coronary vessels, but it has been shown that alcohol does not prevent the electrocardiographic evidences of coronary insufficiency following exercise tolerance.[54] Alcohol may lessen precordial pain, but this action is likely to be exerted on the brain rather than on the coronary vessels. Adverse myocardial responses to alcohol have been demonstrated in animal experiments.[50]

The ingestion of alcohol promotes the secretion of acid gastric juice. It has been postulated that this action may be mediated through the release of histamine or gastrin in the stomach wall.[64]

The diuresis observed in persons who drink alcoholic beverages is partly caused by the ingestion of water. Inhibition of the release of antidiuretic hormone from the posterior pituitary lobe by alcohol has also been demonstrated.

Metabolism

Ingested alcohol is absorbed rapidly from the stomach and the small intestine. The rate of absorption is influenced by the concentration of the alcohol ingested and most importantly by the presence of food in the stomach. On an empty stomach the drinking of an alcoholic beverage produces peak blood levels in less than 1 hour. There may be considerable delay if the stomach is filled with food.

Once absorbed, alcohol is distributed in total body water. The concentration of alcohol in different tissues and body fluids correlates well with the concentration of water at these sites. If the concentration of alcohol in blood is assigned the value of 1.0, the relative values given in Table 26-4 may be expected in the various body fluids, tissues, and alveolar air.

The concentration of alcohol in the blood has great medicolegal importance since it is generally accepted that a blood level of alcohol of 150 mg/100 ml may be taken as evidence that the person is drunk. It is of some importance to know also the relationship between the quantities of alcohol ingested and the blood levels that may be expected. The concentration of alcohol in the blood will depend on the following factors: (1) quantity of alcohol ingested and rate at which it is drunk, (2) speed of absorption, (3) body weight and the percentage of total body water, and (4) rate of metabolism of alcohol.

The blood levels of alcohol that may be expected following the ingestion of various alcoholic beverages may be calculated.[21] Since intoxication occurs when a blood level of 150 mg of alcohol/100 ml of blood is reached (0.15%), it can be calculated that this will occur if approximately 8 fluid ounces of a distilled spirit containing 45% alcohol is drunk rapidly. If a distilled spirit is drunk over a period of several hours, the number of ounces required for producing a blood level of 0.15% may be calculated by the following formula: 8 + H = Number of ounces of distilled spirits re-

TABLE 26-4. Relative concentration of alcohol in various body fluids, tissues, and alveolar air (concentration in blood is 1.0)

Serum	1.15
Urine	1.3
Saliva	1.3
Spinal fluid	1.15
Brain or liver	0.85 to 0.90
Kidney	0.83
Alveolar air	0.0005 of blood concentration[75a]

quired to cause intoxication, where H is the number of hours during which the beverage is drunk.

The corresponding formula for fortified wine (containing 20% alcohol) is 18 + 2H; for ordinary wine (containing 10% alcohol) it is 36 + 4H; for beer (containing 4.5% alcohol) the figure would be 80 + 10H.

The relationships between the ingestion of various beverages, blood levels of alcohol, and prognosis in terms of ability in driving an automobile are shown in Fig. 26-2.

Elimination   The quantity of alcohol excreted in the urine, exhaled through the lungs, or lost in the perspiration ordinarily represents less than 10% of the total ingested. The remainder is metabolized; the end products are carbon dioxide and water.

The steps in the metabolism of alcohol appear to be as shown on p. 322.[28]

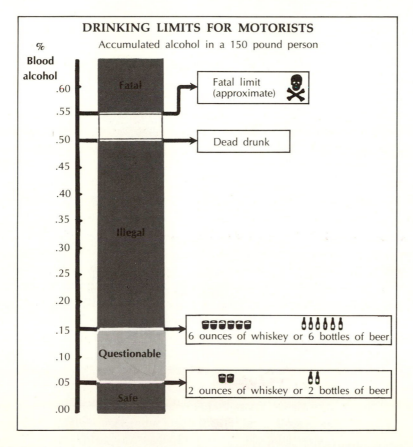

FIG. 26-2. Level of alcohol in blood of an automobile driver relative to his being "under the influence." (From Harger, R. N. In Economos, J. P., and Kreml, F. M., editors: Judge and prosecutor in traffic court, Chicago, 1951, American Bar Association and The Traffic Institute, Northwestern University.)

The liver plays an important role in the metabolic transformation of alcohol. The first step occurs almost entirely in the liver.

The average person metabolizes 6 to 8 g (7.5 to 10 ml) of alcohol per hour. This figure is fairly constant for a given individual and is independent of the quantity present in the body. Habitual drinkers may metabolize alcohol slightly more rapidly than abstainers.[16]

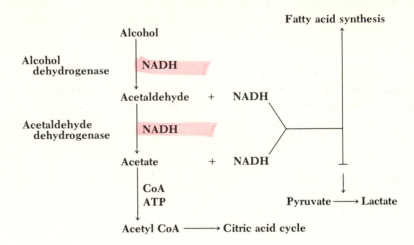

It has been claimed that the administration of glucose and insulin, various vitamins, dinitrophenol, and muscular exercise accelerate the metabolism. However, most of these claims have been denied.

The metabolism of 1 g of alcohol yields 7 calories. Since the maximal amount that can be metabolized in 24 hours is approximately 170 g, it may be calculated that alcohol can contribute up to 1200 calories per day to the metabolic requirements of an individual.

Metabolic effects   The influence of alcohol on carbohydrate and lipid metabolism has received much attention in recent years. Hypoglycemia can be induced in humans by the ingestion of 35 to 50 ml of ethanol after a 2-day fast. Such individuals must have low liver glycogen because they do not respond to glucagon with the characteristic increase in blood glucose.[13] Animal studies indicate that alcohol can inhibit glycogen synthesis, probably by interfering with glyconeogenesis from amino acids.

It is quite likely that acute hyperlipemia following alcohol ingestion and the hyperlipemia of the chronic alcoholic have different mechanisms. The acute hyperlipemia is probably mediated through sympathetic activation, norepinephrine release, and lipolysis from fat depots. This effect of norepinephrine can be prevented by β-adrenergic blocking agents. On the other hand, hyperlipemia in the chronic alcoholic may depend to a large extent on deficient removal of lipid from the blood. Evidence for decreased lipoprotein lipase activity in alcoholic patients has been presented.[36]

Fatty livers are commonly observed in alcoholic patients. The most likely explanations would appear to be (1) increased mobilization from fat depots, (2) increased esterification to triglycerides rather than to phospholipids and cholesterol esters, and (3) decreased triglyceride release from the liver.

Tolerance and addiction

It is commonly known that the experienced drinker shows fewer and less marked effects from moderate amounts of alcohol than does the abstainer. This moderate tolerance cannot be explained on the basis of what is known about absorption, distribution, and metabolism in the chronic alcoholic. It is concluded, therefore, that the experienced drinker has learned to behave and to perform habitual tasks at blood alcohol levels that would seriously disturb the unaccustomed individual. This apparent tolerance probably does not extend to the lethal effect of alcohol, and blood levels exceeding 550 mg/100 ml may produce death in the chronic alcoholic.

The severely intoxicated patient represents a medical emergency and should be managed according to the following recommendations[77]:

1. Respiratory support should be given if necessary.
2. Aspiration of vomitus should be prevented by placing the patient in semi-lateral decubitus position with head forward and mouth down.
3. Fluid needs should be assessed. The patient may be fluid overloaded or may have fluid deficits.
4. Gastric lavage can be helpful.
5. Hypoglycemia is suspected on the basis of unusual neurological findings, such as convulsions or coma. Intravenous glucose and intramuscular thiamine are recommended.
6. Metabolic acidosis, if severe, may require the use of sodium bicarbonate.
7. Hemodialysis may be useful in patients with excessive blood levels of alcohol.
8. Fructose and other measures that supposedly increase the rate of metabolism of alcohol are not recommended.

In alcohol withdrawal, magnesium replacement is often indicated. Intramuscular magnesium sulfate in 2 ml doses of a 50% solution may be given three times a day for 2 days. The benzodiazepines—chlordiazepoxide and diazepam—are commonly used, but their prolonged use can lead to a secondary abstinence syndrome.[77] Propranolol has a favorable effect on alcoholic tremor, but its usefulness in alcohol withdrawal has not been established.

The blood alcohol levels that may be lethal are usually in excess of 0.5% or 500 mg/100 ml. If the person has taken some other CNS depressant such as a barbiturate, even lower blood alcohol levels may result in a lethal outcome.

Chronic alcoholism

A variety of pathological changes occur in the alcoholic with much greater frequency than in the general population. Chronic gastritis, cirrhosis of the liver, and the neuropsychiatric condition known as Korsakoff's syndrome have received considerable attention. The mechanism of production of these abnormalities is difficult to state because the chronic alcoholic often suffers from nutritional deficiencies also. When benefited by psychiatric treatment or the organization known as Alcoholics Anonymous, about 50% of chronic alcoholics may be able to abstain from drinking.

Another approach to the problem has been the administration of drugs that will make the effects of alcohol extremely unpleasant or even dangerous. The best known of these is disulfiram.

Disulfiram. The development of the disulfiram approach (Antabuse) to chronic alcoholism was the consequence of a chance observation.[23] While testing certain new drugs as potential anthelmintics, it was observed that following ingestion of tetraethylthiuram disulfide even a few bottles of beer caused very unpleasant side effects. Careful study of this unusual occurrence led to the discovery of the probable mechanism involved and to the eventual introduction of disulfiram into therapeutics.

From a chemical standpoint, disulfiram is tetraethylthiuram disulfide. Certain other disulfides have similar properties with respect to alcohol intolerance.

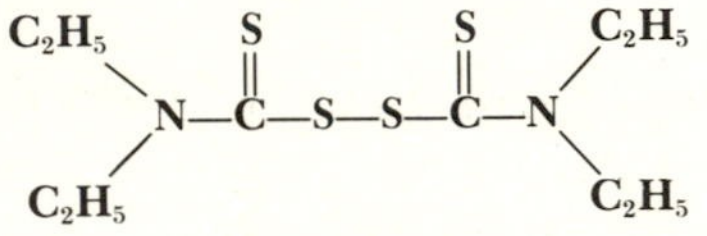

Disulfiram

If alcohol is ingested several hours after taking disulfiram in doses of 1 to 2 g, the individual develops the typical reaction characterized by nausea, vomiting, flushing, palpitation, and headache. There may be lowering of the blood pressure, even to shock levels. These symptoms are so unpleasant that the patient simply cannot drink alcohol while on a maintenance dose of 0.25 to 0.5 g of disulfiram. Even when the drug administration is stopped, it may take a week before the alcohol intolerance disappears. Disulfiram by itself can cause some effects. Dizziness, metallic taste, reduced sexual potency, electroencephalographic changes, and skin reactions have occurred following its use.

It seems reasonable to assume that disulfiram interferes with the metabolism of alcohol, resulting in the accumulation of some toxic intermediate. Indeed, it has been demonstrated that acetaldehyde accumulates in the blood when the patient ingests alcohol while taking disulfiram.[28] Blood acetaldehyde levels under these conditions may be of the order of 1 mg/100 ml. It has also been demonstrated that the intravenous infusion of acetaldehyde, which would produce comparable blood levels, reproduces the manifestations of the "Antabuse reaction." It has also been demonstrated in experimental animals that the administration of disulfiram delays the metabolism of administered acetaldehyde.

On the basis of these facts it may be concluded that disulfiram inhibits the second step in alcohol metabolism: the further utilization of acetaldehyde. This intermediate is a very potent pharmacological agent with vasopressor and vasodepressor properties.

Acetaldehyde apparently can cause the release of catecholamines from the tissues and thus behaves as an indirect-acting sympathomimetic drug.[60] It is quite likely that it releases other amines also, which may account for the symptoms of the "Antabuse reaction."

Disulfiram is usually administered in a dosage of 1 to 2 g the first day, the quantity administered being gradually decreased in 4 days to about 0.5 g, but it may be even further reduced to 0.25 g as a maintenance dose.

Other drugs that create intolerance to alcohol and may elicit an "Antabuse reaction" include the hypoglycemic sulfonylureas, such as **tolbutamide** (Orinase) and **chlorpropamide** (Diabinese); and the antimicrobials, such as **chloramphenicol, furazolidone** (Furoxone), **griseofulvin** (Fulvicin), **isoniazid, metronidazole** (Flagyl), and **quinacrine** (Atabrine).

OTHER ALCOHOLS

The aliphatic alcohols other than ethyl alcohol are of interest in medicine largely because they are sometimes involved in cases of poisoning.

Methanol

Generally the toxicity of the alcohols increases with the chain length. An exception to this statement is methyl alcohol, which is unique in producing marked acidosis and blindness in primates but not in lower animals. As little as 30 ml of methanol has caused serious poisoning, and even death has been attributed to this quantity or even less. In addition to the acidosis, methanol intoxication involves the CNS, with the production of headache, dizziness, delirium, and coma. Blindness, which is a common accompaniment of these effects, may be total or partial.

Although methanol is metabolized in part to formaldehyde and formic acid, the amount of the latter is not sufficient to explain the profound metabolic acidosis that may result from ingestion of relatively small quantities of the alcohol. Blindness is probably a consequence of the toxic effects of formaldehyde on the retina. Interference with adenosine triphosphate generation by uncoupling of oxidation phosphorylation has been postulated.[11]

Metabolism of methyl alcohol in the body is much slower than that of ethyl alcohol, a fact that further complicates the management of methanol poisoning. The treatment of methanol poisoning is based largely on the correction of the acidotic state with appropriate intravenous fluids. Another approach is based on the observation that ethanol delays the metabolic transformation of methanol.[52] Although some investigators favor the use of ethanol in treating methanol poisoning, it must be kept in mind that correction of the acidotic state with sodium bicarbonate given orally or intravenously (500 ml of a 5% solution) is the most important therapeutic procedure.

Isopropyl alcohol

Isopropyl alcohol has some toxicological interest also. It is metabolized to acetone in the body. Severe renal damage is found in patients who have recovered from ingestion of a few ounces of isopropyl alcohol. The fatal dose is estimated as 120 to 240 ml.

REFERENCES

1 Anton, A. H.: Ethanol and urinary catecholamines in man, Clin. Pharmacol. Ther. **6**:462, 1965.

2 Beecher, H. K., and Moyer, C. A.: Mechanisms of respiratory failure under barbiturate anesthesia (Evipal, Pentothal), J. Clin. Invest. **20**:549, 1952.

3 Brodie, B. B., Burns, J. J., Mark, L. C., Lief, P. A., Bernstein, E., and Papper, E. M.: The fate of pentobarbital in man and dog and a method for its estimation in biological material, J. Pharmacol. Exp. Ther. **109**:26, 1953.

4 Burns, J. J.: Implications of enzyme induction for drug therapy, Am. J. Med. **37**:329, 1964.

5 Bush, M. T.: Sedatives and hypnotics. In Root, W. S., and Hofmann, F. G., editors: Physiological pharmacology, vol. 1, New York, 1963, Academic Press, Inc.

6 Butler, T. C.: The metabolic fate of chloral hydrate, J. Pharmacol. Exp. Ther. **92**:49, 1948.

7 Butler, T. C.: The rate of penetration of barbituric acid derivatives into the brain, J. Pharmacol. Exp. Ther. **100**:219, 1950.

8 Butler T. C.: Quantitative studies of the metabolic fate of mephobarbital (N-methyl phenobarbital), J. Pharmacol. Exp. Ther. **106**:235, 1952.

9 Cares, R. M., Newman, B., and Mauceri, J. C.: Poisoning by methylparafynol (Dormison), Am. J. Clin. Pathol. **23**:129, 1953.

10 Clemmesen, C., and Nilsson, E.: Therapeutic trends in the treatment of barbiturate poisoning: the Scandinavian method, Clin. Pharmacol. Ther. **2**:220, 1961.

11 Cooper, J. R., and Kini, M. M.: Biochemical aspects of methanol poisoning, Biochem, Pharmacol. **2**:405, 1962.

12 Essig, C. F.: Addiction to nonbarbiturate sedative and tranquilizing drugs, Clin. Pharmacol. Ther. **5**:334, 1964.

13 Field, J. B., Williams, H. E., and Mortimore, G. E.: Studies on the mechanism of ethanol-induced hypoglycemia, J. Clin. Invest. **42**:497, 1963.

14 Forney, R. B., and Hughes, F. W.: Combined effects of alcohol and other drugs, Springfield, Ill., 1968, Charles C Thomas, Publisher.

15 Friend, D. G.: Sedative hypnotics, Clin. Pharmacol. Ther. **1**:5, 1960.

16 Goldberg, L.: Quantitative studies on alcohol tolerance in man, Acta Physiol. Scand. **5**(Supp. 16):1, 1943.

17 Goldbert, T. M., Sanz, C. J., Rose, H. D., and Leitschuh, H.: Comparative evaluation of treatments of alcohol withdrawal syndromes, J.A.M.A. **201**:99, 1967.

18 Goldestein, A., and Aranow, L.: The duration of action of thiopental and pentobarbital, J. Pharmacol. Exp. Ther. **128**:1, 1960.

19 Goldstein, A., and Judson, B. A.: Alcohol dependence and opiate dependence: lack of relationship in mice, Science **172**:290, 1971.

20 Goldstein, D. B., and Pal, N.: Alcohol dependence produced in mice by inhalation of ethanol: grading the withdrawal reaction. Science **172**:288, 1971.

21 Greenberg, L. A.: The definition of an intoxicating beverage, Q. J. Stud. Alcohol **16**:316, 1955.

22 Hadden, J., Johnson, K., Smith, S., Price, L., and Giardina, E.: Acute barbiturate intoxication, J.A.M.A. **209**:893, 1969.

23 Hald, M., Jacobsen, E., and Larsen, V.: The sensitizing effect of tetraethyl-thiuram disulfide (Antabuse) to ethyl alcohol, Acta Pharmacol. **4**:285, 1948.

24 Hughes, F. W., and Forney, R. B.: Comparative effect of three antihistaminics and ethanol on mental and motor performance, Clin. Pharmacol. Ther. **5**:414, 1964.

25 Isbell, H., and Faser, H. F.: Addiction to analgesics and barbiturates, Pharmacol. Rev. **2**:355, 1950.

26 Israel, Y., Kalant, H., LeBlanc, E., Bernstein, J. C., and Salazar, I.: Changes in cation transport and (Na + K)-activated adenosine triphosphatase produced by chronic administration of ethanol, J. Pharmacol. Exp. Ther. **174**:330, 1970.

27 Isselbacher, K. J., and Greenberger, N. J.: Metabolic effects of alcohol on the liver, N. Engl. J. Med. **270**:351, 1964.

28 Jacobsen, E.: The metabolism of ethyl alcohol, Pharmacol. Rev. **4**:107, 1952.

29 Jouvet, M.: Neurophysiology of the states of sleep, Physiol. Rev. **47**:117, 1967.

30 Kales, A.: Psychophysiological and biochemical changes following use and withdrawal of hypnotics. In Kales, A., editor: Sleep: physiology and pathology, Philadelphia, 1967, J. B. Lippincott Co.

31 Keplinger, M. L., and Wells, J. A.: The effect of disulfiram on the action and metabolism of paraldehyde, J. Pharmacol. Exp. Ther. **119**:19, 1957.

32 Landauer, A. A., Milner, G., and Patman, J.: Alcohol and amitryptiline effects on skills related to driving behavior, Science 163:1467, 1969.

33 Larrabee, M. G., and Holaday, D. A.: Depression of transmission through sympathetic ganglia during general anthesia, J. Pharmacol. Exp. Ther. 105:400, 1952.

34 Lasagna, L.: The pharmacological basis for the effective use of hypnotics, Pharmacol. Phys. 1(2):1, 1967.

35 Levine, H. A., Gilbert, A. J., and Bodansky, M.: The pulmonary and urinary excretion of paraldehyde in normal dogs and in dogs with liver damage, J. Pharmacol. Exp. Ther. 69:316, 1940.

36 Losowsky, M. S., Jones, D. P., Davidson, C. S., and Lieber, C. S.: Studies of alcoholic hyperlipemia and its mechanism, Am. J. Med. 35:794, 1963.

37 Magoun, H. W.: A neural basis for the anesthetic state. In Symposium on sedative and hypnotic drugs, Baltimore, 1954, The Williams & Wilkins Co.

38 Magoun, H. W.: The waking brain, Springfield, Ill., 1958, Charles C Thomas, Publisher.

39 Maher, J. F., Schreiner, G. E., and Westervelt, F. B.: Acute glutethimide intoxication. I. Clinical experience (twenty-two patients) compared to barbiturate intoxication (sixty-three patients), Am. J. Med. 33:70, 1962.

40 Mardones, J.: The alcohols. In Root, W. S., and Hofmann, F. G., editors: Physiological pharmacology, vol. 1, New York, 1963, Academic Press, Inc.

41 Mark, L. C.: Metabolism of barbiturates in man, Clin. Pharmacol. Ther. 4:504, 1963.

42 Mark, L. C.: Archaic classification of barbiturates: commentary, Clin. Pharmacol. Ther. 10:287, 1969.

43 Mark, L. C., and Papper, E. M.: Changing therapeutic goals in barbiturate poisoning, Pharmacol. Phys. 1(3):1, 1967.

44 Marshall, E. K., Jr., and Owens, A. H., Jr.: Absorption, excretion and metabolic fate of chloral hydrate and trichloroethanol, Bull. Johns Hopkins Hosp. 95:1, 1954.

45 Maxwell, J. M., Cook, L., Davis, G. J., Toner, J. J., and Fellows, E. J.: Effects of β-diethylaminoethyldiphenylpropylacetate hydrochloride (SKF No. 525-A) on a series of hypnotics, Fed. Proc. 12:349, 1953.

46 Nilsson, E.: On treatment of barbiturate poisoning; a modified clinical aspect, Acta Med. Scand. 139(Supp. 253):1, 1951.

47 Oswald, I.: Drugs and sleep, Pharmacol Rev. 20:273, 1968.

48 Owens, A. H., Jr., Marshall, E. K., Jr., Broun, G. O., Jr., Zubrod, C. G., and Lasagna, L.: A comparative evaluation of hypnotic potency of chloral hydrate and trichloroethanol, Bull. Johns Hopkins Hosp. 96:71, 1955.

49 Perlman, P. L., Sutter, D., and Johnson, C. B.: Further studies on the metabolic disposition of Dormison (3-methyl-pentyne-ol-3) in dogs and man, J. Am. Pharmacol. Assoc. 42:750, 1953.

50 Regan, T. J., Koroxenidis, G., Moschos, C. B., Oldewurtel, H. A., Lehan, P. H., and Hellems, H. K.: The acute metabolic and hemodynamic responses of the left ventricle to ethanol, J. Clin. Invest. 45:270, 1966.

51 Riegelman, S., Rowland, M., and Epstein, W. L.: Griseofulvin-phenobarbital interaction in man, J.A.M.A. 213:426, 1970.

52 Roe, O.: The metabolism and toxicity of methanol, Pharmacol. Rev. 7:399, 1955.

53 Rubin, E., and Lieber, C. S.: Alcohol-induced hepatic injury in nonalcoholic volunteers, N. Engl. J. Med. 278:869, 1968.

54 Russek, H. I., Urbach, K. F., and Doerner, A. A.: Choice of a coronary vasodilator in clinical practice, J.A.M.A. 153:207, 1053.

55 Schallek, W., Kuehn, A., and Seppelin, D. K.: Central depressant effects of methyprylon, J. Pharmacol. Exp. Ther. 118:139, 1956.

56 Sessions, J. T., Jr., Minkel, H. P., Bullard, J. C., and Ingelfinger, F. J.: The effect of barbiturates in patients with liver disease, J. Clin. Invest. 33:1116, 1954.

57 Sjoquist, F., and Lasagna, L.: The hypnotic efficacy of doxylamine, Clin. Pharmacol. Ther. 8:48, 1967.

58 Strickler, J. C.: Forced diuresis in the management of barbiturate intoxication, Clin. Pharmacol. Ther. 6:693, 1965.

59 Van Dyke, H. B., and Ames, R. G.: Alcohol diuresis, Acta Endocrinol. 7:110, 1951.

60 Walsh, M. J., Hollander, P. B., and Truitt, E. B., Jr.: Sympathomimetic effects of acetaldehyde on the electrical and contractile characteristics of isolated left atria of guinea pigs, J. Pharmacol. Exp. Ther. 167:173, 1969.

61 Weatherall, M.: Drugs and porphyrin metabolism, Pharmacol. Rev. 6:133, 1954.

62 Webb, W. R., and Degerli, I. U.: Ethyl alcohol and the cardiovascular system, J.A.M.A. 191:1055, 1965.

63 Widmark, E. M. P.: Die theoretischen Grundlagen und die praktische Verwendbarkeit der

gerichtlich-medizinischen Alkoholbestimmung, Berlin, 1932, Urban & Schwarzenberg.

64 Woodward, E. R., Slotten, D. S., and Tillmans, V. C.: Mechanism of alcoholic stimulation of gastric secretion, Proc. Soc. Exp. Biol. Med. **89**:428, 1955.

REVIEWS

65 Becker, C. E., and Scott, R.: The treatment of alcoholism, Ration. Drug Ther. **6**:1, 1972.

66 Bueno, F., and Mezey, E.: Management of alcoholism, Ration. Drug Ther. **10**:1, 1976.

67 Hartmann, E.: Drugs for insomnia, Ration. Drug Ther. **11**:1, 1977.

68 Inaba, D. S., Gay, G. R., Newmeyer, J. A., and Whitehead, C.: Methaqualone abuse, J.A.M.A. **224**:1505, 1973.

69 Ismel, Y.: Cellular effects of alcohol, Q. J. Stud. Alcohol **31**(2):293, 1970.

70 Johns, M. W.: Methods for assessing human sleep, Arch. Intern. Med. **127**:484, 1971.

71 Kales, A., and Kales, J. D.: Evaluation, diagnosis, and treatment of clinical conditions related to sleep, J.A.M.A. **213**:2229, 1970.

72 Kales, A., and Kales, J. D.: Sleep laboratory evaluation of psychoactive drugs, Pharmacol. Phys. **4**(9):1, 1970.

73 Kales, A., and Kales, J. D.: Shortcomings in the evaluation and promotion of hypnotic drugs, N. Engl. J. Med. **293**:826, 1975.

74 Koch-Weser, J., and Greenblatt, D. J.: The archaic barbiturate hypnotics, N. Engl. J. Med. **291**:790, 1974.

75 Lokhandwala, M. F., Cavero, I., Buckley, J. P., and Jandhyala, B. S.: Influence of pentobarbital anesthesia on the effect of certain autonomic blocking agents on heart rate, Eur. J. Pharmacol. **24**:274, 1973.

75a Mason, M. F., and Dubowski, K. M.: Alcohol, traffic, and chemical testing in the United States: a resumé and some remaining problems, Clin. Chem. **20**(2):126, 1974.

76 Mendelson, J. H.: Biologic concomitants of alcoholism, N. Engl. J. Med. **283**:24, 71, 1970.

77 Redetzki, H. M.: Treatment of ethanol intoxication, Hosp. Formulary, p. 934, Oct. 1979.

78 Sellers, E. M., and Kalant, H.: Alcohol intoxication and withdrawal. N. Engl. J. Med. **294**:757, 1976.

79 Solomon, F., White, C. C., Parron, D. L., and Mendelson, W. B.: Sleeping pills, insomnia and medical practice, New Engl. J. Med. **300**:803, 1979.

80 Wallgren, H., and Barry, H.: Actions of alcohol, New York, 1970, American Elsevier Publishing Co., Inc.

CHAPTER 27

Central nervous system stimulants of the convulsant type

GENERAL CONCEPT

A variety of drugs raise the reflex excitability of the CNS, stimulation respiration, cause hyperreflexia, and induce convulsions in a dose-dependent fashion. Because of their awakening effect they are often referred to as *analeptics*.

These drugs are mostly of toxicological interest, although they may occasionally be used as respiratory stimulants. Strychnine, picrotoxin, pentylenetetrazol (Metrazol), nikethamide (Coramine), bemegride (Megimide), doxapram (Dopram), and the methylxanthines, such as caffeine, belong to this group.

MECHANISMS OF CONVULSANT ACTION

The various stimulants may act by several different mechanisms. They may cause neuronal excitation, they may block presynaptic inhibition (picrotoxin), and they may block postsynaptic inhibition (strychnine). The antagonism between strychnine and glycine on spinal motoneurons is discussed on p. 129.

CNS STIMULANTS

Only the essential features of the pharmacology of the various CNS stimulants will be considered.

The older analeptics, such as pentylenetetrazol (Metrazol), picrotoxin, and nikethamide (Coramine), have a low margin between analeptic and convulsant doses. The newer analeptics such as doxapram (Dopram) have replaced the older ones because of their more favorable therapeutic index.

Pentylenetetrazol

The structural formula of pentylenetetrazol (Metrazol) is as follows:

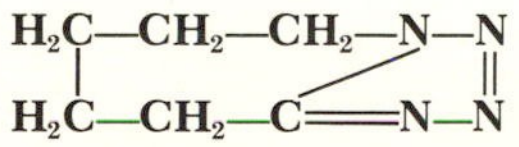

H₂C—CH₂—CH₂—N—N
H₂C—CH₂—C═N—N

Pentylenetetrazol

There is much experience with the convulsant action of pentylenetetrazol in humans because the drug has been used extensively in shock treatment for mental disease. When approximately 5 ml of 10% solution of pentylenetetrazol is injected rapidly by the intravenous route, the individual becomes apprehensive and in a few seconds goes into convulsions and becomes unconscious. The major convulsive movements are tonic at first but rapidly become clonic. The convulsive phase may last only a minute but is followed by exhaustion and sleep.

Muscular contractions may be so powerful that fractures of vertebrae and other bones may occur. For this reason muscle relaxants such as succinylcholine may be administered along with the convulsant.

Pentylenetetrazol is now largely obsolete both as an analeptic and for convulsive therapy.

Picrotoxin   Picrotoxin is a nonnitrogenous compound obtained from an East Indian shrub. It is available in injectable solution containing 3 mg/ml.

The drug is a typical convulsant of the pentylenetetrazol rather than the strychnine type. In normal animals it stimulates respiration only in doses close to the convulsant dose. Barbiturate-anesthetized animals may show significant respiratory stimulation without a convulsant action because the barbiturates antagonize the convulsive tendency.

Picrotoxin, once widely used as an analeptic in barbiturate poisoning, is seldom used today and is largely obsolete.

Nikethamide   Nikethamide (Coramine) is closely related to nicotinamide and is converted to the vitamin in the body. The structural relationships are as follows:

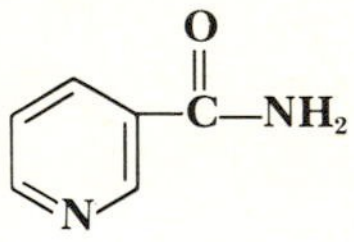

Nicotinamide 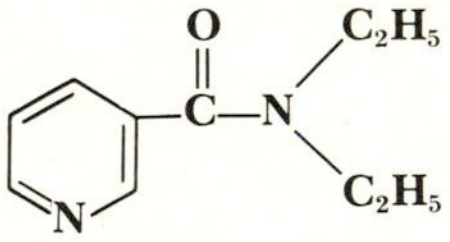   Nikethamide

Nikethamide is available in ampules containing 0.4 g/1.5 ml or 1.25 g/5 ml. The drug is not a cardiac stimulant, and as an analeptic it is seldom used today.

Doxapram   Doxapram (Dopram) is an analeptic that is claimed to have outstanding respiratory stimulant effects.[9] Its therapeutic index, expressed as convulsant dose$_{50}$/respiratory stimulant dose$_{50}$, is higher than that of the older analeptics, as determined in animals. This ratio may be as high as 25. The drug is administered intravenously in doses of 1 to 1.5 mg/kg of body weight.

Doxapram has a very short duration of activity. It is used as a postanesthetic respiratory stimulant. It causes sympathomimetic side effects and may be considered a very short-acting sympathomimetic stimulant.

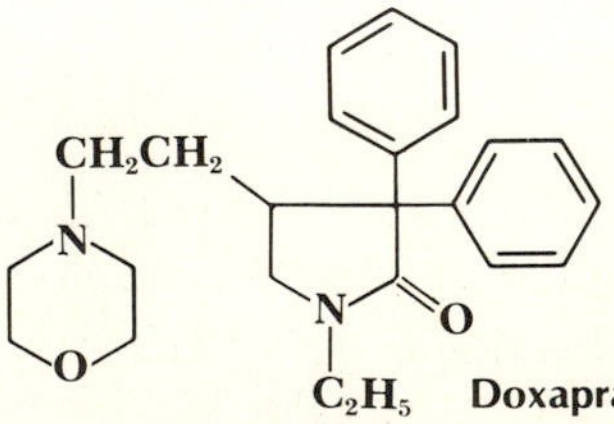

Doxapram

Strychnine is a complex alkaloid obtained from the seeds of the plant *Strychnos nus vomica*.

Strychnine exerts a predominant effect on the spinal cord, in which it lowers the threshold of excitability of various neurons. More recent studies[3] indicate that it opposes the inhibitory influence of Renshaw cells on the motoneurons. Strychnine convulsions differ from pentylenetetrazol seizures in humans by the predominance of the tonic extensor phase, opisthotonos being characteristic of both this type of poisoning and of tetanus. The individual becomes highly susceptible to various stimuli, so that any sudden stimulation such as noise precipitates a tonic extensor seizure.

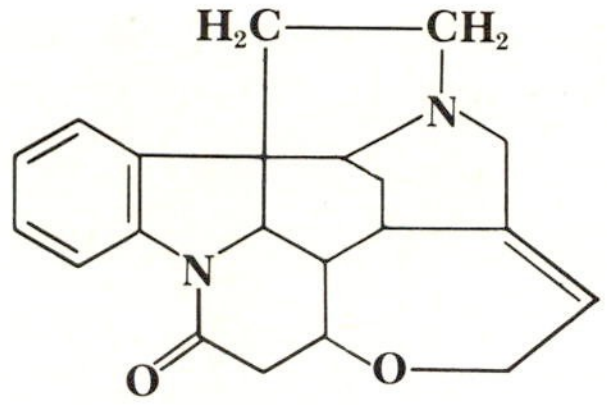

Strychnine

Death in strychnine poisoning probably results from asphyxia or exhaustion after a prolonged series of seizures. Barbiturates are effective antagonists against the convulsant and lethal actions of strychnine. The muscle relaxants such as mephenesin (Tolserol) are also capable of protecting animals against strychnine poisoning.

Treatment of strychnine poisoning is based on the prompt use of intravenous barbiturates. The stomach may be lavaged with a dilute potassium permanganate solution to remove and alter the poison at the early stages of intoxication.

Caffeine (1,3,7-trimethylxanthine) is one of the most widely used stimulants by the lay public and it also has some medical uses. Coffee contains approximately 1.3% caffeine, and a cup of coffee may contain from 100 to 150 mg of the alkaloid. It has been estimated that the annual consumption of caffeine in the United States in the form of coffee is about 7,000,000 kg.

The structural formula of caffeine, a methylated xanthine, is as follows:

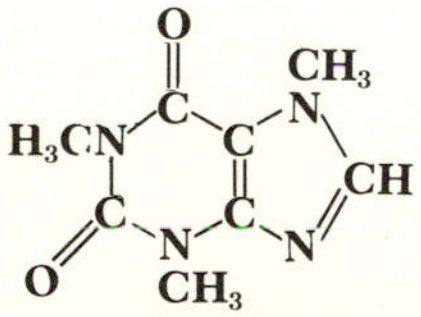

Caffeine 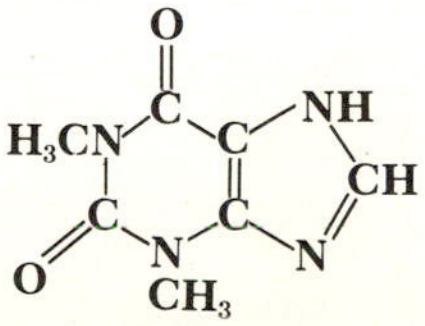   **Theophylline**

This drug is closely related to theophylline but has greater CNS stimulant action.

The main pharmacological actions of caffeine are exerted on the CNS and the cardiovascular system. In addition, the drug is a diuretic and stimulates gastric secretion (Table 27-1).

TABLE 27-1. Relative activity of methylxanthines

Methylxanthine	Source	CNS stimulation	Diuretic potency	Cardiac effects
Caffeine	Coffee, tea, cocoa, cola	1*	3	3
Theophylline	Tea	2	1	1
Theobromine	Cocoa	3	2	2

*1 = most potent; 3 = least potent.

Caffeine stimulates the cerebral cortex and medullary centers. In ordinary doses it causes wakefulness, restlessness, and mental alertness. These actions of caffeine are considered pleasant by most persons, and it is not surprising that wherever a caffeine-containing plant grows, the inhabitants of the area have usually learned to utilize the drug. Some habituation to the use of caffeine occurs, but the drug is not truly addictive.

In larger doses, caffeine can stimulate respiration and can also precipitate clonic convulsions in experimental animals.

Caffeine has some stimulant action on the myocardium and can cause an increase in cardiac output. Increased coronary blood flow is probably a consequence of the increased myocardial work. Systemic blood pressure is not changed by ordinary doses of caffeine, although the drug directly dilates some blood vessels. The cerebral vessels are constricted by caffeine. These effects are similar to those of aminophylline.

The end product of caffeine metabolism in the body appears to be l-methyluric acid and other methyl derivatives of uric acid. It is quite certain that caffeine does not increase the miscible pool or urinary excretion of uric acid itself and is not contraindicated in gout.

For therapeutic use, caffeine is available as caffeine sodium benzoate in ampules of 0.25 and 0.5 g in 2 ml for intramuscular injection. For oral administration, citrated caffeine is available in 60 and 120 mg tablets. In addition, caffeine is often added to headache remedies containing salicylates and acetophenetidin and to ergotamine (Cafergot) for the treatment of migraine.

It has been shown that methylxanthines inhibit the enzyme phosphodiesterase,[8] which inactivates cyclic adenosine-3′,5′-phosphate. Since catecholamines promote the formation of the cyclic nucleotide whereas the methylxanthines inhibit its destruction, a very interesting hypothesis could be constructed for explaining similarities of pharmacological action at many sites such as the heart and the bronchial smooth muscle. The action of methylxanthines and epinephrine on cyclic adenylic acid metabolism is discussed further on pp. 183 and 510.

REFERENCES

1 Adriani, J., Drake, P., and Arens, J.: Use of antagonists in drug-induced coma, J.A.M.A. **179:**752, 1962.

2 Bader, M. E., and Bader, R. A.: Respiratory stimulants in obstructive lung disease, New York, 1964, Academic Press, Inc.

3 Eccles, J. C.: The physiology of nerve cells, Baltimore, 1957, The Johns Hopkins University Press.

4 Eccles, J. C.: The physiology of synapses, Am. J. Med. **38:**165, 1965.

5 Eccles, J. C., Schmidt, R., and Willis, W. D.: Pharmacological studies on presynaptic inhibition, J. Physiol. **168:**500, 1963.

6 Killam, K. F., and Bain, J. A.: Convulsant hydrazides: in vitro and in vivo inhibition of vita-min B_6 enzymes by convulsant hydrazides, J. Pharmacol. Exp. Ther. **119:**255, 1957.

7 Miller, W. F., Archer, R. K., Taylor, H. F., and Ossenfort, W. F.: Severe respiratory depression. Role of a respiratory stimulant, ethamivan, in the treatment, J.A.M.A. **180:**905, 1962.

8 Sutherland, E. W., and Rall, T. W.: The relation of adenosine-3'5'-phosphate to the action of catecholamines. In Adrenergic mechanisms, Ciba Foundation and Committee for Symposium on Drug Action, Boston, 1960, Little, Brown & Co.

9 Wasserman, A. J., and Richardson, D. W.: Human cardiopulmonary effects of doxapram, a respiratory stimulant, Clin. Pharmacol. Ther. **4:**321, 1963.

CHAPTER 28

Antiepileptic drugs

GENERAL CONCEPT   Convulsions are involuntary, general paroxysms of muscular contractions. They are classified as (1) generalized tonic-clonic seizures, (2) partial seizures, and (3) absence seizures (petit mal). The generalized tonic-clonic group includes grand mal epilepsy and certain atypical seizures, such as myoclonic attacks and hypsarrhythmia. Partial seizures may be focal (jacksonian) or complex (psychomotor).

Bromides were the earliest antiepileptic drugs, followed by phenobarbital in 1912 and phenytoin in 1938. Significant newer developments relate to the drugs primidone, carbamazepine, the benzodiazepines diazepam and clonazepam, and valproic acid. Certain oxazolidinediones, such as trimethadione, and succinimides represended by ethosuximide are used in the treatment of absence seizures.

ANTIEPILEPTIC DRUGS
Mode of action

The exact mode of action of antiepileptic drugs is unknown. Nevertheless there are neurophysiological and biochemical mechanisms that characterize various drugs in this group. At the neurophysiological level, the spread of seizure discharge is decreased by phenytoin, phenobarbital, and primidone. Convulsive threshold, as measured by electroshock or pentylenetetrazol convulsions, is elevated by phenobarbital, primidone, and trimethadione. Pentylenetetrazol threshold is elevated also by ethosuximide and diazepam.

Biochemical explanations invoke alterations in neuronal permeability to sodium and potassium. Phenytoin influences sodium permeability, whereas trimethadione, ethosuximide, and diazepam exert an effect on potassium permeability. It appears that drugs that are effective in the treatment of petit mal tend to decrease potassium permeability.

Classes

From a chemical standpoint the various drugs used in epilepsy may be listed in the following categories:

Barbiturates and related drugs
    Phenobarbital (Luminal)
    Mephobarbital (Mebaral)
    Metharbital (Gemonil)
    Primidone (Mysoline)
Hydantoins
    Phenylethylhydantoin (Nirvanol)
    Mephenytoin (Mesantoin)
    Phenytoin (Dilantin)

Oxazolidinediones
    Trimethadione (Tridione)
    Paramethadione (Paradione)
Succinimides
    Phensuximide (Milontin)
    Methsuximide (Celontin)
    Ethosuximide (Zarontin)

Miscellaneous anticonvulsants

Phenacemide (Phenurone)	Diazepam (Valium)
Acetazolamide (Diamox)	Carbamazepine (Tegretol)
Aminoglutethimide (Elipten)	Valproic acid

An examination of the basic structural formulas of the barbiturates, hydantoins, oxazolidines, and succinimides reveals certain obvious similarities.

Whereas barbituric acid is malonylurea, hydantoin has a five-membered ring that may be considered to be a combination of acetic acid and urea. In the oxazolidine derivatives the nitrogen in the hydantoin ring is replaced by oxygen. The succinimides obviously resemble the oxazolidines.

Barbiturates and related drugs

Phenobarbital (Luminal) is one of the oldest antiepileptic drugs. It is administered in a total daily dose of 0.1 to 0.2 g. Phenobarbital differs from most of the other barbiturate hypnotics in possessing a significant antiepileptic effect at does levels that do not cause excessive sedation or sleep. When phenobarbital is used, care must be taken never to withdraw it suddenly because this procedure can precipitate a grand mal attack.

The major usefulness of phenobarbital is in the management of grand mal epilepsy. It has little effect on petit mal but may be advantageous in combination with trimethadione in patients who have both types of epilepsy. Phenobarbital has a long half-life of 50 to 150 hours. Therapeutic blood levels are 10 to 30 μg/ml. Drowsiness and irritability are the main side effects of phenobarbital, and, in children, hyperactivity and interference with learning ability are distinct disadvantages.

Mephobarbital (Mebaral) is N-methylphenobarbital. Its indications and uses are similar to those of phenobarbital. In fact, it has been shown that the compound is demethylated to a significant extent to phenobarbital in the body.[1] As a consequence, the antiepileptic effects of mephobarbital may be due, at least in part, to phenobarbital. The dosage of mephobarbital is 300 to 600 mg/day.

Metharbital (Gemonil) is N-methylbarbital and is probably demethylated in the body to barbital. Its dosage is 100 mg two or three times a day.

Primidone (Mysoline), although not a true barbituric acid, shows considerable similarity in structure to phenobarbital. It may produce considerable drowsiness and vertigo. Because of this, it should be started in small doses, about 50 mg, with a gradual increase to as much as 250 mg three times a day. Primidone is converted into two active metabolites: phenobarbital and phenylethylmalonamide. Therapeutic blood levels are 5 to 10 μg/ml.

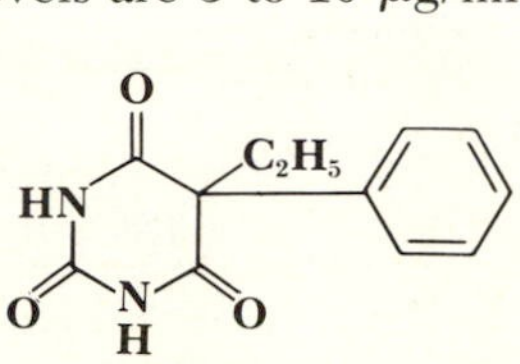

Phenobarbital 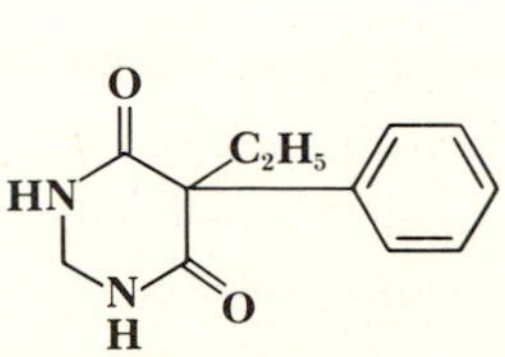   Primidone

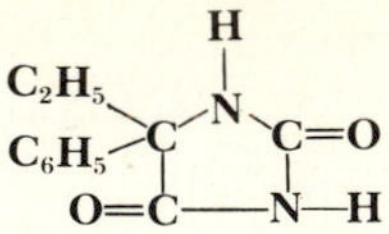

Phenylethylhydantoin

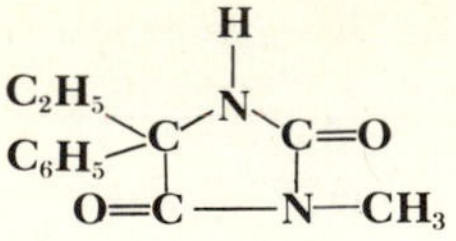

Mephenytoin

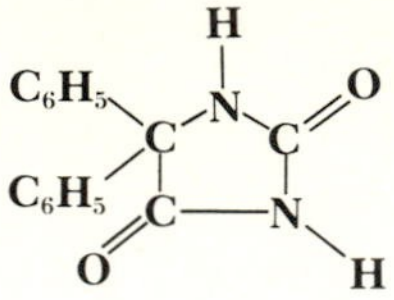

Phenytoin

Hydantoins   **Phenylethylhydantoin** (Nirvanol) was used as a sedative as early as 1916. The drug was abandoned because it tended to produce an extraordinarily high incidence of drug fever, skin sensitization, and eosinophilia. Interestingly, the replacement of the ethyl radical by a phenyl group yielded the highly useful drug phenytoin.

On the other hand, **mephenytoin** (3-methyl-5-ethyl-5-phenylhydantoin; Mesantoin), which is the *N*-methyl derivative of phenylethylhydantoin, is demethylated in the body to this highly toxic and sensitizing drug. It is not surprising, therefore, that a high incidence of drug reactions has been reported following the use of mephenytoin. Some of these are skin rashes and fever, granulocytopenia, and aplastic anemia. Clearly the drug should be used only if other compounds are ineffective.

Phenytoin (Dilantin), introduced in 1938, is still one of the most valuable antiepileptic drugs. It is administered in capsules containing 0.1 g of the drug as its sodium salt. The daily dose in adults varies from 0.2 to 0.6 g.

The main advantage of phenytoin in the management of grand mal and psychomotor epilepsy is that it exerts little sedative action at effective dose levels. However, in large doses it can cause ataxia, tremors, and nausea.

Adverse effects of phenytoin. The unwanted effects of phenytoin are of three categories.[12] It has *toxic effects*, true *side effects*, and *idiosyncratic reactions*. Intoxication is characterized by sedation, ataxia, and nystagmus. These manifestations are dose related and appear at plasma levels of 20 to 40 $\mu g/ml$.

Side effects include osteomalacia hypocalcemia caused probably by an interference with vitamin D metabolism. Long-term use of phenytoin may lead to lowered serum folic acid levels resulting in megaloblastic anemia.

An unusual side effect caused by phenytoin is the hypertrophy of the gums. It occurs in 20% of patients and is generally attributed to a disorder of fibroblastic activity.

Drugs of the hydantoin group may produce blood dyscrasias and rarely a clinical picture resembling malignant lymphoma. Phenytoin has antiarrhythmic effects.[8] Its use as an antiarrhythmic drug is discussed on p. 464.

Pharmacokinetics of phenytoin. Phenytoin is absorbed rapidly from the gastrointestinal tract, and the drug is about 90% protein bound. The half-life of phenytoin is 24 to 30 hours. The therapeutic blood level range is 10 to 20 μg/ml. Phenytoin shows some unusual pharmacokinetic features. Once plasma concentrations of 10 μg/ml are reached, further increases in dosage produce greater than expected plasma levels. It appears that metabolic pathways for the elimination of the drug become saturated. As a consequence the half-time of the drug increases as plasma concentrations rise. For these reasons monitoring of plasma concentrations are quite important, since minor increases in dosage can result in markedly elevated plasma concentrations, leading to toxic manifestations and even paradoxical seizures.

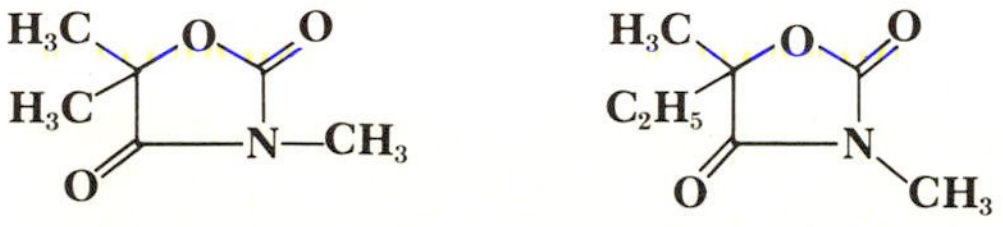

Trimethadione   Paramethadione

Trimethadione (Tridione) and **paramethadione** (Paradione) are useful in the management of petit mal. They are available in capsules containing 0.3 g, and the daily dose varies from 1 to 2 g.

Oxazolidinediones

In clinical use of the oxazolidine derivatives, the following toxic effects have been reported: drowsiness and ataxia, photophobia, and a strange visual disturbance consisting of a white halo around various objects. Bone marrow depression and kidney damage have also been reported following prolonged use of the oxazolidines. Skin rashes and alopecia also have been reported.

Succinimides such as **phensuximide** (Milontin), **methsuximide** (Celontin), and **ethosuximide** (Zarontin) are useful in the management of petit mal. They may be less toxic than the oxazolidones, although dizziness or skin rashes may occur following their use. Rare cases of neutropenia and other blood dyscrasias have also been reported.

Succinimides

Usual dosages of these drugs are phensuximide, 0.5 to 1 g three times a day; methsuximide, 0.3 to 0.6 g three times a day; and ethosuximide, 0.5 g two to four times a day. Ethosuximide is now considered the drug of choice in the treatment of petit mal.

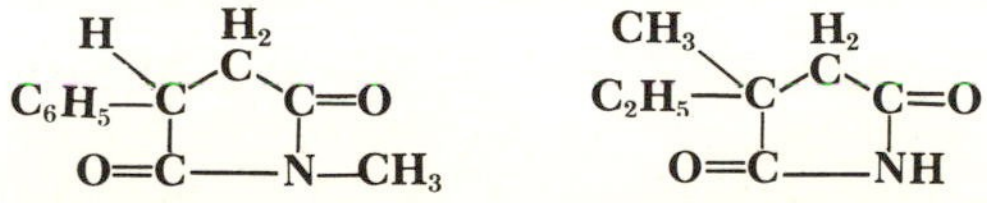

Phensuximide   Ethosuximide

Phenacemide (Phenurone), a very potent but quite toxic anticonvulsant, should be used rarely, if at all, only after all other measures fail. When used in doses of 0.5 g three times a day, it may cause severe bone marrow depression, hepatocellular damage, and toxic psychoses.

Miscellaneous anticonvulsants

Bromides were used extensively at one time but are now obsolete. Their use is associated with mental depression, toxic psychoses, and skin rashes.

Acetazolamide (Diamox), a carbonic anhydrase inhibitor, is used occasionally. Milk metabolic acidosis induced by a ketogenic diet was at one time used in epilepsy. The carbonic anhydrase inhibitors, which produce metabolic acidosis, have been found useful in all types of epilepsy. There is a possibility that their effectiveness is not caused by systemic acidosis but by inhibition of carbonic anhydrase in the CNS. Acetazolamide is given in doses of 250 to 500 mg two or three times a day.

Aminoglutethimide (Elipten) is a drug chemically related to the hypnotic glutethimide (Doriden). Although it is claimed to be effective in all types of epilepsy, it was withdrawn because of its toxicity. Aminoglutethimide blocks cholesterol metabolism in the adrenal cortex.

Carbamazepine (Tegretol) is an iminostilbene derivative related structurally to the tricyclic antidepressants. The drug is useful in the treatment of generalized tonic-clonic seizures and also in partial and complex seizures.[10] Carbamazepine has been used since 1974 as an antiepileptic drug.

The drug is absorbed slowly from the gastrointestinal tract and is 75% protein bound. Its half-life is 12 hours. Adverse effects of carbamazepine include ataxia, dizziness, drowsiness, and, rarely, hepatic damage and bone marrow depression. The drug is available in 200 mg tablets.

Clonazepam (Clonopin) and **diazepam** (Valium) are the two benzodiazepines used as antiepileptic drugs. Clonazepam is useful in the treatment of absence seizures, whereas diazepam, administered intravenously, is indicated in the treatment of status epilepticus.

Therapeutic blood concentrations of clonazepam are from 20 to 80 ng/ml. Adverse side effects produced by the drug include drowsiness, ataxia, and, in children, personality changes.[10] The drug is available in tablets containing 0.5, 1, or 2 mg. Diazepam (Valium) for intravenous use is available in ampules containing 2 ml, 5 mg/ml.

Valproic acid (Depakene) is dipropylacetic acid and is the most recently introduced antiepileptic drug. The drug may act by increasing the concentrations of γ-aminobutyric acid in the brain.[10] The drug is absorbed rapidly from the gastroin-

TABLE 28-1. Clinical classification of seizures*

Type of seizure	Age group	EEG
Grand mal	Any age	Multifocal spikes (may be normal)
Petit mal	8-14 years	3/sec spike-and-wave
Minor motor seizures	Childhood	Multifocal spikes; variable spike-and-wave
Hypsarrhythmia	Infancy	Diffuse, chaotic, high voltage, sharp, and slow
Focal	Any age	Spikes from appropriate region
Motor		
Sensory		
Psychomotor		
Status epilepticus	Any age	Diffuse, continuous spiking

*Courtesy J. E. Walker, M.D.

testinal tract and has a short half-life of 6 to 13 hours. Thus, it must be administered three or four times daily.

Valproic acid is useful in the treatment of generalized seizures, both tonic-clonic and absence, and is indicated also in the treatment of myoclonic seizures.

Adverse effects of valproic acid include drowsiness, gastrointestinal discomfort, transient hair loss, weight gain, and, rarely, hepatotoxicity. Valproic acid interacts with other antiepileptic drugs. It inhibits the metabolism of phenobarbital, and it lowers phenytoin plasma concentrations by competition for protein binding.

Valproic acid (Depakene) is available in 250 mg capsules and as a syrup containing 250 mg/5 ml as the sodium salt. The recommended dose is 30 mg/kg with therapeutic blood concentrations of 50 to 100 μg/ml.

The usefulness of the antiepileptic drugs in various types of seizures[10] is indicated below:

Clinical pharmacology

Generalized tonic-clonic and partial seizures	*Absence seizures*
Phenytoin	Ethosuximide
Phenobarbital	Clonazepam
Primidone	Valproic acid
Carbamazepine	*Status epilepticus*
Valproic acid	Diazepam

Adverse effects and drug interactions

The adverse effects of the antiepileptic drugs depend greatly on the individual drugs, but in general they are gastrointestinal, neurological, cutaneous, mental, hematopoietic, and renal.

Gastrointestinal side effects are usually seen at the initiation of treatment, and they respond to a reduction in dosage.

Drowsiness and ataxia are common side effects. Ataxia is commonly seen following the use of the hydantoins and barbiturates.

Skin eruptions are produced by many of the antiepileptic drugs, and they vary greatly in severity.

Alterations in mood and mental changes in patients treated with the antiepileptic drugs are not uncommon.

Megaloblastic anemias that respond to folic acid may occur following the use of hydantoins, barbiturates, and primidone. Lymphadenopathies resembling malignant lymphomas have been reported in association with the use of phenytoin and mephenytoin, paramethadione, and trimethadione.

Nephropathies have been reported following the use of trimethadione and paramethadione.

Among the miscellaneous adverse effects, gingival hyperplasia following the use of phenytoin has been commented on before. Severe liver damage may be associated with the use of hydantoins, and congenital abnormalities have been reported following the use of trimethadione and paramethadione in pregnant women.

Drug interactions are numerous in connection with the antiepileptic drugs. Phenobarbital speeds up the metabolism of phenytoin, although this interaction seldom creates a serious problem. The metabolism of the coumarin anticoagulants is also increased by phenobarbital. On the other hand, dicumarol inhibits the metabolism of phenytoin.

Isoniazid, aminosalicylic acid, chloramphenicol, and disulfiram potentiate the actions of phenytoin by inhibiting its metabolism. Reserpine may oppose the actions of anticonvulsants by lowering convulsive thresholds.

REFERENCES

1 Butler, T. C.: Quantitative studies of the metabolic fate of mephobarbital (N-methyl phenobarbital), J. Pharmacol. Exp. Ther. 106:235, 1952.

2 Camerman, A., and Camerman, N.: Diphenylhydantoin and diazepam: molecular structure similarities and steric basic of anticonvulsant activity, Science 168:1458, 1970.

3 Geller, M., and Christoff, N.: Diazepam in the treatment of childhood epilepsy, J.A.M.A. 215:2087, 1971.

4 Gunn, C. G., Gogerty, J., and Wolf, S.: Clinical pharmacology of anticonvulsant compounds, Clin. Pharmacol. Ther. 2:733, 1961.

5 Livingston, S.: Drug therapy for epilepsy, Springfield, Ill., 1966, Charles C Thomas, Publisher.

6 Livingston, S., Pauli, L., and Najmabadi, A.: Ethosuximid in the treatment of epilepsy, J.A.M.A. 180:822, 1972.

7 Merritt, H. H., and Putnam, T. J.: Sodium diphenylhydantoinate in the treatment of convulsive disorders, J.A.M.A. 111:1068, 1938.

8 Unger, A. H., and Sklaroff, H. J.: Fatalities following the intravenous use of sodium diphenylhydantoin for cardiac arrhythmias, J.A.M.A. 200:335, 1967.

REVIEWS

9 Booker, H. E.: Clorazepate dipotassium in the treatment of intractable epilepsy, J.A.M.A. 229:550, 1974.

10 Dreifuss, F. E.: Use of anticonvulsant drugs, J.A.M.A. 241:607, 1979.

11 Drugs for epilepsy, Med. Lett. 18:25, 1976.

12 Harris, P., and Mawdsley, C.: Epilepsy, London, 1974, Churchill Livingstone.

13 Kutt, H., and Louis, S.: Untoward effects of anticonvulsants, N. Engl. J. Med. 286:1316, 1972.

14 Livingston, S., Berman, W., and Pauly, L. L.: Anticonvulsant drug blood levels, J.A.M.A. 232:60, 1975.

15 Rose, S. W., Smith, L. D., and Penry, J. K.: Blood level determinations of antiepileptic drugs, Bethesda, Md., 1971, National Institutes of Neurological Diseases and Stroke; National Institutes of Health.

16 Van Horn, G.: Anticonvulsant therapy in adults, Tex. Med. 76:55, 1980.

17 Vasko, M. R., Bell, R. D., Daly, D. D., and Pippenger, C. E.: Inheritance of phenytoin hypometabolism: a kinetic study of one family, Clin. Pharmacol. Ther. 27:96, 1980.

18 Woodbury, D. M., Perry, J. K., and Schmidt, R. P.: Antiepileptic drugs, New York, 1972, Raven Press.

CHAPTER 29

Narcotic analgesic drugs

Relief of pain is one of the great objectives in medicine. Drugs with a predominant pain-relieving action are called *analgesics* and are commonly classified as *narcotic* and *nonnarcotic*. The narcotic analgesics include the alkaloids of opium and many related synthetic drugs. Their use in most instances is regulated by the Federal Controlled Substances Act of 1970.

The opiate analgesics and related compounds are addictive. They produce physical dependence, characterized by withdrawal symptoms. Tolerance develops to most of their effects. The characterization of the opiate receptor and the discovery of endogenous opioid peptides, the endorphins and enkephalins, give the pharmacology of the opiates an entirely new perspective.

Morphine has been available for 200 years, but opium has been used for thousands of years. Opiate antagonists were introduced in 1941.

THE OPIATE RECEPTOR

It has been suspected for some time that there are specific opiate receptors in the brain.[24] First of all, some opiates are extremely potent, etorphine being 10,000 times as potent as morphine. In addition, the actions of opiates are stereospecific, the levo isomers representing the active form. Finally, there are pure opiate antagonists, such as naloxone, which exert no analgesia but block the effect of the opiates.

The concept of specific opiate receptors was greatly strengthened when stereospecific binding of opiates and their antagonists to brain membranes was demonstrated by using labeled compounds. The potencies of these drugs in competing for binding parallel closely their pharmacological activities.[43]

Opiate receptors in the brain are concentrated in the limbic system, the spinoreticular tracts, containing such areas as the periaqueductal gray, medial thalamic nuclei, the hypothalamus, and other pathways involved in pain perception.[43] Opiate receptors are also found in the *substantia gelatinosa* of the spinal cord and spinal trigeminal nucleus, the *nucleus tractus solitarii*, and the vagus nerve. High concentration in these areas may explain their role in the cough reflex, gastric secretion, and orthostatic hypotension.[44] The amygdala is highest in receptor binding, followed by the periaqueductal gray, hypothalamus, and medial thalamus.[42]

Role of sodium

Sodium concentration is an important determinant of the affinity of the receptor for agonists and antagonists. In the opiate series there are pure agonists, which are analgesic and addicting. There are pure antagonists, such as naloxone, which are not analgesic and are nonaddicting. Finally there are partial agonists, such as nalorphine or pentazocine.

It has been shown that sodium concentration greatly influences the affinity of the receptor. It appears that the receptor may exist in two different states. In the presence of sodium the receptor has high affinity for the antagonists. In the absence of sodium the conformation of the receptor favors the binding of the agonists.

Endogenous opioid peptides

Enkephalins and endorphins. The demonstration of specific receptors for the opiates suggested the possiblity of the existence of endogenous morphine-like compounds. Pentapeptides with opiate-like activity[18] such as methionine enkephalin (H-tyrosine-glycine-glycine-phenylalanine-methionine-OH) and leucine enkephalin (H-tyrosine-glycine-glycine-phenylalanine-leucine-OH) have been isolated from brain tissue and appear to act as neurotransmitters.[43]

Other peptides that are opiate-like from the standpoint of competing for the receptor have also been isolated. β-Lipotropin isolated from the pituitary some time ago contains the amino acid sequence of methionine enkephalin in residues 61 to 65. The functions of the compound β-endorphin is not clear. The enkephalins and endorphins will be further discussed on p. 362. Although these discoveries are quite recent, their significance in relation to analgesia, addiction, and behavior is of the greatest importance.

METHODS OF STUDY OF ANALGESIC ACTION

Quantitative studies on analgesics are difficult because the pain experience in humans depends not only on the perception of the painful stimulus but also on psychological factors.

Two types of experimental approaches are commonly used for evaluation of analgesic action. In one, the threshold for pain is determined in humans or animals by the application of painful stimuli of graded intensity. In the other method, analgesics are administered to postoperative patients, and their pain-relieving potency is compared with that of a placebo,[5] which has a distinct analgesic effect.

CHEMISTRY AND CLASSIFICATION

Narcotic analgesics and atagonists can be divided into several categories as follows:

Naturally occurring alkaloids and semisynthetic opiates
Morphine
Codeine (methylmorphine)
Oxymorphone (Numorphan)
Hydromorphone (Dilaudid)
Methyldihydromorphinone (metopon)
Hydrocodone (Dicodid)
Heroin (diacetylmorphine)

Meperidine and related phenylpiperidines
Meperidine (Demerol)
Alphaprodine (Nisentil)
Anileridine (Leritine)
Piminodine (Alvodine)
Diphenoxylate (in Lomotil)
Methadone and related drugs
Methadone
Propoxyphene (Darvon)

Benzomorphans (agonists and partial antagonists)
    Phenazocine (Prinadol)
    Pentazocine (Talwin)
Morphinan derivatives
    Levorphanol (levo-Dromoran)
    Dextromethorphan

Narcotic antagonists (allyl substituted compounds)
    Nalorphine (Nalline)
    Levallorphan (Lorfan)
    Naloxone (Narcan)

Pharmacological studies indicate a basic similarity among the various addictive analgesics. They are all potent against severe pain, all can be substituted for each other in the addict (although great tolerance develops to all of them), and all are antagonized by such drugs as nalorphine or levallorphan. It could be anticipated from these facts that some basic chemical similarity must exist in this series; and, in fact, examination of the formulas of all of these drugs reveals the presence of a common moiety, γ-phenyl-N-methyl-piperidine.

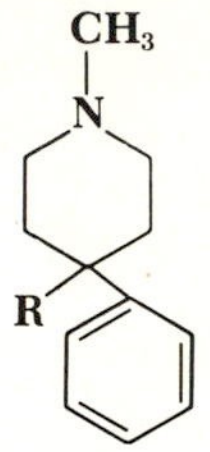

4-R-4-Phenyl-1-methyl-piperidine

Morphine, which has been used extensively for many years, remains the most important narcotic analgesic. its pharmacology will be discussed in some detail, and it will serve as a standard of comparison with the other narcotics.

Morphine is an alkaloid obtained from opium, which is the dried juice of the poppy plant *Papaver somniferum.* The many different alkaloids found in opium fall into two categories: the phenanthrene alkaloids and the benzylisoquinoline compounds. Of the latter group, only papaverine has achieved any medical importance as an antispasmodic and vasodilator. It is not an analgesic.

Morphine and codeine are the only important narcotics obtainable from the phenanthrene group of opium alkaloids. Opium contains 10% morphine and 0.5% codeine.

Morphine, the chief alkaloid of opium, was isolated as early as 1803 by Sertürner but was not totally synthesized until 1952. The synthesis confirmed the structure proposed by Gulland and Robinson in 1925.

The two hydroxyl groups, one phenolic and the other alcoholic, are of great importance, since some of the natural morphine derivatives are obtained by simple modifications of one or both of these groups. For example, codeine is methylmorphine, the substitution being in the phenolic hydroxyl. Heroin is diacetylmorphine. In dihydromorphinone the alcoholic hydroxyl is replaced by a ketonic oxygen and the double bond adjacent to it is removed. Although most of the useful semisyn-

NATURAL OPIATES AND SEMISYNTHETIC DERIVATIVES
Morphine

Chemistry

thetic alkaloids are prepared by substitutions in the hydroxyl groups, the antidotal compound nalorphine is prepared by replacement of the CH_3 group on the nitrogen by the allyl radical $-CH_2CH=CH_2$.

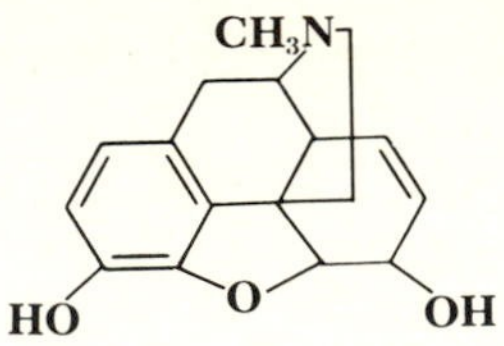

Morphine

Morphine sulfate is the most commonly employed salt. It is available in ampules of 1 ml or in tablets of various sizes for preparing the injectable solution. It is also available in ampules of larger sizes. An ampule is not a dose. The subcutaneous dosage range is 8 to 15 mg.

Analgesic and other CNS effects

When morphine is administered by the subcutaneous route to a normal person in the amount of 10 to 15 mg, it produces drowsiness and euphoria in some but anxiety and nausea in others. The individual may go to sleep, the respiration slows, and the pupils constrict.

There are at least two factors involved in the pain relief afforded by morphine. The drug elevates the pain threshold and alters the reaction of the individual to the painful experience.

The optimal dose of morphine for the average adult is 8 to 15 mg. This dose may elevate the threshold for pain perception by 60% to 70%. It has been shown that 10 mg of morphine gave relief of moderate postoperative pain to at least 90% of the patients.[6] This is reduced to 70% in severe postoperative pain. A dose of 15 mg may raise this to 80%. Interestingly, placebo administration provided relief to 30% of the patients and morphine by the oral route to only 40%.

Respiration

The respiratory center is markedly depressed by morphine, and stoppage of respiration is the cause of death in morphine poisoning. Therapeutic doses of morphine causes some lowering of respiratory minute volume and lessened response to carbon dioxide inhalation without much change in respiratory rate.[23] Larger doses also depress the rate of respiration, and carbon dioxide retention becomes severe. The onset of respiratory depression following injection of morphine depends on the method of administration. Maximal depression of respiration occurs within about 5 minutes following intravenous injection, whereas it may be delayed for 60 minutes or longer if the drug is injected by the intramuscular route. As tolerance develops to the analgesic and euphoric actions of morphine, the respiratory center becomes tolerant also. For this reason the addict may exhibit resistance to otherwise lethal doses of morphine.

Carbon dioxide retention is the probable cause of the cerebral vasodilation and increased intracranial pressure that follow the administration of morphine.

Morphine is not a uniform depressant of neural structures. It does not oppose the action of stimulants such as strychnine or picrotoxin. Indeed, it may be synergistic with such drugs. Also, morphine may enhance monosynaptic reflexes, whereas it depresses multineuronal reflexes. Thus it has been shown by Wikler that the knee and ankle jerks in the cat with spinal cord section was enhanced or not affected, whereas the flexor and crossed extensor reflexes were depressed.[32]

Morphine may actually be excitatory in certain persons and in several species of animals. Some patients may become nauseated and vomit following a morphine injecton and may even become delirious. Similarly, cats and horses are stimulated by morphine. The violent excitement of cats caused by morphine is still present in decortication, requiring experimental lesions in the hypothalamus for its prevention.

Excitation

The emetic effect of morphine may be exerted on the chemoreceptor trigger zone in the medulla.[31] Interestingly, apomorphine, which is obtained from morphine through a major chemical modification, is a most potent stimulant of the chemoreceptor trigger zone.

Emesis

Other effects of morphine include pupillary, gastrointestinal, biliary, cardiovascular, bronchial, antidiuretic, and metabolic influences.

Miscellaneous effects

Effect on pupils. The pupils are constricted by morphine, and this action is antagonized by atropine. Pupillary constriction is a consequence of the CNS action of the drug. Addicts do not develop tolerance to the pupillary constrictor action of morphine, and during withdrawal their pupils become widely dilated. Animals excited by morphine show pupillary dilation.

Gastrointestinal effects. Morphine has a marked constipating effect, and opiates are time-honored remedies in the management of diarrhea.

In general, morphine tends to increase the tone of intestinal smooth muscle and decrease propulsive movements. Morphine delays gastric emptying through decreased gastric motility and contraction of the pylorus and perhaps of the duodenum as well. Atropine tends to partially oppose this spasmogenic action of morphine.

The constipating effect of morphine may result from several factors. The most important ones are (1) increased tone and decreased propulsive activity throughout the gastrointestinal tract and (2) failure to perceive sensory stimuli that would otherwise elicit the defecation reflex.

Effect on biliary tract. Morphine increases intrabiliary pressure as a consequence of constricting the smooth muscles of the biliary tract. Pain relief under these conditions must be caused by its central analgesic action. Atropine may not be effective in relieving severe spasm of the biliary tract induced by morphine.

Cardiovascular effects. Morphine reduces arterial resistance and venous tone. These effects are beneficial in reducing ventricular work, pulmonary congestion, and edema.[1] The hemodynamic effects may be excessive, leading to considerable hypotension, which is posturally related. The depressor response to intravenous morphine is decreased but not abolished by atropine.

In some species histamine release following intravenous morphine administration has been demonstrated; histamine may contribute to severe hypotensive reactions.

Effect on bronchial smooth muscle. The bronchial smooth muscle is contracted by morphine. Since death has occurred in asthmatic patients following morphine injection, many investigators attribute this adverse effect to the bronchoconstrictor action of morphine. It is quite possible, however, that this reaction of the asthmatic patient may be related to the depressant action of morphine on the response of the respiratory center to carbon dioxide. According to this view, carbon dioxide narcosis, rather than bronchial constriction, may be the cause of death; however, the question is not settled.

Effect on genitourinary tract. The smooth muscle of the urinary tract is affected by morphine. The narcotic tends to contract the ureter and the detrusor muscle of the bladder and to cause an increase in the tone of the vesical sphincter. Atropine tends to relieve the ureteral spasm induced by morphine. Despite its smooth muscle effect, morphine is often used in the relief of ureteral colic, where its effectiveness must be a result of its analgesic action.

The urinary retention that may follow administration of morphine results from difficulty in micturition and decreased perception of the stimulus for micturition. Morphine is also an antidiuretic. It causes release of the antidiuretic hormone, and its hemodynamic actions also contribute to this antidiuretic effect.

Uterine contractions during labor are not significantly affected by a therapeutic dose of morphine, although they may be slowed somewhat.

Metabolic effects. One metabolic effect of morphine is some lowering of total oxygen consumption, probably because of decreased activity and muscle tone. Hyperglycemia of varying intensity has been observed after the injection of morphine. It is generally believed that this is a consequence of increased sympathetic activity, since total sympathectomy will prevent the rise in blood sugar.[8]

Metabolism   Morphine is readily absorbed following subcutaneous or intramuscular injection. It is estimated that about 60% of subcutaneously injected morphine is absorbed in the first 30 minutes. Absorption is strongly influenced by cutaneous circulation. Its absorption from the gastrointestinal tract is slow, however, and the drug is not given by this route.

About 90% of an administered dose can be recovered from the urine in a conjugated form, and a small percentage can be recovered from the feces. Biliary excretion may account for the presence of morphine in the feces. It has been shown that a microsomal enzyme in the liver can convert morphine to its glucuronide.

Tolerance   A striking feature of the pharmacology of morphine and related drugs is the gradual tolerance that develops to some of its effects.

If a patient in chronic pain is given 10 to 15 mg of morphine sulfate by the subcutaneous route twice a day, it is often observed that after a week or so he or she will not receive as much pain relief as was received at the beginning. The dose must be gradually increased. This tolerance extends not only to the analgesic but also to the respiratory depressant actions of morphine. On the other hand, no tolerance develops to the gastrointestinal or pupillary constrictor actions of morphine or to the excitatory effects of the drug.

If the administration of morphine is prolonged, both a normal person and an addict will require progressively larger doses of morphine to obtain the same subjective effects. The tolerance may reach almost incredible proportions. Addicts have been known to take as much as 4 g of the drug in 24 hours. This quantity is far greater than the lethal dose in a nontolerant person. The duration of tolerance is 1 to 2 weeks, and following this period of abstinence the individual again responds to a small dose of the drug. Addicts may die as a consequence of taking their usual large dose of morphine after a period of abstinence during which they have lost their tolerance.

Problem 29-1. Could tolerance to morphine be a consequence of altered absorption, increased rate of metabolism, and excretion? Obviously not, because the tolerant addict can administer doses of morphine intravenously that would depress the respiratory center of a nonaddict premanently. There must be a true cellular tolerance of some nervous elements. In agreement with this view, experimental studies[12] failed to show a difference in the metabolism of morphine in tolerant and nontolerant dogs.

Many factors influence the development of tolerance. Regular frequent administration of the drug is more likely to produce tolerance than widely spaced, irregular modes of administration. The administration of the narcotic antagonists nalorphine or naloxone produces acute withdrawal symptoms of individuals who are tolerant to large doses of morphine.

The mechanism of tolerance may become understandable as a consequence of the discovery of the enkephalins. If the enkephalins are neurotransmitters, the continued presence of morphine at the opiate receptor could turn off their production, thus the requirement for larger doses of morphine for analgesia would become a necessity.[43]

In *acute* morphine poisoning the individual is comatose and cyanotic, the respirations are slow, and the pupils are of pinpoint size.

Morphine poisoning

The management of a patient in acute morphine poisoning is quite different from that of the barbiturate-poisoned patient. First, central stimulant drugs such as picrotoxin or pentylenetetrazol (Metrazol) should not be used, since there is experimental evidence for lack of antidotal value. Morphine, in contrast to the barbiturates, has many excitatory actions and may be synergistic with the convulsants.

The major development in the treatment of acute morphine poisoning has been the discovery of the antidotal action of nalorphine. Intravenous injection of 5 to 10 mg of this drug produces striking improvement in respiration and circulation of the acutely poisoned individual. The dosage may be repeated but should not exceed a total of 40 mg. This action of nalorphine does not extend to the barbiturates or general anesthetics but is so specific for morphine and related narcotics that it can be of diagnostic significance.

Naloxone hydrochloride (Narcan) is a new narcotic antagonist of great importance discussed on p. 353.

Codeine
Codeine, or methylmorphine, is a very important analgesic and antitussive drug. In therapeutic doses it is less sedative and analgesic than morphine, but tolerance to the drug develops more slowly, and codeine is less addictive than morphine. It has less effect also on the gastrointestinal and urinary tracts and on the pupil and causes less nausea and constipation than morphine.

Codeine administered orally is not as effective an analgesic as when it is injected subcutaneously. In one study performed on postoperative patients, 60 mg of codeine administered by mouth produced relief in 40% of the patients, whereas a placebo was effective in 33%.[6] On the other hand, administered subcutaneously, the drug was effective in 60% of the patients, whereas 10 mg of morphine provided relief in 71%. Although effective, codeine is not quite as effective an analgesic as morphine, even when its dosage is six times higher.

Codeine phosphate is widely used in oral doses of 15 to 64 mg for moderately severe pain when the nonaddictive analgesics prove to be ineffective. It is given by subcutaneous injection for severe pain.

Codeine is partly demethylated to morphine in the body and is partly changed to norcodeine. The conjugated forms of these compounds are excreted in the urine.

Semisynthetic derivatives
Oxymorphone (Numorphan) is a more potent analgesic than morphine, but it causes more side effects.

Hydromorphone (Dilaudid) is up to ten times as potent as analgesic as is morphine. Its respiratory depressant effect is correspondingly greater, although it may be less nauseating and constipating. Doses for hypodermic injection are about one tenth of the morphine dose, or 1 to 2 mg.

Hydrocodone (Dicodid) resembles codeine but may be a more effective antitussive compound and is also more addictive. The recommended oral dose for adults is 5 to 15 mg, which may be given three to four times a day.

Methyldihydromorphinone, or metopon, is more potent than morphine, but it has no significant advantages over the latter, except that it is effective by oral administration.

Heroin, or diacetylmorphine, is a highly euphoriant and analgesic drug. It is much preferred by the addict, who may take it by the intravenous route in order to obtain a peculiar orgastic sensation. Because of its great addictive liability, heroin may not be legally manufactured in or imported into the United States.

Pantopium (Pantopon) contains the alkaloids of opium in the same proportion as they exist naturally. Since it contains about 50% morphine, its dosage is correspondingly higher. It has no significant advantages over morphine.

MEPERIDINE AND RELATED COMPOUNDS
Meperidine (pethidine; isonipecaine; Demerol; Dolantin) was introduced originally as an antispasmodic of the atropine type.[14]

The analgesic potency of meperidine is such that 50 mg is equivalent to 8 mg of morphine and 100 mg is equivalent to 12 mg of morphine.

Despite early claims, it appears that meperidine is just as depressant to respiration as is morphine when the two drugs are compared in equianalgesic doses.

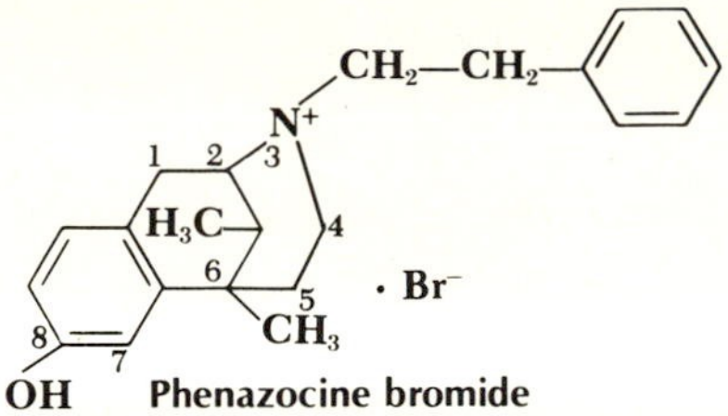

Phenazocine bromide

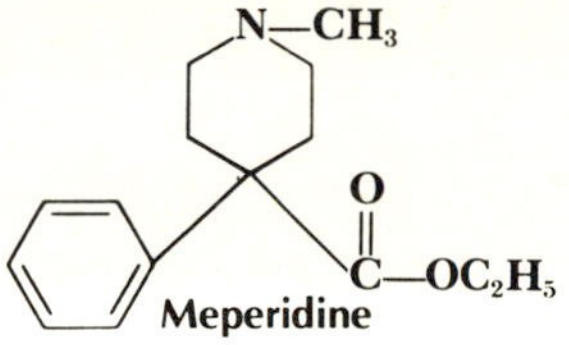

Meperidine

The drug may be slightly less sedative than morphine, but there is no basis for the belief that it has a significantly different action on the gastrointestinal or biliary tract or on the bronchial smooth muscle. Intravenous injection of meperidine may be followed by severe hypotension, caused at least in part by histamine release. Meperidine is definitely addictive.

The liver plays an important role in the metabolism of meperidine, which may be toxic in persons with liver disease.

Alphaprodine (Nisentil) is a piperidine derivative resembling meperidine. Its analgesic action is prompt and of short duration, but its superiority to meperidine remains to be demonstrated.

Anileridine (Leritine) is related to meperidine but is slightly more potent. The oral dose in adults is 25 to 50 mg. It may be given intramuscularly in 40 mg dosage for severe pain.

Piminodine (Alvodine) and **diphenoxylate** (with atropine, as Lomotil) are related chemically to meperidine. Piminodine is used primarily as an analgesic orally or by injection. Diphenoxylate has been recommended for the control of diarrhea in doses of 5 mg three times a day by mouth. It may cause addiction.

Loperamide hydrochloride (Imodium), recently introduced as an antidiarrheal drug, is similar to diphenoxylate, but it is not combined with atropine. It is available in 2 mg capsules.

Methadone (Amidone; dolophine) was discovered in Germany during World War II. Although the structural formula of methadone does not obviously resemble that of morphine, its analgesic potency and some other effects, including the antagonistic action of nalorphine, are quite similar.

The analgesic potency of *dl*-methadone is largely due to the levo isomer. Isomethadone differs from methadone only in the position of the methyl group in the side chain.

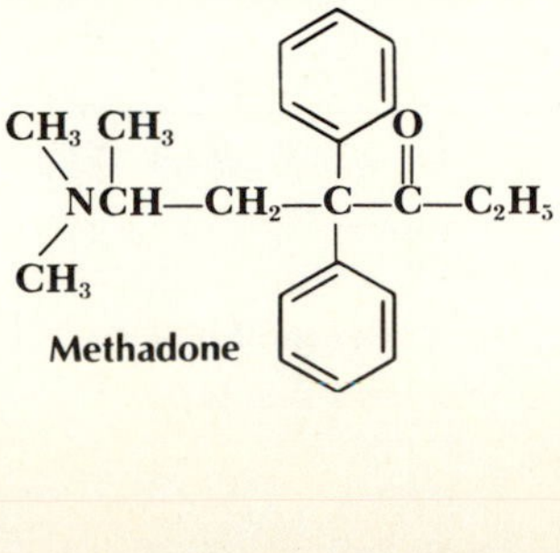

Methadone

The analgesic potency of methadone is about as great as that of morphine but is of longer duration. As a consequence, it is administered in doses of 10 mg and is quite effective following oral administration. It causes considerable respiratory depression, but its emetic and constipating actions are less than those of morphine. Development of tolerance and addiction to methadone are known to occur.

Methadone is widely employed as an analgesic. Sedation and euphoria are slight. A unique application of methadone is in the treatment of morphine addiction.[13] If the drug can be substituted for morphine, subsequent withdrawal will be less severe, but it may be more prolonged. The use of methadone in addicts is discussed in Chapter 30.

BENZOMORPHANS   **Phenazocine** (Prinadol) is a synthetic addictive analgesic that is about four times as active as morphine but is without other significant advantages.

Pentazocine (Talwin) is a synthetic analgesic structurally related to phenazocine.

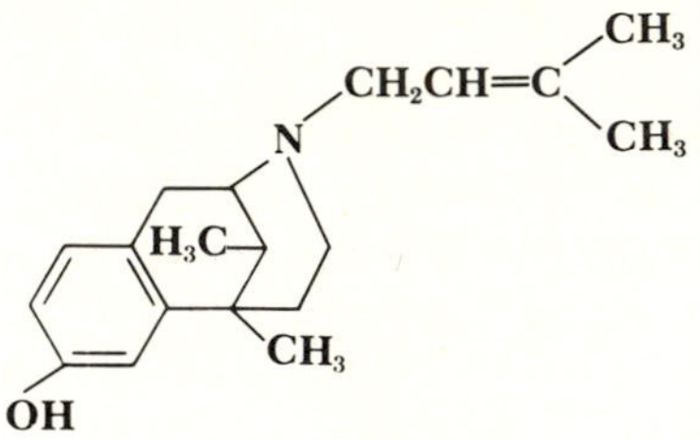

Pentazocine

Pentazocine is actually a weak narcotic antagonist with a significant analgesic effect of its own. Its potency is moderate and of short duration, but its low addiction liability makes it useful in chronic illnesses in which the more addictive drugs would constitute a hazard. Administered in 20 to 40 mg doses by the subcutaneous or intramuscular route,[4] pentazocine may be as effective as 10 mg of morphine. Larger doses do not increase its analgesic power. Pentazocine is also available in tablet form (50 mg) for oral administration. It is difficult to evaluate its analgesic potency compared with that of other drugs by the oral route.

Morphinan derivatives   The **morphinan series** of drugs includes levorphanol, dextrorphan, and dextromethorphan.

Levorphanol (Levo-Dromoran) is a synthetic drug that is closely related chemically to morphine.

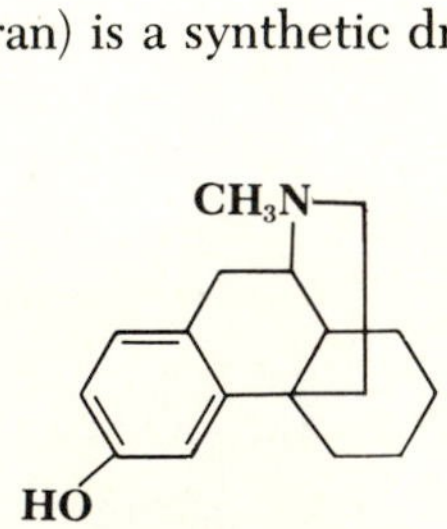

Levorphanol

The levo isomer is about five times as analgesic as morphine and consequently is administered in dosages of 2 mg. Its duration of action is somewhat longer than that of morphine. Respiratory depression and addiction liability are marked, but emetic and constipating actions are only moderate.

The dextro isomer, **dextrorphan,** has little analgesic action but possesses some antitussive properties.

Dextromethorphan (Romilar), the methyl ether of dextrorphan, has about the same antitussive potency as codeine, with no analgesic, euphoric, or respiratory-depressant properties. It is widely used as a cough suppressant, an action that is clearly unrelated to any narcotic analgesic property. It is a fairly harmless drug.[11]

Propoxyphene (Darvon) is widely used, often in combination with aspirin, phenacetin, and caffeine, the so-called Darvon Compound. Its analgesic potency is said to be similar to that of codeine, but this is doubtful. For many of its uses, aspirin contributes an anti-inflammatory analgesic effect to the Darvon Compound, which then may be more potent than codeine for specific applications. Pure propoxyphene is a weaker analgesic than codeine.

When its widespread use is considered, the number of individuals who have become addicted to propoxyphene is very low, although tolerance and addiction to the drug are possible. Doses of 32 or 64 mg of propoxyphene should suffice for most of its indications, but some individuals take the larger dose six or more times a day. In chronic painful conditions it is often difficult to know whether one is dealing with iatrogenic addiction.

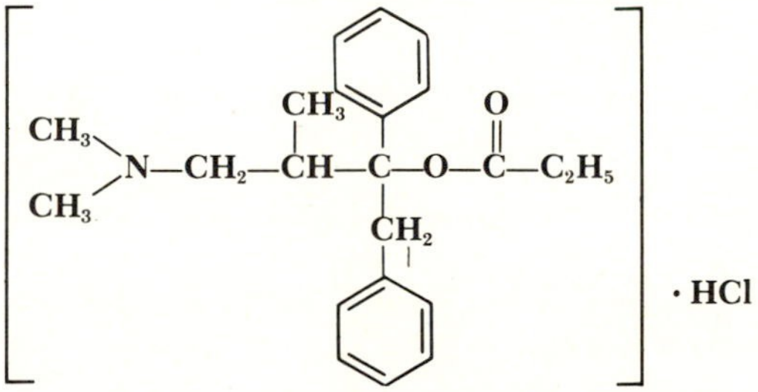

Propoxyphene hydrochloride

Problem 29-2. How does propoxyphene compare in analgesic efficacy with aspirin? In a recent double-blind crossover study,[21] propoxyphene (65 mg) gave no significant evidence of therapeutic activity and aspirin was clearly superior. It should be kept in mind, however, that these studies involved single administration to patients who had definite pain problems caused by cancer. It is conceivable that on continued administration the results would have been different.

Acute propoxyphene intoxication resembles morphine posioning. The respiratory depression responds to the administration of a narcotic antagonist such as nalorphine.

Propoxyphene overdosage causes hundreds of deaths every year in the United States. Although in most instances alcohol and other drugs contribute to the lethal outcome, physicians should be careful in starting a patient on propoxyphene unless the use of the drug is absolutely necessary.[28]

NEW ANALGESICS   Two new analgesics, **butorphanol tartrate** (Stadol) and **nalbuphine hydrochloride** (Nubain) have become available recently. These drugs are mixed agonist-antagonists, and they resemble pentazocine pharmacologically but produce psychotomimetic effects less frequently. The abuse potential of these drugs is lower that that of codeine or propoxyphene. Nevertheless, they should be used with caution since they are opiate-like drugs.[39] These drugs are not classified under the Controlled Substances Act.

Butorphanol tartrate (Stadol) is available as an injectable solution containing 1 or 2 mg/ml. Nalbuphine hydrochloride (Nubain) is available as an injectable solution containing 10 mg/ml.

NARCOTIC ANTAGONISTS   Competitive antagonism of the narcotic analgesics, particularly their respiratory depressant actions, results from certain substitutions on the nitrogen atom of morphine or levorphanol. Nalorphine and levallorphan are important narcotic antagonists. Pentazocin is a weak antagonist and is much more useful as an analgesic of low addiction liability.

Subclassification of opiate receptors   There are differences in the action of agonist-antagonists and morphine-type drugs. These differences led to a subclassification of receptors.[42] There may be two analgesic receptors. At the μ receptor, morphine acts as an agonist and nalorphine as a competitive antagonist. At the κ receptor, nalorphine acts as an agonist and morphine is inactive. Finally, the σ receptor may mediate the dysphoric and psychotomimetic effects of drugs such as pentazocine.

According to this hypothesis, pentazocine is a weak competitive antagonist at the μ receptor, a strong agonist at the κ receptor, and is also a σ receptor agonist.[42] Naloxone is a competitive antagonist at all three receptor sites. Butorphanol and nalbuphine may act like pentazocine, but cause less euphoria and psychotomimetic effects.

Nalorphine (Nalline) is *N*-allylnormorphine. Although there was evidence in the literature for many years that *N*-allyl derivatives of certain opiate drugs might antagonize the respiratory depressant effects of the various narcotics,[29] it was not until 1950 that nalorphine received clinical recognition.

Nalorphine is capable of antagonizing practically all the effects of morphine and other narcotics, including meperidine and methadone. It is a most important antidote in cases of poisoning from these drugs and can also precipitate acute withdrawal symptoms in an addicted person.

Interestingly, in the normal person, nalorphine behaves only as weak morphine. It has been suggested that the antidotal action of the drug may be caused by competitive inhibition with replacement of potent drugs by a weak compound having higher affinity for the receptors.

Nalorphine is administered in doses of 5 to 10 mg, usually by the intravenous route in cases of poisoning. The dosage should not exceed 40 mg.

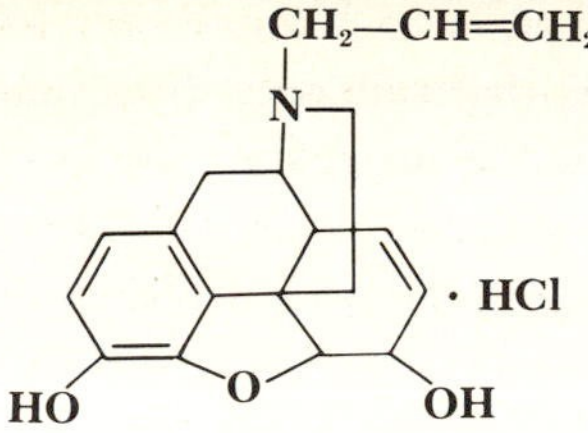

Nalorphine hydrochloride

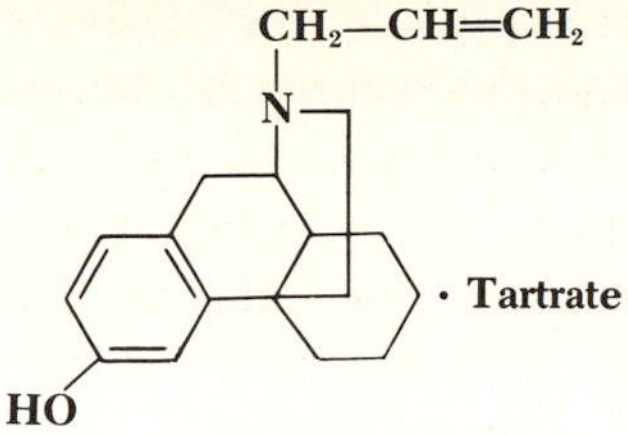

Lorfan, tartrate
of levallorphan

Levallorphan (Lorfan [Lorfan is the tartrate derivative of levallorphan]) is a morphine antagonist that is very similar in indications to nalorphine. From the pharmacological standpoint, it has the same relationship to levorphanol as nalorphine has to morphine. Levallorphan is used in doses of 0.3 to 1.2 mg by injection.

Naloxone hydrochloride (Narcan), the *N*-allyl derivative of oxymorphone hydrochloride (Numorphan), is an important and specific narcotic antagonist. It is available for intravenous, intramuscular, or subcutaneous administration in ampules and vials containing 0.4 mg/ml.

Naloxone reverses the respiratory-depressant action of the narcotics related to morphine, meperidine, and methadone. It differs from the other narcotic antagonists in several important respects. By itself, naloxone *does not cause* respiratory depression, pupillary constriction, sedation, or analgesia. It antagonizes the actions of pentazocine. Although naloxone does not antagonize the respiratory-depressants effects of barbiturates and other hypnotics, it does not aggravate their depressant effects on respiration. Just like the other narcotic antagonists, naloxone precipitates an abstinence syndrome when administered to patients addicted to opiate-like drugs.

The following medical conditions are generally considered to be contraindications to the use of morphine and related drugs:
Head injuries and following craniotomy
Bronchial asthma
Acute alcoholism
Convulsive disorders

CONTRAINDICATIONS TO THE USE OF MORPHINE AND RELATED AGENTS

The important problems of physical dependence to narcotics is discussed in detail in Chapter 30.

PHYSICAL DEPENDENCE

Of considerable interest is a recent finding that opiate withdrawal symptoms are inhibited by the administration of clonidine.[15a] This action of clonidine may be related to its ability to inhibit activity of central noradrenergic neurons by an action on presynaptic α receptors mediating the firing rate of locus coeruleus neurons. Inhibitory receptors in the locus coeruleus become tolerant to opiates, thus allowing excessive neuronal activity following opiate withdrawal.

CLINICAL PHARMACOLOGY OF ANTITUSSIVE DRUGS

From a pharmacological standpoint, cough may be suppressed by action on the neural component of the reflex or by procedures that influence the quantity or viscosity of respiratory tract fluid. Drugs that act on the neural component may act on the CNS or on sensory endings in the mucous membranes of the respiratory tract. The specific effectiveness of antitussives is difficult to determine because nonspecific sedation and placebos can be of benefit. Furthermore, in many of the cough mixtures the demulcent action of vehicles may play a significant part in the effects claimed.

There is little doubt that morphine and synthetic opiate-like drugs are potent cough suppressants. However, because of their addiction liability, they are seldom used for this purpose. Codeine is the traditional cough suppressant, and all nonaddictive antitussives should be compared with codeine in controlled clinical trials. Claims for their effectiveness are often based on uncontrolled clinical trials and experimental studies that may not be relevant.

Codeine is the standard narcotic antitussive. It is highly effective, and its addiction liability is not nearly as great as that of the strong narcotics. Nausea, constipation, and drowsiness are among the common side effects of codeine. In contrast with morphine, excessive doses of codeine may cause convulsions, especially in children. These convulsions are attributed to an effect of codeine on the spinal cord. The usual adult dosage of codeine phosphate USP is 8 to 15 mg three or four times daily.

Hydrocodone bitartrate (Dicodid) is a somewhat more potent antitussive than codeine, but its addiction liability is greater. It is available in 5 mg tablets.

Dextromethorphan (Romilar) is a substituted dextro isomer of the narcotic levorphan (Dromoran). It is not analgesic and is not addictive. It is claimed that it approaches codeine in antitussive potency. The usual dose is 10 to 20 mg by mouth.

Noscapine (Nectadon) is the isoquinoline alkaloid narcotine found in opium. The drug is not addictive and has little analgesic action but is claimed to be antitussive. The dose is 15 to 30 mg by mouth three times a day.

Benzonatate (Tessalon) is a local anesthetic related to tetracaine. It is claimed to be an effective antitussive when used in doses of 100 mg. It is believed to influence the cough reflex both at the stretch receptors in the lungs and within the CNS. It does not depress respiration.

Antihistaminics are also claimed to be of benefit as antitussives. Although there may be some reason for this action in asthmatic bronchitis of allergic etiology, their mode of action in other types of cough is not understood and according to some investigators is not well documented. Drugs of this type include carbetapentane (Toclase), dimethoxanate (Cothera), a phenothiazine, and other antihistaminic drugs.

Levopropoxyphene (Novrad), in contrast to its dextro form (Darvon), is claimed to have antitussive properties without being an analgesic. It may be too early to evaluate these claims on the basis of the evidence presented so far, although the drug is claimed to be as potent as codeine.

In addition to the antitussives that depress the cough reflex, drugs may be beneficial in the treatment of respiratory illnesses associated with coughing because they may reduce the viscosity of thick mucus.

Glyceryl guaiacolate (Guaianesin) apparently increases the volume and decreases the viscosity of bronchial secretions. Its dose is 100 to 200 mg by mouth, which may be repeated in 2 to 4 hours. Its efficacy is in doubt.

$$\text{O—CH}_2\text{—CH—CH}_2\text{—OH}$$

with OH above the central CH, and OCH$_3$ on the benzene ring.

Glyceryl guaiacolate

Iodides are sometimes employed in bronchial asthma. The mode of action of these drugs is not known with certainty, but they may decrease the viscosity of bronchial mucus.

Ipecac and **ammonium chloride** are believed to cause thinning of bronchial mucus, perhaps by some reflex mechanism.

As a general statement, the antitussive drugs may be valuable in reducing a useless cough. They are purely symptomatic medications, and their use should not obviate the necessity of determining the cause of the cough. Claims made for the many nonaddictive antitussives should be examined critically.

REFERENCES

1 Alderman, E. L.: Analgesics in the acute phase of myocardial infarction, J.A.M.A. **229:**1646, 1974.

2 Axelrod, J.: The enzymatic demethylation of narcotic drugs, J. Pharmacol. Exp. Ther. **117:** 322, 1956.

3 Axelrod, J.: Possible mechanism of tolerance to narcotic drugs, Science **124:**263, 1956.

4 Beaver, W. T., Wallenstein, S. L., Houde, R. W., and Rogers A.: A comparison of the analgesic effects of pentazocine and morphine in patients with cancer, Clin. Pharmacol. Ther. **7:**740, 1966.

5 Beecher, H. K.: Appraisal of drugs intended to alter subjective responses, symptoms. Report to Council on Pharmacy and Chemistry, J.A.M.A. **158:**399, 1955.

6 Beecher, H. K.: Measurement of subjective responses, New York, 1959, Oxford University Press.

7 Bickerman, H. A., Cohen, B. M., and German, E.: Cough response of healthy human subjects stimulated by citric acid aerosol: evaluation of antitussive agents, Am. J. Med. Sci. **234:**191, 1957.

8 Bodo, R. C., Cotui, F. W., and Benaglia, A. E.: Studies on the mechanism of morphine hyperglycemia: role of the sympathetic nervous system, with special reference to the sympathetic supply to the liver, J. Pharmacol. Exp. Ther. **62:**88, 1938.

9 Bucher, K.: Pathophysiology and pharmacology of cough, Pharmacol. Rev. **10:**43, 1958.

10 Burks, T. F.: Mediation by 5-hydroxytryptamine of morphine stimulant actions in dog intestine, J. Pharmacol. Exp. Ther. **185:**530, 1973.

11 Cass, L. J., Frederik, W. S., and Andosca, J. B.: Quantitative comparison of dextromethorphan hydrobromide and codeine, Am. J. Med. Sci. **227:**291, 1954.

12 Cochin, J., Haggart, J., Woods, L. A., and Seevers, M. H.: Plasma levels, urinary and fecal excretion of morphine in non-tolerant and tolerant dogs, J. Pharmacol. Exp. Ther. **111:** 74, 1954.

13 Dole, V. P., and Nyswander, M.: A medical treatment for diacetylmorphine (heroin) addiction: a clinical trial with metadone hydrochloride, J.A.M.A. **193:**646, 1965.

14 Eisleb, O., and Schaumann, O.: Dolantin, ein neuartiges Spasmolytikum and Analgetikum (chemisches and pharmakologisches), Deutsch. Med. Wochenschr. **65**:967, 1939.

15 Fraser, H. F., and Harris, L. S.: Narcotic and narcotic antagonist analgesics, Annu. Rev. Pharmacol. **7**:277, 1967.

15a Gold, M. S., Redmond, D. E., and Kleber, H. D.: Clonidine blocks acute opiate-withdrawal symptoms, Lancet **2**:559, 1978.

16 Goldstein, D. B., and Goldstein, A.: Possible role of enzyme inhibition in repression in drug tolerance and addiction, Biochem. Pharmacol. **8**:48, 1961.

17 Gross, E. G.: Effect of liver damage on urinary morphine excretion, Proc. Soc. Exp. Biol. Med. **51**:61, 1942.

18 Hughes, J., et al.: Identification of two related pentapeptides from the brain with potent opiate agonist activity, Nature **258**:577, 1975.

19 Kay, D. C., Gorodetzky, C. W., and Martin, W. R.: Comparative effects of codeine and morphine in man, J. Pharmacol. Exp. Ther. **156**:101, 1967.

20 Lasagna, L.: The clinical evaluation of morphine and its substitutes as analgesics, Pharmacol. Rev. **16**:47, 1964.

21 Moertel, C. G., Ahmann, D. L., Taylor, W. F., and Schwartau, N.: A comparative evaluation of marketed analgesic drugs, N. Engl. J. Med. **286**:813, 1972.

22 Murphree, H. B.: Clinical pharmacology of potent analgesics, Clin. Pharmacol. Ther. **3**:473, 1962.

23 Papadopoulos, C. N., and Keats, A. S.: Studies of analgesic drugs. VI. Comparative respiratory depressant activity of phenazocine and morphine, Clin. Pharmacol. Ther. **2**:8, 1961.

24 Pert, C. B., and Snyder, S. H.: Opiate receptor: demonstration in nervous tissue, Science **179**:1011, 1973.

25 Reynolds, A. K., and Randall, L. O.: Morphine and allied drugs, Toronto, 1957, University of Toronto Press.

26 Sadove, M., Balagot, R. D., and Pecora, F. N.: Pentazocine—a new nonaddicting analgesic, J.A.M.A. **189**:199, 1964.

27 Seevers, M. H., and Woods, L. A.: The phenomena of tolerance, Am. J. Med. **14**:546, 1953.

28 Sengupta, A., and Peat, M. A.: Propoxyphene overdose: a study involving analgesic preparations containing dextropropoxyphene, Arch. Toxicol. **37**:123, 1977.

29 Unna, K.: Antagonistic effect of N-allynor-morphine upon morphine, J. Pharmacol. Exp. Ther. **79**:27, 1943.

30 Vandam, L. D.: Clinical pharmacology of the narcotic analgesics, Clin. Pharmacol. Ther. **3**:827, 1962.

31 Wang, S. C. and Glaviano, V. V.: Locus of emetic action of morphine and hydergine in dogs, J. Pharmacol. Exp. Ther. **111**:329, 1954.

32 Wikler, A.: Sites and mechanisms of action of morphine and related drugs in the central nervous system, Pharmacol. Rev. **2**:435, 1950.

33 Winter, C. A., and Flataker, L.: Antitussive compounds: testing methods and results, J. Pharmacol. Exp. Ther. **112**:99, 1954.

34 Wolff, B. B., Kantor, T. G., Jarvik, M. E., and Laska, E.: Response of experimental pain to analgesic drugs. I. Morphine, aspirin and placebo, Clin. Pharmacol. Ther. **7**:224, 1966.

35 Wolff, H. G., Hardy, J. D., and Goodell, H.: Studies on pain: measurement of the effect of morphine, codeine, and other opiates on the pain threshold and an analysis of their relation to the pain experience, J. Clin. Invest. **19**:659, 1940.

REVIEWS

36 Alderman, E. L.: Analgesics in the acute phase of myocardial infarction, J.A.M.A. **229**:1646, 1974.

37 Edison, G. R.: The drug laws. Are they effective and safe? J.A.M.A. **239**:2578, 1978.

38 Goldstein, A.: Opioid peptides (endorphins) in pituitary and brain, Science **193**:1081, 1976.

38a Ketchum, J. S., and Jarvik, M. E.: Pharmacotherapy for the opioid addict: agonists or antagonists? Ration. Drug Ther. **13**:1, Jan. 1979.

39 Lewis, J. R.: Evaluation of new analgesics. Butorphanol and Nalbuphine, J.A.M.A. **243**:1465, 1980.

40 Lewis, J. W., Bentley, K. W., and Cowan, A.: Narcotic analgesics and antagonists, Annu. Rev. Pharmacol. **11**:241, 1971.

41 Martin, W. R.: Naloxone, Ann. Intern. Med. **85**:765, 1976.

42 Martin, W. R.: History and development of mixed opioid agonists, partial agonists and antagonists, Br. J. Clin. Pharmacol. **7**(Supp. 3):273, 1979.

43 Snyder, S. H.: Opiate receptors in the brain, N. Engl. J. Med. **296**:266, 1977.

44 Snyder, S.: The opiates, opioid peptides (endorphins) and the opiate receptor, Tex. Med. **75**:41, 1979.

45 Way, E. L., and Settle, A. A.: Uses of narcotic antagonists, Ration. Drug Ther. **9**:1975.

CHAPTER 30

Contemporary drug abuse

The term *abuse* implies that a particular application of a drug is more destructive than constructive for society or the individual. Needless to say, it is sometimes difficult to decide whether an application is preponderantly destructive or constructive. Some observers[162] assert that the connotation of "drug abuse" represents solely a cultural value judgment, a biased accusation; it is nevertheless obvious that some drug usage would be considered abusive from almost any cultural frame of reference. Prolonged dependence on amphetamines in high doses, for example, invariably invokes a progressive organic brain syndrome.

It is important to distinguish between *drug abuse* and *drug dependence;* the two concepts are not synonymous. Drug abuse may exist without drug dependence, drug dependence without drug abuse, or both may coexist. A single administration of a hazardous drug may represent abuse without dependence, whereas the maintenance of a diabetic person on insulin represents dependence without abuse. The concept of abuse also depends in part on cultural values, unlike the concept of dependence.

Most abused drugs are drugs with a primary action on the CNS. The reason is obvious: drug users wish to modify their mental state. Abuse of drugs without primary CNS activity is mostly a matter of misuse by medical or paramedical personnel, such as the indiscriminate prescription of penicillin and the "treatment" of obesity with digitalis, thyroid hormone, and diuretics.[90]

Drug dependence has traditionally been conceptualized in terms of a rigid duality: psychological dependence and physical dependence. This duality probably originates in the ancient distinction between mind and body.[27] The dual concepts are still used today and are incorporated into the discussions of individual drugs in this chapter. If a physiologically disruptive withdrawal illness follows the abrupt discontinuation of a drug taken over a prolonged period of time, the drug is said to be physically addicting. Physically addicting drugs include the opiates, barbiturates, antianxiety agents, ethanol, and some nonbarbiturate sedatives. Psychological drug dependence, on the other hand, has been described as a craving for a drug producing a desired effect and to which one has become accustomed by habit; the habit has become a crutch and may assume enormous importance to the individual. It is said that psychological dependence, not physical dependence drives opiate addicts back to their drug after months or years of successful abstinence.

Bridging the gap between psychological and physical dependence would now seem feasible. Studies of central neurotransmitter action have led to the theory that central mediation of reward perception occurs in association with potentiation of catecholamine action at central synapses, although the mechanism of potentiation may differ with different drugs. If the theory is correct, it partially bridges the gap between psychological and physical dependence in that psychological dependence on a drug occurs in association with a physicochemical change at central synapses.[27] The gap is not fully bridged by this theory, however, since psychological dependence also embodies the concept of dependence on established habit patterns; thus one may become dependent on a drug or on any oft-repeated behavior, such as eating a hearty breakfast each morning.

OPIATES AND OPIATE-LIKE DRUGS

In some state statutes the legal category "narcotics" embraces the opiates, opiate-like drugs, marihuana, and cocaine. Medically defined, however, the term *narcotic* refers only to drugs having both a sedative and an analgesic action and is essentially restricted to the opiates and opiate-like drugs. These drugs are classified on p. 342.

Physical dependence and tolerance

Marked physical dependence develops rapidly during continued administration of any of the narcotic drugs. A striking tolerance also develops to all but the miotic action; the addict continues to have constricted pupils, even after low doses. A high degree of cross-tolerance exists among all the opiates and opiate-like drugs in spite of chemical dissimilarities.

Characteristics of abuse

Heroin is generally the opiate most preferred by the drug user, except for physician addicts, who use meperidine more than any other. Many users consider heroin more euphorigenic than any other opiate. In regions of the United States where good-quality heroin is hard to obtain, however, the addict may prefer "drugstore dope" (usually morphine or hydromorphone stolen from drugstores). Until recently narcotic addiction in the United States had been mostly confined to the lower socio-economic classes of the larger cities and to members of the medical profession; it is now spreading alarmingly to youth from all socioeconomic levels.

The veteran heroin addict seeks two principal desired effects from the drug: avoidance of the withdrawal illness and a feeling described most commonly as "relief." These effects are usually more important to the addict than the transitory "kick" or "rush" felt immediately after intravenous injection. The opiates tend to leave the user in a state of drive satiation; everything is "as it should be." Accordingly, sexual drive is usually diminished.

There is no evidence that the opiates produce organic CNS damage or other organ pathology, even after years of continuous use. An 84-year-old physician morphine addict was found to exhibit no evidence of mental or physical deterioration after continuous use for 62 years.[33,80] Complications of parenteral administration, however, are legion and include viral hepatitis, bacterial and fungal endocarditis, nephropathy with massive proteinuria, systemic and pulmonary mycoses, lung abscess, pulmonary fibrosis or granulomatosis, pneumonia, chronic liver disease (of obscure type), transverse myelitis, osteomyelitis (frequently *Pseudomonas*), acute and chronic polyneuropathy, acute and chronic myopathy, acute rhabdomyolysis with myoglobinuria, tetanus, tuberculosis (including tuberculous vertebral osteomyelitis), malaria (now rare in the United States), thrombophlebitis, cellulitis, local abscesses, and sclerosis and occlusion of veins.* In addition, there is a constant risk of overdose and death from an unexpectedly concentrated sample of heroin; the triad of coma (or stupor), respiratory depression, and pinpoint pupils strongly suggests opiate overdose. Death from overdose may be a result of respiratory depression or acute pulmonary edema[164] or both; the mechanism of production of pulmonary edema is obscure. Still another ever present hazard is the masking of pain, which may delay awareness of a serious medical condition; cigarette burns between the fingers of opiate addicts are a common finding. Since 1955, most cases of tetanus in New York City have occurred in heroin addicts.[14]

Additional dangers arise from foreign substances intentionally added to the sample by the supplier. Heroin is commonly "cut" with lactose or quinine; other adulterants include barbiturates, procaine, mannitol, aminopyrine, methapyrilene, and baking soda.[121]

Social consequences of narcotic addiction include crime, interruption of employment, and personal and family neglect. Criminal activity is usually restricted to property offenses and peddling, which may become necessary in the absence of employment in order to support the habit. Some addicts become functionally disabled, spending much of the 24-hour period "nodding" (remaining inactive in a semistuporous state) or suffering withdrawal symptoms; other addicts who have an uninterrupted drug supply and are careful with dosage may lead a seemingly normal life at work and at home. The concept of the opiate addict as a dangerous "dope fiend" is not justified; in contrast to alcohol, the opiates tend to quell aggressive drives. When

---

*See references 34, 57, 77, 113, 121, and 147.

TABLE 30-1. Comparison of commonly abused centrally acting drugs

Drug category	Physical dependence*	Tolerance	Psychotogenic in high doses
Opiates	X	X	
Marihuana		X	X
Ethanol	X	X	
Barbiturates	X	X	
Amphetamines		X	X
Cocaine		X	X
Psychotomimetics		X	X
Phenothiazines			
Antianxiety agents	X		
Inhalants†		?	X

*An abstinence syndrome results from abrupt discontinuation of any drug producing physical dependence.
†See text for details.

an addict's supply of drugs is exhausted, however, violence may be resorted to in order to obtain a continuing supply. Another incentive for assaultive behavior is fear of police detection. A fellow addict suspected of collaborating with the police may be silenced permanently by an overdose of drug, either arranged by a supplier who provides an unusually concentrated sample of heroin to the victim or accomplished more directly by assault and enforced injection. The apparent cause of death in either case is accidental overdose.

Abstinence syndromes   **Morphine or heroin.** Symptoms first appear about 8 hours after the last dose, reaching peak intensity between 36 and 72 hours. Lacrimation, rhinorrhea, yawning, and diaphoresis appear between 8 and 12 hours. Shortly thereafter, at about 13 hours, a restless sleep (the "yen") may intervene. At about 20 hours, gooseflesh, dilated pupils, agitation, and tremors may appear. During the second and third day, when the illness is at its peak, symptoms and signs include weakness, insomnia, chills, intestinal cramps, nausea, vomiting, diarrhea, violent yawning, muscle aches in the legs, severe low back pain, elevation of blood pressure and pulse rate, diaphoresis, and waves of gooseflesh. The skin may have the appearance of a cold plucked turkey, hence the expression "cold turkey," denoting abrupt withdrawal. Fluid depletion during the withdrawal period has at times resulted in cardiovascular collapse and death. At any point during the course of withdrawal, administration of an opiate in adequate dosage will dramatically eliminate the symptoms and restore a state of apparent normalcy. The duration of the syndrome is roughly 7 to 10 days.

Other narcotic drugs. Most narcotic abstinence syndromes are similar to that of morphine or heroin. Narcotics with a shorter duration of action tend to produce a shorter and more severe abstinence syndrome; those with a longer duration of action or slower rate of elimination, such as methadone, usually produce a milder and more prolonged syndrome.

Methadone maintenance   Withdrawal from an opiate may be accomplished simply by administering smaller and smaller doses of the same opiate over a period of days. Rehabilitation of the opiate addict, however, is another matter. The craving for the drug long after withdrawal is one factor in the very low success rate. In 1964 Drs. Vincent P. Dole and Marie E. Nyswander reported that if heroin addicts were maintained on oral methadone they could give up heroin and engage in an active rehabilitation program.[7] Methadone, a synthetic opiate-like drug, substitutes well for most other opiates and is well absorbed from the gastrointestinal tract, unlike morphine or heroin; parenteral administration is thereby avoided. In addition, methadone has a longer duration of action than other opiates, permitting administration only once or twice in a 24-hour period. The total period of drug administration is shortened, since methadone remains in the body for 36 to 72 hours after the last dose.

In the early 1970s methadone maintenance was attempted with federal support on a nationwide scale.[39] It was found to be less effective on a large scale than on the small personal scale initiated by Dole and Nyswander, but more effective than any other known approach. One-year retention rates were found to be about 50% at best. After a period of 12 to 36 months of methadone maintenance, withdrawal of methadone ("methadone detoxification") is attempted. One study has shown a 58% return to narcotic use 6 years after methadone detoxification.[165] The highest recidivism rates appear to be associated with premature detoxification from methadone maintenance.

A synthetic congener of methadone, 1-α-acetylmethadol hydrochloride (methadylacetate), can prevent withdrawal symptoms for more than 72 hours.[88,117] Because of this relative advantage, methadylacetate is currently being evaluated as a substitute for methadone. It appears that the two drugs are equivalent in rehabilitative efficacy, but that one or the other may be more effective with different subsets of the addict population.[156]

An intensive search is now under way for the "ideal" narcotic antagonist, namely, a pharmacological agent that blocks the effects of opiates, has few or no side effects of its own, requires relatively infrequent administration, and is not prohibitively expensive to produce. No drug has yet met these criteria, but some have come close. Naloxone, for example, abolishes the euphoria, respiratory depression, nausea, and gastrointestinal disturbances produced by opiates and produces virtually no side effects; it is expensive, however, and its limited duration of action requires more than one dose per day for the treatment or prevention of addiction.[189] A new experimental drug, naltrexone, has come closer than any other substance to fulfilling the criteria of an ideal narcotic antagonist.[95]

Narcotic antagonists

The earliest known narcotic antagonists were nalorphine (Nalline) and levallorphan (Lorfan). Administration of a narcotic antagonist precipitates a telltale abstinence syndrome if physical dependence on an opiate has become established. A severe abstinence syndrome may be precipitated that cannot be suppressed during the period of action of the antagonists, and some antagonists may further embarrass respiration that has been compromised by alcohol, barbiturates, or other nonnarcotic depressants.

This exciting new area of discovery and theory began with the finding in 1971 that opiates bind to receptors on the cell membrane of some neurons of the CNS.[61,161] The neurons are distributed in brain regions corresponding to anatomical structures and pathways involved in pain perception. Receptor binding has been demonstrated in many vertebrate species, from primitive fish to monkeys and humans, but appears to be absent in invertebrates. The natural question arose: Why should receptors exist in vertebrates for the alkaloids of the poppy? The logical answer was that there may be *endogenous* opiate-like compounds that are recognized by the receptors and serve some purpose in brain function.

Opiate receptors and endogenous opiates

Many drugs, after all, turn out to be mimics of endogenous substances. An accident of molecular shape allows them to fit into our receptors, either activating or blocking them.

The receptor theory of opiate action is supported by several lines of evidence.

First, all natural and some synthetic opiate agonists have basic similarities of structure, suggesting the possibility of common recognition by an opiate receptor. Second, the extraordinary potency of some synthetic opiate agonists can be explained only by considering a highly selective receptor site. Etorphine, for example, is 5000 to 10,000 times more potent than morphine and produces euphoria and analgesia in doses as small as 0.0001 g, making it even more potent than LSD. Third, usually only levorotatory opiate isomers are active, suggesting stereospecific receptor function. Finally, opiate antagonists can be synthesized by effecting very slight molecular modifications of opiates, and the rapid action of these antagonists in reversing the effects of opiates suggests receptor site blockade.

The receptor theory of opiate action provoked a search for endogenous opiate-like compounds. This search has been successful; since 1975 two groups of brain peptides have been found with opiate-like activity: pentapeptides, called *enkephalins*, which appear to be neurotransmitters or neuromodulators with a distribution paralleling that of opiate receptors, and larger peptides, called *endorphins*, all isolated from the hypothalamus and neurohypophysis.[69] Amino acid sequences of the peptides have been found to be identical to sequences in fragments of β-lipotropin, a minor component of pituitary extract isolated in 1964.

The enkephalins and endorphins are indistinguishable from morphine in opiate-binding bioassays. When administered in vivo to laboratory animals, the enkephalins display weak analgesic action, and the endorphins evoke a host of variable effects: α-endorphin produces apparent tranquilization, analgesia of face and neck, and hypothermia; γ-endorphin produces agitation, hyperthermia, and no analgesia; and β-endorphin also produces hypothermia and profound analgesia of the whole body. β-Endorphin also produces prolonged muscular rigidity and immobility similar to a catatonic state.[15] In every case the effects are abolished rapidly by the administration of a narcotic antagonist. The profound behavioral effects of the endorphins have led to speculation that opiate receptors may have functions other than modulating pain sensation. Just as exogenous opiates induce a state of euphoria and emotional detachment from the experience of suffering, endogenous opiates may play some central role in affective and behavioral homeostasis.[61]

Avram Goldstein has asked the following questions: Do opiate addicts suppress or damage their endogenous opioid systems? Are some people more vulnerable to opiate addiction because of a relative deficiency of endogenous opioids?[62]

The analgesic action of some of these biogenic peptides has led to hopes that "natural" nonaddicting analgesics will finally be discovered. One study has failed to support these hopes. A typical morphine withdrawal illness was demonstrated in rats infused with methionine-enkephalin and β-endorphin for 70 hours and subsequently challenged with naloxone.[181] But it is too early to draw conclusions; it still seems feasible that an endogenous opioid, or a mixed agonist-antagonist developed from such an opioid, will provide a superior analgesic with less addiction potential.

ALCOHOL   It is often forgotten that alcoholism is still the most serious form of drug abuse in western society. It is estimated that over 9 million Americans are alcoholics and that over 50% of crimes and over 50% of highway accidents in the United States are alcohol-related.

A marked degree of physical dependence and a moderate degree of tolerance develop to alcohol when ingested regularly and in large amounts. Tolerance may be explained in part by induced hypertrophy of hepatic smooth endoplasmic reticulum with stimulation of alcohol metabolism.[151]

Physical dependence and tolerance

Alcohol is a primary and continuous depressant of the CNS. Even a small amount decreases mental acuity and impairs motor coordination; at times, however, this deficit may be more than compensated for by the improved performance accompanying the induced state of euphoria and release from inhibitory attitudes.

Characteristics of abuse

In chronic alcoholism one may observe organ pathology and clinical syndromes not usually associated with other types of drug abuse, including fatty metamorphosis and cirrhosis of the liver, peripheral polyneuropathy, alcoholic gastritis, Korsakoff's psychosis, Wernicke's encephalopathy, and the complications of portal hypertension. Some of these changes are thought to be the result of nutritional deficiency rather than the direct action of alcohol; unlike other commonly abused drugs, alcohol supplies calories, depressing the appetite and encouraging a dietary deficit in the face of a deceptive maintenance of body weight. It is believed that alcohol is directly incriminated, however, in the pathogenesis of alcoholic fatty liver.[114]

Chronic alcohol consumption leads to hypertrophy of hepatic smooth endoplasmic reticulum, with consequent stimulation of drug metabolism. This finding may explain in part the tolerance of alcoholics, *when sober,* to drugs such as barbiturates. *When inebriated,* alcoholics display a *heightened* sensitivity to barbiturates, not only because of the synergistic action of the two drugs but perhaps also because hepatic metabolism of other drugs is temporarily slowed during the active metabolism of alcohol.[151]

A recent study of blood pressure in relation to drinking habits of over 80,000 men and women of three races strongly suggests that regular use of three or more drinks per day is a significant risk factor predisposing to hypertension.[100]

In the history of many opiate addicts there occurs a turning from alcohol to opiates. The addict recalls that he was frequently "getting into fights" while under the influence of alcohol and that such poorly controlled behavior diminished or disappeared entirely "behind heroin."

Alcoholism appears to be a genetically influenced disorder. This conclusion is strongly suggested by familial incidence, twin studies, genetic marker studies, and adoption studies.[65,133] A higher incidence of elevated blood acetaldehyde levels after an ethanol test dose has also been shown to occur in families of alcoholics.[153]

After prolonged, heavy intake of alcohol, withdrawal symptoms may appear within a few hours after the last dose; these include tremulousness, weakness, anxiety, intestinal cramps, and hyperreflexia. Between 12 and 24 hours the stage of "acute alcoholic hallucinosis" may appear, in which visual hallucinations are re-

Abstinence syndrome

ported, at first only with the eyes closed. By 48 hours an acute brain syndrome may become apparent, with confusion, disorientation, and delusional thinking. When this syndrome is accompanied by gross tremulousness, it is called "delirium tremens." Major convulsive seizures ("rum fits") may occur but are less common than in barbiturate withdrawal. The chronic alcoholic may be in too poor a condition to withstand the stress of withdrawal; if death is not the price, recovery occurs by the fifth to the seventh day.

MARIHUANA

SLANG EQUIVALENTS:
Grass, weed, pot, dope, hemp; marihuana cigarette = joint, "j," number, reefer, root
Cigarette butt = roach

Marihuana is inadequately described by any one drug category, as it possesses properties of a sedative, euphoriant, and hallucinogen.

The source of marihuana is the Indian hemp plant *Cannabis sativa,* an herbaceous annual growing wild in temperate climates all over the world. The plant is dioecious; that is, male and female flowers are borne on separate plants. The active compounds are most concentrated in the resinous exudate of the female flower clusters.

In the United States the term *marihuana* refers to any part or extract of the plant. The smoking mixture termed "bhang" consists only of the cut tops of uncultivated female plants. The most concentrated natural supply of cannabinols is found in the preparations called "hashish" and "charas," which consist largely of the actual resin from the flower clusters of cultivated female plants. The potency of any marihuana preparation varies with the plant strain and the growth conditions.

The principal psychoactive compound in marihuana appears to be *l*-Δ^9-transtetrahydrocannabinol (hereafter referred to as Δ^9THC; Δ^1THC and Δ^9THC represent different systems of nomenclature for the same compound). A varying, usually small, amount of $\Delta^{8(9)}$THC may also be present.[112,128,129]

Black-market samples labeled "THC" virtually never contain THC but are comprised of any number of other psychotomimetic agents.

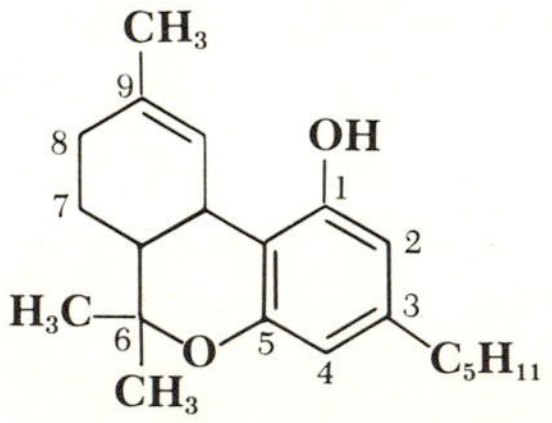

Δ^9THC 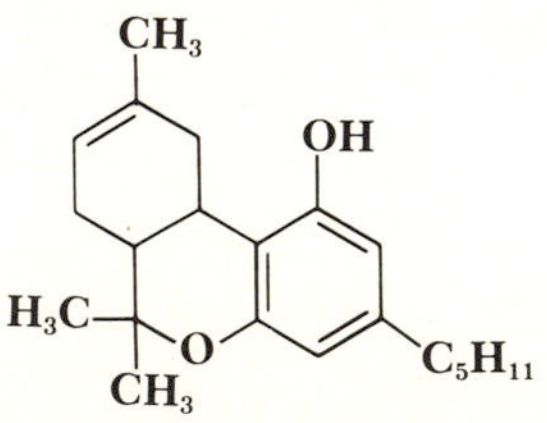 $\Delta^{8(9)}$THC ($\Delta^{1(6)}$THC)

Physical dependence and tolerance

Physical dependence is not known to develop. It is generally conceded that tolerance develops in most species tested; in one study, however, tolerance failed to develop to THC administered to chimpanzees for 63 consecutive days.[53] Two studies have failed to demonstrate cross-tolerance between Δ^9THC and LSD in humans[83] or between Δ^9THC and mescaline in rats.[160] On the other hand, one study has demonstrated a dose-related cross-tolerance between Δ^9THC and ethanol,[138] and the cross-tolerance is symmetric (that is, either drug induces cross-tolerance to the other).

Anecdotal reports. Most users report that marihuana induces a dreamy, euphoric state of altered consciousness, with feelings of detachment, gaiety, and jocularity and preoccupation with simple and familiar things. In the company of others there is a tendency toward laughter and loquaciousness. Perceptual distortion of space and time is regularly reported; distances may be judged inaccurately, and things may seem to be happening very slowly or very rapidly.

Characteristics of intoxication

Dissociative phenomena such as partial amnesia or a feeling of being outside of oneself looking on are frequently reported. Libido is variably affected; since sexual desire may be enhanced, marihuana has gained a reputation as an aphrodisiac. There may be an unusually vivid remembrance or reliving of experiences or mood states of the past. The continuity of a story or movie may be lost, to be replaced by an intense experiencing of individual segments or scenes. Users are sometimes recognized by the characteristic hiliarity of their mutual laughter, which may become prolonged and uncontrolled. Appetite and appreciation of the flavor of food are usually enhanced, and weight gain may accompany regular smoking.

A paranoid state is sometimes reported, in which the smoker is keenly sensitive of others watching him; some forsake marihuana for this reason. Antisocial behavior under the influence of marihuana appears to be rare; users ordinarily withdraw from company that they find unpleasant.

Adverse reactions to unadulterated preparations of marihuana are relatively rare, but they may be serious when they do occur. Such reactions include acute paranoid states, dissociative states, and, less commonly, acute psychotic reactions. Adverse reactions to marihuana appear to be dose related (they are more frequent with hashish) and highly individualized (some users regularly have adverse reactions and some never do). The evaluation of reports of adverse reactions is complicated by the fact that marihuana is frequently adulterated with other drugs; some reports have failed to take this possibility into consideration.[97,141]

Regular use of marihuana may result in a pervasive feeling of apathy, the so-called amotivational syndrome. The user discovers that "things just don't seem important to me any more." This development may be especially damaging to the psychological maturation of the adolescent. Such a syndrome is undoubtedly multidetermined, but in many adolescents undergoing psychotherapy, its development has been observed to coincide temporally with regular use of marihuana.

Clinical studies. An early study by Isbell and co-workers[82] demonstrated that Δ^9THC produces effects similar to those of crude marihuana preparations and that the psychotomimetic effects are dose-related. Isbell subsequently compared the effects of Δ^9THC and LSD and showed that (1) pupillodilatation and hyperreflexia occurred with LSD but not with THC, (2) heart rate was increased markedly by THC, (3) conjunctival injection and pseudoptosis were produced by THC but not

LSD, (4) differences in the subjective states induced by the two drugs were difficult to determine, and (5) no cross-tolerance between the two drugs could be demonstrated.[83]

Hollister[74] has found that perceptual and psychological changes in humans to measured doses of synthetic THC include euphoria, sleepiness (deep sleep followed higher doses), alteration in time sense, visual perceptual distortion, depersonalization, difficulty in concentrating, dreamlike states, and decreased aggressiveness with increasing dose. Psychometric tests demonstrated reduced accuracy in some cases and slowing of performance in other cases to a mild degree. Physiological effects were limited to regular and constant increase in pulse rate, no change or slight decrease in blood pressure, two instances of orthostatic hypotension, regular conjunctival injection (no smoke was present), and muscle weakness (measured in the fingers). For comparison, the synthetic THC homolog, synhexyl, was also administered orally to human subjects; effects were similar to Δ^9THC, but synhexyl was approximately one-third as potent.

THC and alcohol were compared in normal subjects, with each subject serving as his or her own control. After smoking 20 mg of THC, each subject experienced more persecutory feelings and perceptual disturbances than after placebo or doses of alcohol calculated to be as intoxicating as the THC doses.[130]

Marihuana smoking has been shown to produce an increase in pulse rate and limb blood flow with a slight rise in both systolic and diastolic pressure.[186] The fact that an increase in limb flow was unaccompanied by a fall in systemic pressure suggests that circulatory adjustments occur in other vascular beds. Propranolol, a β-adrenergic blocker, prevented both the tachycardia and the increased limb flow; atropine increased the pulse rate but not limb flow. Cooling the hand with ice failed to evoke the normal reduction in blood flow to the hand. It is apparent from this study that marihuana smoking may impair vascular reflex responses and render the individual more vulnerable both to blood loss in the event of peripheral injury and to hypotension in the event of blood loss. The risk of aggravating or prolonging marihuana-induced tachycardia by administration of atropine is also revealed by the study.

A study of the effect of marihuana smoking on cardiovascular function[5] suggests that marihuana increases myocardial oxygen demand and decreases myocardial oxygen delivery, with the result that angina pectoris is experienced sooner and with less exertion. Smoking only one marihuana cigarette decreases exercise tolerance in patients with angina caused by coronary artery disease.

A study of marihuana-induced temporal disintegration was conducted at the Stanford University School of Medicine,[131,132] using doses of 20, 40, and 60 mg of THC (the higher two doses were admittedly larger than the dose to be expected from ordinary social smoking). All three doses significantly impaired serial operations in performing a task requiring sequential cognitive functions. Progressively more errors were made with increasing dose. The subjects reported a feeling of timelessness and uncertainty of how much time had elapsed; the time line extending from past to future seemed discontinuous, and past and future seemed unrelated to the present.

One individual stated: ". . . I can't stay on the same subject. . . . I can't remember what I just said or what I want to say . . . because there are just so many thoughts that are broken in time, one chunk there and one chunk here." Impairment of immediate memory with emergence of loose associations was noted, and the latter was considered to have its probable origin in the former. The serious implications of such an effect over a prolonged period of time are clear.

Apparent overestimation of the passage of time was also reported in chimpanzees to whom Δ^9THC was administered orally.[29] Temporally spaced responses of the chimps came to be made closer and closer together as the dose of THC was increased, suggesting that the chimps perceived shorter and shorter intervals of time as being of the original familiar duration.

In a careful study of aggression in mice, rats, and squirrel monkeys, THC was shown to decrease species-specific attack behavior.[134] Comparatively low doses of THC were administered and did not appear to induce a general depression or incapacitation; other social interactions, such as allogrooming, actually increased in frequency.

It appears that a serious hazard of marihuana smoking is enhancement of a paranoid thought disorder and exacerbation of psychosis in schizophrenic patients.[176]

In contrast to anecdotal reports that marihuana smoking increases interpersonal communication, one study has demonstrated an overall decrease in affective exchange and interpersonal skills during marihuana use.[89]

A study of marihuana and driving skills[101] suggests that marihuana has a detrimental effect on driving ability. This effect is dose related and not uniform for all persons. The author of the study recommends that driving under the influence of marihuana be avoided as stringently as driving under the influence of alcohol. As mentioned previously, marihuana and alcohol are commonly used together; driving performance appears to deteriorate rapidly with simultaneous use of both.

A report of 31 American soldiers who were heavy hashish smokers suggests that respiratory tract irritation may be a prominent feature of hashish smoking. Bronchitis, asthma, rhinopharyngitis, and sinusitis were common findings, with a mild obstructive pulmonary dysfunction in five who underwent pulmonary function studies. It was noted that the uvula becomes swollen and edematous while hashish is smoked and remains so for 12 to 24 hours afterward.

A 3-year study of 720 hashish smokers in an American Army population[175] revealed a marked difference in the effects of light versus heavy hashish smoking. Occasional smoking in small, intermittent doses caused only minor respiratory ailments with no adverse mental effects. Heavier smoking, several times a day, resulted in a chronic intoxicated state with frequent acute adverse effects, such as disorientation, panic reaction, or acute psychotic reaction. Many chronic users become psychotic for long periods of time and were unresponsive to treatment with antipsychotic agents. Symptoms of chronic intoxication were similar to those of long-term dependence on depressant-hypnotic drugs and included apathy, dullness, and lethargy with mild to severe impairment of judgment, concentration, and memory.

The heavy user, dubbed a "hashaholic" in Army jargon, appeared dull and maintained poor hygiene. He rarely resorted to violence or overt criminal behavior. His consumption of hashish reached 500 to 600 g per month, the equivalent of several thousand American marihuana cigarettes. The frequent practice of abusing ethanol and hashish simultaneously was reported to greatly increase the likelihood of adverse reaction and long-term morbidity.

Studies of the acute pulmonary physiological effects of marihuana show that both smoked marihuana and orally administered Δ^9THC produce significant bronchodilatation of relatively long duration (6 hours for the 20 mg dose).[164,178] Another pulmonary function study suggests that occasional social smoking of marihuana does not result in functional respiratory impairment in healthy young men, but that heavy marihuana use for 6 to 8 weeks produces mild but definite *narrowing* of large, medium, and small airways, in spite of the acute bronchodilator action of THC.[170]

Long-term marihuana use may impair the expression of cell-mediated immunity, rendering the host more susceptible to viral and fungal infections and cancer. An in vitro study[135] has demonstrated that blastogenic responses to phytohemagglutinin and allogeneic lymphocytes were depressed in lymphocytes of long-term marihuana smokers; these responses were comparable to those of patients with uremia and patients undergoing immunosuppressive therapy. Other in vitro studies have also suggested that natural cannabinoids inhibit nucleic acid synthesis. One recent study, however, has failed to demonstrate impaired immune response in long-term marihuana smokers.[184] Although this is currently an area of dispute, it appears that immunological suppression does occur in conjunction with marihuana smoking in some instances.

In various studies THC has been shown to impair spermatogenesis, inhibit the synthesis of testosterone, and, in the female, decrease serum levels of follicle-stimulating hormone (FSH), luteinizing hormone (LH), and prolactin.[136] Oral administration of cannabinoids to female mice late in pregnancy and during early lactation produces a permanent alteration in body weight regulation, pituitary-gonadal function, and adult copulatory activity in male offspring.[35] Clearly the cannabinoids exert profound effects on reproductive function, the mechanisms of which are unknown. Dose-related fetal resorptions are produced by administering cannabinoids to rats and mice; the mechanism may involve disruption of placental function.

[^{14}C] Δ^9THC administered to rats was shown to accumulate in tenfold greater concentrations in fat than in other tissues[105]; 11-hydroxy THC, an active metabolite of Δ^9THC, showed a similar distribution, with highest concentration in body fat. The importance of fat localization of drugs in prolonging pharmacological activity is well known; it is conceivable that slow release from fat stores may help explain the phenomenon of "reverse tolerance," in which regular users of marihuana achieve a "high" more quickly and easily than sporadic users.

The psychological effects, disposition, and excretion of [^{14}C] Δ^9THC in humans were compared.[110] High plasma levels of unchanged [^{14}C] Δ^9THC were rapidly achieved after intravenous administration and inhalation, whereas after oral administration plasma levels remained low, requiring several hours to peak. Psychological effects were maximal in all subjects at the times of maximal plasma levels of metabolites, lending support to the suggestion that a metabolite of Δ^9THC is the active compound responsible for the psychological effects of marihuana.

Further evidence in support of this belief was provided by a study in which 11-hydroxy-Δ^9THC was administered intravenously to humans.[108] The metabolite produced tachycardia and a "high" that was difficult to evaluate but was somewhat comparable to a marihuana "high." The disposition and metabolism of 11-hydroxy-Δ^9THC were similar to the disposition and metabolism of THC, as indicated by rate of disappearance from plasma, rate of excretion, and metabolic profile in urine and feces.

Plasma levels of THC fall rapidly to a low value, which remains for days, suggesting penetration into and release from storage sites. One study has demonstrated a half-life in tissues of 7 days; after 5 days, 15% of the THC is found as metabolites excreted by the kidney and 40% to 50% is excreted by the intestines.[136]

Studies comparing absorption of THC from lung and gastrointestinal tract have been conflicting. One study demonstrated 90% to 95% absorption from gastrointestinal tract[110]; low plasma levels were explained by slow absorption. Other studies have demonstrated absorption of only 5% to 10% of an oral dose of THC, with bioavailability being 5 to 10 times greater by the pulmonary route.[136]

Further considerations. Although it is too early to predict, THC and related compounds may become useful drugs.[25] THC reduces intraocular pressure, has a bronchodilator action, may be an effective antiemetic,[152] and has properties of a sedative and an antianxiety agent. Its toxicity in laboratory animals and in humans is low, as is its respiratory-depressant activity.

Marihuana is sometimes said to "lead to other drugs." Many drug users experiment first with marihuana, and in this sense marihuana may serve as a "stepping-stone" to the more potent agents. Most drug users believe strongly, however, that they would have eventually tried other drugs whether or not they had first smoked marihuana.

The potency of street marihuana in the United States has tended to increase so that there is less difference now between marihuana and hashish than formerly. Recent evidence suggests that the THC content of hashish is only twice that of strong marihuana and that the potency of marihuana may continue to increase.

Marihuana is often compared to alcohol. Unlike alcohol, marihuana is not known to be physically addicting and tolerance does not develop to the effects of ordinary marihuana preparations. When inebriated, the alcoholic usually suffers a greater temporary loss of judgment and control than the marihuana user, whose "highs" are usually characterized by mild alterations in perception and mood without marked loss of behavioral control. Hostility and aggression are commonly released by alcohol but rarely by marihuana. The appetite is stimulated by marihuana, whereas calories are provided by alcohol; nutritional deficiency commonly complicates the syndrome of chronic alcoholism. The hangover of the alcoholic is unknown to the "pothead," who awakens the next morning feeling refreshed. Psychological dependence on either drug may develop, and both drugs may impair the physical performance essential to safe automobile driving. Acute paranoid states, dissociative reactions, and near-psychotic reactions are occasionally seen with marihuana use; moderate drinking rarely if ever induces such reactions. There is strong suggestive evidence that chronic marihuana use interferes with motivational and goal-directed thinking; chronic alcoholism may do the same and ultimately result in brain damage and general physical deterioration.

In summary, in the light of our present incomplete knowledge, the principal medical risks in the use of marihuana appear to be (1) the occasional adverse reaction, characterized by paranoid thinking and extreme anxiety, sometimes with an acute psychotic reaction; (2) enhancement of preexisting paranoid thought disorders and exacerbation of psychosis in schizophrenic patients; (3) alteration of time and space perception, with loosening of associations and impairment of driving skills; (4) loss of motivation and drive, associated with regular and frequent use; (5) probable impairment of vascular reflex responses; (6) possible impairment of immune response; and (7) disturbance of hypothalamopituitary function with impairment of reproductive functions.

SLANG EQUIVALENTS:
Dextroamphetamine (Dexedrine) = dexies, co-pilots, oranges
Amphetamine (Benzedrine) = bennies, splash, peaches
Methamphetamine (Methedrine; Desoxyn) = meth, speed, crystal, crank, white cross (tablets)
Dextroamphetamine + amphetamine (Diphetamine; Biphetamine) = footballs

It appears that little if any physical dependence develops to the amphetamines. A change in sleep pattern on abrupt withdrawal has been reported in association with minimal EEG changes,[139] but there is no physiologically disruptive abstinence syndrome. Abrupt withdrawal is physiologically safe and is characterized by the onset of lethargy, somnolence, and often a precipitous depressive reaction; the possibility of suicide should be kept in mind. Some consider the period of lethargy and somnolence an abstinence syndrome in itself.[104]

Tolerance to amphetamines develops slowly and becomes marked. At any level of tolerance the margin between euphoria and toxic psychosis remains narrow.

Characteristics of abuse   The amphetamines are direct CNS stimulants and in ordinary therapeutic doses produce the following effects: euphoria, with increased sense of well-being; heightened mental acuity, until fatigue sets in from lack of sleep; nervousness, with insomnia; and anorexia. Amphetamines are useful in circumstances demanding optimal endurance and mental acuity; they have been prescribed for airmen in the military and for astronauts during difficult maneuvers. They are commonly abused by students, housewives, truck drivers, and all-night workers who self-administer the drugs for extended periods of time. Liberal dispensing by physicians of amphetamines for dietary management has contributed significantly to the abuse of these agents.

Undesirable and potentially hazardous effects accompany the prolonged use of amphetamines. As many a student has learned the hard way, fatigue eventually sets in and blocks coherent thought at inopportune times, such as during an examination. In addition, brief lapses of alertness, with sudden drooping of the head ("nodding"), may occur without warning as fatigue "breaks through"; this phenomenon, like the seizure of the epileptic individual, may result in a catastrophic loss of control in dangerous circumstances.

High doses of amphetamines reduce mental acuity and impair performance of complex acts, even in the absence of fatigue. Behavior may become irrational. A peculiar phenomenon observed among amphetamine users is a condition described as being "hung up." The user may get stuck in a repetitious behavioral sequence, repeating an act ritually for hours; the perseverative behavior may become progressively more irrational.

The "amphetamine psychosis"[112] may develop during long-term or short-term abuse of amphetamines and is characterized by visual and auditory hallucinations and paranoid delusions in the setting of a clear sensorium and full orientation. The psychosis clears within a few days after the drug is discontinued. It has been compared to a severe paranoid state closely resembling paranoid schizophrenia, with fixed, systematized delusions aggravated by attempts at intervention.[67]

The expressions "meth is death" and "speed kills" reflect the belief, widespread among drug users, that brain damage may result from administration of methamphetamine in large doses. In most cases a prolonged acute brain syndrome follows withdrawal.

Tolerance develops to such a degree that the habitual user may come to inject several hundred milligrams of an amphetamine every few hours. A total 24-hour dose of methamphetamine estimated at over 10 g has been reported.[104] Some users report that the subjective effects of intravenous amphetamines are similar to the effects of intravenous cocaine except for the longer duration of action of the amphetamines.

The mechanism behind the "paradoxical" calming effect of amphetamines and methylphenidate in hyperkinetic children remains unknown. A recent study with possible relevance demonstrated that amphetamine administration to preweanling rats appeared to enhance the normal tendency to approach and maintain contact with conspecifics. In contrast, adult rats responded to amphetamines with marked increase in random, nondirected locomotor activity.[19]

Physiological effects of high doses of amphetamines include mydriasis, elevation of blood pressure, hyperreflexia, and hyperthermia. Hypertensive crisis with intracranial hemorrhage has been reported following oral and intravenous administration of methamphetamine.[21,63,96] It is important to recall that amphetamine is an indirectly acting adrenergic drug, promoting the release of dopamine in the CNS (p. 279).

Amphetamines have sometimes been used, and abused, for the relief of pain. It appears that they may have some effectiveness, at least in combination with an analgesic agent. When morphine was administered with 10 mg of dextroamphetamine, it was found to be twice as potent as morphine alone. And the combination with 5 mg was one and one-half times as potent as morphine.[58]

Other sympathomimetic agents that are chemically related to the amphetamines and commonly abused include ephedrine, phenmetrazine (Preludin), mephentermine (Wyamine and Dristan inhalers), and methylphenidate (Ritalin). These drugs all produce central stimulation much like the amphetamines, but generally less marked. As with the amphetamines, physical dependence is not known to develop.

COCAINE

SLANG EQUIVALENTS:
Coke, snow, candy, girl, Charlie, big C

Cocaine is a local anesthetic and vasoconstrictor agent and powerful CNS stimulant. It occurs naturally in the leaves of the coca plant *Erythroxylon coca* and in other species of *Erythroxylon*, which are indigenous to Peru and Bolivia. Coca chewing has been a way of life for centuries for the Inca Indians living in the Andean highlands. Cocaine use at parties, usually by intranasal application, has recently become popular with many who can afford the high price of the drug.

Physical dependence and tolerance

Neither physical dependence nor tolerance is known to develop to the prolonged use of cocaine. It is possible that heightened responsiveness actually develops in some cases.[84]

Characteristics of abuse

Euphoric excitement, often of orgastic proportions, is rapidly produced even when cocaine is sniffed ("snorted" or "horned"). Grandiose feelings of great mental and physical prowess may cause the user to overestimate his or her capabilities. Strong sexual desire is often aroused, and the drug is sometimes used expressly for this effect. After intravenous injection, spontaneous ejaculation in the absence of genital stimulation has been reported; some users joke about letting the drug "replace" a sexual partner (as suggested by the slang names "girl" and "Charlie").

The effect of each injection is fleeting, and to recapture it the user injects repeated doses at 5- to 15-minute intervals, often leaving the needle in place. Users have been known to lock themselves in a room and enjoy 2 days and nights of uninterrupted cocaine euphoria, sharing a large supply of cocaine until it is exhausted.

If dosage is not watched carefully, signs of toxicity may appear, such as rapid heart rate with palpitations, hallucinations (visual, auditory, and tactile), and paranoid delusions. At times delusions have been so compelling that the user has assaulted an innocent party without provocation. The hyperexcited, paranoid state is similar to the amphetamine psychosis, except that it is short-lived in cases of parenteral injection. When the user perceives that a safe dose has been exceeded, he or she often chooses to "come down" comfortably by injecting an opiate and delaying the next dose of cocaine.

It has long been assumed that orally administered cocaine is hydrolyzed in the gastrointestinal tract and rendered ineffective. A recent study in human subjects has demonstrated that cocaine is well absorbed from the gastrointestinal tract, with peak plasma levels occurring 50 to 90 minutes after ingestion.[180]

Smoking of cocaine alkaloid ("free base") is becoming more widespread and appears to be frequently associated with cocaine toxicity.

One complication among cocaine sniffers is perforation of the nasal septum, occurring as a result of ischemic necrosis in the wake of the intense and prolonged vasoconstriction induced by the drug. Plasma concentrations reach a peak between 15 and 60 minutes after intranasal application, and cocaine persists in the plasma for 4 to 6 hours.[179] The long plasma life may result from continuous absorption secondary to the vasoconstrictor action of cocaine and brings about a far more enduring toxic state than does parenteral injection. Cocaine remains on the nasal mucosa for 3 hours after application.

Physiological disturbances from high doses of cocaine include pyrexia, dilated pupils, tachycardia, irregular respiration, abdominal pain, vomiting, and major convulsive seizures. Central stimulation is followed by depression; the higher centers are the first to become depressed, making this transition while the lower centers are still excited. Death results from medullary paralysis and respiratory failure. Acute poisoning may pursue a rapid course. In one survey of deaths from recreational cocaine use, respiratory collapse occurred rapidly after intravenous injection, but occurred suddenly as late as 1 hour after oral or nasal administration.[183]

BARBITURATES

SLANG EQUIVALENTS:
Barbiturates in general = goofballs, fool pills
   Short acting: secobarbital (Seconal) = red birds, red devils, reds; pentobarbital (Nembutal) = yellow jackets
   Intermediate acting: amobarbital (Amytal) = blue heavens
   Long acting: phenobarbital (Luminal) = purple hearts
   Combinations: secobarbital + amobarbital (Tuinal) = tooies, Christmas trees, rainbows

Physical dependence and tolerance

A marked degree of both physical dependence and tolerance develops to all the barbiturates. There is a sharp upper border to the tolerance, so that a slight increase in dosage may precipitate toxic symptoms.

Characteristics of abuse

The effects of ordinary doses of barbiturates include sedation (without analgesia), decreased mental acuity, slowed speech, and emotional lability. Toxic symptoms resulting from overdose include ataxia, diplopia, nystagmus, difficulty in accommodation, vertigo, and a positive Romberg sign. There is risk of overdose as a result of the delayed onset of action of the longer-acting barbiturates and also as a result of perceptual time distortion, which induces users to ingest more than they intended in a short period of time. Death from overdose, as with the opiates, results from respiratory depression; the respiratory depression of barbiturate overdose, however, is not antagonized by nalorphine or levallorphan.

In contrast to opiate addiction, the direct harm to the individual and society stems more from the toxic effects of the drug than from the difficulty of maintaining a continuing supply.

The barbiturates are rapidly becoming archaic drugs in modern medicine because of their disadvantages and hazards. REM rebound commonly follows use for insomnia; toxicity and respiratory-depressant action are great risks of higher doses; and induction of hepatic microsomal enzymes by barbiturates accelerates the biotransformation of many other drugs.

Abstinence syndrome

The barbiturate abstinence syndrome is one of the most dangerous drug withdrawal syndromes. Symptoms progress from weakness, restlessness, tremulousness, and insomnia to abdominal cramps, nausea, vomiting, hyperthermia, blepharoclonus (clonic blink reflex), orthostatic hypotension, confusion, disorientation, and eventually major convulsive seizures. The syndrome is sometimes mistaken for the "delirium tremens" of alcohol withdrawal. The seizures may become prolonged, as in status epilepticus. Agitation and hyperthermia may lead to exhaustion and cardiovascular collapse. With the short-acting barbiturates, convulsions are most likely to appear during the second or third day of abstinence; with the longer-acting barbiturates, convulsions are less likely to occur and usually appear between the third and the eighth day.

The barbiturate type of abstinence syndrome is occasionally observed in an addict being withdrawn from heroin who insists that he or she has used no other drug. In such cases one should suspect that the lot of heroin last used by the patient had been "cut" (diluted) with barbiturates, a practice that is known to exist. A barbiturate withdrawal regimen is then instituted immediately.

Withdrawal from barbiturates

Hospitalization is advisable for the duration of the withdrawal period. Instead of accepting the addict's word for the level of barbiturate to which he or she has become addicted, an objective test is made to determine the level of tolerance to barbiturates.[37] An ordinary therapeutic dose of pentobarbital is administered, and the patient is observed for clinical signs of drug effect. If the sedative action of the drug is not soon apparent, it is concluded that the patient's level of tolerance is higher and that he or she has become accustomed to higher individual doses. Additional increments of pentobarbital are administered until drug effect is evident; at this point the total dose of drug administered is considered the baseline from which subsequent doses are tapered over the ensuing 7 to 14 days. The long withdrawal period is advisable to minimize the likelihood of convulsions.

NONBARBITURATE SEDATIVES

Glutethimide (Doriden): Marked physical dependence develops, resulting in a severe abstinence syndrome characterized by nausea, vomiting, abdominal cramps, tachycardia, pyrexia, hyperesthesia, dysphagia, and major convulsive seizures.[92,118]

Methaqualone (Quaalude; Sopor; Parest): Nicknamed "quaas" and "sopors," methaqualone has become a popular "downer" with the young. Overdose, in contrast to barbiturate overdose, may result in restlessness, hypertonia, and convulsive seizures. Pulmonary edema has been reported with large overdoses. Death may occur from respiratory arrest, pulmonary edema, or other causes. It appears that physical dependence may develop after prolonged use in high doses.

Chloral hydrate (Noctec; Somnos): Moderate physical dependence develops, as manifested by a "chloral delirium" on abrupt withdrawal, characterized by agitation, confusion, disorientation, and hallucinations.[149] Slight to moderate tolerance develops; a "break in tolerance" may result from abrupt impairment of the mechanism of hepatic detoxification, with resulting overdose and death.[64]

Methyprylon (Noludar): Abrupt withdrawal has resulted in confusion, agitation, hallucinations, and generalized convulsions.[13,91]

Paraldehyde: Moderate physical dependence develops, as seen by the withdrawal symptoms of tremulousness, visual and auditory hallucinations, and a state of agitation and disorientation similar to delirium tremens.[64]

Bromides: Physical dependence has not been demonstrated.[64] In low doses bromides act as sedatives; in toxic doses they produce a so-called bromide psychosis characterized by confusion, disorientation, vivid hallucinations, and eventually coma. The slow elimination of bromide from the body may lead to chronic accumulation when it is administered over a period of time, with the subtle onset of the toxic syndrome.

Drugs in this category, unlike the antipsychotic agents, characteristically produce a marked physical dependence of the barbiturate type, as evidenced by the common occurrence of major convulsive seizures after abrupt withdrawal. Barbiturates may, in fact, be substituted for any of the following drugs for purposes of controlled withdrawal. **Antianxiety agents**

Diazepam (Valium): Major convulsive seizures have been reported during the withdrawal illness.[3,75] A recent study suggests that ethanol ingested simultaneously with diazepam accelerates diazepam absorption; plasma diazepam levels from 30 to 240 minutes after ingestion were significantly higher after administration with ethanol than with water alone.[72]

Chlordiazepoxide (Librium): Withdrawal symptoms are reported to progress from agitation and insomnia to major convulsive seizures.[76] Because of slow elimination of the drug, seizures may be delayed as long as 1 week after the last dose.

Meprobamate (Equanil; Miltown; Meprospan): Withdrawal symptoms may progress from insomnia, tremors, ataxia, and vomiting to an acute psychotic reaction, major convulsive seizures, coma, and death.[49,166] Seizures occur between 24 and 48 hours after the last dose.

Ethchlorvynol (Placidyl): Abrupt withdrawal may result in agitation, hallucinations, and generalized convulsions.[18]

It is remarkable that no significant physical dependence develops during long-term administration of the antipsychotic drugs in high doses. One author has de- **Antipsychotic agents** scribed a syndrome characterized by anxiety, insomnia, and gastrointestinal disturbances following the abrupt discontinuation of phenothiazines,[17] but, as in the case of amphetamine withdrawal, there is no gross physiological disturbance. The issue of whether or not to call this an "abstinence syndrome" is largely a matter of semantics.

Moderate tolerance develops to the sedative effects of the phenothiazines; it is not known whether a true tolerance develops to the antipsychotic effects.

The antipsychotic drugs have low abuse potential for drug users, since they do not produce a "high" or pleasurable emotional state.

PSYCHOTOMI-METIC DRUGS   Considered in this category are psychotogenic (hallucinogenic) drugs taken primarily for their psychotomimetic effects. Many other drugs such as the amphetamines and cocaine are also psychotogenic in high doses.

Phencyclidine   SLANG EQUIVALENTS:
PCP, angel dust, DOA, peace pill, hog

Phencyclidine hydrochloride (Sernylan, Sernyl),[4,24,68,157] a veterinary anesthetic agent, since the late 1970s has become increasingly popular as a psychotomimetic drug, in part because it is easily synthesized from readily available precursors. It is administered by ingestion, inhalation (sprinkled on smoking preparations or inhaled directly), and injection.

In low doses, from 1 to 5 mg, phencyclidine may induce euphoria and disinhibition, with release from social inhibitory attitudes and increased emotional lability. Many use the drug for this effect alone. In higher doses a variable clinical picture is produced, with excitement, somatic perceptual distortions, impairment of pain and touch perception, confusion, disorientation, and difficulty speaking. The user may appear agitated or quiet and withdrawn. The clinical syndrome may resemble schizophrenia in many respects and may persist for days or weeks. Posturing, catatonic states and mutism have been reported. Attack behavior, directed or chaotic, has also been observed with large doses.[52]

Phencyclidine produces both sympathomimetic effects (tachycardia, hypertension) and cholinergic effects (flushing, diaphoresis, drooling, meiosis). Increased deep tendon reflexes, clonic movements, nystagmus, ataxia, and dysarthria are common effects. Paresthesias and analgesia may occur. At higher doses major convulsions, status epilepticus, hypertensive crisis,[46] and cardiac or respiratory arrest may occur.

Treatment measures include emesis (if early after ingestion), control of hypertension, ventilatory support, and control of behavioral disturbance.

It is obvious that phencyclidine is one of the most dangerous drugs ever to appear on the street. Like most other street drugs, it is commonly misrepresented by sellers as THC, mescaline, peyote, or other drugs. It appears in powder form or in tablets or capsules, and the color is variable. It is inexpensive to produce and may bring great profits (1 pound may cost $100 to produce and bring $20,000), so its spread across North America and Europe is not surprising.

SLANG EQUIVALENT:
  Acid; many different local names. The term "mikes" refers to micrograms, "clinical mikes" to actual micrograms, "street mikes" to a fictional microgram one-third to one-fourth as potent.

LSD (LSD-25; D-lysergic acid diethylamide tartrate) was first synthesized from the alkaloids of ergot *(Claviceps purpurea)* a fungus that parasitizes rye and other grains in Europe and North America. The ergot alkaloids, which include ergotamine and ergonovine, are active oxytocics and vasoconstrictors. The chance synthesis of LSD was accomplished in 1938 by a research chemist working for Sandoz, Ltd., who attached a diethylamide radical to lysergic acid, the skeletal structure common to all the ergot alkaloids. The sample was set aside until 1943, when it was first tested by the researcher and found to have strange and potent central effects.

Physical dependence is not known to develop. Tolerance, however, develops rapidly and is lost as rapidly after discontinuance of LSD. The usual initial dose of 200 to 400 μg is often raised to several thousand micrograms after a few days of continuous use. Cross-tolerance between LSD, mescaline, and psilocybin has been shown[31]; it appears that cross-tolerance between LSD and DMT (dimethyltryptamine) and between LSD and Δ^9THC does not develop.[47,83]

Physical dependence and tolerance

The nature of the "trip" taken with LSD is not predictable in advance but is influenced to some degree by the state of mind, mood, and expectations at the time the drug is taken. This is also true of one's response to marihuana, which may act as a stimulant, aphrodisiac, or sedative, depending largely on the environment and the state of mind. The usual trip with LSD is characterized by exhilarating feelings of strangeness and newness of experience, vividly colored and changing hallucinations, reveries, "free thinking," and "new insight." Colors become alive and may seem to glow; the space between objects may take on greater subjective importance as a thing in itself; and there is dazed wonderment at the beauty in common things. The introspective experience may be intense and sobering; it has been described as an intellectual earthquake in which conditioned attitudes and feelings are reevaluated and values are reshuffled. To some degree there appears to be a regression to primary process thinking.

Characteristics of abuse

Unpleasant experiences with LSD are relatively frequent and may involve an uncontrollable drift into confusion, dissociative reactions, acute panic reactions, a reliving of earlier traumatic experiences, or an acute psychotic hospitalization.[119,148] Prolonged nonpsychotic reactions have included dissociative reactions, time and space distortion, body image changes, and a residue of fear or depression stemming from morbid or terrifying experiences under the drug.

Catastrophic reactions to LSD are better understood when one conceptualizes the disruption by the drug of psychological defense mechanisms such as repression and denial in an individual precariously defended against confrontation of conflict material. With the failure of the usual defenses, the onslaught of repressed material overwhelms the integrative capacity of the ego, and a psychotic reaction results. It appears that this disruption of long-established patterns of adapting may be a lasting or semipermanent effect of the drug.

It also appears that LSD removes the usual intrinsic restraints on the intensity of affective response. It is well known to LSD users that a specific emotional response, whether it be fear, dread, delight, or sadness, may become rapidly more intense under the influence of the drug until it reaches overwhelming proportions. The users are then virtually in the grip of the reaction; they may indeed derive insight from the introspective experience, as most users report, but they may become so disturbed as to engage in behavior that endangers their own life. Deaths while under the influence of LSD have occurred by drowning, falling from a window,[99] and walking into the path of a car. The meaningless question has been asked: "Was it an accident or suicide?" An instance of homicide by a 22-year-old student during an LSD-induced psychotic reaction has been reported[146]; the student, not previously psychotic except for one other experience with LSD, killed a stranger with a knife in response to persecutory delusions. During 4 years of observation after the episode, the student was not again psychotic.

Disturbing implications are inherent in the finding of many "acid heads" that after 25 to 50 trips the frequency of taking LSD may be reduced progressively without sacrificing the desired state of mind. Users may discover that between trips they begin to feel as they did while under the influence of the drug, until they eventually find themselves on a continuous trip with no further ingestion of the drug. They state that their thinking has become different, and they no longer "need" the drug. Indeed, their changed behavior is apparent to others; with no further drug ingestion, they remain preoccupied with any trivial thing at hand, feel "at one" with all living things, and act as they often did while under the influence of the drug. The ultimate duration of these changes as well as their significance remains unknown.

Symptoms occurring during an LSD trip may recur unpredictably days, weeks, or months after a single dose. Strangest of drug effects, these "flashback" reactions may occur at intervals following the administration of many drugs with CNS activity, but they most commonly follow an LSD reaction. Flashback symptoms vary from gentle mood states to severely disruptive changes in thought and feeling and may occur with or without further administration of the drug. The reaction may be initiated voluntarily in some cases. The mechanism remains unknown, but the existence of the phenomenon suggests a residual impairment of psychological defense mechanisms, with periodic emergence of repressed feelings. Flashback reactions may also be "triggered" by strong affective states or by administration of a drug with CNS activity.

The physiological effects of LSD are few and include mydriasis, hyperreflexia, and muscular incoordination.[73] Grand mal seizures have been observed following ingestion of LSD.[55]

It has been demonstrated that injections of LSD in rats decrease the turnover rate of serotonin (5-hydroxytryptamine).[115] Some investigators suggest that this may in part explain the psychotomimetic effects of LSD.

Numerous studies suggest that LSD may induce mutations, damage chromosomes, or have teratogenic effects.[86,127] The studies are complicated, however, by many etiological variables, such as exposure to other drugs during pregnancy. The question of reproductive hazard remains unanswered though suspected.

Because it is water soluble, odorless, colorless, and tasteless and because by weight it is one of the most potent drugs known, LSD is easily administered to the unwary. At a party it will not be detected in the punch until its effects are evident.

LSD is usually taken by mouth. It is occasionally "mainlined,"[126] however, alone or in combination with other drugs. It is also absorbed through the lungs when marihuana soaked in an LSD solution is smoked.

It was once believed that a transient "model psychosis" resembling schizophrenia could be experimentally induced with LSD. It was soon recognized, however, that the psychotic reaction from LSD differs substantially from most types of schizophrenic reactions. In schizophrenia one usually finds a disordered thought pattern characterized by subtle or flagrant delusions that are systematized and integrated into the personality structure of the individual. The LSD psychosis, on the contrary, is characterized by a chaotic and unpredictable thought disturbance with little or no organization or integration. It resembles an acute brain syndrome more closely than it does most types of schizophrenic reaction, although it differs somewhat from a brain syndrome in the wide range of affective disturbance and in the complex nature of the hallucinatory experiences.

In the opinion of some investigators, LSD may become useful as a psychotherapeutic agent when administered under strictly controlled conditions in the course of psychotherapy.[106,177] Two studies, however, failed to demonstrate superiority of LSD in the treatment of alcoholism.[93,122]

Phenothiazines and barbiturates, singly or in combination, have sometimes been found effective in treating the acutely intoxicated state.[31] The regular LSD user knows this well and may keep a supply of chlorpromazine on hand.

p-**Chlorophenylalanine** ("PCPA") has been found to induce long-lasting sexual excitation in male rats.[60,167] Nicknamed "steam" by drug users, it has gained a reputation as a dangerous drug capable of inducing a prolonged psychotic reaction when taken in high doses. Drug users warn each other that "steam burns."

Dimethyltryptamine (DMT), **Diethyltryptamine** (DET), and **Dipropyltryptamine** (DPT) are commonly abused for their psychotomimetic effects. All three tryptamine derivatives produce a syndrome resembling an LSD reaction but differing in the following ways: the onset is more rapid, increasing the likelihood of panic reaction; the duration of action is only 1 to 2 hours (the experience has been dubbed a "businessman's trip"); and the autonomic effects consisting of pupillodilatation and elevation of blood pressure are more marked than with LSD.[47] DMT is present in several South American snuffs, including cohoba snuff.

The labels "**STP**" and "**DOM**" have been given to the hallucinogenic drug 2,5-dimethoxy-4-methyl amphetamine.[162] It is said to induce an LSD-like reaction lasting

Other psychotomimetic agents

72 hours or longer. Many who have tried the drug dislike the long "come-down" period of 1 to 3 days; perhaps for this reason, among others, it is generally less popular than LSD.

Another psychotomimetic agent related to the amphetamines is "MDA," or the "love pill" (3-methoxy-4,5-methylenedioxy amphetamine),[158] which is said to induce a relatively mild LSD-like reaction lasting 6 to 10 hours. An amphetamine-like effect is also produced and tends to persist longer than the psychotomimetic effect, so that the period of "crashing" or "coming down" may be characterized by euphoria instead of the psychic depression that frequently concludes an LSD trip.

Morning glory seeds

VARIETIES:
1. *Rivea corymbosa:* ololiuqui, Mexican morning glory, Heavenly Blue (used in ceremony by Aztec Indians of Mexico)
2. *Ipomoea versicolor* (alternate names: *I. violacea, I. tricolor*): Pearly Gates

Morning glory seeds, readily purchasable in stores, contain compounds similar to LSD—D-lysergic acid amide among others. Up to several hundred seeds are ingested at a time to produce effects; less commonly an extract is injected intravenously.

Symptoms include drowsiness, perceptual distortion, confusion, lability of affect, and hallucinations; giddiness and euphoria may alternate with intense anxiety.[54,79] Common side effects of oral ingestion include nausea, vomiting, and diarrhea.

An instance of suicide apparently related to a morning glory seed flashback reaction has been described.[23] A 24-year-old college student ingested 300 Heavenly Blue seeds and developed an acute psychotic reaction. Three weeks later the symptoms recurred for no apparent reason, and the student expressed a fear of losing his mind. The symptoms persisted and one morning he awoke, communicated his distress to others, and drove his car at an estimated 90 to 100 miles per hour down a hill to his death.

Mescaline

The dumpling (peyote) cactus, *Lophophora williamsii,* is indigenous to the Rio Grande Valley, Protuberances atop the plant are cut off and dried in the sun to form the peyote or mescal buttons; these contain the active drug, mescaline (peyote; peyotl; 3,4,5,-trimethoxyphenethylamine). The buttons are prepared into cakes, tablets, or powder; the powder is water soluble and may be administered orally or parenterally. Peyote is used in ceremonies by the Indians of northern Mexico and by the Navahos,[1] Apaches, Comanches, and other tribes of the southwestern United States.

Mescaline produces effects similar to those of LSD, but it is less potent. Vivid and colorful hallucinations are reported. Flagrant psychotic reactions are far less common than with LSD.

Mescaline has been found in smaller quantities in another North American cactus, *Pelecyphora aselliformis,*[137] and is known also to occur in some species of South American cacti.

The hallucinogenic agents psilocybin and psilocin, available in powder and liquid form, are extracted from the mushrooms *Stropharia* spp. and *Psilocybe* spp., which occur principally in Mexico.

A native religious cult in which these mushrooms are consumed as a sacrament has deep roots in Mexican tradition.[154] Psilocybin is now popular with drug users in the United States and produces an effect similar to mescaline.

Psilocybin and psilocin

Commonly abused anticholinergic agents include atropine, scopolamine, synthetic atropine substitutes, and preparations or plants containing these agents (such as the over-the-counter preparation Asthmador[98] and the plants jimsomweed[51,66] and angel's trumpet[71] [*Datura* spp.]). In high doses these agents produce a central anticholinergic syndrome characterized by fever, agitation, veridical hallucinations (bugs, spiders, etc.), and confusion. Severe intoxication may result in convulsions, flaccid paralysis, coma, and death. Other signs of anticholinergic intoxication are present, such as mydriasis, tachycardia, decreased salivary secretion, anhidrosis, urinary retention, and warm, flushed skin. Anticholinergic agents abused for their psychotomimetic effects are sometimes falsely marketed as LSD.

Anticholinergics

Nutmeg (*Myristica*), a spice used throughout the world, is the powdered seed kernel of the East Indian tree *Myristica fragrans*. Unknown to many, it contains a hallucinogen thought to be myristicin. Ingestion of large amounts of nutmeg produces euphoria, hallucinations, and an acute psychotic reaction. Side effects, which may be confused with atropine poisoning, include flushing of the skin, tachycardia, and decreased salivary secretion. Unlike atropine, nutmeg may produce early pupillary constriction.[140,182]

Nutmeg

The term *inhalant*, as used here, includes gases and highly volatile organic compounds and excludes liquids sprayed into the nasopharynx (droplet transport required) and substances that must be ignited prior to inhalation (such as marihuana).

This category of drug abuse attracts the youngest customers. Not infrequently one learns of elementary schoolchildren who have experimented dangerously with inhalants for weeks or months before being discovered.

Among the currently most popular inhalants are the volatile nitrites, principally amyl nitrite and isobutyl nitrite.[26,159] They are nicknamed "poppers" and "snappers" because of the sound produced by breaking open the thin glass ampule in which amyl nitrite is marketed. Isobutyl nitrite has been marketed in various containers with trade names such as "Bolt," "Heart-On," "Rush," and "Locker Room." The effects of inhalation of the volatile nitrites are immediate and fleeting and may consist of light-headedness, euphoria (variable), headache, and enhancement of sexual orgasm. The latter effect accounts for the most common usage of the drugs. The basic pharmacological action is relaxation of vascular smooth muscle; complaints of users include a prolonged pulsatile headache and symptoms of orthostatic hypotension, glaucoma, recent head injury, or intracranial hemorrhage. If inhalation is pro-

INHALANTS

longed or practiced regularly, hemoglobin may be converted to methemoglobin; this should be kept in mind in the evaluation of the regular user.

Other popular inhalants include model airplane glues, plastic cements, gasoline, brake and lighter fluids, paint and lacquer thinners, varnish remover, cleaning fluid (spot remover), and nail polish remover. These household agents contain a variety of volatile aliphatic and aromatic hydrocarbons, including benzene, toluene, xylene, carbon tetrachloride, chloroform, acetone, amyl acetate, trichloroethane, naphtha, ethyl alcohol, and isopropyl alcohol. Some of these compounds are depressants of the CNS and may produce anesthesia and death in high concentrations. Some have known toxic effects. Chloroform and carbon tetrachloride, for example, are toxic to the myocardium, liver, and kidney and may produce hepatic or renal failure or cardiac arrhythmias with severe hypotension; mild poisoning with either agent may produce a reversible oliguria of a few days' duration. Exposure to high concentrations of toluene may result in renal tubular acidosis,[168] acute hepatic failure, bone marrow suppression, and permanent encephalopathy.[102] Lead poisoning has resulted from gasoline sniffing.[150]

A case of fatal aplastic anemia secondary to glue sniffing has been reported.[143] A drug user habituated to one inhalant may resort to using another when the first inhalant is unavailable; a gasoline sniffer substituted carbon tetrachloride with near-fatal results.[44]

Symptoms produced by inhalation of the agents just listed are essentially similar for all. A sense of exhilaration and light-headedness are usually reported, progressing to hallucinations. Judgment and reality perception are impaired. Transient ataxia, slurred speech, diplopia, and vomiting have been reported in cases of glue sniffing. If inhalation is not interrupted, coma and death may result.[45,186]

The development of a definite tolerance has been reported.[139] Physical dependence is not known to develop.

Anesthetic agents such as nitrous oxide ("laughing gas"), diethyl ether, cyclopropane, trichloroethylene (Trilene), and halothane (Fluothane) are also subject to abuse. Nitrous oxide, currently a very popular inhalant, represents an exception to the general rule that inhalants are organic compounds.

"Sudden sniffing death" is a new phenomenon associated with inhalant abuse.[9] In the usual reported case a young person inhales a volatile hydrocarbon deeply and gets the urge to run; after sprinting a short distance he or she falls to the ground, dead. The cause of death is assumed to be a cardiac arrhythmia induced by the inhaled agent and intensified by exercise and hypercapnia. Most reported cases have followed inhalation of fluoroalkane gases such as the pressurized propellants of many aerosol sprays. Once called "inert," fluoroalkane gases have been found to sensitize the hearts of mice to asphyxia-induced sinus bradycardia, atrioventricular block, and ventricular T-wave depression.[172] Inhalation of airplane glue or toluene has likewise been shown to sensitize the heart of mice to asphyxia-induced atrioventricular block.[173] Some reported deaths have occurred while running just after sniffing vapors; in one case inhalation of vapors was incidental to siphoning only.[10] Fatal cardiac arrhythmias have been produced in dogs by inhalation of fluorinated hydrocarbons (trichloromonofluoromethane and dichlorodifluoromethane) in the absence of hypoxia, with careful maintenance of normal arterial oxygen tension, carbon dioxide tension, pH, serum carbon dioxide level, and base excess.[56]

Propoxyphene. There is no evidence that significant physical dependence or tolerance develops when propoxyphene (Darvon) is administered in ordinary therapeutic doses. In very large doses, however, both physical dependence and tolerance have been observed to develop.[18,59,187] The withdrawal syndrome is characterized by chills, diaphoresis, rhinitis, yawning, muscle aches, irritability, abdominal cramping, and diarrhea.[48,187] Evidence suggesting that propoxyphene is pharmacologically related to the opiates is provided by the finding that it can suppress the morphine abstinence syndrome to a slight degree.[59,107] Perhaps the most convincing evidence of such a relationship is the finding that the toxic effects of an overdose of propoxyphene (muscular fasciculations, respiratory depression, and convulsive seizures) are antagonized by the narcotic antagonists nalorphine and levallorphan.

In a study at the Addiction Research Center in Lexington, Kentucky,[59] comparison of propoxyphene with codeine was made on the basis of the occurrence of an abstinence syndrome following abrupt withdrawal, suppression of morphine abstinence syndrome, and precipitation of an abstinence syndrome on administration of nalorphine. It was concluded that propoxyphene induces considerably less physical dependence than codeine and has substantially less addiction liability than codeine. The same investigators also found that a toxic psychosis was induced by single doses of propoxyphene in excess of 900 mg. Propoxyphene overdosage may be rapidly fatal. Respiratory depression, convulsions, and pulmonary edema are common terminal events.[188]

Propoxyphene has become a major drug of abuse in the United States. In some cities it is associated with more deaths than either heroin or morphine, and it ranks near the top in drugs mentioned in emergency room visits.

Nicotine. Nicotine is extracted from the tobacco plant *Nicotiana tabacum*, which has been cultivated from remote antiquity and in every country of the world where the climate has permitted. It has never been found as a wild plant and fails to survive outside of cultivation. Nicotine is one of the most toxic of all drugs; the dosage encountered in cigarettes is extremely small. Physiological effects of nicotine include elevation of blood pressure, increased bowel activity, and an antidiuretic action. Apparently a moderate tolerance and a mild to moderate physical dependence develop.[64]

Caffeine. Caffeine occurs naturally in the coffee bean (seeds of *Coffea arabica* and related species), the leaves of the tea plant *(Thea sinensis)*, and the seeds of the chocolate tree *(Theobroma cacao)*. Caffeine is added to many soft beverages and over-the-counter medications. It stimulates the CNS at all levels, beginning with the cortex; a more rapid and clear flow of thought is produced and a sense of fatigue is diminished. Physical dependence on caffeine has not been demonstrated. It appears that a mild degree of tolerance develops during continued use.

Cantharidin. Cantharidin (Spanish fly) is erroneously reputed to have a specific

MISCELLANEOUS DRUGS

aphrodisiac effect, presumably because priapism may result from irritation of the male urethra when the drug is excreted in the urine.[64] Ingestion of cantharidin may be followed by stomatitis, abdominal cramps, vomiting, bloody diarrhea, urinary urgency, dysuria, hematuria, and priapism. Cantharidin is directly toxic to the kidneys; deaths from renal damage and cardiorespiratory collapse have been reported.[145,163]

Catnip. The dried leaves of the catnip plant *(Nepeta Cataria)* are smoked like marihuana or the extract is sprayed over ordinary tobacco. Effects are said to be euphoria and enhanced appreciation of sensory experiences.[85] No definite pharmacological activity has yet been demonstrated. One wonders to what extent the alleged effects of catnip, like those of banana peels,[16] are the result of placebo effect and hyperventilation.

DRUG MIXING

Drug users are aware that the combination of two or more centrally active drugs may provide a novel dimension of feeling unobtainable with a single drug alone. A second drug may be taken to enhance the effects of the first drug, to prevent undesired effects of the first drug, or to reduce the discomfort of discontinuing the first drug. Adulteration is virtually the rule with black-market drug samples.

CLINICAL EVALUA-TION OF THE DRUG USER

When drugs of abuse are classified as they are in this chapter and in Appendix B (p. 763), it is often forgotten that a large percentage of drugs taken by people today are black-market samples and that three unknowns are thereby introduced: dose, actual identity, and purity. Any one of these three unknowns constitutes a serious danger in itself, and all three are present in any black-market sample.[20]

Fundamental to the diagnostic evaluation of the suspected drug user is an attempt to place the apparent drug-related symptoms into one or more of four categories: symptoms occurring during intoxication; symptoms of withdrawal; "flashback" symptoms; and the "masking" of symptoms of illness or injury by a drug.[37]

The lack of symptom specificity in cases of intoxication makes the evaluation tricky even for an experienced observer; manic excitement, panic reaction, dissociative reaction, paranoid reaction, and overt psychotic reactions may occur during a "bad trip" with most of the drugs discussed. An etiological diagnosis is best reached through laboratory analysis of drug sample, gastric aspirate, blood, or urine; even laboratory identification may be difficult, however, because of introduction of new chemical agents in an evolving drug scene.[174] To make matters more complicated, a patient may be simultaneously in withdrawal from one drug and intoxicated with another.

Contrary to earlier thinking, it is now apparent that discontinuing almost any drug after heavy use is likely to result in serious abstinence symptoms. It may be unrealistic to describe the phenomenon of "crashing" (discontinuing a drug after heavy use or a large dose) in either physiological or psychological terms; it is clearly neither the one nor the other alone.

Symptoms of coincident illness or injury may not be reported by intoxicated drug users because of the analgesic action of the drug or because of a mental state in which they are only vaguely aware of the symptoms (or lack the incentive to report them). Heart attack or head injury may thereby escape detection. Systemic infection, metabolic disturbance (especially diabetic crisis), and head injury may contribute to the moribund state of patients who have taken a depressant drug.

It is important to remember that a patient under the influence of, or in withdrawal from, almost any drug may show no obvious symptoms or signs referable to recent drug use.

A syndrome of necrotizing angiitis associated with drug abuse has been described.[22,103] It appears to be pathologically indistinguishable from periarteritis nodosa and is manifest clinically by few or no symptoms in some patients and multiple-system involvement, with pulmonary edema, hypertension, pancreatitis, and renal failure, in others. Although the etiology is unclear, a frequent associated finding has been the intravenous injection of methamphetamine. The actual existence of this syndrome as a new drug-related phenomenon is challenged by some observers.[8]

Injection of oral drug preparations may release a shower of vascular emboli in the form of tablet filler material, which becomes deposited in capillary beds of the retina, lung, endocardium, liver, spleen, and kidney. Pulmonary angiothrombotic granulomatosis has been reported, with consequent pulmonary hypertension and fatal cor pulmonale, as a result of deposition of talc (magnesium trisilicate) in the pulmonary vessels.[78] Ophthalmologic examination may reveal crystals of talc and cornstarch clustered in the macular region.[6] Retinopathy and retinal detachment have resulted.[70] The list of tablet filler materials is endless and includes lactose, colloidal silica, microcrystalline cellulose, magnesium stearate, and dibasic calcium phosphate. The list may be almost as long as that of contaminants added to black-market drugs.

Gangrene of an extremity is a common end result of inadvertent arterial injection of a drug. The mechanism of vascular injury is not known, but chemical damage to the intima by the concentrated drug may play an important role. Tissue ischemia after intra-arterial injection of *oral* drug preparations appears to be more severe than that after injection of parenteral preparations,[116] perhaps because of the presence of the many additives of the filler.

A drug habit carries a proportionately greater risk if (1) black-market drugs are used, (2) the higher-risk drugs such as LSD, amphetamines, or heroin are used, and (3) the route of administration is intravenous. The intravenous route introduces a number of risks of its own, including greater likelihood of adverse reaction or lethal overdose, viral hepatitis, bacterial endocarditis, serious sequelae of injecting filler from oral drug preparations, and development of a "needle habit" (craving for injection of anything by needle).

REFERENCES

1 Aberle, D. F.: The peyote religion among the Navaho, Chicago, 1966, Aldine Publishing Co.
2 Ackerly, W. C., and Gibson, G.: Lighter fluid "sniffing," Am. J. Psychiatry 120:1056, 1964.
3 Aivazian, G. H.: Clinical evaluation of diazepam, Dis. Nerv. Syst. 25:491, 1964.
4 Allen, R. M., and Young, S. J.: Phencyclidine-induced psychosis, Am. J. Psychiatry 135:1081, 1978.

5 Aronow, W. S., and Cassidy, J.: Effect of marihuana and placebo-marihuana smoking on angina pectoris, N. Engl. J. Med. **291**:65, 1974.

6 AtLee, W. E., Jr.: Talc and cornstarch emboli in eyes of drug abusers, J.A.M.A. **219**:49, 1972.

7 Ausubel, D. P.: The Dole-Nyswander treatment of heroin addiction, J.A.M.A. **195**:949, 1966.

8 Baden, M. M.: Angiitis in drug abusers (letter to the editor), N. Engl. J. Med. **284**:111, 1971.

9 Bass, M.: Sudden sniffing death, J.A.M.A. **212**:2075, 1970.

10 Bass, M.: Death from sniffing gasoline (letter to the editor), N. Engl. J. Med. **299**:203, 1978.

11 Beaconsfield, P., Ginsburg, J., and Rainsbury R.: Marihuana smoking: cardiovascular effects in man and possible mechanisms, N. Engl. J. Med. **287**:209, 1972.

12 Bell, D. S.: Comparison of amphetamine psychosis and schizophrenia, Br. J. Psychiatry **111**:701, 1965.

13 Berger, H.: Addiction to methyprylon: report of a case of 24-year-old nurse with possible syngergism with phenothiazine, J.A.M.A. **177**:63, 1961.

14 Berger, S. A., Cherubin, C. E., Nelson, S., and Levine, L.: Tetanus despite preexisting antitetanus antibody, J.A.M.A. **240**:769, 1978.

15 Bloom, F., Segal, D., Guillemin, R., and Ling, N.: Endorphins: profound behavioral effects in rats suggest new etiological factors in mental illness, Science **194**:630, 1976.

16 Bozzetti, L., Jr., Goldsmith, S., and Ungerleider, J. T.: The great banana hoax, Am. J. Psychiatry **124**:678, 1967.

17 Brooks, G. W.: Withdrawal from neuroleptic drugs, Am. J. Psychiatry **115**:931, 1959.

18 Cahn, C. H.: Intoxication by ethclorvynol (Placidyl): report of four cases, Can. Med. Assoc. J. **81**:733, 1959.

19 Campbell, B. A., and Randall, P. J.: Paradoxical effects of amphetamine on preweanling and postweanling rats, Science **195**:888, 1977.

20 Cheek, F. E., Newell, S., and Joffe, M.: Deceptions in the illicit drug market, Science **167**:1276, 1970.

21 Chynn, K. Y.: Acute subarachnoid hemorrhage, J.A.M.A. **233**:55, 1975.

22 Citron, B. P., et al.: Necrotizing angiitis associated with drug abuse, N. Engl. J. Med. **283**:1003, 1970.

23 Cohen, S.: Suicide following morning glory seed ingestion, Am. J. Psychiatry **120**:1024, 1964.

24 Cohen, S.: Angel dust, J.A.M.A. **238**:515, 1977.

25 Cohen, S.: Marijuana: does it have a possible therapeutic use? J.A.M.A. **240**:1761, 1978.

26 Cohen, S.: The volatile nitrites, J.A.M.A. **241**:2077, 1979.

27 Collier, H. O. J.: The experimental analysis of drug dependence, Endeavour **31**:123, 1972.

28 Connell, P. H.: Clinical manifestations and treatment of amphetamine type of dependence, J.A.M.A. **196**:718, 1966.

29 Conrad, D. G., Elmore, T. F., and Sodetz, F. J.: Delta-9-tetrahydrocannabinol: dose-related effects on timing behavior in chimpanzee, Science **175**:547, 1972.

30 Council on Mental Health and Committee on Alcoholism and Drug Dependence: Dependence on cannabis (marihuana), J.A.M.A. **201**:368, 1967.

31 Council on Mental Health and Committee on Alcoholism and Drug Dependence: Dependence on LSD and other hallucinogenic drugs, J.A.M.A. **202**:47, 1967.

32 Crancer, A., Jr., Dille, J. M., Delay, J. C., Wallace, J. E., and Haykin, M. D.: Comparison of the effects of marihuana and alcohol on simulated driving performance, Science **164**:851, 1969.

33 Cutting, W. C.: Morphine addiction for 62 years: a case report, Stanford Med. Bull. **1**:39, 1942.

34 D'Agostino, R. S., and Arnett, E. N.: Acute myoglobinuria and heroin snorting, J.A.M.A. **241**:277, 1979.

35 Dalterio, S., and Bartke, A.: Perinatal exposure to cannabinoids alters male reproductive function in mice, Science **205**:1420, 1979.

36 Deneau, G. A., and Seevers, M. H.: Pharmacological aspects of drug dependence, Adv. Pharmacol. **3**:267, 1964.

37 Dimijian, G. G., and Radelat, F. A.: Evaluation and treatment of the suspected drug user in the emergency room, Arch. Intern. Med. **125**:162, 1970.

38 Dishotsky, N. I., Loughman, W. D., Mogar, R. E., and Lipscomb, W. R.: LSD and genetic damage, Science **172**:431, 1971.

39 Dole, V. P.: Methadone maintenance treatment for 25,000 heroin addicts, J.A.M.A. **215**:1131, 1971.

40 Dole, V. P., and Nyswander, M. E.: Medical treatment of diacetylmorphine (heroin) addiction, J.A.M.A. **193**:646, 1965.

41 Dole, V. P., and Nyswander, M. E.: The treatment of heroin addiction (letter to the editor), J.A.M.A. **195**:188, 1966.

42 Dole, V. P., and Nyswander, M. E.: Heroin addiction—a metabolic disease, Arch. Intern. Med. **120**:19, 1967.

43 Dole, V. P., Nyswander, M. E., and Warner, A.: Successful treatment of 750 criminal addicts, J.A.M.A. **206**:2708, 1968.

44 Durden, W. D., Jr., and Chipman, D. W.: Gasoline sniffing complicated by acute carbon tetrachloride poisoning, Arch. Intern. Med. **119**:371, 1967.

45 Easson, W. M.: Gasoline addiction in children, Pediatrics **29**:250, 1962.

46 Eastman, J. W., and Cohen, S. N.: Hypertensive crisis and death associated with phencyclidine poisoning, J.A.M.A. **231**:1270, 1975.

47 Efron, D. H., editor-in-chief: Ethnopharmacologic search for psychoactive drugs, Public Health Service Publication No. 1645, Washington, D.C., 1967, U.S. Government Printing Office.

48 Elson, A., and Domino, E. F.: Dextro propoxyphene addiction: observations of a case, J.A.M.A. **183**:482, 1963.

49 Essig, C. F.: Newer sedative drugs that cause states of intoxication and dependence of barbiturate type, J.A.M.A. **196**:126, 1966.

50 Expert Committee on Addiction-Producing Drugs, Seventh Report, WHO Techn. Rep. Ser. 116, 1957.

51 Farnsworth, N. R.: Hallucinogenic plants, Science **162**:1086, 1968.

52 Fauman, M. A., and Fauman, B. J.: Violence associated with phencyclidine abuse, Am. J. Psychiatry **136**:1584, 1979.

53 Ferraro, D. P., and Grilly, D. M.: Lack of tolerance to delta-9-tetrahydrocannabinol in chimpanzees, Science **179**:490, 1973.

54 Fink, P. J., Goldman, M. J., and Lyons, I.: Recent trends in substance abuse: morning glory seed psychosis, Int. J. Addictions **2**:143, 1967.

55 Fisher, D. D., and Ungerleider, J. T.: Grand mal seizures following ingestion of LSD-25, Calif. Med. **106**:210, 1967.

56 Flowers, N. C., and Horan, L. G.: Nonanoxic aerosol arrhythmias, J.A.M.A. **219**:33, 1972.

57 Forlenza, S. W., Axelrod, J. L., and Grieco, M. H.: Pott's disease in heroin addicts, J.A.M.A. **241**:379, 1979.

58 Forrest, W. H., Jr., et al.: Dextroamphetamine with morphine for the treatment of postoperative pain, N. Engl. J. Med. **296**:712, 1977.

59 Frazer, H. F., and Isbell, H.: Pharmacology and addiction liability of *dl-* and *d-*propoxyphene, Bull. Narcotics **12**:9, 1960.

60 Gessa, G. L., Tagliamonte, A., and Tagliamonte, P.: Aphrodisiac effect of p-chlorophenylalanine, Science **171**:706, 1971.

61 Goldstein, A.: Opioid peptides (endorphins) in pituitary and brain, Science **193**:1081, 1976.

62 Goldstein, A.: Endorphins: physiology and clinical implications. In Recent developments in chemotherapy of narcotic addiction, vol. 311, New York, 1978, The New York Academy of Sciences, p. 49.

63 Goodman, S. J., and Becker, D. P.: Intracranial hemorrhage associated with amphetamine abuse (letter to the editor), J.A.M.A. **212**:480, 1970.

64 Goodman, L. S., and Gilman, A., editors: The pharmacological basis of therapeutics, ed. 6, New York, 1980, Macmillan Publishing Co., Inc.

65 Goodwin, D. W.: Alcoholism and heredity, Arch. Gen. Psychiatry **36**:57, 1979.

66 Gowdy, J. M.: Stramonium intoxication: review of symptomatology in 212 cases, J.A.M.A. **221**:585, 1972.

67 Griffith, J. D., Cavanaugh, J., Held, J., and Oates, J. A.: Dextroamphetamine: evaluation of psychomimetic properties in man, Arch. Gen. Psychiatry **26**:97, 1972.

68 Grove, V. E.: Painless self-injury after ingestion of 'angel dust', J.A.M.A. **242**:655, 1979.

69 Guillemin, R.: Endorphins, brain peptides that act like opiates, N. Engl. J. Med. **296**:226, 1977.

70 Gunby, P.: Methylphenidate abuse produces retinopathy (editorial), J.A.M.A. **241**:546, 1979.

71 Hall, R. C. W., Popkin, M. K., and McHenry, L. E.: Angel's Trumpet psychosis: a central nervous system anticholinergic syndrome, Am. J. Psychiatry **134**:312, 1977.

72 Hayes, S. L., Pablo, G., Radomski, T., and Palmer, R. F.: Ethanol and oral diazepam absorption, N. Engl. J. Med. **296**:186, 1977.

73 Hollister, L. E.: Human pharmacology of lysergic acid diethylamide (LSD). In Efron, D. H., editor-in-chief: Psychopharmacology: a review of progress, 1957-1967, Public Health Service Publication No. 1836, Washington, D.C., 1968, U.S. Government Printing Office.

74 Hollister, L. E.: Marihuana in man: three years later, Science **172**:21, 1971.

75 Hollister, L. E., Bennett, J. L., Kimbell, I., Savage, C., and Overall, J. E.: Diazepam in newly admitted schizophrenics, Dis. Nerv. Syst. **24**:746, 1963.

76 Hollister, L. E., Motzenbecker, F. P., and

Degan, R. O.: Withdrawal reactions from chlordiazepoxide (Librium), Psychopharmacologia 2:63, 1961.

77 Holzman, R. S., and Bishko, F.: Osteomyelitis in heroin addicts, Arch. Intern. Med. 75:693, 1971.

78 Hopkins, G. B.: Pulmonary angiothrombotic granulomatosis in drug offenders, J.A.M.A. 221:909, 1972.

79 Ingram, A. L., Jr.: Morning glory seed reaction, J.A.M.A. 190: 1133, 1964.

80 Isbell, H.: Medical aspects of opiate addiction, Bull. N.Y. Acad. Med. 33:866, 1955.

81 Isbell, H., and Gorodetzky, C. W.: Effect of alkaloids of ololiuqui in man, Psychopharmacologia 8:331, 1966.

82 Isbell, H., Gorodetzky, C. W., Jasinski, D., Claussen, U., Spulak, F. V., and Korte, F.: Effects of $(-)-\Delta^9$ trans-tetrahydrocannabinol in man, Psychopharmacologia 11:184, 1967.

83 Isbell, H., and Jasinski, D. R.: A comparison of LSD-25 with $(-)-\Delta^9$-trans-tetrahydrocannabinol (THC) and attempted cross tolerance between LSD and THC, Psychopharmacologia 14:115, 1969.

84 Isbell, H., and White, W. M.: Symposium on drug addiction: clinical characteristics of addictions, Am. J. Med. 14:558, 1953.

85 Jackson, B., and Reed, A.: Catnip and the alteration of consciousness, J.A.M.A. 207:1349, 1969.

86 Jacobson, C. B., and Berlin, C. M.: Possible reproductive detriment in LSD users, J.A.M.A. 222:1367, 1972.

87 Jaffe, J. H.: Drug addiction and drug abuse. In Goodman, L. S., and Gilman, A., editors: The pharmacological basis of therapeutics, ed. 4, New York, 1970, The Macmillan Co.

88 Jaffe, J. H., and Senay, E. C.: Methadone and 1-methadyl acetate: use in management of narcotics addicts, J.A.M.A. 216:1303, 1971.

89 Janowsky, D. S., Clopton, P. L., Leichner, P. P., Abrams, A. A., Judd, L. L., and Pechnick, R.: Interpersonal effects of marijuana, Arch. Gen. Psychiatry 36:781, 1979.

90 Jelliffe, R. W., Hill, D., Tatter, D., and Lewis, E., Jr.: Death from weight-control pills, J.A.M.A. 208:1843, 1969.

91 Jensen, G. R.: Addiction to Noludar: a report of two cases, N.A. Med. J. 59:431, 1960.

92 Johnson, F. A., and Van Buren, H. C.: Abstinence syndrome following glutethimide intoxication, J.A.M.A. 180:1024, 1962.

93 Johnson, F. G.: LSD in the treatment of alcoholism, Am. J. Psychiatry 126:481, 1969.

94 Judd, L. L., Brandkamp, W. W., and McGlothlin, W. H.: Comparison of the chromosomal patterns obtained from groups of continued users, former users, and nonusers of LSD-25, Am. J. Psychiatry 126:626, 1969.

95 Julius, D. A.: Research and development of naltrexone: a new narcotic antagonist, Am. J. Psychiatry 136:782, 1979.

96 Kane, F. J., Jr., Keeler, M. H., and Reifler, C. B.: Letter to the editor, J.A.M.A. 210:556, 1969.

97 Keeler, M. H.: Adverse reaction to marihuana, Am. J. Psychiatry 124:128, 1967.

98 Keeler, M. H., and Kane, F. J., Jr.: The use of hyoscyamine as a hallucinogen and intoxicant, Am. J. Psychiatry 124:852, 1967.

99 Keeler, M. H., and Reifler, C. B.: Suicide during an LSD reaction, Am. J. Psychiatry 123:884, 1967.

100 Klatsky, A. L., Friedman, G. D.: Siegelaub, A. B., and Gerard, M. J.: Alcohol consumption and blood pressure: Kaiser-Permanente Multiphasic Health Examination data, N. Engl. J. Med. 296:1194, 1977.

101 Klonoff, H.: Marijuana and driving in real-life situations, Science 186:317, 1974.

102 Knox, J. W., and Nelson, J. R.: Permanent encephalopathy from toluene inhalation, N. Engl. J. Med. 275:1494, 1966.

103 Koff, R. S., Widrich, W. C., and Robbins, A. H.: Necrotizing angiitis in a methamphetamine user with hepatitis B—angiographic diagnosis, five-month follow-up results and localization of bleeding site, N. Engl. J. Med. 288:946, 1973.

104 Kramer, J. C., Fischman, V. S., and Littlefield, D. C.: Amphetamine abuse: pattern and effects of high doses taken intravenously, J.A.M.A. 201:305, 1967.

105 Kreuz, D. S., and Azelrod, J.: Delta-9-tetrahydrocannabinol: localization in body fat, Science 179:391, 1973.

106 Kurland, A. A., Unger, S., Shaffer, J. W., and Savage, C.: Psychedelic therapy utilizing LSD in the treatment of the alcoholic patient: a preliminary report, Am. J. Psychiatry 123:1202, 1967.

107 Lasagna, L.: The clinical evaluation of morphine and its substitutes as analgesics, Pharmacol. Rev. 16:47, 1964.

108 Lemberger, L., Crabtree, R. E., and Rowe, H. M.: 11-Hydroxy-delta-9-tetrahydrocannabinol: pharmacology, disposition, and metabolism of a major metabolite of marihuana in man, Science 177:62, 1972.

109 Lemberger, L., Silberstein, S. D., Axelrod, J., and Kopin, I. J.: Marihuana, studies on the

disposition and metabolism of delta-9-tetrahydrocannabinol in man, Science **170:**1320, 1970.

110 Lemberger, L., Weiss, J. L., Watanabe, A. M., Galantes, I. M., Wyatt, R. J., and Cardon, P. V.: Delta-9-tetrahydrocannabinol: temporal correlation of the psychologic effects and blood levels after various routes of administration, N. Engl. J. Med. **286:**685, 1972.

111 Lemere, F.: The danger of amphetamine dependency, Am. J. Psychiatry **123:**569, 1966.

112 Lerner, P.: The precise determination of tetrahydrocannabinol in marihuana and hashish, Bull. Narcotics **21:**39, 1969.

113 Lewis, R., Gorbach, S., and Altner, P.: Spinal pseudomonas chondro-osteomyelitis in heroin users, N. Engl. J. Med. **286:**1303, 1972.

114 Lieber, C. S.: Liver adaptation and injury in alcoholism, N. Engl. J. Med. **288:**356, 1973.

115 Lin, R. C., Ngai, S. H., and Costa, E.: Lysergic acid diethylamide: role in conversion oif plasma tryptophan to brain serotonin (5-hydroxytryptamine), Science **166:**237, 1969.

116 Lindell, T. D., Porter, J. M., and Langston, C.: Intra-arterial injections of oral medications, N. Engl. J. Med. **287:**1132, 1972.

117 Ling, W., Klett, C. J., and Gillis, R. D.: A cooperative clinical study of methadyl acetate, Arch. Gen. Psychiatry **35:**345, 1978.

118 Lloyd, E. A., and Clark, L. D.: Convulsions and delirium incident to glutethimide (Doriden) withdrawal, Dis. Nerv. System **20:**524, 1959.

119 Louria, D. B.: Lysergic acid diethylamide, N. Engl. J. Med. **278:**435, 1968.

120 Louria, D. B.: Medical complications of pleasure-giving drugs, Arch. Intern. Med. **123:**82, 1969.

121 Louria, D. B., Hensle, T., and Rose, J.: The major medical complications of heroin addiction, Ann. Intern. Med. **67:**1, 1967.

122 Ludwig, A., Levine, J., Stark, L., and Lazar, R.: A clinical study of LSD treatment in alcoholism, Am. J. Psychiatry **126:**59, 1969.

123 Malitz, S., and Hoch, P. H.: Drug therapy: neuroleptics and tranquilizers. In Arieti, S., editor: American handbook of psychiatry, vol. 3, New York, 1966, Basic Books, Inc., Publishers.

124 Martin, W. R., Gorodetzky, C. W., and McClane, T. K.: An experimental study in the treatment of narcotic addicts with cyclazocine, Clin. Pharmacol. Ther. **7:**455, 1966.

125 Massengale, O. N., Glaser, H. H., LeLievré, R. E., Dodds, J. B., and Klock, M. E.: Physical and psychologic factors in glue sniffing, N. Engl. J. Med. **269:**1340, 1963.

126 Materson, B. J., and Barret-Conner, E.: LSD "mainlining": a new hazard to health, J.A.M.A. **200:**1126, 1967.

127 McGlothlin, W. H., Sparkes, R. S., and Arnold, D. O.: Effect of LSD on human pregnancy, J.A.M.A. **212:**1483, 1970.

128 Mechoulam, R.: Marihuana chemistry, Science **168:**1159, 1970.

129 Mechoulam, R., Shani, A., Edery, H., and Grunfeld, Y.: Chemical basis of hashish activity, Science **169:**611, 1970.

130 Melges, F. T.: Tracking difficulties and paranoid ideation during hashish and alcohol intoxication, Am. J. Psychiatry **133:**1024, 1976.

131 Melges, F. T., Tinklenberg, J. R., Hollister, L. E., and Gillespie, H. K.: Marihuana and temporal disintegration, Science **168:**1118, 1970.

132 Melges, F. T., Tinklenberg, J. R., Hollister, L. E., and Gillespie, H. K.: Marihuana and the temporal span of awareness, Arch. Gen. Psychiatry **24:**564, 1971.

133 Mendelson, J. H., and Mello, N. K.: Biologic concomitants of alcoholism, N. Engl. J. Med. **301:**912, 1979.

134 Miczek, K. A.: Δ^9-Tetrahydrocannabinol: antiaggressive effects in mice, rats, and squirrel monkeys, Science **199:**1459, 1978.

135 Nahas, G. G., Suciu-Foca, N., Armand, J. P., and Morishima, A.: Inhibition of cellular mediated immunity in marihuana smokers, Science **183:**419, 1974.

136 Nakas, G. G.: Current status of marijuana research, J.A.M.A. **242:**2775, 1979.

137 Neal, J. M., Sato, P. T., and Howald, W. N.: Peyote alkaloids: identification in the Mexican cactus *Pelecyphora aselliformis* Ehrenberg, Science **176:**1131, 1972.

138 Newman, L. M., Lutz, M. P., Gould, M. H., and Domino, E. F.: Delta-9-tetrahydrocannabinol and ethyl alcohol: evidence for cross-tolerance in the rat, Science **175:**1022, 1972.

139 Oswald, I., and Thacore, V. R.: Amphetamine and phenmetrazine addiction, Br. Med. J. **2:**427, 1963.

140 Payne, R. B.: Nutmeg intoxication, N. Engl. J. Med. **269:**36, 1963.

141 Perna, D.: Psychotogenic effect of marihuana, J.A.M.A. **209:**1085, 1969.

142 Pillard, R. C.: Medical progress: marihuana, N. Engl. J. Med. **283:**294, 1970.

143 Powars, D.: Aplastic anemia secondary to glue sniffing, N. Engl. J. Med. **273:**700, 1965.

144 Press, E., and Done, A. K.: Solvent sniffing: physiologic effects and community control measures for intoxication from the intentional

inhalation of organic solvents, Pediatrics 39: 451, 611, 1967.

145 Presto, A. J., and Muecke, E. C.: A dose of Spanish fly, J.A.M.A. **214**:591, 1970.

146 Reich, P., and Hepps, R. B.: Homicide during a psychosis induced by LSD, J.A.M.A. **219**: 869, 1972.

147 Richter, R. W., et al.: Acute myoglobinuria associated with heroin addiction, J.A.M.A. **216**: 1172, 1971.

148 Robbins, E., Frosch, W. A., and Stern, M.: Further observations on untoward reactions to LSD, Am. J. Psychiatry **124**:393, 1967.

149 Robinson, J. T.: A case of chloral hydrate addiction, Int. J. Soc. Psychiatry **12**:66, 1966.

150 Robinson, R. O.: Tetraethyl lead poisoning from gasoline sniffing, J.A.M.A. **240**:1373, 1978.

151 Rubin, E., and Lieber, C. S.: Alcoholism, alcohol, and drugs, Science **172**:1097, 1971.

152 Sallan, S. E., Zinberg, N. E., and Frei, E.: Antiemetic effect of delta-9-tetrahydrocannabinol in patients receiving cancer chemotherapy, N. Engl. J. Med. **293**:795, 1975.

153 Schuckit, M. A., and Rayses, V.: Ethanol ingestion: differences in blood acetaldehyde concentrations in relatives of alcoholics and controls, Science **203**:43, 1979.

154 Schultes, R. E.: I. The plant kingdom and hallucinogens, Bull. Narcotics **21**:3, 1969.

155 Seevers, M. H.: Drug dependence and drug abuse: a world problem, Pharmacologist **12**: 172, 1970.

156 Senay, E. C., Dorus, W., and Renault, P. F.: Methadyl acetate and methadone, J.A.M.A. **237**:138, 1977.

157 Showalter, C. V., and Thornton, W. E.: Clinical pharmacology of phencyclidine toxicity, Am. J. Psychiatry **134**:1234, 1977.

158 Shulgin, A. T.: 3-Methoxy-4, 5-methylenedioxy amphetamine, a new psychotomimetic agent, Nature **201**:1120, 1964.

159 Sigell, L. T., Kapp, F. T., Fusaro, G. A., Nelson, E. D., and Falck, R. S.: Popping and snorting volatile nitrites: a current fad for getting high, Am. J. Psychiatry **135**:1216, 1978.

160 Silva, M. T. A., Carlini, E. A., Claussen, U., and Korte, F.: Lack of cross-tolerance in rats among (−)-Δ⁹-*trans*-tetrahydrocannabinol (Δ⁹ THC), cannabis extract, mescaline and lysergic acid diethylamide (LSD-25), Psychopharmacologia **13**:332, 1968.

161 Snyder, S. H.: Opiate receptors in the brain, N. Engl. J. Med. **296**:266, 1977.

162 Snyder, S. H., Faillace, L., and Hollister, L.: 2,5-Dimethoxy-4-methyl-amphetamine (STP):

a new hallucinogenic drug, Science **158**:669, 1967.

163 Sollman, T.: A manual of pharmacology and its applications to therapeutics and toxicology, ed. 8, Philadelphia, 1957, W. B. Saunders Co.

164 Steinberg, A. D., and Karliner, J. S.: The clinical spectrum of heroin pulmonary edema, Arch. Intern. Med. **122**:122, 1968.

165 Stimmel, B., Goldberg, J., Rotkopf, E., and Cohen, M.: Ability to remain abstinent after methadone detoxification, J.A.M.A. **237**:1216, 1977.

166 Swanson, L. A., and Okada, T.: Death after withdrawal of meprobamate, J.A.M.A. **184**: 780, 1963.

167 Tagliamonte, A., Tagliamonte, P., Gessa, G. L., and Brodie, B. B.: Compulsive sexual activity induced by p-chlorophenylalanine in normal and pinealectomized male rats, Science **166**:1433, 1969.

168 Taher, S. M., Anderson, R. J., McCartney, R., Popovtzer, M. D., and Schrier, R. W.: Renal tubular acidosis associated with toluene "sniffing," N. Engl. J. Med. **290**:765, 1974.

169 Tashkin, D. P., Shapiro, B. J., and Frank, I. M.: Acute pulmonary physiologic effects of smoked marijuana and oral Δ⁹ tetrahydrocannabinol in healthy young men, N. Engl. J. Med. **289**:336, 1973.

170 Tashkin, D. P., Shapiro, B. J., Lee, Y. E., and Harper, C. E.: Subacute effects of heavy marihuana smoking on pulmonary function in healthy men, N. Engl. J. Med. **294**:125, 1976.

171 Tatum, A. L., and Seevers, M. H.: Theories of drug addiction, Physiol. Rev. **11**:107, 1931.

172 Taylor, G. J., and Harris, W. S.: Cardiac toxicity of aerosol propellants, J.A.M.A. **214**:81, 1970.

173 Taylor, G. J., and Harris, W. S.: Glue sniffing causes heart block in mice, Science **170**:866, 1970.

174 Taylor, R. L., Maurer, J. I., and Tinklenberg, J. R.: Management of "bad trips" in an evolving drug scene, J.A.M.A. **213**:422, 1970.

175 Tennant, F. S., and Groesbeck, C. J.: Psychiatric effects of hashish, Arch. Gen. Psychiatry **27**:133, 1972.

176 Treffert, D. A.: Marijuana use in schizophrenia: a clear hazard, Am. J. Psychiatry **135**: 1213, 1978.

177 Unger, M.: Mescaline, LSD, psilocybin, and personality change, Psychiatry **26**:111, 1963.

178 Vachon, L., FitzGerald, M. X., Solliday, N. H., Gould, I. A., and Gaensler, E. A.: Single-dose effect of marihuana smoke, N. Engl. J. Med. **288**:985, 1973.

179 Van Dyke, C., Barash, P. G., Jatlow, P., and Byck, R.: Cocaine: plasma concentrations after intranasal application in man, Science **191:** 859, 1976.

180 Van Dyke, C., Jatlow, P., Ungerer, J., Barash, P. G., and Bych, R.: Oral cocaine: plasma concentrations and central effects, Science **200:**211, 1978.

181 Wei, E., and Loh, H.: Physical dependence on opiate-like peptides, Science **193:**1262, 1976.

182 Weiss, G.: Hallucinogenic and narcoticlike effects of powdered Myristica (nutmeg), Psychiatr. Q. **34:**346, 1960.

183 Wetli, C. V., and Wright, R. K.: Death caused by recreational cocaine use, J.A.M.A. **241:** 2519, 1979.

184 White, S. C., Brin, S. C., and Janicke, B. W.: Mitogen-induced blastogenic responses of lymphocytes from marihuana smokers, Science **188:**71, 1975.

185 Wickler, A.: Opiate addiction, Springfield, Ill., 1953, Charles C Thomas, Publisher.

186 Winek, C. L., Collom, W. D., and Wecht, C. H.: Fatal benzene exposure by glue-sniffing, Lancet **1:**683, 1967.

187 Wolfe, R. C., Reidenberg, M., and Vispo, R. H.: Propoxyphene (Darvon) addiction and withdrawal syndrome, Ann. Intern. Med. **70:** 773, 1969.

188 Young, D. J.: Propoxyphene suicides, Arch. Intern. Med. **129:**62, 1972.

189 Zaks, A., Jones, T., Fink, M., and Freedman, A. M.: Naloxone treatment of opiate dependence, J.A.M.A. **215:**2108, 1971.

CHAPTER 31

Nonnarcotic analgesics and anti-inflammatory drugs

GENERAL CONCEPT A group of widely used mild analgesics lower body temperature when administered for fever. These *analgesic-antipyretic* drugs belong to several classes: the salicylates, pyrazolones, acetaminophen, and the newer group of anti-inflammatory drugs, such as indomethacin, mefenamic acid, ibuprofen, fenoprofen, naproxen, tolmetin, and sulindac. All but acetaminophen are commonly referred to as *nonsteroidal anti-inflammatory drugs* or *nonsteroidal antirheumatic drugs*. They probably act by inhibiting the synthesis of prostaglandins.

SALICYLATES Salicylic acid, or *o*-hydroxybenzoic acid, is a simple organic compound that exerts remarkable analgesic, antipyretic, anti-inflammatory, anti-rheumatic, and uricosuric effects in humans. Compounds closely related to this drug occur naturally in willow bark as the glycoside *salicin* and in oil of gaultheria (oil of wintergreen).

Since it is believed that compounds related to salicylic acid act either by conversion to this acid or by mechanisms similar to its mode of action, the various preparations related to salicylic acid are referred to as *salicylates*. Most commonly employed are sodium salicylate, aspirin, and salicylamide.

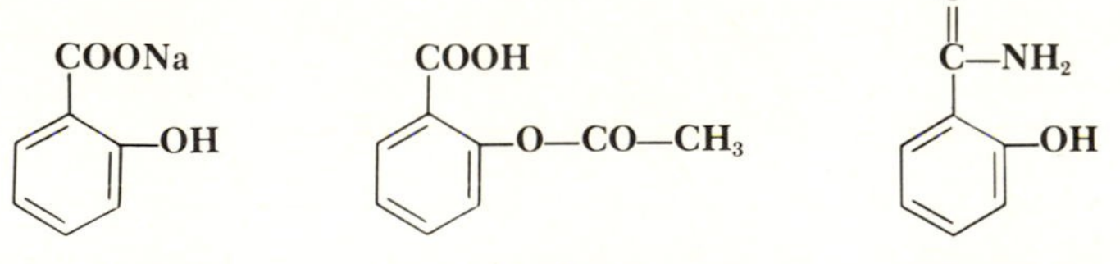

COONa   COOH   O
                                          $\mathrm{C-NH_2}$

        OH $\mathrm{O-CO-CH_3}$ OH

Sodium salicylate   **Aspirin**   **Salicylamide**

Although sodium salicylate, aspirin, and salicylamide are structurally very similar, some of their effects in the body may be quite diverse. Thus aspirin is more potent than sodium salicylate as an analgesic and antipyretic, and salicylamide is much less effective than either.

Pharmacological effects When as much as 600 mg of sodium salicylate, aspirin, or salicylamide is taken orally by a normal adult, the effects are negligible. Some persons may notice slight drowsiness and may complain of gastric irritation, but generally no medically useful property could be anticipated from the effects on a normal person. In disease states or in certain painful conditions, however, the therapeutic actions of the salicylates become quite prominent.

It is well known that the pain of headache, arthralgia, and muscular ache responds remarkably well to aspirin. Opinions on the mechanism of pain relief by these drugs vary considerably. Aspirin has an analgesic effect on the pain-producing actions of bradykinin.[25] In addition it blocks postaglandin synthesis,[42,56] and prostaglandins may sensitize nerve endings to the pain-producing effect of bradykinin.

Analgesic effect

The salicylates decrease the temperature of patients who have fever but do not lower normal temperature. The same phenomenon can be demonstrated in experimental animals. Intravenous injections of bacterial suspensions such as typhoid vaccine can produce fever in rabbits. The salicylates oppose this experimental temperature elevation but do not lower normal body temperature.

Antipyretic effect

Normal body temperature is maintained by the balance between heat production and heat dissipation. Central regulation of this process is accomplished in the hypothalamus. Under normal circumstances, increased heat production, such as is caused by muscular exercise, brings about increased heat dissipation through peripheral vasodilatation and sweating. Thus the constancy of body temperature is maintained within relatively narrow limits.

In fever there appears to be primarily a defect in heat dissipation. Although the production of heat may be increased, it is not followed by a corresponding increase in heat dissipation. The temperature-regulating centers behave under these conditions much as would a thermostat that has been set higher. The salicylates lower the temperature in fever by increasing heat loss through promotion of peripheral vasodilatation and sweating. Sweating is not essential for the antipyretic action, since temperature can be lowered by the salicylates even when sweating is prevented by atropine.

The possibility of the prostaglandins playing a role in temperature regulation is of great interest. Prostaglandins E_1 and E_2 produced hyperthermia when injected into the third ventricle of cats and rabbits.[30] This is especially interesting in view of the inhibitory action of several antipyretics on prostaglandin synthesis.[42,56]

In rheumatic fever the administration of salicylates in large doses results in lowering of fever, relief of joint symptoms, and normalization of the elevated sedimentation rate. It is agreed by most investigators that whereas these drugs are highly effective against the joint manifestations of the disease, they have no effect on rheumatic carditis.

Antirheumatic and anti-inflammatory effects

The antirheumatic effect of the salicylates is probably just a manifestation of their anti-inflammatory action. The latter action can be demonstrated experimentally in studies of inflammation following the injection of irritating compounds such as carrageenin, a sulfated polygalactose. The anti-inflammatory potency of a series of drugs correlates well with their antirheumatic usefulness in humans.[45] The inhibitory action of aspirin on prostaglandin synthesis[42] is of great research interest.

Uricosuric action   Salicylates in large doses increase the excretion of uric acid in the urine, probably by preventing its tubular reabsorption. On the other hand, small doses such as used for analgesia not only are not uricosuric but actually prevent the effects of probenecid on uric acid excretion.

Miscellaneous effects   Salicylates also affect the gastrointestinal tract and respiration, exert an anti-
of salicylates   inflammatory action, and have metabolic effects.

Gastrointestinal effects. Salicylates cause gastric irritation. Furthermore, gastric ulceration has been produced with salicylates in experimental animals, and occult blood can be demonstrated in the stools of patients who are taking salicylates.

Generally, salicylic acid in solid particles is more irritating to the gastric mucosa than is the sodium salt solution. Aspirin completely dissolved by the addition of sufficient alkali is less likely to cause gastric bleeding.

The gastric effects of aspirin create a serious problem for those patients who must take the drug for long periods of time in high doses.

The mechanism of gastrointestinal bleeding induced by aspirin may be quite complex. Lesions of the gastric mucosa are more common after aspirin ingestion when intragastric pH is low. This finding suggests that hydrochloric acid plays an important role in causing the erosions and bleeding. It is likely also that bleeding is aggravated by the striking effect of aspirin on platelet aggregation and stickiness.[32]

In a clinical study using fiberoptic gastroscopy, antral ulceration and acute mucosal lesions were found in seven of fourteen patients with rheumatoid arthritis who were taking aspirin, 4 g/day. Fenoprofen produced such an effect only in one and acetaminophen in none.[26]

Aspirin and platelet aggregation. It has been shown that aspirin, but not sodium salicylate, inhibits platelet aggregation induced by collagen in the test tube.[44] Ingestion of even small analgesic doses of aspirin prolongs the bleeding time in humans, presumably by inhibiting platelet function. Such prolongation of bleeding time by aspirin ingestion has been noted also in a variety of diseases such as von Willebrand's disease, afibrinogenemia, and abnormalities of platelet aggregation.

The mode of action of aspirin in blocking platelet aggregation and its significance in the prevention of thrombosis are being investigated. Aspirin appears to block the release of adenosine diphosphate (ADP) induced by collagen, and this effect may explain its inhibitory action on platelet aggregation.[38] The thromboxanes made by platelets from cyclic endoperoxides may play an important role in platelet aggregation. Aspirin blocks the formation of the endoperoxides and may prevent aggregation by its action on thromboxane synthesis.

The effect of aspirin on platelet aggregation suggested its possible usefulness in preventing strokes and myocardial infarction. In a large-scale clinical trail,[57] the Aspirin Myocardial Infarction Study (AMIS), aspirin did not reduce mortality in heart attack patients. There were suggestions of a favorable effect on strokes and transient ischemic attacks. More recent trials suggest that sulfinpyrazone may have some usefulness in the prevention of death following myocardial infarction.

Effect on respiration. Patients with salicylate poisoning show marked hyperpnea. Large oral doses in humans or intravenous injections in animals result in marked stimulation of respiration. The immediacy of this response following intravenous injection of sodium salicylate suggests that it is a direct effect rather than a consequence of some metabolic alteration in the body. It has been shown experimentally that in cats and rabbits the respiratory stimulant action results from a reflex mediated through vagal afferent nerve fibers not involving the carotid bodies.[15]

Metabolic effects. Salicylates affect intermediary metabolism, thyroid function, carbohydrate metabolism, and handling of water and electrolytes.

Salicylates uncouple oxidative phosphorylation.[3] This may be the reason for the increased heat production and oxygen consumption that can be demonstrated in isolated tissues or in whole animals. These drugs also inhibit biosynthesis of acid mucopolysaccharides.

Interference with thyroid function is more apparent than real. The salicylates interfere with binding of thyroxine by plasma proteins. As a consequence, certain tests of thyroid function, such as the protein-bound iodine test, are altered.

Salicylates lower blood sugar levels in diabetic persons, an effect not mediated by insulin. The drugs can deplete liver glycogen in experimental animals.

In toxic doses the salicylates cause disturbances in acid-base balance. As will be discussed in relation to salicylate poisoning, metabolic acidosis may be caused by these drugs in infants and young children, but respiratory alkalosis is more likely in older children and adults.

Metabolism

Because sodium salicylate and aspirin are rapidly absorbed from the stomach and small intestine. Salicylic acid is poorly ionized at the usual pH of the stomach contents, and its absorption is facilitated by this fact, the nonionized form being more diffusible through membranes.

The absorption of aspirin is greatly influenced by the dissolution characteristics of the tablets. Addition of sufficient alkali to dissolve aspirin would facilitate absorption but could have the disadvantage of inducing systemic alkalosis if large enough doses are administered.

Following absorption, aspirin is hydrolyzed to salicylates, so that the original drug has a half-life of only 20 minutes. On the other hand, salicylate has a half-life that may vary from 6 to 30 hours, depending on the dose. Thus, salicylates have nonlinear pharmacokinetics as a consequence of saturation of the enzymes involved in their metabolism. This means that increases in dosage or frequency of administration can lead to disproportionate increases in plasma levels and serious toxic effects.[58a]

The salicylates are metabolically altered in the body. The various products of biotransformation, together with some unaltered salicylate, can be found in the urine. In humans about 50% of sodium salicylate administered is excreted in 24 hours.[20] The urine contains a variable amount of free salicylate, glucuronides, salicyluric acid (conjugation product with glycine), and gentisic acid (2,5-dihydroxybenzoic acid).

Plasma levels of salicylates are greatly influenced by the pH of the urine, since an acid urine favors tubular reabsorption but an alkaline urine is associated with increased salicylate excretion. The administration of sodium bicarbonate to a group of individuals taking 1 g of aspirin four times a day changed the pH of the urine from between 5.6 and 6.1 to between 6.2 and 6.9. At the same time the mean salicylate plasma levels changed from 27 to 15 mg/100 ml.[23] It has been estimated that if an individual had plasma salicylate levels of 20 to 30 mg/100 ml and a urine pH of 6.5, a change to pH 5.5 would more than double the plasma levels and could be quite hazardous.

Poisoning   Aspirin can cause adverse effects, even death. The most common adverse effect is related to gastric irritation and bleeding. Most efforts at introducing newer aspirin substitues are aimed at a reduction of the gastric effects of the drug.

Some patients show an aspirin intolerance that has all the characteristics of an anaphylactoid reaction, including angioedema and asthma. The intolerance has no immunological basis. Patients having aspirin intolerance cross-react to some other anti-inflammatory drugs and also show reactions to the yellow dye tartrazine, which is present in many foods and pharmaceuticals. The reaction to aspirin can be quite severe.[39,48a]

Salicylate intoxication may be mild or serious. The mild form is often called *salicylism* and is characterized by ringing of the ear, dizziness, headache, and mental confusion. The picture is similar to *cinchonism*, seen after the administration of large doses of quinine.

Serious salicylate intoxication is characterized by hyperpnea, gastrointestinal symptoms, disturbances in acid-base balance, and petechial hemorrhage. The lethal dose of aspirin for adults is about 20 g.

Petechial hemorrhages is salicylate poisoning may be caused by the ability of these drugs to depress the formation of prothrombin in a manner similar to that of the coumarin anticoagulants. Hemorrhages may reflect other mechanisms, and thrombocytopenic purpura has been reported to occur rarely after the use of the salicylates.

The disturbances in acid-base balance caused by toxic doses of salicylates are quite complex. Hyperventilation leads to respiratory alkalosis. Secondarily, and perhaps triggered by the lowered Pco_2, lactic acid is released from the tissues. As a consequence, respiratory alkalosis may lead to metabolic acidosis, particularly in infants.

The treatment of salicylate poisoning is based on the correction of fluid and electrolyte disturbances. Hemodialysis may be useful for removing salicylates from the blood.

Salicylamide is much less effective than aspirin as an analgesic and antipyretic. *Salicylamide* It has some CNS depressant actions, but there is serious question about its clinical usefulness.

Aspirin USP is available in tablets containing 60, 75, 150, and 300 mg; in enteric- *Preparations* coated tablets of 300 and 600 mg; in capsules containing 300 mg; and in rectal suppositories containing 60, 75, 120, 150, 200, 300, and 600 mg and 1 g. Sodium salicylate USP is available in tablets and enteric-coated tablets, both containing 300, 500, and 600 mg. (Aluminum aspirin is poorly absorbed from the gastrointestinal tract; salicylamide is much less effective than aspirin.)

Choline magnesium trisalicylate (Trilisate) contains 293 mg of choline salicylate and 362 mg of magnesium salicylate to provide 500 mg salicylate content. This preparation causes less fecal blood loss than aspirin and it has no effect on platelet aggregation.

Aminopyrine (Pyramidon) is an effective analgesic, antipyretic, and antirheumatic **NONSALICYLATE** drug, but its use has led to the development of agranulocytosis in a significant num- **ANALGESICS** ber of patients. As a result of this disadvantage and the greater safety of other anal- **Pyrazolone** gesics, there is little reason to prescribe aminopyrine. **compounds**
Aminopyrine

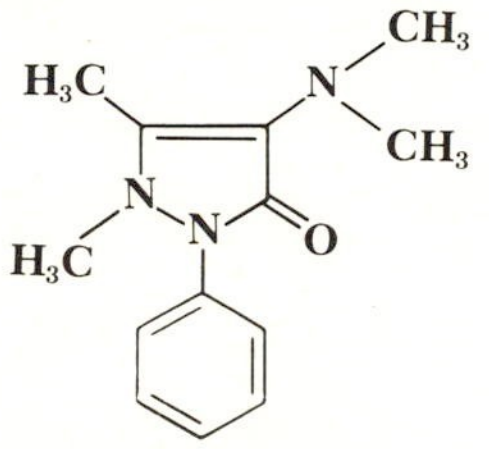

Aminopyrine

The closely related drug dipyrone (Dimethone; Key-Pyone; Narone; Pyrilgin) *Dipyrone* is also quite hazardous because of its capability of producing agranulocytosis.[17] The drug is popular in some circles because it is one of the few *injectable* nonnarcotic analgesics. There is some question, however, about its continued use since the drug has caused several deaths.

Preparations of dipyrone include tablets of 300, 324, 600, and 648 mg; liquid containing 500 mg/5 ml; and solution for injection, 500 mg/ml.

Of much greater interest is another pyrazolone derivative, phenylbutazone (Buta- *Phenylbutazone and* zolidin), as are the related drugs **oxyphenbutazone** (Tandearil) and **sulfinpyrazone** *derivatives* (Anturan).

The discovery of the therapeutic effectiveness of phenylbutazone has an interesting history. In order to increase the solubility of aminopyrine in an injectable preparation, phenylbutazone was added. Not only did this preparation prove very effective in the treatment of rheumatoid arthritis, but the duration of action also appeared much greater than what could be expected from aminopyrine alone. It was subsequently shown that the blood levels of phenylbutazone were higher and could be maintained for a much longer time than those of aminopyrine.

Pharmacological actions. This drug is particularly effective in the treatment of rheumatoid arthritis, ankylosing spondylitis, osteoarthritis, and gout. The effectiveness of the drug is somewhere between that of the salicylates and the anti-inflammatory steroids.

Phenylbutazone has a uricosuric action and may cause sodium retention and edema.

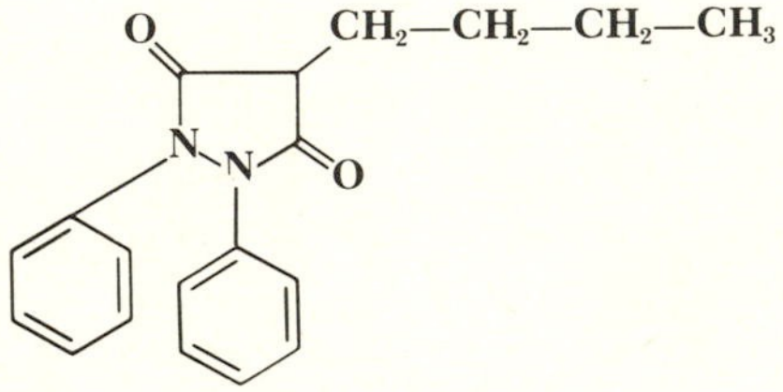

Phenylbutazone

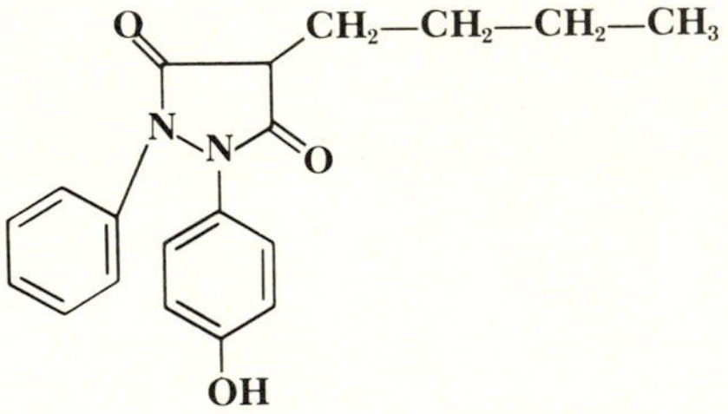

Oxyphenbutazone

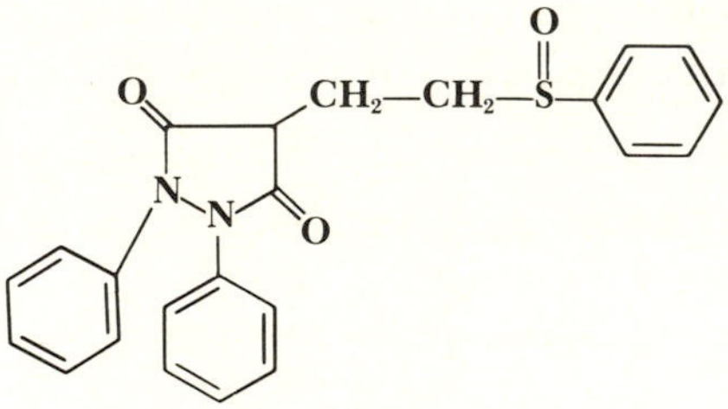

Sulfinpyrazone

Metabolism. The metabolism of phenylbutazone has been studied extensively.[4] The drug is absorbed much more readily from the gastrointestinal tract than from an intramuscular site. It is almost completely altered in the body, but its metabolism is so slow that its half-life in humans may be 72 hours. The drug is bound to plasma proteins and is thus protected from metabolizing enzymes. When large doses are given, the plasma-binding capacity is exceeded and the free drug is metabolized rapidly.[4]

The metabolic alteration of phenylbutazone leads to two active compounds. Oxyphenbutazone, a drug produced by aromatic hydroxylation, has activity and toxicity very similar to those of the parent compounds. Another metabolic product that results from alkyl chain oxidation is strongly uricosuric and is similar to sulfinpyrazone.

Toxic effects. It should be emphasized that phenylbutazone can produce many and varied toxic effects. As a consequence, it should be used only when safer medications do not suffice. It has been estimated that some toxic manifestations may appear in 25% of the patients receiving phenylbutazone treatment. Some of these manifestations are skin rash, gastrointestinal symptoms with activation of peptic ulcer, generalized hypersensitivity reactions similar to the sulfonamide-induced clinical picture, bone marrow depression, bleeding tendency, and jaundice. Thus phenylbutazone is another example of a potent drug that should not be used promiscuously because of the high incidence of adverse effects it may produce.

Drug interactions. Phenylbutazone increases the effect of concurrently administered drugs, such as the oral anticoagulants and the oral hypoglycemic agents. Phenylbutazone is an important cause of drug interactions because it competes with other drugs for plasma protein binding.

Dosage. The optimal blood level of phenylbutazone appears to be 10 mg/100 ml. This level may be obtained by administering an initial dose of 200 mg daily. This dose may have to be increased gradually to 600 mg/day.

Oxyphenbutazone is employed in oral doses of 100 mg three times a day.

Both phenylbutazone (Butazolidin) and oxyphenbutazone (Tandearil) are available in tablets containing 100 mg.

Acetaminophen is a metabolic product of acetophenetidin (Phenacetin). It is an effective analgesic and antipyretic without the uricosuric, anti-inflammatory, and antirheumatic effects of aspirin.[55]

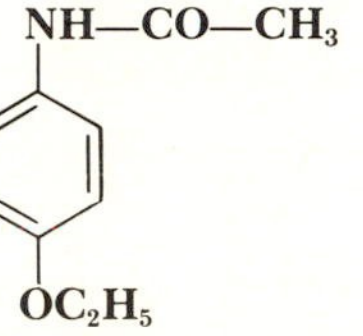

Acetaminophen

$NH-CO-CH_3$ $NH-CO-CH_3$

OC_2H_5 OH

Acetophenetidin 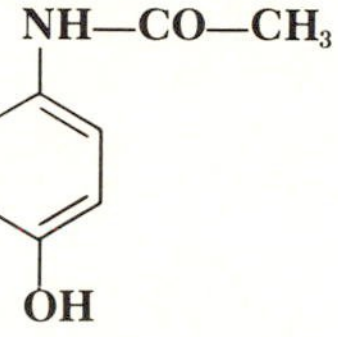 **Acetaminophen**

Pharmacokinetics. Acetaminophen is absorbed rapidly following oral administration with peak serum concentrations developing within 1 to 2 hours. Serum concentrations of 5 to 20 mg/L may be obtained after the administration of analgesic doses. The half-life of elimination is from 1 to 3 hours. If the half-life increases to 4 hours or more, this may be considered an indication of hepatic necrosis, which may be induced by large doses of acetaminophen itself.

Most (80%) of the acetaminophen is eliminated as the glucuronide. Other metabolites are formed by hydroxylation and deacetylation. Drugs that promote or inhibit hepatic drug metabolizing enzymes influence the rate of formation of these metabolites.

Adverse effects. Acetaminophen given in therapeutic doses produces remarkably few adverse effects. The drug does not cause gastric irritation or bleeding, does not interfere with platelet function, does not potentiate the oral hypoglycemic agents, and has no effect on uric acid excretion. This is in contrast with aspirin. Hepatotoxicity is a serious toxic effect, but it occurs only after the ingestion of large doses of the drug.[55]

Acetaminophen is available in tablets of 300 and 325 mg, in drops containing 60 mg/0.6 ml, and in elixir or syrup containing 120 mg/5 ml.

Hypatotoxicity. In large doses acetaminophen is quite hepatotoxic. Although this effect has not received adequate recognition until recently, it represents one of the most common causes of hepatic failure in Britain.[28] Acute hepatic injury may occur after ingestion of 10 g. Acetaminophen is metabolized in the liver to a glucuronide and to a highly hepatotoxic metabolite by the mixed function oxidase system. This compound is normally inactivated by glutathione.

Treatment of acetaminophen poisoning is generally unsatisfactory. Gastric lavage is useful in the early stages. Cysteamine (2-aminoethanethiol) can protect animals experimentally against acetaminophen overdosage. Also pretreatment with cysteine or methionine has some protective value.[55]

NEWER ANTI-INFLAMMATORY DRUGS

A number of potent new anti-inflammatory drugs were developed recently on the basis of screening procedures in experimental animals. Their mode of action is similar to that of aspirin, and they inhibit the synthesis of prostaglandins.

Indomethacin is comparable in effectiveness to phenylbutazone in rheumatoid arthritis. It is also used in the treatment of osteoarthritis, rheumatoid spondylitis, and gout.[16,33] Adverse effects caused by the drug include headache, gastrointestinal symptoms, blood dyscrasias, and peptic ulcer. Indomethacin (Iodocin) is available in capsules containing 25 and 50 mg.

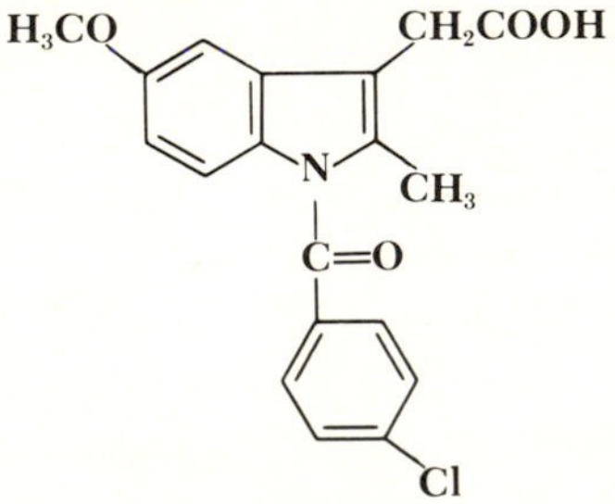

Indomethacin

Mefenamic acid, a mild analgesic, is no more effective than aspirin, and it may produce serious adverse reactions such as diarrhea, gastrointestinal bleeding, impairment of renal function, and blood dyscrasias. Mefenamic acid is available in capsules, 250 mg.

Ibuprofen, one of the newest nonsteroidal anti-inflammatory drugs, shows considerable promise as a substitute for aspirin in patients suffering from rheumatoid arthritis and osteoarthritis. The main advantage of the drug over aspirin is the lower incidence of gastrointestinal toxicity. Nevertheless, some patients do develop gastrointestinal symptoms.[50] In addition, blurred vision and skin rashes have been reported following its use. Ibuprofen (Motrin) is available in 300, 400 and 600 mg tablets. Daily dosage for adults consists of 400 mg every 4 to 6 hours.

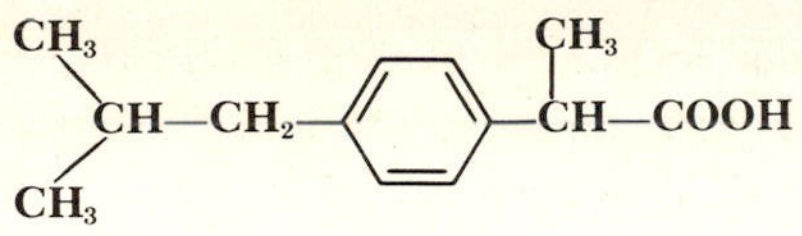

$$CH_3 \quad\quad\quad\quad\quad\quad CH_3$$

CH₃—CH—CH₂—⟨benzene ring⟩—CH—COOH with CH₃ below the left CH

Ibuprofen

Drug interactions with the anticoagulants may be anticipated. Aspirin should not be used concurrently with ibuprofen, since animal experiments indicate a net decrease in inflammatory activity on such a regimen.

In addition to aspirin, phenylbutazone, oxyphenbutazone, and indomethacin, many other drugs may be useful in the treatment of rheumatic diseases. Some of these such as chloroquine and adrenal corticosteroids are discussed in Chapters 59 and 43, respectively. Gold salts such as aurothioglucose (Solganal) and gold sodium thiomalate (Myochrysine), available for intramuscular injection, have some limited usefulness also.

Miscellaneous drugs used in rheumatic diseases

In recent years a large number of arylacetic and propionic acid derivatives have been introduced essentially as aspirin substitutes. Ibuprofen became available in 1975, naproxen (Naprosyn) in 1976. Tolmetin (Tolectin), introduced in 1976, differs chemically from the previous group but is similar pharmacologically. It is believed that all of these aspirin substitutes inhibit prostaglandin synthetase. The efficacy of these drugs is not superior to that of aspirin, but the incidence of adverse reactions, such as gastrointestinal bleeding, may be less following their use.[24]

Sulindac (Clinoril) has some chemical similarity to indomethacin with similar anti-inflammatory properties but lower gastrointestinal toxicity.[49] The drug is indicated for the treatment of osteoarthritis, rheumatoid arthritis, ankylosing spondylitis, and acute gouty arthritis. It is available in 150 and 200 mg tablets.

Penicillamine (Cuprimine) is being used in the treatment of rheumatoid arthritis. In contrast with the nonsteroidal antirheumatic drugs, which control only the inflammatory symptoms, penicillamine, along with gold salts, antimalarials, and immunosuppressive drugs, is believed to induce remission of the disease. Unfortunately, penicillamine causes skin rashes, thrombocytopenia, and proteinuria in a high percentage of patients.[54]

Methotrimeprazine (Levoprome), a phenothiazine closely related to chlorpromazine, has been introduced as a novel nonaddictive analgesic. In a carefully controlled clinical study, 20 mg of methotrimeprazine was approximately equivalent to 10 mg of morphine when both drugs were administered by the intramuscular route.[1] Special advantages claimed for this phenothiazine analgesic are an antiemetic effect and a lack of respiratory-depressant action. On the other hand, marked sedation and possible orthostatic hypotension may limit its usefulness in some patients. The structural formula of methotrimeprazine as contrasted with that of chlorpromazine is shown on p. 402.

NONADDICTIVE PHENOTHIAZINE ANALGESIC

Methotrimeprazine

Chlorpromazine

REFERENCES

1 Beaver, W. T., Wallenstein, S. L., Houde, R. W., and Rogers, A.: A comparison of the analgesic effects of methotrimeprazine and morphine in patients with cancer, Clin. Pharmacol. Ther. 7:436, 1966.

2 Brodie, B. B., and Axelrod, J.: The fate of acetophenetidin (phenacetin) in man and methods for the estimation of acetophenetidin and its metabolites in biological material, J. Pharmacol. Exp. Ther. 97:58, 1949.

3 Brodie, T. M.: Action of sodium salicylate and related compounds on tissue metabolism in vitro, J. Pharmacol. Exp. Ther. 117:39, 1956.

4 Burns, J. J., Rose, R. K., Goodwin, S., Reichenthal, J., Horning, E. C., and Brodie, B. B.: The metabolic fate of phenylbutazone (Butazolidin) in man, J. Pharmacol. Exp. Ther. 113:481, 1955.

5 Cass, L. J., and Frederik, W. S.: The augmentation of analgesic effect of aspirin with phenacetin and caffeine, Curr. Ther. Res. 4:583, 1962.

6 Collier, H. O. J.: The action and antagonism of kinins on bronchioles, Ann. N.Y. Acad. Sci. 104:290, 1963.

7 Cooperating Clinics Committee of the American Rheumatism Association: A three-month trial of indomethacin in rheumatoid arthritis, with special reference to analysis and inference, Clin. Pharmacol. Ther. 8:11, 1967.

8 Croft, D. N., and Wood, P. H. N.: Gastric mucosa and susceptibility to occult gastrointestinal bleeding caused by aspirin, Br. Med. J. 1:137, 1967.

9 Davison, C., Hertig, D. H., and DeVine, R.: Gastric hemorrhage induced by nonnarcotic analgetic agents in dogs, Clin. Pharmacol. Ther. 7:239, 1966.

10 DeKornfeld, T. J., Lasagna, L., and Frazier, T. M.: A comparative study of five proprietary analgesic compounds, J.A.M.A. 182:1315, 1962.

11 Dixon, A. St. J., Martin, B. K., Smith, M. J. H., and Wood, P. H. N., editors: Symposium

on salicylates, London, 1963, J. & A. Churchill, Ltd.

12 Fraser, H. F., and Isbell, H.: Pharmacology and addiction liability of dl- and d-propoxyphene, Bull. Narcotics 12:9, 1960.

13 Gilman, A.: Analgesic nephrotoxicity: a pharmacological analysis, Am. J. Med. 36:167, 1964.

14 Glander, G. W., Chaffee, J., and Goodale, F.: Studies on the antipyretic action of salicylates, Proc. Soc. Exp. Biol. Med. 126:205, 1967.

15 Graham, J. D. P., and Parker, W. A.: The toxic manifestations of sodium salicylate therapy, Q. J. Med. 17:153, 1948.

16 Hart, F. D., and Boardman, P. L.: Indomethacin: a new nonsteroid anti-inflammatory agent, Br. Med. J. 2:965, 1963.

17 Huguley, C. M.: Agranulocytosis induced by dipyrone, a hazardous antipyretic and analgesic, J.A.M.A. 189:938, 1964.

18 Hutchison, H. E., Jackson, J. M., and Cassidy, P.: Drug-induced hemolytic anemia, Lancet 2:1022, 1962.

19 Ingle, D. J.: Effects of aspirin, aminopyrine, and HPC upon glycosuria in the diabetic rat, J. Am. Pharm. Assoc. 42:247, 1953.

20 Kapp, E. M., and Coburn, A. F.: Urinary metabolites of sodium salicylate, J. Biol. Chem. 145:549, 1942.

21 Katz, A. M., Pearson, C. M., and Kennedy, J. M.: A clinical trial of indomethacin in rheumatoid arthritis, Clin. Pharmacol. Ther. 6:25, 1965.

22 Leonards, J. R., and Levy, G.: Reduction of prevention of aspirin-induced occult gastrointestinal blood loss in man, Clin. Pharmacol. Ther. 10:571, 1969.

23 Levy, G., and Leonards, J. R.: Urine pH and salicylate therapy (letter to the editor), J.A.M.A. 217:81, 1971.

24 Lewis, J. R.: New antirheumatic agents, J.A.M.A. 237:1260, 1977.

25 Lim, R. K., Miller, D. G., Guzman, F., Rodgers, D. W., Rogers, R. W., Wang, S. K.,

Chao, P. Y., and Shih, T. Y.: Pain and analgesia evaluated by the intraperitoneal bradykinin-evoked pain method in man, Clin. Pharmacol. Ther. **8**:521, 1967.

26 Loebl, D. H., Craig, R. M., Culic, D. D., Ridolfo, A. S., Falk, J., and Schmid, F. R.: Gastrointestinal blood loss. Effect of aspirin, fenoprofen and acetaminophen in rheumatoid arthritis as determined by sequential gastroscopy and radioactive fecal markers, J.A.M.A. **237**:976, 1977.

27 Mandel, H. G., Rodwell, W. W., and Smith, P. K.: A study of the metabolism of C^{14} salicylamide in the human, J. Pharmacol. Exp. Ther. **106**:433, 1952.

28 McJunkin, B., Barwick, K. W., Little, W. C., and Winfield, J. B.: Fatal massive hepatic necrosis following acetaminophen overdose, J.A.M.A. **236**:1874, 1976.

29 Medical Research Council Report: Treatment of acute rheumatic fever in children: a cooperative clinical trial of A.C.T.H., cortisone, and aspirins, Br. Med. J. **1**:555, 1955.

30 Milton, A. S., and Wendlandt, S.: Effects on body temperature of prostaglandins of the A, E and F series of injection into the third ventricle of unanesthetized cats and rabbits, J. Physiol. (London) **218**:325, 1971.

31 Moolten, S. E., and Smith, I. B.: Fatal nephritis in chronic phenacetin poisoning, Am. J. Med. **28**:127, 1960.

32 O'Brien J. R.: Effects of salicylates on human platelets, Lancet **1**:779, 1968.

33 O'Brien, W. M.: Indomethacin: a survey of clinical trials, Clin. Pharmacol. Ther. **9**:94, 1968.

34 Ross, J. D., and Ciccarelli, R. F.: Acquired methemoglobinemia due to ingestion of acetophenetidin: report of a case in a small infant, N. Engl. J. Med. **266**:1202, 1962.

35 Roth, J. L. A., Valdes-Dapena, A., Pieses, P., and Buchman, E.: Topical action of salicylates, Gastroenterology **44**:146, 1963.

36 Sahud, M. A., and Aggeler, P. M.: Platelet dysfunction—differentiation of a newly recognized primary type from that produced by aspirin, N. Engl. J. Med. **280**:453, 1969.

37 Salassa, R. M., Bollman, J. L., and Dry, T. J.: The effect of para-aminobenzoic acid on the metabolism and excretion of salicylate, J. Lab. Clin. Med. **33**:1393, 1948.

38 Salzman, E. W., Harris, W. H., and DeSanctis, R. W.: Reduction in venous thromboembolism by agents affecting platelet function, N. Engl. J. Med. **284**:1287, 1971.

39 Samter, M.: The acetyl in aspirin, Ann. Intern. Med. **71**:208, 1969.

40 Scott, D.: Aspirin: action on receptor in the tooth, Science **161**:180, 1968.

41 Smith, J. B., and Willis, A. L.: Aspirin selectively inhibits prostaglandin production in human platelets, Nature (New Biol.) **231**:235, 1971.

42 Vane, J. R.: Inhibition of prostaglandin synthesis as a mechanism of action of aspirin-like drugs, Nature **231**:232, 1971.

43 Vignec, A. J., and Gasparik, M.: Antipyretic effectiveness of salicylamide and acetylsalicylic acid in infants, J.A.M.A. **167**:1821, 1958.

44 Weiss, H. J., Aledort, L. M., and Kochwa, S.: The effects of salicylates on the hemostatic properties of platelets in man, J. Clin. Invest. **47**:2169, 1968.

45 Winter, C. A.: Nonsteroid anti-inflammatory agents, Annu. Rev. Pharmacol. **6**:157, 1966.

46 Winter, C. A., Risley, E. A., and Nuss, G. W.: Carrageenin-induced edema in hind paw of the rat as an assay for antiinflammatory drugs, Proc. Soc. Exp. Biol. Med. **111**:544, 1962.

47 Yu, T. F., and Gutman, A. B.: Study of the paradoxical effects of salicylate in low, intermediate, and high dosage on the renal mechanisms for excretion of urate in man, J. Clin. Invest. **38**:1298, 1959.

REVIEWS

48 Abrishami, M. A., and Thomas, J.: Aspirin intolerance—a review, Ann. Allergy **39**:28, 1977.

48a Atkins, E., and Bodel, P.: Fever, N. Engl. J. Med. **286**:29, 1972.

49 Brogden, R. N., Heel, R. C., and Speight, T. M.: Sulindac: a review of its pharmacological properties and therapeutic efficacy in rheumatic disease, Drugs **12**:97, 1978.

50 Brooks, C. D., Schlagel, C. A., Sekhar, N. C., and Sobota, J. T.: Tolerance and pharmacology of ibuprofen, Curr. Ther. Res. **15**:180, 1973.

51 Clark, W. G.: Mechanisms of antipyretic action, Gen. Pharmacol. **10**:71, 1979.

52 Danilevicius, Z.: Medical treatment leads to closure of patent ductus arteriosus, J.A.M.A. **237**:2326, 1977.

53 Davison, C.: Salicylate metabolism in man, Ann. N.Y. Acad. Sci. **179**:249, 1971.

54 Kaye, R. L., and Pemberston, R. E.: Treatment of rheumatoid arthritis, Arch. Intern. Med. **136**:1023, 1976.

54a Ketchum, J. S., and Jarvik, M. E.: Pharmacotherapy for the opioid addict: agonists or antagonists?, Ration. Drug Ther. **13**:1, Jan. 1979.

55 Koch-Weser, J.: Acetaminophen, N. Engl. J. Med. **295:**1297, 1976.

56 Krane, S. M.: Action of salicylates, N. Engl. J. Med. **286:**317, 1972.

57 Marx, J. L.: AMIS negative on aspirin and heart attacks, Science **207:**859, 1980.

58 Mills, J. A.: Nonsteroidal antiinflammatory drugs, N. Engl. J. Med. **290:**781, 1974.

58a Simon, L. S., and Mills, J. A.: Nonsteroidal antiinflammatory drugs, N. Engl. J. Med. **302:** 1179, 1980.

59 Vandam, L. D.: Analgesic drugs—the mild analgesics, N. Engl. J. Med. **286:**20, 1972.

SECTION FIVE

Anesthetics

CHAPTER 32

Pharmacology of general anesthesia

The scope of anesthesiology touches nearly every specialty of medicine. Drugs that allow painless, controlled surgical, obstetric, and diagnostic procedures constitute one of the cornerstones of modern-day pharmacological therapy. It is estimated that 20 million anesthetics are administered annually in the United States alone.

The hallmark of anesthetic drugs is *controllability*. For this reason, most of the potent anesthetics are gases or vapors. Such drugs can be administered at required dosages via the lungs with consequent rapid uptake into the systemic circulation. Elimination of these drugs is also primarily by the pulmonary route. Unlike "fixed" or nonvolatile drugs, elimination and pharmacological termination of action, therefore, do not depend on intrinsic hepatic biotransformation or renal excretion; rather they depend on a pulmonary process, which can be actively controlled by the anesthesiologist. The lungs possess a large surface area, which can be utilized for precise dosage administration or elimination.

Anesthetics are nonspecific, that is, they do not function by means of interaction with specific receptors.[34] As a corollary to this general action, there are no specific antagonists to anesthetics. Inhalation anesthetics should produce all of the following characteristics, although there may be quantitative differences among various drugs: (1) hypnosis, (2) analgesia (freedom from pain), (3) skeletal muscle relaxant properties, and (4) reduction of certain autonomic reflexes.

Selection of a particular anesthetic or combination of anesthetics is predicated on the patient's pathophysiological state and the nature of the anticipated surgical procedure. Anesthetics differ in degrees of depression of various organ systems, in potency, in speed of induction and awakening, in degree of skeletal muscle relaxation, and in other effects. Thus one anesthetic may be superior to another, depending on the clinical circumstances.

Popular potent organohalogen inhalation anesthetics include enflurane and halothane. Nitrous oxide, a weak gaseous anesthetic, is frequently used in combination with these volatile compounds or with fixed intravenous drugs such as barbiturates (for hypnosis), narcotics (for analgesia), and neuromuscular blockers (for skeletal muscle relaxation). Use of nitrous oxide in this latter circumstance is termed *balanced anesthesia*. The older anesthetics, cyclopropane and diethyl ether are used infrequently due to flammability. This feature is inconsistent with modern operating suites loaded with cautery and electronic monitoring gear. Isoflurane represents a potent halogenated anesthetic new to the armamentarium.

The so-called intravenous anesthetics are used for specific purposes or to supplement inhalation anesthetics, but lack controllability and other salutary features of the inhalation anesthetics. Thiobarbiturates (e.g., thiopental) are still highly preferred induction agents as they rapidly and pleasantly produce hypnosis. Lack of analgesic and muscle relaxant properties and slow elimination limit both dose and usefulness. Narcotics such as morphine and the more rapidly eliminated fentanyl are frequently used to supplement nitrous oxide anesthesia. Combinations of narcotic and tranquilizers, such as fentanyl plus droperidol (Innovar), are employed commonly with nitrous oxide. The sobriquet "dissociative anesthesia" has been given to the effect of certain phencyclidine drugs such as ketamine. Such drugs have limited scope, however, as they do not allow for other than superficial procedures and often have prolonged effects including abnormal psychic reactions.

POTENCY AND EFFICACY

Because volatile and gaseous anesthetics distribute and reach equilibrium in the body by virtue of partial pressure, it is convenient to establish potency in terms of this physical characteristic rather than the more conventional ED_{50}. The minimal anesthetic concentration (MAC) is the standard of potency for inhalation anesthetics.[24,27,59] MAC is defined as *that concentration of anesthetic (in v/v percent or mm Hg), which prevents response to a standard painful stimulus in 50% of humans or test animals.* In the clinical situation anesthetics are usually given in multiples of MAC (1.5 to 2.5 × MAC). Several factors change MAC. These include circadian rhythm, body temperature (direct proportional decrease), age (direct proportional decrease), other drugs (sedative, hypnotic, anesthetics, and other central nervous system (CNS) depressants decrease MAC). Factors that do not influence MAC include sex, species, state of oxygenation, acid-base changes, and arterial blood pressure changes.*

SOLUBILITY

Anesthetic gases and vapors are soluble in blood, tissue fluids, and tissues. Anesthetics in general are quite lipophilic. Since various tissues and fluids differ in lipid content, any particular gas or vapor will distribute to an eventual equilibrium with different concentrations in biophases, depending on solubility of the anesthetic.[39] Table 32-1 illustrates this effect with a hypothetical inhalation anesthetic at equilibrium. Note that although the partial pressure of the anesthetic in all phases is the same, the concentration in those tissues varies several hundredfold. This is due to the

*See references 3, 13, 14, 28, and 57.

TABLE 32-1. Distribution of inhalation anesthetic concentrations in various biophases following partial pressure equilibrium

Anesthetic	Biophase		
	Blood	**Lean tissue**	**Fat**
Concentration at equilibrium	3 mM ⇌	6 mM ⇌	660 mM
Partial pressure at equilibrium	8 mm Hg ⇌	8 mm Hg ⇌	8 mm Hg

difference in solubility of the drug in various tissues. Table 32-1 illustrates the large fat storage capacity of an anesthetic due to its high lipophilic nature.

There are three solubility coefficients germane to anesthetic distribution.[25] All are based on Henry's law and are temperature dependent. For clinical purposes these coefficients are measured at 37° C.

1. *Blood-gas partition coefficient* (λ). This is the most important solubility parameter for understanding uptake of inhaled gases and vapors. Fig. 32-1 illustrates how this coefficient is derived. It will be noted from this figure that when equilibrium is reached, the end-tidal concentration of the anesthetic (upward directed arrow) is proportional to the pulmonary blood concentration. Thus end-tidal concentration or partial pressure (abbreviated F_E) can be used as a measure of degree of equilibrium steady-state.[23] The partial pressure of anesthetics being administered to the lungs for uptake by the blood is inspired alveolar partial pressure (F_I). Thus when $F_E/F_I = 1$, blood-gas equilibrium has been reached.

2. *Tissue solubility.* Anesthetics enter the lungs, are picked up by pulmonary arterial blood, and then are distributed to peripheral tissues. Obviously, those organs with the highest degree of blood flow per unit time will receive more anesthetic molecules than organs with lower flow. Richly perfused organs include brain, heart, liver, and kidney; skeletal muscle perfusion is intermediate; lowest perfusion goes to bone, ligaments, and fat. The blood and tissue partition coefficient is usually between

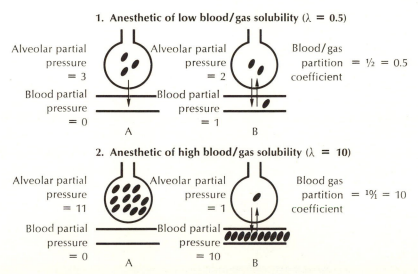

FIG. 32-1. Schematic illustrating derivation of blood-gas solubility coefficient (λ) Gas or vapor is inhaled into lungs perfused with pulmonary arterial blood. Anesthetic partial pressure in lungs is high initially and absent in blood. Anesthetic molecules diffuse into blood and reach partial pressure equilibrium. Due to solubility coefficient, partial pressure equilibrium results in concentration differences in anesthetic. Anesthetic of low blood-gas coefficient will have fewer molecules in blood than in gas phase; high coefficient produces fewer molecules in gas than in blood at equilibrium.

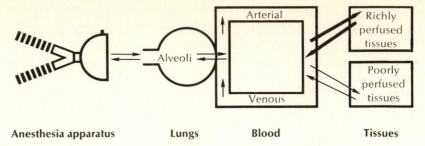

FIG. 32-2. Flow of anesthetic gases and vapors from anesthesia machine to peripheral tissues.

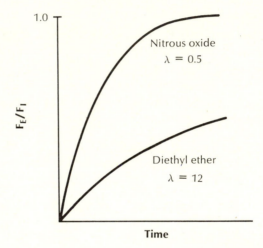

FIG. 32-3. Equilibrium curve for two anesthetics. Note that anesthetic with lower blood-gas solubility approaches equilibrium much faster than anesthetic with higher solubility. Anesthetic with lower solubility will achieve state of anesthesia more rapidly.

TABLE 32-2. MAC, blood-gas, and oil-gas partition coefficients for six general anesthetics

Anesthetic	MAC in humans (v/v%)	Blood-gas (λ)	Oil-gas
Halothane $CF_3CHBrCl$	0.78	2.3	224
Enflurane CF_2HOCF_2CFClH	1.7	1.8	98
Diethyl ether $(C_2H_5)_2O$	2.0	12.1	65
Isoflurane $CF_3CClHOCF_2H$	1.3	1.4	99
Nitrous oxide N_2O	188*	0.4	1.4
Methoxyflurane $CCl_2HCF_2OCH_3$	0.16	12.0	970

*Extrapolated data.

1 and 2 for most anesthetics.[40] Fat solubility is much higher, however. At times it exceeds blood solubility several hundredfold. Due to the combination of low flow and high solubility, it is apparent that body fat requires a long time to achieve complete equilibrium. In Fig. 32-2 transfer of anesthetics from the anesthesia machine to peripheral tissues is demonstrated.

3. *Oil-gas partition coefficient.* This partition coefficient is an artificial one in certain respects because the oil commonly used, olive oil, is not a biological constituent of the body. However, olive oil has certain solubility characteristics similar to body fat and correlates with it. Lipid solubility of anesthetics is proportional to potency. This is the basis of the Meyer-Overton correlation of directly proportional fat solubility to anesthetic potency. Thus a high oil-gas partition coefficient indicates a potent anesthetic (e.g., one with low MAC and low partial pressure required for anesthesia). This correlation does nothing to define mechanism of anesthesia but can be used to predict MAC.

Importance of blood-gas partition coefficient in speed of induction. The lower the blood-gas partition coefficient the faster the anesthetic equilibrium between alveolar gas and pulmonary blood is reached (e.g., the faster $F_E/F_I = 1$). Because such a gas or vapor is relatively insoluble, equilibrium with blood is quickly attained. Thus, induction of anesthesia is rapid with such an agent.[21] On the other hand, a high blood-gas solubility mandates a long time interval before blood-gas equilibrium is attained. This implies a slow induction. Due to the higher solubility, it takes a longer time for the blood to become saturated with molecules of anesthetic. Therefore, attainment of final anesthetizing partial pressure is delayed. The difference between the speed of eventual equilibrium of an inhalation anesthetic of low blood-gas partition coefficient compared to one of high blood-gas partition coefficient is seen in Fig. 32-3. Table 32-2 lists MAC, blood-gas, and oil-gas partition coefficients for six commonly employed inhalation anesthetics.[22]

Ventilation with an inhaled anesthetic causes a rapid rise in alveolar anesthetic partial pressure or concentration (F_I). The rise in F_I is antagonized by uptake into arterial pulmonary blood, removing the gas or vapor from the lungs. Arterial blood containing anesthetic then distributes the anesthetic to peripheral tissues. Uptake of the anesthetic by any tissue is a function of solubility, blood flow to the tissues, and the arterial to tissue anesthetic partial pressure difference. The partial pressure difference acts as the driving force. When the partial pressure difference is zero, no uptake occurs.

Uptake from the lungs (as from any tissue) is directly related to three variables: (1) blood-gas partition coefficient of the anesthetic, (2) cardiac output ($\dot{Q}$), and (3) alveolar to venous anesthetic partial pressure difference.[19] As described before, when equilibrium is attained, uptake falls to zero. The time to such equilibrium depends on the peripheral tissue capacity, which is related to the particular volume and capacity of the tissue concerned. In summary

$$\text{Uptake} = \lambda \cdot \dot{Q} \cdot (P_A - P_V)/BP$$

UPTAKE OF AN ANESTHETIC

where

$$(P_A - P_V) = (\text{Alveolar} - \text{Venous partial pressure of anesthetic})$$
$$Q = \text{Cardiac output}$$
$$\lambda = \text{Blood-gas partition coefficient}$$
$$BP = \text{Barometric pressure}$$

An increase in any of these factors will increase uptake. It is worthwhile noting that if uptake of an anesthetic is plotted graphically, the resulting curve is the reciprocal of the equilibrium curve.

Factors that prevent zero uptake

There are several variables that prevent the equilibrium curve from reaching the $F_E/F_I = 1$ state. Because of these, equilibrium is slowed.

1. *Fat solubility.* Because of the poor perfusion and large storage solubility characteristics of general anesthetics, body fat may take hours, even days to achieve total equilibrium with alveolar anesthetic partial pressure.

2. *Biotransformation of anesthetics.* Inhalation anesthetics interact with microsomal enzyme systems and are metabolized.[64] Actually, the degree of metabolism is small compared to the overabundance of drug molecules given during the course of an anesthetic. Obviously, metabolism limits obtaining complete equilibrium. However, unlike fixed drugs such degradation has little if any effect on the conduct or dosage requirements of the anesthetic. On the other hand, biotransformation of inhalation anesthetics may well be a vector of viscerotoxicity of the halogenated anesthetics.[7]

3. *Diffusion through skin into bowel and air spaces.* Diffusion of anesthetic through the skin into the atmosphere is a source of loss preventing complete equilibrium.[63] Typical losses include nitrous oxide ($F_I = 70\%$) 2.5 ml/min/M^2 and halothane ($F_I = 0.9\%$) 0.006 ml/min/M^2. Anesthetics given at a high F_I such as nitrous oxide, replace nitrogen in bowel and air spaces (e.g., middle ear, pneumothorax, brain ventricular air from pneumoencephalography).[10,65] Since nitrous oxide is more soluble than nitrogen at the same partial pressure, when it passes from a dissolved state in blood to an air space, it expands to a larger volume than the nitrogen it replaces. Enlargement of brain ventricles filled with air from pneumoencephalography can cause herniation through the foramen magnum. Enlargement of a preexisting pneumothorax can occur via the same mechanism.[26] In this manner nitrous oxide anesthesia produces variable increases in bowel volume.[30]

Concentration effect

Basically, the concentration effect stipulates that the higher the inspired concentration of an anesthetic, the faster the rate of rise to equilibrium. In theory, the equilibrium curves in Fig. 32-3 should be independent of the concentration or partial pressure of the anesthetic inspired. In practice, this is not so. High concentrations give a more rapid initial rise toward an equilibrium state than low (subanesthetic) concentrations.[20] To understand this effect, imagine an inspired concentration of an anesthetic to be 100% ($F_I = 1.0$). If this 100% concentration fills the alveoli, regardless of uptake into blood, the remaining end-tidal alveolar concentration will be 100%

(FE = 1.0). Actually, the concentration effect is seen with nitrous oxide given in relatively high concentrations (FI = 0.5 to 0.7). Under these circumstances there is rapid uptake of a significant portion of the anesthetic into the blood. In order to maintain lung volume there is literal sucking of anesthetic mixtures from the reservoir of the anesthesia machine into the lungs. Since the FI of anesthetic from the machine is generally higher during induction than the FE (due to uptake), mixing of the two produces a higher FE than would be expected. With the FE higher, the FE/FI ratio approaches 1.0 sooner than would be expected.

Second gas effect

Uptake of large volumes of a first or primary gas given in high concentrations (the "concentration effect") accelerates the alveolar rate of rise for a second gas given simultaneously.[29,62] Thus the second gas in low concentrations achieves equilibrium faster than if it were given in the absence of the primary, high concentration gas. Clinically, nitrous oxide (the primary gas) is given in high concentrations (FI = 0.5 to 0.7) with low concentrations of a potent anesthetic such as halothane or enflurane (FI = 0.005 to 0.02). Due to the second gas effect, actually a spin-off of the concentration effect, the potent low concentration anesthetic will reach equilibrium faster than if it had been administered in oxygen alone.

Effects of ventilation

An increase in minute alveolar ventilation ($\dot{V}_A$) obviously causes a more rapid rise in FE because more molecules of anesthetic are presented to the alveoli per unit time.[60,66] However, uptake of anesthetics of high solubility is altered more than uptake of anesthetics of low solubility by increases in ventilation.

1. *High solubility anesthetics ($\lambda > 1.0$)*. Increasing $\dot{V}_A$ causes a large increase in FE per unit time. The reason is that the blood has a large capacity for soluble anesthetics. When blood is exposed to more molecules of higher solubility anesthetics, more of these molecules can be taken up. This causes increases in the partial pressure of anesthetics in the blood manifested as an increase in FE partial pressure.

2. *Low solubility drugs ($\lambda < 1.0$)*. An increase in number of anesthetic molecules presented to pulmonary arterial blood per unit time with an agent of low solubility does not increase uptake (hence arterial blood partial pressure and FE) to a great extent. The insoluble anesthetic almost maximally saturates the blood rapidly with a relatively low number of molecules. Being near saturation with the low capacity for these drugs, the blood can pick up only a few of the extra molecules presented to it with an increase in $\dot{V}_A$.

The clinical corollary of uptake changes produced by increases in $\dot{V}_A$ are obvious. Higher solubility anesthetics are taken up rapidly with forced artificial ventilation. They may quickly reach dangerous concentration levels in tissues and blood. On the other hand, it is generally safe to hyperventilate patients with anesthetics of low solubility.

Effects of cardiac output

An increase in cardiac output ($\dot{Q}$) lowers FE, as there is more pulmonary arterial blood available for uptake of the anesthetic per unit time. Low solubility anesthetics are altered to a lesser extent than are high solubility anesthetics. The clinical corollaries of this fact are (1) anesthetic depression of cardiac output can alter its own uptake as the alveolar end-tidal rate of rise (FE) is rapid with decreased cardiac output; and (2) highly soluble anesthetics rapidly reach equilibrium with depressed cardiac output. In shock states, use of soluble anesthetics can thus excessively depress an already compromised circulation if care is not taken.[46,47]

To summarize the salient features of uptake and distribution of inhaled gases and vapors, the blood-gas partition coefficient is the most important physical constant establishing speed of induction of an anesthetic. The lower this coefficient, the faster pulmonary blood reaches saturation and hence the faster the induction of anesthesia. Awakening from anesthesia is similar. The lower the solubility, the faster the awakening as the anesthetic rapidly dissipates from pulmonary venous blood into alveoli. The concentration and second gas effects hasten induction of an inhalation anesthetic. Changes in ventilation and cardiac output have opposite effects—increasing ventilation causes an increase in the rise to equilibrium (more prominent with soluble anesthetics) and increased cardiac output slows the rate of equilibrium. In clinical practice these and factors such as ventilation/perfusion inequalities, alterations of regional blood flow, volume status, degree of circulatory depression, and so on are taken into account during the conduct of general anesthesia.

STAGES AND SIGNS OF ANESTHESIA

Early pioneers in the field of anesthesia such as W. T. G. Morton, John Snow, and Arthur Guedel recognized that there is a progression of predictable physiological changes produced during anesthesia. The signs and stages of diethyl ether anesthesia with increasing depth were characterized by Guedel[33] as follows:

Stage I   Analgesia
Stage II Delirium
Stage III Surgical anesthesia
  Phase 1. Sleep and analgesia. Patient unresponsive to surgical stimulations. Pupils constricted and eyes moist. Intercostal ventilation (arterial blood concentration = 110 mg/100 ml).
  Phase 2. Pupils dilate and eyes dry. Beginning intercostal paralysis with increased diaphragmatic ventilation (arterial blood concentration = 120 mg/100 ml).
  Phase 3. Increasing skeletal muscle relaxation. Intercostal activity markedly decreased; diaphragmatic ventilation predominates. Tidal volume falls. Corneal reflexes absent with dilated pupils. (Arterial blood concentration = 130 mg/100 ml.)
  Phase 4. Onset of complete intercostal paralysis; ends with diaphragmatic paralysis. Circulatory depression. Pupils maximally dilate. (Arterial blood concentration = 140 to 160 mg/100 ml.)
Stage IV Medullary paralysis; failure of ventilation and circulation

Although evaluation of the patient anesthetized with diethyl ether is rather straightforward, newer more potent anesthetics with lower solubilities pass through these various phases faster. In addition the overall pharmacological effects are somewhat different, although the end result is similar. Basically the new, more rapid anesthetics can be categorized into two stages: the stage of analgesia and delirium and the stage of surgical anesthesia. This latter stage is divided into light, moderate, and deep. With progressive deepening of surgical anesthesia there are parallel diminutions in ventilation and circulatory integrity. Death can occur from medullary paralysis and circulatory arrest in the absence of hypoxia with overdosage of potent anesthetics.

The anesthetic gases and vapors are customarily administered to the lungs via an anesthesia machine. The basic components of an anesthesia machine include

METHODS OF ADMINISTRATION OF GENERAL ANESTHETICS

1. Steel cylinders containing anesthetic gases and oxygen under pressure. Reduction valves lower the extremely high pressures of the cylinders to usable pressures conducive to flow gradients.
2. Flowmeters that accurately measure minute flow of gases.
3. Calibrated vaporizers. These are containers of a high capacity metal such as copper, filled with liquid anesthetic. A sintered bronze disk in the bottom of the vaporizer disperses in-flowing oxygen into small bubbles, which vaporize the liquid anesthetic in precision fashion. Volatile anesthetics such as halothane and enflurane are vaporized to permit the administration of precise amounts.
4. A carbon dioxide absorber.

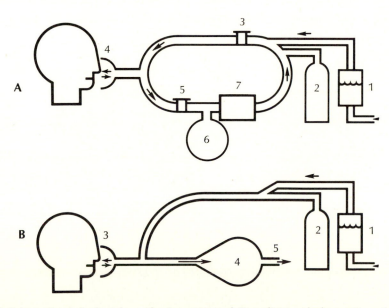

FIG. 32-4. Schematic of, **A,** closed anesthesia system and, **B,** pediatric valveless system. **A,** *1,* Vaporizer for volatile liquid anesthetics; *2,* compressed gas source; *3,* inhalation unidirectional valve; *4,* mask; *5,* unidirectional exhalation valve; *6,* rebreathing bag; and *7,* carbon dioxide absorption chamber. **B,** *1,* Vaporizer for volatile liquid anesthetics; *2,* compressed gas source; *3,* mask; *4,* rebreathing bag; and *5,* gas exhaust port.

5. A rebreathing bag.
6. Connecting tubing.
7. Unidirectional valves.

Although open drop and insufflation techniques were used in the past, they are only of historical interest now. The closed system and the semiclosed systems are used commonly for adult patients at present; the nonrebreathing, nonvalvular systems are used for pediatric patients. A description, including the advantages and disadvantages of these systems, follows:

1. *Closed system:* Economical; prevents excess anesthetics from polluting operating room; conserves heat and respiratory moisture; more difficult to calculate anesthetic dosage.
2. *Semiclosed system:* Easy to calculate anesthetic dose; not economical because gases are expelled into environment and system loses heat and moisture.
3. *Nonrebreathing, nonvalvular system:* Low resistance highly suitable for pediatric patients; loses heat and contributes to operating room pollution of trace anesthetic concentrations.

Fig. 32-4 illustrates the schematics of each of these systems. Administration of gases and vapors from the anesthesia machine is accomplished either by face mask or endotracheal tube.

THEORIES OF GENERAL ANESTHESIA

The mechanism by which anesthetics work is not known. Inhaled anesthetics possess no unique molecular configuration that can be associated with a particular structure-activity relationship. Interaction with cellular components is by means of van der Waals forces only. The anesthetics are nonspecific and change the function of all cellular constituents.[34]

Effects of anesthetics have been attributed to blocks of ionic channels and alterations of neurotransmitter release, but these actions cannot be correlated well enough to evolve a unitary hypothesis of mechanism of action. Several theories of anesthesia have been postulated, but all have been found to be deficient in certain respects.

1. *Biochemical hypothesis.* Quastel[56] theorized that anesthetics depress cellular respiration. This theory was postulated on the finding that certain anesthetics decrease adenosine triphosphate (ATP) production and cellular oxygen utilization in vitro. However, brain ATP concentration is not reduced by anesthetics in vivo.
2. *Hydrate theory.* Pauling and Miller[44,51] postulated that anesthetic molecules form gas hydrates or structured water, which inhibit brain function at crucial sites. However, recent studies have demonstrated that correlation of hydrate formation and potency of inhalation anesthetics is very poor.
3. *Ionic pore theory.* Another theorized mechanism of anesthesia attributes the state to block of ionic channels by interaction of anesthetic molecules with membranes.[1,35] In many cases, high pressures can reverse anesthetics, perhaps by changing membrane structure so that the anesthetics can no longer interact at these sites. However, this theory has poor correlation with the lipid solubility of anesthetics.

The Meyer-Overton correlation with fat solubility[43,50] has stood the test of time. In general, the more lipid soluble an anesthetic, the more potent it is. However, this is a correlation only rather than a mechanism of the anesthesia state. It is difficult to imagine that anesthetics act on lipids only, and many organic solvents are quite fat soluble without appreciable anesthetic effects.

Certain types of fixed drugs are classified as anesthetics, although it should be remembered that they are incomplete and do not have the controllability of the inhaled drugs.

INTRAVENOUS ANESTHETICS

Barbiturates used intravenously to produce or supplement hypnosis during anesthesia are highly lipid-soluble molecules. They follow many of the distribution characteristics of the inhaled anesthetics. It must be remembered that barbiturates are hypnotics only and do not possess analgesic or muscle relaxant activity except with gross overdosage. Two barbiturates, thiopental and methohexital, are commonly employed.

Barbiturates

Thiopental sodium (Pentothal) is a potent ultrashort-acting thiobarbiturate, which is the sulfur analog of pentobarbital (Nembutal). The thio-group gives the drug greater lipid solubility, hence fosters penetration of the blood-brain barrier. Although barbiturates are organic acids, the pH has to be increased to 10 (as the sodium salt) to produce aqueous solubility.

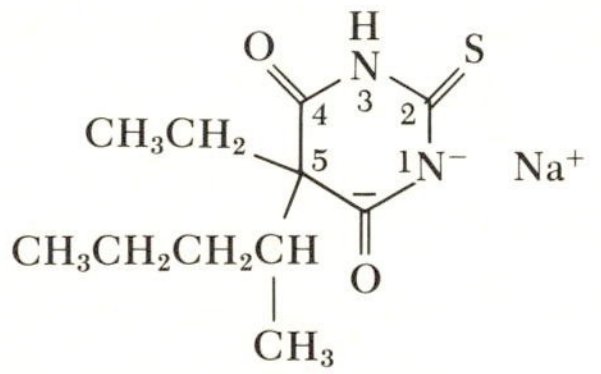

Thiopental sodium

Thiopental is depressive to both circulation and ventilation. The drug is commonly used to produce a smooth, pleasant induction of anesthesia. It has no viscerotoxic effects, and overdosage is marked by an extension of pharmacological effects (i.e., marked circulatory and ventilatory depression with upper airway obstruction).

Termination of action of this, and other intravenously administered barbiturates, is due to both redistribution and metabolism.[53,58] Plasma levels fall rapidly as the drug is taken up by richly perfused organs. It is then distributed to muscle and eventually to fatty tissues. Awakening occurs with normal therapeutic dosages within 15 minutes, about the time skeletal muscle is reaching saturation. Metabolism of the barbiturate is extensive, with less than 5% being excreted unchanged by the kidney. Metabolism begins as soon as the barbiturate is administered but is not as important in terminating activity as redistribution. **Thiamylal** (Surital) is a thiobarbiturate similar to thiopental.

Methohexital (Brevital) is an ultrashort-acting oxybarbiturate. It was designed to have a slightly shorter duration of hypnosis than thiopental, but clinically this difference is not always apparent.

Contraindications to the use of intravenous barbiturates include shock states and asthma. Barbiturates exacerbate the metabolic disease acute intermittent porphyria and should not be used in such patients. Inadvertent intra-arterial injections of barbiturates can induce severe arterial spasm and thrombosis followed by gangrene of the extremities. Barbiturates are given intravenously in 1.0% to 2.5% solutions.

Innovar   Innovar is a trade name for the combination of a narcotic analgesic, fentanyl, and a butyrophenone tranquilizer, droperidol. Each milliliter contains 0.05 mg fentanyl and 2.5 mg droperidol. The drug combination is used as a supplement to nitrous oxide anesthesia. Fentanyl has a relatively short duration of action and is used by itself as a narcotic-analgesic during anesthesia. Droperidol is a potent tranquilizer and antiemetic. However, it has a rather long half-life.

The combination is a useful adjuvant to balanced anesthesia. Fentanyl, like all narcotics, severely depresses ventilation.[18] A peculiar increase in chest wall muscle tone, termed "wooden rigidity," is occasionally observed if the narcotic is injected rapidly intravenously. Rarely droperidol produces a parkinsonian-type extrapyramidal reaction in certain individuals. The anesthetic-like state produced by Innovar has been termed *neurolept-anesthesia*. Innovar, given by the intramuscular route, is also used for preoperative medication in certain patients.

Ketamine   Ketamine hydrochloride is a phencyclidine derivative capable of producing a trance like state with freedom from pain, termed *dissociative anesthesia*. The drug is given either intravenously or intramuscularly. Ketamine produces little to no muscular relaxation. Patients will respond to visceral pain but not to superficial pain under the influence of ketamine. It frequently produces psychic problems when used in adults. These have been described as terrifying dreams and severe distortions of reality. For that reason use of ketamine is usually limited to that of an anesthetic for superficial procedures in infants and children. Ketamine stimulates the sympathetic nervous system so that there may be an increase in blood pressure. It frequently increases salivation. Ketamine raises intracranial pressure and is thus relatively contraindicated in the presence of central nervous system (CNS) tumors or space-occupying lesions. Ketamine is available in solutions of 10 mg/ml for intravenous use and 50 mg/ml for intramuscular administration.

Ketamine

PREANESTHETIC   Several classes of drugs are frequently given prior to the induction of anesthesia.
MEDICATION   The primary objectives are to produce an anxiety-free, sedated patient. Additional

reasons to give such medications include depression of vagal tone and as supplements to the anesthetic drugs. Individual drugs used for preanesthetic medication are described in the following categories:

1. *Anticholinergics:* Atropine, scopolamine, and glycopyrrolate are frequently given intramuscularly prior to anesthesia to decrease vagal cardiac tone and to block bronchial secretions. The value of such muscarinic blockers is less now than when secretion-producing irritant anesthetics such as cyclopropane and diethyl ether were used.

2. *Narcotics:* Analgesics such as meperidine (Demerol), morphine, and fentanyl (Sublimaze) are given to decrease anxiety and as a narcotic supplement to anesthesia. These drugs all produce certain degrees of respiratory depression by themselves, which is increased when combined with anesthetics.

3. *Sedatives:* Barbiturates, primarily the short-acting drugs secobarbital (Seconal) and pentobarbital (Nembutal), are given to allay anxiety and produce a drowsy patient.

4. *Benzodiazepines:* Diazepam (Valium) given orally or intravenously produces sedation and some amnesia without significant detriments to circulation or to ventilation. For this reason, drugs of this class are now quite frequently employed as preanesthetic medications.

All the preanesthetic drugs possess certain disadvantages such as respiratory depression, and so on. Thus, use is dependent on intimate pharmacological and pathological knowledge and clinical judgment. As important as the premedicant drugs are in allaying the patient's anxieties, of equal importance is the psychological rapport made by the anesthesiologist.

PHARMACOLOGICAL EFFECTS OF ANESTHETICS

Because of the ubiquitous nature of anesthetic distribution and the nonspecific effect on all cellular functions, discussion of the specific organ effects from these drugs is frequently incomplete. Although anesthetics in general are depressants to function, there are many quantitative differences in these actions. To add complexity, each of the anesthetics differs qualitatively in this regard.

Nervous system

Central nervous system. Anesthetics depress all portions of the CNS. There is no single site or locus of effect; however, there are considerable regional differences. It is believed that the higher cortical centers and the ascending reticular activating system are the most susceptible portions of the brain to anesthetics. This is a dose-dependent phenomenon. As anesthetic concentration in the brain increases, lower centers are depressed. This eventually leads to respiratory and circulatory arrest, the mechanism of death with overdosage of general anesthetics. The neurons of the reticular activating system are depressed in a differential manner.[15,16,32] For example, in very light planes of anesthesia, one commonly encounters clonus, hyperreflexia, and other neurological signs, which indicate that the depressor neurons of the reticular activating system are inhibited at lower dosages than the excitatory neurons.

Peripheral nervous system. Recent studies have indicated that profound effects on the spinal cord are produced by the general anesthetics. The gating area for pain impulses, the substantia gelantinosa of Rolando, is depressed in function, such that pain impulses ascending via pathways including the lateral, spinal, and thalamic tracts are depressed.[17] Thus fewer pain impulses reach the brain during anesthesia. Many of the general anesthetics also produce skeletal muscle relaxation by an effect on the internuncial pool of the spinal cord. Although there are discernible effects of general anesthetics in the region of the myoneural junction, it is believed that the spinal cord effects are the ones responsible for most of the skeletal muscle relaxation seen with the administration of these drugs.[37]

Autonomic nervous system. Here, there is a wide difference in action spectrum produced by the general anesthetics, differences made more complex by the profound dose relationships involved. Some of the inhalation anesthetics, particularly the older ones, such as diethyl ether and cyclopropane, appear to be sympathetic nervous system stimulants.[52] Actually, rather than a stimulating effect, this may be due to quantitative differences in action on excitatory and inhibitory neurons controlling sympathetic nervous activity.[55] Levels of plasma norepinephrine may increase threefold to tenfold during anesthesia with an anesthetic such as cyclopropane. This is one of the primary reasons that until a decade or so ago, cyclopropane was considered to be the anesthetic of choice in shock states. Due to the release of norepinephrine, blood pressure was maintained with this anesthetic, although flow to organs was consequently diminished because of arteriolar constriction. Other sympathomimetic effects are revealed in the increased glycogenolysis seen with the anesthetic diethyl ether. Blood sugars may reach levels as high as 200 to 250 mg/100 ml with this anesthetic. By contrast, modern halogenated anesthetics such as halothane cause total inhibition of the sympathetic nervous system and a reduced plasma norepinephrine content. These agents also do not produce glycogenolysis. Effects of general inhalation anesthetics on parasympathetic activity are quite variable. Some of the anesthetics, such as cyclopropane and halothane, have been adjudged to be vagal stimulants, particularly in lighter planes of anesthesia. The evidence for this is scanty, but both anesthetics seem to produce a mild degree of bradycardia, which can be overcome by the muscarinic-blocking drug atropine. Further evidence for enhanced vagal activity comes from the clinical reports implicating cyclopropane in possibly triggering bronchial constriction in asthmatics. On the other hand, halothane and the other halogenated hydrocarbon anesthetics do not have this effect on bronchial smooth muscle and are therefore considered to be drugs of choice for the patient with constrictive bronchiolar disease.

Respiration   With deep levels of anesthesia, respiratory depression is common with all general anesthetics.[31,41] Diethyl ether produces a clear-cut depression of tidal volume due to intercostal muscle paralysis and finally diaphragmatic paralysis. With other anesthetics, such as halothane, this differential effect on muscle activity to depress respiration is less clear. Certainly, at all planes of anesthesia there is a graded depression of medullary activity. Classically, ventilation during anesthesia shows lowered tidal volume and increased frequency of respiration with a net reduction in alveolar minute ventilation. Response to arterial and alveolar carbon dioxide tensions is decreased, so that there is a classic rightward shift and decreased slope of the carbon dioxide response curve. This is a dose-dependent phenomenon. In lighter planes of surgical anesthesia, some anesthetics, such as diethyl ether, have less effects on respiration, such that normal or near normal carbon dioxide tension is maintained.[45] However, with most of the halogenated anesthetics, the drop in alveolar ventilation and alveolar minute ventilation ($\dot{V}A$) will produce an increased Pa_{CO_2}. For this reason, the administration of a general anesthetic is frequently performed with assisted or controlled ventilation. This may be done either by manual inflation of the rebreathing bag of the anesthesia machine or by the insertion of a mechanical ventilator into the circuit. Some of the older anesthetics, such as diethyl ether, cause increased bronchial secretions. These can be blocked with atropine, scopolamine, or glycopyrrolate and are one of the reasons why anticholinergics were frequently given as preoperative medications. The present-day anesthetics do not normally cause an increase in pulmonary secretions, so use of the anticholinergics for this reason is waning.

Circulation

Anesthetics affect both the heart and the peripheral circulation. All the drugs in this category affect the heart by producing a dose-related, negative inotropic effect. In isolated animal preparations, this can be seen as a depression of twitch height in isolated papillary muscles and in intact humans by a fall in cardiac output. The anesthetics differ from a quantitative point of view in this action. Halothane, for example, depresses the myocardium to a greater extent in equally anesthetic dosages than does diethyl ether.[5] There are subtle autonomic differences, which change the situation in intact humans also. For example, with those anesthetics that stimulate norepinephrine release from adrenergic nerves, there is less negative inotropic effect because increases in sympathetic transmitter indirectly stimulate the myocardium.[61] The anesthetics, particularly the halogenated ones, depress peripheral sympathetic nerves by affecting the ganglia. For this reason, peripheral vasodilatation usually occurs during anesthesia. The overall effect of the negative inotropic effects and the depression of peripheral circulation is a drop in blood pressure in a dose-dependent fashion. Systolic blood pressure seems to be affected to a greater degree than does diastolic blood pressure, so that during clinical anesthesia there is a tendency for the pulse pressure to narrow.

Changes in cardiac rhythm and conduction are not uncommon during anesthesia. The most common arrhythmia seen is a downward displacement of the pacemaker, progressing from wandering pacemaker to nodal rhythm. This arrhythmia is usually benign. The second most common form of arrhythmias are premature ventricular contractions. Many anesthetics are capable of interacting with plasma epinephrine or norepinephrine concentration elevation to produce the so-called hydrocarbon anesthetic arrhythmias. Probably due to changes in automaticity, the threshold to premature ventricular contractions is lowered by many anesthetics. In light planes of anesthesia, if there is sympathetic stimulation or if exogenous sympathomimetic amines are administered, troublesome ventricular arrhythmias can be produced.[2,54] For example, the cyclopropane-epinephrine sequence is used in pharmacology in testing cardiac antifibrillatory drugs. Since hypercapnia can lead to increased release of catecholamines, these may interact with the myocardium "sensitized" to a lower arrhythmia threshold by hydrocarbon anesthetics to produce ventricular arrhythmias. These arrhythmias are frequently clues to the clinician that ventilation is not adequate. Injection of catecholamines during anesthesia with certain of these anesthetics should be done with caution, if at all. There have been minimal dose schedules of drugs such as epinephrine, which can be safely injected during the course of halothane anesthesia.[38] The agents most likely to produce these catecholamine anesthetic arrhythmias are the straight chain hydrocarbons, namely cyclopropane and halothane. The ether series of anesthetics, halogenated or not, seems to present far fewer problems in this regard.

Uterus   The halogenated anesthetics inhibit the contractile response of the gravid uterus when oxytocic drugs are administered. Thus, they may produce or allow certain degrees of uterine relaxation, which may be advantageous for version extractions or other intrauterine manipulations. This is a two-edged sword, however, as these anesthetics will also permit sufficient degrees of uterine relaxation to increase postpartum bleeding. The gaseous and vapor anesthetics pass the placenta into the fetus with a great deal of ease. These effects must be taken into consideration during obstetric anesthesia.

Hepatic and metabolic actions   Anesthetics have several effects on the liver. Experimental evidence indicates that anesthetics depress mitochondrial function[9] such that total body oxygen consumption is reduced. Actually, this has a certain advantage, since if there is reduction in flow due to altered peripheral circulation and cardiac effects, its use in the anesthetized state will require less oxygen, the delivery of which may be somewhat impaired. Splanchnic blood flow is diminished by most of the anesthetics,[11] such that total hepatic flow is decreased. In addition, the anesthetics seem to have an "anti-insulin effect," which decreases the ability of the liver to take up glucose and incorporate it into glucose-6-phosphate. For example, if an exogenous glucose load is administered during the course of general anesthesia, a diabetic type of prolonged tolerance curve will result because of this effect. The hepatic microsomal enzymes responsible for the biotransformation of various drugs are diminished in activity during clinical anesthesia.[4] Combined with the drop in hepatic blood flow limiting access of drugs to the liver, there will be prolonged half-lives of drugs seen during clinical anesthesia. Recent evidence indicates that during the high dose levels of clinical anesthesia there is impairment of certain synthetic pathways, such as the urea cycle, and of bilirubin conjunction. These effects quickly dissipate as the anesthetic is terminated.

Until 1965 it was thought that the general inhalation anesthetics are inert and are not extensively biotransformed in the body. This concept has proved to be fallacious.[64] The anesthetics are metabolized to various degrees, depending on the molecular structure and partition coefficients. Low partition coefficients limit the time that the anesthetic is in contact with the enzymes of biotransformation. Thus, an anesthetic of rather low partition coefficient would not be expected to undergo as much biotransformation as one that persists in the body for a long period of time. The extremes are seen in the case of isoflurane, which is only 1% to 2% metabolized in the body, as compared to methoxyflurane. Methoxyflurane has a rather high degree of metabolism; over 50% of the drug absorbed by the body is biotransformed.[36] The biotransformation of certain anesthetics may be responsible for cases of viscerotoxicity reported following anesthesia. For example, methoxyflurane is converted to free fluoride ion. High fluoride concentrations greater than 80 μm/L may give rise to renal damage and the so-called high output renal failure syndrome.[48] Biotransformation of chloroform, the older anesthetic no longer clinically employed, has definitely been implicated in hepatic toxicity.[6] The mechanism of this effect is that biotransformation produces free radicals or reactive intermediates, which combine with liver macromolecules to form covalent bonds. The altered proteins and lipoproteins are no longer capable of function and may actually undergo necrosis. Halothane, ordinarily a very safe anesthetic, has been implicated in unpredictable hepatic toxicity.[8] This is a rare, sporadic event, which probably occurs no more often than 1:20,000 administrations. Although there is a possibility that this may represent an allergy, evidence is accumulating that the biotransformation of halothane to reactive intermediates may be the proximate vector of liver damage in these rare individuals.[42] The abnormal biotransformation is via a reductive pathway, which may be controlled by genetic and/or environmental (drug induction) factors.

Biotransformation and toxicity

Reduction in renal function is commonly seen during the course of anesthesia.[12] This occurs primarily by a reduction in renal blood flow and leads to decreases in glomerular infiltration rate. Nausea and vomiting may follow the administration of general anesthetics. Although this effect may have a CNS etiology, it must be kept in mind that surgical pain and stimulation probably play a role in this side effect. Certain of the older anesthetics, such as cyclopropane and diethyl ether, seem to cause postoperative nausea and vomiting to a greater degree than some of the newer anesthetics such as halothane. Because of hypothalamic depression, generally patients' temperatures decrease slightly during anesthesia. Certain anesthetics, such as halothane, seem to trigger a catastrophic disease known as malignant hyperpyrexia in genetically susceptible individuals. This sudden and highly lethal event causes rises in temperatures to 42° C or higher with severe tissue acidosis.

Miscellaneous effects

The inhalation anesthetics are divided into two broad categories: gaseous anesthetics and volatile liquid anesthetics (Table 32-3). The gaseous anesthetics are defined as those with boiling points below room temperature and critical pressures

CLINICAL PHARMACOLOGY OF INDIVIDUAL ANESTHETICS

TABLE 32-3. Clinical characteristics of general anesthetics

Anesthetic	Analgesia	Hypnosis	Skeletal muscle relaxation	Depression of reflexes	Flammability	Compatibility with epi-nephrine
Nitrous oxide	+	+	0	+	No	Yes
Cyclopropane	++	++++	+	++	Yes	No
Diethyl ether	++++	++++	++++	++++	Yes	Yes
Methoxyflurane	++++	++++	++++	++++	No	Yes
Halothane	++	++++	++	++++	No	No
Enflurane	+++	++++	+++	++++	No	Yes
Isoflurane	+++	++++	+++	++++	No	Yes

greater than 760 torr. They are usually marketed as compressed gases, are in the liquid or gaseous state, and are under high pressures in steel cylinders. The cylinders are colored differently for each gas, such as blue for nitrous oxide and orange for cyclopropane. The volatile liquid anesthetics are liquids at room temperature, are usually more potent than the gases, and are ethers or halogenated hydrocarbons. Gaseous anesthetics generally possess blood-air and oil-gas partition coefficients lower than the volatile anesthetics, are consequently faster for induction and recovery, and are less potent. Selection of a particular anesthetic for a particular surgical patient is predicated on the pathophysiology and the type of surgical procedure involved. Selection of the appropriate anesthetic(s) is one of the critical factors involved in the presurgical rounds of the anesthesiologist.

Gaseous anesthetics
Nitrous oxide

Nitrous oxide (N_2O) is a colorless, odorless, tasteless gas, which is not metabolized. It is carried in the body in physical solution only. Nitrous oxide is an impotent anesthetic. It must be supplemented and used in the so-called balanced anesthetic technique, which consists of additional hypnosis (usually by barbiturates or tranquilizers), analgesia, (accomplished by intravenous narcotics), and supplementary muscle relaxants produced by the curariform drugs. Nitrous oxide is not flammable and is compatible with all other drugs, including catecholamines. Analgesia occurs with inspired concentrations of greater than 20% and hypnosis at concentrations of about 40% at sea level. However, because of its lack of potency, it is impossible to achieve complete surgical anesthesia with nitrous oxide without depriving the patient of oxygen. If it were not for its lack of potency, nitrous oxide would be the ideal anesthetic. Nitrous oxide has no significant effects on the respiratory, hepatic, renal, or autonomic nervous systems, except for a very slight myocardial depressant action and sympathomimetic effect.

In addition to use in the so-called balanced technique, nitrous oxide is commonly administered simultaneously with the more powerful anesthetics such as halothane and diethyl ether. This is done to speed the equilibrium attainment of the more powerful agent and to add the analgesic potency of nitrous oxide to that of the more powerful agents without harmful systemic effects. For example, halothane is quite depressive to myocardial contractility. The MAC for halothane with oxygen only is 0.8%. If the halothane is administered in 70% nitrous oxide with 30% oxygen atmosphere, the MAC of halothane is reduced to 0.35%.

Cyclopropane

Cyclopropane (C_3H_6) represents a potent gas, which can produce complete anesthesia without supplementation by intravenous anesthetics. The usual anesthetic dose at equilibrium is 10% to 20% inspired. Cyclopropane is no longer a popular anesthetic because of its flammability and explodability. It does stimulate the sympathoadrenal system and blood pressure is well maintained with this drug. However, this blood pressure maintenance is performed at the expense of critical alterations in peripheral flow. Cyclopropane is the classical drug, which is incompatible with catecholamines.

Volatile liquid anesthetics
Diethyl ether

Diethyl ether ($[C_2H_5]_2O$) is a pungent, volatile liquid, which is irritating to respiratory mucosa and may reflexively stimulate ventilation. Diethyl ether was the first general anesthetic to be employed clinically. It is rarely used now, primarily because of its flammability when mixed with air or oxygen. The hallmark of diethyl ether is that it is more benign to the cardiovascular system than any other complete anesthetic. Although it does cause a certain degree of negative inotropic effect, this is countered in humans by the reflex release of catecholamines. The net effect is only a slight fall in cardiac output. Ether does not lower the threshold of the ventricular myocardium to catecholamines. Diethyl ether produces good skeletal muscle and uterine relaxation. Due to its high partition coefficients and the fact that there are good clinical signs of depth of ether anesthesia, following the planes of anesthesia with this drug is easier than with many of anesthetics of lower solubility. For this reason, ether has often been termed the safest anesthetic.

The major disadvantages of diethyl ether, in addition to its flammability, are the high incidence of nausea and vomiting during recovery and its slow induction and emergence.

Halothane

Halothane (C_2F_3HBrCl) is one of the two most popular general inhalation anesthetics at the present time. It was developed in the 1950s as a nonflammable, potent anesthetic. Halogen substitution decreases flammability. It is a volatile, pleasant smelling liquid, which is well tolerated by patients.

Halothane produces marked depression of alveolar minute ventilation with the classical decrease in tidal volume but increase in inspiratory rate. Therefore, assisted or controlled ventilation is commonly employed when halothane is administered. It is nonirritating to the respiratory tract and does not cause increased pulmonary secretions.

Halothane is an example of an anesthetic with depressant effects on the heart with no increase in sympathetic nervous activity to secondarily augment contractility. Cardiac output, contractile force, and blood pressure all fall during the administration of halothane. Part of the blood pressure fall is due to a decrease in the sympathetic nervous system activity with a decline in peripheral resistance. Some degree of brady-cardia is frequently seen during anesthesia with halothane. Halothane does lower the threshold of ventricular muscle to catecholamine-induced arrhythmias. How-ever, this effect is not as great as with cyclopropane, but still warrants extreme cau-tion when epinephrine or other sympathomimetic amines are to be administered to a patient during the course of halothane anesthesia. Uterine relaxation is good with halothane anesthesia.

Because of its low solubility characteristics, it is considered a rapid anesthetic. It is commonly given together with nitrous oxide, although it may be given alone in oxygen. At the present time, it is regarded as the premier drug for pediatric anesthe-sia due to its ease of induction and rapid awakening characteristics. Although there is the spectre of hepatic damage, which is occasionally reported following its use, this viscerotoxic effect does not seem to occur in infants and children.

Methoxyflurane

Methoxyflurane ($CCl_2HCF_2OCH_3$) is a potent, nonflammable anesthetic, which was one of the first of a series of halogenated ethers. Its hallmark is that it produces excellent skeletal muscle relaxation. A difficulty with it, however, is the rather high solubility characteristics, which make for slow induction and awakening. Unlike halothane, methoxyflurane does not sensitize the myocardium to catecholamines to a very high degree. Again, this may be a function of the ether link of the anesthetic. It is a rather pleasant smelling liquid of low volatility, which is only slightly irritating to the respiratory tracts. Although it does depress ventilation, depression of cardiac contractility is probably less than that of halothane at equally effective dosages.

The great drawback to methoxyflurane, which has decreased its clinical use over the last few years, is its biotransformation to free fluoride ions that contribute to high output renal failure. It has fairly extensive biotransformation due to its molecular configuration and its highly lipophilic nature. To reduce the amount of free fluoride form from biotransformation, it has been suggested that methoxyflurane anesthesia be limited in humans to 2 MAC hours.

Enflurane

Enflurane (CF_2HOCF_2CFClH) is possibly the most popular potent anesthetic in clinical use at this time. It is a halogenated ether, which combines many of the vir-tues of both halothane and methoxyflurane without some of their disadvantages. It is a potent, volatile liquid, which is usually administered with nitrous oxide or solely in oxygen. It produces depression of myocardial contractility to a degree about equal to halothane. However, because of its ether link, it does not sensitize the myocar-dium to endogenous and exogenous catecholamines to the degree that halothane does. This link also gives enflurane its excellent skeletal muscle relaxant properties.

Because of lower solubility parameters, the anesthetic is not extensively bio-transformed in the body. Perhaps 1% to 2%, and no more than 2% to 3%, of an ab-sorbed dose is metabolized. Even though a metabolic product is free fluoride ion, this halogen does not achieve blood levels sufficient to produce renal disease. Its de-gree of sporadic hepatic damage seems to be far less than that of halothane. Clinically, the drug may be a little more difficult to use than halothane, but it seems to be replacing that anesthetic in adult anesthesia.

A major problem associated with enflurane is that the combination of high concentrations of the anesthetic and hypocapnia foster grand mal seizures. Under such circumstances, the EEG reveals classical spike and dome traces. This effect does not seem to be a deleterious one and can be avoided by maintaining normocapnia and employing just those concentrations necessary at the time for the surgery.

Isoflurane ($CF_3CHClOCHF_2$) is an isomer of enflurane. It is the newest in the long line of halogenated ether compounds, so clinical experience with it is not as extensive as with halothane and enflurane. The drug is even more resistant to biotransformation than is enflurane; less than 1% of the total absorbed is metabolized. Therefore, it may have the virtue of less viscerotoxicity than any other commonly employed anesthetic. Many of its features are quite similar to that of enflurane. However, there is evidence to support the fact that its respiratory depressant effect may be slightly greater than that of enflurane but its cardiovascular depressant effect less than that of enflurane. It also does not tend to foster convulsive activity. The drug is nonflammable and is compatible, to a certain degree, with catecholamines similar to enflurane. Skeletal muscle and uterine relaxation properties appear to be good.

Isoflurane

REFERENCES

1 Bangham, A. D., Standish, M. M., and Miller, N.: Cation permeability of phospholipid model membranes: effects of narcotics, Nature **208:** 1295, 1965.

2 Black, G. W., Linde, H. W., Dripps, R. D., and Price, H. L.: Circulatory changes in accompanying respiratory acidosis during halothane (Fluothane) anesthesia in man, Br. J. Anesth. **31:**238, 1959.

3 Bridges, B. E., Jr., and Eger, E. I., II: The effect of hypocapnia on the level of halothane anesthesia in man, Anesthesiology **28:**856, 1967.

4 Brown, B. R., Jr.: The diphasic action of halothane on the oxidative metabolism of drugs by the liver: an in vitro study in the rat, Anesthesiology **35:**241, 1971.

5 Brown, B. R., Jr., and Crout, J. R., Jr.: A comparative study of the effects of five general anesthetics on myocardial contractibility. I. Isometric conditions, Anesthesiology **34:**236, 1971.

6 Brown, B. R., Jr., Sipes, I. G., and Sagalyn, A. M.: Mechanisms of acute hepatic toxicity: chloroform, halothane, and glutathione, Anesthesiology **41:**554, 1974.

7 Brown, B. R., Jr., and Vandam, L. D.: A review of current advances in metabolism of inhalation anesthetics, Ann. N.Y. Acad. Sci. **179:** 235, 1971.

8 Bunker, J. P., Forrest, W. H., Jr., Mosteller, F., and Vandam, L. D.: The National Halothane Study, Bethesda, Md., National Institute of Health, National Institute of General Medical Sciences, 1969.

9 Cohen, P. J., and Marshall, B. E.: Effects of halothane on respiratory control and oxygen consumption of rat liver mitochondria. In Fink, B. R., editor: Toxicity of anesthetics, Baltimore, 1968, The Williams & Wilkins Co.

10 Collan, R., and Iivanainen, M.: Cardiac arrest caused by rapid elimination of nitrous oxide from cerebral ventricles after encephalography, Can. Anaesth. Soc. J. **16:**519, 1969.

11 Cooperman, L. H.: Effects of anesthetics on the splanchnic circulation, Br. J. Anaesth. **44:**967, 1972.

12 Craig, F. N., Visscher, F. E., and Houck, C. R.: Renal function in dogs under ether or cyclopropane anesthesia, Am. J. Physiol. **143:**108, 1945.

13 Cullen, D. J., and Eger, E. I., II: The effects of

hypoxic and isovolemic anemia of the halothane requirement (MAC) of dogs. I. The effect of hypoxia, Anesthesiology **32:**28, 1970.

14 Cullen, D. J., and Eger, E. I., II: The effects of hypoxia and isovolemic anemia on the halothane requirement (MAC) of dogs. III. The effects of acute isovolemic anemia, Anesthesiology **32:**46, 1970.

15 Darbinjar, T. M., Golovchinsky, V. B., and Plehotkina, S. I.: Effects of anesthetics on reticular and cerebral activity, Anesthesiology **34:**219, 1971.

16 Davis, H. S., Collins, W. F., and Ranat, C. F.: Effects of anesthetic agents on evoked central nervous system responses: gaseous agents, Anesthesiology **18:**624, 1957.

17 DeJong, R. H., Robles, R., Corbin, R. W., and Nace, R. A.: Effect of inhalational anesthetics on monosynaptic and polysynaptic transmission in the spinal cord, J. Pharmacol. Exp. Ther. **162:**326, 1968.

18 Downes, J. J., Kemp, R. A., and Lambertson, C. J.: The magnitude and duration of respiratory depression due to fentanyl and meperidine in man, J. Pharmacol. Exp. Ther. **158:**416, 1967.

19 Eger, E. I., II: Applications of a mathematical model of gas uptake. In Papper, E. M., and Kitz, R. J., editors: Uptake and distribution of anesthetic agents, New York, 1963, McGraw-Hill Book Co.

20 Eger, E. I., II: Effect of inspired anesthetic concentration on the rate of rise of alveolar concentration, Anesthesiology **24:**153, 1963.

21 Eger, E. I., II: A mathematical model of uptake and distribution. In Papper, E. M., and Kitz, R. S., editors: Uptake and distribution of anesthetic agents, New York, 1963, McGraw-Hill Book Co.

22 Eger, E. I., II: Uptake of inhaled anesthetics: the alveolar to inspired anesthetic difference. In Eger, E. I., II, editor: Anesthetic uptake and distribution, Baltimore, 1974, The Williams & Wilkins Co.

23 Eger, E. I., II, and Bahlman, S. H.: Is the end-tidal anesthetic partial pressure an accurate measure of the arterial anesthetic partial pressure? Anesthesiology **35:**301, 1971.

24 Eger, E. I., II, Brandstatter, B., Saidman, L. J., Regan, M. J., Severinghaus, J. W., and Munson, E. S.: Equipotent alveolar concentrations of methoxyflurane, halothane, diethyl ether, fluroxene, xenon and nitrous oxide in the dog, Anesthesiology **26:**771, 1965.

25 Eger, E. I., II, and Larson, C. P., Jr.: Anaesthetic solubility in blood and tissues: values and significance, Br. J. Anaesth. **36:**140, 1964.

26 Eger, E. I., II, and Saidman, L. J.: Hazards of nitrous oxide anesthesia in bowel obstruction and pneumothorax, Anesthesiology **26:**61, 1965.

27 Eger, E. I., II, Saidman, L. J., and Brandstatter, B.: Minimum alveolar anesthetic concentration: a standard of anesthetic potency, Anesthesiology **26:**756, 1965.

28 Eger, E. I., II, Saidman, L. J., and Brandstatter, B.: Temperature dependence of halothane and cyclopropane anesthesia in dogs: correlation with some theories of anesthetic action, Anesthesiology **26:**764, 1965.

29 Epstein, R. M., Racknow, H., Salanitre, E., and Wolf, G. L.: Influence of the concentration effect on the uptake of anesthetic mixtures: the second gas effect, Anesthesiology **25:**364, 1964.

30 Foldes, F. F., Kepes, E. R., and Ship, A. G.: Severe gastrointestinal distension during nitrous oxide and oxygen anesthesia, J.A.M.A. **194:**1146, 1965.

31 Fourcade, H. E., Stevens, W. C., Larson, C. P., Jr., Cromwell, T. H., Bahlman, S. H., Hickey, R. F., Halsey, M. J., and Eger, E. I., II: The ventilatory effects of Forane, a new inhaled anesthetic, Anesthesiology **35:**26, 1971.

32 French, J. D., Verzeano, M., and Magoun, H. W.: A neural basis of the anesthetic state, Arch. Neurol. Psychiatr. **69:**519, 953.

33 Guedel, A.: Third stage ether anesthesia: subclassification regarding significance of position and movements of eyeball, Am. J. Surg. **34:**53, 1920.

34 Halsey, M. J.: Mechanisms of general anesthesia. In Eger, E. I., II, editor: Anesthetic uptake and distribution, Baltimore, 1974, The Williams & Wilkins Co.

35 Halsey, M. J., Smith, E. B., and Wood, T. E.: Effects of general anaesthetics on Na^+ transport in human red cells, Nature **225:**1151, 1970.

36 Holaday, D. A., Rudolsky, S., and Treuhaft, P. S.: The metabolic degradation of methoxyflurane in man, Anesthesiology **33:**579, 1970.

37 Karis, J. H., Gissen, A. J., and Nastuk, W. L.: Mode of actions of diethyl ether in blocking neuromuscular transmission, Anesthesiology **27:**42, 1966.

38 Katz, R. L., and Epstein, R. A.: The interaction of anesthetic agents and adrenergic drugs to produce cardiac arrhythmias, Anesthesiology **29:**763, 1968.

39 Kety, S. S.: Theory and applications of exchange of inert gases at lungs and tissues, Pharmacol. Rev. **3:**1, 1951.

40 Larson, C. P., Jr.: Solubility and partition coefficients. In Papper, E. M., and Kitz, R. J., edi-

tors: Uptake and distribution of anesthetics, New York, 1963, McGraw-Hill Book Co.

41 Larson, C. P., Jr., Eger, E. I., II, Muallem, M., Buechel, D. R., Munson, E. S., and Eisele, J. H.: The effects of diethyl ether and methoxyflurane on ventilation, Anesthesiology **30:**174, 1965.

42 McLain, G. E., Sipes, I. G., and Brown, B. R., Jr.: An animal model of halothane hepatotoxicity. Role of enzyme induction and hypoxia, Anesthesiology **51:**321, 1979.

43 Meyer, H. H.: Zur theorie der alkoholnarkose. III. Mit der einfluss wechselnder temperatur auf wirkungstärke und teilungskoefficient der narkotica. Arch. Exp. Pathol. Pharmakol. **46:** 338, 1901.

44 Miller, S. L.: A theory of gaseous anesthetics, Proc. Natl. Acad. Sci. U.S.A. **47:**1515, 1961.

45 Muallen, M., Larson, C. P., Jr., and Eger, E. I., II: The effects of diethyl ether on Pa_{CO_2} in dogs with and without vagal, somatic and sympathetic block, Anesthesiology **30:**185, 1969.

46 Munson, E. S., Eger, E. I., II, and Bowers, D. L.: Effects of anesthetic-depressed ventilation and cardiac output on anesthetic uptake, Anesthesiology **38:**251, 1963.

47 Munson, E. S., Eger, E. I., II, and Bowers, D. L.: The effects of changes in cardiac output and distribution in the rate of cerebral anesthetic equilibrium: calculations using a mathematical model, Anesthesiology **29:**523, 1968.

48 Nazze, R. I., Trudell, J. R., and Cousins, M. J.: Methoxyflurane metabolism and renal dysfunction: clinical correlation in man, Anesthesiology **35:**247, 1971.

49 Niejadik, K., and Galindo, A.: Electrocorticographic seizure activity during enflurane anesthesia, Anesth. Analg. **54:**722, 1975.

50 Overton, E.: Studien uber die narkose zugleich ein beitrag zur algemeinen pharmakologie, Jena, 1901, G. Fischer.

51 Pauling, L.: Molecular theory of general anesthesia, Science **134:**15, 1961.

52 Price, H. L.: Circulatory actions of general anesthetic agents and the homeostatic roles of epinephrine and norepinephrine in man, Clin. Pharmacol. **2:**163, 1961.

53 Price, H. L., Kovnat, P. J., Safer, J. N., Conner, E. H., and Price, M. L.: The uptake of thiopental by body tissues and its relation to the duration of narcosis, Clin. Pharmacol. Ther. **1:** 16, 1960.

54 Price, H. L., Lurie, A. A., Jones, R. E., Price, M. L., and Linde, H. W.: Cyclopropane anes-

thesia. II. Epinephrine and norepinephrine in initiation of ventricular arrhythmias by carbon dioxide inhalation, Anesthesiology **19:**619, 1958.

55 Price, H. L., Warden, J. C., Cooperman, L. H., and Millar, R. A.: Central sympathetic excitation caused by cyclopropane, Anesthesiology **30:**426, 1969.

56 Quastel, J. M.: Effects of drugs on metabolism of the brain *in vitro*, Br. Med. Bull. **21:**49, 1965.

57 Saidman, L. J., and Eger, E. I., II: Effect of nitrous oxide and of narcotic premedication in the alveolar concentration of halothane required for anesthesia, Anesthesiology **25:**302, 1964.

58 Saidman, L. J., and Eger, E. I., II: Uptake and distribution of thiopental after oral, rectal, or intramuscular administration, Clin. Pharmacol. Ther. **14:**12, 1973.

59 Saidman, L. J., Eger, E. I., II, Munson, E. S., Babad, A. A., and Muallem, M.: Minimum alveolar concentration of methoxyflurane, halothane, ether, and cyclopropane in man: correlation with theories of anesthesia, Anesthesiology **28:**994, 1967.

60 Severinghaus, J. W.: Role of lung factors. In Papper, E., and Kitz, R. J., editors: Uptake and distribution of anesthetic agents, New York, 1963, McGraw-Hill Book Co.

61 Shimasato, S., and Etsten, B. E.: Effects of anesthetic drugs on the heart: a critical review of myocardial contractility and its relation to hemodynamics, Clin. Anesth. **2:**17, 1969.

62 Stoelting, R. K., and Eger, E. I., II: An additional explanation for the second gas effect, Anesthesiology **30:**273, 1969.

63 Stoelting, R. K., and Eger, E. I., II: Percutaneous loss of nitrous oxide, cyclopropane, ether and halothane in man, Anesthesiology **30:**278, 1969.

64 Van Dyke, R. A., Chenoweth, M. B., and Van Poznak, A.: Metabolism of volatile anesthetics. I. Conversion in vivo of several anesthetics to $^{14}CO_2$ and chloride, Biochem. Pharmacol. **13:** 1239, 1964.

65 Waun, J. E., Sweitzer, R. S., and Hamilton, W. K.: Effect of nitrous oxide in middle ear mechanics and hearing acuity, Anesthesiology **28:** 846, 1967.

66 Yamamura, H., Wakasugi, B., Okuma, Y., and Maki, K.: The effects of ventilation in the absorption and elimination of inhalation anesthetics, Anaesthesia **18:**427, 1963.

CHAPTER 33

Pharmacology of local anesthesia

GENERAL CONCEPT Local anesthetics are drugs employed to produce a transient and reversible loss of sensation in a circumscribed area of the body. They achieve this effect by interfering with nerve conduction.

In 1884 Köller, who had studied *cocaine* with Sigmund Freud, introduced the drug into medicine as a topical anesthetic in ophthalmology. This was the beginning of the first era in the history of local anesthesia.

The second era began in 1904 with the introduction of *procaine* by Einhorn. This was the first safe local anesthesia suitable for injection. Procaine remained the most widely used local anesthetic until the introduction of *lidocaine* (Xylocaine), which is considered the agent of choice for infiltration at present. Other local anesthetics of importance are *tetracaine, mepivacaine, prilocaine,* and *bupivacaine.* All of these drugs are either esters or amides, and they differ from each other in their toxicity, metabolism, onset, and duration of action. Lidocaine, in addition to being an important local anesthetic, has important uses as an antiarrhythmic agent (p. 463).

Electrophysiological studies indicate that the local anesthetics interfere with the rate of rise of the depolarization phase of the action potential. As a consequence the cell does not depolarize sufficiently after excitation to fire. Thus the propagated action potential is blocked by these drugs.

CLASSIFICATION Local anesthetics may be classified according to their chemistry or on the basis of their clinical usage.

According to chemistry Local anesthetics are either esters or amides. They consist of an aromatic portion, an intermediate chain, and an amine portion. The aromatic portion confers lipophilic properties to the molecule, whereas the amine portion is hydrophilic. The ester or amide components of the molecule determine the characteristics of metabolic degradation. The esters are mostly hydrolyzed in plasma by pseudocholinesterase, whereas the amides are destroyed largely in the liver.

Esters of benzoic acid	*Esters of p-aminobenzoic acid*
Cocaine	Procaine (Novocain)
Tetracaine (Pontocaine)	Butethamine (Monocaine)
Piperocaine (Metycaine)	Chloroprocaine (Nesacaine)
Hexylcaine (Cyclaine)	Proparacaine (Ophthaine)
Ethyl aminobenzoate (Benzocaine)	
Butacaine (Butyn)	

Esters of meta-aminobenzoic acid
Cyclomethycaine (Surfacaine)
Metabutoxycaine (Primacaine)

Amides
Lidocaine (Xylocaine)
Dibucaine (Nupercaine)
Mepivacaine (Carbocaine)
Prilocaine (Citanest)
Bupivacaine (Marcaine)

Local anesthetics have several types of clinical applications, and their suitability for these varies with their pharmacological properties. Some of these applications are (1) infiltration and block anesthesia, (2) surface anesthesia, (3) spinal anesthesia, (4) epidural and caudal anesthesia, and (5) intravenous anesthesia. In the following list the drugs of greatest interest are italicized.

According to clinical usage

Infiltration and block anesthesia: *procaine, chloroprocaine, hexylcaine, lidocaine,* mepivacaine, *bupivacaine,* piperocaine, prilocaine, propoxycaine, and tetracaine; also, in dentistry: butethamine, metabutethamine, isobucaine, meprylcaine, and pyrrocaine

Surface anesthesia: *benzocaine, benoxinate, butacaine, butyl aminobenzoate, cocaine,* cyclomethycaine, dibucaine, dimethisoquin, diperodon, dyclonine, hexylcaine, lidocaine, phenacaine, piperocaine, pramoxine, proparacaine, and tetracaine; also, benzyl alcohol, phenol, and ethyl chloride

Spinal anesthesia (subarachnoid or intrathecal): *tetracaine,* procaine, dibucaine, lidocaine, mepivacaine, and piperocaine

Epidural and caudal anesthesia: *lidocaine, prilocaine,* and *mepivacaine;* also, procaine, chloroprocaine, piperocaine, and tetracaine

Intravenous anesthesia: *lidocaine* and *procaine* (seldom used for anesthesia but for other indications)

Electrophysiological studies indicate that the local anesthetics do not alter the resting membrane potential or threshold potential of nerves. They act on the rate of rise of the depolarization phase of the action potential. Since depolarization does not reach the point at which firing occurs, propagated action potential fails to occur.

MODE OF ACTION

The effects of local anesthetics on ionic fluxes are of great interest, and recent studies emphasize the relationships between these drugs and the calcium ion with secondary effects on sodium fluxes. Although no detailed discussion will be attempted,[29] local anesthetic agents appear to compete with calcium for a site in the nerve membrane that controls the passage of sodium across the membrane. It is believed at present that calcium is bound to phospholipids in the cell membrane. A fair correlation could be found between local anesthetic potency and their ability to prevent the binding of calcium by phosphatidylserine in artificial membranes.

Experimental studies[1] indicate also that an increase in calcium concentration is able to overcome the nerve block produced by local anesthetics.

Problem 33-1. When the hydrochloride of a local anesthetic is injected, which is the active form, the uncharged base or the charged cation? When dealing with an intact isolated nerve, the local anesthetics such as lidocaine are more potent in an alkaline solution, suggesting the uncharged base as the active form.[22] On the other hand, when a desheathed nerve is used, the less alkaline preparations are more efficacious. It is believed at present that the uncharged base

Active form

penetrates better across the nerve sheath, but it is the charged cation that exerts its pharmacological effect.[22] The problem is complicated by the fact that the results are not applicable to all members of the series of local anesthetics.[29]

Action on various nerve fibers

According to diameter, myelination, and conduction velocities, nerve fibers can be classified into three types—A, B, and C fibers.[10] The A fibers have a diameter of 1 to 20 μm, are myelinated, and have conduction velocities up to 100 m/sec. Somatic motor and some sensory fibers fall into this classification. Blockade of these fibers results in skeletal muscle relaxation, loss of thermal and tactile sensation, proprioceptive loss, and loss of the sensation of sharp pain. B fibers vary in diameter from 1 to 3 μm, are myelinated, and conduct at intermediate velocities. Preganglionic fibers fall into this group, and their blockade obviously results in autonomic paralysis. C fibers are usually under 1 μm in diameter and are not myelinated, and conduction velocity is approximately 1 m/sec. Postganglionic fibers as well as more somatic sensory fibers fall into this classification. Blockade results in autonomic paralysis; loss of the sensation of itch, tickle, and dull pain; and loss of much of the thermal sensation.

Clinically the general order of loss of function is as follows: (1) pain, (2) temperature, (3) touch, (4) proprioception, and (5) skeletal muscle tone. If pressure is exerted on a mixed nerve, the fibers are depressed in somewhat the reverse order.

In summary, local anesthetic drugs depress the small, unmyelinated fibers first and the larger, myelinated fibers last. The time for the onset of action is shorter for the smaller fibers, and the concentration of drug required is less.

ABSORPTION, FATE, AND EXCRETION

Absorption of the various local anesthetics depends on the site of injection, the degree of vasodilatation caused by the agent itself, the dose, and the presence of a vasoconstrictor in the solution. Epinephrine added to a procaine hydrochloride solution greatly increases its duration of action as an infiltration agent.

The onset and duration of action of various local anesthetics as determined by a standardized ulnar block technique are shown in Table 33-1.

Local anesthetics of the ester type are hydrolyzed by plasma pseudocholinesterase. Those having the amide linkage are largely destroyed in the liver.

In human beings, procaine is broken down to p-aminobenzoic acid,[6] 80% of which is excreted in the urine, and diethylaminoethanol, 30% of which is excreted in the urine. Only 2% is excreted unchanged in the urine. Only 10% to 20% of lidocaine appears unchanged, the rest being metabolized, presumably mainly in the liver.[12]

Procaine is hydrolyzed in spinal fluid 150 times more slowly than in plasma, there being very little esterase present. The hydrolysis results from the alkalinity of the spinal fluid and is approximately the same as with a buffer having the same pH.[8]

Lidocaine is metabolized in the liver by removal of one or both ethyl groups from the molecule. The resulting metabolites, monoethylglycinexylidide (MEGX) and glycinexilidine (GX), still have pharmacological activity and may contribute to CNS toxicity.[25]

TABLE 33-1. Onset and duration of action of various local anesthetics determined by a standardized ulnar block technique*

Drug	Concentration	Relative potency	Onset in minutes	Duration of action in minutes
Procaine	1	1	7	19
Lidocaine	1	4	5	40
Mepivacaine	1	4	4	99
Prilocaine	1	4	3	98
Tetracaine†	0.25	16	7	135
Bupivacaine†	0.25	16	8	415

*Modified from Covino, B. G.: N. Engl. J. Med. **286:**975, 1035, 1972; based on data from Albert, J., and Löfström, B.: Acta Anesth. Scand. **5:**99, 1961.
†Solutions contain epinephrine 1:200,000.

TABLE 33-2. Relative hydrolysis rates of local anesthetics by plasma esterase

Local anesthetic	Rate of hydrolysis
Piperocaine	6.5
Chloroprocaine	5.0
Procaine	1.0
Tetracaine	0.2
Dibucaine	0

METHODS OF ADMINISTRATION

Local anesthetics may be administered by topical application, by infiltration of tissues to bathe fine nerve elements, by injection adjacent to nerves and their branches, and by injection into the epidural or subarachnoid spaces. Occasionally intravenous injections are utilized to control certain pain situations. The details of subarachnoid and epidural anesthesia are outside the intended scope of this discussion.

SYSTEMIC ACTIONS

Local anesthetics exert their effect largely on a circumscribed area. Nevertheless, they are absorbed from the site of injection and may exert systemic effects, particularly on the cardiovascular system and the CNS and particularly when an excessive dose is utilized.

Cardiovascular effects

Since lidocaine is widely used as an antiarrhythmic drug, much has been learned about its effect on the heart, and this information is generally also applicable to the other local anesthetics. At nontoxic concentrations lidocaine alters or abolishes the rate of slow diastolic depolarization in Purkinje's fibers and may shorten the effective refractory period as well as the duration of the action potential. In toxic doses lidocaine decreases the maximal depolarization of Purkinje's fibers and reduces conduction velocity. Such doses may also have a direct negative inotropic effect.

The local anesthetics tend to relax the vascular smooth muscle, but cocaine can cause vasoconstriction by blocking the reuptake of norepinephrine.[29]

CNS effects   Although the usual local anesthesia produces no CNS effects, increased doses may cause excitatory effects resulting in convulsions and eventually respiratory depression. It is believed on the basis of animal experiments that the local anesthetics may block inhibitory cortical synapses.[29] This leads to excitation. Larger doses depress both inhibitory and facilitory neurons, leading to depression.

Miscellaneous effects   Compared with their actions on the cardiovascular system and the CNS, the local anesthetics have few additional effects. They may depress ganglionic transmission and neuromuscular transmission. These actions are unimportant unless some other potent agent is used concomitantly. For example, lidocaine may enhance the action of neuromuscular blocking agents.

Vasoconstrictors and local anesthetics   Vasoconstrictors, particularly epinephrine, are commonly added to local anesthetic solutions that are to be used for infiltration or nerve block. The purpose is to prevent absorption of the drug and thereby prolong its action locally and reduce systemic reactions. Concentrations of epinephrine used for this purpose in local anesthesia vary from 2 to 10 μg/ml, or 1:500,000 to 1:100,000.

Although the addition of epinephrine to such drugs as procaine is sound, other drugs such as lidocaine, prilocaine, mepivacaine, and bupivacaine may be used without the addition of vasoconstrictors.

Epinephrine may contribute to the systemic effects of local anesthetics and may be responsible for symptoms such as anxiety, tachycardia, and hypertension.

TOXICITY   The ester-type local anesthetics, such as procaine and tetracaine, may produce true allergic reactions manifested as skin rashes or bronchospasm. Allergic reactions to the amides, such as lidocaine, are very rare.

The majority of toxic reactions are a result of overdosage. The figures given in Table 33-3 refer to maximum safe dosages, determined in milligrams per kilogram of body weight, administered to healthy adults without inadvertent intravascular or subarachnoid injection.

In general the true pharmacological signs of toxicity from local anesthetics are CNS stimulation followed by depression and peripheral cardiovascular depression. Salivation and tremor, convulsion, and coma, associated with hypertension and tachycardia and followed by hypotension, all occurring in a few minutes, represent the full-blown picture.

TABLE 33-3. Maximum safe dosages of local anesthetics administered to healthy adults without inadvertent intravascular or subarachnoid injection

Anesthetic	mg/kg of body weight
4% cocaine	1 (topical)
1% procaine	10 (injection)
0.15% tetracaine	1 (injection)
1% lidocaine	5 (injection)

The treatment is symptomatic and essentially involves restoration of normal ventilation and circulation. Barbiturates in doses greater than hypnotic are effective in the *prevention* of CNS stimulation caused by local anesthetics. Diazepam (Valium) is being used increasingly for the same purpose.

Cocaine is too toxic to be injected into the tissues and is therefore used only topically. It produces excellent topical anesthesia and vasoconstriction, which results in shrinkage of mucous membranes. Absorption from the urinary mucous membranes is rapid, and cocaine should not be used in this area. Some clinicians believe that vasoconstriction with 10% cocaine is better than with a 4% solution and that toxicity will be less with the stronger preparation because the cocaine will be more slowly absorbed. This may be dangerous, however. The vasoconstrictor effect of cocaine and potentiation by this local anesthetic of the actions of catecholamines are most likely consequences of inhibition of the uptake of catecholamines by adrenergic nerve terminals. Cocaine abuse is discussed on p. 372. Acute cocaine poisoning is probably best treated with chlorpromazine.

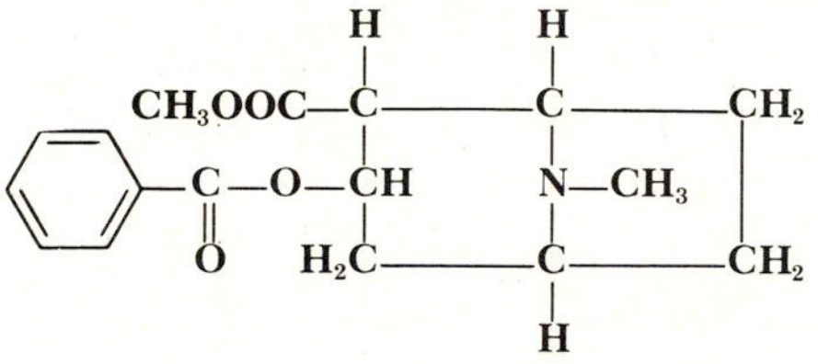

CLINICAL CHARACTERISTICS
Cocaine

Cocaine

Ethyl aminobenzoate (Benzocaine) is so poorly soluble that it is not absorbed from mucous membranes. Ointments containing 5% to 10% concentrations of ethyl aminobenzoate provide potent, safe topical anesthesia.

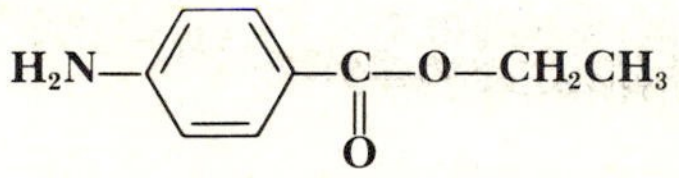

Ethyl aminobenzoate

Ethyl aminobenzoate

Procaine (Novocain) was the standard against which all local anesthetics were compared. However, it has the disadvantage of producing poor topical anesthesia. Its duration of action is approximately 1 hour but can be significantly prolonged by the addition of epinephrine. Onset of anesthesia occurs rapidly. Afterward the patient often notes only the soreness produced by the needle used for injection. Procaine will block small to large nerve fibers in concentrations of 0.5% to 2%.

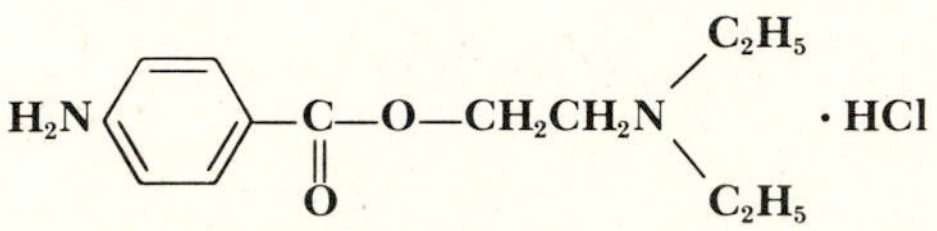

Procaine

Procaine hydrochloride

Chloroprocaine (Nesacaine) is a derivative of procaine that has a much shorter duration of action because of its more rapid hydrolysis.

Lidocaine Lidocaine (Xylocaine) has supplanted procaine as the standard of comparison for local anesthetics. It is more potent and more versatile, being suitable not only for infiltration and nerve block but for surface anesthesia as well. This results in a rapid, potent anesthetic effect. It is used in concentrations of 0.5% to 2% and is more potent than equivalent solutions of procaine. Lidocaine has one other characteristic that distinguishes it from procaine and other local anesthetics—it very often produces sedation along with the local anesthesia. Lidocaine differs from most drugs in this group in being an amide rather than an ester. Lidocaine is metabolized in the liver by N-dealkylation. Two of the metabolites still have pharmacological activity and may contribute to toxic reactions in patients with altered metabolism.[25]

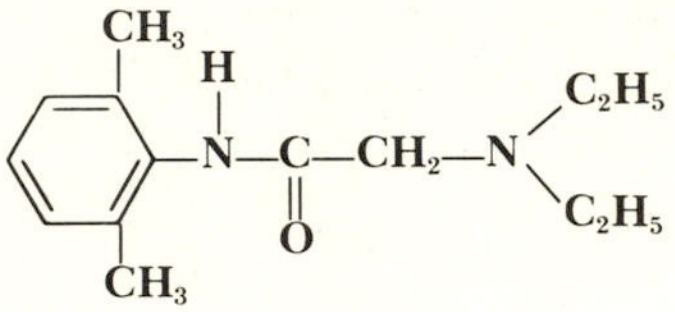

Lidocaine

Tetracaine The chief differences between tetracaine (Pontocaine) and procaine and lidocaine are tetracaine's longer time required for full onset of action (10 minutes or more), longer duration of action (approximately 50%), and greater potency. For injection anesthesia, tetracaine is available in 0.15% solution. For topical anesthesia it is used in 1% to 2% concentrations. Tetracaine should not be sprayed into the airway in concentrations greater than 2%. The total dose should be carefully calculated and probably should not, in this situation, exceed 0.5 mg/kg of body weight. It is rapidly absorbed topically and has resulted in several fatalities from topical misuse. The chief disadvantage of tetracaine is slowness in onset of action.

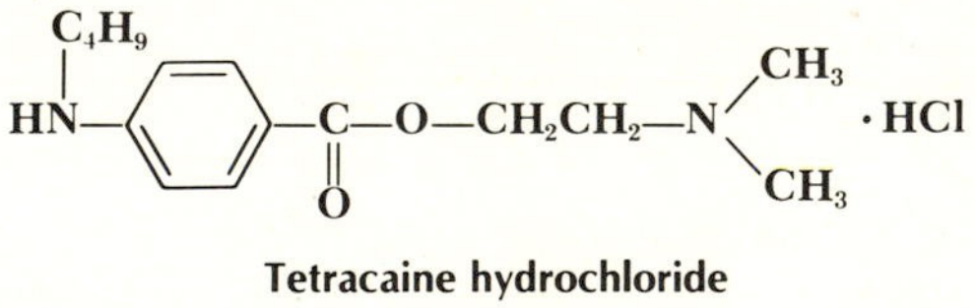

Tetracaine hydrochloride

Mepivacaine Mepivacaine (Carbocaine) has essentially the same clinical effects as lidocaine except for two particular points. It does not spread in the tissues quite as well, and its duration of action is longer.

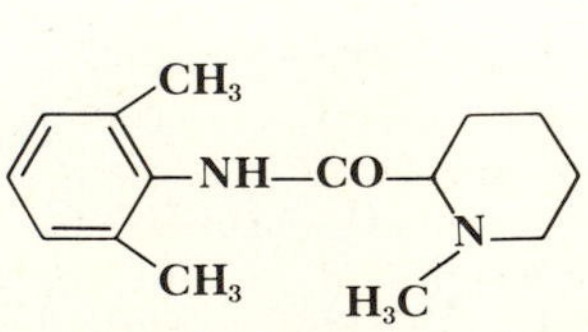

Mepivacaine

Bupivacaine (Marcaine) is an amide chemically related to mepivacaine. It has a long duration of action and its potency is four times greater than that of mepivacaine. Bupivacaine is used for infiltration, nerve block, and peridural anesthesia. Adverse effects of bupivacaine are similar to those produced by other local anesthetics. Bupivacaine is available in solutions containing 0.25%, 0.5%, and 0.75% of the drug. **Bupivacaine**

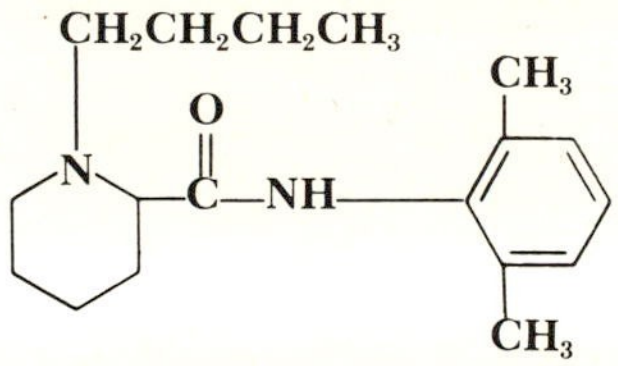

$CH_2CH_2CH_2CH_3$

CH_3

CH_3

Bupivacaine

Dibucaine (Nupercaine) is a very potent local anesthetic having a long duration of action. It is from 10 to 20 times as active and toxic as procaine. As a consequence, it is employed in a more dilute solution for injection than procaine (0.05% to 0.1%). It is suitable for topical use and also for spinal anesthesia. **Dibucaine**

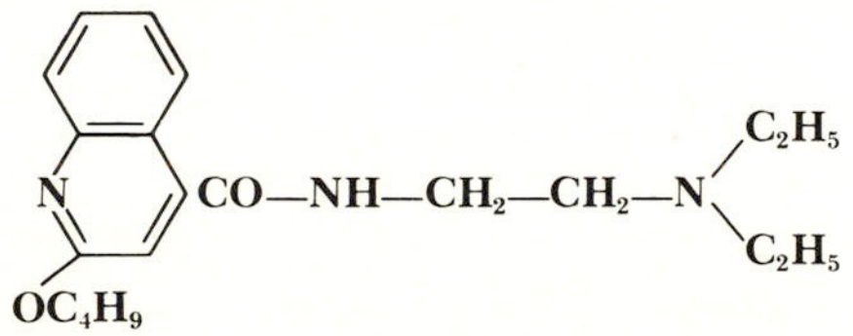

$CO-NH-CH_2-CH_2-N$

C_2H_5

C_2H_5

OC_4H_9

Dibucaine

The needs of most physicians can be met by a few of the available local anesthetics. For infiltration lidocaine and bupivacaine are preferred. For spinal anesthesia, tetracaine appears to be the best. It has a duration of action of 2 hours or more and is hydrolyzed by plasma cholinesterase. For epidural anesthesia lidocaine (short duration) or bupivacaine (long duration) are often employed. Cocaine still has some uses for topical anesthesia. **CHOICE OF LOCAL ANESTHETICS**

REFERENCES

1 Aceves, J., and Machne, X.: The action of calcium and of local anesthetics on nerve cells, and their interaction during excitation, J. Pharmacol. Exp. Ther. **140:**138, 1963.

2 Adriani, J.: Pharmacology of anesthetics, ed. 3, Springfield, Ill., 1952, Charles C Thomas, Publisher.

3 Adriani, J., and Zepernick, R.: Some recent studies on the clinical pharmacology of local anesthetics of practical significance, Ann. Surg. **158:**666, 1963.

4 Adriani, J., and Zepernick, R.: Clinical effectiveness of drugs used for topical anesthesia, J.A.M.A. **188:**711, 1964.

5 Albert, J., and Löfström, B.: Bilateral ulnar nerve blocks for the evaluation of local anesthetic agents: tests with procaine, Xylocaine and Carbocaine, Acta Anesth. Scand. **5:**99, 1961.

6 Brodie, B. B., Lief, P. A., and Poet, R.: The fate of procaine in man following its intravenous administration and methods for the estimation of procaine and diethylaminoethanol, J. Pharmacol. Exp. Ther. **94:**359, 1948.

7 Crampton, R. S., and Oriscello, R. G.: Petit and grand mal convulsions during lidocaine hydrochloride treatment of ventricular tachycardia, J.A.M.A. **204:**201, 1968.

8 Foldes, F. F., and Aven, M. A.: The hydrolysis

of procaine and 2-chloroprocaine in spinal fluid, J. Pharmacol. Exp. Ther. **105**:259, 1952.

9 Foldes, F. F., Davidson, G. M., Duncalf, D., and Shigeo, K.: The intravenous toxicity of local anesthetic agents in man, Clin. Pharmacol. Ther. **6**:328, 1965.

10 Galley, A. H.: Caudal analgesia—clinical applications in vasospastic diseases of the legs and in diabetic neuropathy, Proc. R. Soc. Med. **45:**748, 1952.

11 Geddes, I. C.: A review of local anesthetics, Br. J. Anaesth. **26**:208, 1954.

12 Gray, T. C., and Geddes, I. C.: A review of local anesthetics, J. Pharmacol. Physiol. **6**:89, 1954.

13 Hille, B.: Common mode of action of three agents that decrease the transient change in sodium permeability in nerves, Nature **210:**1220, 1966.

14 de Jong, R. H., and Wagman, I. H.: Physiological mechanisms of peripheral nerve block by local anesthetics, Anesthesiology **24**:6484, 1963.

15 Kalow, W.: Hydrolysis of local anesthetics by human serum cholinesterase, J. Pharmacol. Exp. Ther. **104**:122, 1952.

16 Luduena, F. P.: Duration of local anesthesia, Annu. Rev. Pharmacol. **9**:503, 1969.

17 Nordqvist, P.: The action of histamine on procaine block in frog nerves, Acta Pharmacol. **8**:183, 1952.

18 Nordqvist, P.: The action of hyaluronidase on frog sciatic nerve with special reference to penetration of procaine, Acta Pharmacol. **8**:195, 1952.

19 Nordqvist, P.: Influence of acetylcholine, decamethonium, and histamine on frog nerves, Acta Pharmacol. **8**:233, 1952.

20 Pizzolato, P., and Renegari, O. J.: Histopathologic effects of long exposure to local anesthetics on peripheral nerves, Anesth. Analg. **38**:138, 1959.

21 Ritchie, J. M., and Greengard, P.: On the active structure of local anesthetics, J. Pharmacol. Exp. Ther. **133**:241, 1961.

22 Ritchie, J. M., and Greengard, P.: On the mode of action of local anesthetics, Annu. Rev. Pharmacol. **6**:405, 1966.

23 Shanes, A. M.: Drugs and nerve conduction, Annu. Rev. Pharmacol. **3**:185, 1963.

24 Skou, J. C.: Local anesthetics: relation between blocking potency and penetration of a monomolecular layer of lipoids from nerves, Acta Pharmacol. **10**:325, 1954.

25 Strong, J. M., Parker, M., and Atkinson, A. J.: Identification of glycinexylidide in patients treated with intravenous lidocaine, Clin. Pharmacol. Ther. **146**:67, 1973.

26 Tapia, L., Cheigh, J. S., David, D. S., Sullivan, J. F., Saal, S., Reidenberg, M. M., Stenzel, K. H., and Rubin, A. L.: Pruritus in dialysis patients treated with parenteral lidocaine, N. Engl. J. Med. **296**:261, 1977.

27 Toman, J. E. P.: Neuropharmacology of peripheral nerve, Pharmacol. Rev. **4**:168, 1952.

REVIEWS

28 Alper, M. H.: Toxicity of local anesthetics, N. Engl. J. Med. **295**:1432, 1976.

29 Covino, B. G.: Local anesthesia, N. Engl. J. Med. **286**:975, 1035, 1972.

30 Dykes, M. H. M.: Evaluation of a local anesthetic agent: bupivacaine hydrochloride (Marcaine), J.A.M.A. **224**:1035, 1973.

SECTION SIX

Drugs used in cardiovascular disease

Although many drugs exert an effect on the heart, five groups of agents will be discussed in this section either because they act selectively on the heart or because they are particularly useful in the treatment of cardiac disease: digitalis glycosides, antiarrhythmic drugs, coronary vasodilator drugs, anticoagulant drugs, and diuretic drugs. In addition, the hypocholesterolemic agents will be briefly discussed. Antihypertensive drugs were considered in Chapter 18.

CHAPTER 34

Digitalis

William Withering, 1785   *It has the power over the motion of the heart to a degree yet unobserved in any other medicine, and this power may be converted to salutary ends.*

GENERAL CONCEPT

Certain steroids and their glycosides have characteristic effects on the contractility and electrophysiology of the heart. Most of these glycosides are obtained from the leaves of the foxglove, *Digitalis purpurea* or *Digitalis lanata*, or from the seeds of *Strophanthus gratus*. These cardioactive steroids are widely used in the treatment of heart failure and in the management of certain arrhythmias. They are collectively referred to as digitalis.

Although catecholamines, methylxanthines, and glucagon also increase the contractility of the myocardium, digitalis must accomplish its effect by a unique mechanism and is an important drug in the treatment of heart failure.

At the molecular level digitalis is a powerful inhibitor of sodium–potassium–adenosine triphosphatase (Na^+-K^+-ATPase). It is possible, although not proved, that the cardiac effects of the glycosides are a consequence of ATPase inhibition with changes in ion distribution.

Digitalis exerts striking effects on the *electrophysiology* of the heart. These effects are not the same in all portions of the organ. Most significant are more rapid repolarization of the ventricles (shortened electric systole) and, in higher concentrations, increased automaticity or increased rate of diastolic depolarization with appearance of ectopic activity. The atrioventricular (A-V) node is markedly affected by the glycosides. Digitalis slows conduction and prolongs the refractory period of this node.

Digitalis poisoning is surprisingly common in current practice.[3] The therapeutic index of the drug is small, and it is dangerous in certain circumstances. For example, either hypopotassemia or hypercalcemia greatly increases the possibility of fatal arrhythmias during digitalis administration.

HISTORY

The history of digitalis is a remarkable example of the discovery of an important drug in a folk remedy. William Withering,[56] having heard of a mixture of herbs that an old woman of Shropshire used successfully in the treatment of dropsy (congestive heart failure), suspected that its beneficial properties must have been caused by the foxglove. In testing it in patients with congestive failure, Withering was greatly impressed with the diuretic effect of the foxglove and believed that the drug probably acted on the kidney. On the other hand, he also stated that the drug had a remarkable "power over the heart."

Over the years digitalis has become the most important drug in the treatment of congestive failure, atrial flutter, and fibrillation. Its position is being challenged by the more intensive use of diuretics, by reduction of afterload and preload, and by newer inotropic agents. Nevertheless, digitalis remains one of the most important drugs in medicine.[64,69]

EFFECTS ON HEART   Digitalis increases the contractility of the heart muscle and influences its electrophysiological properties such as conductivity, refractory period, and automaticity. It is increasingly recognized that the effectiveness of digitalis in the treatment of congestive failure is a consequence of its positive inotropic effect. On the other hand, some of its electrophysiological influences make the drug highly useful in the treatment of a variety of arrhythmias.

Contractility is influenced by digitalis in both the normal and the failing heart. As shown in Fig. 34-1, it has been demonstrated in humans by attaching a Walton-

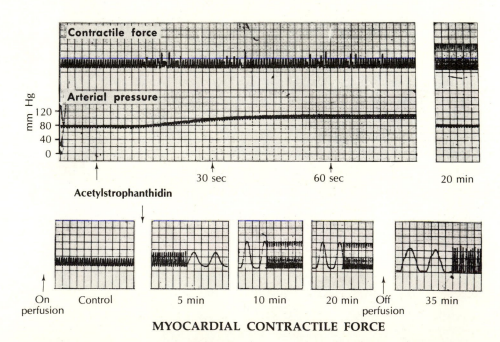

FIG. 34-1. Contractile force and arterial pressure recordings immediately and 20 minutes after injection of 1.4 mg acetylstrophanthidin in a 28-year-old woman with an atrial septal defect. The lower tracings show contractile force recordings before injection and at intervals after acetylstrophanthidin. Note that the drug augments the contractile force of the nonfailing human heart and constricts the systemic vascular bed. (From Braunwald, E., Bloodwell, R. D., Goldberg, L. I., and Morrow, A. G.: J. Clin. Invest. **40:**52, 1961.)

Brodie strain gauge arch to the right ventricular myocardium of patients undergoing cardiac surgery. It has also been shown in the isolated heart (Fig. 34-2).

Digitalis increases both the force and the velocity of myocardial contraction, and it shortens the duration of systole. It promotes more complete emptying of the ventricles and decreases the size of the heart in failure.

Problem 34-1. Although digitalis increases the contractility of the normal as well as the failing heart, its effect on cardiac output is much greater in congestive failure. In fact, its ability to increase cardiac output in normal individuals has been questioned for many years.

The explanation of this paradox is related to hemodynamic adjustments. In the normal individual, digitalis not only increases cardiac contractility but it also causes constriction of peripheral vessels. It may also decrease venous pressure and may slow the sinus rate. Under these circumstances no increase in cardiac output can be demonstrated despite the positive inotropic effect.

The situation is different in the failing heart. In patients with congestive failure, the periphreral resistance is already high because the falling cardiac output leads to increased sympathetic

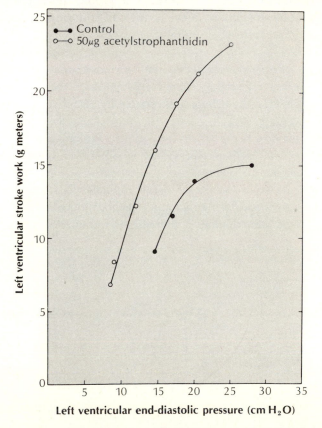

FIG. 34-2. Left ventricular curves before and after injection of 50 μg acetylstrophanthidin into the left coronary artery in the isolated supported heart preparation. Mean aortic pressure constant at 65 mm Hg; heart rate constant at 162 beats/min. Stroke work was varied by varying stroke volume. In response to the injection of acetylstrophanthidin the ventricular function curve shifted upward and to the left; that is, myocardial contractility increased. (From Sarnoti, S. J., Gilmore, J. P., Wallace, A. G., Skinner, N. S., Mitchell, J. H., and Daggett, W. M.: Am. J. Med. **37**:3, 1964.)

tone. Under these circumstances the positive inotropic effect of digitalis increases cardiac output because the tone of peripheral vessels is lowered as a result of decreased sympathetic tone.

Problem 34-2. Does digitalis increase the *efficiency* of the failing heart? It has been observed that digitalis will increase cardiac output in the failing heart without a corresponding increase in oxygen consumption. At first glance this could be interpreted as an increase in efficiency, since more work is performed by the heart per unit of oxygen consumed.[6]

The problem is much more complicated, however. The ventricular radius of the failing heart is reduced by digitalis. Oxygen consumption should be reduced as the ventricular radius becomes smaller. It is becoming clear that if heart size remained constant, digitalis would increase oxygen consumption as it increased contractility. On the other hand, the reduction of ventricular radius leads to a decrease in oxygen utilization, and the two effects cancel each other out.

Electrophysiological effects

The electrophysiological effects of digitalis provide the basis of its actions on *conductivity*, *refractory period*, and *automaticity*. These effects must be examined separately on the conducting tissue and the ventricular and atrial muscle cells. The problem is made complex by the existence of both *autonomic* and *direct* actions of the glycosides and by differences in the sensitivity of normal and diseased heart to the electrophysiological effects of digitalis.

Conducting tissue

The low-dose effects of digitalis in the atrioventricular conduction, which is slowed, are commonly referred to as *vagal effects*, since they are reversed by atropine. The direct effect of the drug not reversible by atropine becomes evident with higher doses.

A-V node conduction is prolonged by digitalis. Prolongation of the P-R interval and varying degrees of block are electrocardiographic evidences of this action when the supraventricular rate is slow.

A-V refractory period is also prolonged by digitalis. This action becomes important when the supraventricular rate is rapid, such as in atrial flutter and fibrillation when the purpose in using digitalis is to decrease the number of impulses reaching the ventricles.

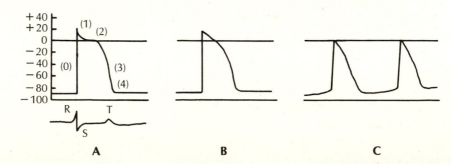

FIG. 34-3. Diagram of the effect of a digitalis glycoside on isolated Purkinje's fibers. **A,** Control before digitalis. **B,** Decrease in duration of action potential as digitalis shortens the plateau. Refractory period in Purkinje's fibers is shortened. **C,** Increased rate of diastolic depolarization with development of ectopic pacemaker activity. (Modified from Hoffman, B. F., and Singer, D. H.: Prog. Cardiovasc. Dis. **7:**226, 1964, by permission of Grune & Stratton, Inc.)

Purkinje's fibers and, to a lesser extent, ventricular muscle respond to digitalis with a shortening of the action potential, decreased refractory period, and the appearance of pacemaker activity as a result of increased rate of diastolic depolarization (Fig. 34-3). Recent evidence suggests that increased automaticity is more likely if the fibers are stretched or potassium is low.[67]

Although it is generally accepted that digitalis increases ventricular automaticity in normal hearts, there are some observations that indicate an antiarrhythmic action of the drug in patients with ventricular premature beats.[31] Further studies are needed on this point.

In the ventricle, digitalis shortens the refractory period and the duration of the action potential. Thus the Q-T interval shortens. Isolated tissue studies show that low concentrations of digitalis increase contractility prior to a significant change in transmembrane action potential.

Ventricular and atrial muscle

In the atrium, the actions of digitalis are complicated by vagal effects. Digitalis may increase the release of acetylcholine and may also increase the sensitivity of the fibers to the released mediator.[37] In a normally innervated atrium without atropine, digitalis shortens the refractory period. On the other hand, in the denervated or atropine-treated atrium, digitalis may cause an increase in the refractory period.

In normal individuals, digitalis has little effect on heart rate. In congestive failure, digitalis slows the rapid sinus rhythm primarily by an indirect mechanism. The tachycardia in this case is a consequence of increased sympathetic activity brought about by decreased cardiac output. As digitalis increases cardiac output, the sympathetic drive to the sinoatrial node is reduced. Digitalis is not useful in the treatment of sinus tachycardia caused by fever and other conditions, since it has essentially no effect on the S-A node.

EFFECT ON HEART RATE

Other factors that may play a role in the cardiac slowing caused by digitalis are (1) prolongation of the refractory period of the A-V node when atrial rate is rapid, (2) slowing of A-V conduction (a partial block may be converted to complete block), and (3) reflex vagal stimulation elicited by digitalis. These mechanisms will be discussed further in connection with the antiarrhythmic drugs.

The effects of digitalis reflect the more rapid repolarization of the ventricle, changes in A-V nodal conduction and refractory period, and increased ectopic activity. They are characterized by S-T segment depression, inversion of the T wave, shortened Q-T interval, prolongation of the P-R interval, A-V dissociation, and ventricular arrhythmias such as premature ventricular contractions, bigeminal rhythm, and ventricular fibrillation.

Electrocardiographic effects

Digitalis has two striking effects that are probably related to its inotropic, electrophysiological, and toxic actions. One is related to Na^+-K^+-ATPase inhibition, the other to calcium metabolism.

FUNDAMENTAL CELLULAR EFFECTS

Inhibition of the Na^+-K^+-ATPase should increase intracellular sodium. This sodium in turn may exchange with extracellular calcium.[63] It is possible, however, that the enzyme inhibition decreases the outward pumping of both sodium and calcium, thus increasing the calcium pool available for excitation-contraction coupling.

There are many reasons to believe that some connection exists between the digitalis effect and calcium. The two drugs are synergistic,[28] and calcium administration is dangerous in digitalized patients. Digitalis may increase the availability of intracellular calcium for the process of excitation-contraction coupling.

EXTRACARDIAC
EFFECTS

When used in therapeutic doses, the effects of digitalis are exerted largely on the heart. Some of the extracardiac effects may be important, however, as an aid to recognizing impending digitalis-induced cardiac toxicity.

The *gastrointestinal effects* manifest themselves commonly in the form of nausea and anorexia. These effects are central or reflex in origin when the purified glycosides are used. With powered digitalis or digitalis tincture, a local effect contributes to nausea and anorexia. The intravenously administered glycosides exert their emetic effect by acting on the chemoreceptor trigger zone.[7]

The *neurological effects* consist of blurred vision, paresthesias, and toxic psychosis. These symptoms are often misdiagnosed in elderly patients.

Endocrinological changes such as gynecomastia occur rarely. Allergic reactions are extremely uncommon.

The *diuretic effect* is mostly a consequence of an improvement of renal circulation, although in large doses the various glycosides cause some inhibition of sodium reabsorption directly in the renal tubules.[41]

Some experiments suggest that an action of digitalis on the central nervous system (CNS) contributes to arrhythmia and ventricular fibrillation.[17,50,51] For example, the intravenous administration of large doses of digitalis glycoside induces ventricular fibrillation in the dog. Ventricular fibrillation did not occur, however, after bilateral cardiac sympathectomy and ligation of the adrenal glands.[36] In some definitive experiments,[17] electric activity was monitored in sympathetic, parasympathetic, and phrenic nerves before and after ouabain administration in cats. Ouabain increased traffic in these nerves. Spinal transection prevented these effects and increased the dose of ouabain needed for producing ventricular arrhythmias. It appears, then, that neural activation, probably at the level of the brain stem, plays a role in the development of ouabain-induced arrythmias.

SOURCES AND
CHEMISTRY

The cardioactive steroids and their glycosides are widely distributed in nature. Since their effects on the heart are qualitatively the same, it is sufficient to utilize only a few of these in therapeutics. Some believe that most physicians would do well to utilize only one such as digoxin, an intermediate acting glycoside, which can be given orally or intravenously. Nevertheless, there are several digitalis glycosides in current use, and their sources and chemistry will be briefly summarized.

The glycosides most commonly used are obtained from the foxglove or *Digitalis purpurea*, *Digitalis lanata*, or the seeds of the African tree, *Strophanthus gratus*. The most important glycosides obtained from these plants are as follows:

Digitalis purpurea	*Digitalis lanata*	*Strophanthus gratus*
Digitoxin	Digoxin	Ouabain
Digoxin	Lanatoside C	
Digitalis leaf	Deslanoside	

The structure of digitoxin is characterized by a steroid nucleus with an unsaturated lactone attached in the C-17 position. The three sugars attached to the C-3 position are unusual deoxyhexoses. The molecule without the sugars is called an *aglycone* or *genin*. The steroidal structure and the unsaturated lactone are essential for the characteristic cardioactive effect. The removal of the sugars results in generally weaker and more evanescent activity.

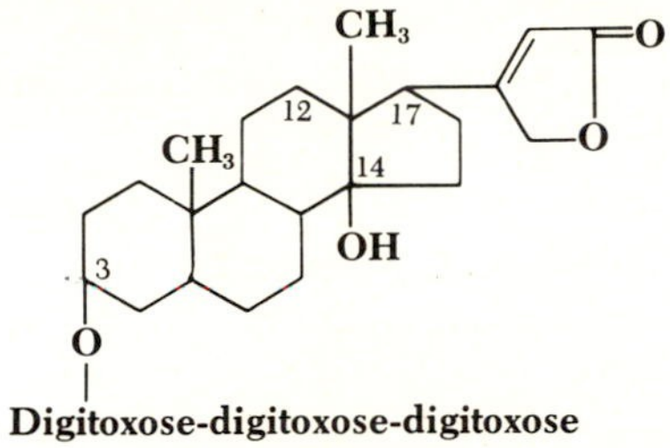

Digitoxose-digitoxose-digitoxose

Digitoxin

(Digoxin differs only in having an OH at C-12)

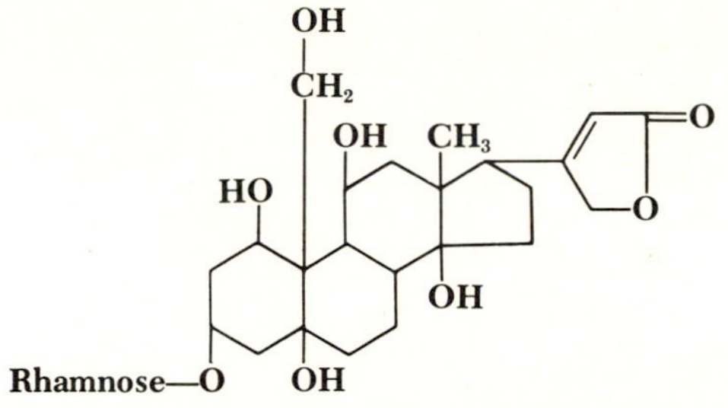

Ouabain

Digoxin differs from digitoxin only in the presence of an OH at the C-12 position. Lanatoside C (Cedilanid) is the parent compound of digoxin and differs only from the latter by having an additional glucose molecule and an acetyl group on the oligosaccharide side chain. Removal of the acetyl group by alkaline hydrolysis yields the deslanoside, and the further removal of glucose by enzymatic hydrolysis gives digoxin.

Ouabain, obtained from the seeds of *Strophanthus gratus*, differs somewhat in its steroidal portion from the previously discussed compounds. Its aglycone is known as G-strophanthidin, and the sugar to which it is attached in the glycoside is rhamnose.

The various clinically useful glycosides and genins differ mainly in their pharmacokinetic characteristics, which are reflections of their water or lipid solubility, gastrointestinal absorption, metabolism, and excretion. Digitoxin is highly lipid soluble, digoxin is less so, and ouabain is water soluble. As expected from their solubilities, digitoxin is completely absorbed from the gastrointestinal tract and persists in the body for a long time, having a half-life of 7 days. Digoxin is not as well absorbed and has a biological half-life of 1.5 days. Ouabain, a highly polar compound,

TABLE 34-1. Properties of digitalis preparations*

Preparation	Gastro-intestinal absorption	Onset of action†	Half-life‡	Peak effect	Excretion or metabolism	Digitalizing dose (mg) Oral	Digitalizing dose (mg) Intravenous	Oral maintenance dose (mg)
Digoxin	75%	15-30 min	36 hr	1½-5 hr	Renal; some GI	1.25-1.5	0.75-1.0	0.25-0.5
Digitoxin	95%	25-120 min	5 days	4-6 days	Hepatic§	0.7-1.2	1.0	0.1
Ouabain	Unreliable	5-10 min	21 hr	½-2 hr	Renal; some GI	—	0.3-0.5	—
Deslanoside	Unreliable	10-30 min	33 hr	1-2 hr	Renal	—	0.8	—

*Modified from Smith, T. W.: N. Engl. J. Med. **288**:721, 1973.
†Intravenous administration.
‡For normal subjects.
§Enterohepatic circulation exists.

is not well absorbed from the gastrointestinal tract and has a short duration of action (Table 34-1).

Digitoxin is highly bound to plasma proteins and is metabolized in the liver. It also undergoes enterohepatic circulation, being excreted in the bile and subsequently reabsorbed. Experimentally, hepatectomy increases the half-life of digitoxin, whereas renal failure increases the half-life of digoxin.

The essential feature of the pharmacokinetics of various digitalis compounds depends on the observation[61] that the total glycoside losses from the body are proportional to the total amount present; that is, the disappearance is a first-order reaction. The more glycoside there is in the body, the more is lost each day.

In the case of digoxin in a patient having normal renal function, the half-life of the drug is 1.6 days. This means that when such a patient is given a *loading dose* of digoxin, 65% of it will still be in the body 1 day later and 35% will be lost. Since the purpose of subsequent *maintenance doses* is to replace losses, the daily maintenance dose will be 35% of the loading dose. The loading dose is usually 0.75 to 1.5 mg of digoxin given in three divided doses approximately 5 hours apart.[61] The loading dose sets the total glycoside in the body to a desired level. Since the glycoside disappears logarithmically, after five glycoside half-lives only one thirty-second of the loading dose remains in the body. The purpose of the maintenance doses, then, is to keep the total amount of glycoside at the desired level. In the case of digoxin, urinary losses represent 86% of the total loss, and changes in renal function will greatly influence its dosages.

If no loading dose is given and the patient is placed on a fixed daily maintenance dose, the body stores of the glycoside will accumulate until the amount lost daily equals the maintenance dose. The curve of accumulation is a mirror image of the

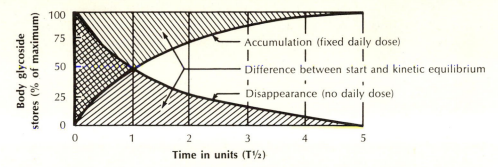

FIG. 34-4. Accumulation of a digitalis glycoside on a fixed daily dose compared with its disappearance after dosage is stopped. Time is expressed in units of half-times. (From Jeliffe, R. W.: Ann. Intern. Med. **69**:703, 1968.)

disappearance curve, and kinetic equilibrium will be reached in approximately 5 half-lives. Ninety percent of maximum will be reached in 3.3 half-lives (Fig. 34-4).

Digoxin may be looked on as the prototype of digitalis glycosides. There are experts who believe that most physicians could limit themselves to this drug whenever a digitalis preparation is needed. Nevertheless, there are several glycosides in current use that differ largely in speed of onset, duration of action, gastrointestinal absorption, and suitability for intravenous administration.

PREPARATIONS

It is essential to remember that all digitalis glycosides exert the same qualitative effects on the myocardium and that the therapeutic to toxic ratios are the same. Some are clearly more dangerous than others by virtue of differences in their durations of action. The patient poisoned with acetylstrophanthidin is not in jeopardy for as long a period as is one with digitoxin.

The modern trend is to use pure glycosides rather than the older digitalis powdered leaf or other impure compounds, which must be standardized by bioassay. In the bioassay techniques, the unknown preparation is compared with a USP reference standard with regard to lethal potency on cats, frogs, or pigeons or using the emetic effect on pigeons. The pure glycosides are measured spectrophotometrically.

Digoxin is becoming the most widely used digitalis glycoside.

Pharmacokinetics. Digoxin has an intermediate duration of action with a biological half-life of 36 hours. The drug may be administered orally or intravenously. When administered orally about 75% of it is absorbed. There may be some variation in bioavailability of digoxin tablets,[25] but the products of the largest suppliers are reliable.

Gastrointestinal absorption of digoxin is influenced by several conditions. Patients with malabsorption syndromes may absorb the drug poorly. Cholestyramine and other resins interfere with digoxin absorption. Also, various antacids, kaolin, and pectin reduce the oral absorption of the glycoside.[9]

Digoxin is excreted by glomerular filtration and is not significantly reabsorbed by the tubules. Only 20% of the drug is bound by plasma proteins. The loss of digoxin from the body takes place in an exponential fashion. In other words, the loss of the glycoside is proportional to the amount present in the body. The half-life of tritiated digoxin is 1.6 days, which increases to 4.4 days in anuric patients.[11,26]

Oral preparations of digoxin (Lanoxin) include tablets of 0.125, 0.25, and 0.5 mg and an elixir of 0.05 mg/ml. It is also available in solution for injection, 0.1 and 0.25 mg/ml.

Like digoxin, deslanoside (Cedilanid-D) is derived from *D. lanata*. It is similar in action to digoxin, and its usual digitalizing intravenous dose is 1.4 mg. Deslanoside is a derivative of lanatoside C (Cedilanid), which is poorly absorbed from the gastrointestinal tract and is rarely used.

Digitoxin is the main active glycoside in digitalis leaf *(D. purpurea)*. On a weight basis it is a thousand times as active as the powdered leaf, so that 1 mg of digitoxin is equivalent to 1 g of the leaf.

Digitoxin is the least polar of the useful cardiac glycosides, and it is highly bound to plasma proteins (97%). In contrast with digoxin, digitoxin is largely metabolized by the liver, with renal excretion being a minor factor in its disposition. Digitoxin undergoes enterohepatic circulation and cholestyramine interferes with its reabsorption.

The physiological half-life of digitoxin is approximately 5 to 7 days. Anuria prolongs the half-time to 8 days. This prolongation is obviously relatively less than in the case of digoxin, which depends much more on renal excretion for its elimination.

A patient receiving digitoxin therapy loses about 10% of the amount in the body in a day. The drug accumulates until the peak stores represent 10 times the daily maintenance dose. A loading dose is generally given at the beginning of treatment, since on a daily maintenance dose a long time would be required for full digitalization. Because of its slow metabolic degradation, its toxic effects continue for a long time after the drug is discontinued. This is one of the reasons for the increasing popularity of digoxin in preference to digitoxin, although there is no unanimity on this question. The metabolic degradation of digitoxin is accelerated by drugs that stimulate the activity of hepatic microsomal enzymes, such as phenobarbital.

Transition from digoxin to digitoxin in a patient may lead to difficulties because of their different pharmacokinetics.[61] Transition from digoxin maintenance to digitoxin maintenance would lead to underdigitalization, whereas changing from digitoxin to digoxin without careful adjustment of dosages may lead to digitalis poisoning.

Oral preparations of digitoxin (Crystodigin; Digitalin Nativelle; Purodigin) include oral tablets containing 0.05, 0.1, 0.15, and 0.2 mg; elixir, 0.5 mg/ml; and injectable solution, 0.2 mg/ml.

Ouabain, a crystalline glycoside, is obtained from *S. gratus*. It is a highly polar glycoside, suitable for intravenous injection only, because it is poorly absorbed from the gastrointestinal tract. It is commonly used in experimental work. Its plasma half-life is 21 hours.

Gitalin is a mixture of glycosides obtained from *D. purpurea*. It has no advantages, although a more favorable therapeutic index has been claimed for it.

Acetylstrophanthidin is an experimental drug of extremely short duration of action. It has been proposed for a therapeutic test to determine the completeness of digitalization. Its use should be reserved for the experts and for clinical investigations only.[33]

Digitalis is the principal drug of choice in the treatment of congestive failure and in certain arrhythmias. Some of the latter indications are absolute and others are controversial.

THERAPEUTIC INDICATIONS

Congestive failure caused by a variety of underlying mechanisms responds well to digitalis treatment. By increasing contractility, the drug increases cardiac output and relieves the elevated ventricular pressures, pulmonary congestion, and venous pressure. Diuresis is brought about with relief of edema.

Congestive failure

Controversy exists in relation to the use of digitalis in myocardial infarction with failure. The drug may aggravate the arrhythmias that commonly accompany the infarction. Some experts believe that this danger has been overemphasized.[32] Other areas of controversy relate to the prophylactic use of digitalis, which is avoided by most clinicians.

Arrhythmias of certain types represent important indications for the use of digitalis. Among these the most prominent are atrial fibrillation, atrial flutter, and paroxysmal atrial tachycardia.

Arrhythmias

Atrial fibrillation. The main purpose of using digitalis in atrial fibrillation in the absence of congestive failure is to slow the ventricular rate. This is achieved by the prolongation of the refractory period of the A-V node, which allows fewer of the supraventricular impulses to get through. Digitalis does not generally stop the atrial fibrillation itself.

Atrial flutter. In atrial flutter, the rapid atrial rate is accompanied by a 2:1 or 3:1 A-V block. Digitalis further increases the magnitude of the A-V block, thus slowing the ventricular rate. As to the atrial flutter itself, digitalis tends to convert flutter to fibrillation. This effect is probably a consequence of decreasing the refractory period of the atria. Occasionally, after flutter is converted to fibrillation by digitalis and the drug is stopped, normal sinus rhythm may result.

Paroxysmal atrial tachycardia. Paroxysmal atrial tachycardia often responds to increased vagal activity, which can be elicited by pressure on the carotid sinus. Digitalis may act by a similar mechanism, since it has a definite vagal effect.

Intoxication with digitalis is common and hazardous. In a survey carried out in a general hospital, digitalis intoxication was found to be the most common adverse drug reaction.[40]

DIGITALIS POISONING

The symptoms of digitalis poisoning include both extracardiac and cardiac manifestations. In mild to moderate intoxication, the symptoms consist of anorexia, ventricular ectopic beats, and bradycardia. These may progress to nausea and vomiting, headache, malaise, and ventricular premature beats. In severe intoxication, the symptoms are characterized by blurring of vision, disorientation, diarrhea, ventricular tachycardia, and sinoatrial and A-V block. This may progress to ventricular fibrillation.

There are several reasons for the frequency of digitalis intoxication. The therapeutic index of digitalis is low and highly variable in different patients. The common use of thiazide diuretics leads to hypopotassemia, which aggravates digitalis toxicity.

The development of methods for determining serum concentrations of digoxin and digitoxin by radioimmunoassay may be important in the prevention of some cases of digitalis intoxication (Fig. 34-5). It should be stressed, however, that such determinations should not replace good clinical judgment because numerous factors influence the significance of a given serum concentration. Some of these factors are the underlying heart disease, the serum concentration of potassium and magnesium, and endocrine factors.

The electrocardiographic changes observed in digitalis poisoning can be explained on the basis of the drug's electrophysiological effects. Ventricular arrhyth-

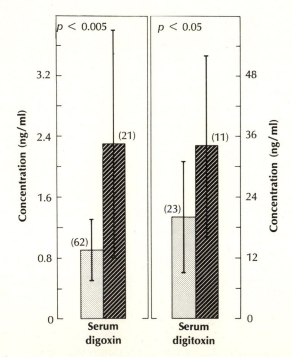

FIG. 34-5. Serum digoxin and serum digitoxin concentrations determined by radioimmunoassay. Stippled bars refer to patients without toxic effects, and crosshatched bars refer to patients with definite toxic effects. Numbers of patients are shown in parentheses. (From Beller, G. A., Smith, T. W., Abelmann, W. H., Haber, E., and Hood, W. B.: N. Engl. J. Med. **284:**989, 1971.)

mias are related to increased automaticity (increased rate of diastolic depolarization). A-V dissociation is related to the actions of digitalis on conduction and refractory period at the A-V node. The lowering of the S-T segment and inversion of the T wave commonly observed after digitalis may reflect rapid repolarization of the ventricle and perhaps a change in the initiation of the repolarization process.

Drug interactions and digitalis intoxication

In addition to the potassium-losing diuretics that predispose to digitalis toxicity, there are other drug interactions of clinical significance. Calcium (parenteral) and catecholamines or sympathomimetic drugs may promote ectopic pacemaker activity in digitalized patients. Barbiturates such as phenobarbital may accelerate the metabolism of digitoxin. Cholestyramine resin binds digitoxin in the intestine and thus interferes with its enterohepatic circulation. Digitalis can be used in reserpinized patients, since the glycosides still exert their characteristic cardiotonic effect. On the other hand, the administration of parenteral reserpine to a digitalized patient may cause arrhythmias, probably as a consequence of sudden catecholamine release.[10]

Digoxin toxicity is enhanced by quinidine. The plasma concentrations of digoxin increase significantly when quinidine is administered along with the glycoside, despite the fact that the elimination half-life of digoxin is not changed appreciably.[23]

Treatment of digitalis poisoning

The most important measure in the treatment of digitalis poisoning is the discontinuation of the drug administration. Potassium chloride by mouth or by slow intravenous infusion may be helpful in stopping the ventricular arrhythmias. It should be remembered, however, that elevated potassium concentrations may aggravate A-V block, although potassium may improve it if serum potassium is low. It is believed by many investigators that the infusion of potassium in a digitalized patient may produce abnormally high serum concentrations because of the effect of the glycosides on the membrane ATPase in various tissues. Other drugs that are used occasionally in digitalis poisoning are the antiarrhythmic drugs such as phenytoin, lidocaine, and procainamide.

DIGITALIZATION AND MAINTENANCE

The principles behind the loading dose and the maintenance dose have already been discussed in relation to pharmacokinetics of digitalis (p. 448). For practical purposes, initial digitalization is accomplished by either a *rapid method* or a *cumulative (slow) method*.

In the rapid method, the estimated loading dose is administered in a single dose or in two or three divided doses given a few hours apart, depending on the response. In the cumulative method, smaller doses are employed at greater intervals until full digitalization take place by cumulation. For example, digitoxin may be given for initial digitalization in a single dose of 1.2 or 0.4 mg every 8 hours for three doses. This initial digitalization is followed in subsequent days by the maintenance dose, which in the case of digitoxin is 0.1 to 0.2 mg daily.

For details on digitalizing and maintenance doses of the various glycosides see Table 34-1.

**NEWER
INOTROPIC
AGENTS**

Dobutamine hydrochloride (Dobutrex) is a synthetic derivative of isoproterenol. It increases myocardial contractility but causes less tachycardia or peripheral arterial effects.[69] Administered by intravenous infusion, the drug may be useful in relatively acute heart failure without severe hypotension. In cardiogenic shock with severe hypotension, dobutamine is not sufficient to elevate blood pressure adequately, since it does not increase peripheral resistance. Since the electrophysiological effects of dobutamine are similar to those of isoproterenol, the drug may cause an increase in heart rate, and in the presence of coronary artery disease ischemia may be aggravated.

Amrinone is a new investigational inotropic agent which differs in its mode of action from digitalis and the β-adrenergic agonists.[62] It does not act on the sodium pump, and it does not alter cyclic AMP levels. It probably influences excitation-contraction coupling. Although preliminary studies[4] indicate a favorable effect in patients with severe congestive failure, the ultimate position of amrinone in relation to digitalis cannot be predicted. Amrinone is a bipyridine derivative.

REFERENCES

1 Allen, J. C., and Schwartz, A.: A possible biochemical explanation for the insensitivity of the rat to cardiac glycosides, J. Pharmacol. Exp. Ther. **168:**42, 1969.

2 Areskog, N. H.: Effects of two rapid acting cardiac glycosides on dog's heart-lung preparation, Acta Physiol. Scand. **55:**139, 1962.

3 Beller, G. A., Smith, T. W., Abelmann, W. H., Haber, E., and Hood, W. B.: Digitalis intoxication: a prospective clinical study with serum level correlations, N. Engl. J. Med. **284:**989, 1971.

4 Benotti, J. R., Grossman, W., Braunwald, E., Davolos, D. D., and Alousi, A. A.: Hemodynamic assessment of amrinone, a new inotropic agent, N. Engl. J. Med. **299:**1373, 1978.

5 Bernstein, M. S., Neschis, M., and Collini, F.: Treatment of acute massive digitalis poisoning by administration of a chelating agent, N. Engl. J. Med. **261:**961, 1959.

6 Bing, R. J., and Danforth, W. H.: Physiology of the myocardium, J.A.M.A. **172:**438, 1960.

7 Borison, H. L.: Role of gastrointestinal innervation in digitalis emesis, J. Pharmacol. Exp. Ther. **104:**396, 1952.

8 Braunwald, E., Bloodwell, R. D., Goldberg, L. I., and Morrow, A. G.: Studies on digitalis. IV. Observations in man on the effects of digitalis preparations on the contractility of the nonfailing heart and on total vascular resistance, J. Clin. Invest. **40:**52, 1961.

9 Brown, D. D., and Juhl, R. P.: Decreased bioavailability of digoxin due to antacids and kaolin-pectin, N. Engl. J. Med. **295:**1034, 1976.

10 Dick, H. L. H., McCawley, E. L., and Fisher, W. A.: Reserpine-digitalis toxicity, Arch. Intern. Med. **109:**503, 1962.

11 Doherty, J. E.: The clinical pharmacology of digitalis glycosides: a review, Am. J. Med. Sci. **255:**382, 1968.

12 Doherty, J. E., Flanigan, W. J., Patterson, R. M., and Dalrymple, G. V.: The excretion of tritiated digoxin in normal human volunteers before and after unilateral nephrectomy, Circulation **50:**555, 1969.

13 Doherty, J. E., and Perkins, W. H.: Studies with tritiated digoxin in human subjects after intravenous administration, Am. Heart J. **63:**528, 1962.

14 Dunham, E. T., and Glynn, I. M.: Adenosine triphosphatase activity and the active movements of alkali metal ions, J. Physiol. **156:**274, 1961.

15 Edman, K. A. P.: Drugs and properties of heart muscle, Annu. Rev. Pharmacol. **5:**99, 1965.

16 Friend, D. G.: Current concepts in therapy: cardiac glycosides, N. Engl. J. Med. **266:**402, 1962.

17 Gillis, R. A., et al.: Neuroexcitatory effects of digitalis and their role in the development of cardiac arrhythmias, J. Pharmacol. Exp. Ther. **183:**154, 1972.

18 Glynn, I. M.: The action of cardiac glycosides on ion movements, Physiol. Rev. **16:**381, 1964.

19 Gold, H.: Pharmacologic basis of cardiac therapy, J.A.M.A. **132:**547, 1946.

20 Gold, H., and Cattell, M.: Mechanism of dig-

italis action in abolishing heart failure, Arch. Intern. Med. **65**:263, 1940.

21 Gold, H., Kwit, N. T., Otto, H., and Fox, T.: On the vagal and extra-vagal factors in cardiac slowing by digitalis in patients with auricular fibrillation, J. Clin. Invest. **18**:429, 1939.

22 Gubner, R. S., and Kallman, H.: Treatment of digitalis toxicity by chelation of serum calcium, Am. J. Med. Sci. **234**:136, 1957.

23 Hager, W. D., Fenster, P., Mayersohn, M., Perrier, D., Graves, P., Marcus, F. I., and Goldman, S.: Digoxin-quinidine interaction, N. Engl. J. Med. **300**:1238, 1979.

24 Hoffman, B. F., and Singer, D. H.: Effects of digitalis on electrical activity of cardiac fibers, Prog. Cardiovasc. Dis. **7**:226, 1964.

25 Huffman, D. H., and Azarnoff, D. L.: Absorption of orally given digoxin preparations, J.A.M.A. **222**:957, 1972.

26 Jeliffe, R. W.: An improved method of digoxin therapy, Ann. Intern. Med. **69**:703, 1968.

27 Katz, A. I., and Epstein, F. H.: Physiologic role of sodium-potassium-activated triphosphatase in the transport of cations across biologic membranes, N. Engl. J. Med. **278**:253, 1968.

28 Koch-Weser, J.: Mechanism of digitalis action on the heart, N. Engl. J. Med. **277**:417, 469, 1967.

29 Kreidberg, M. B., Chernoff, H. L., and Lopez, W. L.: Treatment of cardiac failure in infancy and childhood, N. Engl. J. Med. **268**:23, 1963.

30 Langer, G. A.: Ion fluxes in cardiac excitation and contraction and their relation to myocardial contractility, Physiol. Rev. **48**:708, 1968.

31 Lown, B., Graboys, T. B., Podrid, P. J., Cohen, B. H., Stockman, M. B., and Gaughan, C. E.: Effect of digitalis drug on ventricular premature beats, N. Engl. J. Med. **296**:301, 1977.

32 Lown, B., Klein, M. D., Barr, I., Hagemejer, F., Kosowsky, B. D., and Garrison, H.: Sensitivity to digitalis drugs in acute myocardial infarction, Am. J. Cardiol. **30**:388, 1972.

33 Lown, B., and Levine, S. A.: Current concepts in digitalis therapy, Boston, 1954, Little, Brown & Co.

34 Marks, B. H.: Effects of drugs on the inotropic property of the heart, Annu. Rev. Pharmacol. **4**:155, 1964.

35 McMichael, J., and Sharpey-Schafer, E. P.: The action of intravenous digoxin in man, Q. J. Med. **13**:123, 1944.

36 Mendez, C., Aceves, J., and Mendez, R.: The antiadrenergic action of digitalis on the refractory period of the A-V transmission system, J. Pharmacol. Exp. Ther. **131**:199, 1961.

37 Mendez, R., and Mendez, C.: The action of cardiac glycosides on the refractory period of heart tissues, J. Pharmacol. Exp. Ther. **107**:24, 1953.

38 Moe, G. K., and Mendez, R.: The action of several cardiac glycosides on conduction velocity and ventricular excitability in the dog heart, Circulation **4**:729, 1951.

39 Morrow, D. H., Gaffney, T. E., and Braunwald, E.: Studies on digitalis. VIII. Effect of autonomic innervation and of myocardial catecholamine stores upon the cardiac action of ouabain, J. Pharmacol. Exp. Ther. **140**:236, 1963.

40 Nechay, B. R., and Nelson, J. A.: Renal ouabain-sensitive ATP-ase activity and Na^+ reabsorption, J. Pharmacol. Exp. Ther. **175**:717, 1970.

41 Ogilvie, R. I., and Ruedy, J.: An educational program on digitalis therapy, J.A.M.A. **222**:50, 1971.

42 Rasmussen, K., Jervell, J., Storstein, L., and Gjerdrum, K.: Digitoxin kinetics in patients with impaired renal function, Clin. Pharmacol. Ther. **13**:6, 1972.

43 Robertson, D. M., Hollenhorst, R. W., and Callahan, J. A.: Ocular manifestations of digitalis toxicity, Arch. Ophthalmol. **76**:640, 1966.

44 Rosenblum, H.: Maintenance of digitalis effects after rapid parenteral digitalization, J.A.M.A. **182**:192, 1962.

45 Sarnoff, S. J., Gilmore, J. P., Wallace, A. G., Skinner, N. S., Mitchell, J. H., and Daggett, W. M.: Effect of acetyl strophanthidin therapy on cardiac dynamics, oxygen consumption and efficiency in the isolated heart with and without hypoxia, Am. J. Med. **37**:3, 1964.

46 Schmidt, D. H., and Butler, V. P.: Immunological protection against digoxin toxicity, J. Clin. Invest. **50**:866, 1971.

47 Schwartz, A., Allen, J. C., and Harigaya, S.: Possible involvement of cardiac Na^+, K^+-adenosine triphosphatase in the mechanism of action of cardiac glycosides, J. Pharmacol. Exp. Ther. **168**:31, 1969.

48 Skou, J. C.: Enzymatic basis for active transport of Na^+ and K^+ across cell membrane, Physiol. Rev. **45**:596, 1965.

49 Spann, J. F., Sonnenblick, E. H., Cooper, T., Chidsey, C. A., Willman, V. L., and Braunwald, E.: Studies on digitalis. XIV. Influence of cardiac norepinephrine stores on the response of isolated heart muscle to digitalis, Circ. Res. **19**:326, 1966.

50 Standaert, F. G., Levitt, B., Roberts, J., and Raines, A.: Antagonism of ventricular arrhythmias induced by digitalis—a neural phenomenon, Eur. J. Pharmacol. **6**:209, 1969.

51 Stickney, J. L., and Lucchesi, B. R.: The effect of sympatholytic agents on the cardiovascular responses produced by the injection of acetyl-strophanthidin into the cerebral ventricles, Eur. J. Pharmacol. 6:1, 1969.

52 Sulakhe, P. V., and Dhalla, N. S.: Excitation-contraction coupling in heart. VII. Calcium accumulation in subcellular particles in congestive heart failure, J. Clin. Invest. 50:1019, 1971.

53 Weissler, A. M., Snyder, J. R., Schoenfeld, C. D., and Cohen, S.: Assay of digitalis glycosides in man, Am. J. Cardiol. 17:768, 1966.

54 West, T. C., and Toda, N.: Cardiovascular pharmacology, Annu. Rev. Pharmacol. 7:145, 1967.

55 Williams, J. F., Klocke, F. J., and Braunwald, E.: Studies on digitalis. XIII. A comparison of the effects of potassium on the inotropic and arrhythmia-producing actions of ouabain, J. Clin. Invest. 45:346, 1966.

56 Withering, W.: An account of the foxglove, and some of its medicinal uses: with practical remarks on dropsy, and other diseases, London, 1785, C. G. J. & J. Robinson. (Reprinted in Medical Classics 2:305, 1937.)

57 Wood, E. H., and Moe, G. K.: Correlation between serum potassium changes in the heart-lung preparation and the therapeutic and toxic effects of digitalis glycosides, Am. J. Physiol. 129:499, 1940.

REVIEWS

58 Braunwald, E.: Vasodilator therapy—a physiologic approach to the treatment of heart failure, N. Engl. J. Med. 297:331, 1977.

59 Butler, V. P.: Digoxin: immunologic approaches to measurement and reversal of toxicity, N. Engl. J. Med. 283:1150, 1970.

59a Cohn, J. N., and Franciosa, J. A.: Vasodilator therapy of cardiac failure, N. Engl. J. Med. 297:27, 1977.

60 Huffman, D. H., and Azarnoff, D. L.: The use of digitalis, Ration. Drug Ther. 8:1, 1974.

61 Jeliffe, R. W.: An improved method for replacing one digitalis glycoside with another, Med. Times 98:105, 1970.

62 Katz, A. M.: A new inotropic drug: its promise and a caution, N. Engl. J. Med. 299:1409, 1978.

63 Langer, G. A.: The mechanism of action of digitalis, Hosp. Pract., p. 49, Aug., 1970.

64 Langer, G. A.: Relationship between myocardial contractility and the effects of digitalis on ionic exchange, Fed. Proc. 36:2231, 1977.

65 Lemberg, L.: Digitalis in congestive heart failure. Fact or fancy. Arch. Intern. Med. 138:451, 1978.

66 Marks, B. H., and Weissler, A. M.: Basic and clinical pharmacology of digitalis: proceedings of a symposium, Springfield, Ill., 1972, Charles C Thomas, Publisher.

66a Mason, D. T., Awan, N. A., and DeMaria, A. N.: Afterload reduction in the management of congestive failure, Hosp. Formulary, p. 641, June, 1979.

67 Rosen, M. R., Gelband, H., Merker, C., and Hoffman, B. F.: Mechanisms of digitalis toxicity: effects of ouabain on phase four of canine Purkinje fiber transmembrane potentials, Circulation 47:681, 1973.

67a Smith, T. W.: Digitalis: ions, inotropy and toxicity, N. Engl. J. Med. 299:545, 1978.

68 Smith, T. W., and Haber, E.: Digitalis, N. Engl. J. Med. 289:945, 1125, 1973.

69 Sonnenblick, E. H., Frishman, W. H., and LeJemtel, T. H.: Dobutamine: a new synthetic cardioactive sympathetic amine, N. Engl. J. Med. 300:17, 1979.

70 Tobin, J. R.: The treatment of congestive heart failure. Digitalis glycosides are still the primary mode of therapy, Arch. Intern. Med. 138:453, 1978.

CHAPTER 35

Antiarrhythmic drugs

GENERAL CONCEPT

The antiarrhythmic drugs are useful in the prevention and treatment of disorders of cardiac rhythm, which manifest themselves as tachyarrhythmias or bradyarrhythmias. Tachyarrhythmias represent the major problem, since bradyarrhythmias are readily treated with atropine or isoproterenol. Major advances have taken place in our understanding of the mode of action of drugs used in the treatment of tachyarrhythmias, and many new antiarrhythmic drugs have been developed, some with novel mechanism of action.

The mechanisms underlying the arrhythmias are attributed to increased automaticity, reentry, and altered excitability. The antiarrhythmic drugs are classified into four groups on the basis of their electrophysiological effects. Class I drugs are local anesthetics, and they include quinidine, procainamide, disopyramide, lidocaine, tocainide, mexiletine, aprindine, and phenytoin. Class II drugs are β-adrenergic blocking drugs, exemplified by propranolol. Class III agents, represented by bretylium, prolong the action potential and refractory period. Finally, Class IV drugs inactivate the slow calcium channel; verapamil is a representative of this new series.[43]

ELECTROPHYSIOLOGICAL BASIS OF ANTIARRHYTHMIC ACTION

The classification of antiarrhythmic drugs is shown in Table 35-1.

Most tachyarrhythmias are consequences of two basic mechanisms[40]: (1) ectopic focal activity and (2) reentry. In ectopic focal activity a potential pacemaker fires independently because of an increase in the slope of diastolic depolarization, the threshold potential being more negative, or because of a decrease in the maximum diastolic potential.[43] If the diastolic depolarization is rapid, phase 0 of the action

TABLE 35-1. Classification of antiarrhythmic drugs

I	II	III	IV
Quinidine Procainamide Disopyramide Lidocaine Tocainide* Mexiletine* Aprindine* Phenytoin	Propranolol	Bretylium	Verapamil

* Investigational drug.

potential is sodium dependent. If it is slow, it may be dependent on the slow inward current.

The conditions necessary for reentry to occur are as follows[41]: (1) the conduction pathway must be blocked, (2) there must be slow conduction over an alternate route to a point beyond the block, and (3) there must be delayed excitation beyond the block. With a sufficient delay in excitation beyond the block, the tissue proximal to the site of block may be excited from the opposite direction and the circuit is then established.[41]

The various classes of antiarrhythmic drugs have characteristic electrophysiological effects on the myocardium, modified in some instances by extracardiac effects.

Class I drugs have local anesthetic properties. They reduce the maximal rate of depolarization, increase the threshold of excitability, depress conduction velocity, prolong the effective refractory period, and reduce the spontaneous diastolic depolarization in pacemaker cells. These effects are shown in quinidine in Fig. 35-1. The decrease in diastolic depolarization tends to suppress ectopic focal activity. Prolongation of refractory periods tends to abolish reentry. These drugs generally prolong the duration of the action potential with simultaneous prolongation of the effective refractory period. Lidocaine and phenytoin differ from other members of the class in shortening the action potential. The actions of quinidine, procainamide, and disopyramide are modified by their anticholinergic activity.

Class II antiarrhythmic drugs are β-adrenergic blocking agents, such as propranolol. Their β-blocking effect is much more important than any local anesthetic activity they may have. Their mode of action is related to a depression of the slope of the spontaneous diastolic depolarization.

Class III drugs, represented mainly by bretylium, appear to act by prolonging the action potential that is associated with a prolongation of the effective refractory period.

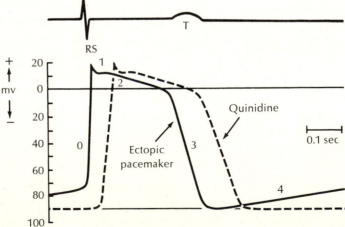

FIG. 35-1. Diagrammatic representation of the effect of quinidine on the transmembrane electrical potential of a spontaneously depolarizing conductive fiber in the ventricular myocardium. (Modified from Mason, D. T., et al.: Clin. Pharmacol. Ther. **11**:460, 1970.)

Class IV antiarrhythmic drugs are relatively new, but verapamil has been found valuable already in treatment of atrial tachyarrhythmias and in the management of angina pectoris.[43] Verapamil blocks the inward current carried by calcium and perhaps the slow current carried by sodium.[25] This concept is very significant. It appears that the rapid current or "fast response" is carried by sodium and the slow current or "slow response" by calcium. The latter mediates pacemaker potentials and may be significant in pathological conditions, such as ischemia or digitalis toxicity.

Quinidine is the dextrorotatory isomer of quinine and has the following structure:

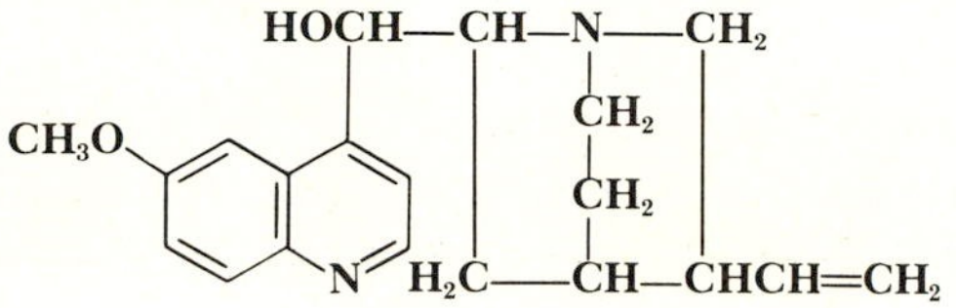

ANTIARRHYTHMIC DRUGS
Quinidine

Quinidine

The introduction of quinidine into therapeutics is one of the classical stories of medical history. In 1914 the Viennese cardiologist Wenckebach[31] had a Dutch sea captain as a patient. The captain had a completely irregular pulse as a consequence of atrial fibrillation. Wenckebach described the situation in this way.

He did not feel great discomfort during the attack, but, as he said, being a Dutch merchant, used to good order in his affairs, he would like to have good order in his heart business also, and asked why there were heart specialists if they could not abolish this very disagreeable phenomenon. On my telling him that I could promise him nothing, he told me that he knew himself how to get rid of his attacks, and as I did not believe him, he promised to come back the next morning with a regular pulse, and he did. It happens that quinine in many countries, especially in countries where there is a good deal of malaria, is a sort of drug for everything, just as one takes acetylsalicylic acid today if one does not feel well or is afraid of having taken a cold. Occasionally, taking the drug during an attack of fibrillation, the patient found that the attack was stopped within from twenty to twenty-five minutes, and later he found that a gram of quinine regularly abolished his irregularity.*

In 1918 Frey[6] tried drugs related to quinine in patients with atrial fibrillation and introduced quinidine, the dextro isomer of quinine, into cardiac therapy. During the succeeding years the antifibrillatory action of quinidine was confirmed, but its widespread use led to a number of sudden deaths.

Eventually it was recognized that there are definite contraindications to use of the drug. In the presence of conduction defects it may produce cardiac standstill and should be avoided. Once the mode of action of the drug was understood and contraindications to its use were recognized, quinidine obtained its present position in cardiac therapy.

---

*From Beckman, H.: Treatment in general practice, Philadelphia, 1934, W. B. Saunders Co.

Cardiac effects   Quinidine is a Class I antiarrhythmic drug. Thus it reduces the maximal rate of depolarization, increases the threshold of excitability, depresses conduction velocity, prolongs the effective refractory period, and reduces the spontaneous diastolic depolarization in pacemaker cells (Fig. 35-1), thus depressing automaticity. The drug is useful in both supraventricular and ventricular tachyarrhythmias. Quinidine can convert atrial tachyarrhythmias to normal sinus rhythm, but cardioversion is replacing this use of the drug.

A complicating factor in the action of quinidine is its "vagolytic" or anticholinergic effect. This may counteract its direct effect and may explain the acceleration of heart rate that may be caused by the drug. The anticholinergic effect may also explain the paradoxical tachycardia that may be seen in some cases during the treatment of atrial flutter with block.

Electrocardiographic effects. Quinidine in higher doses prolongs the P-R, QRS, and Q-t intervals (Fig. 35-2). Widening of the QRS complex is related to slowing conduction in the His-Purkinje system and in the ventricular muscle. Changes in the Q-T interval and alteration in T waves are related to changes in repolarization. The direct effect of the drug on A-V conduction and refractoriness of the A-V system explains the prolongation of the P-R interval.

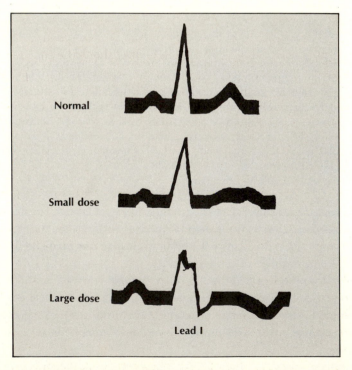

FIG. 35-2. Effect of quinidine on electrocardiogram. Note changes in P wave, QRS complex, and T wave at varying dosage levels. (From Burch, G. E., and Winsor, T.: A primer of electrocardiography, Philadelphia, 1960, Lea & Febiger.)

Quinidine tends to depress all muscle tissue, including vascular smooth muscle and skeletal muscle. Particularly when injected intravenously, the drug can cause profound hypotension and shock. Its effect on skeletal muscle becomes particularly evident in patients with myasthenia gravis, in whom it causes profound weakness.

Extracardiac and adverse effects

Cinchonism caused by quinidine is characterized by ringing of the ears and dizziness and is similar to what may be observed after the administration of quinine or salicylates.

Quinidine thrombocytopenia appears to occur on an allergic basis. In a typical case, a patient taking quinidine for several weeks notices the development of petechial hemorrhages in the buccal mucous membranes. The symptoms disappear when the drug is discontinued and reappear after reinstitution of therapy. A positive Ackroyd test can usually be demonstrated in vitro.

Quinidine may cause ventricular arrhythmias and even ventricular fibrillation. The so-called quinidine syncope is probably a consequence of ventricular fibrillation.[48]

Cardiotoxicity and its treatment

It may seem paradoxical that an antiarrhythmic drug can cause ventricular arrhythmias. Since quinidine depresses automaticity, the clinically observed ventricular arrhythmias after excessive doses of quinidine are probably caused by reentry mechanism rather than by increased automaticity.[44]

Quinidine is particularly dangerous in patients having conduction defects. In such patients when conduction is further impaired and automaticity of the Purkinje system is depressed, the ventricles may not take over when A-V conduction fails, and cardiac standstill may ensue. The administration of the drug should be stopped when significant increases in P-R interval or QRS widenings supervene during treatment.

In addition to stopping the drug administration, quinidine intoxication is treated supportively with maintenance of blood pressure, oxygen, and bed rest. Sodium bicarbonate and sodium lactate have also been recommended.

When given orally, quinidine produces its peak effect in 2 to 4 hours. Its half-life is about 4 to 6 hours. Therapeutic plasma levels are 3 to 6 μg/ml.

Pharmacokinetics

About 10% to 50% of administered quinidine is excreted in unchanged form in the urine. The rest is transformed in the liver by hydroxylation. The amount excreted is influenced by the pH of the urine. Alkalinization with molar sodium lactate tends to decrease the excretion of quinidine, although it may improve some toxic effects of the drug.

Quinidine is bound to plasma proteins, a fact that may account for some lack of correlation between blood levels and therapeutic effect. Nevertheless, toxic manifestations correlate better with serum levels than with the dose of the drug.[40]

Drug interactions occur with quinidine and will be discussed in Chapter 63.

Preparations of quinidine include the following: quinidine sulfate in tablets containing 200 and 300 mg and timed-release tablets of 300 mg; and quinidine gluconate (Quinaglute) in tablets containing 300 mg.

Preparations, administration, and dose

The usual adult dosage of quinidine is 200 to 400 mg three to five times daily for 1 to 3 days. Larger doses should be used only in the hospital.

Quinidine gluconate is available for intramuscular injection. Intravenous administration is dangerous and should not be undertaken without monitoring the electrocardiogram.

Blood levels of quinidine have been studied by several investigators. A single dose of 200 to 400 mg of quinidine sulfate given on an empty stomach will produce a plasma level of 2 to 4 mg/L in about 2 hours. The level tends to decline fairly rapidly, and at the end of 24 hours little quinidine remains in the blood. If the same dose is given every 4 hours or at shorter intervals, definite accumulation occurs. It is the opinion of some investigators that there is a relationship between the height of the blood level of quinidine and success in converting auricular fibrillation.[24] The level necessary could not be predicted in a given patient, but most patients require 4 to 8 mg/L. This level is attained by deliberately producing a cumulation through the frequent administration of the drug.

Procainamide
Development as cardiac drug

The commonly used local anesthetic procaine was shown by Mautz[17] in 1936 to elevate the threshold to electric stimulation when applied to the myocardium of animals. In subsequent years thoracic surgeons and anesthesiologists frequently used topical procaine in surgery to reduce premature ventricular and atrial contractions during surgery. Procaine was even administered intravenously for this purpose.

Procaine hydrochloride

Procainamide hydrochloride

Encouraged by these studies, investigators studied the antifibrillatory activities of compounds related to procaine, including the effects of the two hydrolysis products of procaine, *p*-aminobenzoic acid and diethylaminoethanol. The most fruitful consequence of these studies was the finding that if the ester linkage in procaine was replaced by an amide linkage, the resulting compound had distinct advantages as an antiarrhythmic drug. The main advantages consist of greater stability in the body and fewer central nervous system (CNS) effects. The greater stability results from the fact that the drug is an amide rather than an ester.

Cardiac effects

Procainamide is so similar in its actions to quinidine that the two drugs could be used interchangeably. Quinidine is preferred for prolonged oral use because procainamide can cause lupus erythematosus. On the other hand, procainamide is safer when used intravenously and is beneficial in the treatment of ventricular tachyarrhythmias that do not respond to lidocaine.

Procainamide is absorbed well from the gastrointestinal tract and is 15% protein bound. It is metabolized in the liver to its major metabolite N-acetylprocainamide, which has antiarrhythmic activity. The rate of acetylation is genetically conditioned, and patients may be fast or slow acetylators. Renal disease prolongs the half-life of procainamide.

Pharmacokinetics

Procainamide hydrochloride (Pronestyl) is available in 250, 375, and 500 mg tablets and in injectable solutions containing 100 and 500 mg/ml.

Procainamide may cause a marked fall of blood pressure after the administration of large intravenous doses. This is probably a consequence of its action on vascular smooth muscle and on contractility of the myocardium, although ganglionic blocking effects have also been described. The drug has local anesthetic properties but is not useful for nerve block.

Extracardiac effects and toxicity

Nausea, anorexia, mental confusion, hallucinations, skin rashes, agranulocytosis, chills, and fever have been reported after the use of procainamide. A lupus erythematosus–like syndrome has also been observed in patients taking procainamide.[23]

Disopyramide phosphate (Norpace) is a Class I antiarrhythmic drug, which resembles quinidine and procainamide in its action. It is used for the prevention of ventricular premature beats and also atrial tachyarrhythmias. The drug has anticholinergic activity. Disopyramide is absorbed well from the gastrointestinal tract and has a plasma half-life of 4 to 5 hours. Renal impairment prolongs the half-life.

Disopyramide

Adverse effects of disopyramide include its anticholinergic effects, tachycardia in patients with atrial flutter and fibrillation. More rarely, the drug can cause headache, psychosis, hypoglycemia, hepatic damage and skin rashes.

Disopyramide phosphate (Norpace) is available in 100 and 150 mg capsules, which are administered every 6 hours in patients with normal renal function.

Lidocaine hydrochloride (Xylocaine hydrochloride) is a Class I antiarrhythmic drug, which has become the most widely used agent for the treatment and prevention of ventricular ectopic activity associated with myocardial infarction.

Lidocaine

Lidocaine differs in some important aspects from most other members of the Class I antiarrhythmic drugs. Although it depresses automaticity and diastolic depolarization, it does not slow conduction and has little effect on atrial function. It does not prolong the action potential and refractory period.

Lidocaine must be injected intravenously or intramuscularly because given orally it shows the first-pass effect, with the liver inactivating it very rapidly. For the same reason, liver damage or impaired hepatic blood flow increases the half-life of lidocaine.

Adverse effects of lidocaine include drowsiness, convulsions, and coma. Very large doses have adverse effects on the heart, manifested by depression of A-V conduction and a negative inotropic effect.

Lidocaine hydrochloride is available as Xylocaine Intravenous Injection in solution containing 20, 40, or 200 mg/ml. A loading dose of 50 to 100 mg is recommended, given over a period of 2 to 5 minutes. The dose may be repeated after 5 minutes without exceeding 300 mg/hour.

Pharmacokinetics

The distribution half-life of lidocaine is 8.3 minutes. Its disposition half-life is 107 minutes. The volume of distribution is 530 ml/kg, and its clearance is 10 ml/kg/min.

If 1 mg/kg is given as a loading dose, a plasma concentration of 2 μg/ml will result. If lidocaine infusion follows the loading dose, a plasma concentration of 1 μg/ml is achieved by administering 10 μg/kg/min. If an arrhythmia responds to 4 μg/ml plasma concentration, it can be calculated that the patient should receive 4 mg/min as a maintenance dose.[47]

Tocainide

Tocainide is an analog of lidocaine that is orally active, since it is not subject to rapid hepatic inactivation or "first-pass effect."[43]

Mexiletine

Mexiletine is very similar to lidocaine in its effects, differing mainly in its suitability for oral administration, its pharmacokinetics, and its side effects. Adverse effects of mexiletine include dizziness, disorientation, tremors, and cardiovascular toxicity, such as His-Purkinje refractoriness.[43]

Aprindine

Aprindine is a powerful Class I antiarrhythmic drug, which may be effective in both supraventricular and ventricular arrhythmias. It is orally active and has a very long half-life but may cause neurological side effects in a small percentage of patients.[43]

Phenytoin

The antiepileptic drug phenytoin (Dilantin) was found to decrease ventricular arrhythmias in dogs after coronary ligation in 1950.[11] More recently it has become widely used as an antiarrhythmic drug, especially in digitalis-induced tachyarrhythmias, which may be its only real indication.[47]

Phenytoin depresses automaticity in ventricular and atrial tissues and may actually improve A-V conduction. Generally it is not a useful antiarrhythmic drug, and even in digitalis toxicity lidocaine is usually preferred.

The effective level of phenytoin for antiarrhythmic activity is about 6 to 18 μg/ml, which is about the same as for its anticonvulsant effectiveness.

Pharmacokinetics

Phenytoin is absorbed slowly when given by mouth, and peak levels are not obtained for several hours. The drugs should not be given intramuscularly, since its absorption is erratic.[48] The drug is metabolized by liver microsomal enzymes, being parahydroxylated. The disappearance of phenytoin does not follow first-order kinetics because of saturation of the microsomal enzymes at therapeutic serum levels. With this reservation, it is useful to know that within the usual therapeutically effective concentration, serum levels fall to one half in 18 to 24 hours.

For oral administration to obtain a prompt effect, phenytoin may be administered in a dose of 1000 mg the first day, 500 to 600 mg the second and third days, and 400 to 500 mg thereafter.[48]

Intravenous phenytoin should be given by infusion only to severely ill patients. Infusion rate should be 25 to 50 mg/min. A total dose of 500 mg to 1 g should not be exceeded.

Dosage

Phenytoin (Dilantin) is available in capsules containing 100 mg. It is also available as a powder to make a solution for injection, 50 mg/ml.

Preparations

Propranolol exerts its anitarrhythmic activity by acting on β-adrenergic receptors. Its membrane stabilizing effect is not as important because plasma concentrations are not high enough to achieve such an effect.

Propranolol depresses automaticity, prolongs A-V conduction, reduces heart rate, and also decreases contractility. The drug is particularly effective in the treatment of tachyarrhythmias caused by increased sympathetic activity. It prevents the reflex tachycardia caused by vasodilator antihypertensive drugs. Along with digitalis it slows ventricular rate in atrial flutter and fibrillation. It has been used in digitalis toxicity, but lidocaine or phenytoin are preferred.

Adverse effects of propranolol include bronchospasm, congestive failure, and cardiac arrest. Bradycardia is common but is not a contraindication to the continued use of propranolol. Sudden withdrawal of propranolol may lead to a recurrence of angina and even sudden death. It is tempting to speculate about the possibility of β-receptor up-regulation caused by prolonged exposure to the blocking agent.

Propranolol

Propranolol (Inderal) may be given orally or intravenously. The oral dose is 10 to 40 mg two to three times a day. Intravenously, 0.1 to 0.15 mg/kg should be administered in divided doses of 0.5 to 0.75 mg every 1 or 2 minutes with appropriate monitoring. The patient should be observed for myocardial depression and bradycardia. Atropine or isoproterenol will reverse excessive bradycardia. It may require relatively large doses of isoproterenol by intravenous infusion to counteract the bradycardia, since propranolol blocks the β-receptors.

Dosage

Bretylium tosylate (Bretylol) is an adrenergic neuronal blocking drug, which was originally developed as an antihypertensive agent. Troublesome side effects made it essentially useless as an antihypertensive drug, but its antiarrhythmic properties brought it back into clinical use.

Bretylium exerts its effect as an antiarrhythmic by prolonging the action potential

Bretylium tosylate

with simultaneous prolongation of the effective refractory period. The drug is used to treat severe ventricular tachyarrhythmias that are unresponsive to other drugs. Even after intravenous injection, the effect of the drug may be delayed for several minutes or hours. Initially, the drug causes norepinephrine release and an increase in blood pressure. This is followed by a fall in blood pressure.

Adverse effects of bretylium include, in addition to changes in blood pressure, nausea, bradycardia, angina, diarrhea, skin rash, and others. The drug should be administered slowly.

Bretylium tosylate is a quaternary ammonium compound, and it is eliminated unchanged by the kidney.

Bretylium tosylate (Bretylol) is available in solution containing 50 mg/ml. The drug is administered intravenously or intramuscularly.

Verapamil   Verapamil is a papaverine derivative, which although still investigational, appears to be of value in certain atrial tachyarrhythmias and also in the management of angina pectoris. The drug has a unique mechanism of action and may represent the first of a series of new arrhythmic drugs. Verapamil inhibits transmembrane fluxes of calcium[43] and acts on the slow channel. Since the slow channel is involved in the action potential in pacemaker cells, verapamil acts on the S-A node, prolongs A-V refractoriness, depresses potential or latent pacemaker cells, and produces vasodilatation. The drug appears to have value in atrial fibrillation and atrial tachycardias. Verapamil is available for investigational purposes in the form of oral preparations and injectable solutions. Contraindications to its use include advanced heart failure, unstable A-V block, cardiogenic shock, and low blood pressure states.

SELECTION OF DRUGS   There are several principles that should be remembered before selecting a drug for the treatment of a cardiac arrhythmia. (1) Many arrhythmias do not require drug treatment. (2) Most antiarrhythmic drugs can be dangerous. (3) Cardioversion (DC countershock) has changed many of the indications for the use of antiarrhythmic medications.

With these limitations, the use of antiarrhythmic drugs in various arrhythmias will be briefly summarized.

Supraventricular arrhythmias
Paroxysmal atrial tachycardia   Paroxysmal atrial tachycardia may occur in otherwise normal individuals. It may terminate spontaneously but may recur. It may also occur as a manifestation of digitalis toxicity.

Vagal maneuvers, such as carotid massage, may terminate the attack. Anticholinesterase drugs, such as edrophonium and neostigmine may be used. Vasoconstrictors, such as methoxamine or phenylephrine, may terminate an attack by causing reflex vagal activity as a consequence of elevation of the blood pressure. Digitalis may be effective and is commonly used in atrial tachycardias of children. Verapamil is being used as an investigational drug, and, finally, propranolol may be used for certain types of supraventricular tachyarrhythmias.

Digitalis is the most important drug in the treatment of atrial flutter. It acts primarily by increasing the degree of A-V block, thereby decreasing the ventricular rate. As to the flutter itself, digitalis tends to convert it to fibrillation. The explanation resides in the ability of digitalis to shorten the refractory period in the atrial muscle.[42] Occasionally quinidine is used for the conversion of flutter to normal sinus rhythm. In this case digitalis should be employed first to prevent excessive tachycardia, a consequence of the vagolytic action of quinidine. Cardioversion finds increasing usefulness in the treatment of atrial flutter.

If digitalis is not effective, the addition of propranolol may be useful.

Atrial flutter

Digitalis is the most important drug in the treatment of atrial fibrillation. It does not convert atrial fibrillation to normal sinus rhythm, but it slows the ventricular rate by increasing A-V block, and it corrects cardiac failure if it is present. Quinidine can convert atrial fibrillation to normal sinus rhythm, but the newer tendency is to use cardioversion for this purpose. Even when DC countershock is employed, quinidine may be helpful in preventing the recurrence of atrial fibrillation.

When quinidine is added to digoxin treatment, the plasma level of the glycoside may rise to dangerous levels.[34] Administration of quinidine is often started before cardioversion, and it may terminate the fibrillation by itself. Disopyramide may be used in the same manner.

Atrial fibrillation

Occasional premature ventricular contractions generally do not require drug treatment. On the other hand, ventricular tachycardia may be a serious condition that requires intensive treatment. Although DC countershock is now commonly used for stopping ventricular tachycardia, it should not be employed if the arrhythmia is caused by digitalis.[20]

For premature ventricular beats lidocaine is the drug of choice, but procainamide may also be tried. For chronic treatment quinidine procainamide, propranolol, or disopyramide are suitable. Lidocaine, procainamide, and propranolol are also commonly used in attempts at terminating ventricular tachycardia. Bretylium is also employed occasionally.

Digitalis-induced arrhythmias may be treated with lidocaine, phenytoin, or propranolol. Antibody fractions to digitalis have been used on an investigational basis.

Digitalis is generally considered to be dangerous in the management of ventricular arrhythmias. This concept is being challenged by some recent investigations.[20]

Ventricular arrhythmias

REFERENCES

1 Beckman, H.: Treatment in general practice, Philadelphia, 1934, W. B. Saunders Co.
2 Bernstein, J. G., and Koch-Weser, J.: Effectiveness of bretylium tosylate against refractory ventricular arrhythmias, Circulation **45**:1024, 1972.
3 Bolton, F. G.: Thrombocytopenic purpura due to quinidine: serologic mechanisms, Blood **11**: 547, 1956.
4 Cheng, T. O.: Atrial flutter during quinidine therapy of atrial fibrillation, Am. Heart J. **52**: 273, 1956.

5 Conn, R. D.: Diphenylhydantoin sodium in cardiac arrhythmias, N. Engl. J. Med. **272:**277, 1965.

5a Doering, W.: Quinidine-digoxin interaction, N. Engl. J. Med. **301:**400, 1979.

6 Frey, W.: Weitere Erfahrungen mit Chinidin bei absoluter Herzunregelmässigkeit, Klin. Wochenschr. **55:**849, 1918.

7 Frieden, J.: Antiarrhythmic drugs. VII. Lidocaine as an antiarrhythmic agent, Am. Heart J. **79:**713, 1965.

8 Gertler, M. M., Kream, J., Hylin, J. W., Robinson, H., and Neidle, E. G.: Effect of quinidine on intracellular electrolytes of the rabbit heart, Proc. Soc. Exp. Biol. Med. **92:** 629, 1956.

9 Greenblatt, D. J., Bolognini, V., Koch-Weser, J., and Harmatz, J. S.: Pharmacokinetic approach to the clinical use of lidocaine intravenously, J.A.M.A. **236:**273, 1976.

10 Grossman, J. I., et al.: Lidocaine in cardiac arrhythmias, Arch. Intern. Med. **121:**396, 1968.

11 Harris, A. S., and Kokernot, R. H.: Effects of diphenylhydantoin sodium (Dilantin sodium) and phenobarbital sodium upon ectopic ventricular tachycardia in acute myocardial infarction, Am. J. Physiol. **163:**505, 1950.

12 Harrison, D. C., Griffin, J. R., and Fiene, T. J.: Effects of beta adrenergic blockade with propranolol in patients with atrial arrhythmias, N. Engl. J. Med. **27:**410, 1965.

13 Hoffman, B. F., and Cranefield, P. F.: The physiological basis of cardiac arrhythmias, Am. J. Med. **37:**670, 1964.

14 Hoffman, B. F., Cranefield, P. F., and Wallace, A. G.: Physiological basis of cardiac arrhythmias. I and II. Mod. Conc. Cardiovasc. Dis. **35:**103, 1966.

15 Johnson, E. A., and McKinnon, M. G.: The differential effect of quinidine and pyrilamine on the myocardial action potential at various rates of stimulation, J. Pharmacol. Exp. Ther. **120:** 460, 1957.

16 Kayden, H. J.: Pharmacology of procaine amide, Am. Heart J. **70:**423, 1965.

17 Koch-Weser, J.: Antiarrhythmic prophylaxis in ambulatory patients with coronary heart disease, Arch. Intern. Med. **129:**763, 1972.

18 Koch-Weser, J., and Klein, S. W.: Procainamide dosage schedules, plasma concentrations and clinical effects, J.A.M.A. **215:**1454, 1971.

19 Koch-Weser, J., Klein, S. W., Foo-Canto, L. L., Kastor, J. A., and DeSanctis, R. W.: Antiarrhythmic prophylaxis with procainamide in acute myocardial infarction, N. Engl. J. Med. **281:**1253, 1969.

20 Lown, B., Grabays, T. B., Podrid, P. J., Cohen, B. H., Stockman, M. B., and Gaughan, C. E.: Effect of digitalis drug on ventricular premature beats, N. Engl. J. Med. **296:**301, 1977.

21 Manning, J. W., Cotten, M. D., Kelly, W. N., and Johnson, C. E.: Mechanism of cardiac arrhythmias induced by diencephalic stimulation, Am. J. Physiol. **203:**1120, 1962.

22 Morrelli, H. F., and Melmon, K. L.: Pharmacologic basis for the clinical use of antiarrhythmic drugs, Pharmacol. Phys. **1**(7):1, 1967.

23 Paine, R.: Procainamide hydrochloride and lupus erythematosus, J.A.M.A. **194:**23, 1965.

24 Scherf, D.: Studies on auricular tachycardia caused by aconitine administration, Proc. Soc. Exp. Biol. Med. **64:**233, 1947.

25 Shigenobu, K., Schneider, J. S. A., and Sperelakis, N.: Verapamil blockade of slow Na$^+$ and Ca^{++} responses in myocardial cells, J. Pharmacol. Exp. Ther. **190:**280, 1974.

26 Sokolow, M., and Edgar, A. L.: Blood quinidine concentrations as guide in treatment of cardiac arrhythmias, Circulation **1:**576, 1950.

27 Sokolow, M., and Perloff, D.: Clinical pharmacology and use of quinidine, Prog. Cardiovasc. Dis. **3:**316, 1961.

28 Strong, J. M., Parker, M., and Atkinson, A. J.: Identification of glycinexylidide in patients treated with intravenous lidocaine, Clin. Pharmacol. Ther. **14:**67, 1973.

29 Unger, A. H., and Sklaroff, H. J.: Fatalities following intravenous use of sodium diphenylhydantoin for cardiac arrhythmias, J.A.M.A. **200:** 335, 1967.

30 Wedd, A. M., Blair, H. A., and Warner, R. S.: The action of procaine amide on the heart, Am. Heart J. **42:**399, 1951.

31 Wenckebach, K. F.: Die unregelmässige Herztätigkeit und ihre klinische Bedeutung, Leipzig, 1914, W. Engelmann.

REVIEWS

32 Aronow, W. S.: The treatment of supraventricular tachyarrhythmias, Ration. Drug Ther. **14:**1, Aug. 1980.

32a Bassett, A. L., and Hoffman, B. F.: Antiarrhythmic drugs: electrophysiological actions, Annu. Rev. Pharmacol. **11:**143, 1971.

33 Bigger, J. T.: Antiarrhythmic drugs in ischemic heart disease, Hosp. Pract., p. 69, Nov., 1972.

34 Bigger, J. T.: The quinidine-digoxin interaction. What do we know about it? N. Engl. J. Med. **301:**779, 1979.

35 Bigger, J. T., and Giardina, E.-G. V.: The pharmacology and clinical use of lidocaine and

procainamide, Med. Coll. Va. Quart. **9:**65, 1973.

36 Escher, D. J. W., and Furman, S.: Emergency treatment of cardiac arrhythmias, J.A.M.A. **214:**2028, 1970.

37 Guyton, A. C.: Textbook of medical physiology, ed. 4, Philadelphia, 1971, W. B. Saunders Co.

38 Hayes, A. H.: The actions and clinical use of the newer antiarrhythmic drugs, Ration. Drug Ther. **6:**1, 1972.

38a Katz, A. M.: Arrhythmias, Hosp. Pract. p. 15, May, 1980.

39 Lee, W. K.: The rational use of drugs in the management of heart block, Ration. Drug Ther. **9**(11):1, 1975.

40 Mason, D. T., Spann, J. F., Zelis, R., and Amsterdam, E. A.: The clinical pharmacology and therapeutic applications of the antiarrhythmic drugs, Clin. Pharmacol. Ther. **11:**460, 1970.

41 Moe, G.: Reentry, Med. Coll. Va. Quart **9:**33, 1973.

42 Moe, G. K., and Mendez, C.: Physiologic basis of premature beats and sustained tachycardias, N. Engl. J. Med. **288:**250, 1973.

42a Pine, M. B., and Aronow, W. S.: The treatment of ventricular premature complexes, Ration. Drug Ther. **14:**1, Nov., 1980.

43 Singh, B. N., Collett, J. T., and Chew C. Y. C.: New perspectives in the pharmacologic therapy of cardiac arrhythmias, Prog. Cardiovasc. Dis. **22:**243, 1980.

44 Surawicz, B.: Ventricular tachyarrhythmias, Med. Coll. Va. Quart. **9:**48, 1973.

45 Surawicz, B.: Arrhythmias and atiarrhythmic therapy in context, Hosp. Pract., p. 59, June, 1976.

46 Valentine, P. A., Frew, J. L., Mashford, M. L., and Sloman, J. G.: Lidocaine in the prevention of sudden death in the pre-hospital phase of acute infarction, N. Engl. J. Med. **291:**1327, 1974.

47 Waller, E. S.: Appropriate lidocaine doses—science added to the art, Tex. Med. (In press).

48 Wasserman, A. J., and Proctor, J. D.: Pharmacology of antiarrhythmias: quinidine, beta-blockers, diphenylhydantoin, bretylium, Med. Coll. Va. Quart. **9:**53, 1973.

49 Yeh, B. K., and Gosselin, A. J.: Current status of antidysrhythmic drugs, Ration. Drug Ther. **9:**1, 1975.

CHAPTER 36

Antianginal drugs

GENERAL CONCEPT

It is an old empiric observation that amyl nitrite (1867) and nitroglycerin (1879) relieve the pain of angina pectoris. Since nitrates and nitrites dilate blood vessels, including the coronary arteries, the role of coronary vasodilatation in the relief of angina has been generally assumed.

The problem is much more complex, however. Angina results from an imbalance between oxygen demand and supply in ischemic areas of the myocardium. Drugs may improve angina theoretically by reducing the demand or by increasing the supply of oxygen. There is increasing evidence for a reduction of demand by an action on the peripheral circulation as a primary mechanism for the antianginal effect of the nitrates and nitrites. On the other hand, drugs that increase myocardial oxygen demand, such as the catecholamines, have adverse effects in patients with coronary disease.

The simple view that coronary vasodilatation is sufficient to explain the antianginal effect of the rapidly acting nitrites has been made untenable by the discovery of drugs (such as dipyridamole) that are potent coronary vasodilators but are not effective as antianginal drugs.

In addition to the short-acting nitrites and nitrates, there are several longer-acting drugs. These prevent anginal attacks also when administered sublingually. However, their prophylactic value when administered orally is controversial.

The use of propranolol, a β-adrenergic blocking drug, emphasizes the importance of reduction of cardiac work in the relief of angina. The drug should not be used in unstable angina caused by coronary spasm. Verapamil and other blockers of the slow calcium channel are investigational drugs in the treatment of coronary spasm.

CORONARY VASO-DILATORS
Nitrates and nitrites

A variety of nitrites and nitrates are useful in medicine because of their relaxing effect on various smooth muscles. The coronary blood vessels are so susceptible to this action that minute doses can cause an increase in coronary blood flow.

Chemistry and preparations

The clinically useful nitrites and nitrates exert qualitatively similar effects. The most interesting compounds in the group and their formulas are as follows:

Nitrates

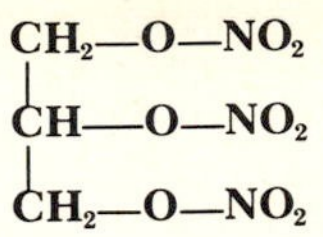

$$CH_2\!-\!O\!-\!NO_2$$
$$CH\!-\!O\!-\!NO_2$$
$$CH_2\!-\!O\!-\!NO_2$$

Glyceryl trinitrate

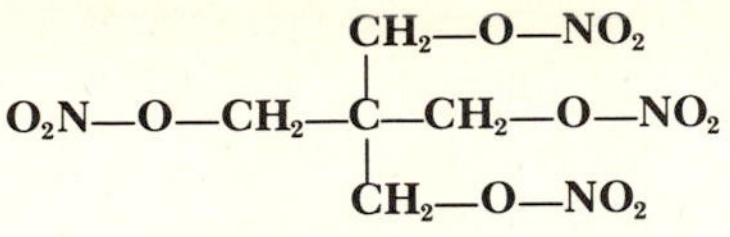

$$O_2N\!-\!O\!-\!CH_2\!-\!\overset{\displaystyle CH_2\!-\!O\!-\!NO_2}{\underset{\displaystyle CH_2\!-\!O\!-\!NO_2}{C}}\!-\!CH_2\!-\!O\!-\!NO_2$$

Pentaerythritol tetranitrate

$$N\!\begin{cases} CH_2\!-\!CH_2\!-\!O\!-\!NO_2 \\ CH_2\!-\!CH_2\!-\!O\!-\!NO_2 \cdot 2H_3PO_4 \\ CH_2\!-\!CH_2\!-\!O\!-\!NO_2 \end{cases}$$

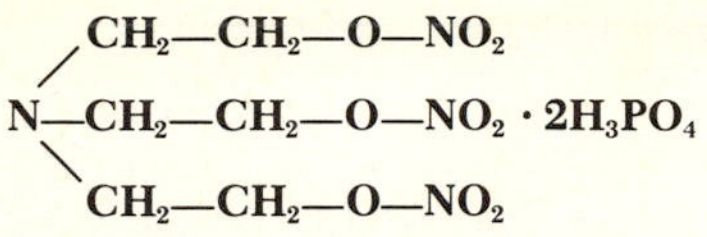

Triethanolamine trinitrate biphosphate

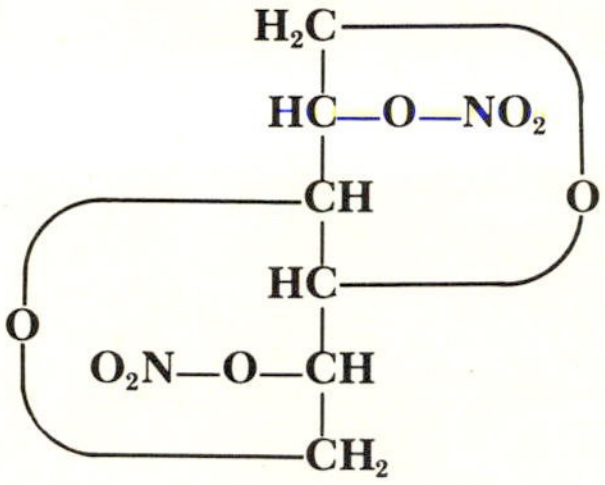

Isosorbide dinitrate

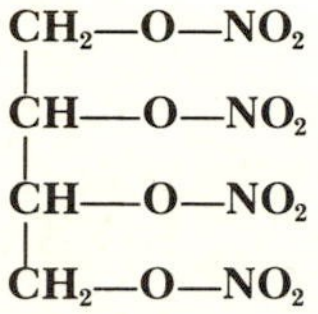

$$CH_2\!-\!O\!-\!NO_2$$
$$CH\!-\!O\!-\!NO_2$$
$$CH\!-\!O\!-\!NO_2$$
$$CH_2\!-\!O\!-\!NO_2$$

Erythrityl tetranitrate

Nitrites

$$NaNO_2$$

Sodium nitrite

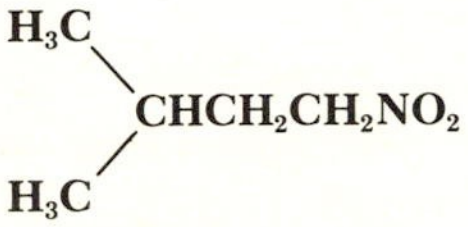

$$\begin{matrix} H_3C \\ {} \\ H_3C \end{matrix}\!\!\!\!CHCH_2CH_2NO_2$$

Amyl nitrite

The nitrates are classified as *sublingual* and *oral*. The sublingual nitrates include nitroglycerin, isosorbide dinitrate, and erythrityl tetranitrate. Oral nitrates include, in addition to the ones previously mentioned, mannitol hexanitrate and pentaerythritol tetranitrate. Nitroglycerin is available also in an ointment form.

Effects of nitroglycerin

If a patient suffering from an attack of angina pectoris places a small 0.3 mg tablet of nitroglycerin under the tongue, the attack frequently subsides in a matter of minutes. Furthermore, the drug is often effective if taken prophylactically before the performance of some task that ordinarily produces angina.

This is not a placebo effect. Although a large proportion of patients suffering from angina pectoris claim benefit from placebo tablets, a significantly greater number derive benefit from nitroglycerin. Furthermore, if a patient between anginal attacks is asked to perform a standard exercise tolerance test such as the Master two-step test, precordial pain and T-wave inversion on the electrocardiogram may be developed, generally interpreted as consequences of myocardial ischemia. If the same patient has received prophylactic nitroglycerin, he or she is often protected against both the pain and the electrocardiographic alterations during exercise.

TABLE 36-1. Effect of nitrites and β-blocking drugs on myocardial oxygen requirements and supply*

	Nitrites	β blockade
Determinants of myocardial oxygen requirements		
Heart rate	↑	↓†
Left ventricular pressure	↓	↓†
Left ventricular volume and radius	↓	↑
Velocity of contraction	↑	↓†
Systolic ejection period	↓	↑
Determinants of myocardial oxygen supply		
Coronary vascular bed	↑†	↓

*Courtesy Dr. Lawrence Cohen.
†Most significant effects.

The simplest interpretation of this remarkable effect of nitroglycerin would be that the drug improves blood flow to ischemic areas in the myocardium by dilating coronary vessels. This interpretation, however, appears to be untenable.

Problem 36-1. Would nitroglycerin administered directly into a coronary artery relieve angina? This has been tested by two clinical investigators.[5] In 25 patients undergoing cardiac catheterization as possible candidates for revascularization surgery, 0.075 mg of nitroglycerin was injected into the left coronary artery through the angiographic catheter at a time when angina was induced by pacing. The intracoronary injection was ineffective despite a significant increase in coronary sinus blood flow in many of the patients. Intravenous injection of 0.2 mg of nitroglycerin relieved the angina that was unaffected by the preceding intracoronary injection. This study indicates that it is the action of nitroglycerin on the systemic circulation that is responsible for its antianginal effect.

The antianginal effect of nitroglycerin is believed to result from reduction of venous tone, diminished venous return, some peripheral arterial dilatation, and to a questionable extent from dilatation of those coronary arteries that are capable of responding to the drug.[25]

In addition to the coronary vessels, certain other vascular areas are quite susceptible to the action of nitrites. The skin vessels of the face and neck, the so-called blush areas, may be markedly dilated. Meningeal vessels are dilated also, and this is the probable cause of the headache that may be produced by the nitrites.

Effects of nitroglycerin and nitrites on other smooth muscles

Probably all smooth muscles can be made to relax by the nitrites, and some minor therapeutic applications of this effect have been made. The biliary tract can be relaxed with sublingual nitroglycerin, as evidenced by a measured decrease in biliary pressure. The nitrites also can relax the ureter. Although they have been shown to relax the bronchial smooth muscle, much more effective medications are available for this purpose.

Amyl nitrite is a volatile liquid that is available in small glass pearls containing 0.2 ml. These are crushed in a handkerchief by the patient and inhaled. Amyl nitrite has a short onset of action, less than 1 minute, but its duration of action is also short, not exceeding 10 minutes. It is particularly prone to cause cutaneous vasodilatation, marked lowering of systemic pressure, and even syncope and tachycardia. In addition, its odor is objectionable, particularly when used by ambulatory patients. For these reasons nitroglycerin is preferred.

Comparison of nitro-glycerin with other nitrites and nitrates

Sodium nitrite has more toxicological than therapeutic importance. Although its smooth muscle effects are similar to those of other nitrites, its irritant effects on the gastric mucosa and its tendency to produce methemoglobin make it unsuitable as a coronary vasodilator.

Isosorbide dinitrate (5 mg) and erythrityl tetranitrate (5 mg) given sublingually are effective, and their duration of action is longer than that of nitroglycerin. Their onset of action is slower also, 2 to 5 minutes.[26] Nitroglycerin ointments applied to the skin may produce a more prolonged effect than the sublingual tablets. Tolerance to the longer-acting nitrates given sublingually may occur. This problem is not significant with nitroglycerin.

Tolerance develops to headache produced by nitrates. Thus, munitions workers when first exposed to nitrates complain of headaches, but they become tolerant in a few days. They may also develop nitrate dependence, since some workers, when they terminate their exposure to the chemical, may develop anginal attacks. Despite these observations, tolerance to the antianginal effects of the nitrates and nitrites apparently does not occur, and nitrate dependence is not a problem in patients who take these drugs by the oral route for long periods of time.

Tolerance to vascular actions of nitrites

The toxic effects of nitrites and nitrates are generally predictable from known pharmacological actions of these compounds. Severe fall of blood pressure with syncope, headaches, glaucoma, and elevated intracranial pressure can result from excessive dosage or unusual susceptibility of the patient. In addition, the nitrites can produce methemoglobinemia by oxidizing the iron of the hemoglobin molecule from the ferrous to the ferric state. This ability is used to advantage in the treatment of cyanide poisoning.[2]

Toxic effects of nitrites and nitrates

Nitrite poisoning may be acute or chronic. It may result from the therapeutic or accidental intake of nitrites or from the ingestion of some nitrate that may be converted to nitrites by intestinal bacteria, as has occurred following the ingestion of bismuth subnitrate. Increasing attention is paid to the fact that well water in some rural areas may contain enough nitrate to cause chronic intoxication with methemoglobinemia. Chronic poisoning from nitrates and nitrites is an industrial hazard, particularly in the explosives industry.

There is increasing concern also about the addition of nitrites and nitrates to meat products. The nitrites may be converted in the stomach to nitrosamines, which are carcinogenic.

Metabolism of organic nitrates

Organic nitrates are changed in the body to nitrites.[12] Blood levels of nitrites, however, do not correlate well with antiginal activity. It has been suggested that coronary dilator activity depends on the intact molecule of the organic nitrate and not on reduction to nitrite. Thus isosorbide dinitrate, although it did not undergo hydrolysis and reduction, evoked increased coronary blood flow in the perfused rabbit heart.[8]

The degradation of nitroglycerin occurs primarily in the liver[11] by means of a glutathione-dependent organic nitrate reductase. The activity of the liver is largely responsible for the ineffectiveness of orally administered nitrates compared with the sublingually given tablets.

Therapeutic aims in use of nitrites and nitrates

The most important indication for the use of these compounds is the management of angina pectoris. Experimental uses include also the treatment of left ventricular failure and a possible reduction of ischemic injury.[23] The nitrates are occasionally used also in the management of biliary colic and ureteral spasm.

Papaverine and related drugs

Papaverine is an alkaloid of opium. Its formula indicates that it is a benzylisoquinoline compound, differing from the morphine group of opium alkaloids both chemically and pharmacologically. Papaverine is not a narcotic and is not addictive.

Papaverine hydrochloride is available for oral administration and for injection. The average dose is 100 mg.

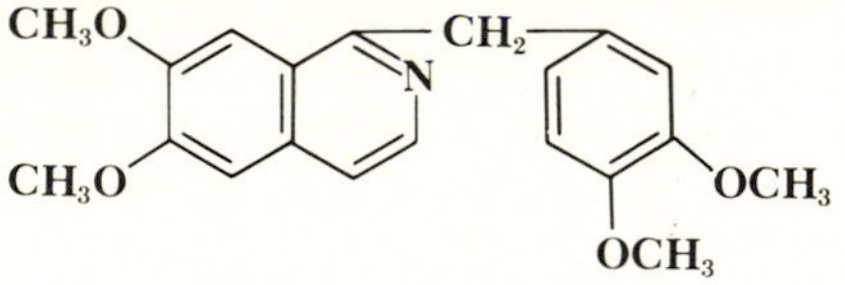

Papaverine

The main pharmacological effect of papaverine is smooth muscle relaxation. In addition, it has a moderate quinidine-like effect on the heart.

Papaverine has been tried in the treatment of angina pectoris and in peripheral vascular diseases, but its effects are not convincing.

Aminophylline and other theophylline compounds

In angina patients the evidence for the usefulness of theophylline compounds is quite conflicting. Several investigators have been unable to demonstrate any benefit from theophylline in reducing the incidence of anginal attacks.[5]

The greatest usefulness of aminophylline is in the treatment of bronchial asthma. It is used occasionally also as an adjunct to certain diuretics such as the mercurials.

Other drugs

Ethyl alcohol has the undeserved reputation of being a coronary vasodilator. Studies of Russek and associates[18] show that although the drug can prevent pain in angina patients following the standard exercise test, it does not prevent electrocardiographic changes in the T waves and RS-T segments. The conclusion seems to be that alcohol acts on the brain rather than on the coronary arteries.

Dipyridamole (Persantine), or 2,6-bis(diethanolamino)-4,8-dipiperidinopyrimido[5,4-*d*] pyrimidine, has been introduced for coronary insufficiency. It is claimed that the drug has dual action, dilating coronary arteries and also influencing myocardial metabolism. Interestingly, although the drug is claimed to increase the oxygen supply to the heart, it is of little or no value in the treatment of angina pectoris.[3] Dipyridamole inhibits platelet aggregation, an action discussed on p. 485.

The overall impression of clinical pharmacologists may be summarized by saying that nitroglycerin is an excellent antianginal drug, particularly for prophylactic therapy. Other coronary vasodilators are recommended by some investigators, but their usefulness is questioned by others.

The usefulness of the long-acting dilators, such as isosorbide dinitrate, in patients with ischemic heart disease has been controversial. Administered sublingually, isosorbide dinitrate improves exercise ability. It has been claimed, however, that the oral administration is not effective because of rapid inactivation of the drug in the liver.[13] Recent studies performed in patients with acute coronary insufficiency tend to indicate effectiveness of isosorbide dinitrate by both the sublingual and oral route of administration.[14]

The experimental use of β-adrenergic blocking agents as antianginal drugs represents a radically new approach to the problem.[7] Propranolol must be used cautiously because it may induce congestive failure and hypotension. It may also increase airway resistance in asthmatic patients. The β blockers reduce the oxygen requirement of the heart and may be effective for 6 hours. Newer β blockers such as practolol, sotalol, and alprenolol may be more selective than propranolol and have been used in the United Kingdom.

CLINICAL PHARMACOLOGY OF ANTIANGINAL DRUGS

Variant angina, or Prinzmetal's angina, is characterized by chest pain at rest rather than following exercise. Coronary artery spasm appears to be the cause of the chest pain and S-T segment elevation.[22]

Attacks may be precipitated by the administration of epinephrine, norepinephrine, and sympathomimetic drugs in general. Propranolol may aggravate variant angina. Ergonovine maleate, a constrictor of vascular smooth muscle, is being used as a diagnostic agent for variant angina. However, the drug is not without danger, since it can cause prolonged spasm of the coronary arteries. Nitroglycerin may relieve the spasm produced by ergonovine maleate.

Variant angina should be treated with sublingual or oral nitrates. Propranolol should not be used, since blockade of β receptors may lead to coronary vasoconstriction by unopposed α-receptor activity.

DRUGS IN VARIANT ANGINA

REFERENCES

1 Amsterdam, E. A., Gorlin, R., and Wolfson, S.: Evaluation of long-term use of propranolol in angina pectoris, J.A.M.A. **210:**103, 1969.

2 Chen, K. K., Rose, C. L., and Clowes, G. H. A.: Comparative values of several antidotes in cyanide poisoning, Am. J. Med. Sci. **188:**767, 1934.

3 DeGraff, A. C., and Lyon, A. F.: Evaluation of dipyridamole (Persantin), Am. Heart J. **65:**423, 1963.

4 Epstein, S. E.: Treatment of angina pectoris by electrical stimulation of the carotid sinus nerves; results in 17 patients with severe angina, N. Engl. J. Med. **280:**971, 1969.

5 Ganz, W., and Marcus, H. S.: Failure of intracoronary nitroglycerin to alleviate pacing-induced angina, Circulation **46:**880, 1972.

6 Haddy, F. J.: Physiology and pharmacology of the coronary circulation and myocardium, particularly in relation to coronary artery disease, Am. J. Med. **47:**274, 1969.

7 Hamer, J.: The effect of propranolol (Inderal) in angina pectoris, Br. Med. J. **2:**720, 1964.

8 Krantz, J. C., Lu, G. G., Bell, F. K., and Cascorbi, H. F.: Nitrites. XIX. Studies of the mechanism of action of glyceryl trinitrate, Biochem. Pharmacol. **2:**1095, 1962.

9 Mason, D. T., Spann, J. F., Zelis, R., and Amsterdam, E. A.: Physiologic approach to the treatment of angina pectoris, N. Engl. J. Med. **281:**1225, 1969.

10 Needleman, P.: Tolerance to the vascular effects of glyceryl trinitrate, J. Pharmacol. Exp. Ther. **171:**98, 1970.

11 Needleman, P., Blehm, D. J., Harkey, A. B., Johnson, E. M., and Lang, S.: The metabolic pathway in the degradation of glyceryl trinitrate, J. Pharmacol. Exp. Ther. **179:**347, 1971.

12 Needleman, P., and Krantz, J. C., Jr.: The biotransformation of nitroglycerin, Biochem. Pharmacol. **14:**1225, 1965.

13 Needleman, P., Lang, S., and Johnson, E. M.: Organic nitrates: relationship between biotransformation and rational angina pectoris therapy, J. Pharmacol. Exp. Ther. **181:**489, 1972.

14 Poliner, L. R., Ritter, W., Wohl, A. J., Nixon, J. V., and Willerson, J. T.: Hemodynamic effects of oral and sublingual forms of isosorbide dinitrate in patients with acute coronary insufficiency, Tex. Med. **73:**53, 1977.

15 Rowe, G. G.: Effects of drugs on the coronary circulation of man, Clin. Pharmacol. Ther. **7:**547, 1966.

16 Russek, H. I.: Propranolol and isosorbide dinitrate synergism in angina pectoris, Am. J. Cardiol. **24:**44, 1968.

17 Russek, H. I., and Howard, J. C.: Glyceryl trinitrate in angina pectoris, J.A.M.A. **189:**108, 1964.

18 Russek, H. I., Naegele, C. F., and Regan, F. D.: Alcohol in the treatment of angina pectoris, J.A.M.A. **143:**355, 1950.

19 Sjoerdsma, A., Axelrod, J., Shofer, R., King, W. M., and Davidson, J. D.: Fate of papaverine, Fed. Proc. **154:**58, 1956.

20 Winbury, M. M.: Experimental approaches to the development of antianginal drugs, Adv. Pharmacol. **3:**2, 1964.

21 Winbury, M. M., Howe, B. B., and Hefner, M. A.: Effect of nitrates and other coronary dilators on large and small coronary vessels; an hypothesis for the mechanism of action of nitrates, J. Pharmacol. Exp. Ther. **168:**70, 1969.

REVIEWS

22 Aronow, W. S.: The treatment of variant angina pectoris, Ration. Drug Ther. **13:**1, 1979.

23 Epstein, S. E., Kent, K. M., Goldstein, R. E., Borer, J. S., and Redwood, D. R.: Reduction of ischemic injury by nitroglycerin during acute myocardial infarction, N. Engl. J. Med. **292:**29, 1975.

23a Karlsberg, R. P., and Aronow, W. S.: Reduction of myocardial infarct size; approach for the 1980s, Arch. Intern. Med. **140:**616, 1980.

24 Melville, K. I.: The pharmacological basis of antianginal drugs, Pharmacol. Phys. **4:**1, 1970.

25 Oglesby, P.: Angina pectoris, Ration. Drug Ther. **6:**1, 1972.

26 Parmley, W. W.: Therapy of angina pectoris, Ration. Drug. Ther. **9:**1, 1975.

27 Reichek, N.: Long-acting nitrates in the treatment of angina pectoris, J.A.M.A. **236:**1399, 1976.

28 Thadani, U., Davidson, C., Singleton, W., and Taylor, S. H.: Comparison of the immediate effects of five β-adrenoreceptor-blocking drugs with different ancillary properties in angina pectoris, N. Engl. J. Med. **300:**750, 1979.

CHAPTER 37

Anticoagulant drugs

Anticoagulants prevent the development or propagation of a thrombus. Their value is clear in venous thromboembolism but is somewhat less certain in the management of arterial thrombosis.

Heparin inhibits the action of thrombin by activation of antithrombin III. The orally administered anticoagulants, derivatives of 4-hydroxycoumarin and indandione, produce a delayed decrease in the activity of vitamin K–dependent coagulation factors, such as factors VII, IX, X, and II.

Theoretically, inhibitors of platelet aggregation and adhesion should have a favorable effect in the prevention of thrombosis. Dipyridamole, aspirin, and a number of other drugs are effective in vitro, but further experience is needed for demonstrating their in vivo usefulness.

There are additional approaches to the treatment of thrombosis. Streptokinase and urokinase activate plasminogen and may dissolve some intravascular thrombi. The venom of the Malayan pit viper causes fibrinogen depletion by direct conversion of fibrinogen to fibrin. Its use is experimental.

Heparin is antagonized by protamine sulfate and coumarin anticoagulants by vitamin K. Heparin therapy may be monitored by whole blood-clotting time, whereas the coumarin and indandione anticoagulants require prothrombin time determinations, most commonly by the Quick one-stage procedure.

GENERAL CONCEPT

A schematic picture of current views of coagulation is as follows:

CLOTTING PROCESS AND DRUG ACTION

Phase I —Formation of activated thromboplastin

Interaction of Hageman factor, glasslike surface, antihemophilic factor, Christmas factor, plasma thromboplastin antecedent, platelets, and calcium lead to plasma thromboplastin; plasma thromboplastin may be acted on by tissue thromboplastin, Stuart factor (factor X), and serum prothrombin conversion accelerator (SPCA or factor VII) in the presence of calcium to form activated thromboplastin.

Phase II —Activated thromboplastin

$$\text{Prothrombin} \xrightarrow{\text{Calcium and proaccelerin (factor V)}} \text{Thrombin}$$

Phase III —Thrombin

$$\text{Fibrinogen} \longrightarrow \text{Fibrin}$$

Phase IV —Fibrinolysin (plasmin)

$$\text{Fibrin} \longrightarrow \text{Lysed fibrin}$$

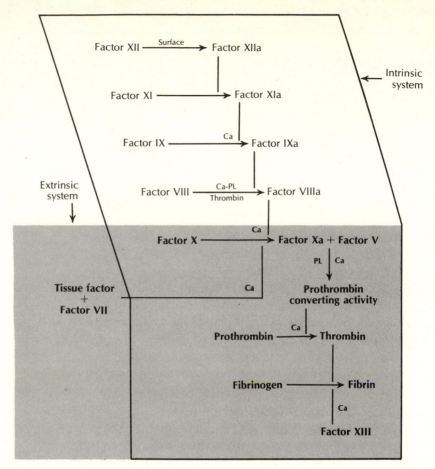

FIG. 37-1. Scheme of blood coagulation. Reactions enclosed by solid lines are of the "intrinsic system," whereas those within the shaded box are of the "extrinsic system." *PL,* Phospholipid; *Ca,* calcium. (From Williams, W. J.: Res. Staff Phys. **15:**39, 1969.)

The clotting process according to this scheme may be divided into four stages. Thromboplastin is generated in the first stage, thrombin in the second, and fibrin in the third. The fourth stage is that of fibrin and fibrinolysin. A more up-to-date scheme of coagulation is shown in Fig. 37-1, and the blood coagulation factors are listed on p. 480.

Coagulation is vulnerable to drug action at several points. In vitro, inactivation of calcium by oxalate, citrate, or ethylenediaminetetraacetic acid (EDTA) will prevent clotting. This approach is not effective in vivo because ionized calcium levels sufficiently low to accomplish an anticoagulant effect are incompatible with life. Heparin and similar highly charged molecules can block clotting both in vitro and in vivo. Finally, compounds that block the production of some of the proteins that are essential in the scheme will prevent clotting in vivo but not in the test tube. This is the mode of action of the coumarins.

ANTICOAGULANTS
Heparin

Heparin is a sulfated mucopolysaccharide containing fractions varying in molecular weight between 6000 and 25,000. Commercial heparin is obtained from beef lung or hog intestinal mucosa.

From a chemical standpoint, heparin is a sulfated mucopolysaccharide composed of repeating units of sulfated glucosamine and glucuronic acid. It is a strong acid and is available in the form of its sodium salt.

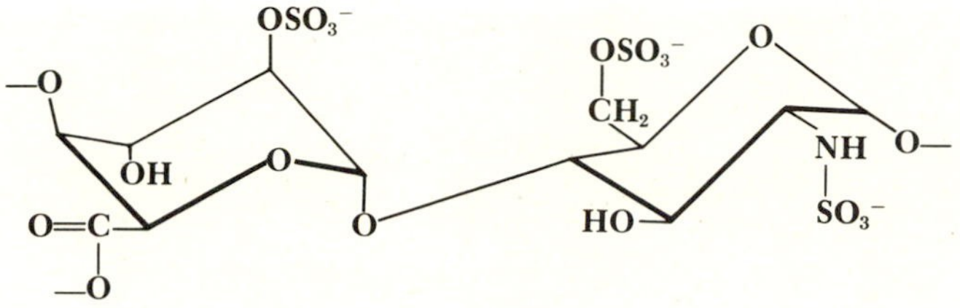

Configuration of disaccharides in heparin

Anticoagulant effect

Heparin inhibits clotting both in vitro and in vivo. It activates antithrombin III in plasma. This α_2 globulin binds heparin and undergoes a change that increases the rate of its inactivating effect on thrombin.

The anticoagulant half-life of heparin injected intravenously varies from 1 to 2 hours. In extensive intravascular thrombosis, an antiheparin, platelet factor 4, is released, which leads to increased heparin requirements.[45]

In addition to its direct anticoagulant effect, heparin may be taken up by endothelial cells, altering the properties of the blood vessels.[47]

Monitoring of anticoagulant activity following heparin administration has been done traditionally by the Lee-White clotting time. This is being abandoned because of poor reproducibility. Instead, the partial thromboplastin time and the thrombin clotting time are being used.[45]

Lipemia-clearing effect

Injected heparin has the remarkable ability of decreasing the turbidity of plasma following alimentary hyperlipemia.[15] Interest in this phenomenon has been growing steadily.

When heparin is added in vitro to lipemic plasma, it causes no clearing. On the other hand, when lipemic plasma is added to clear plasma from an animal that has received heparin, clearing takes place.

The actual clearing factor appears to be a lipase that catalyzes the hydrolysis of triglycerides. The triglycerides of plasma are associated with proteins in the chylomicrons. Neutral fats that are split off by the enzyme from the chylomicrons are gradually dissolved in the plasma. Probably through the same mechanism, the β lipoproteins, which are of high molecular weight and low density, are transformed into α lipoproteins of lower molecular weight and high density.[14]

BLOOD COAGULATION FACTORS*

Factor I	Fibrinogen
Factor II	Prothrombin
Factor III	Tissue factor, tissue thromboplastin, thrombokinase
Factor IV	Calcium
Factor V	Proaccelerin, labile factor, plasma Ac-globulin
Factor VI	
Factor VII	Proconvertin, stable factor, serum prothrombin conversion accelerator (SPCA)
Factor VIII	Antihemophilic globulin (AHG), antihemophilic factor (AHF)
Factor IX	Plasma thromboplastin component (PTC), Christmas factor
Factor X	Stuart-Prower factor
Factor XI	Plasma thromboplastin antecedent (PTA), antihemophilic factor C
Factor XII	Hageman factor
Factor XIII	Fibrin-stabilizing factor, fibrinase

*Modified from Williams, W. J.: Res. Staff Phys. **15**:39, 1969.

The clearing factor is present in various tissues and appears to be released from its binding sites by heparin. Heparin is most probably an integral part of the lipase and may provide a link between enzyme and substrate.

The lipemia-clearing effect of heparin requires much smaller doses than those necessary for significant anticoagulant action. Lipemia is cleared by doses of less than 1 μg/kg in the rat and as little as 2 mg in humans. Larger doses of heparin, however, will release greater enzyme activity.

Administration and dosage

Heparin is not absorbed from the gastrointestinal tract. In order to obtain an anticoagulant effect the sodium salt of heparin is injected intravenously or subcutaneously.

The usual intravenous dose of heparin is an initial 5000 units, followed by doses of 5000 to 10,000 units every 4 hours for a total of 25,000 units daily. Recent studies indicate that small subcutaneous doses of 5000 units may be useful in the prevention of deep vein thrombosis.[11]

Commercial preparations of heparin are bioassayed on the basis of anticoagulant action in comparison with a standard preparation. One hundred USP units corresponds to about 1 mg of heparin.

Preparations

Heparin sodium USP is available as a suspension for injection, 1000, 5000, 10,000, 20,000, and 40,000 units/ml, and as a gel for repository injection, 20,000 units/ml.

Toxicity

Except for its anticoagulant effect, heparin is quite inert pharmacologically. An intravenous injection of 5 mg/kg is used routinely in experimental animals, and this large quantity has no significant effects on blood pressure, heart rate, or respiration. In its clinical use heparin may promote bleeding from open wounds and mucous membranes, especially when dosage is excessive. Some believe that cerebral hemorrhage may be precipitated in susceptible patients. Elderly women are especially susceptible to heparin.[20]

In humans, long-term heparin treatment may result in osteoporosis.[19] Also, symptoms suggesting hypersensitivity and inhibition of aldosterone secretion have been reported.

Heparin antagonists

The effects of heparin overdosage will last only a relatively short time because the drug is metabolized in a few hours. If hemorrhage threatens during even a short waiting period, chemical antidotes are available.

Protamine sulfate will combine with heparin milligram for milligram to block its anticoagulant effect both in the test tube and in the patient.

Toluidine blue and **hexadimethrine** (Polybrene) have also been used clinically as heparin antagonists but are now considered obsolete.

Metabolism and excretion

After intravenous injection, blood levels of heparin decline exponentially with a half-life of about 1 hour. Although most of the heparin is metabolized in the body, as much as 50% of a large intravenous dose may be excreted in the urine.[50]

Coumarin and indandione anticoagulants
Development

The story of the introduction of the coumarin compounds into therapeutics is unusually interesting. It has been known for many years that cattle can develop a hemorrhagic disease when they eat spoiled sweet clover. It has also been known that the hemorrhages are caused by lowered prothrombin levels in the animals. In 1941 Link[26] and associates at the University of Wisconsin showed that a coumarin compound was responsible for this hemorrhagic disease of cattle. They synthesized dicumarol, which has been used quite extensively in clinical practice and was the forerunner of a number of coumarin and indandione derivatives.

The various coumarin anticoagulants act by the same basic mechanism. They inhibit the formation of prothrombin, factor VII (proconvertin), factor IX (Christmas), and factor X (Stuart-Prower factor).

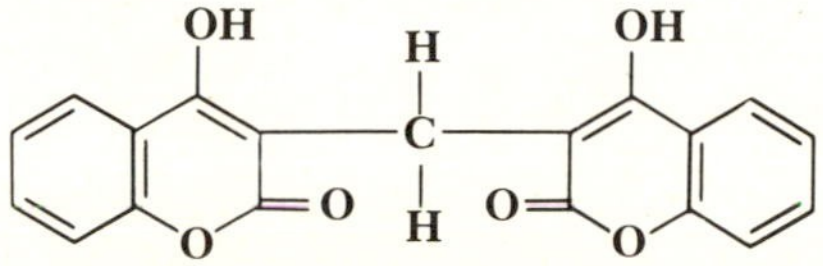

Dicumarol

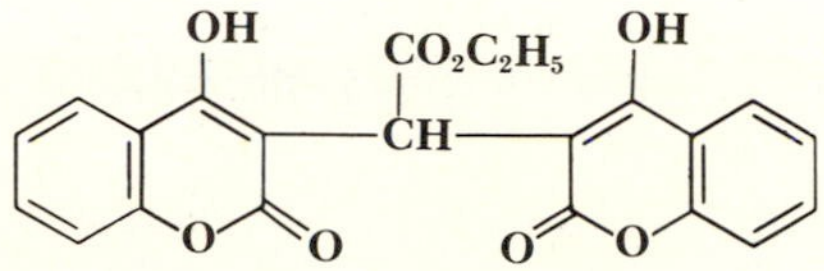

Ethyl biscoumacetate

The coumarin anticoagulants include, in addition to dicumarol, warfarin sodium (Coumadin sodium), warfarin potassium (Athrombin-K), acenocoumarol (Sintrom),

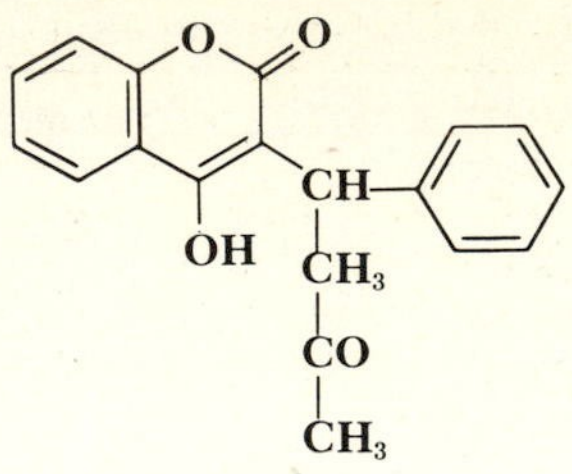

Warfarin

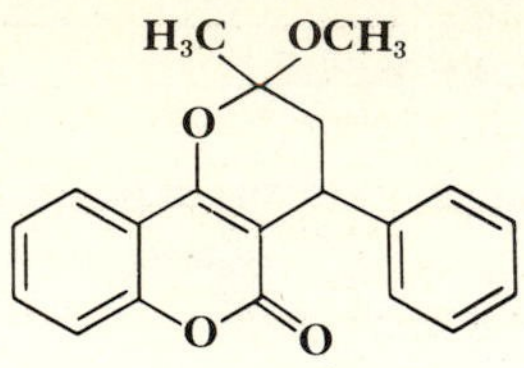

Cyclocumarol

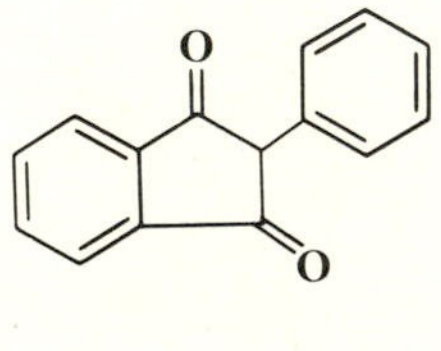

Phenindione

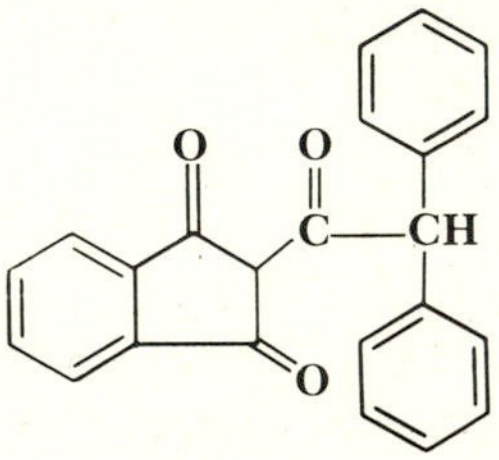

Diphenadione

and phenprocoumon (Liquamar). The indandione derivatives are phenindione (Danilone, eridione, Hedulin), diphenadione (Dipaxin), and anisindione (Miradon).

Mode of action   There is a characteristic delay in the action of these compounds. This is understandable because the normal prothrombin content of the plasma must decline before the evidence of deficient synthesis can manifest itself. The coumarin compounds vary in speed of onset and duration of action, probably because of their varying speeds of absorption and metabolic degradation.

The administration of vitamin K can reverse the coumarin-induced hypoprothrombinemia. This fact and the structural similarities between these compounds suggest that the coumarins act as antimetabolites of vitamin K.

The exact mode of action of the coumarin anticoagulants is not known. Studies suggest that these drugs inhibit the transport of vitamin K to its site of action in liver cells.[27]

It has also been suggested that the coumarins lead to the synthesis of abnormal forms of the clotting factors, which do not function effectively.[45]

Variations in susceptibility   There is great individual variation in susceptibility to the coumarin anticoagulants. The variation is a consequence of many factors. Absorption from the intestine, metabolic transformation, diet, and genetically conditioned resistance[26] may all contribute.

Prothrombin concentration during coumarin therapy is measured by comparing the prothrombin time of the patient's plasma with that of normal plasma. In the usual one-stage prothrombin test, thromboplastin is added to citrated plasma at 37° C. Calcium chloride is then added in excess and the time for clotting is recorded. It is

TABLE 37-1. Average doses of various coumarin and indandione anticoagulants

Preparation	Average initial dose (mg)	Average maintenance dose (mg)
Dicumarol	300	100-200
Warfarin sodium (Coumadin sodium)	60	10
Acenocoumarin (Sintrom)	15-25	2-10
Phenprocoumon (Liquamar)	20-30	1-5
Phenindione (Hedulin; Danilone)	100-200	25-50
Diphenadione (Dipaxin)	20-30	15

known now that the test measures not only prothrombin but also such other components as factor VII.

During therapy with the coumarin drugs it is desirable to maintain prothrombin concentration at 20% of normal, and dosage is adjusted to achieve this aim. Without such laboratory control, use of the coumarins would be dangerous. Severe depression of prothrombin concentration may be associated with bleeding, which can manifest itself as microscopic hematuria or even such severe bleeding as cerebral hemorrhage.

Two methods are available for counteracting the action of the coumarin drug and their congeners: fresh whole blood transfusion and use of vitamin K preparations.

Vitamin K as antidote to prothrombin-depressant drugs

Among the most effective antidotes for coumarin poisoning is phytonadione (vitamin K_1; Mephyton), which is water soluble and may be administered intravenously in doses of 100 to 200 mg. Vitamin K_1 oxide and phytonadione are administered as emulsions. When used in large doses as antidotes, the vitamin K preparations have prolonged action and prevent reinstitution of coumarin or indandione therapy for as long as 2 weeks. Some advocate the use of much smaller doses for this reason. Vitamin K preparations have no effect on the anticoagulant action of heparin.

Anticoagulants are indicated for the prevention and treatment of deep venous thrombosis and pulmonary embolism, in some stages of myocardial infarction, in prevention of arterial embolism in mitral stenosis, in patients with prosthetic heart valves (when the simultaneous use of aspirin may be beneficial), in cardioversion, in cerebrovascular disease, in systemic coagulopathy, and during cardiovascular operations.[45]

CLINICAL PHARMACOLOGY AND DRUG INTERACTIONS

Heparin is the most effective and safest anticoagulant. On the one hand, the necessity for frequent injections and its high cost are disadvantages. On the other hand, the effectiveness of small subcutaneous doses of heparin in the prevention of venous thrombosis is of great current interest.[11] Disadvantages of the coumarins and the indandiones are delay in action and need for careful laboratory control for adjustment of dosage.

Phenindione has caused serious toxic effects such as agranulocytosis and liver damage. Many clinical investigators in the United States prefer the coumarins and find that warfarin is one of the best from the standpoint of ease of regulation. According to one survey, there is no justification for the preference of heparin over warfarin for anticoagulation following myocardial infarction.[35] It is a good rule for physicians to use the anticoagulant with which they are thoroughly familiar and only if they have facilities for one-stage prothrombin time determinations.

Drug interactions in the clinical use of coumarin anticoagulants are of great importance. (See also Chapter 63.) Some drugs stimulate the metabolic degradation of the coumarins and thus decrease their effectiveness. Other drugs increase the effectiveness of the anticoagulants by blocking their metabolism or by interfering with their binding to plasma proteins.

Drug effects on the response to coumarin anticoagulants are as follows:

Drugs that increase the effect of coumarin anticoagulants
- Antibiotics affecting the intestinal flora
- Phenylbutazone and some other acidic drugs
- Salicylates (large doses)
- Chloral hydrate
- Clofibrate
- Disulfiram
- Adrogenic anabolic steroids
- Methylphenidate
- Propylthiouracil
- *d*-Thyroxine

Drugs that decrease the effect of coumarin anticoagulants
- Barbiturates
- Ethchlorvynol
- Glutethimide
- Griseofulvin

Coumarin potentiation of other drugs
- Tolbutamide
- Phenytoin

FIBRINOLYSIN   Blood has the inherent capacity of dissolving clots by means of the fibrinolytic system. There are reasons to believe that this system functions under normal circumstances to remove minor fibrin depositions that occur in small vessels. Clotted blood may be injected repeatedly into rabbits without being demonstrable at autopsy. It is presumably dissolved through fibrinolysis.

Fibrinolysin, also called *plasmin* by some investigators, is a proteolytic enzyme that attacks a variety of proteins but has a great affinity for fibrinogen or fibrin. A schematic representation of the human fibrinolytic system is shown below.

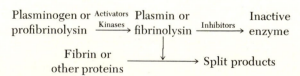

Plasminogen, or profibrinolysin, occurs in plasma as the inactive precursor of fibrinolysin. Among those substances that may activate it directly or indirectly in humans is streptokinase.

Streptokinase-streptodornase (Varidase) is a mixture of enzymes used topically for dissolving blood clots (streptokinase) and the viscous nucleoproteins of pus (streptodornase). It is useful in evacuating the contents of hemothorax and empyema and as an aid in surgical debridement.

Adverse effects to the enzyme mixture include fever and local irritation. Active hemorrhage is a contraindication to its use. The usefulness of streptokinase-streptodornase in the form of buccal tablets or the intramuscular route for a systemic anti-inflammatory effect is not certain.

Streptokinase-streptodornase is available as a powder for topical use containing 100,000 units of streptokinase and 25,000 units of streptodornase per vial. Streptokinase-streptodornase should not be injected intravenously because of hazardous impurities present in the preparation.

ε-Aminocaproic acid (Amicar) inhibits plasminogen activators and to a lesser extent plasmin. The drug has been used to decrease hemorrhage associated with certain surgical procedures. In one study it lowered fibrinolytic activity and suppressed urokinase excretion in cirrhotic patients at a dosage of 10 g daily for 7 days.[25]

Urokinase, the naturally occurring activator of the fibrinolytic enzyme system in human urine, is being investigated. It has many advantages over bacterial products such as streptokinase, although its preparation is quite difficult. Preliminary results in pulmonary embolism are promising.[44]

Prostaglandins and related compounds appear to play an important role in platelet function. The platelets can synthesize thromboxanes from endoperoxides. The thromboxanes cause platelet aggregation. At the same time another derivative of endoperoxides, the prostacyclines, which may be synthesized by the vascular emdothelium, are powerful inhibitors of platelet aggregation. Aspirin, indomethacin, and some other anti-inflammatory drugs block the formation of endoperoxides by inhibiting the enzyme cyclooxygenase. Dipyridamole (Persantine) is a powerful inhibitor of platelet aggregation and may prevent thromboembolic phenomena in patients with artificial heart valves.[50]

Prostaglandins and platelet aggregation

In contrast with these inhibitors of platelet aggregation, intravenously administered arachidonic acid can cause massive thrombosis in animals, presumably because it is converted to endoperoxides and eventually thromboxanes.

Antiplatelet drugs should theoretically be useful in patients with vascular disease. Aspirin and sulfinpyrazone are useful in cerebrovascular disease, but data are not sufficient to prove the usefulness of these drugs in patients with coronary disease. Nevertheless, clinical trials in this area are continuing.[48]

REFERENCES

1 Advisory Committee on Coagulation Products: Investigations of fibrinolysis and labeling changes in fibrinolysin products, J.A.M.A. **180:** 536, 1962.

2 Astrup, T., and Buluk, K.: Thromboplastic and fibrinolytic activities in vessels of animals, Circ. Res. **13:**253, 1963.

3 Brodie, B. B., Weiner, M., Burns, J. J., Simson, G., and Yale, E. K.: The physiological disposition of ethyl biscoumacetate (Tromexan) in man and a method for its estimation in biological material, J. Pharmacol. Exp. Ther. **106:**453, 1952.

4 Burns, J. J., Weiner, M., Simson, G., and Brodie, B. B.: The biotransformation of ethyl biscoumacetate (Tromexan) in man, rabbit and dog, J. Pharmacol. Exp. Ther. **108:**33, 1953.

5 Coon, W. W., and Willis, P. W.: Some side effects of heparin, heparinoids, and their antagonists, Clin. Pharmacol. Ther. **7:**379, 1966.

6 Cucuianu, M. P., Nishizawa, E. E., and Mus-

tard, J. F.: Effect of pyrimido-pyrimidine compounds on platelet function, J. Lab. Clin. Med. **77:**958, 1971.

7 Deykin, D.: The use of heparin; current concepts, N. Engl. J. Med. **280:**937, 1969.

8 Deykin, D.: Warfarin therapy, N. Engl. J. Med. **283:**691, 801, 1970.

9 Ebert, R. V.: Long-term anticoagulant therapy after myocardial infarction, J.A.M.A. **207:**2263, 1969.

10 Fletcher, A. P., and Sherry, S.: Thrombolytic agents, Annu. Rev. Pharmacol. **6:**89, 1966.

11 Gallus, A. S., Hirsch, J., Tuttle, R. J., Trebilbock, R., O'Bryan, S. E., Carroll, J. J., Minden, J. H., and Hudecki, S. M.: Small subcutaneous doses of heparin in prevention of venous thrombosis, N. Engl. J. Med. **288:**545, 1973.

12 Gaston, L. W.: The blood clotting factors, N. Engl. J. Med. **270:**236, 290, 1964.

13 Glynn, M. F., Murphy, E. A., and Mustard, J. F.: Platelets and thrombosis, Ann. Intern. Med. **64:**715, 1966.

14 Graham, D. M., Lyon, T. P., Gofman, J. W., Jones, H. B., Yankley, A., Simonton, J., and White, S.: Blood lipids and human atherosclerosis: influence of heparin upon lipoprotein metabolism, Circulation **4:**666, 1951.

15 Hahn, P. F.: Abolishment of alimentary lipemia following injection of heparin, Science **98:**19, 1943.

16 Harlan, W. R., Jr., Winesett, P. S., and Wasserman, A. J.: Tissue lipoprotein lipase in normal individuals and in individuals with exogenous hyperglyceridemia and the relationship of this enzyme to assimilation of fat, J. Clin. Invest. **46:**239, 1967.

17 Holemans, R.: Enhancement of fibrinolysis in the dog by injection of vasoactive drugs, Am. J. Physiol. **208:**511, 1965.

18 Howell, W. H.: The purification of heparin and its chemical and physiological reactions, Bull. Johns Hopkins Hosp. **42:**199, 1928.

19 Jaffee, M. D., and Willis, P. W., III: Multiple fractures associated with long-term sodium heparin therapy, J.A.M.A. **193:**158, 1965.

20 Jick, H., Slone, D., Borda, I. T., and Shapiro, S.: Efficacy and toxicity of heparin in relation to age and sex, N. Engl. J. Med. **279:**284, 1968.

21 Jorpes, J. E.: Heparin in the treatment of thrombosis: an account of its chemistry, physiology, and application in medicine, ed. 2, London, 1946, Oxford University Press.

22 Jorpes, J. E.: Heparin: its chemistry, pharmacology, and clinical use, Am. J. Med. **33:**692, 1962.

23 Kazmier, F. J., Spittell, J. A., Thompson, J. J., and Owen, C. A.: Effect of oral anticoagulants on factors VII, IX, X, and II, Arch. Intern. Med. **115:**667, 1965.

24 Lee, C. C., Trevoy, L. W., Spinks, J. W. T., and Jacques, L. B.: Dicumarol labeled with C^{14}, Proc. Soc. Exp. Biol. Med. **74:**151, 1950.

25 Lewis, J. H., and Doyle, A. P.: Effects of epsilon aminocaproic acid on coagulation and fibrinolytic mechanisms, J.A.M.A. **188:**56, 1964.

26 Link, K. P.: The anticoagulant from spoiled sweet clover hay, Harvey Lect. **39:**162, 1944.

27 Lowenthal, J., and Birnbaum, H.: Vitamin K and coumarin anticoagulants: dependence of anticoagulant effect on inhibition of vitamin K transport, Science **164:**181, 1969.

28 O'Reilly, R. A., Aggeler, P. M., Hoag, M. S., Leong, L. S., and Kropatkin, M. L.: Hereditary transmission of exceptional resistance to coumarin anticoagulant drugs, N. Engl. J. Med. **271:**809, 1964.

29 Packham, M. A., Warrior, E. S., Glynn, M. F., Senyi, A., and Mustard, J. F.: Alteration of the response of platelets to surface stimuli by pyrazole compounds, J. Exp. Med. **126:**171, 1967.

30 Ratnoff, O. D.: Epsilon aminocaproic acid—a dangerous weapon, N. Engl. J. Med. **280:**1124, 1969.

31 Robinson, D. S., and French, J. E.: Heparin, the clearing factor, lipase, and fat transport, Pharmacol. Rev. **12:**241, 1960.

32 Seaman, A. J., Griswold, H. E., Reaume, R. B., and Ritzmann, L.: Long-term anticoagulant prophylaxis after myocardial infarction, N. Engl. J. Med. **281:**115, 1969.

33 Sellers, E. M., and Koch-Weser, J.: Potentiation of warfarin-induced hypoprothrombinemia by chloral hydrate, N. Engl. J. Med. **283:**827, 1971.

34 Sherry, S., Fletcher, A. P., and Alkjaersig, N.: Fibrinolysis and fibrinolytic activity in man, Physiol. Rev. **39:**343, 1959.

35 Sodium heparin versus sodium warfarin in acute myocardial infarction (cooperative study), J.A.M.A. **189:**555, 1964.

36 Spinks, J. W. T., and Jaques, L. B.: Tracer experiments in mammals with Dicumarol labeled with carbon^{14}, Nature **166:**184, 1950.

37 Stirling, M., and Hunter, R. B.: Pharmacology of bis 3-3'-(4-oxycoumarinyl) ethyl acetate (Tromexan), Lancet **2:**611, 1951.

38 Tow, D. E., Wagner, H. N., and Holmes, R. A.: Urokinase in pulmonary embolism, N. Engl. J. Med. **277:**1161, 1967.

39 Vietti, T. J., Stephens, J. C., and Bennett,

K. R.: Vitamin K$_1$ prophylaxis in the newborn, J.A.M.A. **176**:791, 1961.

40 Weiner, M.: The rational use of anticoagulants, Pharmacol. Phys. **1**(11):1, 1967.

41 Weiner, M., Shapiro, S., Axelrod, J., Cooper, J. R., and Brodie, B. B.: The physiological disposition of Dicumarol in man, J. Pharmacol. Exp. Ther. **99**:409, 1950.

42 Wright, I. S., Marple, C. D., and Beck, D. F.: Myocardial infarction: its clinical manifestations and treatment with anticoagulants. A study of 1031 cases, New York, 1954, Grune & Stratton, Inc.

REVIEWS

43 Anticoagulants in acute myocardial infarction: results of a cooperative clinical trial, J.A.M.A. **225**:724, 1973.

44 Bell, W. R., and Meek, A. G.: Guidelines for the use of thrombolytic agents, N. Engl. J. Med. **301**:1266, 1979.

45 Coon, W. W.: Use of anticoagulant drugs, Ration. Drug Ther. **13**:1, 1979.

46 Davis, F. B., Estruch, M. T., Samson-Corvera, E. B., Voigt, G. C., and Tobin, J. D.: Management of anticoagulation in outpatients, Arch. Intern. Med. **137**:197, 1977.

47 Jaques, L. B.: Heparin: an old drug with a new paradigm, Science **206**:528, 1979.

48 Mehta, J., and Mehta, P.: Status of antiplatelet drugs in coronary heart disease, J.A.M.A. **241**:2649, 1979.

49 Modan, B., Shani, M., Schor, S., and Modan, M.: Reduction of hospital mortality from acute myocardial infarction by anticoagulant therapy, N. Engl. J. Med. **292**:1359, 1975.

50 Ogston, D., and Douglas, A. S.: Anticoagulant and thrombolytic drugs, Drugs **1**:228, 1971.

51 O'Reilly, R. A., and Aggeler, P. M.: Determinants of the response to oral anticoagulant drugs in man, Pharmacol. Rev. **22**:35, 1970.

CHAPTER 38

Diuretic drugs

GENERAL CONCEPT   Diuretics are drugs that increase the net renal excretion of solute and water. The renal tubule utilizes numerous transport processes for the reabsorption of most of the glomerular filtrate. Diuretics inhibit some of these transport processes, and their site of action within the nephron determines the quantitative and qualitative influence they exert on water and solute excretion.

Although the *mercurial diuretics* are looked on by many as having mainly historical interest, they still have important clinical uses. They produce predictable diuresis without excessive potassium loss and are given by intramuscular injection.

The *carbonic anhydrase inhibitors* are somewhat ineffective in edematous states but are used in other conditions, such as glaucoma and as adjuncts in conditions in which alkaline urine may be of benefit.

The *thiazide diuretics* are administered orally and are especially useful in hypertensive patients with congestive failure. They have disadvantages such as the induction of hypokalemic alkalosis, occasional hyperglycemia, and hyperuricemia.

Furosemide and *ethacrynic acid* are powerful diuretics, and their potent action requires close supervision of the patient.

The *osmotic diuretics* such as mannitol are effective in restoring glomerular filtration after transient hypotension. They must be injected intravenously.

Spironolactone and *triamterene* conserve potassium. They are not potent when used alone but may increase the degree of diuresis obtained by other drugs.

DIURETICS   The diuretic action of inorganic mercury salts such as calomel has been known for
Development   centuries, but the discovery that organic mercurials are highly potent in reducing edema came accidentally from their former use in the treatment of syphilis. One compound, merbaphen (Novasurol), was noted to have a powerful diuretic action.[48]

The development of the carbonic anhydrase inhibitors was an outgrowth of investigations on sulfanilamide. It was observed that sulfanilamide tended to produce metabolic acidosis. Pitts and co-workers[37] traced this effect to inhibition of the acidification of urine. This observation, coupled with knowledge that the compound was an inhibitor of carbonic anhydrase led to the hypothesis that other inhibitors of this enzyme might prove to be useful diuretics. Synthetic work in this direction led to the introduction of acetazolamide.

TABLE 38-1. Functional subdivisions of various renal segments*

Segment	% Na reabsorbed	C_{H_2O}	T^CH_2O	K secretion
Proximal	70	−	−	−
Ascending limb of inner medullary segment	$\geqq 10$	−	−	−
Medullary diluting segment	5	+	+	−
Cortical diluting segment	10	+	−	−
Distal	5	±	−	+
Collecting duct	1-2	±	−	+

*From Seldin, D. W., Eknoyan, G., Suki, W., and Rector, F. C., Jr.: In Proceedings of the Third International Congress on Nephrology, vol. 1, Basel, 1967, S. Karger.

Further work on carbonic anhydrase inhibitors produced other compounds such as chlorothiazide, which has additional effects in decreasing tubular reabsorption of electrolytes. These compounds were found to be highly effective in management of both congestive failure and hypertensive cardiovascular disease. Because of their effectiveness and ease of administration by the oral route, they have essentially replaced all other diuretics for major clinical uses.

More recently, two very powerful diuretics were introduced. One, furosemide, is a sulfonamide and is related to the thiazides. The other, ethacrynic acid, is chemically unrelated to the other diuretic drugs.

Renal handling of salt and water

Normally 180 L of plasma is filtered through the glomeruli and 99% of the filtrate is reabsorbed by the tubules. The transport of sodium is an active process in the proximal tubules, distal convoluted tubules, and the collecting ducts. There is active chloride reabsorption in the thick ascending limb of Henle's loop, also known as the "diluting segment."[52]

About 60% to 70% of the filtered sodium is reabsorbed iso-osmotically in the proximal tubules. Henle's loop is most important in the concentration and dilution of the urine. About 15% to 20% of the filtered sodium is reabsorbed in the ascending loop, which is not permeable to water. The actively reabsorbed chloride along with sodium is deposited in the medulla, establishing a hypertonic medullary interstitium. The resulting hypotonic tubular fluid is further influenced by reabsorption of water from the collecting ducts under the control of the antidiuretic hormone. In the distal tubules and collecting ducts, sodium is reabsorbed in exchange for potassium and hydrogen ions, a process that is controlled by aldosterone.

Renal handling of sodium

The anatomical and functional subdivisions of the nephron are shown schematically in Fig. 38-1. Sodium reabsorption in the proximal tubule may be measured by micropuncture in rats and dogs and is about 70% of the filtered load. Indirect methods must be used for the estimation of sodium reabsorption at other segments of the nephron.

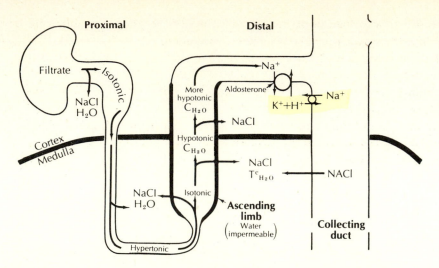

FIG. 38-1. Anatomical and functional subdivisions of the nephron. (From Seldin, D. W., Eknoyan, G., Suki, W., and Rector, F. C., Jr.: In Proceedings of the Third International Congress on Nephrology, vol. 1, Basel, 1967, S. Karger.)

The site of action of the various diuretics may be summarized in the following manner:

Proximal tubules
    Carbonic anhydrase inhibitors: acetazolamide, metolazone
    Osmotic diuretics: mannitol
    Vasodilators: aminophylline
Thick ascending limb (medullary)
    Loop diuretics: furosemide, ethacrynic acid, mercurials
Thick ascending limb (cortical)
    Thiazides, mercurials
Distal tubule
    Spironolactone, triamterene, amiloride

The most potent diuretics act on the medullary thick ascending limb or diluting segment by inhibition of active chloride transport. Although the proximal tubule reabsorbs most of the glomerular filtrate, diuretics acting at this site are not very potent because solutes that are retained by the proximal tubules are effectively reabsorbed in the diluting segment.

The mercurial diuretics inhibit active chloride transport in the thick ascending limb of Henle's loop. At one time the parenterally administered mercurial diuretics were commonly used and were very effective. They have been replaced by the loop diuretics, such as furosemide. Oral mercurial diuretics are no longer available.

Toxicity   When properly used, mercurial diuretics are quite safe. Their safety is a consequence of their selective localization in the kidney, where their concentration may be

100 times greater than in plasma. Cardiac toxicity develops only following intravenous injection, which may be considered an improper use.

True mercury poisoning may develop if the diuretics are given in excessive doses or too frequently. The most frequent cause of mercury poisoning with diuretics is their administration to patients whose renal blood flow is severely impaired.

Mercaptomerin sodium (Thiomerin) is still used occasionally, but the loop diuretics are more convenient and less toxic. Mercaptomerin sodium is available for intramuscular or subcutaneous administration as an injectable solution containing 125 mg, equivalent to 40 mg/ml of mercury.

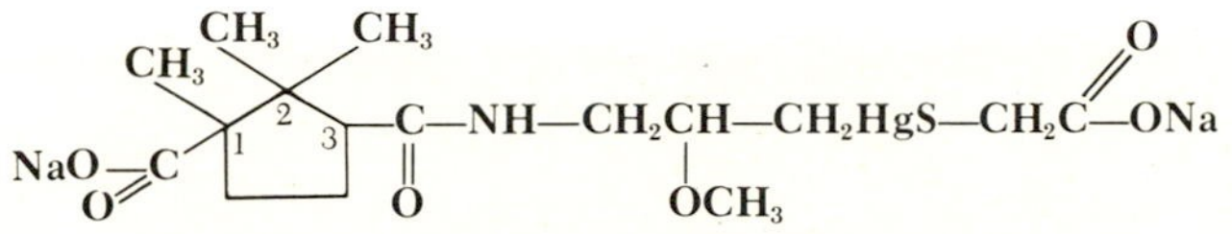

Mercaptomerin sodium

Although obsolete as diuretics, the carbonic anhydrase inhibitors are employed in the treatment of other conditions such as glaucoma. They represent interesting examples of the therapeutic application of enzyme inhibitors.

When sulfanilamide was introduced into therapeutics, its use was observed to lead to the development of acidosis, a drop in plasma CO_2, a rise in urinary pH, and a loss of Na^+, K^+, and H_2O into the urine. The compound was also demonstrated to be a specific inhibitor of carbonic anhydrase. The role of H^+ transport in renal acidification was established by Pitts and co-workers.[37]

Further studies on the sulfonamides have shown that their carbonic anhydrase inhibition is associated with a free $-SO_2NH_2$ group. The various sulfonamides that were later introduced as chemotherapeutic agents contained substitutions in the sulfonamide nitrogen to inhibit their action on carbonic anhydrase.

A large number of sulfonamides were synthesized for the purpose of finding potent inhibitors of carbonic anhydrase. This work led to the development of acetazolamide (Diamox) and eventually to the discovery of the chlorothiazide diuretics, which have additional diuretic actions not explained by their inhibitory effect on carbonic anhydrase. The structure of acetazolamide is shown along with that of sulfanilamide for comparison.

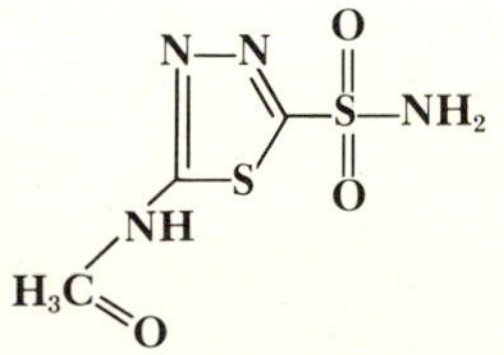

Carbonic anhydrase inhibitors

Acetazolamide 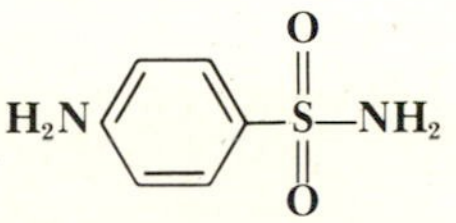   **Sulfanilamide**

The carbonic anhydrase inhibitors block the catalysis of the reaction $CO_2 + H_2O \rightleftharpoons H \cdot HCO_3$. Even though the enzyme is widely distributed in the body, therapeutic doses of acetazolamide exert their principal effect on the kidney. Effects on

Mode of action

other systems are also demonstrable, particularly when large doses of the drug are given.

The carbonic anhydrase inhibitors reduce the absorption of sodium bicarbonate in the proximal tubules. The excess chloride and sodium are reabsorbed in the thick ascending limb. The urine contains increased amounts of sodium bicarbonate and potassium, and the pH of the urine becomes elevated. Some hyperchloremic acidosis may develop.

Extrarenal effects of acetazolamide

Carbonic anhydrase is present in red cells, but therapeutic doses of acetazolamide do not interfere with the transport of carbon dioxide in the blood. The carbonic anhydrase inhibitors may have a CNS effect, causing drowsiness and disorientation in some patients. A favorable action has been claimed in the treatment of epilepsy, although the mode of action of the drug in this case is not clear. It may be a consequence of the acidosis, which has been reported to have a beneficial effect in epilepsy.

Glaucoma is the main indication for the use of carbonic anhydrase inhibitors. The aqueous humor has a high concentration of bicarbonate, and the beneficial effect of the carbonic anhydrase inhibitors may be related to an action on the secretion of bicarbonate.

Newer carbonic anhydrase inhibitors

Ethoxzolamide (Cardrase) is similar in action to acetazolamide. It is administered in doses of 62.5 to 250 mg one or more times daily. Its administration should be intermittent rather than continuous.

Dichlorphenamide (Daranide) is one of the most potent carbonic anhydrase inhibitors. The dose must be individualized and may range from 25 to 100 mg.

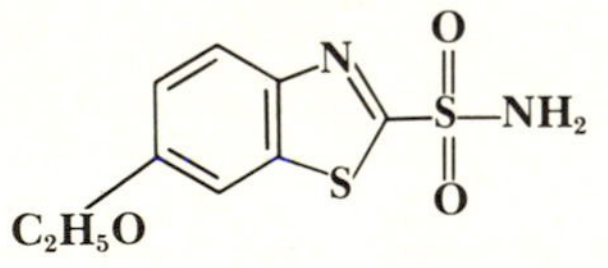

Ethoxzolamide 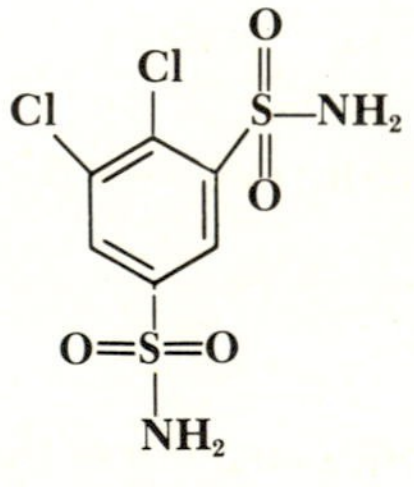   **Dichlorphenamide**

Thiazide diuretics

One of the most important developments in the diuretic field has been the introduction of chlorothiazide (Diuril) and its derivatives. The discovery of the thiazide diuretics is an outgrowth of studies on the carbonic anhydrase inhibitors. The thiazides have some inhibitory actions on carbonic anhydrase. They differ from the parent compounds in having additional effects on sodium reabsorption. Although they tend to cause loss of potassium, uric acid retention, and some impairment of carbohydrate tolerance, they have become very popular in the treatment of edematous states and also as antihypertensive medications.

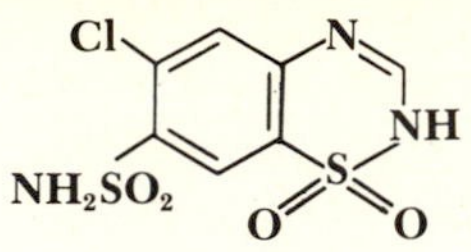

Chlorothiazide 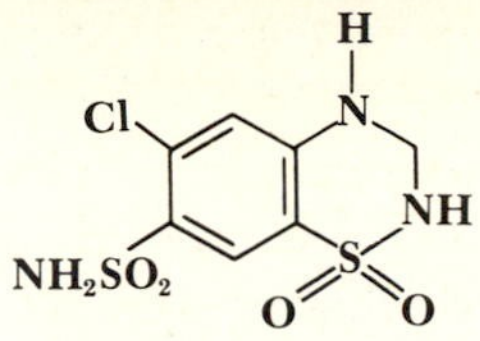   Hydrochlorothiazide

The thiazides and related compounds act on the cortical segment of the thick ascending limb to inhibit the reabsorption of sodium chloride. They interfere with urinary dilution without affecting the concentrating mechanisms. Although they have some carbonic anhydrase inhibitory activity, this is probably unimportant in their diuretic action. The thiazides promote the excretion of potassium by delivering increased amounts of sodium to the tubular exchange sites. Hypokalemia and some hypochloremic alkalosis may result.

Renal effects

Aldosterone levels may increase in patients who are taking thiazides. This is probably a consequence of decreased plasma volume, which stimulates the renin-angiotensin system. In the presence of increased aldosterone concentrations, hypokalemia may become quite significant and dangerous in patients receiving digitalis.

The thiazides are secreted by the renal tubules, utilizing the transport mechanism for organic acids.[5] Probenecid alters the time course of secretion without altering the total amount secreted and without altering the effectiveness of the diuretic. This is important because the two drugs may be used simultaneously, and the thiazides exert their effect from the luminal surface. The overall effect of chlorothiazide may even be increased by probenecid.[6]

Chlorothiazide can cause a significant reduction in urine volume when administered to patients having diabetes insipidus. The mechanism of this apparently paradoxical effect is not completely understood, but there is no reason to believe that there is any similarity between the actions of thiazides and the antidiuretic hormone.

The thiazides have a small but definite antihypertensive action, and they increase the effectiveness of other antihypertensive medications.[16]

Antihypertensive action

The nondiuretic congener of the thiazides, *diazoxide,* lowers blood pressure without having a renal effect. This is often used as an argument for some undefined action of the thiazides, perhaps on vascular smooth muscles. It is more likely, however, that the diuretic effect does play an important role in the lowering of the blood pressure by the thiazides.

The thiazides may cause hypokalemia, hyperglycemia, hyperuricemia, and, rarely, hypercalcemia, hyperlipidemia, and blood dyscrasias.

Adverse effects

Hypokalemia may become significant if the patient has diarrhea and vomiting or if the sodium intake is excessive. Hypokalemia is dangerous in digitalized patients. Hyperglycemia is generally unimportant unless the patient has subclinical diabetes.

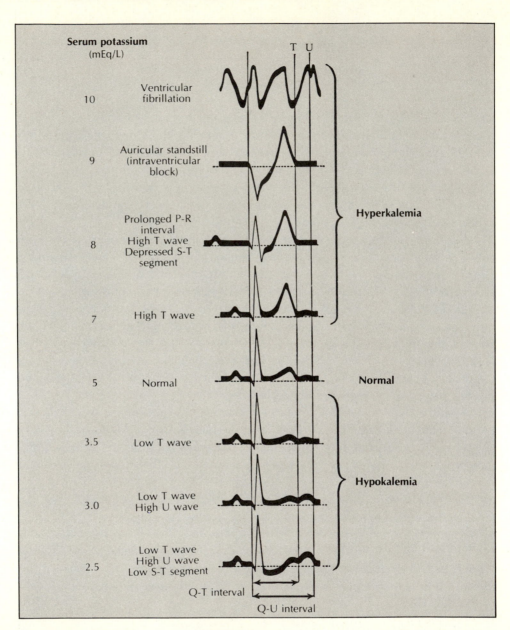

FIG. 38-2. Effect of varying serum potassium levels on electrocardiogram. (From Burch, G. E., and Winsor, T.: A primer of electrocardiography, Philadelphia, 1960, Lea & Febiger.)

Hyperuricemia is generally asymptomatic, but if the patient develops gouty attacks, the addition of colchicine and uricosuric drugs may be advisable.[19]

A number of patients taking hydrochlorothiazide in the form of enteric-coated capsules that also contain potassium chloride developed ulcerations of the small bowel.[29] Thorough study of this problem led to the tentative conclusion that this adverse effect was caused by this particular form of potassium chloride.

Adverse effects of potassium supplements

Other potassium salts such as gluconate are also widely used by patients who receiving thiazide therapy. Recent evidence indicates that if hypopotassemia is associated with hypochloremic alkalosis, only potassium *chloride* is effective in restoring normal acid-base balance.[25]

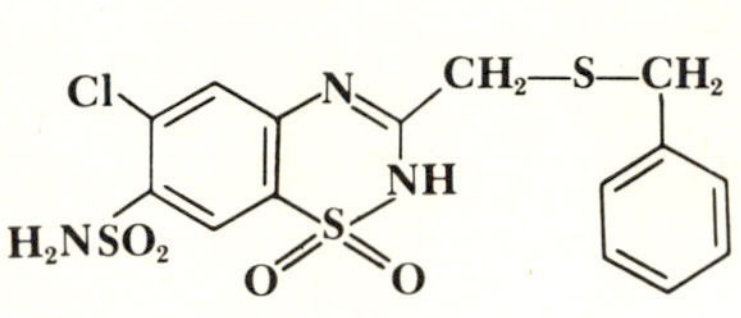

Benzthiazide

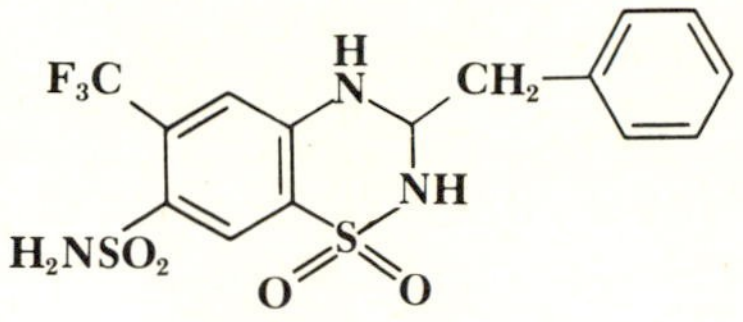

Bendroflumethiazide

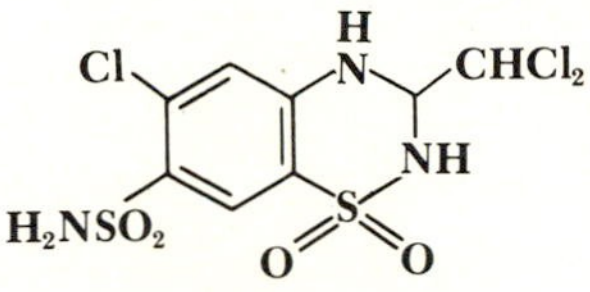

Trichlormethiazide

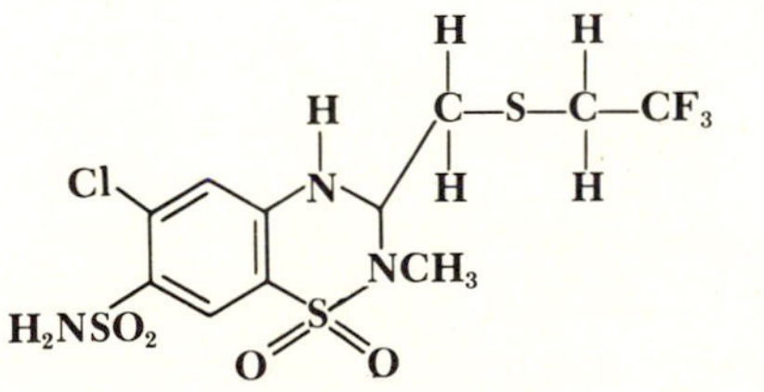

Polythiazide

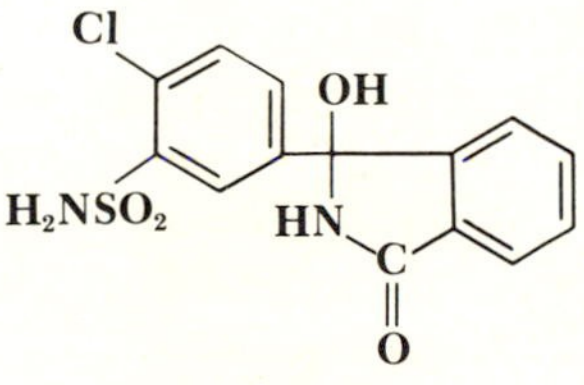

Chlorthalidone

Examination of the formulas of the various thiazide diuretics show that they are very closely related to each other and to chlorthalidone, which is not truly a benzo-thiadiazine.

Comparison of the various thiazide diuretics

Flumethiazide (Ademol) has the same structural formula as chlorothiazide, except that F_3C replaces Cl.

Hydroflumethiazide (Saluron) has the same structural fromula as hydrochloro-thiazide, except that F_3C replaces Cl.

Chlorthalidone, quinethazone, and **metolazone** are not thiazides but sulfon-amides with diuretic properties very similar to those of the thiazides. They differ from the thiazides mainly in their duation of action. Chlorthalidone (Hygroton) is

TABLE 38-2. Comparable daily doses and duration of action of thiazide diuretics

Preparation	Dose (mg)	Duration of action (hours)
Chlorothiazide (Diuril)	1000	9
Hydrochlorothiazide (HydroDiuril)	100	15
Hydroflumethiazide (Saluron)	100	21
Benzthiazide (ExNa)	100	15
Methyclothiazide (Enduron)	5-10	More than 24
Bendroflumethiazide (Naturetin)	5-10	More than 18
Trichlormethiazide (Naqua)	4-8	More than 24
Polythiazide (Renese)	4-8	More than 24
Chlorthalidone (Hygroton) (not a thiazide but resembles one)	200	More than 24
Quinethazone (Hydromox) (not a thiazide but resembles one)	50-100	21

available in 50 and 100 mg tablets, quinethazone (Hydromox) in 50 mg tablets, and metolazone (Zaroxolyn) in 2.5, 5, and 100 mg tablets.

There is some confusion about the relative advantages of one thiazide over another, promoted perhaps by commercial competition. It is often said, for example, that one thiazide is more potent than another. This is certainly true if *potency* is defined as activity per unit weight, as reflected in the various dosages given in Table 38-2. A different picture appears if the diuretic *efficacy* of these drugs is compared on the basis of what percentage of the filtered sodium is excreted under their maximum influence. If viewed in this manner, the percentage for most thiazides is about 10. For the newer sulfonamide furosemide it may be as high as 30. For ethacrynic acid the figure is about 20.

Furosemide and ethacrynic acid   These highly potent diuretics have many similar properties and indications, although they are quite different chemically. Furosemide is a sulfonamide related to the thiazides. Ethacrynic acid was developed on the basis of rational drug design. Since the mercurials owe their diuretic action to an affinity for sulfhydryl groups, the chemist combined an unsaturated ketone, which tends to combine with sulfhydryl groups, and an aryloxyacetic acid, which is known to concentrate in the kidney. The result was ethacrynic acid.

Both drugs are not only more potent than the thiazides but also have a greater *efficacy*. They promote the excretion of a higher percentage of filtered salt than is the case for other diuretics. This percentage is of the order of 20 to 30, compared with 10 for the thiazides.

It is believed that furosemide and ethacrynic acid exert their major action on the ascending limb of the loop of Henle (p. 490).

Compared to thiazides   Except for their much greater efficacy, furosemide and ethacrynic acid resemble the thiazides in their pharmacology. Both drugs are excreted unchanged into the urine. Their mechanism of excretion is the organic acid secretory system of the proximal tubules. Since uric acid is secreted by the same mechanism, both drugs tend to cause retention of urate. Probenecid is useful in preventing hyperuricemia caused by these drugs.

Both furosemide and ethacrynic acid cause potassium loss and impaired glucose tolerance. Potassium loss is greatly augmented in the presence of increased aldosterone secretion. Under these circumstances the potassium-retaining diuretics triamterene or spironolactone are useful adjuncts to furosemide or ethacrynic acid therapy.

The greatest dangers associated with the use of furosemide or ethacrynic acid are excessive diuresis with circulatory collapse and severe hypokalemia. Ototoxicity has also been described after the use of these diuretics.

Furosemide (Lasix) is available for oral administration in tablets containing 40 mg and in solution for injection, 10 mg/ml. *Preparations and dosage*

The usual oral dosage for adults initially is 40 to 80 mg, which may be increased gradually. Excessive doses may cause hypotension and vascular collapse. Dosage for intravenous administration in adults is 20 to 40 mg, given slowly. The same dosage may be used for intramuscular administration. The immediate diuretic effect may be an advantage in the treatment of acute pulmonary edema and hypertensive crisis.

Preparations of **ethacrynic acid** (Edecrin) include tablets containing 25 and 50 mg for oral administration and, for injection, Edecrin sodium powder, 50 mg.

The usual dosage by mouth for adults is 50 mg initially, with careful adjustment subsequently. The intravenous dose is 50 mg for adults, or 0.5 mg/kg. The rapid and potent diuretic action may be useful, just as that of furosemide, in the treatment of acute pulmonary edema and hypertensive crisis. The drug may cause hypotension, vascular collapse, potassium depletion, hyperuricemia, and transient deafness.

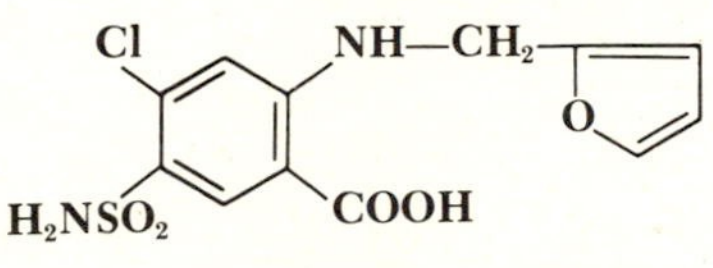

Furosemide 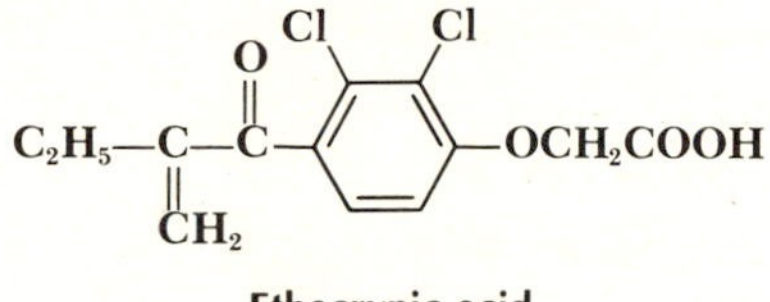   Ethacrynic acid

Triamterene and spironolactone, and also the investigational drug **amiloride**, are potassium-sparing diuretics. They are not potent when used alone but may be useful in combination with the thiazides. They may cause hyperkalemia. **Triamterene and spironolactone**

Triamterene is not a true aldosterone antagonist; nevertheless, it causes some sodium excretion associated with potassium retention. Spironolactone is a competive inhibitor of aldosterone. Thus it blocks the reabsorption of sodium in exchange for potassium and hydrogen. The different mechanisms of action of triamterene and spironolactone are evident by the demonstration that a combination of the two drugs has a greater effect than the sum of the maximal actions of the drugs when given alone.[26]

Triamterene (Dyrenium) is supplied in capsules containing 100 mg. Dosage must be carefully regulated, but the usual dose is 100 mg twice daily. The drug is contra-indicated in severe kidney disease and in the presence of hyperkalemia. Triamterene and a thiazide diuretic are sometimes used in the same patient. The rationale for using such a combination is that the natriuresis resulting from thiazide therapy promotes a compensatory aldosterone secretion. Aldosterone tends to antagonize the sodium-excreting action of the thiazide, while aggravating potassium loss. Addition of triamterene provides the opposite effect.

Spironolactone (Aldactone) is supplied in 25 mg tablets. The daily dosage is 50 to 100 mg. The main contraindication to the use of the drug is hyperkalemia. Potassium supplementation should be avoided when spironolactane or triamterene is prescribed. Spironolactone can cause tumors in rats.

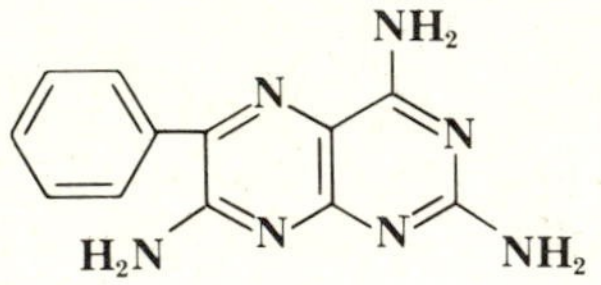

Triamterene

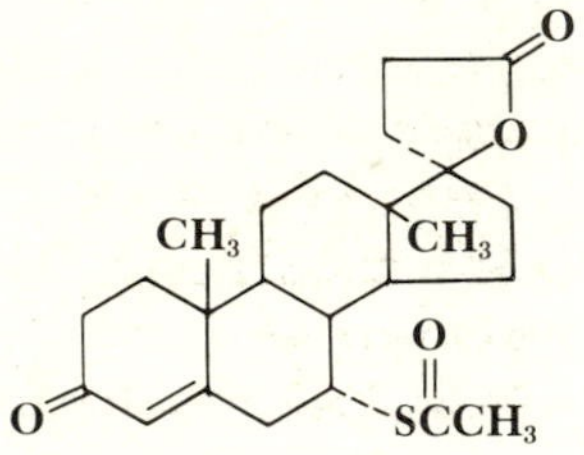

Spironolactone

Mannitol

Mannitol is not reabsorbed by the tubules and may be considered to be the prototype of the osmotic diuretics. Its site of action is the proximal tubule, leading to a greater delivery of sodium and chloride to the loop of Henle. The drug must be injected intravenously.

Mannitol is available as a 25% solution for intravenous injection in 50 ml containers. It is also available as a 5%, 10%, 15%, and 20% solution in 1000 ml containers. In addition to its use as a diuretic adjunct, mannitol finds some usefulness in neurosurgery for reduction of cerebrospinal fluid pressure and for the reduction of intraocular pressure. It is contraindicated in patients with severe renal disease.

Minor diuretics
Xanthines

The previously discussed major diuretics primarily affect the tubular reabsorptive processes of the kidney. The xanthines—theophylline, theobromine, and caffeine—have a combined effect on renal hemodynamics and tubular reabsorptive capacity.

Of the three xanthines, theophylline is the most potent diuretic.

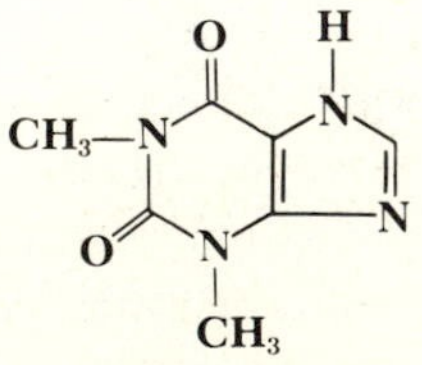

Theophylline

The ability of theophylline to inhibit tubular reabsorption of electrolytes has been shown experimentally. It is most effective when injected intravenously as one of its soluble salts, *aminophylline*. In addition, the compound increases cardiac output and can produce increased glomerular filtration. When aminophylline and a mercurial are administered simultaneously, the combined diuretic effect is greater than what could be expected from one of these drugs alone. This may be advantageous when the effectiveness of mercurials is decreased as a result of impaired glomerular filtration.

Ammonium chloride

Ammonium salts produce metabolic acidosis because ammonium is converted to urea by the liver, thus leaving an excess of chloride.

The renal tubules respond to metabolic acidosis by increasing their production of ammonia from glutamine and other amino acids. There is a delay of several hours to days, however, before the kidney can fully develop this capacity to form ammonia. During this period of delay, sodium in the urine is excreted in combination with chloride, and true diuresis ensues. Once the kidney is able to produce nearly as much ammonia as the amount ingested, the diuretic action of ammonium chloride ceases because chloride in tubular urine can then be balanced with ions of ammonium rather than sodium. Thus refractoriness to ammonium chloride diuresis develops within a few days.

Ammonium chloride is seldom used by itself as a diuretic, but it is helpful in potentiating the action of the mercurials.

Ammonium chloride is administered in large doses, 6 to 10 g/day. It can cause considerable gastric irritation, and for this reason enteric-coated tablets are occasionally used. The compound is given intermittently to avoid development of refractoriness. It may induce hepatic coma in liver disease, in which case L-lysine monohydrochloride may be substituted.

REFERENCES

1 Baer, J. E., and Beyer, K. H.: Renal pharmacology, Annu. Rev. Pharmacol. **6:**261, 1966.

2 Bank, N., Koch, K. M., Aynedjian, H. S., and Aras, M.: Effect of changes in renal perfusion pressure on the suppression of proximal tubular sodium reabsorption due to saline loading, J. Clin. Invest. **48:**271, 1969.

3 Berliner, R. W., Levinsky, N. G., Davidson, D. G., and Eden, M.: Dilution and concentration of the urine and the action of antidiuretic hormone, Am. J. Med. **24:**730, 1958.

4 Beyer, K. H.: Electrolyte adjustments in modern diuretic therapy, Pharmacol. Phys. **1**(8):1, 1967.

5 Beyer, K. H., and Baer, J. E.: Physiological basis for the action of newer diuretic agents, Pharmacol. Rev. **13:**517, 1961.

6 Brater, D. C.: Increase in diuretic effect of chlorothiazide by probenecid, Clin. Pharmacol. Ther. **23:**259, 1978.

7 Bricker, N. S.: The control of sodium excretion with normal and reduced nephrone populations, Am. J. Med. **43:**313, 1967.

8 Brickman, A. S., Massry, S. G., and Coburn, J. W.: Changes in serum and urinary calcium during treatment with hydrochlorothiazide; studies on mechanisms, J. Clin. Invest. **51:**945, 1972.

9 Bryant, J. M., Yü, T. F., Berger, L., Schwartz, N., Torosdag, S., Fletcher, L., Fertig, H., Schwartz, M. S., and Quan, R. B. F.: Hyperuricemia induced by the administration of chlorthalidone and other sulfonamide diuretics, Am. J. Med. **33:**408, 1962.

10 Cafruny, E. J.: The site and mechanism of action of mercurial diuretics, Pharmacol. Rev. **20:**89, 1968.

11 Calesnick, B., Christensen, J. A., and Richter, M.: Absorption and excretion of furosemide-S^{35} in human subjects, Proc. Soc. Exp. Biol. Med. **123:**17, 1966.

12 Cornish, A. L., McClellan, J. T., and Johnston,

D. H.: Effects of chlorothiazide on the pancreas, N. Engl. J. Med. **265**:673, 1961.

13 Davidow, M., Kakaviatos, N., and Finnerty, F. A.: Intravenous administration of furosemide in heart failure, J.A.M.A. **200**:824, 1967.

14 Dirks, J. H., Cirksena, W. J., and Berliner, R. W.: Effects of saline infusion on sodium reabsorption by proximal tubule of dog, J. Clin. Invest. **44**:1160, 1965.

15 Earley, L. E.: Diuretics, N. Engl. J. Med. **276**:966, 1967.

16 Earley, L. E., and Orloff, J.: Thiazide diuretics, Annu. Rev. Med. **15**:149, 1964.

17 Ehrlich, E. N.: Aldosterone, the adrenal cortex and hypertension, Annu. Rev. Med. **19**:373, 1968.

18 Frazier, H. S.: Renal regulation of sodium balance, N. Engl. J. Med. **279**:868, 1968.

19 Freis, E. D., and Sappington, R. F.: Long-term effect of probenecid on diuretic-induced hyperuricemia, J.A.M.A. **198**:127, 1966.

20 Giebisch, G.: Measurements of electrical potentials and ion fluxes in single renal tubules, Circulation **21**:879, 1960.

21 Ginsberg, D. J., Saad, A., and Gabuzda, G. J.: Metabolic studies with the diuretic triamterene in patients with cirrhosis and ascites, N. Engl. J. Med. **271**:1229, 1964.

22 Gottschalk, C. W.: Osmotic concentration and dilution of the urine, Am. J. Med. **36**:670, 1964.

23 Haber, E.: Recent developments in pathophysiologic studies in the renin-angiotensin system, N. Engl. J. Med. **280**:148, 1969.

24 Hagedorn, C. W., Kaplan, A. A., and Hulet, W. H.: Prolonged administration of ethacrynic acid in patients with renal disease, N. Engl. J. Med. **272**:1152, 1965.

25 Kassirer, J. P., Berkman, P. M., Lawrenz, D. R., and Schwartz, W. B.: The critical role of chloride in the correction of hypokalemic alkalosis in man, Am. J. Med. **38**:172, 1965.

26 Kessler, R. H.: The use of furosemide and ethacrynic acid in the treatment of edema, Pharmacol. Phys. **1**:(9):1, 1967.

27 Kessler, R. H.: The treatment of noncardiac edema, Pharmacol. Phys. **2**:(7):1, 1968.

28 Komorn, R. M., and Cafruny, E. J.: Ethacrynic acid: diuretic property coupled to reaction with sulfhydryl groups in renal cells, Science **143**:133, 1964.

29 Lawrason, F. D., Alpert, E., Mohr, F. L., and McMahon, F. G.: Ulcerative-obstructive lesions of the small intestine, J.A.M.A. **191**:641, 1965.

30 Levinsky, N. G., and Lalone, R. C.: Mechanism of sodium diuresis after saline infusion in the dog, J. Clin. Invest. **42**:1261, 1963.

31 Liddle, G. W.: Sodium diuresis induced by steroidal antagonists of aldosterone, Science **126**:1016, 1957.

32 Martz, B. L.: A diuretic assay utilizing normal subjects, Clin. Pharmacol. Ther. **3**:340, 1962.

33 Mathog, R. H., and Klein, W. J.: Ototoxicity of ethacrynic acid and aminoglycoside antibiotics in uremia, N. Engl. J. Med. **280**:1223, 1969.

34 Parfitt, A. M.: Chlorothiazide-induced hypercalcemia in juvenile osteoporosis and hyperparathyroidism, N. Engl. J. Med. **281**:55, 1969.

35 Pitts, R. F.: The physiological basis of diuretic therapy, Springfield, Ill., 1959, Charles C Thomas, Publisher.

36 Pitts, R. F.: Renal production and excretion of ammonia, Am. J. Med. **36**:720, 1964.

37 Pitts, R. F., Alexander, R. S., and Fagan, K.: The nature of the renal tubular mechanism for acidifying the urine, Am. J. Physiol. **144**:239, 1945.

38 Ramos, G., Rivera, A., and Pena, J. C.: Mechanism of the antidiuretic effect of saluretic drugs, Clin. Pharmacol. Ther. **8**:557, 1967.

39 Rocha, A. S., and Kokko, J. P.: Sodium chloride and water transport in the medullary thick ascending limb of Henle: evidence for active chloride transport, J. Clin. Invest. **52**:612, 1973.

40 Schwartz, W. B., and Relman, A. S.: Effects of electrolyte disorders on renal structure and function, N. Engl. J. Med. **276**:383, 452, 1967.

41 Seldin, D. W., Eknoyan, G., Suki, W., and Rector, F. C., Jr.: The physiology of modern diuretics. In Proceedings of the Third International Congress on Nephrology, vol. 1, Basel, 1967, S. Karger.

42 Shenkin, H. A., Goluboff, B., and Haft, H.: The use of mannitol for the reduction of intracranial pressure in intracranial surgery, J. Neurosurg. **19**:897, 1962.

43 Stahl, W. M.: Effect of mannitol on the kidney: changes in intrarenal hemodynamics, N. Engl. J. Med. **272**:381, 1965.

44 Steinmetz, P. R.: Excretion of acid by the kidney—functional organization and cellular aspects of acidification, N. Engl. J. Med. **278**:1102, 1968.

45 Suki, W., Rector, F. C., Jr., and Seldin, D. W.: The site of action of furosemide and other sulfonamide diuretics in the dog, J. Clin. Invest. **44**:1458, 1965.

46 Thurau, K.: Renal hemodynamics, Am. J. Med. **36**:698, 1964.

47 Timmerman, R. J., Springman, F. R., and

Thomas, R. K.: Evaluation of furosemide, a new diuretic agent, Curr. Ther. Res. **6**:88, 1964.

48 Vogl, A.: The discovery of the organic mercurial diuretics, Am. Heart J. **39**:881, 1950.

49 Weiner, I. M., and Mudge, G. H.: Renal tubular mechanisms for excretion of organic acids and bases, Am. J. Med. **36**:743, 1964.

50 Wirz, H.: Kidney, water and electrolytes, Annu. Rev. Physiol. **23**:577, 1961.

51 Wolff, F. W., Parmley, W. W., White, K., and Okun, R.: Drug-induced diabetes: diabetogenic activity of long-term administration of benzothiadiazines, J.A.M.A. **185**:568, 1963.

REVIEWS

52 Burg, M. B.: Tubular chloride transport and the mode of action of some diuretics, Kidney Int. **9**: 189, 1976.

53 Gantt, C. L.: Diuretic therapy, Ration. Drug Ther. **6**:1, 1972.

54 Giebisch, G.: Coupled ion and fluid transport in the kidney, N. Engl. J. Med. **287**:913, 1972.

55 Jacobson, H. R., and Kokko, J. K.: Diuretics: sites and mechanisms of action, Annu. Rev. Pharmacol. Toxicol. **16**:201, 1976.

56 Jamison, R. L., and Maffly, R. H.: The urinary concentrating mechanism, N. Engl. J. Med. **295**:1059, 1976.

57 Klahr, S., and Slatopolsky, E.: Renal regulation of sodium excretion, Arch. Intern. Med. **131**: 780, 1973.

57a Kokko, J. P.: Renal concentrating and diluting mechanisms, Hosp. Pract. p. 110, Feb. 1979.

58 Krumlovsky, F. A.: Hyponatremia, Ration. Drug Ther. **9**:1, 1975.

59 Landon, E. J., and Forte, L. R.: Cellular mechanisms in renal pharmacology, Annu. Rev. Pharmacol. **11**:171, 1971.

60 Newmark, S. R., and Dluhy, R. G.: Hyperkalemia and hypokalemia, J.A.M.A. **231**:631, 1975.

61 Orloff, J., and Burg, M.: Kidney, Annu. Rev. Physiol. **33**:83, 1971.

62 Porter, G. A.: The role of diuretics in the treatment of heart failure, J.A.M.A. **244**:1614, 1980.

63 Seely, J. F., and Dirks, J. H.: Site of action of diuretic drugs, Kidney Int. **11**:1, 1977.

64 Sweadner, K. J., and Goldin, S. M.: Active transport of sodium and potassium ions, N. Engl. J. Med. **302**:777, 1980.

CHAPTER 39

Pharmacological approaches to atherosclerosis

Research on atherosclerosis is dominated by concepts that envision some connection between hyperlipoproteinemias and the arterial disease. A major new concept invokes a receptor-mediated control of cholesterol metabolism.[7] According to this concept, mammalian cells have a low-density lipoprotein (LDL) receptor on their surface, which mediates the internalization of the cholesterol-rich lipoprotein. Cholesterol is then removed and utilized within the cell. In familial hypercholesterolemia the receptor is deficient and atherosclerosis is common.[6] In other approaches the high-density lipoproteins are viewed as protective and useful cholesterol carriers.

Although there is no conclusive evidence for a beneficial effect of correction of hyperlipoproteinemia, several drugs have been introduced for the purpose of lowering abnormally elevated serum lipid concentrations.

Clofibrate may inhibit the release of lipoproteins from the liver and does inhibit cholesterol biosynthesis. *Cholestyramine* and *colestipol* are resins that bind bile acids and prevent their absorption. *Dextrothyroxine* increases the catabolism of apoprotein B. *Nicotinic acid* depresses the synthesis of LDL and apoprotein B. *Estrogens* are no longer used in the treatment of hyperlipidemias, but *norethindrone acetate*, a progestational agent and some anabolic steroids are used in some patients investigationally. *Sitosterols* from plants compete with cholesterol for absorption and *probucol* reduces LDL concentrations. In addition, neomycin sulfate precipitates cholesterol in the intestine and prevents its absorption.

Clofibrate

Clofibrate (*p*-chlorophenoxyisobutyrate; Atromid S) is becoming the most important lipid-lowering drug, and favorable results have been reported in the long-term treatment of hyperlipidemia.[3] It was first used in combination with, or as a vehicle for, androsterone, which is known to decrease cholesterol synthesis in the liver. Further studies revealed that clofibrate alone, when administered orally in doses of 500 mg four times daily, lowers the concentration of triglycerides, lipoproteins, and cholesterol in plasma in a few weeks.

The mode of action of clofibrate is probably related to an inhibition of hepatic cholesterol synthesis and to a decrease in the rate of lipoprotein release from the liver.[2,29] The drug is useful in hyperlipidemia types III, IV, and V and is less effective in type II.

Although clofibrate is the drug of choice for type III hyperlipoproteinemia, its gastrointestinal effects and other side effects and its many drug interactions limit its usefulness. The drug should be given only to patients who are at risk for myocardial infarction and whose hyperlipidemia responds to the drug.

Clofibrate is available in 500 mg capsules. The usual dose is one capsule four times a day.

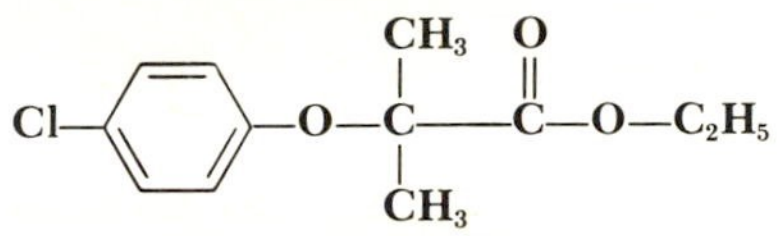

$$Cl-\!\!\!\!\bigcirc\!\!\!\!-O-\underset{\underset{CH_3}{|}}{\overset{\overset{CH_3}{|}}{C}}-\overset{\overset{O}{\|}}{C}-O-C_2H_5$$

Clofibrate

Cholestyramine (Questran; Cuemid) is a quaternary ammonium anion exchange resin that binds bile acids in the intestinal lumen, exchanging them for chloride. Since the resin is not absorbed, it promotes the excretion of bile acids. Increased fecal excretion of bile acids may lower serum cholesterol because there is a continual conversion of the sterol to bile acids, which are in large part reabsorbed under normal circumstances. Cholestyramine is used primarily for the relief of pruritus associated with biliary tract obstruction. The drug may interfere with the absorption of numerous drugs and fat-soluble vitamins.[11]

Cholestyramine

Cholestyramine may be useful in hyperlipoproteinemia type II. Side effects of the drug include constipation and nausea. A similar drug, **colestipol**,[13] has been introduced.

Cholestyramine is available in granular form. It is administered in doses of 4 g three times a day.

It is generally known that a reciprocal relationship exists between thyroid function and serum cholesterol. Among the thyroxine analogs that have been synthesized, dextrothyroxine (Choloxin) has received the most attention in the treatment of hyperlipoproteinemias. It is estimated that levothyroxine is 10 to 20 times as calorigenic as dextrothyroxine, but the latter has about 20% of the hypocholesterolemic action of levothyroxine.

Dextrothyroxine

Dextrothyroxine may promote the catabolism of apoprotein B, thus reducing LDL. The drug is probably useful in type II hyperlipoproteinemia.

Side effects of dextrothyroxine are a consequence of its metabolic stimulating action. They include angina and arrhythmias. In the large Coronary Drug Research Project,[23] dextrothyroxine at 6 mg/day produced sufficient adverse effects and suspicion of excess mortality that the drug was eliminated from the study.

Nicotinic acid and aluminum nicotinate when used in large doses inhibit the synthesis of LDL and apoprotein B. The drugs may be effective in all types of hyperlipoproteinemias except type I. The usefulness of nicotinic acid and aluminum nicotinate is limited by troublesome side effects. Flushing occurs in all patients

Nicotinic acid

initially and may persist in some. Activation of peptic ulcer and hepatic dysfunction are other toxic effects of large doses of these drugs.

Sitosterols

Absorption of cholesterol from the gastrointestinal tract is interfered with by certain plant sterols, known as sitosterols (Cytellin). These sterols are not significantly absorbed but have many disadvantages. They must be administered frequently and they are unpalatable. As a consequence they have not become widely used.

Female sex hormones

Although estrogens may lower serum cholesterol, they elevate serum triglycerides. Studies of women taking oral contraceptives often reveal an elevation of serum triglycerides.

Some reports claimed that conjugated estrogenic substances (Premarin) increased the chances of survival of men having coronary disease. Other studies in which ethinyl estradiol was used failed to show any benefit in patients who had a previous myocardial infarction.

Norethindrone acetate and oxandrolone

Norethindrone acetate (Norlutate), a progestational agent, may be useful in some women with type V hyperlipoproteinemia. The drug apparently decreases the concentrations of LDL and apoprotein A.

Oxandrolone (Anavar) may be useful in some men for the reduction of triglyceride concentrations. This drug, which is an anabolic steroid, is a derivative of testosterone.

Probucol

Probucol (Lorelco) may block some early step in cholesterol biosynthesis, and it reduces LDL concentrations. The drug appears to be effective in some forms of type II hyperlipoproteinemia.

Neomycin sulfate

This aminoglycoside given orally is not well absorbed from the gastrointestinal tract. It precipitates cholesterol and prevents its absorption; thus it acts in a manner similar to cholestyramine. The drug may be useful in some forms of type II hyperlipoproteinemia.

Classification and management of hyperlipoprotein-emias

Atherosclerosis is common and severe in some types of hyperlipoproteinemia, and the aim of management is to lower the concentration of lipids. The use of lipid-lowering agents depends on the type of hyperlipoproteinemia. The Fredrickson classification[10] recognizes five different lipoprotein patterns, which are designated *types I* through *V*.

Type I   This type is characterized by elevated chylomicrons with normal β lipoproteins. None of the drugs is useful in its treatment, although reduction of dietary fat may be helpful.

Type II   Patients in this group have elevated serum cholesterols and normal triglycerides. In addition to a low cholesterol diet and substitution of polyunsaturated fats for saturated ones, the following drugs are helpful: clofibrate, dextrothyroxine (Choloxin), nicotinic acid, and cholestyramine.

Type III   Patients in this group show abnormalities in the composition of their lipoproteins. Response to diet and drugs is much better than in type II patients. Clofibrate is effective, and dextrothyroxine and nicotinic acid are also useful.

Type IV   Patients in this group are usually obese and show a prebeta band on electrophoresis. Diet therapy with carbohydrate restriction, the use of polyunsaturated fats, and clofibrate are effective therapeutic measures.

Type V   This group has the characteristics of a combination of types I and IV. Weight reduction, clofibrate, and nicotinic acid are recommended.

REFERENCES

1 Ahrens, E. H., Jr., Hirsch, J., Insull, W., Jr., Tsaltas, T. T., Blomstrand, R., and Peterson, M. L.: Dietary control of serum lipids in relation to atherosclerosis, J.A.M.A. **164**:1905, 1957.

2 Avoy, D. R., Swyryd, E. A., and Gould, R. G.: Effects of *p*-chlorophenoxyisobutyryl ethyl ester (CPIB) with and without androsterone on cholesterol biosynthesis in rat liver, J. Lipid Res. **6**:369, 1965.

3 Berkowitz, D.: Treatment of hyperlipidemia with clofibrate, J.A.M.A. **218**:1002, 1971.

4 Best, M. M., and Duncan, C. H.: Effects of clofibrate and dextrothyroxine singly and in combination on serum lipids. Arch. Intern. Med. **118**:97, 1966.

5 Boyd, G. S.: Effect of linoleate and estrogen on cholesterol metabolism, Fed. Proc. **21**:86, 1962.

6 Brown, M. S., and Goldstein, J. L.: Familial hypercholesterolemia: a genetic defect in the low-density lipoprotein receptor, N. Engl. J. Med. **294**:1386, 1976.

7 Brown, M. S., and Goldstein, J. L.: Receptor-mediated control of cholesterol metabolism, Science **191**:150, 1976.

8 Christensen, N. A., Achor, R. W. P., Berge, K. G., and Mason, H. L.: Nicotinic acid treatment of hypercholesteremia, J.A.M.A. **177**:546, 1961.

9 Fredrickson, D. S., and Lees, R. S.: Familial hyperlipoproteinemia. In Stanbury, J. B. Wyngarden, J. B., and Fredrickson, D. S., editors: The metabolic basis of inherited disease, New York, 1965, McGraw-Hill Book Co.

10 Fredrickson, D. S., Levy, R. I., and Lees, R. S.: Transport in lipoproteins: an integrated approach to mechanisms and disorders, N. Engl. J. Med. **276**:34, 94, 148, 215, 273, 1967.

11 Gallo, D. G., Bailey, K. R., and Sheffner, A. L.: The interaction between cholestyramine and drugs, Proc. Soc. Exp. Biol. Med. **120**:60, 1965.

12 Garattini, S., and Paoletti, R.: Drugs in lipid metabolism, Ann. Rev. Pharmacol. **3**:91, 1963.

13 Glueck, C. J., Ford, S., Scheel, D., and Steiner, P.: Colestipol and cholestyramine resin, J.A.M.A. **222**:676, 1972.

14 Oliver, M. F., and Boyd, G. S.: Influence of reduction of serum lipids on prognosis of coronary heart disease, Lancet **2**:499, 1961.

15 Oliver, M. F., Roberts, S. D., Hayes, D., Pantridge, J. F., Suzman, M. M., and Bersohn, I.: Effect of atromid and ethylchlorophenoxyisobutyrate on anticoagulant requirements, Lancet **1**:143, 1963.

16 Parsons, W. B., Jr.: Studies on nicotinic acid use in hypercholesterolemia, Arch. Intern. Med. **107**:653, 1961.

17 Spritz, N., Ahrens, E. H., Jr., and Grundy, S.: Sterol balance in man as plasma cholesterol concentrations are altered by exchanges of dietary fats, J. Clin. Invest. **44**:1482, 1965.

18 Steiner, A., Howard, E. J., and Algun, S.: Importance of dietary cholesterol in man, J.A.M.A. **181**:186, 1962.

19 Wessler, S., and Avioli, L. A.: Classification and management of familial hyperlipoproteinemia, J.A.M.A. **207**:929, 1969.

20 Wilens, S. L., and Plair, C. M.: Blood cholesterol, nutrition, and atherosclerosis, Arch. Intern. Med. **116**:373, 1965.

REVIEWS

21 Cathcart-Rake, W. F., and Dujovne, C. A.: The treatment of hyperlipoproteinemias, Ration. Drug Ther. **13**:1, 1979.

22 The Coronary Drug Project Research Group: The coronary drug project, J.A.M.A. **214**:1303, 1970.

23 The Coronary Drug Project Research Group: The coronary drug project, J.A.M.A. **220**:996, 1972.

23a Goldstein, J. L., and Brown, M. S.: The low density lipoprotein pathway and its relation to atherosclerosis, Annu. Rev. Biochem. **46**:897, 1977.

24 Lees, R. S., and Wilson, D. E.: The treatment of hyperlipidemia, N. Engl. J. Med. **284**:186, 1971.

25 Minnick, C. R., and Murphy, G. E.: Experimental production of atheroarteriosclerosis by the synergy of allergic injury to arteries and lipid-rich diet, Am. J. Pathol. **73**:265, 1973.

26 Ross, R., and Harker, L.: Hyperlipidemia and atherosclerosis, Science **193**:1094, 1976.

27 Spaet, T. H.: Optimism in the control of atherosclerosis, N. Engl. J. Med. **291**:576, 1974.

28 Thompson, G. R.: Management of familial hypercholesterolemia and new approaches to atherosclerosis, Atherosclerosis Rev. **5**:67, 1979.

29 Weiss, P.: The treatment of hyperlipidemia, Ration. Drug Ther. **6**:1, 1972.

Drug effects on the respiratory and gastrointestinal tracts

CHAPTER 40

Drug effects on the respiratory tract

Numerous drugs, along with other measures, contribute to the effective management of pulmonary disorders, particularly in chronic obstructive lung disease. The *bronchodilators* are helpful in opening blocked airways; the *mucolytic drugs* aid in altering the characteristics of respiratory tract fluid; the *antibiotics* are useful in dealing with infections; the *corticosteroids* reduce the inflammatory process. In addition to these useful drug effects, the hazardous nature of sedative drugs and oxygen at high concentration is increasingly recognized. It is also becoming clear that the lung is a metabolic organ that contributes to the elaboration and destruction of a variety of endogenous compounds of great pharmacological activity. Drug-induced pulmonary diseases are also receiving increased attention.

The groups of drugs that will be discussed at this point are the bronchodilators, expectorants, and mucolytic agents. In addition, current concepts on the metabolic functions of the lung of pharmacological interest and drug-induced pulmonary diseases will also be considered.

Numerous drugs are capable of causing contraction or relaxation of the bronchial smooth muscle. The more important ones are enumerated in Table 40-1.

The bronchial constrictors listed in Table 40-1 are of experimental interest only and have no therapeutic importance. Histamine and methacholine are said to have a greater constrictor effect in asthmatic than in normal individuals, and these compounds are sometimes used by clinical investigators for testing the potency of bronchodilator drugs.

The bronchodilators listed in Table 40-1 vary greatly in their usefulness. Atropine and other anticholinergics traditionally have been avoided because they decrease bronchial secretions, leading to inspissated mucus. However, recent studies indicate that atropine or its N-isopropyl derivative, ipratropium, may be quite effective when given by inhalation.[12] At the present time the useful bronchodilators are limited to the β-adrenergic agonists and the methylxanthines.

The effectiveness of epinephrine, sympathomimetic drugs, and theophylline derivatives such as aminophylline in bronchial asthma has been known for many years. Increased knowledge of the mode of action of these compounds is of more recent origin, and schemes of their influence on the bronchi are shown in Fig. 40-1.

PHARMACOLOGY OF BRONCHIAL SMOOTH MUSCLE

BRONCHODILATORS
β-Adrenergic agonists and methylxanthines

509

With the postulation of α and β receptors[7] it became clear that the β receptor agonists and the methylxanthines or phosphodiesterase inhibitors are especially potent in dilating the bronchial smooth muscle. It is most likely that the effectiveness of both groups of drugs is based on their common property of increasing the levels of adenosine 3':5'-cyclic phosphate (cyclic AMP) in the smooth muscle of the bronchioles (Fig. 40-1).

The pure, direct-acting β-adrenergic agonist isoproterenol has become one of the most widely used bronchodilators. Its administration by a specially constructed inhaler has contributed to its popularity. It has some disadvantages, however. As expected from its pharmacology, isoproterenol causes considerable cardiac stimulation and its action is short. Furthermore, it has been suggested[13] that the use of isoproterenol may have contributed to the annual increase in mortality of asthmatic individuals in England and Wales. The deaths have been attributed to various

TABLE 40-1. Drugs acting on bronchial smooth muscle

Causing contraction	Causing relaxation or opposing contraction
Acetylcholine and related drugs	Atropine and other anticholinergic drugs
Histamine	Antihistaminics
β-adrenergic blockers	β-adrenergic agonists
α-adrenergic agonists	Dimethylxanthine (theophylline)
Slow-reacting substance of anaphylaxis	Inhibitors of the immunological release of mediators of anaphylaxis
Bradykinin	Prostaglandins E
Prostaglandin $F_{2\alpha}$	Antagonists of slow-reacting substances of anaphylaxis and prostaglandins F

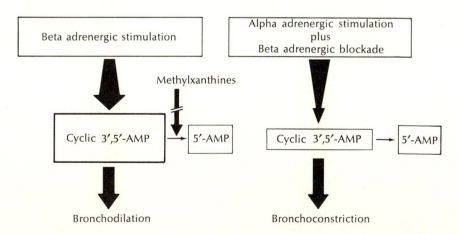

Fig. 40-1. Bronchodilation and bronchoconstriction as influenced by cyclic 3'5' AMP tissue concentrations. (Schematic representation of a working hypothesis. For details see Problem 40-2.)

causes, such as alterations in the viscosity of bronchial secretions, decreased arterial oxygen tensions, and increased ventricular irritability with arrhythmias.[13]

With the postulation by Lands[7] of two types of β-adrenergic receptors, efforts have been directed at synthesizing drugs that would have a more specific effect on the bronchial smooth muscle and would also have a more prolonged action, thus avoiding the disadvantages of isoproterenol.

Lands termed β_1 those receptors responsible for cardiac stimulation and lipolysis, whereas those responsible for bronchodilation and vasodepression were referred to as β_2. If two types of β receptors indeed exist, it should be possible to synthesize β agonists that have marked bronchodilator activity without much cardiac stimulation. Salbutamol and terbutaline appear to have such characteristics.

Problem 40-1. Is it possible to increase bronchodilator activity without a corresponding increase in cardiac stimulant effect in β-adrenergic agonists? Salbutamol and isoproterenol were compared on asthmatic subjects and in normal individuals in a double-blind trial to compare bronchodilator and cardiovascular activity.[14]

Aerosols containing salbutamol (100 γg/inhalation) or isoproterenol (500 γg/inhalation) were provided for a double-blind trial in identical containers. Forced expiratory spirograms were analyzed for forced expiratory volume in 1 second (FEV_1) and forced vital capacity (FVC) as well as by other criteria. Heart rate was measured from a continuous electrocardiogram.

In asthmatic subjects the FEV_1 showed a similar increase with both drugs initially, but 3 and 4 hours later the values were significantly higher for salbutamol. Heart rate did not increase with salbutamol but showed a rise with isoproterenol. In normal subjects, salbutamol produced a small increase in heart rate, whereas isoproterenol increased heart rate on the average by 33 beats a minute and caused palpitation.

It may be concluded from this clinical study that for comparable bronchodilator activity salbutamol produces much less cardiac stimulation. It appears, then, that the β receptors in bronchial smooth muscle and the heart are somewhat different. Animal experiments[5] point to the same conclusion.

Since β adrenergic receptors mediate bronchodilatation, the question remains: are there α-adrenergic receptors in the bronchial smooth muscle and do they have any function in drug effects?

Problem 40-2. Do α-adrenergic receptors play a role in drug-induced bronchoconstriction? In a recent experimental study,[8] isolated strips of human bronchi were tested for their response to a variety of drugs. The bronchodilating effect of epinephrine was abolished by propranolol. After β-receptor blockade, epinephrine produced bronchoconstriction. However, the dose of epinephrine required for the constrictor effect was 10 times greater than the dose that caused bronchial dilatation prior to β-receptor blockade. The constriction caused by epinephrine could be abolished by phentolamine, an α-adrenergic blocking drug. It may be concluded from this study and from other evidence that α-adrenergic agonists may cause bronchoconstriction in high doses. Such bronchoconstriction becomes evident after the β receptors are blocked. Whether the α-receptor–mediated bronchoconstriction has any clinical significance remains to be demonstrated. It is not known, for example, if it is related to tachyphylaxis to epinephrine, the so-called *epinephrine fastness* in asthmatic individuals.

Although the adrenergic drugs are most effective, the methylxanthines such as theophylline and its double salt aminophylline are useful. This is especially true in patients in whom some contraindication exists to the adrenergic drugs or in those who are tolerant to them. Intravenously administered aminophylline may be effective in terminating an asthmatic attack.

In addition to the adrenergic drugs and the methylxanthines, the adrenal corticosteroids are used in severe asthma. The mode of action of the corticosteroids remains unknown, although it is probably related to their anti-inflammatory effect. Several other drugs are used experimentally as bronchodilators, such as the prostaglandins of the E series. Other drugs are useful in combination with bronchodilators, such as disodium cromoglycate (p. 718) and the mucolytic agents that will be discussed later (p. 513).

Adverse effects   Epinephrine and isoproterenol have all the cardiovascular side effects predictable from their pharmacology, and patients may manifest tachycardia, palpitations, and arrhythmias. Ephedrine, which acts by releasing endogenous catecholamines, crosses the blood-brain barrier and causes nervousness and wakefulness in addition to the peripheral sympathomimetic effects.

Orally administered theophylline or aminophylline causes gastric irritation, and these drugs are irregularly absorbed from the gastrointestinal tract. It is claimed that theophylline in 20% alcohol is less likely to cause gastric irritation and is better absorbed. Aminophylline suppositories are irregularly absorbed and may lead to rectal irritation. Intravenously administered aminophylline may lead to central nervous system (CNS) stimulation and convulsions.

Individual bronchodilators   **Epinephrine** is highly effective in the treatment of acute asthma. It may be injected subcutaneously for a short duration of action, intramuscularly, or as a suspension in oil. It may be administered as an inhalant. When issued frequently, it may produce tachyphylaxis, the mechanism of which is not understood. Perhaps it is a rebound phenomenon.

Ephedrine is highly useful in the prevention and treatment of asthma. It is effective when given orally, and it has a duration of action that last several hours. It acts by releasing endogenous catecholamines, and tachyphylaxis may develop to its continued use. CNS stimulation is a common side effect caused by ephedrine. For this reason there are combinations of ephedrine and phenobarbital available. The latter is usually present in doses too small to counteract the wakefulness caused by ephedrine. The usual dosage of ephedrine for adults is 15 to 50 mg, which may be given as often as every hour if needed. **Pseudoephedrine hydrochloride** (Sudafed) is an active stereoisomer of ephedrine used in a manner similar to the latter.

Isoproterenol as the hydrochloride or sulfate is administered preferably by inhalation. The drug may also be given intravenously. Sublingual tablets of the drug are available, but absorption of these is irregular. Cardiovascular side effects are common after the administration of isoproterenol. Sudden death has occurred under these circumstances.

Salbutamol is one of a series of selective stimulants of the β_2 receptors. Its cardiovascular effects are less than its bronchodilator actions, and the duration of action of the drug is considerably greater than that of isoproterenol.

Metaproterenol sulfate, also known as orciprenaline, is a β receptor agonist with a moderately long duration of action. It differs from isoproterenol only in its two hydroxyl groups attached in meta position on the benzene ring.

It is claimed that the oral administration of a single dose of 20 mg exerts a bronchodilator effect that may last up to 4 hours. Its main contraindications are in patients with cardiac arrhythmias associated with tachycardia.

Metaproterenol sulfate (Alupent) is available in tablets, 20 mg, and in metered dose inhalers. Each metered dose delivers at the mouthpiece approximately 0.65 mg of metaproterenol sulfate.

Terbutaline sulfate (Brethine) is closely related to metaproterenol and may have a greater preference for β_2 receptors.[21] It is available in 5 mg tablets.

Aminophylline (theophylline ethylenediamine) may be administered by slow intravenous injection, orally, or rectally. Its absorption from the gastrointestinal tract is variable. Irritation of the rectum may result from suppositories. Excessive blood levels such as may occur from intravenous injections may lead to convulsions, shock, and death. About 85% of aminophylline is theophylline. For blood levels of theophylline after its intravenous injection, see Mitenko and Ogilvie.[9]

Oxtriphylline (Choledyl) is the choline salt of theophylline containing 64% theophylline. It is more soluble than theophylline and may be better absorbed after oral administration.

Dyphylline (Dilor, Lufyllin, Neothylline) is 7(2,3-dihydroxypropyl) theophylline, a neutral derivative. It corresponds to 70% anhydrous theophylline. It is more soluble than the parent compound and is less irritating. It may even be injected intramuscularly.

Theophylline is also available in timed-release tablets (Theo-Dur) and timed-release capsules (Slo-Phyllin).

Pharmacokinetics of theophylline. Ideal serum concentrations of theophylline vary from 5 to 20 μg/ml. The drug is adequately absorbed from the gastrointestinal tract, and dosage is determined by the clearance rate. Half-life of the drug varies from 3 to 13 hours and is more rapid in children than in adults.

Although widely used, the expectorants and mucolytic drugs hardly constitute one of the brilliant chapters of pharmacology. These drugs presumably alter the viscosity of the sputum, change the volume of respiratory tract fluid, and facilitate expectoration. The mode of action of some of these drugs is understood. In many cases, however, there is much doubt about their mechanism of action and their effectiveness.

Acetylcysteine (Mucomyst) reduces the viscosity of sputum, presumably by depolymerizing mucopolysaccharides. It is used by nebulization or by instillation of the upper respiratory tract and the mouth. The drug reacts with rubber and metals.

Terpin hydrate is volatile oil believed to act on bronchial secretory cells. It is commonly used as a vehicle for cough mixtures in the form of the elixir.

EXPECTORANTS AND MUCOLYTIC DRUGS

A number of expectorants are believed to stimulate respiratory tract secretion by a reflex through irritation of the stomach. These include **potassium iodide, syrup of ipecac, glyceryl guaiacolate,** and **ammonium chloride.** Proof for the effectiveness of these drugs is hard to find.

Pancreatic dornase is pancreatic deoxyribonuclease that hydrolyzes the deoxyribonucleoprotein of purulent sputum and thereby reduces its viscosity.

It is the belief of competent authorities that the inhalation of nebulized water, sodium chloride solutions, and hygroscopic agents may be more valuable than the use of other inhalants in the treatment of diseases of the respiratory tract complicated by difficulties in expectoration.

ELABORATION AND DESTRUCTION OF PHARMACOLOGICAL AGENTS BY THE LUNGS

It is increasingly recognized that the lungs are involved in the elaboration and destruction of a variety of pharmacological agents. Histamine has long been known to be present in high concentration in the mast cells of the lungs, and its release by anaphylaxis has been studied by many workers.

In addition to histamine, other pharmacological agents are released during anaphylaxis. According to a study on the perfused guinea pig lung,[16] in addition to histamine, the lipid slow-reacting substance, prostaglandins, serotonin, and certain polypeptides such as bradykinin may also be released or elaborated.

The prostaglandins are receiving much attention for a number or reasons. The lungs are a major site of prostaglandin synthesis. In addition, mechanical stimulation of the lungs or simply hyperinflation[10] may lead to increased synthesis or release of prostaglandins. The significance of this is still not clear. In addition to the prostaglandins, a number of peptides such as bradykinin and others[16] may be elaborated by the lungs.

The potential of the lung for synthesizing hormonal agents is best seen in cases of bronchogenic carcinoma, which may lead to endocrine syndromes with elaboration of many different polypeptide hormones.

The lungs are highly efficient in inactivating a number of pharmacologically active compounds. PGE and PGF are rapidly removed and inactivated during one circulation through the lungs. Bradykinin is almost completely removed in one circulation through the lungs. This is achieved by kininases, which act on the nonapeptide by splitting off a C-terminal dipeptide.

DRUG-INDUCED PULMONARY DISEASES

Drugs may influence pulmonary function directly or indirectly. An example of a direct adverse effect is oxygen toxicity. Drugs alter pulmonary function indirectly by various mechanisms. Sedative drugs are an important cause of acute ventilatory failure. Pulmonary edema may be caused by salt and water overload or by depression of cardiac output. Intravenous medications causing thrombophlebitis contribute to pulmonary embolism. Finally, drug allergies may cause bronchospasm.

The directly acting drugs that may induce pulmonary disease encompass a variety of classes, such as inhalants, cancer chemotherapeutic agents, analgesics, antimicrobial drugs, and a miscellaneous category.

Several inhalants may lead to altered pulmonary function. They include oxygen, acetylcysteine, and isoproterenol. In addition, aspiration of mineral oil and iodinated oils used for bronchography can lead to adverse effects.

It may seem surprising that *oxygen* is toxic in high concentrations, but the tendency of premature infants to develop retrolental fibroplasia and blindness after the prolonged administration of the gas at greater than 40% concentration is well documented. In addition, adults who inhale oxygen at greater than 60% concentrations may develop pulmonary irritation, congestion, atelectasis, and decreased vital capacity. CNS changes manifested by paresthesias also occur. The pulmonary toxic effect of oxygen in humans under hyperbaric conditions has been studied in great detail.[3] Breathing oxygen at 2 atmospheres, symptoms began within 3 to 8 hours and consisted of mild tracheal irritation and decreased vital capacity. After 8 to 10 hours, symptoms were characterized by uncontrollable coughing, dyspnea at rest, and a tracheobronchial burning sensation. Recovery of vital capacity occurred generally in 1 to 3 days.

Mineral oil, when aspirated, causes acute or chronic pneumonitis. *Iodinated oils* employed in bronchography may have adverse effects on a pulmonary reserve that is already impaired.

The bronchoconstrictor effect of acetylcysteine has already been mentioned (p. 513). *Isoproterenol* has been implicated by association in cases of sudden death in asthmatic persons. It has been suggested that in some individuals the drug is converted to 3-methoxyisoproterenol, which is a weak antagonist of the β-adrenergic receptor. *Disodium cromoglycate* may also cause some bronchospasm when given by nebulization.

Cancer chemotherapeutic agents may in some cases cause pulmonary diseases. Diffuse pulmonary disease has been associated with the use of *busulfan* and *cyclophosphamide*.[11] *Methotrexate* has also been implicated in some cases of pulmonary disease.

The narcotic analgesics *heroin* and *methadone* may produce pulmonary edema by mechanisms that are obscure (p. 359). *Propoxyphene* poisoning has also been associated with pulmonary edema.

Aspirin may cause bronchoconstriction in some individuals. Although this is often referred to as aspirin allergy, its immunological basis is unlikely. Often aspirin-sensitive persons fail to show similar reactions to sodium salicylate, whereas they may react to chemically unrelated anti-inflammatory drugs such as indomethacin. The mechanism of this aspirin hypersensitivity remains a mystery.

A variety of antimicrobial drugs may cause pulmonary diseases. *Nitrofurantoin* administration may lead to a pleuropneumonic reaction. *Sulfonamides* may cause vasculitis, which may include the pulmonary vessels. Sulfonamides, para-amino-salicylate, and penicillin may produce pulmonary infiltration with eosinophilia,

Inhalants

Cancer chemotherapeutic agents

Analgesics

Antimicrobial drugs

usually referred to as Löffler's syndrome. The *aminoglycosides* may cause muscle weakness, which with involvement of respiratory muscles may lead to respiratory paralysis. *Polymyxin B* given by aerosol can cause bronchospasm. This antibiotic is a well-known histamine releaser.

Miscellaneous drugs causing pulmonary disease   *Methysergide* can produce chronic pleural effusion. *Corticosteroids* may lead to the development of opportunistic pulmonary infections, particularly *Pneumocystis carinii* pneumonia.

REFERENCES

1 Bianco, S., Griffin, J. P., Kamburoff, P. L., and Prime, F. J.: The effect of thymoxamine on histamine induced bronchospasm in man, Br. J. Dis. Chest. **66:**27, 1972.

2 Choo-Kang, Y. F. J., Simpson, W. T., and Grant, I. W. B.: Controlled comparison of the bronchodilator effects of three β-adrenergic stimulant drugs administered by inhalation to patients with asthma, Br. Med. J. **2:**287, 1969.

3 Clark, J. M., and Lambertsen, C. J.: Rate of development of pulmonary O_2 toxicity in man during O_2 breathing at 2.0 Ata, J. Appl. Physiol. **30:**739, 1971.

4 Henderson, W. R., Shelhamer, J. H., Reingold, D. B., Smith, L. J., Evans, R., and Kaliner, M.: Alpha-adrenergic hyper-responsiveness in asthma, N. Engl. J. Med. **300:**642, 1979.

5 Hinds, L., and Katz, R. L.: Dissociation of tracheobronchial and cardiac effects of some beta-adrenergic stimulants, Anesthesiology **34:**445, 1971.

6 Igic, R., Erdos, E. G., Yeh, H. S. J., Sorrels, K., and Nakajima, T.: The angiotensin I converting enzyme of the lung, Circ. Res. **31**(Supp. 2):51, 1972.

7 Lands, A. M., et al.: Differentiation of receptor systems activated by sympathomimetic amines, Nature **214:**597, 1967.

8 Mathé, A. A., Aström, A., and Persson, N. A.: Some bronchoconstricting and bronchodilating responses of human isolated bronchi: evidence for the existence of α-adrenoceptors, J. Pharm. Pharmacol. **23:**905, 1971.

9 Mitenko, P. A., and Ogilvie, R. I.: Rational intravenous doses of theophylline, N. Engl. J. Med. **289:**600, 1973.

10 Piper, P., and Vane, J. R.: The release of prostaglandins from lung and other tissues, Ann. N.Y. Acad. Sci. **180:**363, 1971.

11 Rosenow, E. C.: The spectrum of drug-induced pulmonary disease, Ann. Intern. Med. **77:**977, 1972.

12 Ruffin, R. E., Wolff, R. K., and Dolovich, M. B.: Aerosol therapy with Sch 1000, Chest **73:**501, 1978.

13 Speizer, F. E., Doll, R., and Heaf, P.: Observations on recent increase in mortality prone asthma, Br. Med. J. **1:**339, 1968.

14 Tattersfield, A. E., and McNicol, M. W.: Salbutamol and isoproterenol; a double-blind trial to compare bronchodilator and cardiovascular activity, N. Engl. J. Med. **281:**1323, 1969.

15 Tinkelman, D. G., and Avner, S. E.: Ephedrine therapy in asthmatic children, J.A.M.A. **237:**553, 1977.

16 Vane, J. R.: Mediators of the anaphylactic reaction, in identification of asthma, Ciba Foundation Study Group No. 38, Edinburgh, 1971, Churchill Livingstone.

17 Vane, J. R.: Prostaglandins and the aspirin-like drugs, Hosp. Pract. **7:**61, 1972.

18 Wolfe, J. D., Tashkin, D. P., Calvarese, B., and Simmons, M.: Bronchodilator effects of terbutaline and aminophylline alone and in combination in asthmatic patients, N. Engl. J. Med. **298:**363, 1978.

19 Zaske, D. E., Miller, K. W., Strem, E. L., Austrian, S., and Johnson, P. B.: Oral aminophylline therapy: increased dosage requirements in children, J.A.M.A. **237:**1453, 1977.

REVIEWS

20 Barton, A. D., and Lourenco, R. V.: Bronchial secretions and mucociliary clearance, Arch. Intern. Med. **131:**140, 1973.

21 Geumei, A., Miller, W. F., Paez, P. N., and Gast, L. R.: Evaluation of a new oral β_2-adrenoceptor stimulant bronchodilator, Pharmacology **13:**201, 1975.

22 Gillis, C. N., and Roth, J. A.: Pulmonary disposition of circulating vasoactive hormones, Biochem. Pharmacol. **25:**2547, 1976.

22a Greenberger, P. A.: Theophylline, Ration. Drug Ther. **14:**1, Sept. 1980.

23 Irwin, R. S., Rosen, M. J., and Braman, S. S.: Cough—a comprehensive review, Arch. Intern. Med. **137**:1186, 1977.

24 Miller, W. F.: Aerosol therapy in acute and chronic respiratory disease, Arch. Intern. Med. **131**:148, 1973.

24a Piafsky, K. M., and Ogilvie, R. I.: Dosage of theophylline in bronchial asthma, N. Engl. J. Med. **292**:1218, 1975.

25 Stolley, P. D.: Asthma mortality, Am. Rev. Respir. Dis. **105**:883, 1972.

26 Weinberger, M.: Theophylline for treatment of asthma, J. Pediatr. **92**:1, 1978.

27 Weinberger, M., and Riegelman, S.: Rational use of theophylline for bronchodilatation, N. Engl. J. Med. **291**:151, 1974.

28 Wilson, A. F.: Drug treatment of acute asthma, J.A.M.A. **237**:1141, 1977.

29 Zelis, R., and Cross, C. E.: Management of pulmonary edema, Ration. Drug Ther. **8**:1, 1974.

CHAPTER 41

Drug effects on the gastrointestinal tract

Drugs that exert a useful effect on the gastrointestinal tract may be best grouped according to their therapeutic indications. Since the most common medical problems in relation to the gastrointestinal tract are the management of peptic ulcer, constipation, diarrhea, and deficiencies of digestive factors, the various drugs used in gastroenterology will be discussed under the following headings: anticholinergics, gastric antacids, and cathartics, laxatives, and antidiarrheal agents. The histamine H_2-receptor antagonists are discussed on p. 253.

ANTICHOLIN-ERGICS
An effective dose of an anticholinergic drug decreases nocturnal acid secretion by about 50%.[20] It also decreases gastric acid secretion stimulated by histamine or pentagastrin or a meal by about 30% to 50%. The duration of action of an anticholinergic drug is longer if it is administered 1 hour after a meal, but effectiveness can be demonstrated even when it is given 30 minutes before a meal. Dosage should be carefully titrated in each patient by increasing the dose until side effects such as dryness of the mouth are noted. Contraindications to the use of anticholinergic drugs include glaucoma, prostatic hyperplasia, and gastric retention.

Some of the most commonly used antispasmodics are propantheline (Pro-Banthine), diphemanil (Prantal), oxyphenonium (Antrenyl), penthienate (Monodral), tricyclamol (Co-Elorine), methscopolamine bromide (Pamine), dicyclomine (Bentyl), and glycopyrrolate (Robinul). Although none of these drugs is perfect, their administration to the point of tolerance along with antacids provides dramatic relief of pain in ulcer patients.

GASTRIC ANTACIDS
Many experimental and clinical observations suggest that antacids are among the most important drugs in the treatment of peptic ulcer. Although used for many years, important aspects of their pharmacology have only been worked out recently.[20]

When administered during the fasting state, the duration of action of the antacids is only 30 minutes. However, when administered after meals, their action may last 3 to 4 hours. The buffering action of the various antacids varies greatly depending on the preparation and the patient.

As shown in Table 41-1, the potency of the antacids varies considerably as does

TABLE 41-1. Characteristics of various antacids*

Antacid	Composition	Buffering capacity (mEq of hydrochloride per ml)	Sodium content (mg/5 ml)
Aludrox	Magnesium and aluminum hydroxides, simethicone	2.81	4.5
Amphojel	Aluminum hydroxide gel	1.93	8.1
Gelusil	Aluminum hydroxide gel, magnesium trisilicate	1.33	6.5
Gelusil M	Aluminum hydroxide gel, magnesium hydroxide, and trisilicate	2.23	5.7
Maalox	Aluminum hydroxide gel, magnesium hydroxide	2.58	2.5
Magaldrate (Riopan)	Magnesium and aluminum hydroxides	2.23	0.7
Mylanta	Magnesium and aluminum hydroxides, simethicone	2.38	3.9
WinGel	Aluminum hydroxide gel, magnesium hydroxide, stabilized with hexitol	2.25	1.25

*Modified from Fordtran, J. S., Morawski, S. G., and Richardson, C. T.: N. Engl. J. Med. **288:**923, 1973.

their sodium content. Effective doses require 75 to 150 mEq buffer. In addition, the hypersecretors, such as patients with duodenal ulcer, require larger quantities of antacid than patients who are not hypersecretors, such as persons with a gastric ulcer.

Gastric antacids are generally classified as *systemic* and *nonsystemic,* depending on the amount of systemic absorption of the cation responsible for the neutralization of gastric hydrochloric acid. Sodium bicarbonate (baking soda) is the only systemic antacid that has been used medically. It is now entirely abandoned except for its use by the lay public. Sodium bicarbonate is a very effective and rapid-acting neutralizer of gastric acid. Its disadvantage is that systemic absorption of the sodium ion causes alkalosis, which is characterized by elevated carbon dioxide content and pH of the plasma, loss of appetite, weakness, mental confusion, and, rarely, tetany. Renal insufficiency and calcinosis have been described in patients who have been taking systemic antacids for long periods of time.

The gastric antacids preferred at present are the drugs whose cationic portion is not absorbed from the intestine and that raise the pH of the gastric contents only to about 4. These drugs are often referred to as *nonsystemic buffer antacids.* Various aluminum and magnesium salts have this property. The antacids containing calcium carbonate are very potent but they cause an increase in gastric secretion after their action is terminated. For this reason, the antacids that do not contain calcium are preferable.

Inhibition of gastric secretion by H_2-receptor antagonists is of great interest. Burimamide, metiamide, and cimetidine are discussed on p. 253.

Nonsystemic gastric antacids

Among the poorly absorbed gastric antacids, calcium carbonate is the most effective but has many disadvantages, such as hypercalcemia, constipation, and acid rebound. Magnesium compounds are potent and useful in counteracting the constipating effects of calcium carbonate and aluminum hydroxide. Aluminum hydroxide is not absorbed and is constipating. It is useful in removing phosphate when such measure is indicated.

Aluminum hydroxide gel and dihydroxyaluminum aminoacetate. Aluminum hydroxide gel (Amphojel) is a colloidal suspension that is available in a liquid preparation or in tablets. In the acid stomach, aluminum chloride is formed, but in the alkaline intestine, aluminum hydroxide is again formed and the chloride reabsorbed. As a consequence, no alteration in systemic acid-base balance occurs. This drug has been widely used in liquid and tablet form and also by continuous drip through a gastric tube in treating peptic ulcer.

$$Al(OH)_3$$

Aluminum hydroxide

$$(HO)_2Al-O-\overset{\overset{\textstyle O}{\|}}{C}CH_2NH_2$$

Dihydroxyaluminum aminoacetate

Aluminum hydroxide gel will raise the pH of the stomach contents to only about 4. Its only disadvantages are a constipating effect and the possibility of causing some loss of phosphate in the feces. The former difficulty may be prevented by the addition of certain magnesium salts. The phosphate loss is not likely to be serious with moderate doses in patients receiving an adequate diet. However, aluminum phosphate gel may be used, which will obviate this difficulty, although it has a lesser capacity to neutralize acid. The binding of phosphate by aluminum salts may be beneficial in the management of patients with renal phosphatic calculi.[12]

Dihydroxyaluminum aminoacetate is comparable to aluminum hydroxide gel on the basis of available clinical experience. In the test tube the buffering action of this antacid in a solid form is comparable to that of liquid preparations of aluminum hydroxide gel. There is not enough clinical evidence to allow a clear-cut decision on the possible superiority of one of these drugs over the others.

Magnesium trisilicate. In the stomach this drug is changed to magnesium chloride and silicon dioxide. In the alkaline intestine, magnesium remains as the carbonate, whereas chloride is reabsorbed.

In contrast to the aluminum salts, magnesium trisilicate not only does not cause constipation but in large doses may even produce some diarrhea. In many very popular preparations, aluminum hydroxide gel and magnesium trisilicate are combined in a single tablet. One of the most popular contains 0.5 g of magnesium trisilicate and 0.25 g of aluminum hydroxide. Apparently some silica may be absorbed, since in rare cases kidney stones containing silicon compounds have been reported.[5]

Other nonabsorbed antacids. Magnesium oxide, magnesium hydroxide, and calcium carbonate are gastric antacids that differ from the previous group in that they can elevate the pH of the gastric contents to 7 or above. An 8% aqueous suspension of magnesium hydroxide, widely known as milk of magnesia, is probably the most potent antacid in common practice. The addition of aluminum hydroxide to magnesium hydroxide tends to decrease the neutralizing power of the magnesium salt.[22]

The absorption of magnesium may be of significance. As much as 15% to 30% of the magnesium chloride formed is available for absorption. The absorbed magnesium is rapidly cleared through the kidney and represents no danger to a normal person. However, magnesium salts should not be given to patients with poor renal function since dangerous toxicity may occur.

Magaldrate (Riopan) is a hydrated magnesium aluminate, a buffer-antacid that is not absorbed. Among advantages claimed for it is its low sodium content. Some of the commonly used antacids have a surprising amount of sodium, a disadvantage in some patients.

In contrast with older concepts, cathartic and laxative action is being attributed to an increase in fecal water excretion, resulting in most instances from alterations in the transport of fluid and electrolytes in the intestine.[16]

Constipation, when not due to organic causes, is generally attributed today to poor dietary habits, lack of bulk-producing foods, and inattention to the stimulus for defecation. Correction of these poor habits will often take care of the problem of chronic constipation without the necessity of prescribing laxatives.

Nevertheless, cathartics and laxatives have some valid uses in medicine. Soft stools and lack of straining during defecation are desirable after hemorrhoidectomy and in persons with myocardial infarction. Cathartics are also prescribed for the purpose of speeding the elimination of various toxic materials such as some of the anthelmintics. By itself, however, chronic constipation should not be an indication for continual use of cathartics.

In diarrheal states the correction of fluid and electrolyte changes is today considered to be the primary therapeutic goal. Small doses of opiates in the form of paregoric (camphorated tincture of opium) or codeine may be employed to slow intestinal motility. Astringents and absorbents are also used but are not very effective. Determination of the cause of the diarrheal state—whether bacterial, parasitic, or toxic—is most important, and the specific cause should be corrected whenever possible.

CATHARTICS, LAXATIVES, AND ANTIDIARRHEAL AGENTS

Cathartics

Cathartics may be classified on the basis of their mode of action as follows:
1. Bulk cathartics—magnesium sulfate, magnesium hydroxide, sodium sulfate, sodium phosphate, methylcellulose, psyllium seeds, agar, and other nonabsorbed salts and hydrophilic colloids
2. Irritant cathartics—anthraquinone compounds such as cascara sagrada, aloe, senna, rhubarb, castor oil, and phenolphthalein
3. Surface-active agents—dioctyl sodium sulfosuccinate

This classification is probably not based on the true mode of action of the cathartics.[16] The irritant cathartics probably alter mucosal permeability.

Bulk cathartics   Bulk cathartics promote intestinal evacuation because they are not significantly absorbed from the intestine. As a consequence, they retain a considerable amount of water, distend the colon, and promote the expulsion of liquid stools.

Magnesium sulfate is widely used in medicine. It is generally administered in doses of 15 g. Little of it is absorbed under normal circumstances, and the effects of the small amount absorbed are minimized by rapid renal excretion. If there is prolonged intestinal retention of the drug and renal function is simultaneously impaired, some systemic effects such as CNS depression may occur. It may be estimated that 15 g of magnesium sulfate requires 400 ml of water in order to make an isotonic solution. If the drug is given in a more concentrated form, it will abstract water from the tissues.

Magnesium hydroxide, usually administered as magnesia magma (milk of magnesia), is considerably more pleasant than the bitter sulfate. It is also considerably less effective.

The hydrophilic colloids are not absorbed from the gastrointestinal tract and retain considerable quantities of water. They are widely used, but simple dietary measures such as inclusion of prunes and bran-containing cereals can generally serve the purpose equally well.

Irritant cathartics   **Anthraquinone cathartics,** also known as emodin compounds, are commonly used in proprietary mixtures and less frequently by the medical profession. The active principles in such drugs as cascara, aloe, senna, and rhubarb are glycosides of anthracene compounds. Their effect is exerted on the large intestine, and there is usually a delay of about 6 to 8 hours in obtaining defecation following the use of these compounds. Injected emodin drugs produce an effect in less than 1 hour. Therefore the delay in their action may result from the time required for their reaching the large bowel, although other explanations have also been advanced.

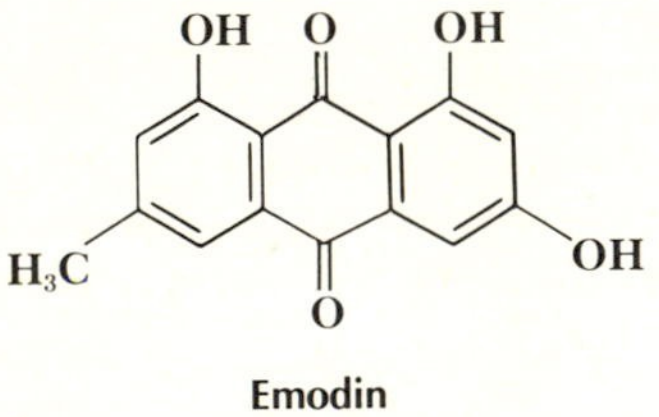

Emodin

Anthraquinone cathartics are partially absorbed from the intestine and may cause discoloration of the urine. One of the breakdown products, chrysophanic acid, behaves as an indicator, being yellow in acid urine and changing to red upon alkalinization.

The highly irritant, drastic **cathartic resins** such as jalap and podophyllum have no valid use in the treatment of constipation. The same may be said of croton oil.

Phenolphthalein is also more commonly used in proprietary preparations than on a physician's prescription. The history of the discovery of the cathartic action of phenolphthalein is interesting. It was used for making adulterated wine in Hungary, and its cathartic properties were soon appreciated.

There is a delay of some 6 to 8 hours in the cathartic action of phenolphthalein, although the time may be less in children. The drug is believed to act on the large intestine, its exact mode of action being unknown. It is partially absorbed, and although its toxicity is low, it can cause very undesirable skin eruptions and persistent discoloration. The phenomenon of fixed eruption caused by phenolphthalein probably has a true allergic basis because the involved areas of skin flare up again when doses of phenolphthalein are taken that would exert no effect in a normal person.

Oxyphenisatin and its acetate salt are related to phenolphthalein. They can cause hepatic damage and should not be used.

Castor oil is obtained from the seeds of *Ricinus communis*, or castor bean. The oil itself is nonirritating, but when it is hydrolyzed in the intestine to ricinoleic acid, a cathartic effect is produced. This action is exerted especially on the small intestine. The usual dose of castor oil is 15 ml.

Bisacodyl (Dulcolax) in the form of oral tablets and suppositories appears to be useful for bowel evacuation. It stimulates the contraction of the large intestine and is apparently not absorbed from the intestine.

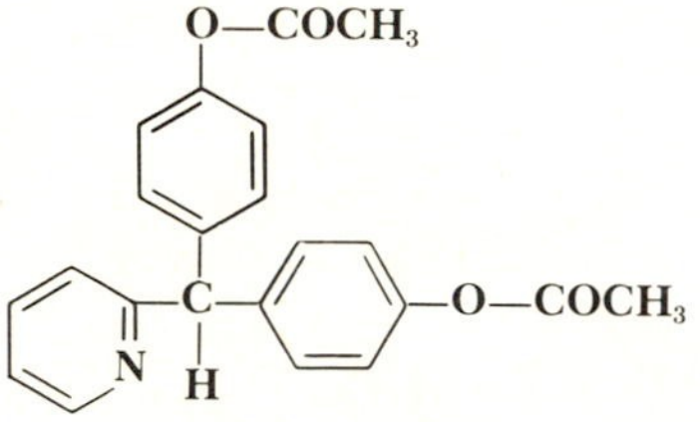

Bisacodyl

Bisacodyl has an effect on fluid and electrolyte absorption in the intestine[16]; its exact mechanism of action is not well understood.

Preparations of bisacodyl (Dulcolax) include enteric-coated tablets containing 5 mg that should be swallowed whole and suppositories containing 10 mg. The suppositories should not be used in patients in whom absorption may be facilitated by the presence of fissures or ulcerations.

Surface-active agents

Dioctyl sodium sulfosuccinate (Doxinate; Colace) was introduced as a fecal softener. The drug acts as a dispersing or wetting agent and appears to be inert from a pharmacological standpoint. It is used in daily doses of 10 to 20 mg in children and in larger doses in adults.[14]

Antidiarrheal agents

The management of diarrhea is based on elimination of the cause when possible and administration of proper fluids and electrolytes. In addition, a variety of absorbent compounds is employed, largely on an empiric basis. Some of these are bismuth subcarbonate, kaolin, activated charcoal, and pectin. Considerably more effective in stopping diarrhea and making the patient comfortable are the opiates. It should be kept in mind, however, that the narcotics may obscure the diagnosis. This is a serious disadvantage if the diarrhea is caused by a major organic disease that may be curable, such as amebic dysentery. The camphorated tincture of opium (paregoric) has been used traditionally in the treatment of diarrhea. The usual dose is 4 ml. Codeine sulfate may be used also in doses of 16 to 32 mg. It is important to keep in mind that the opiates represent only symptomatic treatment, and efforts for detecting and correcting the underlying disturbances should not be neglected.

In severe diarrhea, when antibiotic treatment is needed, antidiarrheal agents should be avoided. Many of these agents may adsorb the antibiotic and may prolong the infection.

The opiate-like drug **diphenoxylate** (with atropine sulfate as Lomotil) has considerable efficacy as an antidiarrheal agent. A relatively low daily dosage (2.5 to 7.5 mg) usually gives good results. Diphenoxylate has been particularly recommended for chronic diarrhea when the more addictive opiates are undesirable.[1] Each Lomotil tablet and each 5 ml of liquid contains 2.5 mg of diphenoxylate and 0.025 mg of atropine sulfate. Diphenoxylate has a low potential for producing physical dependence, but it may increase the effect of other CNS depressants. It should be used with caution in persons with liver disease as well as in those who have severe colitis.

Loperamide hydrochloride (Imodium) has recently been introduced as an antiperistaltic antidiarrheal agent. In contrast with Lomotil, the drug does not contain atropine but has some opiate-like properties, since it can cause morphine-like dependence in monkeys, and naloxone is recommended as a possible antidote. The drug is available in 2 mg capsules. Loperamide is a very effective drug, but it should not be used in persons with infectious diarrheas where the causative organism may invade the intestinal wall.

Cholestyramine may be an effective antidiarrheal agent whenever there is malabsorption of bile acids that contribute to the diarrhea. Such conditions include ileal resection[6] or the irritable bowel syndrome.[11] Cholestyramine therapy proved ineffective in tropical diarrhea in Vietnam.[8]

REFERENCES

1 Barowsky, H., and Schwartz, S. A.: Methods for evaluating diphenoxylate hydrochloride: comparison of its antidiarrheal effect with that of camphorated tincture of opium, J.A.M.A. **180**:1058, 1962.

2 Fordtran, J. S., and Collyns, J. A. H.: Antacid pharmacology in duodenal ulcer—effect of antacids on postcibal gastric acidity and peptic activity, N. Engl. J. Med. **274**:921, 1966.

3 Fordtran, J. S., Morawski, S. G., and Richardson, C. T.: In vivo and in vitro evaluation of liquid antacids, N. Engl. J. Med. **288**:923, 1973.

4 Hammerlund, E. R., and Rising, L. W.: A further study of the comparative buffering capacities of various commercially available gastric antacids, J. Med. Pharm. Assoc. **41**:295, 1952.

5 Herman, J. R., and Goldberg, A. S.: New type of urinary calculus caused by antacid therapy, J.A.M.A. **174**:1206, 1960.

6 Hofmann, A. F., and Poley, J. R.: Cholestyramine treatment of diarrhea associated with ileal resection, N. Engl. J. Med. **281**:397, 1969.

7 Kirsner, J. B., Rubio, C. E., Mlynaryk, P., and Reed, P. I.: Problems in the evaluation of gastrointestinal drugs, Clin. Pharmacol. Ther. **3**:510, 1962.

8 McCloy, R. M., and Hofmann, A. F.: Tropical diarrhea in Vietnam—a controlled study of cholestyramine therapy, N. Engl. J. Med. **284**:139, 1971.

9 McHardy, G., and Balart, L. A.: Jaundice and oxyphenisatin, J.A.M.A. **211**:83, 1970.

10 Roth, J. L. A.: Role of drugs in production of gastroduodenal ulcer, J.A.M.A. **187**:418, 1964.

11 Rowe, G. G.: Control of diarrhea by cholestyramine administration, Am. J. Med. Sci. **255**:84, 1968.

12 Shorr, E., and Carter, A. C.: Aluminum gels in management of renal phosphatic calculi, J.A.M.A. **144**:1549, 1950.

13 Texter, E. C., Smith, H. W., and Barborka, C. L.: Evaluation of newer anticholinergic agents, Gastroenterology **30**:772, 1956.

14 Wilson, J. L., and Dickinson, D. G.: Use of dioctyl sodium sulfosuccinate (aerosol O. T.) for severe constipation, J.A.M.A. **158**:261, 1955.

REVIEWS

15 Barreras, R. F.: The carbonate affair—is calcium indictable? N. Engl. J. Med. **289**:587, 1973.

16 Binder, H. J.: Pharmacology of laxatives, Annu. Rev. Pharmacol. Toxicol. **17**:355, 1977.

17 Christensen, J.: The controls of gastrointestinal movements: some old and new views, N. Engl. J. Med. **285**:85, 1971.

18 Cohen, S., and Snape, W. J.: The pathophysiology and treatment of gastroesophageal reflux disease, Arch. Intern. Med. **138**:1398, 1978.

19 Grady, G. F., and Keusch, G. T.: Pathogenesis of bacterial diarrheas, N. Engl. J. Med. **285**: 831, 891, 1971.

20 Isenberg, J. I.: Therapy of peptic ulcer, J.A.M.A. **233**:540, 1975.

21 McCarthy, D. M.: Peptic ulcer: antacids or cimetidine? Hosp. Prac. p. 52, Dec. 1979.

22 Morrissey, J. F., and Barreras, R. F.: Antacid therapy, N. Engl. J. Med. **290**:550, 1974.

23 Netchvolodoff, C. V., and Hargrove, M. D.: Recent advances in the treatment of diarrhea, Arch. Intern. Med. **139**:813, 1979.

24 Sparberg, M.: The therapy of peptic ulcer disease, Ration. Drug. Ther. **7**:1, 1973.

CHAPTER 42

Insulin, glucagon, and oral hypoglycemic agents

Insulin, the hormone elaborated by the β cells of the pancreas, is a key regulator of metabolic processes. Although its action on carbohydrate metabolism has received the most attention, its absolute or relative deficiency results in many other serious metabolic consequences. *Glucagon*, the hormone produced by the α cells of the pancreatic islets, has some actions such as glycogenolysis and hyperglycemia that are opposed to those of insulin. The ratio of the two hormones may determine their overall effect on the liver. Glucagon has positive inotropic effects on the heart, probably as a consequence of stimulating cyclic AMP production. The *hypoglycemic sulfonylureas* promote the release of insulin from β cells. *Phenformin* is also used occasionally for lowering the blood sugar in diabetic persons, but the drug acts by some mechanism other than the promotion of insulin release.

Insulin is elaborated in the β cells as part of a larger peptide known as *proinsulin*. The release of insulin is stimulated not only by glucose but also by certain amino acids, gastrointestinal hormones, ketone bodies, and α-receptor blockers such as phentolamine. Inhibitors of insulin release include α-adrenergic agonists such as norepinephrine and epinephrine, unusual sugars (mannoheptulose), and diazoxide. The action of insulin is exerted on specific receptors in cell membranes.

Although diabetes mellitus is defined as a relative or absolute deficiency of insulin, increasing attention is being paid to the role of a defect in the insulin receptors on the surface of cells as a major factor in the pathogenesis of the disease.

GENERAL CONCEPT

In 1889 the surgical removal of the pancreas in the dog was shown to result in experimental diabetes,[30] and in 1922 insulin was isolated from a dog's pancreas.[1] The introduction of insulin revolutionized the treatment of diabetes and greatly prolonged the lives of juvenile diabetic patients. Subsequent work was directed at developing injectable forms of insulin that would delay the absorption of the hormone and would thereby prolong its action in the body. Protamine zinc insulin and other insulin protein complexes were introduced. Finally, isophane insulin suspension (NPH) and insulin zinc suspension (lente) received wide clinical application because their administration only once each day proved very convenient.

Studies on insulin and diabetes were facilitated by the demonstration that alloxan could selectively destroy the β cells of the pancreas.[9] This discovery provided a

INSULIN
Development of current concepts

simple method for making experimental animals diabetic, compared with the previous and more laborious procedure of almost complete pancreatectomy.

Hand in hand with these investigations, work has proceeded on the chemistry and mode of action of insulin. The chemical structure of this protein hormone was established by Sanger and co-workers in 1954. More recently, insulin has been synthesized.

Studies on insulin were greatly aided by methods for determining the concentration of the hormone. This can be done by measuring its influence on glucose uptake by the isolated diaphragm of the rat or by immunoassay.

In addition to its effect on glucose entry into muscle and fat, insulin exerts important influences on the liver.[18] In this organ, insulin inhibits the hepatic release of glucose and regulates directly or indirectly the level of certain enzymes such as those involved in gluconeogenesis and glycolysis. However, in the liver the effect of insulin is not simply on the entry of glucose into cells.

Glucagon, the hormone produced by the α cells of the pancreatic islets, is looked on by many as a physiological antagonist to insulin.[45] In large doses, glucagon causes glycogenolysis and hyperglycemia. It also promotes gluconeogenesis in the liver from amino acids. Hypoglycemia results in high glucagon and low insulin levels, a hormonal ratio that favors glycogenolysis and gluconeogenesis. The ingestion of carbohydrates produces high insulin and low glucagon levels. Such a ratio would favor glycogen deposition, glycolysis, and fat synthesis.[34] Somatostatin inhibits glucagon release.

Glucagon is available as the hydrochloride for the treatment of insulin reactions. It is administered subcutaneously or intramuscularly in doses of 0.5 to 2 mg.[28] Glucagon has some uses also as a cardiac drug. It has a positive inotropic effect probably mediated by increased cyclic AMP production. Its positive inotropic action differs from those of the catecholamines in that it is not accompanied by ventricular irritability or increased peripheral resistance.[22] Glucagon may be useful in the treatment of acute heart failure.[22]

Chemistry and standardization   The complete amino acid sequence of insulin has now been worked out.[26] The molecule consists of two chains of polypeptides, the A and B chains, joined by two disulfide bridges. In addition, the A chain contains another disulfide bridge. Insulins of various animal species have similar biological activity and differ only in the sequence of three amino acids in the A chain. When the disulfide bonds are broken by reduction, the biological activity of insulin disappears.

Proinsulin, the biosynthetic precursor of insulin, is a single-chain polypeptide. Its molecular weight is about 1.5 times that of insulin. Cleavage of proinsulin occurs within the β cells, resulting in insulin and the connecting fragment known C-peptide.[29,43]

Proinsulin is important in two clinical situations. Normally about 6% to 8% of plasma insulin consists of proinsulin. In some islet cell adenomas this concentration is much higher. The other clinical situation is related to the C-peptide. The C-pep-

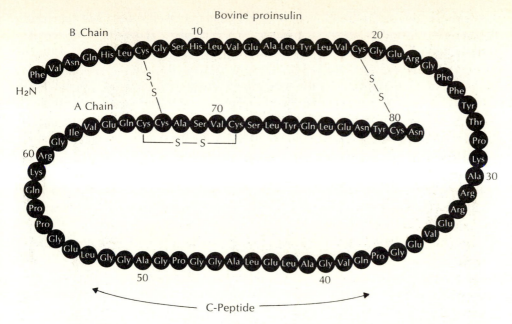

FIG. 42-1. Structure of bovine proinsulin showing A and B chains and C-peptide. Human proinsulin differs in three amino acids in the chains and several amino acids in the C-peptide. (From Steiner, D. F.: TRIANGLE, the Sandoz Journal of Medical Science, vol. II, no. 2, 1972, p. 52.)

tide has no biological activity but can be measured. This is important in individuals who develop antibodies to insulin after taking it for a long time. In these individuals the antibodies interfere with the determination of plasma insulin. On the other hand, the C-peptide can be measured as an indicator of endogenous insulin release, since it is released along with insulin and no antibodies are formed to it in humans.

Insulin is *standardized* on the basis of its ability to lower the blood sugar in experimental animals, usually in the rabbit. An international unit of insulin should lower the blood sugar to 45 mg/100 ml when injected into a fasting 2 kg rabbit. The international standard insulin contains 22 IU/mg.

Electron microscopic studies indicate that insulin is present in β cells of the pancreas in a particulate form. The most important stimulus for insulin release is *glucose*, but there are many other factors that can increase or decrease the release of insulin.

Release and metabolism

Factors that *promote* the release of insulin are *glucose, leucine, arginine* or a mixture of amino acids, *glucagon, ketone bodies, sulfonylureas, gastrin, secretin, pancreozymin, isoproterenol,* and *α-receptor blockers,* such as phentolamine.

Factors that *inhibit* the release of insulin are *norepinephrine* and *epinephrine*[24] (*α*-adrenergic effects), unusual sugars such as *mannoheptulose,* and *diazoxide*[19] (p. 221).

Once released, insulin reaches the liver first, where much of it is retained.

Mechanisms involved in the ultimate destruction are not well known, but apparently both enzymatic and nonenzymatic processes are at play. There probably is not a specific insulin-binding protein in plasma.[4]

Mode of action   When insulin is injected into a normal or diabetic individual, the following changes may be observed in the blood chemistry: (1) blood sugar decreases, (2) blood pyruvate and lactate increase, (3) inorganic phosphate decreases, and (4) potassium decreases.

Lowering of the blood sugar may be explained on the basis of an increased uptake of sugar by tissues such as muscle and fat. There is evidence indicating a decreased hepatic output of glucose through the action of insulin.[18] It has been shown by hepatic vein catheterization in humans that the injection of insulin causes decreased hepatic output of glucose.[2,18]

Increases in blood pyruvate and lactate are generally attributed to the increased rate of glucose utilization. As more glucose-6-phosphate is produced, more will pass through the various triose states to pyruvate and lactate.

Fall of inorganic phosphate levels may be assumed to reflect the increased rate of phosphorylation of glucose, which results in greater consumption of phosphate. Finally, for reasons that are not well understood, whenever glycogen is deposited in the liver, potassium is also deposited. This would explain the *lowering of the plasma potassium.*

In addition to these effects, insulin causes a fall in free amino acids in the plasma. It has also been shown that the incorporation of ^{35}S-labeled methionine into muscle was reduced in diabetic dogs but could be restored to normal with insulin. Thus insulin has an effect on protein metabolism also.

When insulin is inadequate, as in most diabetic persons, counterregulatory events occur that seem to have a purpose of providing the fuels needed, such as glucose, free fatty acids, and ketone bodies. Thus low insulin plasma levels lead to an increase in epinephrine, glucagon, growth hormone, and cortisol. These hormones mobilize free fatty acids, which are converted into ketone bodies by the liver. They also accelerate gluconeogenesis in the liver.

Glucagon plasma concentrations are consistently elevated in diabetic individuals in relation to insulin, and diabetes is increasingly viewed as a bihormonal disease.

It appears likely from studies on the red cell that a nonlipid-soluble compound such as glucose is transported across the cell membrane through some carrier mechanism.[21] Certain tissues such as muscle differ from erythrocytes in having a superimposed mechanism that opposes the penetration of glucose. This appears to be the site at which insulin acts. As a consequence, insulin promotes the entry of glucose into skeletal and heart muscle, fat, and leukocytes, whereas it is not required for sugar transport into the red cells, brain, or liver.

Preparations and clinical uses   Various insulin preparations differ mainly in their rate of absorption following subcutaneous injection. The rapidly absorbed regular insulin has been modified to

TABLE 42-1. Insulin preparations

| Action | Preparation | Hours after subcutaneous injection | | Units/ml |
		Peak action	Duration of action	
Rapid	Insulin injection (regular, crystalline zinc)	2-3	5-7	40, 80, 100, 500
	Prompt insulin zinc suspension (semilente)	4-6	12-16	40, 80
Intermediate	Isophane insulin suspension (NPH)	8-12	18-24	40, 80, 100
	Insulin zinc suspension (lente)	8-12	18-24	40, 80, 100
	Globin zinc insulin injection (globin)	6-10	12-18	40, 80
Long	Protamine zinc insulin suspension	16-18	24-36	40, 80, 100
	Extended insulin zinc suspension (ultralente)	16-18	24-36	40, 80, 100

form suspensions by two different procedures. The basic protamine has been added to raise the isoelectric point of the acidic insulin. In the newer procedure, the use of high concentrations of zinc and acetate buffer made it possible to prepare insulin suspensions having varying particle size. The most widely used insulins are regular insulin, which is rapid-acting, and isophane insulin suspension (NPH) or insulin zinc suspension (lente), which are intermediate-acting. The various properties of the available insulins are summarized in Table 42-1.

In addition to the USP insulins, which are not pure and may contain 6% proinsulin, there are single peak and single component insulins available, which are more than 99% pure and have 26 to 30 units of activity per milligram. The single component insulins are not as likely to induce the formation of antibodies, thus reducing the likelihood of insulin resistance.

Adverse effects

Adverse effects of insulin include hypoglycemia; allergic reactions, systemic and local; insulin resistance; visual changes caused by changes in the properties of the lens; and interactions with many hormones and drugs. Hypoglycemia should be avoided since it causes brain damage. Lipodystrophy results from the absorption of subcutaneous fat at the site of injection.

ORAL ANTIDIABETIC DRUGS
Hypoglycemic sulfonylurea compounds

The introduction of the hypoglycemic sulfonylurea compounds represents a notable development in the management of diabetes. Loubatières[17] observed in 1942 in France that certain sulfonamides, when administered experimentally to patients suffering from typhoid fever, produced symptoms and signs of hypoglycemia. Extensive investigations done subsequently in many laboratories established the fact that certain sulfonylureas can indeed produce hypoglycemia in normal animals but not in those made diabetic through the administration of alloxan. The most commonly used preparations in the United States are tolbutamide, chlorpropamide, acetohexamide, and tolazamide.

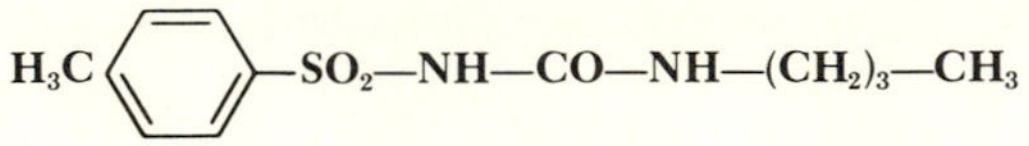

$$H_3C \langle \bigcirc \rangle - SO_2-NH-CO-NH-(CH_2)_3-CH_3$$

Tolbutamide

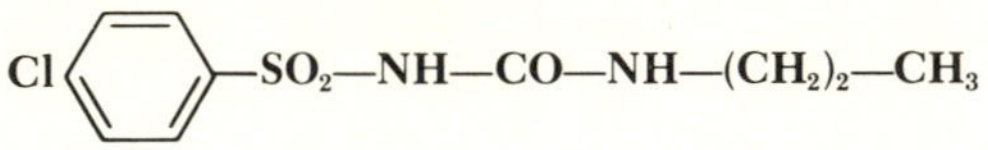

$$Cl \langle \bigcirc \rangle - SO_2-NH-CO-NH-(CH_2)_2-CH_3$$

Chlorpropamide

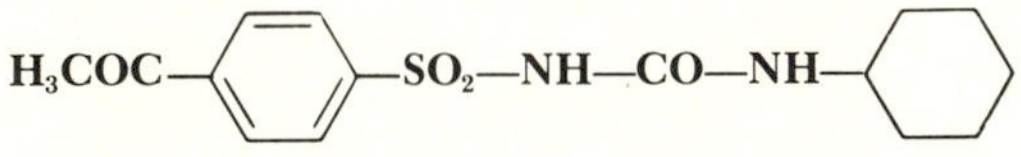

$$H_3COC - \langle \bigcirc \rangle - SO_2-NH-CO-NH - \langle \bigcirc \rangle$$

Acetohexamide

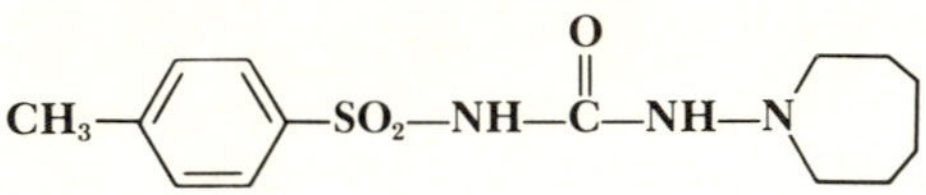

$$CH_3 - \langle \bigcirc \rangle - SO_2-NH-\overset{\overset{O}{\|}}{C}-NH-N \langle \bigcirc \rangle$$

Tolazamide

Mode of action   Despite earlier arguments to the contrary, the pancreas is essential for the hypoglycemic action of the sulfonylureas.[12] The degree of granulation of the islet cells is related to the insulin content of the pancreas, and the sulfonylureas cause a decrease in the granulation of the β cells.[7]

Advantages of the hypoglycemic sulfonylureas over insulin in the management of diabetes are as follows:

1. *Ease of administration.* The sulfonylureas are taken in tablet form, whereas insulin must be injected.
2. *Endogenous release.* Release of insulin by the sulfonylureas resembles the physiological process in that the hormone first reaches the liver, where much of it is retained and exerts an effect on hepatic output of glucose. In contrast, injected insulin floods the peripheral tissues before it reaches the liver.
3. *Less allergic reaction.* Patients who are allergic to exogenous insulin obtained from animal sources or who have antibodies against such insulins may be managed more satisfactorily by promoting endogenous insulin release by means of the sulfonylureas.

Tolbutamide   In a recent cooperative study at 12 university medical centers, a group of more
controversy   than 800 diabetic persons was followed on one of four treatment schedules for 3 to 8 years. During that time 89 patients died, 61 of them from heart attacks or other cardiovascular causes. Of the deaths, 30 occurred in the tolbutamide-treated group. The findings were interpreted as an indication that diet and tolbutamide therapy

TABLE 42-2. Characteristics of oral hypoglycemic drugs

Chemical type	Name	Half-life (hours)	Duration of action (hours)	Tablet size (mg)
Sulfonylurea	Tolbutamide (Orinase)	4-6	6-12	500
	Acetohexamide (Dymelor)	6-18	12-24	250, 500
	Chlorpropamide (Diabenese)	30-36	60	100, 250
	Tolazamide (Tolinase)	7	10-14	100, 250
Biguanide	Phenformin hydrochloride (DBI)	3	4-6	25
	Phenformin hydrochloride, timed-release (DBI-TD)	3	8-14	50 (capsules)

are no more effective than diet alone in prolonging life or even that diet and tolbutamide may be less effective than diet and insulin or diet alone insofar as cardiovascular mortality is concerned. Because of these findings, it has been recommended to physicians that sulfonylurea agents be used only in patients with adult-onset, nonketotic diabetes that cannot be controlled by diet or weight loss and in whom the use of insulin is impractical.

Many competent diabetologists have criticized the study and the conclusions on the basis of deficiencies in design, and it is quite possible that a more extensive study would not support the same conclusions. Until such information is available, some caution in the use of the sulfonylureas is advisable.

The major characteristics of the oral hypoglycemic drugs are shown in Table 42-2. The differences in oral agent activity are determined by their fate in the body. Thus tolbutamide and tolazamide are rapidly metabolized. Acetohexamide is also rapidly metabolized, but its metabolite is more potent than the original drug. Chlorpropamide is long-acting because it is metabolized to a negligible extent.

Preparations and clinical uses

Hypoglycemia with sulfonylureas is generally not as great a danger as that after the use of insulin, but it may be serious and of long duration. An intolerance to alcohol similar to the disulfiram (Antabuse) reaction may occur, and gastrointestinal and allergic skin reactions have been reported.

Adverse effects

Phenformin (phenethylbiguanide; DBI) has been used in the management of some diabetic persons. It lowers blood sugar by some unknown mechanism, probably by decreasing the hepatic output of glucose. Since the drug in larger than recommended doses has caused lactic acidosis that was often fatal, efforts are being made to remove it from the market.

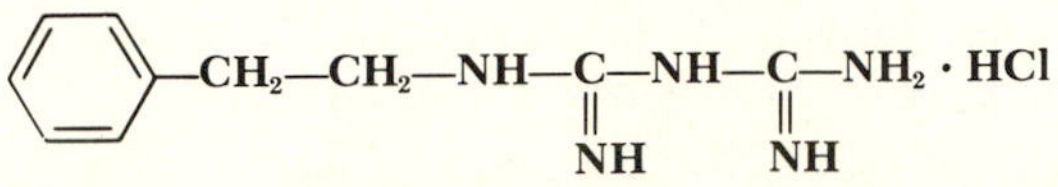

Phenformin

$$\text{—CH}_2\text{—CH}_2\text{—NH—}\overset{\displaystyle \text{NH}}{\underset{}{\overset{\|}{\text{C}}}}\text{—NH—}\overset{\displaystyle \text{NH}}{\underset{}{\overset{\|}{\text{C}}}}\text{—NH}_2 \cdot \text{HCl}$$

Phenformin hydrochloride

Clinical
pharmacology

Extensive clinical experience indicates that the sulfonylureas just discussed are of about equal effectiveness in the treatment of adult-onset ketosis-resistant diabetic persons. These drugs differ from each other mainly in duration of action and in recommended dosage.

The *oral hypoglycemic agents* should be used only in maturity-onset, nonketotic diabetic persons whose blood glucose cannot be controlled by diet alone and in whom insulin cannot be used.

Drug interactions complicate the clinical use of the sulfonylureas. Tolbutamide is strongly bound to plasma proteins, where it can displace dicumarol, thus leading to an increased anticoagulant effect.[31] The interactions of tolbutamide and anticoagulants in patients may be quite complex. Although some reports indicate that administration of tolbutamide to patients on dicumarol therapy resulted in an increased anticoagulant effect,[6] others find that diabetic patients on long-term tolbutamide treatment reacted normally to dicumarol and warfarin.[25] Perhaps the order of administration is important.[31] Thiazide diuretics oppose the action of the sulfonylureas.[11]

REFERENCES

1 Banting, F. G., and Best, C. H.: The internal secretion of the pancreas, J. Lab. Clin. Med. **7:**251, 1922.

2 Bearn, A. G., Billing, B. H., and Sherlock, S.: The response of the liver to insulin in normal subjects and in diabetes mellitus: hepatic vein catheterization studies, Clin. Sci. **11:**151, 1952.

3 Berson, S. A., and Yalow, R. S.: Plasma insulin in health and disease, Am. J. Med. **31:**874, 1961.

4 Berson, S. A., and Yalow, R. S.: Insulin in blood and insulin antibodies, Am. J. Med. **40:** 676, 1966.

5 Brotherton, P. M., Grieveson, P., and McMartin, C.: A study of the metabolic fate of chlorpropamide in man, Clin. Pharmacol. Ther. **10:**505, 1969.

6 Chaplin, H., and Cassell, M.: Studies on the possible relationship of tolbutamide to Dicumarol in anticoagulant therapy, Am. J. Med. Sci. **235:**706, 1958.

7 Colwell, A. R., Jr., Colwell, J. A., and Colwell, A. R., Sr.: Intrapancreatic perfusion of the antidiabetic sulfonylureas, Metabolism **5:**727, 1956.

8 Dear, H. D., Buncher, C. R., and Sawayama, T.: Changes in electrocardiogram and serum potassium values following glucose ingestion, Arch. Intern. Med. **124:**25, 1969.

9 Dunn, J. S., and McLetchie, N. G. B.: Experimental alloxan diabetes in rat, Lancet **2:**383, 1943.

10 Fajans, S. S., Floyd, J. C., Jr., Knopf, R. F.,

Rull, J., Guntsche, E. M., and Conn, J. W.: Benzothiadiazine suppression of insulin release from normal and abnormal islet tissue in man, J. Clin. Invest. **45:**481, 1966.

11 Goldner, M. G., Zarowitz, H., and Akgun, S.: Hyperglycemia and glycosuria due to thiazide derivative administered in diabetes mellitus, N. Engl. J. Med. **262:**403, 1960.

12 Houssay, B. A., Penhos, J. C., Teodosio, N., Bowkett, J., and Apelbaum, J.: Action of the hypoglycemic sulfonyl compounds in hypophysectomized, adrenalectomized, and depancreatized animals, Ann. N.Y. Acad. Sci. **71:** 12, 1957.

13 Johnson, R. D.: The management of coma in the diabetic patient—hypoglycemia, ketoacidosis, and the hyperosmolar state, Pharmacol. Phys. **2**(5): 1968.

14 Levine, R.: The action of insulin at the cell membrane, Am. J. Med. **40:**691, 1966.

15 Levine, R., Goldstein, M., Huddlestun, B., and Klein, S. P.: Action of insulin on the permeability of cells to free hexoses, as studied by its effect on the distribution of galactose, Am. J. Physiol. **163:**70, 1950.

16 Long, C. N. H., and Lukens, F. D. W.: The effects of adrenalectomy and hypophysectomy upon experimental diabetes in the cat, J. Exp. Med. **63:**465, 1936.

17 Loubatières, A.: The hypoglycemic sulfonamides: history and development of the problem from 1942 to 1955, Ann. N.Y. Acad. Sci. **71:**4, 1957.

18 Madison, L. L., Combes, B., Adams, R., and

Strickland, W.: The physiological significance of the secretion of endogenous insulin into the portal circulation. III. Evidence for a direct, immediate effect of insulin on the balance of glucose across the liver, J. Clin. Invest. 39:507, 1960.

19 Mereu, T. R., Kassoff, A., and Goodman, A. D.: Diazoxide in the treatment of infantile hypoglycemia, N. Engl. J. Med. 275:1455, 1966.

20 Mirsky, I. A., and Broh-Kahn, R. H.: Inactivation of insulin by tissue extracts: distribution and properties of insulin inactivating extracts (insulinase), Arch. Biochem. 20:1, 1949.

21 Park, C. R., Reinwein, D., Henderson, M. J., Cadenas, E., and Morgan, H. E.: The action of insulin on the transport of glucose through the cell membrane, Am. J. Med. 26:674, 1959.

22 Parmely, W. W., Glick, G., and Sonnenblick, E. H.: Cardiovascular effects of glucagon in man, N. Engl. J. Med. 279:12, 1968.

23 Perley, M., and Kipnis, D. M.: Effect of glucocorticoids on plasma insulin, N. Engl. J. Med. 274:1237, 1966.

24 Porte, D., Jr.: A receptor mechanism for the inhibition of insulin release by epinephrine in man, J. Clin. Invest. 46:86, 1967.

25 Poucher, R. L., and Vecchio, T. J.: Absence of tolbutamide effect on anticoagulant therapy, J.A.M.A. 197:1069, 1966.

26 Sanger, F., and Thompson, E. O. P.: Amino-acid sequence in the glicyl chain of insulin, Biochem. J. 53:353, 1953.

27 Seltzer, H. S., and Allen, E. W.: Hyperglycemia and inhibition of insulin secretion during administration of diazoxide and trichlormethiazide in man, Diabetes 18:19, 1969.

28 Sokal, J. E.: Glucagon—an essential hormone, Am. J. Med. 41:331, 1966.

29 Steiner, D. F., Hallund, O., Rubenstein, A., Cho, S., and Bayliss, C.: Isolation and properties of proinsulin, intermediate forms, and other minor components from crystalline bovine insulin, Diabetes 17:725, 1968.

30 Von Mering, J., and Minkowski, O.: Diabetes mellitus nach Pankreas Extirpation, Centralbl. Klin. Med. 10:393, 1889.

31 Welch, R. M., Harrison, Y. E., Conney, A. H., and Burns, J. J.: an experimental model in dogs for studying interactions of drugs with bishydroxycoumarin, Clin. Pharmacol. Ther. 10:817, 1969.

REVIEWS

32 Arky, R. A., and Knopp, R. H.: Evaluation of islet-cell function in man, N. Engl. J. Med. 285:1130, 1971.

33 Bressler, R., and Galloway, J. A.: The insulins, Ration. Drug Ther. 5:1, 1971.

34 Cahill, J. F.: Glucagon, N. Engl. J. Med. 288:157, 1973.

35 Cuatrecasas, P.: Insulin receptor of liver and fat cell membranes, Fed. Proc. 32:1838, 1973.

36 Cuatrecasas, P.: Hormone-receptor interactions and the plasma membrane, Hosp. Pract. July, 1974.

37 Flier, J. S., Kahn, R., and Roth, J.: Receptors, antireceptor antibodies and mechanisms of insulin resistance, N. Engl. J. Med. 300:413, 1979.

38 Goodner, C. J.: Somatostatin leads to glucagon's renaissance, N. Engl. J. Med. 292:1022, 1975.

39 Knatterud, G. L., Meinert, C. L., Klimt, C. R., Osborne, R. K., and Martin, D. B.: Effects of hypoglycemic agents on vascular complications in patients with adult-onset diabetes. IV. A preliminary report on phenformin results, J.A.M.A. 217:777, 1971.

40 McGarry, J. D., and Foster, D. W.: Hormonal control of ketogenesis, Arch. Intern. Med. 137:495, 1977.

41 Poffenbarger, P. L., and Deiss, W. P.: Insulin therapy for diabetic ketoacidosis, Tex. Med. 75:42, 1979.

42 Shen, S. W., and Bressler, R.: Clinical pharmacology of oral antidiabetic agents, N. Engl. J. Med. 296:787, 1977.

43 Steiner, D. F.: Proinsulin, Triangle 11:51, 1972.

44 Unger, R. H.: Glucagon physiology and pathophysiology, N. Engl. J. Med. 285:443, 1971.

45 Unger, R. H., and Lefebre, P. J.: Glucagon: molecular physiology, clinical and therapeutic implications, New York, 1972, Pergamon Press, Inc.

CHAPTER 43

Adrenal steroids

GENERAL CONCEPT   Since the observation by Hench in 1949 of a dramatic response to cortisone in a patient with rheumatoid arthritis, adrenal steroids and synthetic corticosteroids have become widely used and sometimes overused in medicine. *Cortisone* and related corticosteroids owe their popularity to their anti-inflammatory effect. More rarely, these drugs are useful for substitution therapy in adrenal insufficiency, which is often iatrogenic.

   Aldosterone, the main mineralocorticoid of the adrenal gland, is largely of research interest. On the other hand, the *aldosterone antagonists* have important therapeutic applications.

DEVELOPMENT OF IDEAS   During the decade following 1930 there was an intensive search for the active principles that could account for the essential role of the adrenal glands. In 1937 Reichstein and von Euw[19] prepared desoxycorticosterone synthetically and later demonstrated it in the adrenal glands. Although this steroid had powerful effects on salt and water metabolism and became useful in the management of Addison's disease, it was obvious that extracts of adrenal cortex also contained some other compounds that could influence not only salt metabolism but also the handling of carbohydrates and proteins as well. Among the many steroids that were being isolated were some that indeed had marked glucocorticoid activity, as opposed to the mineralocorticoid desoxycorticosterone.

   World War II stimulated interest in the glucocorticoids, previously isolated by Kendall at the Mayo Clinic. It was suspected that such compounds might be valuable in the treatment of shock and exhaustion,[21] although the scarcity of these compounds did not permit their evaluation in humans. Intense efforts were made to synthesize adequate amounts of the glucocorticoids for clinical trial.

   A milestone in the history of the adrenal steroids was the report of Hench and co-workers[13] on the effectiveness of cortisone and corticotropin in rheumatoid arthritis. Hench had been impressed for years with the potential reversibility of rheumatoid arthritis on the basis of the observation that patients tended to improve when jaundiced and also during pregnancy. It seemed possible that these improvements were associated with the production or retention of some "antirheumatic substance." Although Hench planned to try cortisone (compound E of Kendall) as early as 1941, it was not until 1948 that partial synthesis provided sufficient material for a clinical trial.

Results of the clinical trials in rheumatoid arthritis were dramatic, and soon cortisone and also corticotropin were found to cause symptomatic improvement in an amazing number of disease conditions. It was recognized at the same time that cortisone was not a cure for these many diseases. It seemed to "provide the susceptible tissues with a shieldlike buffer against the irritant."[12]

Although cortisol was largely responsible for the glucocorticoid activity of adrenal extracts, it was suspected that the amorphous fraction of such extracts still contained some material whose mineralocorticoid activity was much greater than that of desoxycorticosterone. The compound responsible for this was isolated in 1953 and was named *aldosterone.*

Subsequent research on the glucocorticoids led to the development of a variety of new steroids that have significantly greater anti-inflammatory potency than cortisone, although their influence on carbohydrate metabolism generally parallels their anti-inflammatory activity. A significant advantage of the newer steroids such as prednisone, methylprednisolone, triamcinolone, and dexamethasone is that these anti-inflammatory steroids exert little effect on renal sodium reabsorption while possessing potent anti-inflammatory activity.

Corticotropin (adrenocorticotropic hormone; ACTH) from the anterior pituitary gland stimulates adrenal steroid synthesis from cholesterol and is necessary for normal cortical structure and function. Although corticotropin stimulates primarily the formation of glucocorticoids, it has a basic influence on the formation of all adrenal steroids.

PITUITARY-ADRENAL RELATIONSHIPS
Corticotropin

Corticotropin release from the anterior pituitary gland is promoted by polypeptides isolated from the hypothalamus, sometimes referred to as corticotropin-releasing factor (CRF).

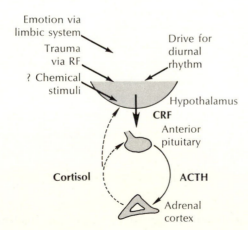

FIG. 43-1. Diagrammatic summary of the principal factors regulating ACTH secretion. (From Ganong, W. F., Alpert, L. C., and Lee, T. C.: Review of medical physiology, ed. 6, Los Altos, Calif., 1973, Lange Medical Publications.)

Regulation of corticotropin release is determined largely by the influence of cortisol levels on CRF production through a negative feedback. Stressful stimuli, including drugs such as epinephrine, can override the feedback inhibition and elevate cortisol blood levels. In addition to these important regulatory influences, there is a diurnal variation in corticotropin release that will be discussed subsequently.

The basic effect of corticotropin on the adrenal cortex is mediated by adenosine 3':5'-cyclic phosphate (cyclic AMP). Cyclic AMP acts similarly to corticotropin both in vitro and on the perfused dog adrenal gland, whereas phosphorylase activity of beef adrenal slices is increased by corticotropin. Corticotropin may stimulate steroid synthesis by the system involving adenyl cyclase.

The polypeptide corticotropin was isolated from the anterior pituitary and eventually synthesized. Human corticotropin consists of 39 amino acids, but not all amino acids are essential for biological activity, since the first 19 (counting from the N-terminal end) are sufficient for stimulating cortisol production. The first 13 amino acids in corticotropin are the same as those in melanocyte-stimulating hormone (α-MSH), so it is not surprising that corticotropin exerts an effect on melanocytes.

Preparations of corticotropin are available for intravenous and intramuscular administration. Oral administration is ineffective. When injected intravenously, corticotropin is rapidly destroyed in a matter of minutes. For this reason the hormone is administered either by intravenous infusion or by the intramuscular route as a repository corticotropin injection USP or sterile corticotropin zinc hydroxide suspension USP. In the latter preparation, slow absorption is achieved by the addition of zinc hydroxide, whereas in the former preparation, gelatin retards absorption. Neither is suitable for intravenous use. Some preparations of corticotropin injection USP are available for intravenous injection.

Corticotropin has some valid uses in the diagnosis of disturbed adrenocortical function. An intravenous infusion of the hormone will result in an increase in the excretion of cortisol metabolites if the adrenal glands are normal or hyperplastic.

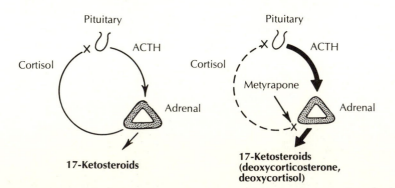

FIG. 43-2. Pituitary-adrenal feedback system and its inhibition by metyrapone. (Modified from Coppage, W. S., Jr., Island, D., Smith, M., and Liddle, G. W.: J. Clin. Invest. **38:**2101, 1959.)

Lowering of the 11-oxygenated (11-oxy) adrenal steroids in the body promotes corticotropin release by removal of the negative feedback. An interesting application of this knowledge is a test for anterior pituitary function by means of metyrapone (Fig. 43-2).

Metyrapone (Metopirone) inhibits the 11-β hydroxylation in the biosynthesis of cortisol, corticosterone, and aldosterone. The decrease in these 11-oxy steroids leads to intense corticotropin release from the anterior pituitary gland in normal individuals. Under these circumstances corticotropin stimulates the production of precursors of the 11-oxy steroids, 11-desoxyhydrocortisone (compound S) and 11-desoxycorticosterone (DOC). The metabolites of these steroids, 17-hydroxycorticosteroids and 17-ketogenic steroids, may be measured in the urine. In deficient anterior pituitary function, metyrapone administration will not increase these urinary metabolites.

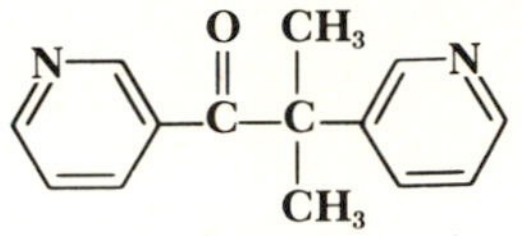

Metyrapone

In adults, metyrapone is administered orally in doses of 750 mg every 4 hours for six doses. Urinary steroids are determined in the following 24 hours.

The metyrapone test is useless if adrenocortical function is defective. This is ascertained previously by determining the influence of corticotropin infusion on steroid output in the urine. Although the metyrapone test is still experimental, it is a remarkable example of the utilization of a new drug for probing body chemistry.

Androgens

In addition to the glucocorticoids and aldosterone, the adrenal cortex produces androgenic steroids such as dehydroepiandrosterone. The production of androgenic steroids is greatly increased in the adrenogenital syndrome, in which an enzymatic defect channels much of the steroid production toward androgens. Exogenous glucocorticoid administration tends to depress the androgen output through pituitary inhibition.

Adrenal suppressants

Certain toxic compounds such as amphenone B and the insecticide tetrachlorodiphenylethane (DDD) may damage the adrenal cortex. Amphenone B blocks several hydroxylations in addition to the one inhibited by metyrapone. Aminoglutethimide (Elipten) also blocks steroidogenesis by interfering with the conversion of cholesterol to pregnenolone.

GLUCOCORTICOIDS
Cortisol and corticosterone

Cortisol (hydrocortisone) and corticosterone are the principal glucocorticoids of the adrenal cortex.

In the human adrenal cortex, cortisol predominates, whereas in some species such as the rat, corticosterone has greater quantitative importance. Human adrenal glands contain 2.3 to 5.5 μg of cortisol per gram of wet tissue. In the plasma of normal

$$CH_2OH$$
$$C=O$$

HO $\quad$ CH₃ ---OH

CH₃

O

Cortisol

$$CH_2OH$$
$$C=O$$

HO $\quad$ CH₃

CH₃

O

Corticosterone

persons its concentration is about 8 μg/100 ml. The rate of secretion shows a characteristic rhythm or diurnal variation. Secretion begins in the early hours of the morning, before the individual awakens, and gradually declines toward late evening. The reasons for this anticipatory secretion before daily activities begin are not known. Normal daily output of cortisol in human beings is about 25 mg.

Pharmacological effects

Cortisol binds to a cytosolic receptor and is translocated to the nucleus where it stimulates transcription of messenger RNA and ultimately protein synthesis.

The three major effects of the steroid are on (1) carbohydrate, protein, and fat metabolism; (2) mineral metabolism; and (3) inflammation.

Effect on carbohydrate, protein, and fat metabolism. Cortisol increases gluconeogenesis and also tends to inhibit peripheral glucose utilization. As a consequence, it causes marked accumulation of glycogen in the liver and can produce hyperglycemia and glycosuria. Because of these effects, it tends to aggravate diabetes and may bring out an insulin-resistant disturbance of carbohydrate metabolism in latent diabetes.

The hormone corrects the disturbances of carbohydrate metabolism seen in adrenalectomized animals or in patients having Addison's disease, as shown in Table 43-1. Adrenalectomy improves experimental diabetes.[13]

Cortisol not only promotes the breakdown of proteins but also tends to inhibit their anabolism or synthesis. When large doses of the hormone are administered to children and young animals, they fail to grow and wounds heal much more slowly. Inhibition of antibody production in some species may also be a consequence of an antianabolic action.[7]

Little is known about the basic action of cortisol on fat metabolism. Unusual accumulations of fat (buffalo hump) occur in the patient treated with glucocorticoids. The adrenal glucocorticoids promote fat mobilization[13] and exert complex effects on ketone metabolism. Cortisol has a *permissive* effect on free fatty acid release from adipose tissue by catecholamines.

Effect on electrolyte and water metabolism. Although the glucocorticoids exert much less effect on renal handling of electrolytes than do desoxycorticosterone and aldosterone, administration of cortisol or cortisone still results in increased sodium retention, increased potassium excretion, and hypokalemic alkalosis in pa-

TABLE 43-1. Effects of bilateral adrenalectomy

Circulatory	Decreased blood pressure
	Decreased blood volume
	Hyponatremia, hypochloremia, hypoglycemia, and hyperkalemia
	Increased nonprotein nitrogen
Renal	Increased excretion of sodium and chloride
	Decreased excretion of potassium
Digestive	Loss of appetite, nausea, and vomiting
Muscular	Weakness
	Decreased sodium and increased potassium and water in muscle
Miscellaneous	Decreased resistance to all forms of stress
	Hypertrophy of lymphoid tissue and thymus
	Death unless treatment is instituted

tients receiving prolonged treatment. On the other hand, patients with Addison's disease cannot be kept in electrolyte balance with glucocorticoids alone.

The adrenalectomized animal cannot excrete a large water load. Cortisone will restore this particular function.

In addition to an influence on renal handling of electrolytes, adrenal steroids may influence the distribution of electrolytes between cells and extracellular fluid.[3]

Calcium metabolism is also affected by cortisol. It promotes the renal excretion of calcium, and it may reduce calcium absorption from the intestine.

Anti-inflammatory action. Most of the clinical uses of the glucocorticoids and of ACTH may be attributed to the remarkable ability of the steroids to inhibit the inflammatory process.

The *mechanism of the anti-inflammatory action* of the corticosteroids remains mysterious, although there is no lack of theories on this subject. The anti-inflammatory action has been attributed to suppression of migration of polymorphonuclear leukocytes, suppression of reparative processes and functions of fibroblasts, reversal of enhanced capillary permeability, and lysosomal stabilization.

Problem 43-1. Since there are both steroidal and nonsteroidal anti-inflammatory drugs, do they act by the same mechanism? This is not likely for several reasons. Clinical experience indicates that the corticosteroids are much more effective in asthma, whereas the nonsteroidal drugs are efficacious in rheumatoid arthritis. Experimentally, the nonsteroidal anti-inflammatory drugs such as aspirin or indomethacin inhibit prostaglandin synthesis, whereas cortisone has no such effect.

Although cortisol does not block the synthesis of prostaglandins from arachidonic acid, it prevents the release of arachidonic acid itself from phospholipids.[14] Thus, its effect is most likely on phospholipase A_2 or on the production of a peptide, which then blocks the enzyme.[6]

Miscellaneous effects. The cortisone-like steroids exert a striking effect on the number of circulating eosinophils. These elements may completely disappear from the blood following the administration of the glucocorticoids or on the injection of corticotropin.

In addition to the eosinopenic effect, cortisone produces a marked decrease in circulating lymphocytes and an involution of lymphoid tissue.

There is little doubt that cortisone exerts effects on the central nervous system (CNS). Euphoria and other behavioral abnormalities may occur that cannot be explained by the clinical improvement of the primary disease. There is also evidence that glucocorticoid treatment may lower convulsive thresholds.

The glucocorticoids improve muscle strength in adrenalectomized animals. On the other hand, they can cause muscle weakness in prolonged treatment, which perhaps results from potassium loss and other metabolic actions on the muscle.

The effect of corticosteroid treatment on infections is quite complex.[23] Animal experiments suggest that cortisone exerts an adverse effect on the course of a variety of experimental infections, particularly fungal diseases. It must be remembered, however, that very large doses of the steroids are used in such experiments. With reasonable doses, antibody production is not decreased, opsonins remain normal, and leukocytes ingest and destroy microorganisms, even in experimental infections. In humans, varicella and herpes of the eye may be more severe, and fungal diseases may develop after prolonged steroid therapy. On the other hand, there is every reason to believe that the danger of using corticosteroids in infections has been exaggerated. Infection must be viewed as an added factor, rather than as an absolute contraindication, when the risks of using corticosteroids are appraised.[25]

Adverse effects. Excessive doses of glucocorticoids after prolonged administration produce the various manifestations of Cushing's disease, including moon face, hirsutism, acne, amenorrhea, osteoporosis, muscle wasting, variable hyeprnatremia and hypokalemia, hypertension, aggravation of diabetes mellitus, necrotizing arteritis in rheumatoid patients, aggravation of peptic ulcer, psychotic manifestations, and adrenal atrophy. The *most serious* systematic complications that may result from the clinical use of high doses of steroids are the diabetogenic and ulcerogenic effects; dissolution of supporting tissues such as bone, muscle, and skin; the hypertensive effect; and impairment of defense mechanisms against serious infections.

Metabolism   Cortisone and other synthetic corticosteroids are absorbed rapidly and completely from the gastrointestinal tract. After oral administration, maximal plasma concentrations are reached in 1 to 2 hours. Hepatic degradation of the corticosteroids leads to a fairly rapid fall in plasma levels so that after 8 hours only 25% of the peak value can be demonstrated and the active drugs disappear completely in about 12 hours.[29]

Drugs that promote the activity of microsomal enzymes in the liver tend to accelerate the metabolism of the corticosteroids. These drugs, which include phenobarbital, phenytoin, and others, may make it necessary to increase the dosage of the corticosteroids.

Cortisol is available in oral tablets containing 10 or 20 mg. It is also available for intravenous injection and in various lotions and ointments for topical application.

Cortisone is used almost entirely in the tablet form or in suspension for intramuscular injection.

The large number of diseases in which cortisone and cortisol have been tried may be classified as follows on the basis of the degree of beneficial effect that may be expected from existing experience.

Favorable responses	*Transient beneficial effects*
Addison's disease	Acute leukemia
Hypopituitarism	Multiple myeloma
Adrenogenital syndrome	Lymphosarcoma
Severe bronchial asthma	Chronic lymphatic leukemia
Acute ocular inflammations	
Rheumatoid arthritis	
Acute bursitis	
Acute rheumatic fever	
Acute gouty arthritis	
Acquired hemolytic anemia	
Severe atopic dermatitis	
Acute lupus erythematosus	
Severe penicillin reactions	

Certain principles may be derived from the accumulated experience in the therapeutic use of the adrenal steroids.

1. These drugs do not cure any disease. They do not represent replacement therapy, as does insulin in diabetes, except in the rare case of Addison's disease or induced hypoadrenocorticism.
2. The anti-inflammatory adrenal steroids are particularly useful in disease processes that occur in episodes and so require no extended therapy. They are also very useful in conditions in which topical application may suffice.
3. Every effort should be made to use other drugs or procedures before prolonged steroid treatment is undertaken. With continued use, hyperadrenocorticism resembling Cushing's syndrome may be inevitable. Cessation of treatment with these steroids may precipitate acute exacerbations of various diseases. Their suppression of the function of the adrenal glands may represent a serious danger if the patient meets with stressful situations.
4. Despite their many disadvantages, the adrenal glucocorticoids are of great therapeutic importance in self-limiting diseases and in chronic disabling processes that fail to respond to any other treatment. The systemic use of these drugs is always a calculated risk that is often worth taking in the presence of incapacitating and otherwise incurable disease.

Several glucocorticoids have been introduced into therapeutics on the basis of having anti-inflammatory potency greater than cortisol without also having a corresponding increase in their tendency to retain sodium.

The chemical relationships among these newer glucocorticoids may be summarized in comparison with the structural formula of cortisone.

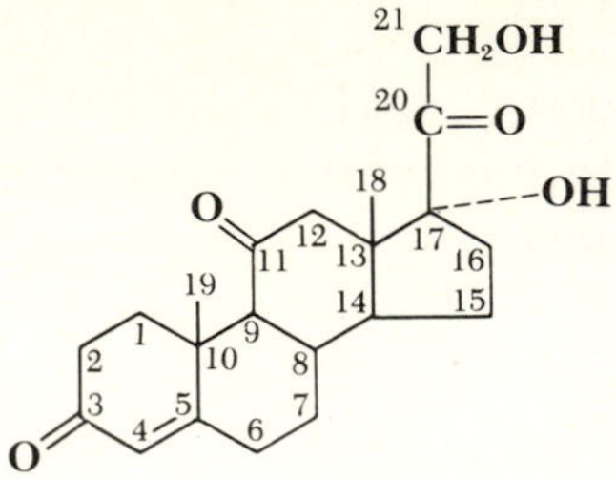

Cortisone

Cortisol has the same structural formulin as cortisone except that OH is in position 11.

Prednisone (Meticorten) is the same as cortisone except that there is a double bond between positions 1 and 2.

Prednisolone (Meticortelone) is the same as prednisone except that OH is in position 11.

Methylprednisolone (Medrol) is the same as prednisolone except that CH_3 is in position 6.

Triamcinolone (Aristocort) is the same as prednisolone except that F (α) is in position 9 and there is an additional α OH in position 16.

Dexamethasone (Decadron) is the same as triamcinolone except that α CH_3 instead of OH is in position 16.

Betamethasone (Celestone) is the same as dexamethasone except that CH_3 is in position 16 β instead of in α.

Fludrocortisone (9-α-fluorohydrocortisone) is the same as cortisol except that α F is in position 9.

Paramethasone (Haldrone) is the same as dexamethasone except that α F moves to position 6.

Halcinonide acetonide differs from triamcinolone acetonide by substitution of chlorine for the hydroxyl group in position 21 and reduction of a double bond at positions 1 and 2 in ring A. The new steroid has dermatological applications.

The introduction of prednisone and prednisolone into therapeutics was of great practical importance since their high anti-inflammatory action was not coupled with a correspondingly high sodium-retaining potency. This separation of effects allowed the physician to use these compounds without special salt-free diets and potassium supplementation.

The synthetic analogs of cortisol are usually administered in the form of oral tablets. Suspensions of some of the drugs are available for intramuscular and intra-articular administration. Although they are of low solubility, water-soluble preparations of some of the steroids are available for intravenous use, such as the succinates or 21-phosphates.

TABLE 43-2. Comparison of potencies of various steroids

Steroid	Anti-inflammatory potency	Daily dose (mg)	Sodium retention
Cortisone acetate (Cortone)	0.8	50-100	0.8
Cortisol (Cortef)	1	50-100	1
Prednisone (Meticorten)	2.5	10-20	0.8
Prednisolone (Meticortelone)	3	10-20	0.8
Methylprednisolone (Medrol)	4	10-20	0
Triamcinolone (Aristocort)	5	5-20	0
Dexamethasone (Decadron)	20	0.75-3	0
Paramethasone (Haldrone)	6	4-6	0
Betamethasone (Celestone)	20	0.6-3	0
Desoxycorticosterone (DOC)	0	1-3	10-25
Fludrocortisone (Florinef)	12	0.1	100
Aldosterone	0.2		250

Dermatological applications

The topical treatment of dermatological diseases has been revolutionized by the introduction of the anti-inflammatory corticosteroids. These drugs applied to the skin cause vasoconstriction,[17] and this effect has been useful in developing dermatological preparations.[31] The percutaneous absorption, particle size, and vehicle composition are important determinants of topical activity of corticosteroids.[31]

Beclomethasone

Beclomethasone dipropionate (Vanceril) was recently introduced for inhalation in asthmatic persons. The drug is related to prednisolone. Vanceril inhaler is a metered-dose aerosol unit, which delivers 50 μg of the drug on each actuation. The usual dosage is two inhalations (100 μg) three or four times a day. The drug appears to be a satisfactory alternative to systemic glucocorticoids in patients with chronic bronchial asthma.[2]

MINERALO-CORTICOIDS
Aldosterone

Aldosterone is the main mineralocorticoid of the adrenal cortex. Extensive studies have been carried out on the role of this hormone in health and disease. A new disease entity, *primary aldosteronism*, has been described as a consequence of such studies.[4] Despite the great interest of such investigations, aldosterone has no therapeutic importance since desoxycorticosterone is available for the correction of electrolyte abnormalities in adrenal insufficiency.

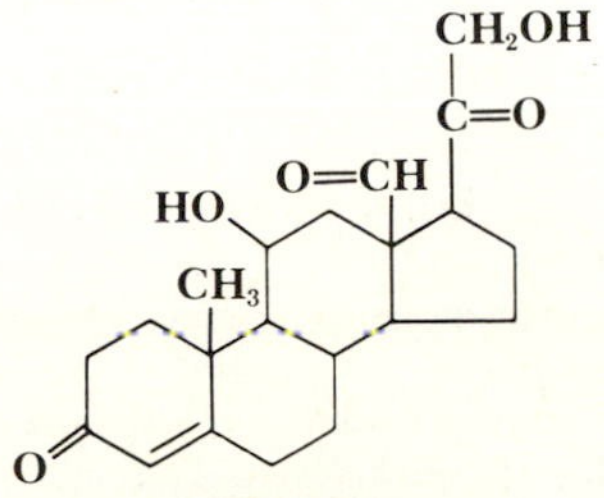

Aldosterone 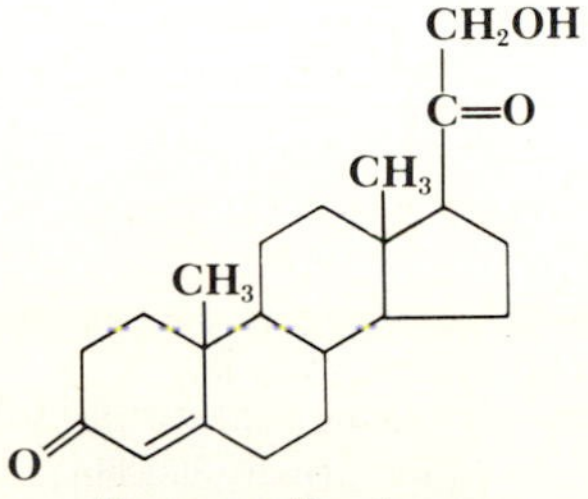   Desoxycorticosterone

Aldosterone has an oxygen atom in position 11 and produces some effect on carbohydrate metabolism. However, its salt-retaining potency is so great and its concentration in the blood so small in relation to cortisol that its physiological function must have little to do with organic metabolism.

Release of aldosterone is promoted by a decrease in circulating blood volume. Stimulation of aldosterone release by angiotensin is of great interest and suggests a connection between aldosterone secretion and the kidney with its juxtaglomerular apparatus. This problem is discussed in Chapter 18. ACTH is necessary for aldosterone synthesis, but the final modulation of its production must be under the influence of other humoral factors, perhaps angiotensin.

Conditions in which aldosterone production is increased are as follows:

1. Primary aldosteronism, characterized by arterial hypertension, muscular weakness, tetany, hypokalemic alkalosis, negative potassium balance, hypomagnesemia, high serum sodium levels, and alkaline urine. This may be caused by adenoma or hyperplasia of the adrenal glands.

2. Secondary hyperaldosteronism, occurring in renal artery constriction with hypertension, malignant hypertension, pregnancy and toxemia of pregnancy, cirrhosis of the liver, nephrotic edema, and less certainly essential hypertension. In many patients with congestive heart failure, aldosterone output is within normal limits.

Aldosterone antagonists. Spironolactone (Aldactone) and triamterene antagonize aldosterone at the level of the renal tubules.

Spironolactone is a synthetic steroid that competes with aldosterone for the distal tubular receptor involved in sodium-potassium exchange. Triamterene, on the other hand, does not compete with aldosterone but has a direct effect on the renal tubules. Both drugs favor sodium excretion and potassium retention (p. 498).

Desoxycortico-sterone   Desoxycorticosterone acetate is available in solution in sesame oil for intramuscular injection. There are also microcrystalline suspensions of desoxycorticosterone trimethyl acetate for the same purpose. Pellets are available for subcutaneous implantation, which allows release of the steroid over a period of several months.

The main effect of desoxycorticosterone is exerted on the renal tubules. It promotes increased reabsorption of sodium and loss of potassium. Prolonged, intensive treatment with desoxycorticosterone in experimental animals can produce hypertension and necrotic changes in the heart and skeletal muscle. It is believed that these actions result from potassium loss and sodium retention.[5]

REFERENCES

1 Bogdonoff, M. D., Estes, E. H., Jr., Friedberg, S. J., and Klein, R. F.: Fat mobilization in man, Arch. Intern. Med. 55:328, 1961.
2 Bondarevsky, E., Shapiro, M. S., Schey, G., Shahor, J., and Bruderman, I.: Beclomethasone dipropionate use in chronic asthmatic patients, J.A.M.A. 236:1969, 1976.
3 Bush, I. E.: Chemical and biological factors in the activity of adrenal steroids, Pharmacol. Rev. 14:317, 1962.

4 Conn, J. W.: Presidential address. Painting background: primary aldosteronism, a new clinical syndrome, J. Lab. Clin. Med. 45:3, 1955.
5 Darrow, D. C., and Miller, H. C.: Production of cardiac lesions by repeated injections of desoxycorticosterone acetate, J. Clin. Invest. 21:601, 1942.
6 Flower, R. J., and Blackwell, G. J.: Anti-inflammatory steroids induce biosynthesis of a phospholipase A_2 inhibitor which prevents prostaglandin generation, Nature 278:456, 1979.

7 Germuth, F. G., Jr., Oyama, J., and Ottinger, B.: Mechanism of action of 17-hydroxy-11-dehydrocorticosterone (compound E) and of adrenocorticotropic hormone in experimental hypersensitivity in rabbits, J. Exp. Med. **94**:139, 1951.

8 Greaves, M. W.: The pharmacological basis for the rational use of topically applied corticosteroids, Pharmacol. Phys. 3(10):1, 1969.

9 Greengard, O., Weber, G., and Singhal, R. L.: Glycogen deposition in the liver induced by cortisone: dependence on enzyme synthesis, Science **141**:160, 1963.

10 Harrison, T. S., Chawla, R. C., and Wojtalik, R. S.: Steroidal influence on catecholamines, N. Engl. J. Med. **279**:136, 1968.

11 Harter, J. G., Reddy, W. J., and Thorn, G. W.: Studies on an intermittent corticosteroid dosage regimen, N. Engl. J. Med. **269**:591, 1963.

12 Hench, P. S.: Introduction: cortisone and ACTH in clinical medicine, Mayo Clin. Proc. **25**:474, 1950.

13 Hench, P. S., Slocumb, C. H., Barnes, A. R., Smith, H. L., Polley, H. L., and Kendall, E. C.: The effects of adrenal cortical hormone 17-hydroxy-11-dehydro-corticosterone (compound E) on the acute phase of rheumatic fever, Mayo Clin. Proc. **24**:277, 1949.

14 Hong, S. L., and Levine, L.: Inhibition of arachidonic acid release from cells as the biochemical action of anti-inflammatory corticosteroids, Proc. Natl. Acad. Sci. U.S.A. **73**:1730, 1976.

15 Kadowitz, P. J., and Yard, A. C.: Influence of hydrocortisone on cardiovascular responses to epinephrine, Eur. J. Pharmacol. **13**:281, 1971.

16 Liddle, G. W., Duncan, L. E., Jr., and Bartter, F. C.: Dual mechanism regulating adrenocortical function in man, Am. J. Med. **21**:380, 1956.

17 McKenzie, A. W., and Stoughton, R. B.: Method of comparing percutaneous absorption of steroids, Arch. Dermatol. **86**:608, 1962.

18 Mills, L. C.: Corticosteroids in endotoxic shock, Proc. Soc. Exp. Biol. Med. **138**:507, 1971.

19 Reichstein, T., and von Euw, J.: Constituents of the adrenal cortex: isolation of substance Q (desoxycorticosterone) and R with other materials, Helv. Chim. Acta **21**:1181, 1938.

20 Schayer, R. W., Smiley, R. L., and Davis, K. J.: Inhibition of cortisone of the binding of new histamine in rat tissues, Proc. Soc. Exp. Biol. Med. **87**:590, 1954.

21 Selye, H.: General adaptation syndrome and diseases of adaptation, J. Clin. Endocrinol. **6**:117, 1946.

22 Soyka, L. F., and Saxena, K. M.: Alternate-day steroid therapy for nephrotic children, J.A.M.A. **192**:225, 1965.

23 Sparberg, M., and Kirsner, J. B.: Steroid therapy and infections, J.A.M.A. **188**:680, 1964.

24 Walton, J., Watson, B. S., and Ney, R. L.: Alternate-day vs shorter interval steroid administration, Arch. Intern. Med. **126**:601, 1970.

25 Weber, G., Singhal, R. L., and Stamm, N. B.: Actinomycin: inhibition of cortisone-induced synthesis of hepatic gluconeogenic enzymes, Science **142**:390, 1963.

REVIEWS

26 Ballin, J. C.: Evaluation of a new aerosolized steroid for asthma therapy. Beclomethasone dipropionate (Vanceril Inhaler), J.A.M.A. **236**:2891, 1976.

27 Cline, M. J.: Drugs and phagocytosis, N. Engl. J. Med. **291**:1187, 1974.

28 David, D. S., Grieco, M. H., and Cushman, P.: Adrenal glucocorticoids after twenty years, J. Chron. Dis. **22**:637, 1970.

29 Fries, J. F., and McDevitt, H. O.: Systemic corticosteroid therapy in rheumatic diseases, Ration. Drug Ther. **6**:1, 1972.

30 Ganong, W. F., Alpert, L. C., and Lee, T. C.: ACTH and the regulation of adrenocortical secretion, N. Engl. J. Med. **290**:1006, 1974.

31 Leibsohn, E., and Bagatell, F. K.: Halcinonide in the treatment of corticosteroid responsive dermatoses, Br. J. Dermatol. **90**:435, 1974.

32 Melby, J. C.: Assessment of adrenocortical function, N. Engl. J. Med. **285**:735, 1971.

33 O'Malley, B. W.: Mechanisms of action of steroid hormones, N. Engl. J. Med. **284**:370, 1971.

CHAPTER 44

Thyroid hormones and antithyroid drugs

GENERAL CONCEPT

The normal thyroid gland stores 15 times as much thyroxine (T_4) as triiodothyronine (T_3). It releases about 1% of the stored hormones daily, which are bound to a thyroid hormone–binding globulin and albumin. Only the free, unbound hormones are active and the ratio of free T_4 to T_3 is about 10:1. All of the circulating T_4 originates from the thyroid, whereas about 80% of T_3 is the product of deiodination of T_4 in the tissues.

The main effects of the thyroid hormones are exerted on metabolism and growth. They have calorigenic and protein anabolic effects.

Hypothyroidism is treated with replacement therapy, for which levothyroxine sodium (T_4) and desiccated thyroid (thyroid USP) are commonly employed. Occasionally Liothyronine (T_3) is useful. *Hyperthyroidism* is treated with the thioamide drugs, propylthiouracil or methimazole, which inhibit the incorporation of iodine into thyroglobulin. Radioactive iodine ^{131}I and surgery have important indications also. Finally, propranolol is beneficial in the management of hyperthyroidism.

THYROID HORMONES
Nature and synthesis

In normal subjects the secretion of the thyroid hormones, thyroxine (T_4) and triiodothyronine (T_3), is regulated by the hypothalamus and the pituitary gland. The hypothalamus produces thyrotropin-releasing hormone (TRH), which stimulates the pituitary gland to synthesize and release the thyroid-stimulating hormone (TSH). The thyroid-stimulating hormone promotes the uptake of iodide by the thyroid, the synthesis of thyroglobulin and the release of T_4 and T_3. Increased concentrations of the thyroid hormones reduce TSH secretion by a negative feedback mechanism.

In hyperthyroidism the thyroid functions at an excessive rate and does so autonomously. Under these circumstances TSH levels become very low and the pituitary becomes unresponsive to TRH.

Steps in synthesis of thyroxine

The structural formulas of the various organic iodine compounds of the thyroid gland are shown on p. 551.

The following steps may be distinguished in the elaboration of thyroxine: (1) concentration of inorganic iodide (iodide trapping), (2) oxidation of iodide to free iodine or hypoiodite, (3) formation of monoiodotyrosine and diiodotyrosine, and (4) coupling of two diiodotyrosines to form thyroxine, or tetraiodothyronine.

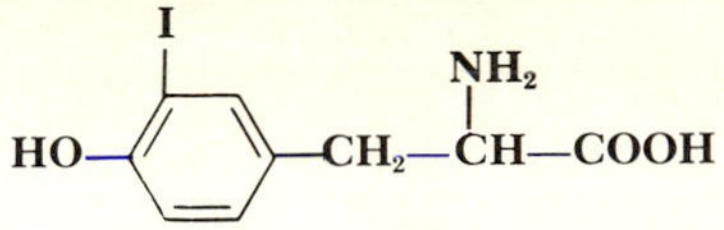

Monoiodotyrosine

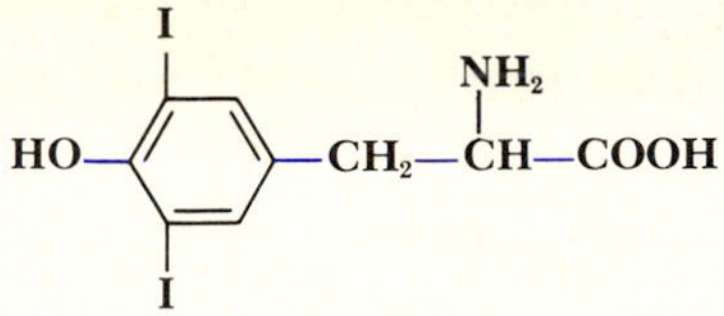

Diiodotyrosine

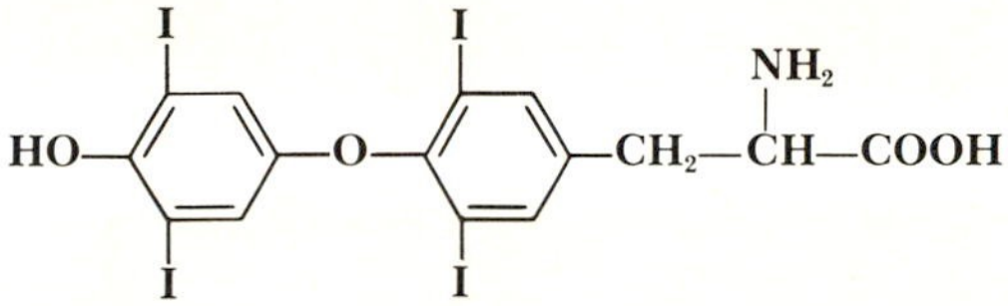

Tetraiodothyronine

The ability of the thyroid gland to concentrate iodide can be demonstrated if the rapid formation of organic iodine compounds is simultaneously blocked by such antithyroid drugs as propylthiouracil or methimazole. Under these conditions the concentration of iodide in the gland may be 30 to 200 times greater than that in plasma. This iodide-trapping mechanism can be blocked by thiocyanate or perchlorate.

The oxidation of iodide to free iodine is believed to be an enzymatic step that may be blocked by antithyroid drugs of the thiourea or thioamide type.

It is believed that tyrosine is iodinated while it is attached in peptide linkage to thyroglobulin. The release of thyroxine from the storage protein probably involves the activity of a proteolytic enzyme.

Iodine cycle

Some of the features of the metabolism of iodine are shown schematically in Fig. 44-1.

The daily intake of iodine is about 150 μg. This quantity plus about 70 μg from the daily thyroxine secretion and degradation enter the inorganic pool of iodine. The thyroid gland takes up about 70 μg of iodine a day. The rest is removed by renal excretion, except for small quantities excreted in the feces. Thus the thyroid gland and the kidney compete with each other with respect to the clearance of inorganic iodide.

Effects

A deficiency of thyroid hormones results in decreased metabolic rate, alterations in growth and development, disturbances in water and electrolyte metabolism, altered functions of the CNS, skeletal muscles, and circulation, and changes in cholesterol metabolism. Clinical conditions that may be attributed to thyroid deficiency are cretinism and myxedema of the adult and juvenile types.

The actions of the thyroid hormones may be exerted on the following functions[2]:
1. Calorigenesis and thermoregulation
2. Metabolism of lipids, proteins, and carbohydrates

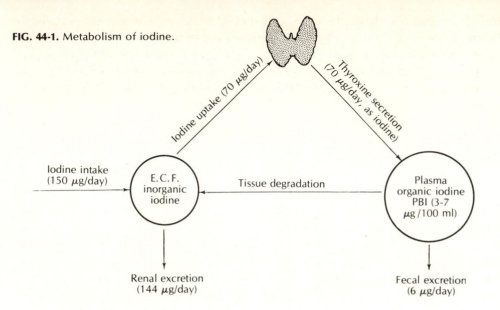

FIG. 44-1. Metabolism of iodine.

3. Reproduction
4. Growth and development
5. Cardiovascular system
6. Water and electrolyte handling
7. Nervous system

An excess of thyroid hormones produces many of the symptoms and signs of thyrotoxicosis such as nervousness and mental instability, tachycardia, elevated pulse pressure, sweating, and hypersusceptibility to epinephrine. The basal metabolic rate is elevated, the plasma PBI is above normal limits, and ^{131}I uptake by the thyroid is increased. By radioimmunoassay, serum T_3 and T_4 concentrations are shown to be elevated, the former more than the latter. The T_3 concentration falls more rapidly during the treatment of thyrotoxicosis.

The thermogenic effect of the thyroid hormones may be mediated at the level of RNA synthesis.[21] A speculative postulate of the events is as follows[31]: binding of the thyroid hormone to a receptor, augmented synthesis of specific classes of RNA, induction of a protein that may be a part of the sodium pump or may activate the sodium pump in the membrane. The result is an increased ATP hydrolysis, increased formation of ADP and inorganic phosphate, and a higher mitochondrial oxidative phosphorylation.

Thyroxine and catecholamines

It is a common belief in medicine that hyperthyroidism makes patients more sensitive to epinephrine. With the availability of numerous catecholamine depleters and adrenergic blocking agents, the traditional view of a thyroxine-catecholamine synergism could be reexamined.

Reserpine and guanethidine have beneficial effects on the symptoms of thyrotoxicosis.[18] In exogenous hyperthyroidism, guanethidine caused a return of heart rate to control values and a disappearance of palpitation and tremor.[8] The drug had no effect on serum cholesterol, body weight, or PBI levels. The amelioration of the symptoms of hyperthyroidism by catecholamine-depleting agents would fit the hypothesis that some end organs are more susceptible to the amines or that the metabolism is altered.

The β-adrenergic blocking drugs, such as propranolol, have become very important in the treatment of hyperthyroidism and are more effective than reserpine and guanethidine.[31]

Thyrotropic hormone

The activities of the thyroid gland are greatly influenced by the thyrotropic hormone of the anterior lobe of the pituitary body, which promotes the synthesis and release of thyroxine by the thyroid gland.

The rate of secretion of the thyrotropic hormone is normally inhibited by increased levels of thyroxine or triiodothyronine. When the synthesis of thyroxine is inhibited by the goitrogenic drugs, the thyroid gland becomes enlarged and its vascularity is increased; these changes are attributed to increased levels of circulating thyroid-stimulating hormone as a consequence of lower thyroxine levels.

There is evidence for a role of a long-acting thyroid stimulator (LATS) in Graves' disease.[16] This substance is unrelated to thyrotropin in regard to chemistry or source. It is a 7S gamma globulin and its mode of action is not understood. If it is an antibody, it may act against some constituent of the thyroid that normally exerts an inhibitory action on the gland. Even more recent evidence indicates the immune factors participate in the pathogenesis of toxic diffuse goiter, and LATS may only be one of the manifestations of such a process.[44]

Clinical uses and preparations

Indications for the use of thyroid preparations include hypothyroidism and conditions in which suppression of thyrotropin secretion is desirable. These include nontoxic goiter and chronic thyroiditis (Hashimoto's disease). Thyroid preparations may also have various diagnostic uses. Their employment in the treatment of obesity and dysmenorrhea is not based on good evidence.

Several preparations are available when treatment with thyroid hormones is indicated.

Thyroid USP is the cleaned, dried, and powdered thyroid gland of animals used for food by humans. It is standardized only by chemical and not by biological assay. It should contain 0.17% to 0.23% of iodine in organic combination. Variability in response may result from reliance on chemical assay alone.

Preparations include tablets containing 15, 30, 60, 120, 200, 250, and 300 mg and enteric-coated tablets of 30, 60, 120, and 200 mg.

Thyroid extract (Proloid) is a purified extract of the thyroid gland, assayed chemically and biologically. It is available in tablets containing 15, 30, 60, 100, 200, and 300 mg.

Levothyroxine sodium (Synthroid sodium) is the synthetic sodium salt of levothyroxine, with actions and uses similar to those of thyroid extract except that it may be injected intravenously in emergencies such as myxedema coma.[41] The potency of 0.1 mg of levothyroxine is equal to that of 60 mg of thyroid USP from the standpoint of a clinical response.

Preparations include tablets containing 0.025, 0.05, 0.1, 0.15, 0.2, 0.3 mg and powder to make an injectable solution, 0.05 mg/ml.

Liothyronine sodium (Cytomel) is the synthetic sodium salt of levotriiodothyronine. It may be injected intravenously in myxedema coma, for which it is the drug of choice. Other uses are similar to those of thyroid extracts. The potency of 0.025 mg of liothyronine sodium is equivalent to that of 60 mg of thyroid USP.

Preparations include tablets containing 5, 25, and 50 μg and powder to make injectable solution, 114 μg/ml.

Liotrix (Euthyroid; Thyrolar) is a mixture of levothyroxine sodium and liothyronine sodium in the ratio of 4:1.

Thyrotropin-releasing hormone (TRH)

The tripeptide pyroglutamylhistidyl-prolinamide or TRH has been synthesized and is undergoing various clinical applications.[33] The drug causes release of thyrotropin and prolactin in normal persons. It may be useful as a diagnostic agent in evaluation of pituitary reserve and differentiation of hypothalamic hypothyroidism from that resulting from pituitary destruction and as a substitute for the thyroid suppression test and others. Hypothyroid patients respond to TRH with a marked elevation of serum thyrotropin. Patients with hyperthyroidism do not respond to TRH.

ANTITHYROID DRUGS

The development of the antithyroid drugs is the result of a series of interesting experimental observations. Perhaps the first indication of antithyroid action was the finding that rabbits on a cabbage diet developed goiter. Numerous studies followed on the antithyroid principles in plants of the *Brassica* genus. Interest in this field was further stimulated when it was found that rats on sulfaguanidine administration also developed hyperplastic thyroid glands. A systematic study of this problem led eventually to the clinical trial of thiourea and thiouracil in thyrotoxicosis.

Classification

Drugs that depress thyroid function can be placed in one of several categories on the basis of their mode of action.

Inhibitors of thyroxine synthesis
  Thiourea (obsolete)
  Thiouracil (obsolete)
  Propylthiouracil
  Methylthiouracil
  Methimazole

Inhibitors of iodide trapping
  Thiocyanates (obsolete)
  Perchlorate (obsolete)
Drugs whose mode of action is uncertain
  Iodides
Drugs that destroy thyroid tissue
  Radioactive iodine (^{131}I)

Inhibitors of thyroxine synthesis

Drugs in this category do not prevent the iodine-concentrating ability of the thyroid gland but block formation of the iodinated amino acids. These drugs inhibit thyroid peroxidase, the iodide-oxidizing enzymes. They block the reactions that require free iodine.

When these inhibitors of thyroxine formation are administered to humans or experimental animals, the preformed thyroxine continues to be secreted. However, thyroxine secretion diminishes as the stored organic iodine becomes exhausted because of a lack of resynthesis. This brings forth increased secretion of the thyroid-stimulating hormone, which produces a hyperplastic, highly vascularized thyroid gland that has a greatly increased capacity for iodide trapping. The individual becomes myxedematous.

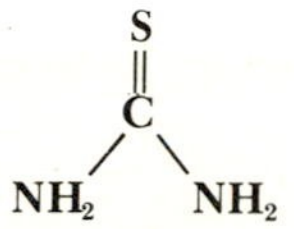

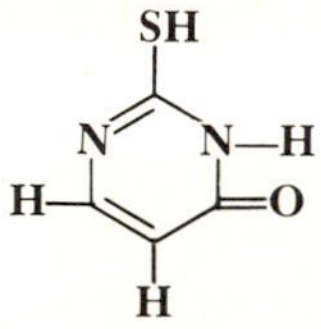

Thiouracil was the first antithyroid drug used extensively. Its use led to numerous cases of drug allergy and agranulocytosis, and it was soon replaced by propylthiouracil. This drug is used in doses of 50 to 100 mg three or four times a day in tablet form. It causes allergic reactions and blood dyscrasias much less frequently than does thiouracil and is one of the most popular antithyroid drugs. Methylthiouracil has about the same potency as propylthiouracil but is less desirable in view of the more frequent allergic side effects observed following its use. Methimazole (Tapazole) is a highly potent antithyroid drug with a long duration of action. It is used in the form of 5 to 10 mg tablets, which are administered three times a day.

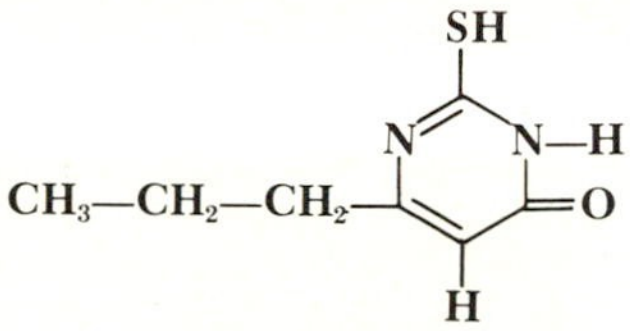

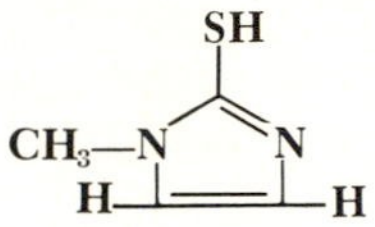

Considering thiouracil as 100, the activity of these drugs in humans is compared as follows: *Activity*

Thiouracil	100
6-N-Propylthiouracil	75
6-Methylthiouracil	100
Methimazole	1000

All these thioamide drugs are absorbed rapidly from the gastrointestinal tract. *Metabolism* They are also excreted and metabolized fairly rapidly, necessitating frequent administration. The distribution of thiouracil in the body is unequal, with several organs, including the thyroid gland, containing more of the drug than the average of other tissues.

Propylthiouracil and methimazole have the following indications: preparation of *Clinical applications* patients for surgery, chronic treatment of hyperthyroidism until spontaneous remission occurs, and management of thyrotoxic crisis (thyroid storm) along with propranolol and other drugs.

The thioamide drugs have a short half-life, about 1½ hours. As a consequence they must be administered several times a day. In long-term therapy it may be possible to reduce the frequency of administration, and the drugs may be given once a day.

The usual daily oral dosages for adults of the inhibitors of thyroxine synthesis are 200 to 300 mg of propylthiouracil, 15 to 30 mg of methimazole (Tapazole), and 200 mg of methylthiouracil.

Inhibitors of iodide trapping   Drugs such as thiocyanate, perchlorate, and nitrate can block the iodide-concentrating ability of the thyroid gland. Perchlorate has undergone clinical trial.[6] It is quite effective, but agranulocytosis has been reported following its use.

Iodides   Although a daily intake of about 150 μg of iodide is essential for normal thyroxine synthesis and although low intakes of iodide lead to goiter and cretinism, in large doses iodides can decrease the functional activity of the thyroid in Graves' disease.

Recent evidence suggests that iodide administered to thyrotoxic patients causes an abrupt inhibition of the release of thyroxine, an effect that may be causally related to its beneficial therapeutic action.[25]

Radioactive iodine   Radioactive iodine (^{131}I) emits γ and β radiation and has a half-life of 8 days. Since it is handled by the body in the same manner as ordinary iodine, it has become extremely useful in the diagnosis of thyroid disease and in the treatment of hyperthyroidism and carcinoma of the thyroid.

The destructive effect of ^{131}I on thyroid tissue is caused by the β radiation. The gamma rays are useful for estimating the quantity of the radioactive material in the gland by placing suitable counting equipment in front of the neck.

The isotope is available as sodium radioiodide. It is generally taken orally, but intravenous preparations are available. For diagnostic purposes the drug is given in doses of about 30 microcuries (μCi), whereas in the treatment of hyperthyroidism about a thousand times as much radioactivity is administered, in other words, 15 to 30 millicuries (mCi). The purpose of the treatment is the same as that of subtotal thyroidectomy.

^{131}I is contraindicated in pregnancy. It is customarily used in patients over 20 years of age. Thyroidectomy is preferred in younger hyperthyroid patients unless surgery represents an unusual hazard, for example, in the presence of heart disease. The most important complication following the use of radioiodine is hypothyroidism.

REFERENCES

1 Astwood, E. B.: Management of thyroid disorders, J.A.M.A. **186**:585, 1963.
2 Barker, S. B.: Peripheral actions of thyroid hormones, Fed. Proc. **21**:635, 1962.
3 Beall, G. N., and Solomon, D. H.: Inhibition of long-acting thyroid stimulator by thyroid particulate fractions, J. Clin. Invest. **45**:552, 1966.
4 Buccino, R. A., Spann, J. F., Jr., Pool, P. E., Sonnenblick, E. H., and Braunwald, E.: Influ-

ence of the thyroid state on the intrinsic contractile properties and energy stores of the myocardium, J. Clin. Invest. **46:**1669, 1967.

5 Cairoli, V. J., and Crout, J. R.: Role of the autonomic nervous system in the resting tachycardia of experimental hyperthyroidism, J. Pharmacol. Exp. Ther. **158:**55, 1967.

6 Crooks, J., and Wayne, E. J.: A comparison of potassium perchlorate, methylthiouracil, and carbimazole in the treatment of thyrotoxicosis, Lancet **1:**401, 1960.

7 DeGroot, L. J.: Current views on formation of thyroid hormones, N. Engl. J. Med. **272:**243, 297, 1965.

8 Gaffney, T. E., Braunwald, E., and Kahler, R. L.: Effects of guanethidine on tri-iodothyronine-induced hyperthyroidism in man, N. Engl. J. Med. **265:**16, 1961.

9 Greer, M. A., Meihoff, W. C., and Studer, H.: Treatment of hyperthyroidism with a single daily dose of propylthiouracil, N. Engl. J. Med. **272:**888, 1965.

10 Gross, J., and Pitt-Rivers, R.: Tri-iodothyronine: isolation from thyroid gland and synthesis, Biochem. J. **53:**645, 1953.

11 Harrington, C. R., and Barger, G.: Thyroxine: constitution and synthesis of thyroxine, Biochem. J. **21:**169, 1927.

12 Harrison, M. J.: The prevention and treatment of thyroid storm, Pharmacol. Phys. **2**(1):1, 1968.

13 Hershman, J. M., Guiens, J., Cassidy, C. E., and Astwood, E. B.: Long term outcome of hyperthyroidism treated with antithyroid drugs, J. Clin. Endocrinol. **26:**803, 1966.

14 Kendall, E. C.: The isolation in crystalline form of the compound containing iodine which occurs in the thyroid: its chemical nature and physiological activity, Trans. Assoc. Am. Phys. **30:**420, 1915.

15 MacGregor, A. G.: Why does anybody use thyroid B. P.? Lancet **1:**329, 1961.

16 McKenzie, J. M.: Review: pathogenesis of Graves' disease: role of the long-acting thyroid stimulator, J. Clin. Endocrinol. **25:**424, 1965.

17 Ochi, Y., and DeGroot, L. J.: Long acting thyroid stimulator of Graves' disease, N. Engl. J. Med. **278:**718, 1968.

18 Oppenheimer, J. H.: Role of plasma proteins in the binding, distribution and metabolism of the thyroid hormones, N. Engl. J. Med. **278:**1153, 1968.

19 Plummer, H. S.: Results of administering iodine to patients having exophthalmic goiter, J.A.M.A. **80:**1955, 1923.

20 Selenkow, H. A., Garcia, A. M., and Bradley, E. B.: An autoregulatory effect of iodide in diverse thyroid disorders, Ann. Intern. Med. **62:**714, 1965.

21 Tata, J. R., et al.: The action of the thyroid hormones at the cell level, Biochem. J. **86:**408, 1963.

22 Taurog, A., Tong, W., and Chaikoff, I. L.: Effects of hypophysectomy on organic iodine formation in rat thyroids. In Wolstenholme, G. E. W., and Millar, E. C. P., editors: Regulation and mode of action of thyroid hormones, Ciba Foundation Colloquia On Endocrinology, Boston, 1957, Little, Brown & Co.

23 Taurog, A., Wheat, J. D., and Chiakoff, I. L.: Nature of the I^{131} compounds appearing in the thyroid vein after injection of iodide I^{131}, Endocrinology **58:**121, 1956.

24 Waldstein, S. S.: Thyroid-catecholamine interrelations, Annu. Rev. Med. **17:**123, 1966.

25 Wartofsky, L., Ransil, B. J., and Ingbar, S. H.: Inhibition by iodine of the release of thyroxine from the thyroid glands of patients with thyrotoxicosis, J. Clin. Invest. **49:**78, 1970.

26 Weiss, W. P., and Sokoloff, L.: Reversal of thyroxine-induced hypermetabolism by puromycin, Science **140:**1324, 1963.

27 Werner, S. C., and Nauman, J. A.: The thyroid, Annu. Rev. Physiol. **30:**213, 1968.

28 Wilson, I. C., Prange, A. J., McClane, T. K., Rabon, A. M., and Lipton, M. A.: Thyroid-hormone enhancement of imipramine in nonretarded depressions, N. Engl. J. Med. **282:**1063, 1970.

29 Wilson, W. R., Theilen, E. O., and Fletcher, F. W.: Pharmacodynamic effects of beta-adrenergic receptor blockage in patients with hyperthyroidism, J. Clin. Invest. **43:**1697, 1964.

REVIEWS

30 Blum, A. S.: The medical management of hyperthyroidism, Ration. Drug. Ther. **8:**1, 1974.

31 Edelman, I. S.: Thyroid thermogenesis, N. Engl. J. Med. **290:**1303, 1974.

32 Haibich, H.: Hyperthyroidism in Graves disease, Arch. Intern. Med. **136:**725, 1976.

33 Hershman, J. M.: Clinical application of thyrotropin-releasing hormone, N. Engl. J. Med. **290:**886, 1974.

34 Hoch, F. L.: The pharmacologic basis for the clinical use of thyroid hormones, Pharmacol. Phys. **4**(4):1, 1970.

35 Ingbar, S. H.: Management of emergencies, IX. Thyroid storm, N. Engl. J. Med. **274:**1252, 1966.

36 Levy, G. S.: Catecholamine sensitivity, thyroid hormone and the heart, Am. J. Med. **50:**413, 1971.

37 Liberti, P., and Stanbury, J. B.: The pharmacology of substances affecting the thyroid gland, Annu. Rev. Pharmacol. **11:**113, 1971.

38 Oppenheimer, J. H.: Thyroid hormone action at the cellular level, Science **203**:971, 1979.

39 Reynolds, L. R., and Kotchen, T. A.: Antithyroid drugs and radioactive iodine. Fifteen years' experience with Graves' disease, Arch. Intern. Med. **139**:651, 1979.

40 Rosenberg, I. N.: Evaluation of thyroid function, N. Engl. J. Med. **286**:924, 1972.

41 Senior, R. M., and Birge, S. J.: The recognition and management of myxedema coma, J.A.M.A. **217**:61, 1971.

42 Sterling, K.: Thyroid hormone action at the cell level, N. Engl. J. Med. **300**:117, 1979.

43 Taurog, A.: The mechanism of action of the thioureylene antithyroid drugs, Endocrinology **98**:1031, 1976.

44 Volpe, R.: The immunologic basis of Graves' disease, N. Engl. J. Med. **287**:463, 1972.

CHAPTER 45

Parathyroid extract and vitamin D

The concentration of ionized calcium in plasma is maintained by rapid exchange with bone calcium, excretion by the kidney, and absorption from the intestine. Parathyroid hormone, vitamin D, and calcitonin contribute in a major way to calcium homeostasis.

A fall in plasma calcium promotes a parathyroid secretion, whereas a rise in calcium inhibits it. The parathyroid hormone not only influences osteoclastic and osteocytic activity, but also stimulates the renal reabsorption of calcium and the formation of 1,25-dihydroxyvitamin D_3, a major regulator of intestinal absorption of calcium and phosphate.

Hypercalcemia is treated with furosemide and saline, phosphate, calcitonin, and glucocorticoids. Hypocalcemia is treated with calcium salts intravenously or orally, vitamin D, or its metabolite calcitriol (1,25-dihydroxyvitamin D_3). The diphosphonate, etidronate sodium has some uses in hypercalcemia also.

The parathyroid hormone is a polypeptide that is seldom used because it is antigenic. It mobilizes calcium from bone, promotes the renal reabsorption of calcium, decreases the renal reabsorption of phosphate, and stimulates the synthesis of 1,25-dihydroxyvitamin D_3.

The secretion of parathyroid is under negative feedback regulation by the serum ionized calcium concentrations.

As shown in Fig. 45-1, the injection of parathyroid extract in patients having idiopathic hypoparathyroidism results in phosphaturia, lowering of serum phosphorus, and gradual elevation of serum calcium. This sequence of events has been interpreted by Albright and Ellsworth[1] as indicative of a primary action of the parathyroid extract on phosphate excretion.

Although parathyroid extract does promote renal excretion of phosphate, there is much experimental evidence to indicate that the most important action of the parathyroid hormones is direct mobilization of calcium from bones. The action of parathyroid extract on serum calcium has been demonstrated in nephrectomized animals.[7] In addition, it has been shown that parathyroid transplants exert a local resorptive effect on bone. This effect has also been demonstrated in tissue cultures.

A variety of factors contribute to the maintenance of extracellular calcium within narrow limits. The daily diet contributes about 1 g of calcium, the absorption of

Calcium homeostasis and parathyroid extract

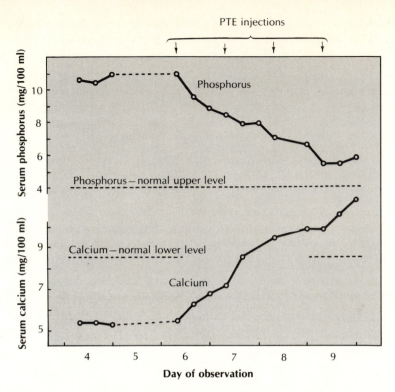

FIG. 45-1. Effect of parathyroid extract *(PTE)* on serum inorganic phosphorus and calcium in patient with idiopathic hypoparathyroidism. (From Munson, P. L.: Fed. Proc. **19:**593, 1960.)

which is influenced by vitamin D and to some extent by parathyroid hormone. Also, the phosphate, oxalate, and phytate content of the diet will decrease calcium absorption. Antacids containing $Al(OH)_3$ promote calcium absorption by binding phosphate in the intestine.

Extracellular calcium is in equilibrium with the exchangeable calcium of bone. When extracellular calcium falls, the exchangeable portion of bone calcium aids in returning it toward normal. In addition, renal reabsorption of calcium, renal excretion of phosphate, and resorption of nonexchangeable bone are important in opposing decreases in extracellular calcium levels. Bone resorption is promoted by the parathyroid hormone and by some steroids related to vitamin D. The release of parathyroid hormone is under the influence of the level of extracellular calcium.

The effects of the parathyroid hormone on bone reabsorption and phosphate excretion are mediated by the adenyl cyclase system and cyclic AMP.

Calcitonin, or thyrocalcitonin, is a second hormone involved in calcium homeostasis. Calcitonin is secreted by the parafollicular cells of the thyroid. These cells originate from the ultimobranchial body, a separate organ in some animals. Calcitonin produces hypocalcemia by inhibiting bone resorption. Calcitonin also promotes the urinary excretion of calcium and phosphate.[4]

Calcitonin is normally present in the blood, and its concentration increases when calcium salts are administered. Its concentration is greatly increased in patients having medullary carcinoma of the thyroid.[6] The function of calcitonin may be a protective one against hypercalcemia induced by increased calcium intake.

Calcitonin has been used clinically in Paget's disease, hypercalcemia, and osteoporosis. Its usefulness is limited by its short duration of action. In addition, resistance develops to its continued use, perhaps because of compensatory increase in the secretion of parathyroid hormone.[19]

VITAMIN D
Current nomenclature

It was discovered more than 40 years ago that irradiation of plant sterols could yield antirachitic compounds. The active sterol produced by irradiation of ergosterol became known as vitamin D_2 or *ergocalciferol*. What was previously called vitamin D_1 was a mixture of active and inactive products. The vitamin that is produced in the skin by irradiation of 7-dehydrocholesterol was named vitamin D_3 or *cholecalciferol*. Although both vitamins D_2 and D_3 are active and undergo similar metabolic transformations, most of the circulating and stored vitamin D is ergocalciferol. This is a consequence of the high dietary intake of irradiated ergosterol. Vitamin D_3 differs from vitamin D_2 only in lacking a double bond between C-22 and C-23.

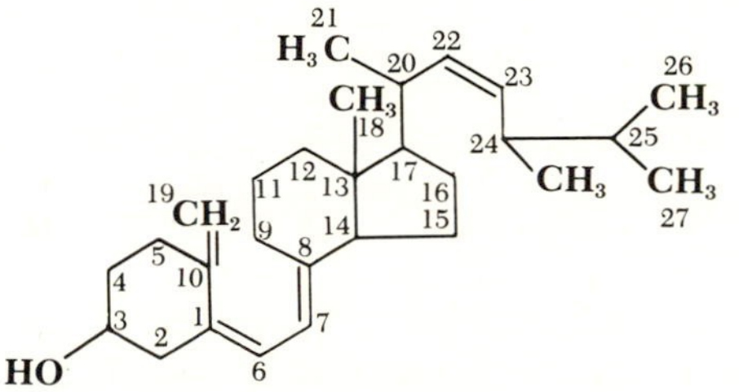

Vitamin D_2 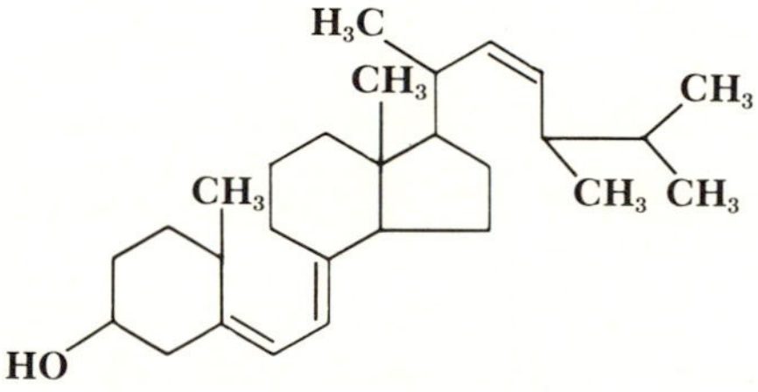   Dihydrotachysterol

Metabolic activation

Both vitamins D_2 and D_3 must be hydroxylated in the C-25 position by the liver to become active. The resulting compounds are referred to as 25-hydroxyergocalciferol and 25-hydroxycholecalciferol, respectively. These compounds are carried in the circulation by a binding protein. Eventually, the microsomal enzymes of the liver convert them to inactive polar metabolites.

A further activating step occurs in the kidney for vitamin D_3. The 25-hydroxycholecalciferol is further hydroxylated to 1,25-hydroxycholecalciferol, which may be the final active form of vitamin D_3.

The first enzymatic hydroxylation of cholecalciferol in the liver is under feedback inhibition by the 25-hydroxylated compound. This feedback inhibition prevents overproduction of this metabolite. The second hydroxylation, which takes place in the kidney, yields the product, 1,25-hydroxycholecalciferol, which is most potent in causing calcium reabsorption from the intestine and reabsorption from the bone. In severe renal disease it is possible to administer the dihydroxylated cholecalciferol, thus bypassing its lack of production by the failing kidney.

Dihydrotachysterol is also hydroxylated in the liver, but the 25-hydroxyl derivative does not exert feedback inhibition on the reaction. The 25-hydroxyl derivative of dihydrotachysterol is the active form of the compound and does not require further activation in the kidney. For these reasons the drug is much more effective in promoting bone reabsorption than cholecalciferol and is commonly used in the treatment of hypoparathyroidism.

Drug interactions   Phenobarbital and phenytoin are known to increase microsomal hydroxylase activity in the liver. It is possible that the great frequency of rickets and osteomalacia in patients taking anticonvulsants is a consequence of increased enzymatic transformation of vitamin D_2 and D_3 to inactive metabolites.[20]

The main function of vitamin D is to promote absorption of calcium and phosphorus from the intestine. Deficiency of the vitamin in children leads to rickets, which may be prevented by the daily requirement of 800 units. Very rarely, osteomalacia can occur in adults following vitamin D deficiency.

In the treatment of hypoparathyroidism, vitamin D_2 may be administered in large doses (400,000 IU) initially, and maintenance doses may vary from 100,000 to 200,000 IU/day. Dihydrotachysterol may be administered initially in doses of 3 to 8 mg (compared with 10 mg or more of vitamin D_2), and for maintenance a dose of about 1 mg/day is usually sufficient.

TOXIC EFFECTS OF PARATHYROID EXTRACT AND VITAMIN D

Toxic effects of parathyroid injection and of vitamin D are manifested as (1) hypercalcemia with numerous clinical consequences, (2) demineralization of bones, and (3) renal calculi and metastatic calcifications in soft tissues.

Hypercalcemia is associated with a number of clinical manifestations such as weakness, vomiting, diarrhea, and lack of muscle tone. The electrocardiographic changes that may occur at various levels of serum calcium are shown in Fig. 45-2. Serious toxic manifestations may be seen at calcium blood levels of 15 mg/100 ml. Signs of hypocalcemia are tetany, cataracts, and mental lethargy.

OTHER DRUGS INFLUENCING SERUM CALCIUM CONCENTRATIONS

Phosphates, sodium sulfate, sodium citrate and **disodium edetate** (Endrate), when given by intravenous infusion, can lower calcium levels in the blood. Their administration should not be undertaken without considering their adverse effects.

Glucocorticoids antagonize the effects of vitamin D on calcium absorption from the intestine. They are useful in hypercalcemia caused by sarcoidosis or hypervitaminosis D. **Salmon calcitonin** (Calcimar) is a polypeptide, which is injected subcutaneously or intramuscularly for the occasional initial treatment of hyperparathyroidism, Paget's disease, and some malignancies. It loses its effectiveness in a few weeks.

Etidronate disodium (EHDP; Didronel) is a diphosphonate used in the treatment of Paget's disease. The drug seems to slow osteoblastic and osteoclastic activity. The drug lowers serum alkaline phosphatase and urinary hydroxyproline. The most serious adverse effect of etidronate is osteomalacia with fractures. Etidronate di-

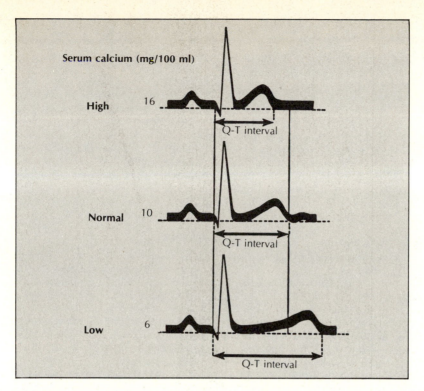

FIG. 45-2. Effect of varying calcium levels on electrocardiogram. (From Burch, G. E., and Winsor, T.: A primer of electrocardiography, Philadelphia, 1960, Lea & Febiger.)

sodium (Didronel) is available in 200 mg tablets. The loop diuretics, such as **furo-semide** (Lasix), tend to promote calcium excretion, whereas the **thiazides** cause hypercalcemia with chronic administration.

Mithramycin, an antibiotic used in the treatment of testicular neoplasms, lowers calcium concentration, perhaps by a toxic effect on osteoclasts.

For the initial treatment of *hypocalcemia,* the intravenous injection of a 10% solution of **calcium gluconate** is highly effective. **Calcium gluceptate** may also be given intravenously or intramuscularly. Calcium salts used orally include calcium gluconate, calcium phosphate dibasic, calcium phosphate tribasic, calcium lactate, and calcium carbonate precipitated.

Calcitriol (Rocaltrol) is 1,25-dihydroxyvitamin D_3, a renal hormone. It promotes intestinal calcium absorption, and it may mobilize calcium from bone. It is used in hypocalcemic patients with chronic renal failure. Calcitriol (Rocaltrol) is available in 0.25 and 0.5 μg tablets.

REFERENCES

1 Albright, F., and Ellsworth, R.: Studies on the physiology of the parathyroid glands: calcium and phosphorus studies in a case of idiopathic hypoparathyroidism, J. Clin. Invest. **7:**183, 1929.

2 Arnaud, C. D., Sizemore, G. W., Oldham, S. B., Fischer, J. A., Tsao, H. S., and Littledike, E. T.: Human parathyroid hormone: glandular and secreted molecular species, Am. J. Med. **50:**630, 1971.

3 Bijvoet, O. L. M., Veer, J. V., De Vries, H. R., and Van Koppen, A. T. J.: Natriuretic effect of calcitonin in man, N. Engl. J. Med. **284:**681, 1971.

4 Copp, D. H.: Parathyroids, calcitonin, and control of plasma calcium, Recent Prog. Hormone Res. **20:**59, 1964.

5 DeLuca, H. F.: 25-Hydroxycholecalciferol, Arch. Intern. Med. **124:**442, 1969.

6 Foster, G. V.: Calcitonin (thyrocalcitonin), N. Engl. J. Med. **279:**349, 1968.

7 Grollman, A.: The role of the kidney in the parathyroid control of the blood calcium as determined by studies on the nephrectomized dog, Endocrinology **55:**166, 1954.

8 Haddad, J. G., Birge, S. J., and Avioli, L. V.: Effects of prolonged thyrocalcitonin administration of Paget's disease of bone, N. Engl. J. Med. **283:**549, 1970.

9 Harrison, H. E., Lifshitz, F., and Blizzard, R. M.: Comparison between crystalline dihydrotachysterol and calciferol in patients requiring pharmacologic vitamin D therapy, N. Engl. J. Med. **276:**894, 1967.

10 Hirsch, P. F., and Munson, P. L.: Thyrocalcitonin, Physiol. Rev. **49:**548, 1969.

11 Kenny, A. D., Draskóczy, P. R., and Goldhaber, P.: Citric acid production by resorbing bone tissue culture, Am. J. Physiol. **197:**502, 1959.

12 Kimberg, D. V.: Effects of vitamin D and steroid hormones on the active transport of calcium by the intestine, N. Engl. J. Med. **280:**1396, 1969.

13 Lukert, B. P.: Vitamin D metabolism in man: effect of corticosteroids, Arch. Intern. Med. **136:**1241, 1976.

14 McLean, F. C., and Hastings, A. B.: The state of calcium in the fluids of the body: the conditions affecting the ionization of calcium, J. Biol. Chem. **108:**285, 1935.

REVIEWS

15 Broadus, A. E., Horst, R. L., Lang, R., Littledike, E. T., and Rasmussen, H.: The importance of circulating 1,25-dihydroxyvitamin D in the pathogenesis of hypercalciuria and renalstone formation in primary hyperparathyroidism, N. Engl. J. Med. **302:**421, 1980.

16 DeLuca, H. F., and Suttie, J. W.: The fat-soluble vitamins, Madison, 1970, University of Wisconsin Press.

17 Juan, D.: Hypocalcemia. Differential diagnosis and mechanisms. Arch. Intern. Med. **139:**1166, 1979.

18 Newmark, S. R.: Hypercalcemic and hypocalcemic crises, J.A.M.A. **230:**1438, 1974.

19 Raisz, L. G.: The pharmacology of bone, Ration. Drug Ther. **5:**1, 1971.

20 Raisz, L. G.: A confusion of Vitamin D's, N. Engl. J. Med. **287:**926, 1972.

21 Tashjian, A. H.: Soft bones, hard facts and calcitonin therapy, N. Engl. J. Med. **283:**593, 1970.

22 Wills, M. R.: Intestinal absorption of calcium, Lancet, **1:**820, 1973.

CHAPTER 46

Posterior pituitary hormones— vasopressin and oxytocin

The posterior lobe of the pituitary body, the neurohypophysis, contains hormones having vasoactive, antidiuretic, and oxytocic properties. The original material was separated into two fractions.[9] One contained most of the vasoactive and antidiuretic portion, whereas the other was predominantly oxytocic. Both active fractions, vasopressin and oxytocin, have been synthesized.[5,6]

Chemistry and preparations

Both vasopressin and oxytocin are polypeptides containing eight amino acids. Vasopressin (in several species) contains the following amino acids: tyrosine, cystine, aspartic acid, glutamic acid, glycine, proline, arginine, and phenylalanine. In vasopressin obtained from hog pituitary, arginine is replaced by lysine.

Oxytocin resembles vasopressin in having six identical amino acids but contains leucine and isoleucine instead of arginine and phenylalanine.

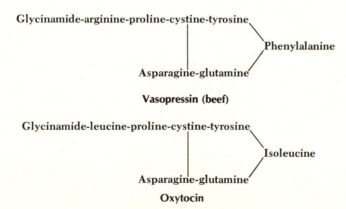

Glycinamide-arginine-proline-cystine-tyrosine

Phenylalanine

Asparagine-glutamine

Vasopressin (beef)

Glycinamide-leucine-proline-cystine-tyrosine

Isoleucine

Asparagine-glutamine

Oxytocin

Preparations of these hormones are standardized by bioassay. Vasopressin preparations are standardized on the basis of the action of such preparations on the blood pressure of the dog. One USP unit is the activity present in 0.5 mg of standard powder of posterior pituitary. Oxytocic potency is determined by the depressor effect of oxytocin preparations on the blood pressure of the chicken.

VASOPRESSIN

The most significant effect of vasopressin is exerted on the kidney. In addition, the hormone can constrict various blood vessels, including the coronary vessels. The only clearly established physiological function of vasopressin is its antidiuretic action.

The antidiuretic potency of vasopressin is very great. The infusion of less than 0.1 μg of vasopressin per hour produces maximal antidiuresis in humans. It is believed that the antidiuretic action of vasopressin is exerted on water reabsorption by the distal tubule and also by the collecting ducts. In physiological doses the hormone does not influence electrolyte absorption. Larger doses in some experiments have shown increased output of sodium and chloride, probably an indirect effect.

The antidiuretic hormone is elaborated by certain hypothalamic structures such as the supraoptic nuclei and is then transported to the neurohypophysis where it is stored. The release of the antidiuretic hormone is influenced by the osmolarity of the extracellular fluid and by many drugs. Endogenous neurohumoral agents also may play an important role in the release of antidiuretic hormones, since pain and emotions have important influences. It is generally accepted that some hypothalamic structures are sensitive to changes in the osmolarity of the extracellular fluid and act as osmoreceptors.[17] Thus the ingestion of water and dilution of the extracellular fluid lead to inhibition of antidiuretic hormone secretion, whereas hypertonic solutions promote this process.

Diabetes insipidus, occurring spontaneously or produced experimentally by pituitary stalk section, is characterized by failure of distal tubular water reabsorption. As a consequence, persons with diabetes insipidus excrete large amounts of dilute urine and drink large quantities of water.

The mode of action of the antidiuretic hormone is now generally attributed to an increase in the size of pores or channels for the flow of water along osmotic gradients.[3] There is evidence for this action on isolated systems such as the skin of toads and frogs.[1]

The mechanism of action of vasopressin involves the activation of the adenyl cyclase system with the increase in the concentration of cyclic AMP.[13]

Other drugs with antidiuretic effects in diabetes insipidus include clofibrate, chlorpropamide, and also the thiazides. Most of these are more likely to be useful in moderate forms of the disease, and the thiazides are useful especially in nephrogenic diabetes insipidus.

Effects on antidiuretic hormone release

In addition to changes in osmolarity of the extracellular fluid, release of the antidiuretic hormone is influenced by a variety of drugs. The existence of a cholinergic mechanism for this process has been suggested on the basis of experiments showing that injections of *acetylcholine* or diisopropyl fluorophosphate into the supraoptic nuclei caused release of antidiuretic hormone. *Nicotine* has been shown to inhibit water diuresis in humans, probably through the release of antidiuretic hormone. *Alcohol* inhibits the release of antidiuretic hormone in response to dehydration and produces inappropriate water diuresis in a dehydrated individual.[10] Alcohol does not block the action of nicotine on the release of the hormone.[10]

Antidiuresis that occurs during general anesthesia[2] and following the injection of histamine, morphine, and barbiturates (but not thiopental[2]) has also been attributed to the release of antidiuretic hormone. Since muscular exercise, pain, and emotional excitement also cause inhibition of water diuresis, it is likely that some central control mechanism of antidiuretic hormone release is very susceptible to neural or neurohumoral influences. Of the large variety of drugs that can influence antidiuretic hormone release, many are known to alter neural activity or to act as stressful stimuli.

Certain hyponatremic syndromes are associated with "inappropriate" secretion of the antidiuretic hormone. They are characterized by primary water retention unassociated with sodium retention and edema. Some of the underlying diseases are bronchogenic carcinoma, head injury, and tuberculous meningitis.[4]

Extrarenal effects

Although the main therapeutic advantage of vasopressin is its antidiuretic action, the hormone has a stimulant effect on the smooth muscles of the blood vessels, intestine, and uterus. This action appears to be a direct musculotropic effect, not mediated by nerves or neurohumoral agents. When posterior pituitary preparations are used in the treatment of diabetes insipidus, the smooth muscle effects are undesirable side effects and usually indicate overdosage.

Preparations containing vasopressin constrict the coronary arteries and are therefore dangerous in persons who suffer from coronary disease. Although intravenous injection of posterior pituitary extract into animals causes marked peripheral vasoconstriction, blood pressure often increases only moderately. This is attributed to the fact that the coronary arteries are also constricted. Tachyphylaxis develops to the pressor action of vasopressin.

Antidiuretic preparations

Posterior pituitary USP is available as a powder for topical application, administered by inhalation or directly to the nasal mucosa. It may cause mucosal irritation. The duration of its antidiuretic effect is such that the drug must be used several times a day. Posterior pituitary is contraindicated in pregnancy and should be used with caution in patients with coronary artery disease. The dose is 40 to 60 mg topically three or four times daily.

Posterior pituitary injection is obsolete, being replaced by vasopressin injection.

Vasopressin injection (Pitressin) produces an antidiuretic effect lasting 2 to 8 hours when administered by subcutaneous or intramuscular injection. The solution may also be used topically. Vasopressin may cause fluid retention, hypertension, myocardial ischemia, gastrointestinal and uterine contractions, and allergic reactions. The available solution for injection contains 10 pressor units/ml.

Vasopressin tannate injection (Pitressin tannate) is a suspension in peanut oil of the insoluble tannate of the hormone, suitable for intramuscular administration. The duration of action is 2 to 3 days. Vasopressin tannate injection is available in oil, 5 pressor units/ml.

Desmopressin acetate (DDAVP) is a vasopressin analog, which has a prolonged action, and its antidiuretic effect in relation to its vasopressor effect is much greater than is the case for the other vasopressins. The drug is used topically by a nasal calibrated catheter. Its antidiuretic effect lasts 10 to 20 hours, and it may replace the other vasopressins in the management of severe diabetes insipidus. The drug is available in solutions containing 0.1 mg/ml of DDAVP.

Lypressin (Diapid) is a synthetic lysine vasopressin. It is administered by intranasal spray.

Clofibrate has an antidiuretic effect, probably by increasing the release of vasopressin from the neurohypophysis. **Chlorpropamide** apparently increases the sensitivity of the renal tubules to the action of vasopressin. The **thiazides** are generally ineffective in central diabetes insipidus but may be useful in the nephrogenic form of the disease.

OXYTOCIN

Oxytocin is a polypeptide amide that consists of eight amino acids and ammonia. Its molecular weight is 1007. Although the physiological functions of the hormone seem to be related to reproductive function in the female, its presence in the male suggests that it must have other functions also.

The separation of posterior pituitary extracts into the oxytocic and vasopressor-antidiuretic fractions was accomplished as early as 1928. More recently, oxytocin has been purified, chemically identified, and synthesized.[6]

Oxytocin differs from vasopressin in the following respects:

1. It contains leucine and isoleucine instead of phenylalanine and arginine; the other six amino acids are identical in the two hormones.
2. It has no effect on water diuresis.
3. It is a potent stimulant of the gravid uterus at term and postpartum.
4. It does not produce vasoconstriction and may even lower blood pressure in certain species.
5. It may produce milk letdown during the postpartum period.
6. It has little effect on intestinal smooth muscle and coronary arteries.

Bioassay

Oxytocin preparations are bioassayed on the basis of the vasodepressor activity in chickens. The oxytocic activity associated with vasopressin preparations is assayed on the guinea pig uterus.

Preparations

Oxytocin injection, synthetic (Pitocin; Syntocinon; Uteracon) is a synthetic preparation and used for induction of labor. It is also used to control postpartum uterine atony, but for the latter indication, ergonovine is often preferred. The drug is available in solutions containing 5 units/0.5 ml or 10 units/ml. Dosage varies according to the indication. To control postpartum bleeding, oxytocin may be administered intramuscularly, 3 to 10 units. When given by intravenous injection for the same indication, its dosage should be reduced to 0.6 to 1.8 units. For intravenous infusion by the drip method, oxytocin, 2 units, is added to 500 ml of normal saline.

Ergonovine maleate (Ergotrate Maleate) and **methylergonovine maleate** (Methergine) are used to decrease uterine bleeding by causing contraction of the uterine muscle after delivery of the placenta.

Prostaglandin preparations are used for producing abortions by the induction of uterine contractions. Carboprost tromethamine (Prostin/M15) is the 15-methyl derivative of prostaglandin F_2-α. It is injected intramuscularly and is effective from the thirteenth to the twentieth week of pregnancy. Dinoprost tromethamine (Prostin F_2-α) is usually administered intra-amniotically. Dinoprostone (Prostin E_2) is available in the form of vaginal suppositories.

OTHER UTERINE STIMULANTS

β-Adrenergic agonists, intravenous alcohol, and prostaglandin synthesis inhibitors, such as indomethacin, may be useful for the prevention of premature delivery.

Ritodrine hydrochloride (Yutopar), a β-adrenergic agonist, has been approved recently as an effective uterine relaxant for premature labor.

UTERINE RELAXANTS

REFERENCES

1 Anderson, B., and Ussing, H. H.: Solvent drag on non-electrolytes during osmotic flow through isolated toad skin and its response to antidiuretic hormone, Acta Physiol. Scand. **39:**228, 1957.

2 Aprahamian, H. A., Vanderveen, J. L., Bunker, J. P., Murphy, A. J., and Crawford, J. D.: The influence of general anesthetics on water and solute excretion in man, Ann. Surg. **150:**122, 1959.

3 Berliner, R. W., Levinsky, N. G., Davidson, D. G., and Eden, M.: Dilution and concentration of the urine and the action of antidiuretic hormone, Am. J. Med. **24:**730, 1958.

4 Clift, G. V., Schletter, F. E., Moses, A. M., and Streeten, D. H. P.: Syndrome of inappropriate vasopressin secretion, Arch. Intern. Med. **118:**453, 1966.

5 du Vigneaud, V.: The isolation and proof of structure of the vasopressins and the synthesis of octapeptide amides with pressor-antidiuretic activity. In Liébecq, C., editor: Proceedings of the Third International Congress on Biochemistry, New York, 1956, Academic Press, Inc.

6 du Vigneaud, V., Ressler, C., Swan, J. M., Roberts, C. W., Katsoyannis, P. G., and Gordon, S.: The synthesis of an octapeptide amide with the hormonal activity of oxytocin: enzymatic cleavage of glycinamide from vasopressin and a proposed structure for this pressor-antidiuretic hormone of the posterior pituitary, J. Am. Chem. Soc. **75:**4879, 1953.

7 Earley, L. E., and Orloff, J.: The mechanism of antidiuresis associated with the administra-

tion of hydrochlorothiazide to patients with vasopressin-resistant diabetes insipidus, J. Clin. Invest. **41:**1988, 1962.

8 Farrell, G., Fabre, L. F., and Rauschkolb, E. W.: The neurohypophysis, Annu. Rev. Physiol. **30:**557, 1968.

9 Kamm, O. H., Aldrich, T. B., Grottee, I. W., Rowe, L. W., and Bugbee, E. P.: The active principles of the posterior lobe of the pituitary gland, J. Am. Chem. Soc. **50:**573, 1928.

10 Kleeman, C. R., Rubini, M. E., Lamdin, E., and Epstein, F. H.: Studies on alcohol diuresis. II. The evaluation of ethyl alcohol as an inhibitor of the neurohypophysis, J. Clin. Invest. **34:**448, 1955.

11 Leaf, A.: Membrane effects of antidiuretic hormone, Am. J. Med. **42:**745, 1967.

12 Milne, M. D.: Renal pharmacology, Annu. Rev. Pharmacol. **5:**119, 1965.

13 Orloff, J., and Handler, J. S.: The cellular mode of action of antidiuretic hormone, Am. J. Med. **36:**686, 1964.

14 Poisner, A. M., and Douglas, W. W.: A possible mechanism of release of posterior pituitary hormones involving adenosine triphosphate and an adenosine triphosphatase in the neurosecretory granules, Molc. Pharmacol. **4:**531, 1968.

15 Reichlin, S.: Functions of the median-eminence gland, N. Engl. J. Med. **275:**600, 1966.

16 Silva, Y. J., Moffat, R. C., and Walt, A. J.: Vasopressin effect on portal and systemic hemodynamics, J.A.M.A. **210:**1065, 1969.

17 Verney, E. B.: The antidiuretic hormone and

the factors which determine its release, Proc. R. Soc. Biol. **135:**25, 1947.

18 Wakim, K. G.: Reassessment of the source, mode and locus of action of antidiuretic hormone, Am. J. Med. **42:**394, 1967.

REVIEWS

19 Hays, R. M.: Antidiuretic hormone, N. Engl. J. Med. **295:**659, 1976.

20 Kosman, M. E.: Evaluation of a new antidiuretic agent, desmopressin acetate (DDAVP), J.A.M.A. **240:**1896, 1978.

21 Taylor, A., Mamelak, M., Reaven, E., and Maffly, R.: Vasopressin: possible role of microtubules and microfilaments in its action, Science **181:**347, 1973.

CHAPTER 47

Anterior pituitary gonadotropins and sex hormones

The anterior pituitary gland produces several polypeptide and glycoprotein hormones. The polypeptides are growth hormone (somatotropin), prolactin, corticotropin, and lipotropin. The glycoproteins are thyrotropin, luteinizing hormone (LH), and follicle-stimulating hormone (FSH). The cells of the anterior pituitary gland may secrete one or more of these hormones.[41]

The secretion of these hormones is stimulated by hypothalamic-releasing factors (Fig. 47-1), also known as *hypophysiotropic hormones*, such as thyrotropin-releasing hormone (TRH), gonadotropin-releasing hormone (GnRH), prolactin-inhibiting factors (PIF), corticotropin-releasing factor (CRF), growth hormone–releasing factor (GHRF), and growth hormone release-inhibitory factor (somatostatin).

GENERAL CONCEPT

Several neuropharmacological agents alter anterior pituitary secretions by acting on the elaboration of hypothalamic releasing factors. It is believed that the neurons that secrete the releasing factors are located in the ventral hypothalamus,[32] and various neurotransmitters regulate their functional activities. Among the possible transmitters, dopamine, norepinephrine, and serotonin have received the most consideration. Many drugs influence the elaboration of various releasing factors by interactions with their neurotransmitters. A brief summary based on a more extensive review[32] will be attempted, classifying these drug effects according to the individual releasing factors.

Protirelin (TRH) is the thyroid-stimulating hormone (TSH)–releasing factor. It is a synthetic tripeptide (pyroglutamyl-histidyl-proline amide) available under the trade names Relefact or Thypinone in a solution containing 0.5 mg/ml of the hormone. Protirelin is used in the diagnosis of thyroid and pituitary disorders and in prolactinemic states, since it also stimulates prolactin secretion.

Corticotropin-releasing factor (CRF). Dextroamphetamine stimulates the release of CRF, which is blocked by an α-adrenergic blocking agent. Reserpine causes a transient increase in basal secretion. The phenothiazines such as chlorpromazine reduce the responses of CRF secretion to hypoglycemia, metyrapone, and pyrogens. These actions could be caused by an antiadrenergic, antidopaminergic, or antiserotoninergic effect of the phenothiazines.

NEUROPHARMA-COLOGICAL AGENTS AND HYPOTHALAMIC RELEASING FACTORS

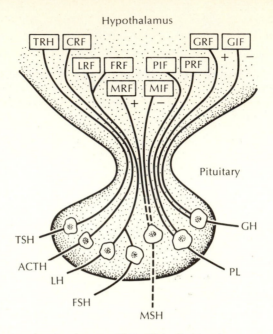

FIG. 47-1. Hypothalamic releasing factors. *TRH,* TSH-releasing hormone; *CRF,* ACTH-releasing factor; *LRF,* LH-releasing factor; *FRF,* FSH-releasing factor; *MRF* and *MIF,* MSH-releasing and -inhibiting factors; *PIF* and *PRF,* prolactin-inhibiting and -releasing factors; *GRF* and *GIF,* GH-releasing and -inhibiting factors; *TSH,* thyroid-stimulating hormone; *ACTH,* adrenocorticotropic hormone; *LH,* luteinizing hormone; *FSH,* follicle-stimulating hormone; *MSH,* melanocyte-stimulating hormone; *PL,* prolactin; *GH,* growth hormone. (From Frohman, L. A.: N. Engl. J. Med. **286:** 1391, 1972.)

Luteinizing hormone- (LH) and follicle-stimulating hormone (FSH)–releasing factors. Experimental studies indicate that dopamine is a stimulatory and serotonin is an inhibitory neurotransmitter involved in the release of LRF and FRF. The abministration of L-dopa leads to a rise in plasma FSH and a more variable rise in plasma LH. The phenothiazines have been claimed to inhibit LRF secretion, whereas FRF was unaffected or even stimulated.

The semisynthetic ergot alkaloid **bromocriptine** (2-bromo-α-ergocryptine) is a drug that acts on dopamine receptors. It is being tried in the treatment of galactor-rhea as well as in puerperal lactation, hyperprolactinemia, hypogonadism, acromeg-aly, and parkinsonism.[44]

Bromocriptine mesylate (Parlodel) is available in 2.5 mg tablets. As a dopaminer-gic drug, it lowers serum prolactin levels, and it is used in the management of repro-ductive disorders associated with hyperprolactinemia and suppression of postpartum lactation and in acromegaly. The drug is used also in the treatment of Parkinson's disease.

Prolactin-inhibiting factor (PIF). Galactorrhea is produced by a variety of psychotropic drugs, such as the phenothiazines, reserpine, methyldopa, and imipra-mine. It is believed that dopamine promotes the secretion of a PIF. The problem is complicated, however, and the previously mentioned effect of imipramine could not be explained on the basis of such a simple hypothesis. On the other hand, prolactin-lowering effect of L-dopa has been reported, an observation that would favor the basic hypothesis of a dopaminergic control.

Growth hormone–releasing factor (GHRF). There is a strong suspicion of an adrenergic control of GHRF secretion. Dextroamphetamine stimulates GHRF, the effect being enhanced by propranolol. GHRF appears to be stimulated by α-adrenergic and inhibited by β-adrenergic mechanisms. Reserpine and chlorpromazine reduce the GHRF hypoglycemia. In an acromegalic patient, chlorpromazine caused a decrease in growth hormone levels.

Somatostatin, a tetradecapeptide, is found not only in the hypothalamus but also in the gastrointestinal tract and the pancreatic islets.[29] It inhibits the secretion of growth hormone, thyrotropin, glucagon, insulin, and some other hormones.

GROWTH HORMONE

Human growth hormone, also known as *somatotropin* (Asellacrin), although very scarce, is available for the treatment of hypopituitary dwarfism. It is administered by intramuscular injection. Growth hormone produces gigantism or acromegaly, depending on the individual's age.

The growth hormone has anti-insulin effects and is diabetogenic. Some of its actions, however, are similar to those of insulin; for example, both promote the cellular uptake of amino acids.

Many of the actions of growth hormone are exerted on factors known as *somatomedins*, which are elaborated largely by the liver.

GONADOTROPINS AND SEX HORMONES

Gonadotropin secretion is regulated by hypothalamic centers that communicate with the anterior pituitary by means of releasing factors. Dopamine plays an important role in these central regulations.[22] FSH promotes the growth of the follicle and the secretion of estrogens. LH, which is identical to the interstitial cell–stimulating hormone (ICSH), produces ovulation and promotes secretion of progesterone from the corpus luteum. Estrogens and progesterone exert a negative feedback on the secretion of gonadotropins.

Estrogens promote the growth of the reproductive organs in the female. They promote growth and cornification of the vaginal epithelium and stimulate cervical mucous secretion. Progesterone contributes to the differentiation in the female reproductive organs and is responsible for the secretions of the endometrium during the luteal phase of the menstrual cycle.

In the male, testosterone is secreted by the interstitial cells of Leydig. The anterior pituitary gland stimulates the activities of Leydig's cells by means of the hormone LH, also known as ICSH in the earlier literature.

OVULATORY CYCLE

The traditional schema of the hormonal control of menstruation is shown in Fig. 47-2, whereas the actual measurements of the serum concentrations of various hormones in normal women are depicted in Fig. 47-3.

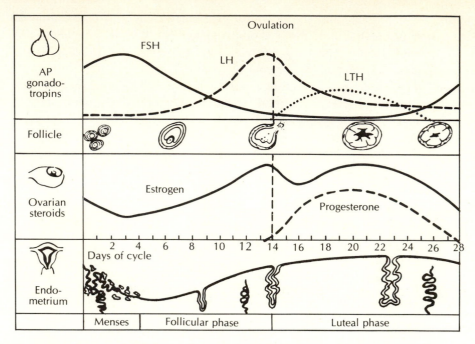

FIG. 47-2. Hormonal control of menstruation. (From Riley, G. M.: Gynecologic endocrinology, New York, 1959, Harper & Row, Publishers.)

The rise of serum FSH and LH concentrations in the early phase of the cycle is probably responsible for the initial growth and development of the follicles. FSH and LH act synergistically with regard to follicular maturation.

Ovulation is preceded by a surge of LH and also FSH. The LH surge is of primary importance in causing rupture of the follicle.[26] Progesterone secretion follows the LH surge.

Estrogens, progesterone, and menstruation

The administration of estrogen to a woman without ovarian function can lead to withdrawal bleeding, breakthrough bleeding, or no bleeding, depending on dose and timing. Withdrawal bleeding occurs when the estrogen is employed in low doses for weeks and is suddenly stopped. Bleeding is like normal menstruation except that it is painless and more prolonged. Withdrawal bleeding can also be produced by administration of a single dose of estrogen.

Breakthrough bleeding occurs during the continued administration of a dose of estrogen that is *larger* than the amount necessary to induce withdrawal bleeding. Breakthrough bleeding is unpredictable in onset or amount. If the dose of estrogen is further increased, breakthrough bleeding will cease.

If progesterone is added to the continued administration of estrogen for a few days and then is stopped, menstruation that resembles normal menses will occur.

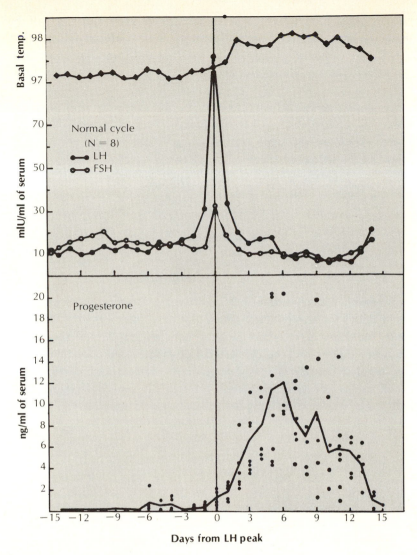

FIG. 47-3. Serum concentrations of progesterone plotted against mean concentrations of FSH and LH determined in normal women. Centered according to day of LH peak (day 0). (From Yen, S. S. C., Vela, P., Rankin, J., and Littell, A. S.: J.A.M.A. **211:**1513, 1970.)

Bleeding is predictable and painful and occurs 3 days after progesterone administration is stopped.

Human chorionic gonadotropin (HCG) is obtained from the urine of pregnant women. It has essentially the same activity as LH and is used for the treatment of cryptorchidism and for some diagnostic purposes. HCG may also be used in the treatment of infertility. Another drug used for the same purpose is **menotropins** (human menopausal gonadotropin [HMG]; Pergonal), which is extracted from the

CHORIONIC GONADOTROPIN

urine of postmenopausal women and contains both FSH and LH activity. Also, **clomiphene citrate** (Clomid), an antiestrogen may induce ovulation. **Danazol** (Danocrin), a derivative of ethisterone, is used for the treatment of endometriosis. It probably acts as an antigonadotropin.

Biosynthesis of steroids

The gonadotropins are believed to promote the synthesis of enzymes, which in turn catalyze the various steps in steroidal biosynthesis. These steps in the formation of androstenedione are the same in testis, ovary, and adrenal cortex and may be summarized in the following manner:

Acetate ⟶ Cholesterol ⟶ Δ^5-Pregnenolone

Δ^5-Pregnenolone ↙ Progesterone ↓ 17α-OH-progesterone ↘ Androstenedione

Δ^5-Pregnenolone ↘ 17α-OH-pregnenolone ↓ Dehydroepiandrosterone ↙ Androstenedione

Androstenedione is converted by the ovary to testosterone and is then aromatized and demethylated to estrogens, the major product being estradiol. Estrone is also secreted by the ovary, with estriol being a metabolic product of the ovarian estrogens. Androstenedione may be converted to estrone in adipose tissue also, which may be a significant source of estrogens in premenopausal and particularly in postmenopausal women. In postmenopausal women, the source of androstenedione is principally the adrenal cortex. Estradiol and estrone are interconvertible in the body.

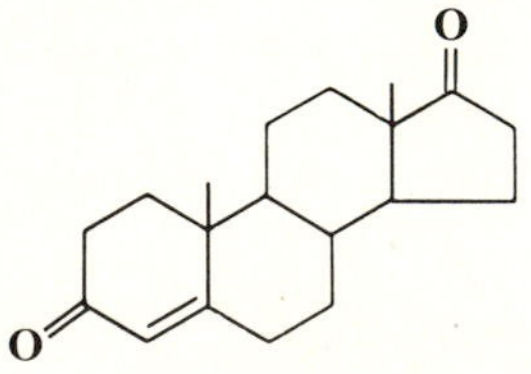

Androstenedione

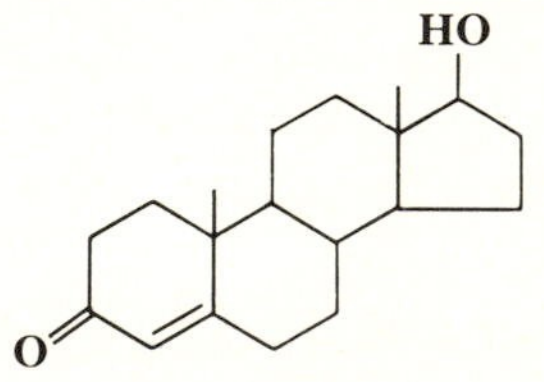

Testosterone

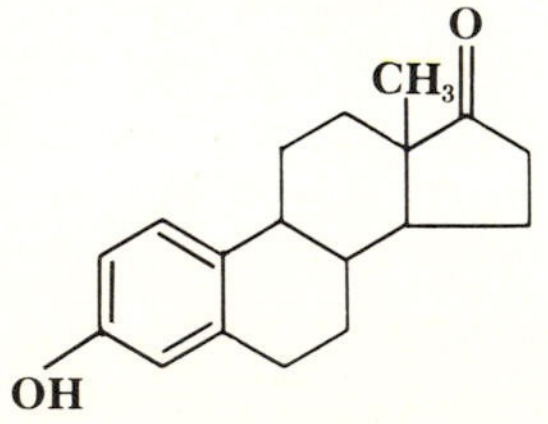

Estrone

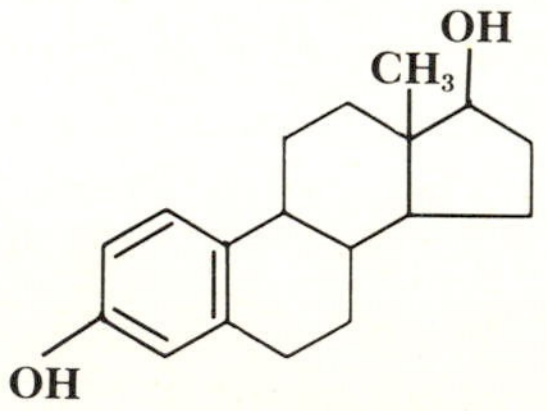

Estradiol

Testosterone may be formed not only in the testis but also in the ovary and the adrenal cortex. Testosterone in women originates from these nontesticular sources. Plasma testosterone levels are about 10 times higher in males than in females.[13]

ESTROGENS

The estrogens have important effects on uterine development and cyclic endometrial changes associated with ovulation. They are also responsible for secondary sex characteristics in the female. Study of the estrogens has been greatly facilitated by the early development of a bioassay method[1] based on changes the estrogens produce in the vaginal smear of the rat. The first estrogen isolated and synthesized was estrone, originally called *theelin*.

Estrogens are bound and retained in their target organs by combining with a specific macromolecule—the estrogen receptor. High concentrations of estrogen-binding protein may be found in the uterus, vagina, and mammary gland, and the receptor is also present in many other tissues. It is believed that the receptor is in the cytosol fraction of cells.[31]   **Estrogen receptor**

Since regulation of protein synthesis in the target tissue is the principal action of steroid hormones, the hormone-receptor complex must be transferred to the nucleus where it causes increased RNA synthesis followed by increased protein synthesis.

In metastatic breast cancer estrogen receptors are measured in the neoplasm to determine hormone sensitivity. Without estrogen receptors the tumor metastases will not respond to hormonal treatment. Response is more probable if receptors can be demonstrated in the tumor.

The available estrogens are of two types: the natural and semisynthetic compounds and the synthetic estrogens. The members of the first group either occur naturally or represent slight chemical modifications of such natural compounds.   **Types**

The synthetic drugs such as diethylstilbestrol appear to be quite different chemically.

Natural and semisynthetic estrogens. Estradiol, also known as α-estradiol or 17β-estradiol, is the most potent estrogen produced by the ovary. It is used in doses of 0.1 to 0.5 mg three times a day in the form of tablets. It is also available in pellets of 0.4 mg for vaginal suppositories. Oily preparations can also be obtained for intramuscular injection.

Estradiol benzoate, estradiol cyclopentylpropionate, and estradiol dipropionate are available in solution in oil for intramuscular injection.

Estrone is used for intramuscular injection and vaginal suppositories.

Estrogenic substances, conjugated, contain a mixture of estrogens obtained from the urine of pregnant mares. The estrogens are in a conjugated form and are water soluble, whereas the previously mentioned preparations have low water solubility. This mixture is commonly used in the form of tablets, but solutions for parenteral administration are also available. These preparations contain sodium estrone sulfonate and equine estrogens. Their activity is expressed in terms of an equivalent amount of sodium estrone sulfonate. An example of this type of preparation is Premarin. Tablets of this preparation contain amounts varying from 0.3 to 2.5 mg. A synthetic conjugated estrogen is piperazine estrone sulfate.

Ethinyl estradiol is a semisynthetic estrogen of high potency. It is available in tablets and is administered in doses of 0.02 to 0.05 mg one to three times a day. The 3-methyl ether of ethinyl estradiol, known as *mestranol*, is commonly used in contraceptive progestin-estrogen combinations.

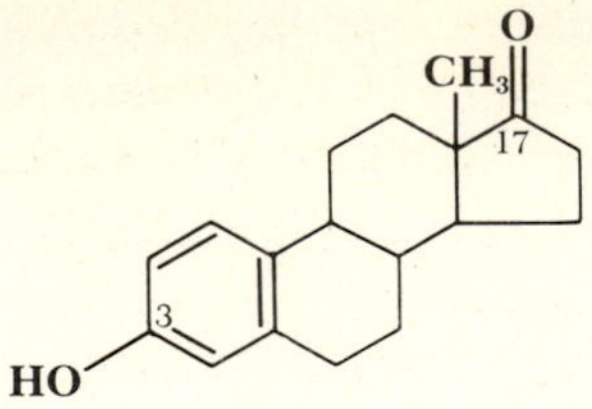

Estrone

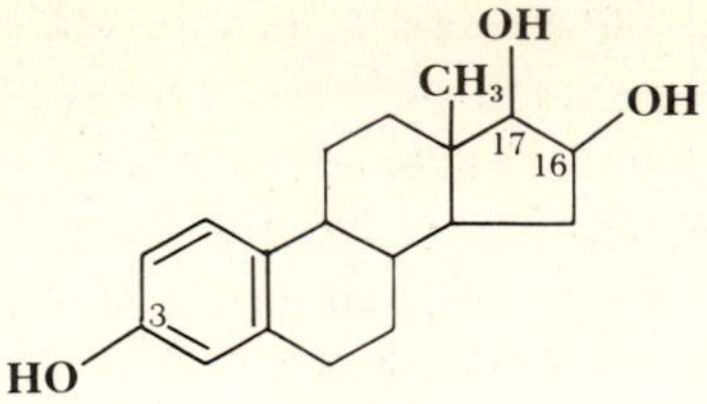

Estriol

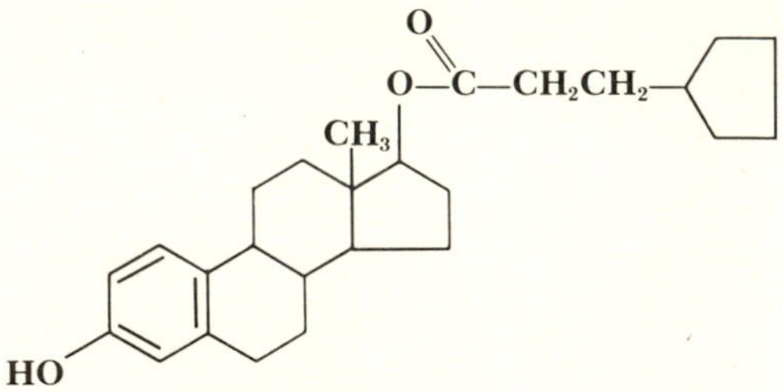

Estradiol cyclopentylpropionate

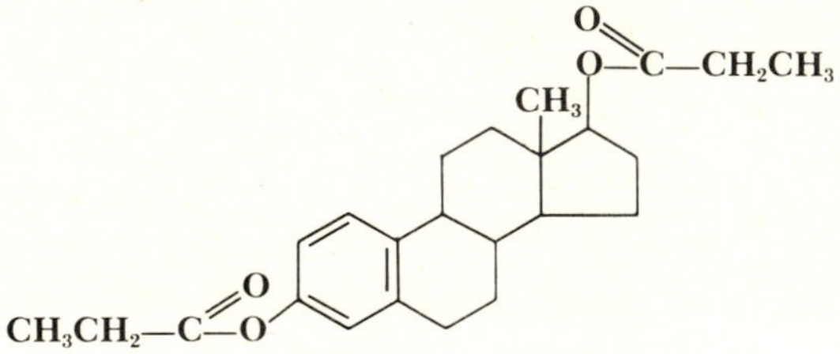

Estradiol dipropionate

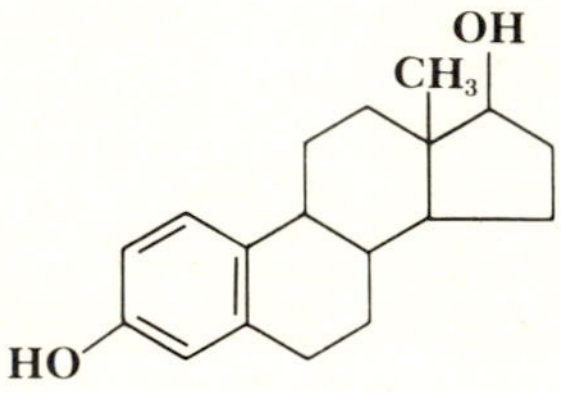

Estradiol

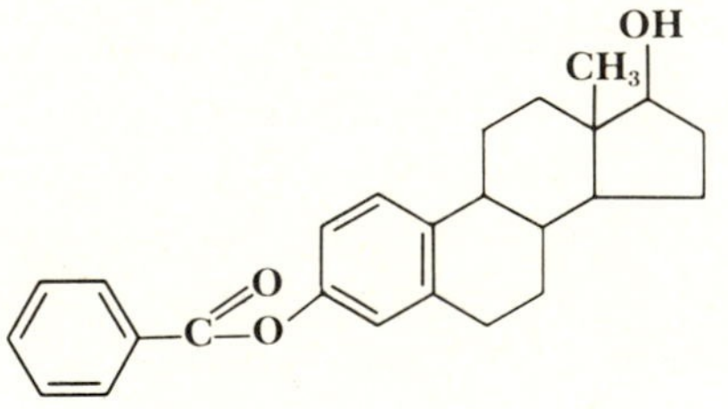

Estradiol benzoate

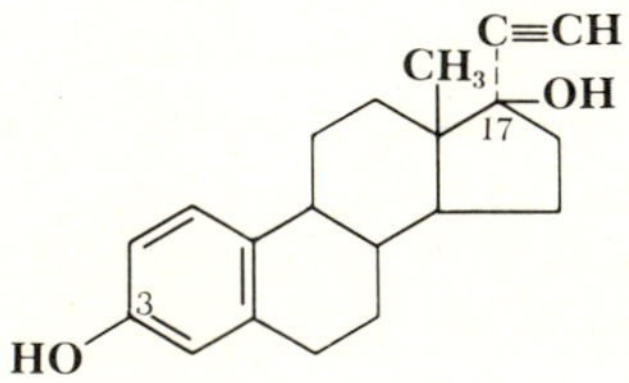

Ethinyl estradiol

Estriol may be a conversion product of estradiol. It is available in tablet form and is administered in doses of 0.06 to 0.12 mg one to four times a day.

Synthetic (nonsteroidal) estrogens. The synthesis of diethylstilbestrol[5] led to recognition of the fact that simple derivatives of stilbene can produce all the effects of naturally occurring estrogens in the body. In addition, they are highly effective when administered by mouth. Many of the synthetic estrogens can be visualized as having basic structural similarities to estradiol. Others, termed proestrogens, must undergo metabolic alteration before they become active in the body. A prime example of a proestrogen is chlorotrianisene.

Diethylstilbestrol is used in tablet form, in ointments and suppositories, and in oily solutions for intramuscular injection. The usual dose is 0.5 to 1 mg/day.

Diethylstilbestrol administration during pregnancy is *strictly contraindicated*. A number of daughters of women who received diethylstilbestrol during pregnancy have developed vaginal adenosis or adenocarcinoma after puberty.

Other synthetic estrogens are dienestrol, hexestrol, benzestrol, and promethestrol dipropionate. The doses of these are of the same order of magnitude as those of diethylstilbestrol.

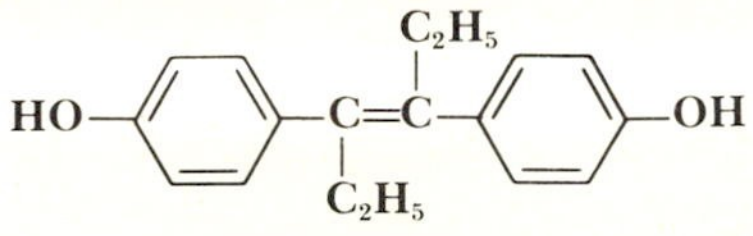

Diethylstilbestrol

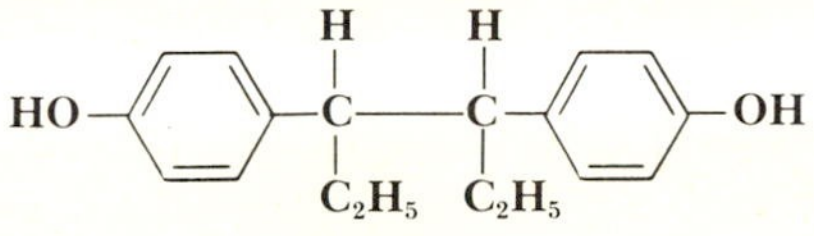

Hexestrol

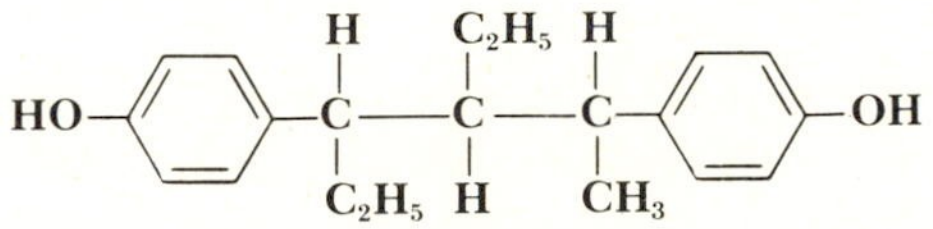

Benzestrol

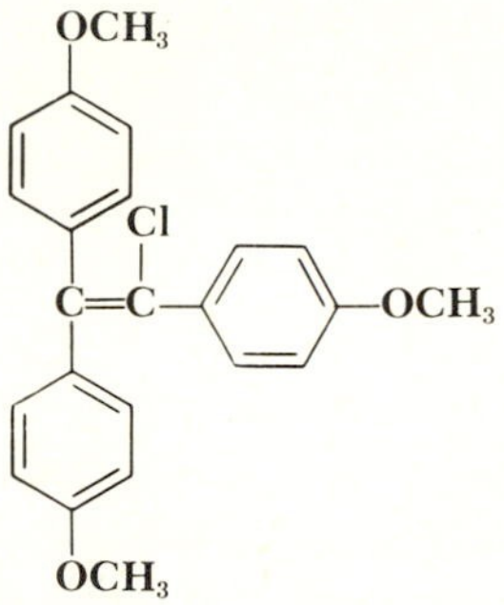

Chlorotrianisene

Chlorotrianisene (Tace) has a very long duration of action, probably as a consequence of its storage in body fat. It is believed to be converted to an active compound in the body. It is available in capsules containing 12 mg in corn oil.

Clomiphene (Clomid), a drug structurally related to chlorotrianisene, appears to stimulate pituitary gonadotropin output in women, although it inhibits the pituitary gland in the rat. It is being tried with some success in treatment of some types of infertility. Clomiphene has been termed an *antiestrogen*. Its stimulant effect on gonadotropin output in women may be a consequence of removal of inhibition exerted by estrogens.

Clomiphene, available in 50 mg tablets, is used for promoting ovulation. Administered in courses of several days, the drug is highly effective. It can also have adverse effects, causing menopausal symptoms (hot flashes), enlargement of the ovaries, and multiple pregnancies that are more common than in normally ovulating women. This incidence has been estimated at 5% to 10%.

Other fertility drugs. It is of considerable investigational interest that extracts of the human pituitary gland or of menopausal urine (human menopausal gonadotropins) are highly effective in promoting ovulation. Given by injection, these investigational drugs cause considerable enlargement of the ovary and an abnormally high incidence of multiple pregnancies.

The preparation of **human menopausal gonadotropins (menotropins)** contains large amounts of FSH and LH. Its mode of action involves the ovary directly, whereas clomiphene acts indirectly as an antiestrogen on the production of the gonadotropins. Enlargement of the ovary occurs within 2 weeks after the administration of menotropins and may lead to ascites, bleeding, and rupture of ovarian cysts. Multiple births may occur in 20% of women who become pregnant after the use of menotropins.

The preparation is injected intramuscularly and is administered daily for 10 days. Menotropins (Pergonal) are available as a powder containing 75 IU of FSH and 75 IU of LH to make a solution for intramuscular injection.

Effects   The estrogens are responsible for the proliferative changes of the endometrium during the ovulatory cycle. In rodents their effects are recognizable by the appearance of the vaginal smear, since induction of estrus is associated with cornification of the vaginal epithelium. The international unit for the estrogens is the activity of 0.1 μg of estrone. This small quantity is sufficient to produce changes in the vaginal smear of a castrated mouse. It may be estimated that the quantity of estrogen necessary for replacing normal ovarian activity in the human female over a period of weeks may be as much as 1 million units. This apparently large quantity is equivalent to 100 mg of estrone and considerably less of the more potent estrogens.

The activity of the various estrogens in the human female may be estimated on the basis of withdrawal bleeding that takes place when the estrogen is administered to amenorrheic women for about 2 weeks and is then suddenly discontinued. When assayed in this manner on ovariectomized women, the various estrogens could be placed in the following order according to their potency: ethinyl estradiol (oral), estradiol dipropionate (intramuscular), diethylstilbestrol (oral), estrone (intramuscular), hexestrol (oral), estradiol (oral), and estrone (oral).

The high activity of oral ethinyl estradiol may be attributed to the protection that this chemical modification of estradiol confers against gastrointestinal and hepatic inactivation of the ingested hormone.

Several extrauterine actions of the estrogens have also received attention. These compounds depress the secretion of FSH. The urinary excretion of FSH is increased in ovariectomized women, but this elevation is abolished by the administration of estrogens. The ability of estrogens to inhibit ovulation with chronic administration is probably due to this interaction with FSH.

Estrogens can also cause salt and water retention and an increase in transcortin and thyroxine-binding proteins in the serum and can exert complex effects on plasma lipoproteins. Plasma cortisol and protein-bound iodine levels become elevated.

Metabolism   Persons with liver damage, as in cirrhosis, may excrete a much higher percentage of an estrogen than do normal persons. This hepatic inactivation is also the probable reason for the greater effectiveness of the natural estrogens when administered parenterally. Estrone, for example, may be 10 times as effective by the intramuscular route as by mouth. On the other hand, the synthetic estrogens are highly effective by mouth. This and other evidence indicate that synthetic estrogens are not degraded as rapidly or as completely as are the natural forms. Chlorotrianisene has a prolonged action because it is stored in body fat.

The only adverse effects of the estrogens observed in a significant number of patients are anorexia, nausea, and vomiting. These symptoms are more likely to develop following the use of the synthetic compounds, diethylstilbestrol being the worst offender in this respect. It is likely, however, that some women become nauseated following the use of any of the estrogens.   *Toxicity*

Estrogens are widely used for the management of amenorrhea, uterine bleeding, endometriosis, and in girls for the suppression of growth. They are also used for menopausal disturbances and osteoporosis.   *Therapeutic applications*

Commonly used estrogens and their daily doses for the menopausal syndrome are as follows: esterified or conjugated equine estrogens, 1.25 mg; ethinyl estradiol, 0.05 mg; dienestrol, 0.5 mg; methallenestril (Vallestril), 3 mg; diethylstilbestrol, 0.2 mg.

The use of estrogens in osteoporosis is based on the belief that in postmenopausal patients there is an osteoblastic defect attributable to estrogen deficiency. More recent studies indicate that osteoporosis results from excessive bone resorption. Furthermore, estrogens or high calcium intake may slow down the progress of the disease but will not bring bone density back to normal, even in postmenopausal patients. Despite this fact, estrogens clearly prevent osteoporosis in women who have had an oophorectomy and also to some extent after menopause. The importance of vitamin D and calcium in the management of osteoporosis is increasingly emphasized.

Progesterone is produced by the corpus luteum and has also been prepared synthetically.   **PROGESTERONE**

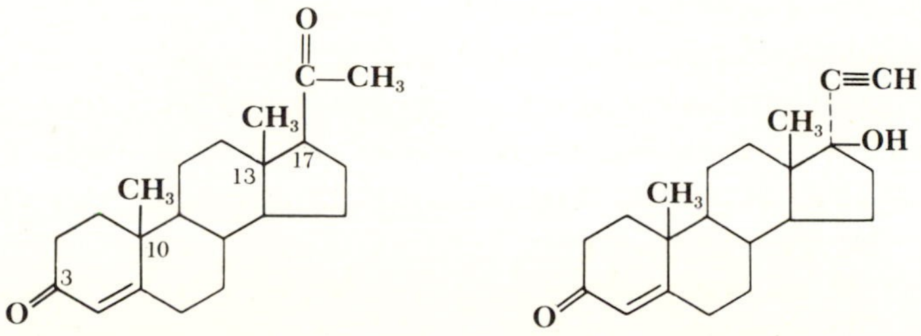

Progesterone   Ethisterone

Progesterone is responsible for the secretory phase of endometrial development. Its effects on the vaginal epithelium and on cervical mucous secretions are the opposite of those of the estrogens. Withdrawal of progesterone results in menstruation. Progesterone is metabolically degraded to pregnanediol, which appears in the urine.

Pharmacological effects of large doses of progesterone include suppression of ovulation, inhibition of the contractility of the uterus, increased sodium excretion, and negative nitrogen balance.

The hormone is assayed in the rabbit on the basis of its progestational effect on the endometrium; the international unit is 1 mg of purified progesterone.

Metabolism   Progesterone is not well absorbed from the gastrointestinal tract following oral administration. It is much more effective when injected intramuscularly or administered sublingually. The intramuscular dose is 10 mg. Similar or even larger doses are used sublingually. Progesterone is metabolically altered in the body, the liver playing an important role in this respect. The urinary excretory products of progesterone are pregnanediol and pregnanolone.

Clinical uses   Progesterone and particularly the *progestogens* find applications in numerous clinical situations. The progestogens are synthetic derivatives of 19-nortestosterone or progesterone. In contrast with progesterone, they are effective when given orally. They differ also in that some preparations are androgenic, but others have estrogenic activity.

Progesterone and the progestogens are used for the cyclic treatment of amenorrhea and dysmenorrhea in addition to antifertility effects. These hormones may also be useful in the treatment of threatened abortions and as replacement therapy in infertile women.

Progesterone itself is available in the form of parenteral preparations in water or oil for intramuscular injection. The drug is ineffective when given by mouth.

The following progestogens are used for purposes other than contraception.

Hydroxyprogesterone caproate (Delalutin) is a progesterone derivative without estrogenic activity and without masculinizing effect on the fetus. It is available as an injectable solution in oil, 125 mg/ml, administered intramuscularly.

Dydrogesterone (Duphaston; Gynorest) is a progesterone derivative that is active by oral administration. The drug has no estrogenic or androgenic activity. It is available in tablets containing 5 and 10 mg.

Norethindrone (Norlutin) and **norethindrone acetate** (Norlutate) are derivatives of 19-nortestosterone, having some androgenic activity. They should not be used in threatened abortion because of masculinizing effect on the fetus. Both drugs are available in tablets containing 5 mg.

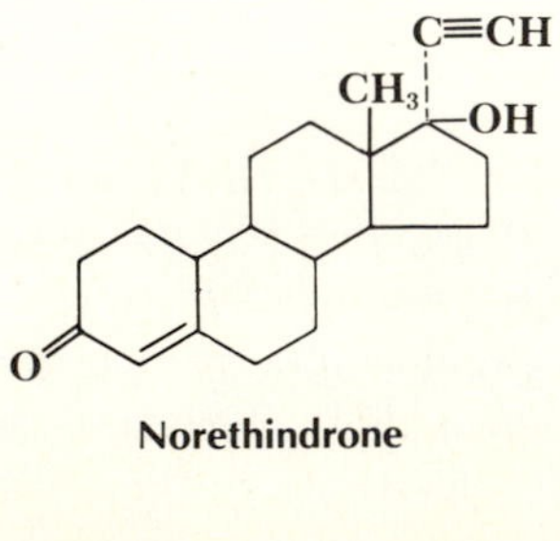

Norethindrone

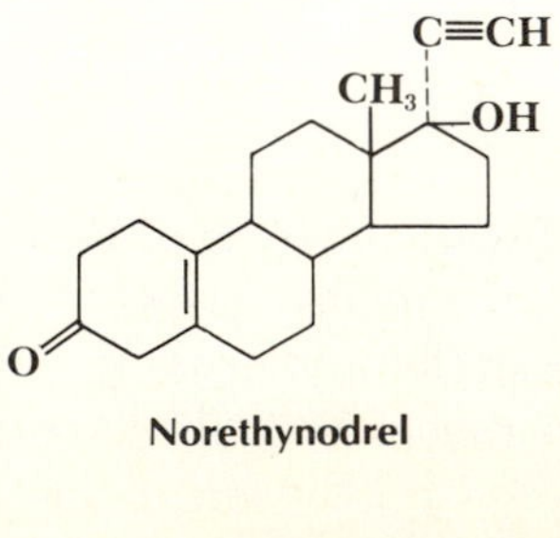

Norethynodrel

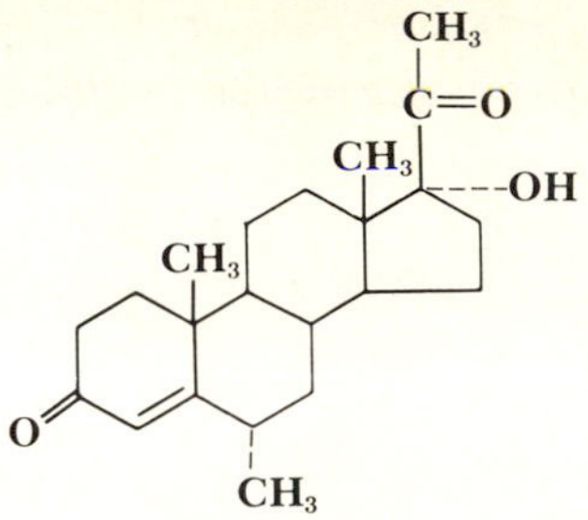

CH₃
$$C=O$$
CH₃ ----OH

CH₃

O

CH₃

Medroxyprogesterone

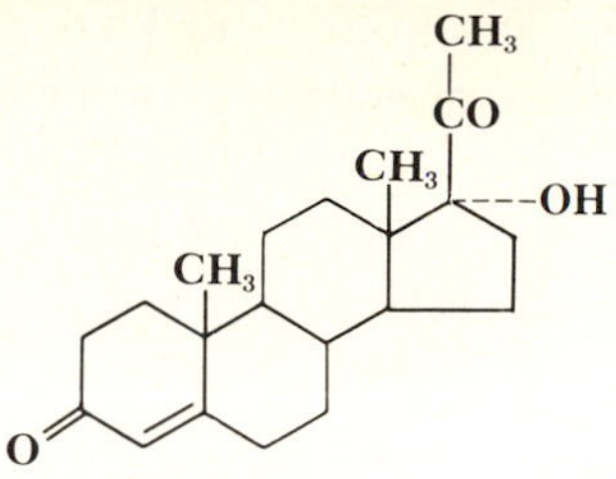

CH₃
CO
CH₃ ----OH

CH₃

O

17α-Hydroxyprogesterone

The first report on the successful inhibition of ovulation by orally administered norethynodrel-mestranol appeared in 1956. Just 10 years later more than 7 million women were taking oral contraceptives. Results indicate that such drugs are the most effective means of controlling fertility, although all the ultimate consequences of such a mass medication are not completely known.

The oral contraceptives contain either a mixture of a synthetic estrogen and progestin or, less frequently, progestin alone ("minipills"). The combination products may contain a "regular" or "low dose" of the estrogen.

Progestogen-estrogen combinations. The mode of action of the combined administration of progestogens and estrogens involves the inhibition of ovulation by an interference with hypothalamic-pituitary mechanisms. They may also have additional sites of action. There is good evidence for an alteration of the characteristics of cervical mucus by the combined treatment. It is possible also that the changes in the endometrium or the secretions of the fallopian tubes are such as to interfere with fertilization.

The progestogen-estrogen combinations are used in the following manner. A single dose a day is taken from the fifth through the twenty-fourth day of the cycle, counting from the first day of menstruation. Withdrawal bleeding occurs within 3 to 4 days after the last dose.

Low-dosage progestogens. Continued low-dosage progestogen is also being tried as an approach to the control of fertility. Chlormadinone, an analog of medroxyprogesterone, has antifertility effects in very small doses. This form of treatment does not prevent ovulation. The mode of action of low-dosage progestogen is not clear. It may put the endometrium out of phase with ovulation or it may alter cervical mucus or tubal physiology.

The "minipills" containing only progestin cause menstrual irregularities and are not popular. They are also less effective than the combination products.

Adverse effects

A number of adverse effects may occur during the administration of the oral contraceptives. Breakthrough bleeding is not uncommon and may call for an increase in dosage or discontinuation of medication to allow withdrawal bleeding to take place. Enlargement of the breast and mastalgia are common. Increases in transcortin and thyroxine-binding protein interfere with tests for thyroid and adrenal function. Disturbances in liver function and glucose tolerance have been observed, but sodium retention has not been found. Headache and cerebral and visual disturbances may be seen occasionally.

Other adverse effects of oral contraceptives are nausea and vomiting, elevation of blood pressure, skin reactions, and a drug interaction with the coumarin drugs, requiring an increase in dosage of the anticoagulants.

The possible relationship between oral contraceptives and thromboembolic disorders is receiving increasing attention. The British Committee on the Safety of Drugs recommended to all practicing physicians (December, 1969) that the lower-dose estrogen products be used instead of the high-dose products. It is believed by competent authorities in the United States that oral contraceptives and estrogens per se increase the risk of thromboembolic disorders. It is also believed that a higher estrogen dose is correlated with increased risk and therefore the lowest estrogen dose is preferable. Although the risk of thromboembolic disorders is not as great in women who take oral contraceptives as in those who become pregnant, it nevertheless does exist and should be taken into consideration by the physician in making a therapeutic decision.

ANDROGENS   The principal testicular hormone is testosterone. Its isolation and synthesis from
Testosterone   testicular extracts were preceded by the isolation of one of its metabolic products, androsterone.

Esterification of testosterone results in compounds with certain advantages. For example, methyltestosterone is effective when given in tablet form by mouth, whereas testosterone is destroyed rapidly when given by the same route. Testosterone propionate is available in buccal tablets for absorption from the oral cavity.

The most widely used androgens are testosterone, methyltestosterone propionate, and testosterone cyclopentylpropionate.

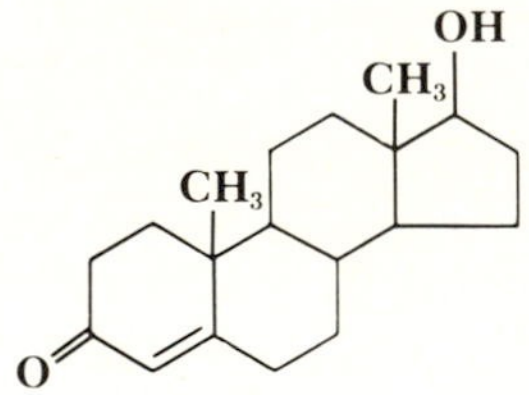

Testosterone 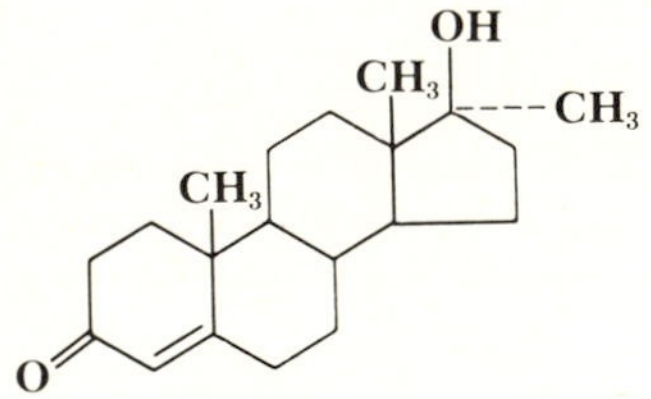   Methyltestosterone

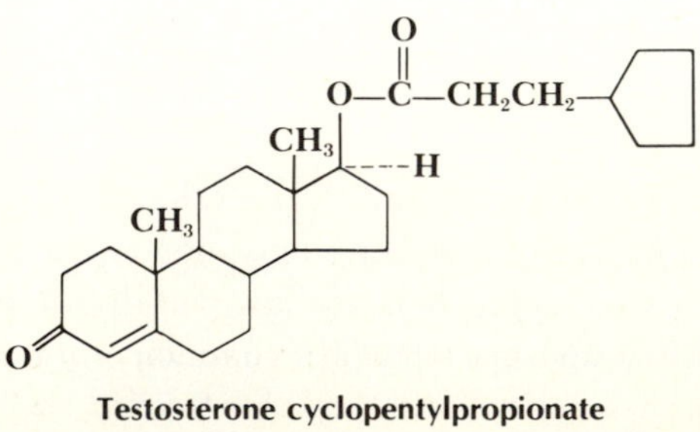

Testosterone cyclopentylpropionate

The main effect of the androgens is on the development of secondary sexual characteristics in males with stimulation of anabolism, growth, and muscular development. Some synthetic analogs of the androgens may have relatively greater anabolic than androgenic effects, and they are termed anabolic steroids. Despite this claim, they may cause some virilization.

Effects

Testosterone is metabolized in the liver and is excreted in the urine as androsterone and etiocholanolone. Methyltestosterone and fluoxymesterone are not inactivated readily by the liver because they are substituted in the 17-position. As a consequence, they can be administered orally. Esters of testosterone, such as the propionate are administered parenterally, and they are absorbed slowly from the intramuscular site, having a long duration of action.

Metabolism

Indications for the use of androgens include hypogonadism in the male, metastatic breast carcinoma, and delayed puberty.

After the anabolic effects of testosterone were administered, efforts were made to dissociate them from the androgenic effects. This research has resulted in a group of drugs known as *anabolic steroids*. Although these steroids have a greater effect on nitrogen retention than their virilizing action would predict, the separation of these effects is not complete. As a consequence, they should be used with great caution in children with growth problems.

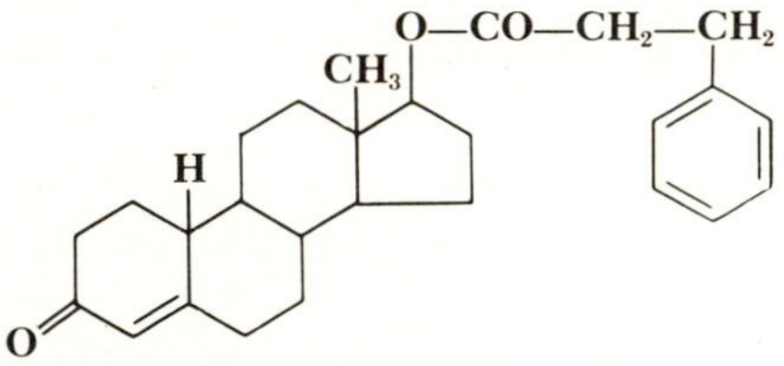

ANABOLIC STEROIDS

Nandrolone phenpropionate 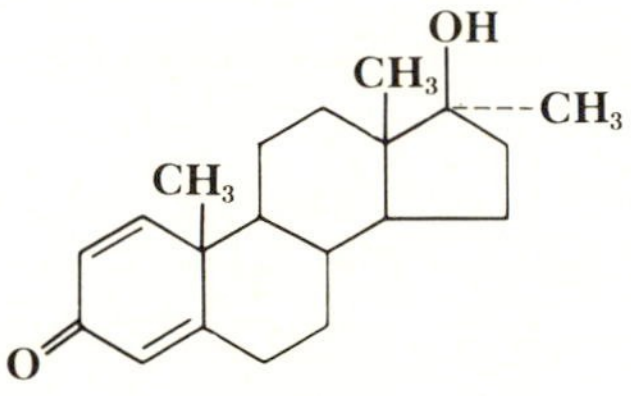   Methandrostenolone

The anabolic steroids are used sometimes in the treatment of osteoporosis and various conditions in which a negative nitrogen balance exists.

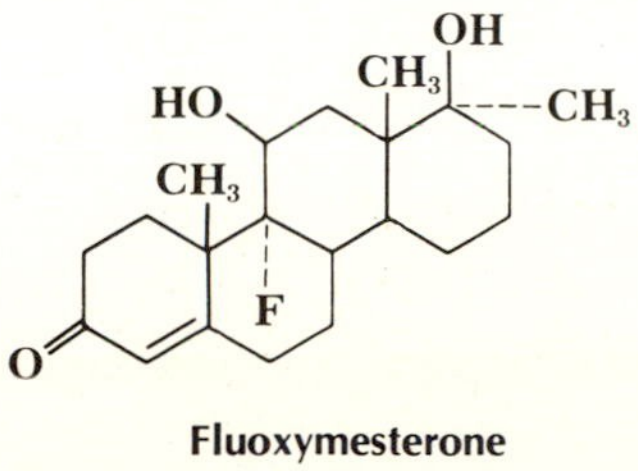

Fluoxymesterone

The anabolic steroids available for oral administration are ethylesternol (Maxibolin), methandrostenolone (Dianabol), norethandrolone (Nilevar), oxandrolone (Anavar), oxymetholone (Adroyd; Anadrol), and stanozolol (Winstrol). Anabolic steroids for intramuscular use include nandrolone phenpropionate (Durabolin), nandrolone decanoate (Deca-Durabolin), and norethandrolone injection (Nilevar). Fluoxymesterone (Halotestin; Ora-Testryl; Ultandren) is used not only as an anabolic steroid but also for androgen deficiency.

The anabolic steroids have numerous disadvantages. They may cause sodium retention, masculinization of the fetus if used in pregnant women (a definite contra-indication), and aggravation of carcinoma of the prostate. Their use is hazardous in children because of their virilizing effect. In addition, androgens or estrogens may actually lead to premature epiphyseal closure when used in children to stimulate their growth. Another adverse effect caused by anabolic steroids that resemble methyltestosterone (17-alkyl-substituted steroids) is cholestatic jaundice.

REFERENCES

1 Allen, E., and Doisy, E. A.: An ovarian hormone: preliminary report on its localization, extraction and partial purification, and action in test animals, J.A.M.A. **81**:819, 1923.

2 Berczeller, P. H., Young, I. S., and Kupperman, H. S.: The therapeutic use of progestational steroids, Clin. Pharmacol. Ther. **5**:216, 1964.

3 Clinical aspects of oral gestogens, No. 326, WHO Technical Report Series, 1966.

4 DeCosta, E. J.: Those deceptive contraceptives, J.A.M.A. **181**:122, 1962.

5 Dodds, E. C., Goldberg, L., Lawson, W., and Robinson, R.: Oestrogenic activity of alkylated stilboestrols, Nature **142**:34, 1938.

6 Evaluation of oral contraceptives, J.A.M.A. **199**:650, 1967.

7 Hazzard, W. R., Spiger, M. J., Bagdade, J. D., and Bierman, E. L.: Studies on the mechanism of increased plasma triglyceride levels induced by oral contraceptives, N. Engl. J. Med. **280**:471, 1969.

8 Herbst, A. L., Ulfelder, H., and Proskanzer, D. C.: Adenocarcinoma of the vagina: association of maternal stilbestrol therapy with tumor appearance in young women, N. Engl. J. Med. **284**:878, 1971.

9 Kamberi, I. A., Mical, R. S., and Porter, J. C.: Lutenizing hormone-releasing activity in hypophysial stalk blood and elevation by dopamine, Science **166**:388, 1969.

10 Kobayashi, Y., Kupelian, J., and Maudsley, D. V.: Ornithine decarboxylase stimulation in rat ovary by luteinizing hormone, Science **172**:379, 1971.

11 Lednicer, D.: Contraception: the chemical control of fertility, New York, 1969, Marcel Dekker, Inc.

12 Lin, T. J., Durkin, J. W., Jr., and Kim, Y. J.: The control of reproduction and of functions of certain endocrine organs as reflected by biochemical and biological assay, Curr. Ther. Res. **6**:225, 1964.

13 Lipsett, M. B., and Korenman, S. G.: Androgen metabolism, J.A.M.A. **190**:757, 1964.

14 Lloyd, C. W., and Weisz, J.: Some aspects of reproductive physiology, Annu. Rev. Physiol. **28**:267, 1966.

15 Masi, A. T., and Dugdale, M.: Cerebrovascular disease associated with the use of oral contraceptives, Ann. Intern. Med. **72**:65, 1970.

16 McCann, S. M., and Porter, J. C.: Hypothalamic pituitary stimulating and inhibiting hormones, Physiol. Rev. **49**:240, 1969.

17 Nalbandov, A. V., and Cook, B.: Reproduction, Annu. Rev. Physiol. **30**:245, 1968.

18 Pincus, G.: The physiology of ovarian hormones. In Pincus, G., and Thimann, K. V., editors: The hormones: physiology, chemistry and applications, vol. 2, New York, 1950, Academic Press, Inc.

19 Pincus, G., and Bialy, G.: Drugs used in control of reproduction, Adv. Pharmacol. **3**:285, 1964.

20 Rudel, H. W.: Mechanisms of action of hormonal antifertility agents, Pharmacol. Phys. **2**(2):1, 1968.

21 Saruta, T., Saade, G. A., and Kaplan, N.: A possible mechanism for hypertension induced by oral contraceptives, Arch. Intern. Med. **126**:621, 1970.

22 Schneider, H. P. G., and McCann, S. M.: Release of LH-releasing factor (LRF) into the peripheral circulation of hypophysectomized rats by dopamine and its blockade by estradiol, Endocrinology **87**:249, 1970.

23 Tyler, E. T.: Antifertility agents, Annu. Rev. Pharmacol. **7**:381, 1967.

24 Tyler, E. T.: Treatment of anovulation with menotropins, J.A.M.A. **205:**16, 1968.

25 Wilson, J. D.: Localization of the biochemical site of action of testosterone on protein synthesis in the seminal vesicle of the rat, J. Clin. Invest. **41:**153, 1962.

26 Yen, S. S. C., Vela, P., Rankin, J., and Littel, A. S.: Hormonal relationships during the menstrual cycle, J.A.M.A. **211:**1513, 1970.

REVIEWS

27 Adlercreutz, H.: Hepatic metabolism of estrogens in health and disease, N. Engl. J. Med. **290:**1081, 1974.

28 Bogdanove, E. M.: Hypothalamic-hypophysial interrelationships: basic aspects. In Balin, H., and Glasser, S., editors: Reproductive biology, Amsterdam, 1972, Excerpta Medica Foundation.

29 Brazeau, P., and Guillemin, R.: Somatostatin: newcomer from the hypothalamus, N. Engl. J. Med. **290:**963, 1974.

30 Cassar, J., Mashiter, K., and Joplin, G. F.: Bromocryptine treatment of acromegaly, Metabolism **26:**539, 1977.

31 Chan, L., and O'Malley, B. W.: Mechanism of action of the sex steroid hormones, N. Engl. J. Med. **294:**1322, 1976.

32 Frohman, L. A.: Clinical neuropharmacology of hypothalamic releasing factors, N. Engl. J. Med. **286:**1391, 1972.

33 Goldgien, A.: Estrogen replacement therapy in postmenopausal women, Ration. Drug Ther. **11**(1):1, 1977.

34 Griffin, J. E., and Wilson, J. D.: The syndromes of androgen resistance, N. Engl. J. Med. **302:**198, 1980.

35 Jensen, E. V., and DeSombre, E. R.: Estrogen-receptor interactions, Science **182:**126, 1973.

36 Kellie, A. E.: The pharmacology of the estrogens, Annu. Rev. Pharmacol. **11:**97, 1971.

37 Kirby, R. W., Kotchen, T. A., and Rees, D.: Hyperprolactinemia—a review of recent clinical advances, Arch. Intern. Med. **139:**1415, 1979.

38 McGuire, W. L.: Steroid receptors and breast cancer, Hosp. Pract., April, 1980, p. 83.

39 Phillips, L. S., and Vassilopoulou-Sellin, R.: Somatomedins, N. Engl. J. Med. **302:**371, 438, 1980.

40 Quigley, M. M., and Hammond, C. B.: Estrogen-replacement therapy—help or hazard, N. Engl. J. Med. **301:**646, 1979.

41 Reichlin, S.: Anterior pituitary—six glands and one, N. Engl. J. Med. **287:**1351, 1972.

42 Schally, A. V., Kastin, A. J., and Arimura, A.: Hypothalamic hormones: the link between brain and body, Am. Sci. **65:**712, 1977.

43 Turkington, R. W.: Prolactin secretion in patients treated with various drugs, Arch. Intern. Med. **130:**349, 1972.

44 Vaisrub, S.: The many faces of bromocriptine (editorial), J.A.M.A. **235:**2854, 1976.

45 Van Wyk, J. J., and Underwood, L. E.: Growth hormone, somatomedins and growth failure, Hosp. Pract., Aug., 1978, p. 57.

46 Weindling, H., and Henry, J. B.: Laboratory test results altered by "The Pill," J.A.M.A. **229:**1762, 1974.

47 Wilson, J. D.: Recent studies on the mechanism of action of testosterone, N. Engl. J. Med. **287:**1284, 1972.

CHAPTER 48

Pharmacological approaches to gout

Gout is characterized by hyperuricemia and arthritis. The disease may be *primary*—caused by overproduction or defective renal excretion of uric acid. The *secondary* form develops during some other disease, such as leukemia, or is caused by drugs such as the thiazide diuretics.

In general, patients with gout may be divided into those who overproduce uric acid and those who underexcrete it.[23] The overproducers excrete about 1 g of uric acid daily in the urine and have a large increase in their body pool of uric acid. The underexcreters have only a moderately increased body pool of uric acid. The daily urinary excretion of more than 750 mg indicates overproduction.[23]

The pharmacological approach to an acute attack is different from the management of the chronic disease. The acute attack is a form of acute arthritis that responds best to *colchicine*, although *phenylbutazone*, *oxyphenbutazone*, *indomethacin*, or *adrenal corticoids* may also be effective. The aim of management of the chronic form of the disease is to reduce the uric acid content of the body with uricosuric drugs such as *probenecid* or *sulfinpyrazone*. The use of *allopurinol*, a xanthine oxidase inhibitor, may have advantages over the uricosuric drugs in some cases.

COLCHICINE

Colchicine is an alkaloid obtained from *Colchicum autumnale*, or meadow saffron, a plant belonging to the lily family. Colchicum has been used for centuries for althralgia that is presumably of gouty origin.

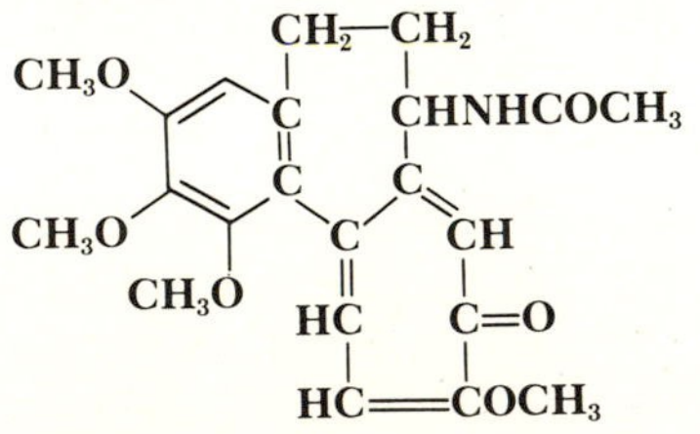

Colchicine

Colchicine is well absorbed from the gastrointestinal tract and has a short half-life in plasma. However, it may remain for a longer period in cells such as the leukocytes. Also, patients with renal disease retain colchicine longer.

When colchicine is given in doses of 0.5 to 1 mg every hour to a patient having an attack of acute gouty arthritis, relief occurs in 2 to 3 hours, but in severe attacks a somewhat longer period is required. It is quite common for gastrointestinal disturbances such as anorexia, nausea, vomiting, diarrhea, and abdominal pain to appear with about the same dosage as the one required for relief. As a consequence, colchicine is administered every hour until relief is obtained or until significant gastrointestinal symptoms develop. In addition to gastrointestinal side effects, colchicine may also cause, although rarely, fever, alopecia, liver damage, and neural and hepatopoietic complications.[3]

Colchicine is known to interfere with the microtubular system in various cells.[24] In the case of gout, it is believed that the effect of colchicine is exerted on leukocytes, which accumulate in the joints and ingest the sharp urate crystals.[14] It is quite possible, however, that the effect of colchicine is also exerted on synovial cells.

In chronic gout the administration of colchicine appears to have prophylactic value with regard to the incidence of acute exacerbations. In addition, it is generally believed that the promotion of uric acid excretion through the use of the uricosuric drugs is beneficial in the gouty patient. The most effective uricosuric agents are probenecid and sulfinpyrazone.

PROBENECID

Probenecid (Benemid) was developed for the purpose of inhibiting tubular secretion of penicillin. Although effective, it is seldom used for this purpose because it is simpler to increase the dosage of penicillin rather than to use two drugs to achieve a higher blood level of the antibiotic.

$$CH_3CH_2CH_2 \diagdown$$
$$NSO_2 - \langle \text{benzene ring} \rangle - COOH$$
$$CH_3CH_2CH_2 \diagup$$

Probenecid

Probenecid causes marked increase in excretion of uric acid in gouty patients. The drug has been given in doses of 0.5 g three or four times daily for years to gouty patients and has produced significant lowering of serum uric acid. In fact, increased urinary concentration of uric acid may lead to development of urate stones, and therefore alkalinization of the urine may be desirable in the early stages of therapy.

Renal handling of uric acid apparently involves glomerular filtration, tubular reabsorption, and tubular secretion. Organic anions such as salicylates and probenecid cause retention of uric acid at low doses but are uricosuric at high doses.[17] It is likely that in small doses they compete with uric acid for secretion.

The ability of thiazide diuretics and pyrazinamide to cause uric acid retention may be explained also by an interference with uric acid secretion.[5] For the same reason, salicylates should not be used when probenecid is prescribed for a hyperuricemic patient.

In addition to uricosuric effect, probenecid inhibits tubular secretion of penicillin, iodopyracet (Diodrast), and p-aminohippurate. It also blocks conjugation of benzoic acid with glycine and increases the blood levels of *p*-aminosalicylate by some unknown mechanism.

Probenecid is rapidly absorbed from the stomach, giving peak plasma concentrations in 4 hours. The urinary excretion of the drug is pH-dependent, being higher at higher pH values. Treatment should begin with small doses, 250 mg twice a day, to decrease the probability of renal stone formation. Dosage must be gradually increased to the 1 or 1.5 g maintenance level, the ultimate dosage being determined by the serum uric acid determinations. Colchicine is often administered concurrently with probenecid to decrease the likelihood of gouty attacks.

During the use of probenecid for chronic gout, adverse effects may occur in a small percentage of patients. The figure generally given is less than 2%, but in some series adverse reactions or side effects have occurred in 8% of patients.[2] Nausea and vomiting, skin rash, and drug fever may occur. Urate stones may cause renal colic.

SULFINPYRAZONE   Sulfinpyrazone (Anturan), which is structurally related to phenylbutazone, is an effective uricosuric agent. This drug prevents tubular reabsorption of uric acid. Its action is antagonized by salicylates but not by probenecid. The marked increase in urate excretion may predispose to urolithiasis. An acute gouty attack may occur at the beginning of treatment, and epigastric distress has been seen. The similarity in structure between sulfinpyrazone and phenylbutazone suggests caution with regard to hematological disturbances. The usual dose is 50 mg four times daily initially, which may be gradually increased until as much as 400 mg is given daily.

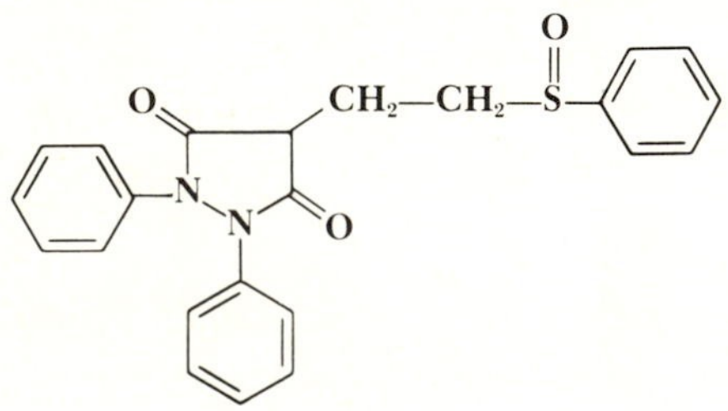

Sulfinpyrazone

Sulfinpyrazone appears to be effective in reducing cardiac deaths during the first year after myocardial infarction.[18] The mode of action of the drug is not clear and some experts doubt its effectiveness. Only additional large-scale trials will settle the question.

ALLOPURINOL   An interesting approach to the treatment of gout is the use of an inhibitor of xanthine oxidase. Allopurinol (Zyloprim) was developed originally for the purpose of protecting 6-mercaptopurine against rapid inactivation in the body. The drug causes a marked decrease in plasma uric acid concentration and in urinary uric acid excretion. Although the oxypurines xanthine and hypoxanthine replace uric acid under these circumstances, renal clearance of the oxypurines is much greater than that of uric acid.

Allopurinol is rapidly oxidized in the body to alloxanthine; 90% to 95% of allopurinol administered is excreted as alloxanthine, the remainder as the original allopurinol. The renal clearance of allopurinol is rapid, while that of alloxanthine is slow—only two or three times the clearance of uric acid. Probenecid promotes the excretion of oxypurinol.

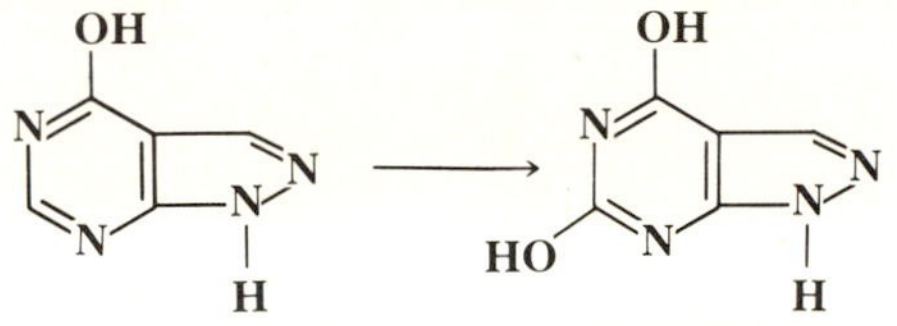

Allopurinol   Oxypurinol

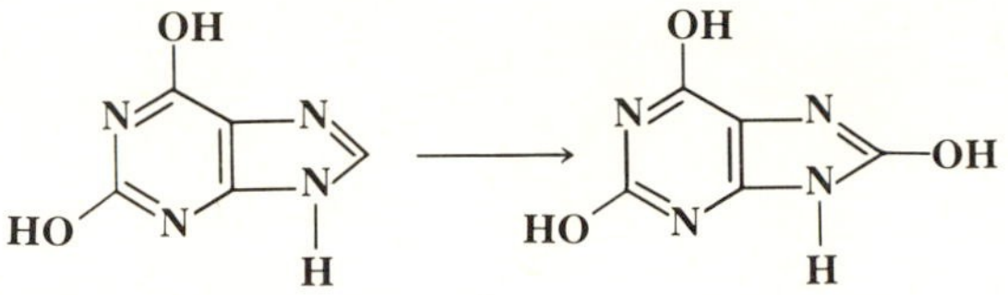

Xanthine   Uric acid

In a series of gouty patients who showed an intolerance to uricosuric agents or failed to respond to them, normal serum urate levels were achieved with doses of 200 to 600 mg/day of allopurinol.[12]

A summary of the present position of allopurinol in the treatment of gout is as follows. Although uricosuric agents are effective in controlling hyperuricemia in most gouty patients, allopurinol may prove to be more useful for a number of reasons. Gouty nephropathy and the formation of urate stones are less likely with allopurinol therapy because the drug *reduces* the amount of uric acid excreted. Colchicine is still the treatment of choice in acute gout and is helpful in the prevention of acute attacks. In severe cases associated with impaired renal function and urate stones, allopurinol appears to be the agent of choice. In addition, the anti-inflammatory drugs phenylbutazone and indomethacin may be very useful in the treatment of acute gout.

Reactions to allopurinol have been mild or moderate, although about 3% of patients taking the drug may develop skin eruptions, fever, hepatomegaly, leukopenia, gastrointestinal distress, diarrhea, pruritus, skin rash, headache, fever, leukopenia, and alterations of liver function.

REFERENCES

1 Beyer, K. H., and associates: "Benemid," p-(di-n-propylsulfamyl)-benzoic acid: its renal affinity and its elimination, Am. J. Physiol. 166:625, 1951.

2 Boger, W. P., and Strickland, S. C.: Probenecid (Benemid): its uses and side effects in 2502 patients, Arch. Intern. Med. 95:83, 1955.

3 Carr, A. A.: Colchicine toxicity, Arch. Intern. Med. 115:29, 1965.

4 DeConti, R. C., and Calabresi, P.: Use of allopurinol for the prevention and control of hyperuricemia in patients with neoplastic disease, N. Engl. J. Med. 274:481, 1966.

5 Demartini, F. E., Wheaton, E. A., Healey, L.

A., and Laragh, J. A.: Effect of chlorothiazide on the renal excretion of uric acid, Am. J. Med. 32:572, 1962.

6 Goldfinger, S., Klinenberg, J., and Seegmiller, J. E.: The renal excretion of oxypurines, J. Clin. Invest. 44:623, 1965.

7 Gutman, A. B., and Yu, T.-F.: Uric acid metabolism in normal man and in primary gout, N. Engl. J. Med. 273:252, 1965.

8 Gutman, A. B., and Yu, T.-F.: Urinary ammonia excretion in primary gout, J. Clin. Invest. 44:1474, 1965.

9 Klinenberg, J. R., Goldfinger, S. E., and Seegmiller, J. E.: The effectiveness of the xanthine oxidate inhibitor allopurinol in the treatment of gout, Ann. Intern. Med. 62:639, 1965.

10 Krakoff, I. H.: Clinical pharmacology of drugs which influence uric acid production and excretion, Clin. Pharmacol. Ther. 8:124, 1967.

11 Pagliara, A. S., and Goodman, D.: Elevation of plasma glutamate in gout; its possible role in the pathogenesis of hyperuricemia, N. Engl. J. Med. 281:767, 1969.

12 Rundles, R. W., Metz, E. N., and Silberman, H. R.: Allopurinol in the treatment of gout, Ann. Intern. Med. 64:229, 1966.

13 Rundles, R. W., and Wyngaarden, J. B. L.: Drugs and uric acid, Annu. Rev. Pharmacol. 9:345, 1969.

14 Seegmiller, J. E., Howel, R. R., and Malawista, S. E.: The inflammatory reaction to sodium urate: its possible relationship to the genesis of acute gouty arthritis, J.A.M.A. 180:469, 1962.

15 Steele, T. H., and Boner, G.: Origins of the uricosuric response, J. Clin. Invest. 52:1368, 1973.

16 Wallace, S. L., Omokoku, B., and Ertel, N. H.: Colchicine plasma levels, Am. J. Med. 48:443, 1970.

17 Yu, T.-F., and Gutman, A. B.: Study of the paradoxical effects of salicylate in low, intermediate and high dosage on the renal mechanisms for excretion of urate in man, J. Clin. Invest. 38:1298, 1959.

REVIEWS

18 The Anturane Reinfarction Trial Research Group: Sulfinpyrazone in the prevention of cardiac death after myocardial infarction, N. Engl. J. Med. 298:289, 1978.

19 Boss, G. R., and Seegmiller, J. E.: Hyperuricemia and gout, N. Engl. J. Med. 300:1459, 1979.

20 Bryan, J.: Biochemical properties of microtubules, Fed. Proc. 33:152, 1974.

21 Calkins, E.: The treatment of gout, Ration. Drug Ther. 5:1, 1971.

22 Goldfinger, S. E.: Treatment of gout, N. Engl. J. Med. 285:1303, 1971.

23 Rastegar, A., and Thier, S. O.: The treatment of hyperuricemia in gout, Ration. Drug Ther. 8:1, 1974.

24 Sorensen, L. B., and Pepe, P.: Hypoxanthine-guanine phosphoribosyltransferase deficiency, Bull. Rheum. Dis. 21:621, 1970.

25 Steele, T. H.: Control of uric acid secretion, N. Engl. J. Med. 284:1193, 1971.

CHAPTER 49

Antianemic drugs

The maintenance of normal red cell mass and the synthesis of hemoglobin are normally adjusted to take care of the physiological loss of the blood elements. Anemia results when there is excessive loss or diminished replacement of red cells.

Most anemias are deficiency diseases resulting from inadequate tissue concentrations of *iron*, *vitamin B₁₂*, or *folic acid*. Correction of the deficiency is highly successful provided an accurate diagnosis is made. In addition, other drugs such as *anabolic steroids* and *pyridoxine* may be useful in some forms of anemia. *Erythropoietin* may be of great importance but is currently only of research interest.

Iron is contained in the body in various forms, principally as hemoglobin. Normal blood contains about 15 g of hemoglobin/100 ml, and each gram of hemoglobin contains 3.4 mg of iron. It may be calculated then that the total normal blood volume contains about 2.6 g of iron, and each milliliter of blood contains 0.5 mg.

In addition to hemoglobin, iron is contained in ferritin, the storage form for iron in the tissues, and in the serum attached to the carrier substance, the globulin transferrin. Minute quantities are also present in the cytochrome enzymes and myoglobin of muscle. Quantitatively, hemoglobin and ferritin contain the bulk of the iron in the body, amounting to a total of about 4 to 5 g.

Under normal circumstances red cells are broken down at a steady rate, their lifespan being on the order of 120 days. Most of the iron released from the breakdown of hemoglobin is reutilized. As a consequence, the daily iron requirement in a normal adult is quite low, about 1 mg. Growth, menstruation, and pregnancy increase the iron requirement.

Perhaps the most remarkable fact about the metabolism of iron is the inability of the body to get rid of significant quantities of this element. Only minute quantities are excreted into the feces, and the urinary loss of iron is even less. This is the reason for the very low iron requirement of normal persons.

Since the body does not readily eliminate iron, there must be a mechanism that limits its absorption. Otherwise the iron content of the body would steadily increase and hemochromatosis would develop. The mechanism that limits the absorption of iron from the intestine is often referred to as the mucosal block.

GENERAL CONCEPT

IRON
Metabolism and effects

Absorption and excretion

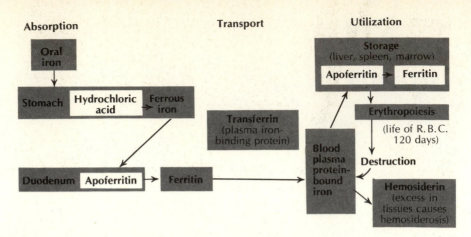

FIG. 49-1. Metabolism of iron. (Courtesy Lederle Laboratories, American Cyanamid Co., Pearl River, N.Y.)

Mucosal block

The mucosal cells of the duodenum and proximal jejunum take up iron but transfer only a variable portion of it to the blood. The remainder stays in the cells probably as ferritin and is eventually lost as the cells are sloughed. Iron absorption has the characteristics of a facilitated or active transport. Other metals such as cobalt and manganese may cause competitive inhibition.

Iron absorption is altered by various derangements. Increased absorption occurs in iron deficiency and enhanced bone marrow activity. Iron overload and decreased marrow activity may cause lowered rates of iron absorption. The exact mechanism of the control of iron absorption is unknown.

The iron-binding globulin transferrin, or siderophilin, is present in normal blood at such a concentration that when fully saturated it can carry 300 μg of iron/100 ml of blood. Since the normal serum iron level is about 100 μg/100 ml, this means that transferrin is only one-third saturated. The globulin combines with two molecules of iron per protein molecule.

The normal daily diet contains approximately 20 mg of iron. Of this, only about 10% is absorbed, but this quantity is adequate for taking care of the very small daily losses of iron. In iron-deficiency anemia, however, the dietary iron is quite insufficient for reasonably rapid correction of the hemoglobin deficit, even though the mucosal block is greatly diminished.

In addition to the mucosal block, other factors influence the absorption of iron. It is generally believed that ferrous iron is more effectively absorbed than the ferric form.[9] On the other hand, a diet rich in phytate, phosphate (milk), or alkalinizing agents such as used for patients with peptic ulcer tends to decrease absorption of iron.

Therapeutic preparations

Dosages of therapeutic iron preparations should be calculated on the basis of their elemental iron content. For the treatment of iron-deficiency anemias in adults a dose of 50 to 100 mg of elemental iron three times daily is recommended.

Iron preparations can be administered both orally and parenterally.

Oral. There are many iron preparations, both organic and inorganic, that may be utilized in treatment of hypochromic anemias. These drugs differ in absorption from the gastrointestinal tract. It is customary to administer a large excess because not more than 15% of an oral dose is absorbed of even the most effective preparation, ferrous sulfate. The percentage of absorption is considerably less when certain other preparations such as reduced iron are administered. The recommended dosages of the various preparations are such that they may be expected to provide absorption of 15 to 25 mg of iron a day in an individual suffering from hypochromic anemia. The following doses are often used:

Preparation	Dosage
Ferrous sulfate tablets	0.3 g three times a day
Ferric ammonium citrate	1.0 g three times a day
Reduced iron	0.5 g three times a day
Ferrous gluconate	0.6 g three times a day
Ferrous fumarate	0.5 g three times a day
Ferrocholinate	0.5 g three times a day

Parenteral. Because of the low degree of efficiency of gastrointestinal absorption of iron, several injectable forms of iron have been introduced.

Iron dextran complex (Imferon) is a useful preparation when parenteral administration of iron is mandatory. It was temporarily withdrawn when carcinogenicity in rats and mice and one questionable case in a human being were reported. The preparation contains 50 mg of iron/ml. The dose is 1 to 4 ml daily intramuscularly. Occasional anaphylactoid and allergic reactions have been reported following its use. Nevertheless, it is less likely to produce severe shocklike states and phlebitis, which may follow the use of the intravenous preparations of iron.

Iron sorbitex (Jectofer) is another intramuscular preparation with characteristics similar to iron dextran.

Dextriferron (Astrafer) is an iron-dextrin complex containing 20 mg/ml of iron. It is replacing saccharated iron oxide (Proferrin) as an intravenous dosage form. The intravenous iron preparations should be used only with the realization of their dangers. They may cause hypotension, vascular collapse, headache, nausea, and anaphylactoid reactions.

The oral iron preparations tend to produce nausea and vomiting through a local irritant effect on the stomach. For this reason the preparations are generally administered immediately after meals. Large doses of ferrous sulfate and of ferrous gluconate have produced poisoning in children. If large amounts of iron are absorbed, it seems that symptoms resembling those of heavy metal poisoning may result.[4]

Adverse effects

Parenteral iron should not be used unless oral preparations cannot be tolerated by the patient. Serious reactions may occur, particularly in patients who are also receiving oral iron preparations. Under these circumstances, transferrin is saturated, and the administration of parenteral iron will produce elevated concentrations of unbound metal.

Claims for lower gastrointestinal toxicity of some iron salts are not based on good evidence. It is the amount of ionized iron in a preparation that determines its toxicity.

Chelating agents in treatment of iron poisoning

The potent and specific iron chelating agent deferoxamine (Desferal) has been used with apparent benefit both in treatment of acute toxic reactions to ferrous gluconate[10] and for removal of iron in patients with overload.[14]

Deferoxamine, also known as desferrioxamine B, is a water-soluble substance of three molecules of trihydroxamic acid. Its molecular weight is 597, and one molecule chelates one molecule of Fe^{+++} ions. The drug is derived from the microbial product ferrioxamine B by removal of iron.

Deferoxamine can bind 8.5 mg iron/100 mg. It removes not only free iron but also iron combined with ferritin and hemosiderin. Transferrin-bound iron is less susceptible to chelation by deferoxamine, and hemoglobin and cytochrome iron are not affected.

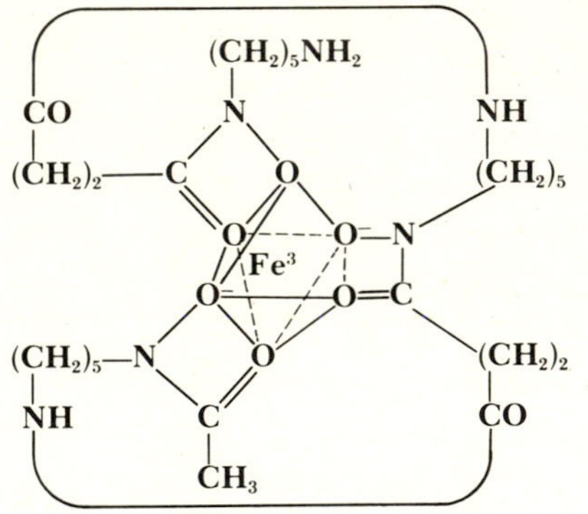

Deferoxamine (in combination with iron)

In acute iron poisoning, deferoxamine, 8 to 12 g, is administered by gastric tube. In addition, 1 to 2 g of the drug may be injected intramuscularly or intravenously. In a small child, repeated doses of deferoxamine (92 mg/kg) have been used with apparent benefit. Smaller doses, 400 to 600 mg daily, are sufficient for promotion of iron excretion in hemochromatosis.

Use of iron in anemias

Iron is effective in the treatment of iron-deficiency anemias.[18] In these states the mean corpuscular volume is below 80 μ^3, and the mean corpuscular hemoglobin concentration is below 30%. These anemic states are generally caused by chronic blood loss or by a deficient dietary supply of iron. The latter is more likely to occur in a growing child.

In most instances ferrous sulfate is quite adequate for the treatment of iron deficiency. Its main disadvantages are gastric irritation, diarrhea, and constipation. It may be advisable to use small doses at first and to increase the dose gradually over a period of 1 to 2 weeks. In general there is no advantage in the addition of cobalt, other metals, or folic acid to preparations whose purpose is to supply iron.

The effectiveness of therapy with ferrous sulfate manifests itself in a rise of the reticulocyte count within 7 days, an increase in hemoglobin levels by 1 to 2 g/100 ml within 3 weeks, and evidence of clinical improvement in 2 to 3 weeks.

VITAMIN B₁₂

Vitamin B_{12} (cyanocobalamin) is a cobalt-containing compound having a molecular weight of 1400. Its isolation from liver[19] brought to a successful conclusion more than 20 years of investigation aimed at finding the cause of *pernicious anemia.*

Until 1926 pernicious anemia was entirely incurable. At that time the key observation was made that large amounts of liver had a beneficial effect in the treatment of the disease.[13] Subsequent work was aimed at purification of the liver factor responsible for the curative effect. Soon injectable purified liver extracts of great potency were available.

The problem of pernicious anemia appeared more complex, however, than a simple deficiency of a liver factor. Clinical experiments showed that normal gastric juice contained an intrinsic factor that had to interact with a dietary extrinsic factor in order for the erythrocyte maturation factor present in liver to be obtained.[3]

When folic acid was isolated in 1943, it was believed at first that the compound was in some way related to the etiology of pernicious anemia. It was soon found, however, that whereas folic acid could remedy the hematological manifestations of the disease, it either had no effect or aggravated the neurological symptoms. Since liver extract was effective against both these aspects of pernicious anemia, it was clear that folic acid could not represent the liver factor.

The picture became clarified when vitamin B_{12} was isolated in 1948. It appears that the absorption of vitamin B_{12} requires the presence of the intrinsic factor of Castle. This is lacking in true addisonian pernicious anemia. Furthermore, injected vitamin B_{12} remedies both hematological and neurological disturbances in pernicious anemia. When reasonable doses of the vitamin are administered by mouth to patients with pernicious anemia, they are ineffective unless some normal gastric juice is given simultaneously. Thus there is little doubt at present that vitamin B_{12} represents both the extrinsic factor and the erythrocyte maturation factor. The function of the intrinsic factor has to do with the absorption of vitamin B_{12}.

Chemistry

The vitamin has been called cyanocobalamin and is only one member of several cobalamins, all of which have vitamin B_{12} activity. The compound has been isolated not only from liver but also from fermentation liquors of *Streptomyces griseus,* the organism that produces streptomycin.

Unlike many other vitamins, vitamin B_{12} is not present in higher plants but can be synthesized by certain microorganisms. Human liver contains at least 400 μg of the vitamin/kg, and beef liver may contain up to 100 μg/kg. Cow's milk contains more than human milk, up to 4 μg/L.[14]

Indication for use

The vitamin is indicated in treatment of megaloblastic states caused by a deficient supply or absorption of vitamin B_{12}. In the majority of cases the deficiency is in the absorption. This is certainly the case in pernicious anemia and following gas-

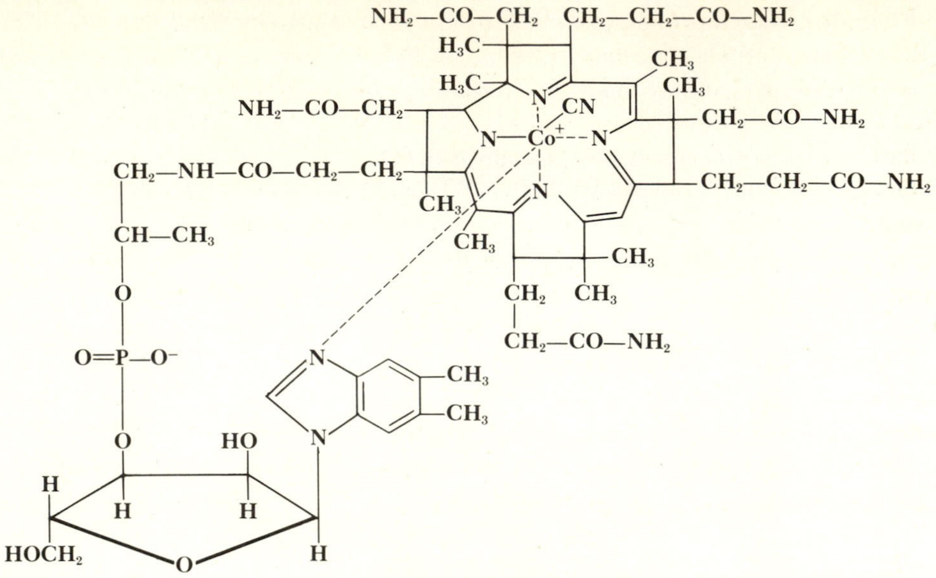

Vitamin B$_{12}$

trectomy. In *Diphyllobothrium latum* (fish tapeworm) infestation the worm itself may concentrate much of the vitamin supplied in the diet.

There are other megaloblastic states in which a deficiency of folic acid exists, and treatment should be based on correction of the deficiency rather than on administration of vitamin B$_{12}$. Some of these megaloblastic states are nutritional macrocytic anemia, certain cases of sprue, megaloblastic anemia of pregnancy, megaloblastic anemia of infants, and certain cases of adult scurvy.

Absorption and fate   When 0.5 μg of labeled vitamin B$_{12}$ was administered orally to normal persons, about 31% was excreted in the feces. In patients with pernicious anemia the fecal excretion averaged 88%.[2] When an intrinsic factor preparation was administered simultaneously, the excretion of the vitamin in patients with pernicious anemia decreased to normal levels. Fecal excretion of the labeled vitamin was also very high in patients following gastrectomy. On the other hand, in megaloblastic anemia of pregnancy there is no deficiency in the absorption of vitamin B$_{12}$.

Vitamin B$_{12}$ does not appear in urine under normal circumstances, probably because the compound is bound to plasma proteins. However, if a large dose of nonlabeled vitamin B$_{12}$ (1000 μg) is injected intramuscularly following oral administration of the labeled compound, normal individuals excrete as much as 30% of the radioactivity in the urine within 24 hours. Apparently the nonradioactive material displaces the labeled compound from its binding sites. This observation has been adapted to the diagnosis of pernicious anemia, since under similar circumstances a patient suffering from the disease will excrete only insignificant quantities in the urine, usually less than 2.5% of the administered dose.

Following intramuscular injection of large doses, much of vitamin B_{12} is excreted in the urine, both in normal individuals and in patients with pernicious anemia. The percentage of the dose excreted increases with the quantity administered. Thus when 40 μg is injected, 7.5% appears in the urine, whereas 60% of the dose may be similarly excreted when 100 μg of the vitamin is injected.

Oral administration of very large doses of vitamin B_{12} (such as 3000 μg) may result in some absorption, even in patients with pernicious anemia. This may indicate that the deficiency of intrinsic factor is not absolute or that there is some other mechanism of absorption.

Vitamin B_{12} and folic acid correct megaloblastosis by influencing DNA synthesis. *Basic mode of action* The characteristic delayed nuclear maturation in megaloblastosis results from inadequate DNA synthesis, a consequence of deficiencies of vitamin B_{12} and/or folic acid.

The pathway affected by vitamin B_{12} and folic acid is that leading to the synthesis of DNA thymine from deoxyuridylate (dUMP) through the following steps:

$$\text{Deoxyuridine} \longrightarrow \text{Deoxyuridylate} \longrightarrow \text{Thymidylate} \longrightarrow \text{DNA thymine}$$

The methylation of deoxyuridylate to thymidylate requires 5, 10-methylenetetrahydrofolic acid. This requirement explains the role of folic acid in DNA synthesis.

The role of vitamin B_{12} is in the regeneration of tetrahydrofolic acid from 5-methyltetrahydrofolic acid by homocysteine transmethylation:

$$\text{5-Methyltetrahydrofolic acid} \longrightarrow \text{Tetrahydrofolic acid}$$

These relationships and the possible role of pyridoxal phosphate are shown in Fig. 49-2.

Vitamin B_{12} contains 10 or 15 μg of the vitamin/ml. Injectable liver extracts are *Preparations and* now standardized on the basis of their vitamin B_{12} content rather than in terms of *clinical uses* USP units, which were based on the hematological response of patients in relapse with pernicious anemia.

In a severely anemic patient, vitamin B_{12} is injected intramuscularly in a dosage of 15 μg. The injection may be repeated every 2 hours for three or four doses. Following this initial treatment, injections of 30 μg of vitamin B_{12} are usually given once a week. In megaloblastic anemias caused by vitamin B_{12} deficiency, a characteristic reticulocyte response appears within 10 days. Some signs of improvement in the general condition of the patient may develop within 48 hours.

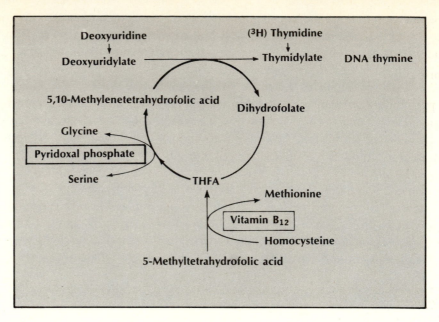

FIG. 49-2. Pathways for DNA thymine synthesis. (From Waxman, S., Corcino, J., and Herbert, V.: J.A.M.A. **214**:101, 1970, copyright 1970, American Medical Association.)

FOLIC ACID
Chemistry and
nomenclature

Folic acid is pteroylglutamic acid.

Folic acid

The compound may be looked upon as a combination of pteridine, *p*-amino-benzoic acid, and glutamic acid. In natural materials such as green vegetables the compound occurs in a conjugated form, being attached to six additional glutamic acid residues.

Folic acid is a growth factor for certain microorganisms such as *streptococcus faecalis* R. Its deficiency causes anemia and leukopenia in monkeys and in humans. Folic acid has been synthesized.

Folinic acid (citrovorum factor; Leucovorin) is closely related to folic acid.

Folinic acid

Folic acid is converted in the body to folinic acid. It has been shown that rats fed folic acid excrete some folinic acid in the urine. It has also been demonstrated that rat liver can convert folic acid to folinic acid in vitro,[16] a conversion accelerated by ascorbic acid.

Functions

The reactions in which folic acid participates are important in the synthesis of DNA (Fig. 49-2). As a consequence, deficiency of folic acid, whether induced by dietary means or by administration of the folic acid antagonists such as methotrexate, leads to damage in those tissues in which DNA synthesis and turnover are rapid. These include the hematopoietic tissues, the mucosa of the gastrointestinal tract, and the developing embryo.

Preparations and clinical uses

Folic acid is available in capsules and tablets containing 5 mg. The vitamin is well absorbed from the gastrointestinal tract, and injectable preparations, although available, are generally unnecessary.

The main use for folic acid is in nutritional macrocytic anemia, certain cases of sprue, megaloblastic anemia of pregnancy, certain cases of megaloblastic anemia in infancy, and scurvy.

It is contraindicated in pernicious anemia. It should not be used in multiple vitamin preparations because it would obscure the diagnosis of unrecognized pernicious anemia. Although it improves the megaloblastic anemia in this instance, it does not protect against the nervous system manifestations of the disease and may even aggravate them.

ERYTHROPOIETIN

There is evidence for the existence of a circulating erythropoiesis-stimulating factor. This factor, called erythropoietin or hemopoietin, has been detected in the plasma of animals made anemic, exposed to lowered pressures, or treated with cobalt. Such a factor has also been demonstrated in the plasma and urine of anemic human beings. Although this factor is of no therapeutic importance at present, it is of great experimental interest and may eventually become important in treatment of certain anemias.

The kidney has been suggested as the site of erythropoietin formation, on the basis of experiments on nephrectomized rats whose response to severe anemia and hypoxia was strikingly reduced. In humans, however, there must be extrarenal sources of erythropoietin, since nephrectomy reduces but does not abolish erythropoiesis.[15] It has also been suggested that the kidney elaborates an erythropoietic factor (REF), the release of which is stimulated by anoxia.[7] This REF acts on a plasma globulin to form erythropoietin.

REFERENCES

1 Brown, E. B.: Clinical pharmacology of drugs used in the treatment of iron deficiency anemia, Pharmacol. Phys. 2(11):1, 1968.

2 Callender, S. T., Turnbull, A., and Wakisaka, G.: Estimation of intrinsic factor of Castle by use of radioactive vitamin B$_{12}$, Br. Med. J. 1: 10, 1954.

3 Castle, W. B.: Etiology of pernicious anemia

and related macrocytic anemias, Ann. Intern. Med. 7:2, 1933.

4 Charney, E.: A fatal case of ferrous sulfate poisoning, J.A.M.A. **178**:326, 1961.

5 Desforges, J. F.: Anemia in uremia, Arch. Intern. Med. **126**:808, 1970.

6 Glass, G. B. J.: Gastric intrinsic factor and its function in the metabolism of vitamin B_{12}, Physiol. Rev. **43**:529, 1963.

7 Gordon, A. S., Cooper, G. W., and Zangani, E. D.: The kidney and erythropoiesis, Semin. Hematol. **4**:337, 1967.

8 Granick, S.: Ferritin: increase of the protein apoferritin in the gastrointestinal mucosa as a direct response to iron feeding. The function of ferritin in the regulation of iron absorption, J. Biol. Chem. **164**:737, 1946.

9 Hahn, P. F., Jones, E., Lowe, R. C., Meneely, G. R., and Peacock, W.: The relative absorption and utilization of ferrous and ferric iron in anemia as determined with the radioactive isotope, Am. J. Physiol. **143**:191, 1945.

10 Henderson, F., Vietti, T. J., and Brown, E. B.: Desferrioxamine in the treatment of acute toxic reaction to ferrous gluconate, J.A.M.A. **186**:1139, 1963.

11 Hwang, Y. F., and Brown, E. B.: Evaluation of deferoxamine in iron overload, Arch. Intern. Med. **114**:741, 1964.

12 Mendel, G. A.: Iron metabolism and etiology of iron storage diseases: an interpretative formulation, J.A.M.A. **189**:45, 1964.

13 Minot, G. R., and Murphy, W. P.: Treatment of pernicious anemia by special diet, J.A.M.A. **87**:470, 1926.

14 Moeschlin, S., and Schnider, U.: Treatment of primary and secondary hemochromatosis and acute iron poisoning with a new, potent iron-eliminating agent (desferrioxamine-b), N. Engl. J. Med. **269**:57, 1963.

15 Nathan, D. G., Shupak, E., Stohlman, F., Jr.,

and Merrill, J. P.: Erythropoiesis in anephric man, J. Clin. Invest. **43**:2158, 1964.

16 Nichol, C. A., and Welch, A. D.: Synthesis of citrovorum factor from folic acid by liver slices: augmentation by ascorbic acid, Proc. Soc. Exp. Biol. Med. **74**:52, 1950.

17 Nieweg, H. O., Faber, J. G., de Vries, J. A., and Kroese, W. F. S.: The relationship of vitamin B_{12} and folic acid in megaloblastic anemias, J. Lab. Clin. Med. **44**:118, 1954.

18 Pritchard, J. A., and Mason, R. A.: Iron stores of normal adults and replenishment with oral iron therapy, J.A.M.A. **190**:897, 1964.

19 Rickes, E. L., Brink, N. G., Koniuszy, F. R., Wood, T. R., and Folkers, K.: Comparative data on vitamin B_{12} from liver and from a new source, Streptomyces griseus, Science **108**:634, 1948.

20 Schade, S. G., Cohen, R. J., and Conrad, M. E.: Effect of hydrochloric acid on iron absorption, N. Engl. J. Med. **279**:672, 1968.

REVIEWS

21 Erslev, A. J.: The search for erythropoietin, N. Engl. J. Med. **284**:849, 1971.

22 Fisher, J. W.: Erythropoietin: pharmacology, biogenesis and control of production, Pharmacol. Rev. **24**:459, 1972.

23 Hallberg, L., Harwerth, H. G., and Vannotti, A.: Iron deficiency, New York, 1970, Academic Press, Inc.

24 Krantz, S. B., and Jacobson, L. O.: Erythropoietin and the regulation of erythropoiesis, Chicago, 1970, University of Chicago Press.

25 Propper, R. D., Shurin, S. B., and Nathan, D. G.: Reassessment of the use of desferrioxamine B in iron overload, N. Engl. J. Med. **294**:1421, 1976.

26 Savin, M. A.: A practical approach to the treatment of iron deficiency, Ration. Drug Ther. **11**:1, 1977.

CHAPTER 50

Vitamins

The early discoveries of vitamins followed observations on naturally occurring diseases such as scurvy and beriberi. The improvement noted in these diseases when modifications were made in the diet suggested that a deficiency of some sort was the cause of the pathological process. Discoveries came much more rapidly when feeding experiments were performed on experimental animals, and soon the essential nature of many vitamins was recognized.

GENERAL CONCEPT

Many of the water-soluble vitamins are coenzymes or essential parts of a coenzyme and thus have an essential function in the enzymatic machinery of cells.

WATER-SOLUBLE VITAMINS

Thiamine in the form of thiamine pyrophosphate or cocarboxylase has been shown to play an important role in the decarboxylation of α-keto acids such as pyruvate.

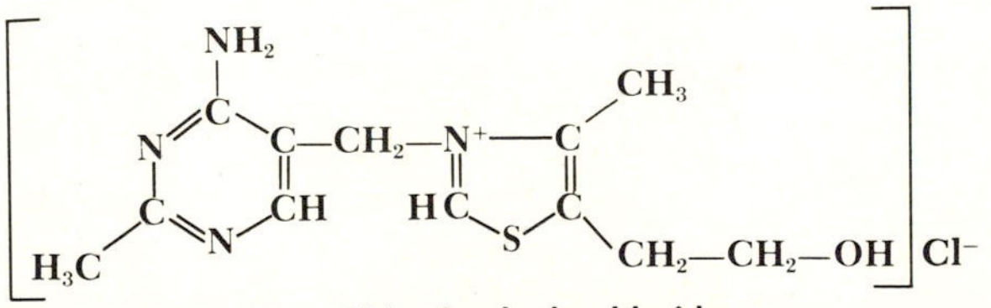

Thiamine

Thiamine hydrochloride

Severe deficiency results in the disease beriberi, characterized by high-output heart failure and peripheral polyneuritis. Other symptoms include anorexia, nausea, intestinal atony, disturbances of peripheral nerves, and mental disorders.

Deficiency

Thiamine is present in sufficient quantities in yeast, wheat germ, and pork. One international or USP unit is equal to 3 μg of thiamine hydrochloride.

Occurrence

Nicotinic acid (niacin) is an integral part of at least two important coenzymes, nicotinamide adenine dinucleotide (NAD), formerly called diphosphopyridine nucleotide (DPN), and nicotinamide adenine dinucleotide phosphate (NADP), formerly called triphosphopyridine (TPN).

NAD and NADP can exist in an oxidized or reduced state and can thus act as hydrogen acceptors or donors in many enzymatic reactions of intermediary metab-

Nicotinic acid

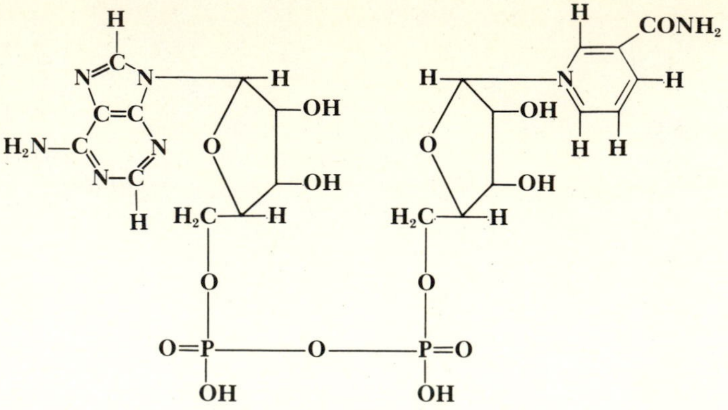

Nicotinamide adenine dinucleotide

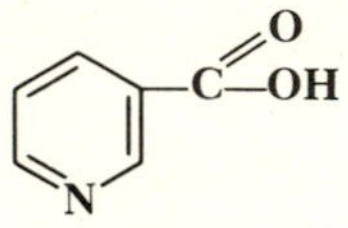

Nicotinic acid 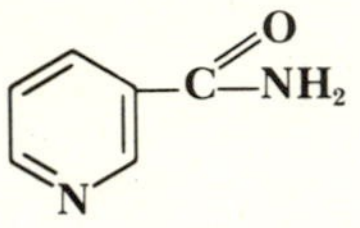   Nicotinamide

olism. Microsomal enzymes requiring NADP play an important role also in the metabolism of many drugs.

Deficiency   Pellagra is the disease caused by niacin deficiency. It is characterized by skin lesions, gastrointestinal mucosal changes with diarrhea, and neurological symptoms including mental disorders.

Occurrence   Nicotinic acid is found in significant amounts in yeast, rice, bran, and liver and other meats. Mammals can synthesize nicotinic acid from tryptophan. Pellagra can occur in patients having carcinoid tumor as a consequence of utilization of tryptophan for serotonin (5-hydroxytryptamine) synthesis.

Pharmacology   Nicotinic acid, but not nicotinamide, produces marked dilatation of small vessels, an effect that is transient but that may be severe on parenteral administration. On a purely empiric basis, nicotinic acid is used experimentally for lowering serum cholesterol and as a vasodilator, but it is not definitely useful.

Riboflavin   Riboflavin is present in flavin adenine dinucleotide (FAD), which is a coenzyme of flavoprotein enzymes. There is also a flavin mononucleotide (FMN).

Deficiency   A deficiency of riboflavin will cause cheilosis, stomatitis, and keratitis.

Occurrence   Riboflavin is present in significant quantities in yeast, green vegetables, liver and other meats, eggs, and milk.

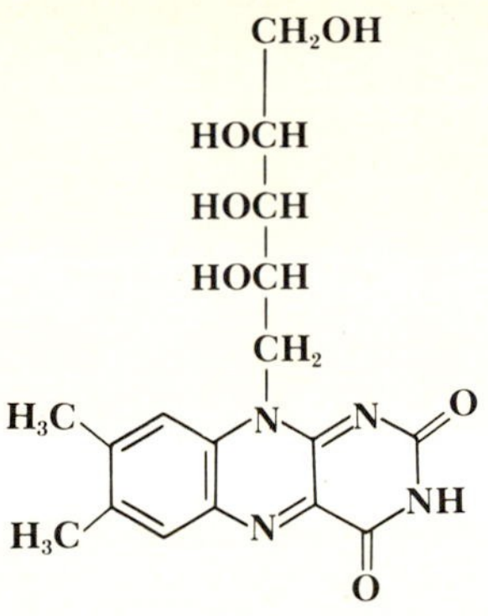

Riboflavin

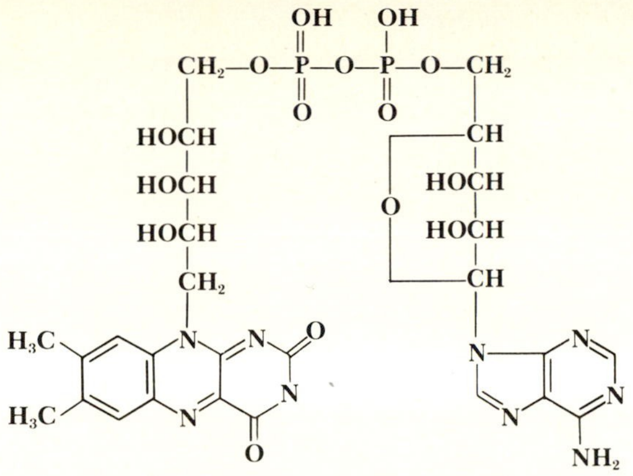

Flavin adenine dinucleotide

Pyridoxine

Pyridoxine and also pyridoxal and pyridoxamine are various forms of vitamin B_6. Pyridoxal phosphate functions as a coenzyme in many reactions such as the decarboxylation of amino acids and transamination reactions between amino acids and keto acids.

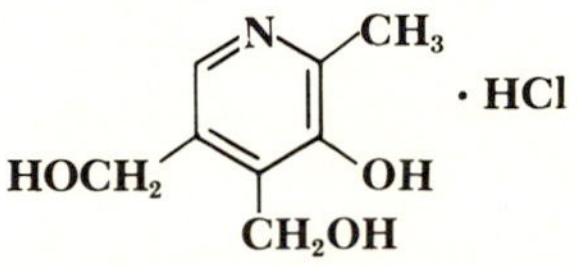

Pyridoxine hydrochloride

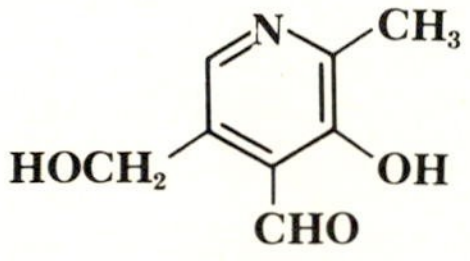

Pyridoxal

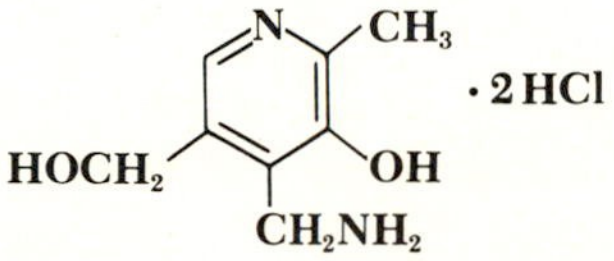

Pyridoxamine dihydrochloride

Deficiency

A deficiency of pyridoxine results in dermatitis and convulsions. Thiosemicarbazide may act as a convulsant by this mechanism. Isoniazid may also cause pyridoxine deficiency.

Occurrence

Pyridoxine is present in significant amounts in yeast, liver, rice, bran, and wheat germ.

Pantothenic acid

Pantothenic acid is a part of a very important coenzyme known as coenzyme A.

Coenzyme A in the form of acetylcoenzyme A is essential for a variety of acetylation reactions such as the formation of acetylcholine from choline and the acetylation of *p*-amino compounds. The coenzyme plays an important role in the Krebs cycle since citric acid is formed from oxaloacetic acid, acetyl coenzyme A, and water, the reaction regenerating coenzyme A. The coenzyme also plays an important role in fatty acid metabolism.

Deficiency

Pantothenic acid deficiency is not well recognized in humans. In animals it may cause dermatitis, adrenal degeneration, and central nervous system (CNS) symptoms.

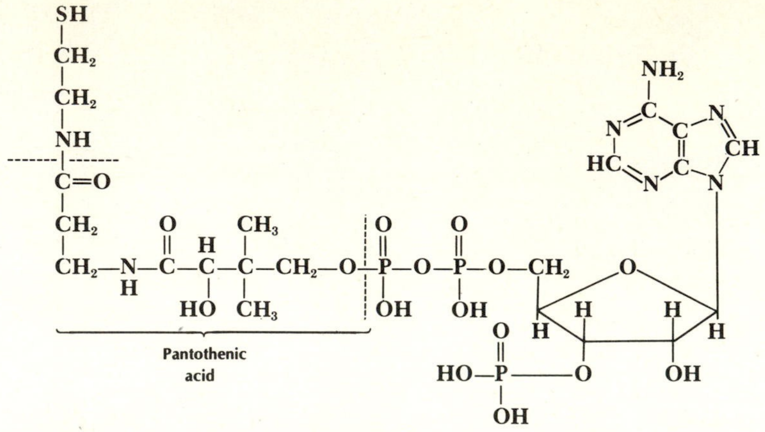

SH
|
CH_2
|
CH_2
|
NH
|
C=O
|
CH_2 O CH_3 O   O NH_2
| || H | || ||
CH_2—N—C—C—C—CH_2—O—P—O—P—O—CH_2
   | | | | |
   H   HO CH_3 OH   OH

Pantothenic acid

Coenzyme A

Occurrence	Pantothenic acid is found particularly in yeast, bran, egg yolk, and liver.
Ascorbic acid	Ascorbic acid is a reducing agent whose exact biological function is not understood. It may be a cofactor for the transformation of folic to folinic acid and may be necessary for adrenal cortical function and maintenance of normal connective tissue. The recent claim for ascorbic acid in the prevention of the common cold is not based on convincing evidence, although large-scale, controlled clinical trials are not available for proving or disproving its efficacy.
Deficiency	The classical disease scurvy is characterized by abnormalities in the connective tissue with capillaries and bone being severely affected.
Occurrence	Ascorbic acid is present in large quantities in citrus fruits, green peppers, tomatoes, and fruits and vegetables in general.
Other water-soluble vitamins	There are several other water-soluble factors essential for experimental animals and presumably for humans. These include biotin, folic acid, choline, and inositol.
	The exact biochemical functions of the other water-soluble vitamins are not known, although there is much information available on the clinical consequences of their deficiency.
FAT-SOLUBLE VITAMINS Vitamin A	Vitamin A performs an important function in connection with dark adaptation, being part of the visual purple of the retina. It also maintains the integrity of various epithelial structures.
	Deficiency of vitamin A produces night blindness, keratinization of the conjunctiva (xerophthalmia), and ulcerations of the cornea (keratomalacia). The skin becomes rough because of hyperkeratosis. Respiratory infections occur in animals deficient in vitamin A, perhaps due to changes in the bronchial epithelium, but there is no good evidence to indicate any connection between vitamin A deficiency and respiratory infection in human beings.

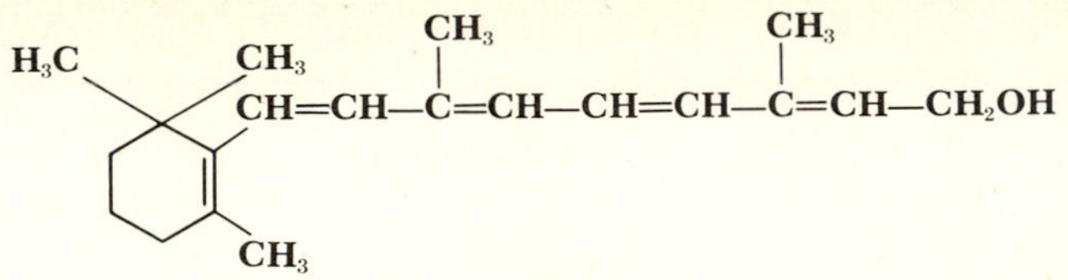

H₃C
CH₃
CH₃
CH₃

CH=CH—C=CH—CH=CH—C=CH—CH₂OH

CH₃

Vitamin A

The assay for vitamin A is based on saponification of the oil (palmitate or acetate) by potassium hydroxide, extraction with ethyl ether, and the measurement of the absorbance of ultraviolet light through an isopropanol dilution in a quartz cell at wavelengths of 310, 325, and 334 mμ.

Vitamin A occurs particularly in eggs, milk, vegetables, and fish liver oils.   *Occurrence*

Vitamin A is stored in the liver. In large quantities the vitamin may cause toxic   *Pharmacology and* effects such as anorexia, hepatomegaly, loss of hair, and periosteal thickening of   *toxicity* long bones.

Cod liver oil contains 850 IU of vitamin A per gram, a unit being equal to 0.6 μg of β-carotene. Both percomorph liver oil and a water-miscible vitamin A preparation contain 50,000 IU/g. The administration of more than 25,000 IU/day is seldom justified.

Vitamin D refers to one of several sterols. Vitamin D_2 (calciferol) is obtained by   **Vitamin D** irradiation of ergosterol. The striking new developments in relation to vitamin D metabolism are discussed on p. 561.[24]

Vitamin D_3 is present in fish liver oils and is produced in the skin by the action of sunlight on 7-dehydrocholesterol. Dihydrotachysterol has actions resembling those of the parathyroid hormone and was discussed in connection with that subject.

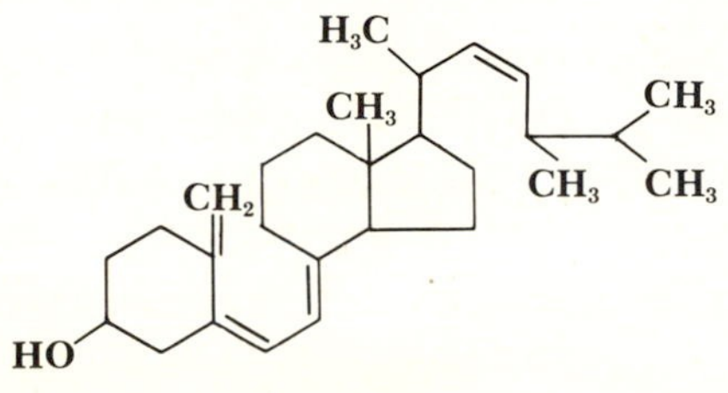

H₃C
CH₃
CH₃
CH₂
CH₃   CH₃

HO

Vitamin D₂

Deficiency of vitamin D brings forth the various manifestations of rickets in growing children and animals. There is a disturbance in calcification of bones and teeth. The bones may become soft. Swollen epiphyses and lack of normal calcification are demonstrable by radiological examination.

The main function of vitamin D appears to be exerted on the intestinal absorption of calcium and phosphate. In large quantities the vitamin may exert an effect on bone dissolution similar to the action of the parathyroid hormone.

The daily requirement of vitamin D depends on the calcium needs of the individual. Growing children and pregnant or lactating women require more of the vitamin because their daily calcium absorption must be greater.

Vitamin D preparations are standardized by determining their effect of calcification in rats maintained on a diet deficient in vitamin D. The international unit is 0.025 μg of vitamin D_3.

Adults require 400 units of vitamin D in 24 hours. Infants, children, and also pregnant or lactating women may require as much as twice this amount. It may be administered in the form of fish liver oils, as calciferol (Drisdol), or as synthetic oleovitamin D. Dihydrotachysterol (Hydracalciferol) is used in hypoparathyroidism to raise the serum calcium level.

Vitamin D is hydroxylated in the liver in the 25-position. It is further hydroxylated in the 1 position in the kidney. The implications of the availability of 1,25-hydroxycholecalciferol may be great in therapeutics (p. 561).

Toxicity   Excessive doses of the D vitamins cause hypercalcemia, with anorexia and metastatic calcifications in the kidney.

Vitamin E   Vitamin E is present in wheat-germ oil and in many foods. Its role in animal reproduction has been well established, and the term *tocopherol* implies its importance in childbearing. There are several tocopherols, but α-tocopherol has the highest activity.

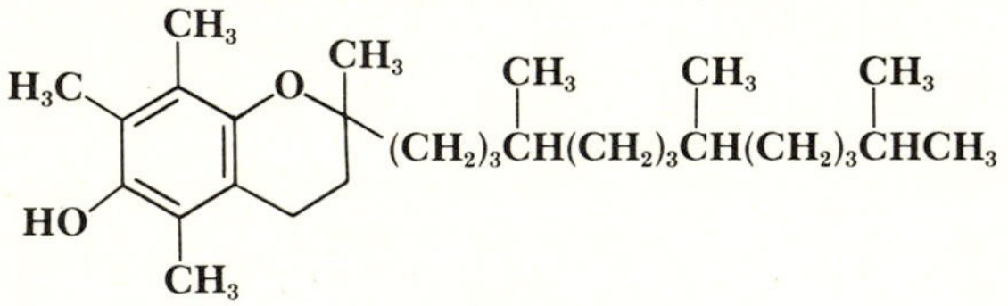

α-Tocopherol

Deficiency of vitamin E produces abortion in the female animal and degeneration of the germinal epithelium in the male animal. Muscular dystrophy also develops in animals on a vitamin E–deficient diet. Many other functions have been claimed for α-tocopherol, and many of its therapeutic applications have been suggested largely on the basis of uncritical clinical observations. The exact daily requirements of vitamin E in humans are not known, but quantities of 5 to 30 mg or more have been used in many clinical series.

The feeding of large amounts of unsaturated fats may increase the tocopherol requirements. It has been suggested that tocopherol functions as a biological antioxidant whose function becomes particularly important when tissues contain peroxidizable lipids.

Vitamin K   Vitamin K is essential for production of prothrombin by the liver, and in its absence hemorrhagic manifestations occur. Various 1,4-naphthoquinones have vitamin K activity. Vitamin K_1 is 2-methyl-3-phytyl-1,4-naphthoquinone.

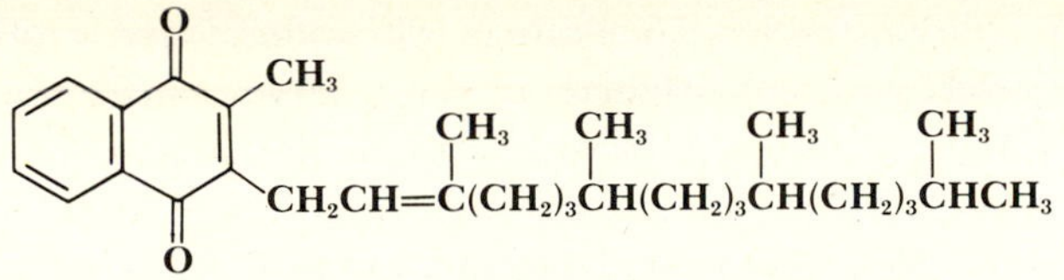

Vitamin K₁

These naphthoquinone compounds are very insoluble in water and are suitable primarily for oral administration. Emulsions of vitamin K_1, however, can be injected intravenously in hemorrhagic emergencies caused by hypoprothrombinemia.

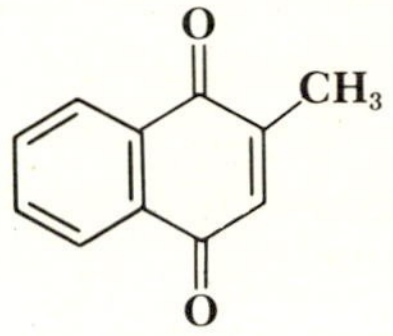

Menadione

Water-soluble derivatives of naphthoquinones have also been prepared. The structural formulas of two such compounds, menadiol sodium diphosphate and menadione sodium bisulfite, are shown below:

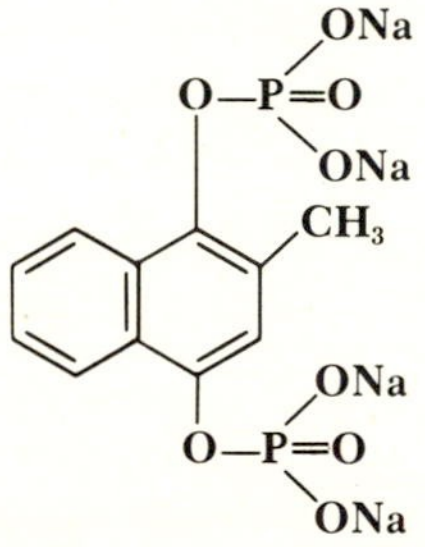

Menadiol sodium diphosphate 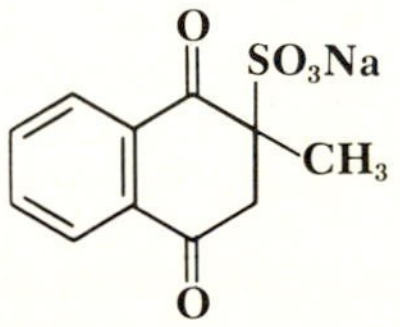   **Menadione sodium bisulfite**

Vitamin K preparations are useful in bleeding caused by hypoprothrombinemia. Causes of hypoprothrombinemia are severe liver disease, biliary obstruction, malabsorption syndromes, coumarin and indandione drugs, salicylates in large doses, reduction of intestinal flora by chemotherapeutic agents, and hypoprothrombinemia of small infants.

Commonly used preparations are vitamin K_1 (phytonadione; Mephyton) and various forms of vitamin K_3 (menadione; menadiol sodium diphosphate, water soluble, or Synkayvite; and menadione sodium bisulfite or Hykinone, also water soluble).

The daily requirement for vitamin K cannot be stated because considerable quantities are synthesized by the bacterial flora of the intestine. The dosage varies greatly, depending on the nature and severity of prothrombin deficiency. Doses of 1 to 2 mg by mouth or injection may suffice. On the other hand, very large doses may have to be administered in emergency situations when prothrombin levels have been depressed by the anticoagulant drugs. As much as 100 mg or more of vitamin K_1 emulsion has been used in this situation by the intravenous route.

Toxicity   Individuals who are subject to primaquine-sensitive anemia may react with hemolysis to large doses of vitamin K. Such doses can also aggravate liver disease and produce jaundice, particularly in infants.

MEDICAL USES   Vitamins should be used in medicine in (1) individuals with a poor dietary history, (2) deficiency diseases, (3) special disease states, or (4) hereditary vitamin dependency states.[21]

Individuals with a poor dietary history include vegetarians who do not consume dairy products, individuals who do not consume fruits and green vegetables, pregnant or lactating women, and infants. Vegetarians develop vitamin B_{12} deficiency and require supplementation with 10 μg daily doses. Ascorbic acid, 50 mg daily, should be given to persons who do not eat fruits and green vegetables. Folate supplementation (0.5 mg) and pyridoxine should be given to pregnant women. Lactating women should probably take at least 80 mg of ascorbic acid daily, and their increased thiamine requirements should be met by proper food intake. Infants fed cow's milk should receive about 35 mg ascorbic acid daily, and the newborn should receive a single intramuscular injection of 0.5 to 1 mg of vitamin K, since vitamin K deficiency develops until the intestinal flora is established.[24]

Deficiency diseases include alcoholism, pernicious anemia, total or partial gastrectomy, chronic pancreatitis (fibrocystic disease), celiac disease (nontropical sprue), tropical sprue, short bowel syndrome, and dietary deficiencies.[24] Detailed discussion of the supplementation required in each of these conditions is beyond the scope of this review.

Additional special disease states include infection with *Diphyllobothrium latum*, hypoparathyroidism, and the carcinoid syndrome. The corresponding supplementations are vitamin B_{12}, vitamin D_2, and niacin.

Hereditary vitamin dependency states have been recognized in which the apoenzyme fails to react normally with the coenzyme, the condition being partially overcome by large doses of the corresponding vitamins. For example, an inborn error in the apoenzyme pyruvate carboxylase can produce lactic acidosis and is treated with 20 mg of thiamine daily. There are several rare diseases of this type, which provide some justification for the search for conditions that might be benefited by the megavitamin concept.[24] It should be remembered that the effectiveness of levodopa in parkinsonism would not have been discovered without someone trying unusually large doses of the drug. This, however, should not be considered an endorsement of the megavitamin therapy, which in most cases is ineffective and is not based on sound theory or controlled clinical trials.

ADVERSE EFFECTS   Although slight excesses of vitamin intake are more wasteful than dangerous, large doses of several of the vitamins can produce adverse effects.

TABLE 50-1. Recommended daily dietary allowances and therapeutic doses of vitamins

Vitamin	Average daily adult requirement	Therapeutic dose
Thiamine	1.5 mg	2-10 mg
Nicotinamide	20 mg	100-300 mg
Riboflavin	2 mg	2-10 mg
Pyridoxine	2 mg	10 mg
Ascorbic acid	60 mg	100-150 mg
Vitamin A	4000 units	25,000 units
Vitamin D	400 units	5000 units or more
Vitamin E	Unknown	30 units

The water-soluble vitamins are generally harmless except in special circumstances. Thiamine injected intravenously has produced a shocklike state, and an anaphylactic-type sensitization to it has been suspected. Nicotinic acid is a fairly potent vasodilator, and for that reason nicotinamide, which does not affect the blood vessels, is preferred. Folic acid may be dangerous in persons who have pernicious anemia, since it may aggravate the neurological manifestations of the disease. For this reason the modern tendency is to eliminate folic acid from multiple vitamin preparations. Ascorbic acid is remarkably nontoxic. When given in large quantities, the vitamin is rapidly cleared by the kidney. Pyridoxine promotes the peripheral decarboxylation of levodopa and thus decreases its effectiveness in the treatment of parkinsonism.

The fat-soluble vitamins are more likely to produce distinct pathological changes when given in excessive quantities.

Hypervitaminosis A has been described as occurring in children when doses of the order of 100,000 units or more are administered for many days. Changes in skeletal development, hepatomegaly, anemia, loss of hair, and other symptoms have been described in these patients.

When used in large quantities, vitamin D can produce hypercalcemia with metastatic calcification in the kidney and blood vessels. This is not likely to happen in the treatment of rickets, but occasionally large amounts of vitamin D_2 are used in other diseases such as lupus vulgaris in which there is no reason to suspect a deficiency.

Hemolytic anemia and jaundice have been reported following parenteral use of large doses of the various vitamin K preparations.

The occurrence of these adverse reactions is an additional reason for maintaining a rational attitude toward the use of vitamins in cases in which their indications are not clear.

REFERENCES

1 Almquist, H. J.: Vitamin K, Physiol. Rev. **21:** 194, 1941.

2 Axelrod, A. E.: Immune processes in vitamin deficiency states, Am. J. Clin. Nutr. **24:**265, 1971.

3 DeLuca, H. F.: Vitamin D, N. Engl. J. Med. **281:**1103, 1969.

4 Elvehjem, C. A.: The vitamin B complex: Council on Foods and Nutrition, J.A.M.A. **138:**960, 1948.

5 Finkel, M. J.: Vitamin K_1 and vitamin K analogues, Clin. Pharmacol. Ther. **2:**794, 1961.

6 Gribetz, D., Silverman, S. H., and Sobel, A. E.: Vitamin A poisoning, Pediatrics **7:**372, 1951.

7 Sebrell, W. H., and Harris, R. S., editors: The vitamins, New York, 1954, Academic Press, Inc.

8 Streif, R. R., and Little, A. B.: Folic acid deficiency in pregnancy, N. Engl. J. Med. **276:** 776, 1967.

9 Suttie, J. W.: Mechanisms of action of vitamin K: demonstration of a liver precursor of prothrombin, Science **179:**192, 1973.

10 Symposium on the detection of nutrition deficiencies in man, Am. J. Clin. Nutr. **20:**513, 1967.

11 Symposium on some findings and observations on the nutritional status of residents of the U.S.A., Am. J. Clin. Nutr. **17:**189, 1965.

12 Unglaub, W. G., and Hunter, F. M.: Essential fatty acids, Am. J. Med. Sci. **233:**90, 1957.

13 Vietti, T. J., Murphy, T. P., James, J. A., and Pritchard, J. A.: Observations on the prophylactic use of vitamin K in the newborn infant, J. Pediatr. **56:**343, 1960.

14 Wald, G.: The chemistry of rod vision, Science **113:**287, 1951.

15 Youmans, J. B.: Deficiencies of the water-soluble vitamins, J.A.M.A. **144:**386, 1950.

REVIEWS

16 DeLuca, H. F.: Vitamin D endocrinology, Ann. Intern. Med. **85:**367, 1976.

17 DeLuca, H. F., and Suttie, J. W.: The fat-soluble vitamins, Madison, 1970, University of Wisconsin Press.

18 Fliss, D. M., and Lamy, P. P.: Trace elements and total parenteral nutrition, Hosp. Formulary **14:**698, 1979.

18a Goodman, D. S.: Vitamin A metabolism, Fed. Proc. **39:**2716, 1980.

19 Rivlin, R. S.: Riboflavin metabolism, N. Engl. J. Med. **283:**463, 1970.

20 Rosenberg, L. E.: Vitamin-dependent genetic disease, Hosp. Pract. **5:**59, 1970.

21 Schnoes, H. K., and DeLuca, H. F.: Recent progress in vitamin D metabolism and the chemistry of vitamin D metabolites, Fed. Proc. **39:**2723, 1980.

22 Scott, M. L.: Advances in our understanding of vitamin E, Fed. Proc. **39:**2736, 1980.

23 Suttie, J. W.: The metabolic role of vitamin K, Fed. Proc. **39:**2730, 1980.

24 Taylor, K. B.: Uses and abuses of vitamin therapy, Ration. Drug Ther. **9**(10):1, 1975.

SECTION NINE

Chemotherapy

CHAPTER 51

Introduction to chemotherapy; mechanisms of antibiotic action

Prior to 1935 systemic bacterial infections could not be effectively treated with drugs. There were many *antiseptics* and *disinfectants* that could eradicate infections when applied topically, but their systemic use was precluded by their unfavorable therapeutic index. Certain parasitic infections such as malaria, amebiasis, and spirochetal infections could be treated effectively. This was an indication that the concept of "chemotherapy" as invisioned by Ehrlich was not unreasonable. Still, systemic bacterial infections, whether seen in patients or produced experimentally in animals, seemed to be hopelessly beyond the reach of existing drugs.

In 1935 a paper appeared in the German medical literature claiming that the red azo dye Prontosil was able to protect mice against a systemic streptococcal infection and was curative in patients suffering from such infections.[5] This was a milestone in the history of chemotherapy. In the test tube, Prontosil was ineffective against the bacteria.

It was soon demonstrated that Prontosil is broken down in the body to *p*-amino-benzenesulfonamide, known later as sulfanilamide.[13] It was also demonstrated that the chemotherapeutic activity of Prontosil was a result of the breakdown product sulfanilamide.

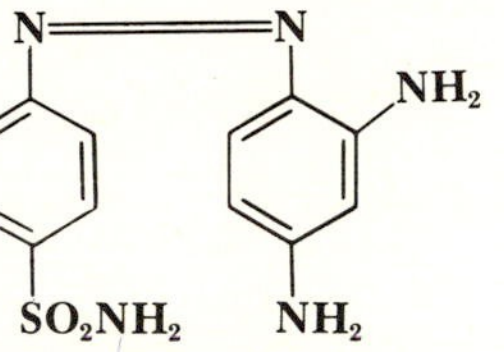

Prontosil 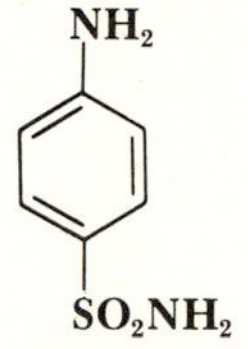   **Sulfanilamide**

These observations initiated a new era in medicine. Numerous derivatives of sulfanilamide were synthesized, and soon a considerable number of systemic infections could be controlled by these drugs. Not only was the treatment of many infectious diseases revolutionized, but study of these drugs led to many great discoveries about bacterial metabolism, opening many new fields in pharmacology. The study of biological antagonism and the discovery of the carbonic anhydrase inhibitors, antithyroid drugs, and many other agents were greatly influenced by basic studies on the sulfonamides.

The successes obtained with the new sulfonamides revived interest in observations on *antibiotics*, or compounds produced by some microorganisms that inhibit the growth of other microorganisms. There were several isolated observations on the phenomenon of antibiosis. One of the most remarkable of these was Fleming's discovery that a mold of the genus *Penicillium* prevented multiplication of staphylococci and that culture filtrates of this mold had similar properties.[7] A concentrate of this antibacterial factor was eventually prepared, and its remarkable activity and lack of toxicity were demonstrated by a team at Oxford, led by Florey.[1,4]

The enormous potency and lack of toxicity of penicillin turned the attention of many investigators in the direction of the antibiotics as potential sources of useful chemotherapeutic agents. Soon hundreds of antibiotics were discovered. The great majority of these were too toxic for clinical use, but a few represented welcome additions to therapeutics. Streptomycin, the tetracyclines, chloramphenicol, polymyxin, bacitracin, neomycin, and several newer antibiotics have greatly increased the range of effectiveness of antibacterial chemotherapy.

Currently, interest is centered on the newer penicillins, cephalosporins, newer aminoglycosides, and combinations of sulfamethoxazole with trimethoprim.

GENERAL CONCEPTS   With the availability of large numbers of effective antimicrobial agents many general principles have evolved that must guide the physician in the selection and dosage of the most appropriate agent to be used in a given patient. Selection and dosage depend not only on the bacteriological diagnosis, but on host factors, such as renal function, age, and disease states. Thus susceptibility tests do not automatically dictate the kind of antimicrobial agent that must be used.[19]

A number of important concepts have been derived from the extensive studies on antibacterial chemotherapy.

Antibacterial spectrum refers to the range of activity of a compound. A broad-spectrum antibacterial agent is one capable of inhibiting a wide variety of microorganisms, including usually both gram-positive and gram-negative bacteria.

Potency, or activity per milligram, of a chemotherapeutic agent is usually expressed on the basis of the lowest concentration at which a chemotherapeutic agent is capable of inhibiting the multiplication of one of the susceptible microorganisms.

Bacteriostatic activity refers to the ability of a compound to inhibit multiplication of microorganisms. *Bactericidal activity* means an actual killing effect, which can only be demonstrated by techniques that are more complex than the usual plate or tube-dilution methods used for the demonstration of bacteriostatic activity. It is an interesting generalization that those antibacterial substances that disturb the synthesis or function of the microbial cell wall or the cell membrane are usually the ones that are bactericidal.

The necessity of maintaining *blood levels* varies greatly. This is important in the case of the sulfonamides, but it may be less so in the case of some of the antibiotics such as penicillin. Blood levels in a given situation can generally be predicted from the dose and the weight of the patient. Determinations of blood levels are important only in some conditions such as renal failure that make it impossible to predict blood levels on the basis of the dose administered.

The terms *antibiotic synergism* and *antibiotic antagonism* usually refer to the magnitude of *bactericidal* activity when combinations of chemotherapeutic agents are used. The *bacteriostatic* activities of such drug combinations are usually additive. For example, if two antibiotics such as penicillin and streptomycin exert greater bactericidal activity when given together rather than singly, a phenomenon of *antibiotic synergism* is said to exist. If a bacteriostatic antibiotic interferes with the killing effect of a bactericidal antibiotic, the phenomenon is *antibiotic antagonism.* These concepts are discussed further in connection with penicillin.

Indications for the combined use of antibiotics are to increase the effectiveness of therapy against a resistant organism and to take advantage of a possible synergistic killing effect, to delay the development of resistance, and to broaden the antibacterial spectrum in mixed infections or in cases in which reliable bacteriological diagnosis is unavailable.

There are many disadvantages to the combined use of antibiotics, which may be entirely unnecessary and wasteful. Combinations expose the patient to the adverse effects of the various members, superinfection may develop, and in rare instances, antibiotic antagonism may be promoted.

RESISTANCE

Resistance to antibiotics may be *genetic* or *nongenetic*. Genetic resistance may be of chromosomal origin or may be transmitted by extrachromosomal *plasmids*. The chromosomal resistance may arise from spontaneous mutations.

Nongenetic resistance is usually associated with nonmultiplying bacteria, the so-called persisters. Many antibiotics, particularly penicillin, act only on rapidly multiplying organisms. For example, penicillin is much more bactericidal at 37° C, when bacteria are actively synthesizing their cell walls, than at refrigerator temperatures. This means that bacteria in the body that are not multiplying or are not synthesizing their cell walls (L forms) are not killed by penicillin.

The way resistant bacteria escape the antibiotic takes many forms. Bacteria may destroy the antibiotic, for example, by developing an enzyme, such as β-lactamase, which destroys penicillin. In other instances, bacteria may become less permeable to the antibiotic, develop alternate metabolic pathways, or undergo some change that allows them to live in the presence of the drug.

Infectious drug resistance

It was recognized in Japan in 1959 that bacterial resistance to several unrelated antibiotics can be transferred to susceptible organisms by cell-to-cell contact or conjugation.[14]

Bacteria contain extrachromosomal genetic elements called R factors that are made up of DNA and act like viruses without coats. Transfer of resistance by RTF, a portion of the R factor, can occur among *Shigella, Salmonella, Klebsiella, Vibrio, Pasteurella,* and *Escherichia coli.* The last-named may be a great reservoir for the transmission of bacterial resistance.

In addition to the gram-negative organisms, staphylococci may also contain extrachromosomal particles called *plasmids*, which may be transferred from cell to cell by phages, a form of *transduction*.

ANTIBACTERIAL CHEMOTHERA- PEUTIC AGENTS
Mechanism of action

Most of the commonly used antibacterial chemotherapeutic agents act by one of the following basic mechanisms: competitive antagonism of some metabolite, inhibition of bacterial cell wall synthesis, action on cell membranes, inhibition of protein synthesis, or inhibition of nucleic acid synthesis.

Competitive antagonism. There are a few examples in which antibacterial substances act as antimetabolites. The sulfonamides compete with *p*-aminobenzoic acid for the synthesis of folic acid in bacteria. This concept of competitive antagonism arose from studies on substrates that tended to inhibit the activity of the sulfonamides in vitro. It was shown that the antagonistic effect of yeast extract was probably caused by the presence of *p*-aminobenzoic acid.[8]

It has subsequently been shown that folic acid, a noncompetitive inhibitor of the sulfonamides, contains *p*-aminobenzoic acid. It now appears that certain bacteria require *p*-aminobenzoic acid for the synthesis of folic acid and that the sulfonamides prevent this synthesis by substrate competition.

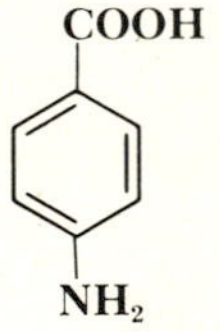

p-Aminobenzoic acid 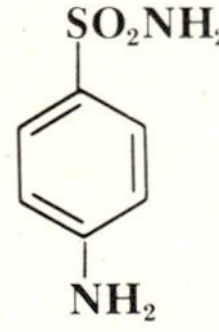   Sulfanilamide 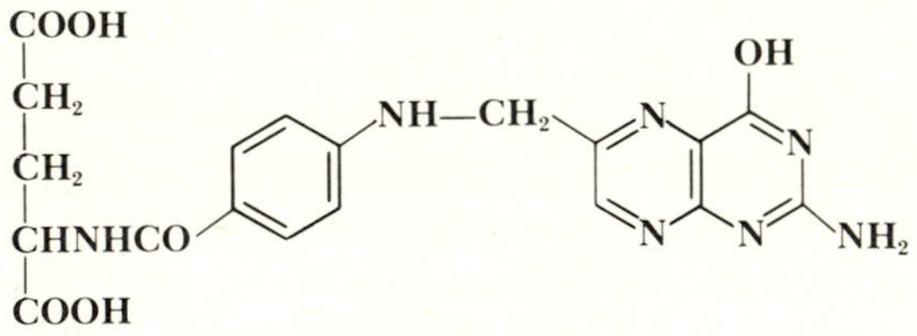   Folic acid

Since mammalian organisms do not synthesize folic acid but require it as a vitamin, the sulfonamides are not expected to interfere with the metabolism of mammalian cells. This difference between microorganisms and mammals explains the favorable therapeutic index of the sulfonamides in the treatment of various infections.

There are other examples of competitive antagonism in antibacterial chemotherapy. *p*-Aminosalicylate also competes with *p*-aminobenzoic acid. Interestingly, *p*-aminosalicylate is ineffective against bacteria other than the tubercle bacillus, although these bacteria may require *p*-aminobenzoic acid and are inhibited by the sulfonamides. A reasonable explanation for this invokes a difference in the receptive mechanisms in the two types of microorganisms.

Inhibition of bacterial cell wall synthesis. Several antibiotics including penicillin, the cephalosporins, cycloserine, and bacitracin act by inhibiting the synthesis of the rigid bacterial cell wall. This cell wall, in contrast with mammalian cell membranes, is rigid, making it possible for bacteria to maintain a very high internal osmotic pressure. If the synthesis of the cell wall is blocked, the high osmotic pressure leads to an extrusion of bacterial protoplasm through defects in the supporting structure and eventually to lysis of the cell when exposed to the isosmotic environment present in mammalian tissues.

The structural element of the bacterial cell wall is known as *murein*. The synthesis of murein is divided into three phases[16]: (1) synthesis of nucleotide intermediates, UDP-*N*-acetylglucosamine and UDP-*N*-acetylmuramyl-pentapeptide, terminating in D-alanyl-D-alanine; (2) assembly of the disaccharide intermediate and its incorporation into murein; and (3) the cross-linking of the peptides by transpeptidation with release of D-alanine.

It was known for many years that penicillin is particularly effective against rapidly multiplying bacteria. It was also known that the antibiotic produced morphological changes in bacteria, such as swelling, large body formation, and lysis. Subsequently it was shown by Lederberg[10] that *E. coli* cells were converted to protoplasts in the presence of penicillin and sucrose. Protoplasts are believed to represent cellular units deprived of their rigid cell wall.

Problem 50-1. Since both penicillin G and ampicillin act on a transpeptidase to block cell wall synthesis, why is ampicillin so much more potent against gram-negative bacilli, such as *E. coli?* It has been shown[16] that in cell-free systems both antibiotics were nearly equally active against the transpeptidase. On the other hand, in the case of penicillin G about 10 times as much was required for growth inhibition of *E. coli* as for transpeptidase inhibition in cell-free systems. This finding suggests permeability as the explanation for the different antibacterial spectrum of the two antibiotics.

Action on cell membranes. Some antibiotics act on cell membranes, altering their permeability. This mode of action is sometimes referred to as a detergent-like action. The best examples of this mechanism are provided by the polymyxins and the antifungal polyene antibiotics.

Although antibiotics acting on cell membranes have some selective toxicity for microorganisms, they may be quite toxic for mammalian cells also. For example, the polymyxins cause renal tubular damage when administered in doses somewhat larger than therapeutic. They can also cause histamine release from mast cells both in vitro and in vivo (p. 240).

There are polyene antibiotics such as amphotericin B that complex with sterols in the cell wall. Fungi, but not bacteria, possess such sterols in their cell membranes; this explains the selective toxicity of the polyenes for fungi. However, mammalian cells also possess sterols in their cell membranes, and the polyenes can lyse red cells and cause numerous toxic effects.

Inhibition of protein synthesis. Most of the commonly used antibiotics inhibit protein synthesis. The list includes the tetracyclines, chloramphenicol, streptomycin, erythromycin, and lincomycin. In addition, the highly toxic experimental tools puromycin and cycloheximide (Actidione) are potent inhibitors of protein synthesis both in microorganisms and in mammals.

The selective toxicity of a protein synthesis for microorganisms is understood only in a few instances. Chloramphenicol interferes with the attachment of amino acids to the ribosomes in bacteria. In mammalian organisms, on the other hand, it only prevents the attachment of *new* messenger RNA to ribosomes. As a conse-

TABLE 51-1. Mechanism of action of antibiotics*

Mechanism	Antibiotic	Site of action	Mode of action
Cell wall synthesis	Penicillin and cephalosporins	Phase 3†	Inhibition of a transpeptidase
	Cycloserine	Phase 1†	Competitive inhibition of alanine racemase and dipeptide synthetase
	Vancomycin (ristocetin)	Phase 2†	Blockade of murein polymerase
	Bacitracin	Phase 2†	Inhibition of a lipid pyrophosphatase
Protein synthesis	Tetracyclines	30 S subunit	Blockade of A site that binds tRNA where mRNA attaches
	Chloramphenicol	50 S subunit	Competitive inhibition of binding aminoacyl-tRNA to ribosome
	Aminoglycosides	30 S subunit	Unclear
	Macrolides	50 S subunit	Inhibition of translocation from A to P site
	Puromycin	50 S subunit	Substitution for aminoacyl-tRNA; transfer to peptide causing its release
	Lincomycin	50 S subunit	Inhibition of peptidyl transferase
DNA synthesis	Mitomycins	Double-stranded DNA	Bifunctional alkylation causing cross-linkages between DNA strands
RNA synthesis	Rifamycins	DNA-dependent RNA polymerase	Binding to polymerase with inhibition
	Actinomycin	DNA segment	Blockade of transcription by binding to DNA

*Based on data from Hash, J. H.: Annu. Rev. Pharmacol. **12:**35, 1972.
†The three phases in cell wall synthesis are as follows: *Phase 1*—synthesis of the nucleotide intermediates; *Phase 2*—assembly and modification of the disaccharide intermediate; *Phase 3*—the cross-linking of the peptide chains by transpeptidation.

quence, chloramphenicol exerts an effect on the synthesis of new antibodies in animals without influencing protein synthesis in general.

Inhibition of nucleic acid synthesis. Some highly toxic antibiotics such as actinomycin complex with DNA at the deoxyguanosine level. As a consequence, messenger RNA formation is blocked. The drug is highly toxic and is used only experimentally and rarely against some forms of malignancies (Wilms' tumor).

Idoxuridine (5-iodo-2'-deoxyuridine) blocks the synthesis of DNA and is used by topical application in the treatment of herpes keratitis. Rifampin blocks RNA synthesis in susceptible organisms (Table 51-1).

REFERENCES

1 Abraham, E. P., et al.: Further observations on penicillin, Lancet 2:177, 1941.
2 Anderson, E. S., and Lewis, M. J.: Drug resistance and its transfer in Salmonella typhimurium, Nature 206:579, 1965.
3 Burchall, J. J., Ferone, R., and Hitchings, G. H.: Antibacterial chemotherapy, Annu. Rev. Pharmacol. 5:53, 1965.
4 Chain, E. B.: The development of bacterial chemotherapy, Antibiot. Chemother. (Basel) 4:215, 1954.

5 Domagk, G.: Ein Beitrag zur Chemotherapie der bakteriellen Infektionen, Deutsch. Med. Wochenschr. **61**:250, 1935.

6 Feingold, D. S.: Antimicrobial chemotherapeutic agents: the nature of their action and selective toxicity, N. Engl. J. Med. **269**:900, 957, 1963.

7 Fleming, A., editor: Penicillin: its practical application, Philadelphia, 1946, The Blakiston Co.

8 Hayes, W.: Conjugation in *Escherichia coli*, Br. Med. Bull. **18**:36, 1962.

9 Jawetz, E., and Gunnison, J. B.: Antibiotic synergism and antagonism: an assessment of the problem, Pharmacol. Rev. **5**:175, 1953.

10 Lederberg, J.: Bacterial protoplasts induced by penicillin, Proc. Natl. Acad. Sci. **42**:574, 1956.

11 McCormack, R. C., Kaye, D., and Hook, E. W.: Resistance of Group A streptococci to tetracycline, N. Engl. J. Med. **267**:323, 1962.

12 Park, J. T., and Strominger, J. L.: Mode of action of penicillin: biochemical basis for the mechanism of action of penicillin and for its toxicity, Science **125**:99, 1957.

13 Trefouel, J., Trefouel, Mme. J., Nitti, F., and Bovet, D.: Activité du p-aminophénylsulfamide sur les infections streptococciques expérimentales de la souris et du lapin, C. R. Soc. Biol. **120**:756, 1942.

14 Watanabe, T.: Infective heredity of multiple drug resistance in bacteria, Bact. Rev. **27**:87, 1963.

15 Weinstein, L., and Dalton, A. C.: Host determinants of response to antimicrobial agents, N. Engl. J. Med. **279**:467, 524, 1968.

REVIEWS

16 Hash, J. H.: Antibiotic mechanisms, Annu. Rev. Pharmacol. **12**:35, 1972.

17 Lorian, V.: The mode of action of antibiotics on gram-negative bacilli, Arch. Intern. Med. **128**: 623, 1971.

18 Seneca, H.: Biological basis of chemotherapy of infections and infestations, Philadelphia, 1971, F. A. Davis Co.

19 Weinstein, L.: Some principles of antimicrobial therapy, Ration. Drug Ther. **11**:1, 1977.

CHAPTER 52

Sulfonamides

GENERAL CONCEPT

Despite the availability of numerous antibiotics, the sulfonamides still have important therapeutic uses, particularly in the treatment of acute urinary tract infections. In addition to a discussion of the pharmacology of the sulfonamides, reference will be made in this chapter to other drugs also that find applications chiefly in infections of the urinary tract (Table 52-2).

The usefulness of the sulfonamides has increased greatly with the introduction of trimethoprim-sulfamethoxazole mixtures, which represent a synergistic combination of antibacterial agents.

SULFONAMIDE DRUGS
Chemistry

The majority of clinically useful sulfonamides may be looked on as derivatives of sulfanilamide. As a rule, only those sulfonamides that have a free *p*-amino group show antibacterial activity. Compounds that are substituted in the amino group become active only if the substituent is removed in the body. This was the reason for the lack of activity of Prontosil in vitro, whereas it had considerable effectiveness in vivo.

Substitutions in the amide group have produced some of the most important sulfonamides, whose advantages over sulfanilamide consist of greater potency, wider antibacterial spectrum, and greater therapeutic index. The structural formulas of some of the most important sulfonamides for systemic use and those for local use are depicted in Table 52-1.

The sulfonamides currently used are short-acting (half-life of 4 to 8 hours) or intermediate-acting (half-life of 11 hours). There are long-acting sulfonamides also, but these are not popular. In addition, there are topical sulfonamides, such as silver sulfadiazine and mafenide (not a true sulfonamide), and there is one poorly absorbed sulfonamide available, phthalylsulfathiazole.

Antibacterial spectrum

The sulfonamides are effective against many gram-positive organisms, against some gram-negative diplococci and bacilli, and against actinomyces, nocardia, chlamydiae, and some protozoa.

The short-acting sulfonamides are among the drugs of choice for the treatment of acute urinary tract infections caused by susceptible bacteria, such as *Escherichia coli* and some strains of *Proteus*. The short-acting sulfonamides are also highly useful in the treatment of nocardiosis, trachoma, and chancroid. Other infections, includ-

TABLE 52-1. Structures of sulfonamides

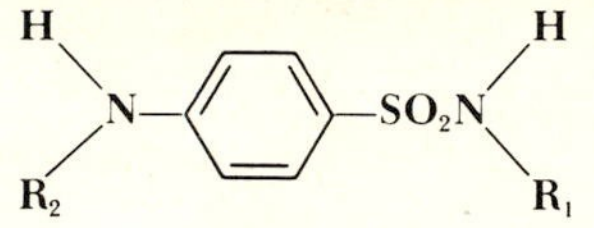

Sulfanilamide

	R_1 substitutions	R_2 substitutions
For systemic use		
Sulfadiazine	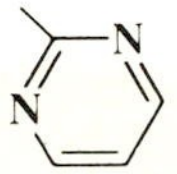	———
Sulfamerazine	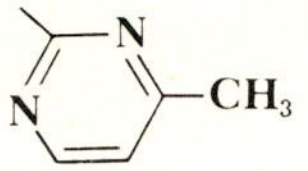	———
Sulfamethazine	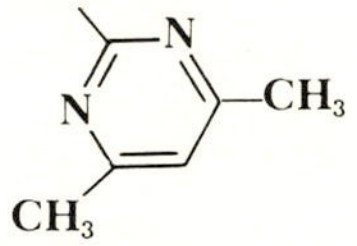	———
Sulfisomidine (Elkosin)	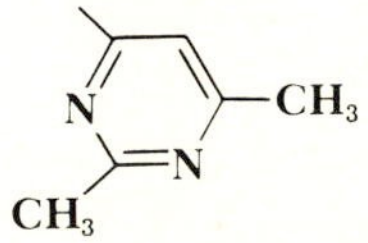	———
Sulfacetamide (Sulamyd)	—COCH$_3$	———
Sulfisoxazole (Gantrisin)	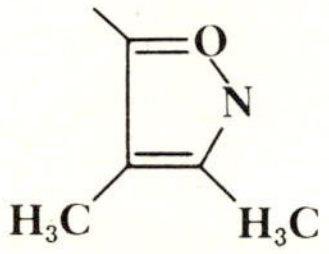	———
Sulfamethizole (Thiosulfil)	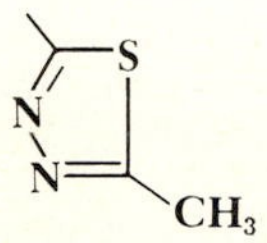	———
Sulfachloropyridazine (Sonilyn)	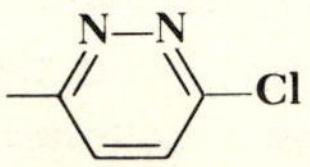	———

Continued.

TABLE 52-1. Structures of sulfonamides—cont'd

	R₁ substitutions	R₂ substitutions

Sulfamethoxypyridazine (Kynex; Midicel)	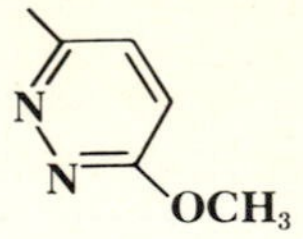	———
Sulfadimethoxine (Madribon)	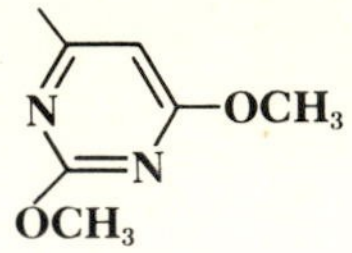	———

For intestinal use

Succinylsulfathiazole (Sulfasuxidine)	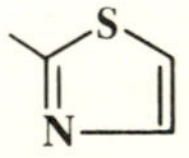	$-\overset{O}{\overset{\|}{C}}-CH_2CH_2-COOH$
Phthalylsulfathiazole (Sulfathalidine)	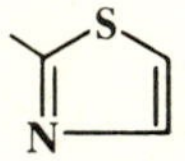	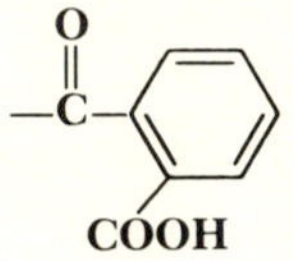

ing otitis media and respiratory infections, may respond to sulfonamide treatment, but some of the antibiotics are more effective.

The *potency* of these drugs is such that growth inhibition may be achieved in simple media at a concentration of about 0.1 to 1 mg/ml and at blood levels of the order of 10 mg/100 ml. The potency of these drugs in the test tube is greatly influenced by the nature of the culture medium. Thus enrichment with yeast extract, pus, or *p*-aminobenzoic acid causes marked decrease in the effectiveness of these drugs. Even in a simple synthetic medium the potency or activity per milligram of the sulfonamides is much smaller than that of the most clinically useful antibiotics. For this reason, when compared with most antibiotics, relatively large doses of the sulfonamides must be administered.

Mode of action   The sulfonamides compete with *p*-aminobenzoic acid for incorporation into folic acid in susceptible bacteria (p. 618).

A study of the in vitro activity of various sulfonamides and the ionization and electron density of their SO_2 group led to the concept that a definite relationship exists between this physical property and activity in the test tube. Activity appeared maximal at around pK_a 6.5 and was less either below or above this figure.[1] Since the pK_a of sulfadiazine was close to the optimal figure, it was thought unlikely that any sulfonamide acting by competition with *p*-aminobenzoic acid would have greater activity than sulfadiazine. This means that newer sulfonamides are more likely to offer advantages on the basis of solubility, metabolism, renal handling, or lack of sensitizing properties than by having a significantly greater antibacterial potency.

Sulfonamides are bacteriostatic. However, they may become bactericidal if the microorganisms are grown in a low thymine medium. For the same reason, it is conceivable that in some infections sulfonamides may exert bactericidal effects also.

The short-acting sulfonamides are absorbed rapidly from the gastrointestinal tract. These drugs include sulfadiazine (although it has a longer half-life than others in this group), sulfisoxazole (Gantrisin), sulfamethizole (Thiosulfil), and sulfachlorpyridazine (Sonilyn). All of these drugs are given in doses of 1 to 4 g initially to adults, followed usually by 1 g every 4 to 8 hours to maintain blood concentrations of approximately 10 mg/100 ml. The half-life of these drugs is from 4 to 7 hours, with sulfadiazine having a somewhat shorter half-life.

Pharmacokinetics

The volume of distribution of most sulfonamides approaches that of total body water, and the drugs penetrate cells. Metabolism of these drugs involves acetylation of the free *p*-amino group. The acetylated metabolite has no antimicrobial activity and may be less soluble in the urine.

In plasma, the sulfonamides are partially bound to proteins, and only the free fraction is active on bacteria. The kidney filters the free fraction through the glomeruli, and the tubules reabsorb a portion of the filtered drug. The concentration of the sulfonamides in the urine is much higher than in plasma. In fact, it may be 25 to 50 times higher, a circumstance that contributes to the usefulness of these drugs as urinary antimicrobials.

The intermediate-acting sulfonamides, such as sulfamethoxazole have a longer half-life than the short-acting compounds, up to 12 hours. Some longer-acting sulfonamides were introduced also but were removed from the market when severe and long-lasting hypersensitivity reactions were found to be associated with their use.

The relationship between the pH and the solubility of the various sulfonamides results from the fact that these compounds behave as weak acids because of the dissociation of the sulfamyl group ($-SO_2NH-$). Substitutions of the sulfamyl nitrogen can produce considerably stronger acids than sulfanilamide. The salts (ions) of the sulfonamides are much more soluble than the molecular form; thus the solubility of these drugs increases greatly when the pH is above the pK_a of the drug.

The implications of these findings are obvious. The urinary volume must be adequate. Alkalinization with sodium bicarbonate may be necessary. Another approach consists of using mixtures of sulfonamides.

It has been shown that when several sulfonamides are dissolved in water or urine, the presence of one does not influence the solubility of the others.[6,7] The antibacterial effects of such mixtures are additive. Such a therapeutic procedure can produce a higher total sulfonamide concentration in the urine, with diminished tendency for crystal formation.

Although the toxicity of the sulfonamides is very low, the drugs can produce hypersensitivity reactions, such as urticaria, rashes, contact dermatitis, and the Stevens-Johnson syndrome.

Toxicity and hypersensitivity

Gastrointestinal effects are fairly common, but central nervous system (CNS) toxicity is rare. Renal toxicity is manifested by nephrosis, crystalluria, and hematuria. Maintenance of adequate urinary output and alkalinization of the urine are important in the prevention of renal toxicity of the sulfonamides.

These drugs can also cause blood dyscrasias and, rarely, hepatic damage. Periarteritis nodosa has been attributed to sulfonamide therapy in some cases.

Drug interactions   Sulfonamides and methenamines should not be administered simultaneously for the treatment of urinary tract infections, since formaldehyde liberated from methenamine in acid urine forms a precipitate with some of the sulfonamides. The binding of sulfonamides by plasma proteins leads to displacement of other drugs and may cause increased drug effects. Thus the actions of tolbutamide may be intensified, and kernicterus may be caused by the sulfonamides. The action of coumarins may also be intensified.

Clinical uses   Sulfadiazine is usually administered in the form of 0.5 g tablets. The daily adult dose is 4 to 6 g. The soluble sodium salt of sulfadiazine is available for intravenous injection.

Bacteria can develop resistance to the sulfonamides. The mechanism of resistance may be related to the ability of the bacteria to produce antagonists to the drug. In some cases increased production of p-aminobenzoic acid by the resistant organism has been demonstrated.

Comparison of sulfonamides   The earlier sulfonamides, **sulfapyridine** and **sulfathiazole,** have been largely eliminated from clinical use because of greater toxicity and much greater incidence of hypersensitivity reactions.

Sulfamerazine and **sulfamethazine** resemble sulfadiazine in most respects, except for the fact that they are excreted more slowly by the kidney and are bound to plasma proteins to a much greater extent. The main usefulness of these methylated sulfadiazines is their inclusion in the **triple-sulfonamide mixtures.**

In minimizing the renal complications caused by insolubility of the drugs, the physician has a choice between using the triple-sulfonamide mixtures and using some of the new sulfonamides that are more soluble.

Sulfisoxazole (Gantrisin) has similar antibacterial properties to those of sulfadiazine. Its solubility at pH 6 is much greater than that of sulfadiazine. In fact, it is more than 10 times as soluble. At pH 5.5 its solubility in human urine is only about 120 mg/100 ml, which is still four times as great as the solubility of sulfadiazine but is no guarantee against crystal formation. Sulfisoxazole is cleared rather rapidly from the blood and produces high urinary levels.

Acetyl sulfisoxazole (Gantrisin acetyl) differs from sulfisoxazole mainly in being tasteless and suitable for liquid oral preparations. The drug is deacetylated in the intestine, and the active drug is absorbed. **Sulfisoxazole diolamine** (Gantrisin diolamine) is less irritating and is thus suitable for topical use. **Sulfamethoxazole**

(Gantanol), a congener of sulfisoxazole, is more slowly absorbed and excreted than the parent drug. It may cause crystalluria.

Other soluble sulfonamides that are used primarily for urinary tract infections are **sulfamethizole** (Thiosulfil), **sulfisomidine** (Elkosin), and **sulfachloropyridazine** (Sonilyn). **Sulfacetamide** (Sulfamyd) is quite soluble also but is useful primarily as a topical drug in ophthalmic infections, being less effective for the treatment of urinary tract infections.

The slowly excreted sulfonamides such as sulfamethoxypyridazine (Kynex) and sulfadimethoxine (Madribon) are no longer used in this country because of the hypersensitivity reactions associated with them. The slow excretion of these drugs is a consequence of their high protein binding.

Trimethoprim-sulfamethoxazole

The **trimethoprim-sulfamethoxazole** preparation (co-trimoxazole; Bactrim, Septra) exerts a truly synergistic effect on bacteria. The sulfonamide in the combination inhibits the utilization of p-aminobenzoic acid in the synthesis of folic acid, while trimethoprim blocks the conversion of dihydrofolic acid to tetrahydrofolic acid by the enzyme dihydrofolate reductase. Thus the preparation blocks two consecutive steps in bacterial metabolism. Trimethoprim has a much greater affinity for the bacterial than the mammalian enzyme.

Trimethoprim-sulfamethoxazole (Bactrim, Septra) is effective against a large variety of gram-positive and gram-negative microorganisms. Acute and chronic urinary tract infections are prime indications. The drug preparation is effective also in the treatment of typhoid and paratyphoid fever, bacterial infections of the upper respiratory tract, uncomplicated gonorrhea, vivax and falciparum malaria, and others.[17]

Absorption of trimethoprim-sulfamethoxazole is rapid, and effective concentrations of the drugs may be present in plasma for 6 to 8 hours. Both drugs are excreted mostly unchanged in the urine, although most of the sulfamethoxazole is secreted in the acetylated form.

All the adverse effects reported following the use of the sulfonamides may occur when trimethoprim-sulfamethoxazole is used. Skin rashes, mild CNS disturbances, and blood dyscrasias have been reported. Crystalluria may occur but is not likely. The preparation is contraindicated in patients with blood dyscrasias, hepatic damage, and severe renal impairment. It should probably not be used in pregnant women, since folic acid inhibitors are teratogenic experimentally. The drug combination should be used cautiously in patients who have a low folic acid level such as malnutrition states or as a consequence of the ingestion of phenytoin or some other drugs.

Bactrim and Septra are available in tablets containing trimethoprim, 80 mg, and sulfamethoxazole, 400 mg.

Topical sulfonamides

The topical application of sulfonamides is generally undesirable because the effectiveness of the drugs is antagonized by pus and sensitization is common. An exception to this statement is **mafenide** (Sulfamylon).

Mafenide acetate (Sulfamylon acetate) and **mafenide hydrochloride** (Sulfamylon hydrochloride) are used when applied topically to infected wounds and for the treatment of burns. These drugs are not inactivated by pus or p-aminobenzoic acid. The acetate is available as a cream and the hydrochloride as a topical solution. Structurally mafenide differs from all other useful sulfonamides in that it is α-amino-p-toluenesulfonamide rather than a benzenesulfonamide.

Silver sulfadiazine is another topical preparation that is used effectively in patients with second and third degree burns.[16]

Problem 52-1. Ten burned patients were treated with topical mafenide acetate cream. The urine became persistently alkaline in nine of the ten patients. What was the probable mechanism? Mafenide is absorbed in part and acts as a carbonic anhydrase inhibitor.[12]

Sulfonamides as intestinal antiseptics

Sulfonamides that are poorly absorbed from the intestine may be used for decreasing intestinal bacterial flora.

Succinylsulfathiazole (Sulfasuxidine) and **phthalylsulfathiazole** (Sulfathalidine) are substituted in the p-amino portion of the sulfathiazole molecule. As a consequence, they have no antibacterial activity in the test tube. However, when they are swallowed and reach the large intestine, they are hydrolyzed, and the free sulfathiazole reaches high local concentrations. The sulfathiazole is not well absorbed from the large intestine.

The coliform and clostridia organisms are markedly decreased in the intestine, and the volume and character of the feces change when these intestinal antiseptic sulfonamides are administered for several days. Certain organisms such as *Proteus*, *Pseudomonas*, *Salmonella*, and enterococci may be resistant to the action of these drugs.

The usual doses for adults are 0.125 to 0.25 g/kg. The antibiotic neomycin, given orally, has largely replaced the sulfonamides in intestinal antisepsis.

Sulfonamides for special uses

Sulfapyridine has only one indication. The drug is useful in dermatitis herpetiformis by a mechanism unrelated to its antibacterial activity. Similarly, **sulfasalazine** (salicylazosulfapyridine; Azulfidine) is commonly used in the treatment of ulcerative colitis. In this condition, the drug apparently does not act as an antimicrobial agent, or at least, its effect on the intestinal flora cannot explain its usefulness.

ANTIBACTERIAL AGENTS FOR URINARY TRACT INFECTIONS

In addition to the sulfonamides, a number of antibacterial agents are used almost exclusively in the treatment of urinary tract infections. Their major characteristics are summarized in Table 52-2.

Nitrofurantoin (Furadantin) is one of a series of nitrofurans that have been introduced as antibacterial agents.

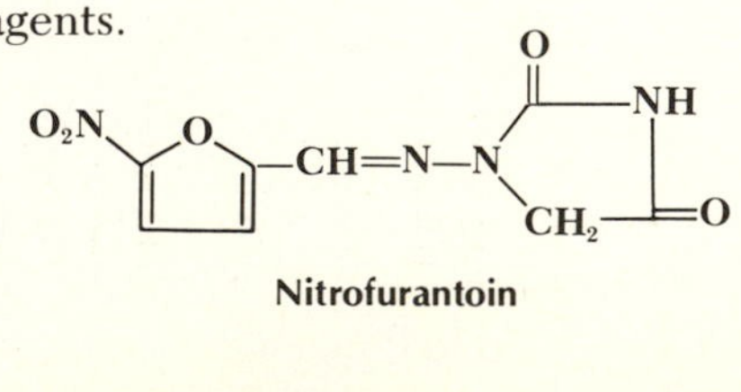

Nitrofurantoin

TABLE 52-2. Antibacterial agents used principally for urinary tract infections*

Drug	Activity spectrum and characteristics	Dosage	Route	Side effects
Sulfonamides	Short-acting sulfonamides are best because of high urinary concentration and good solubility at acid pH; more active in alkaline urine; especially effective against *E. coli* and *P. mirabilis*; many strains of *Klebsiella, Aerobacter, Proteus,* and *Pseudomonas* are resistant Sulfisoxazole (Gantrisin) Sulfamethizole (Thiosulfil) Sulfisomidine (Elkosin) Sulfachloropyridazine (Sonilyn) Sulfamethoxazole (Gantanol) Trimethoprim-sulfamethoxazole	Varies with drug	Oral	Allergic reactions; skin rash, drug fever, pruritus, photosensitization; periarteritis nodosa, S.L.E., Stevens-Johnson syndrome, serum sickness syndrome, myocarditis; neurotoxicity (psychosis, neuritis); hepatotoxicity; blood dyscrasias, usually agranulocytosis; crystalluria; nausea and vomiting, headache, dizziness, lassitude, mental depression, acidosis, sulfhemoglobin; hemolytic anemia in G6PD-deficient individuals; possible teratogenic effects; should not be used in newborn infants or in women near term
Nitrofurantoin (Furadantin)	Many gram-positive and gram-negative organisms; as relates to urinary tract, nitrofurantoin is effective against likely pathogens except *Pseudomonas* and some *Klebsiella-Enterobacter* and *Proteus* species; high urinary concentration (ineffective in renal failure); increased activity in acid urine; action much reduced at pH 8 or over	100 mg q6h (5-7 mg/kg)	Oral Intravenous	Nausea and vomiting, hypersensitivity, peripheral neuropathy, pulmonary infiltrate, intrahepatic cholestasis, hemolytic anemia in G6PD deficiency; contraindicated in renal failure; should not be used in infants less than 1 month of age
Methenamine mandelate (Mandelamine)	Combination effect against most organisms in vitro; methenamine has no action per se but in acid medium is slowly decomposed with liberation of formaldehyde; mandelic acid also requires acid pH; effective only when acid urine (preferably about pH 5) can be maintained; limited place in therapy; should not be used in tissue infection (pyelonephritis)	1 g q6h	Oral	Nausea and vomiting; contraindicated in renal failure because it leads to acidosis; should not be used with sulfonamides
Nalidixic acid (NegGram)	Gram-negative urinary tract pathogens (*Enterobacteriaceae*) except *Pseudomonas*; high degree of resistance may develop rapidly during therapy	1 g q6h	Oral	GI hypersensitivity, fever, eosinophilia, photosensitivity, neurological disturbances (malaise, drowsiness, dizziness, visual disturbances); convulsions pseudomotor cerebri (?); mild leukopenia, thrombocytopenia, hemolytic anemia; can produce false elevations of 17-ketosteroids and 17-ketogenic steroids in urine

*Courtesy Dr. Jay P. Sanford, Washington, D.C.

The drug is absorbed rapidly, and much of it is excreted unchanged in the urine. It has a wide antibacterial spectrum, and both gram-positive and gram-negative bacteria can be inhibited at levels that are obtainable in the urine following the daily oral administration of 5 to 10 mg/kg. It may cause a variety of sensitivity reactions: nausea and vomiting, skin sensitization, peripheral neuritis, and cholestatic jaundice. A macrocrystalline preparation (Macrodantin) may be less nauseating. The sodium salt of nitrofurantoin may be administered intravenously.

Preparations of **nitrofurantoin** as Furadantin include tablets containing 50 and 100 mg and a suspension, 25 mg/5 ml; and as Macrodantin, capsules containing 50 and 100 mg. **Nitrofurantoin sodium** (Furadantin sodium) is available for intravenous injection as a powder, 180 mg in 20 ml containers.

No bacteriostatic blood levels are produced following oral administration of nitrofurantoin. Its use in systemic infections is not supported by the available evidence.[10]

Drugs related to nitrofurantoin are available for special applications. **Nitrofurazone** (Furacin) is used topically for infections of the skin, but it may cause sensitization. **Furazolidone** is used orally for bacterial and giardial intestinal infections. Furazolidone is an inhibitor of monoamine oxidase, and foods rich in tyramine should be avoided when the drug is used. It may also cause disulfiram-like reactions when alcohol is ingested. **Furazolidone** (Furoxone) is available in tablets containing 100 mg.

Methenamine mandelate (Mandelamine) is a combination of two fairly old urinary antiseptics, methenamine (Urotropin) and mandelic acid.

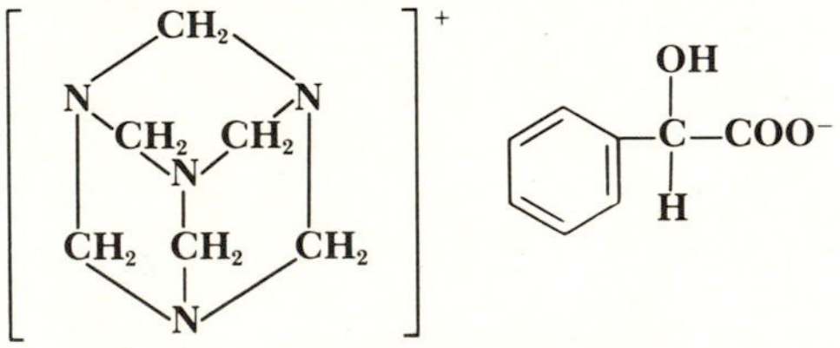

Methenamine mandelate

Methenamine, or hexamethylenetetramine,, liberates *formaldehyde* in acid urine. Mandelic acid also is bactericidal if the pH of the urine is low. If the pH of the urine is higher than 6, it is necessary to administer ammonium chloride in amounts of 0.5 to 1 g three or four times daily.

Methenamine mandelate is relatively nontoxic, but gastric irritation may occur following its use. This is probably related to production of some formaldehyde in the acid gastric juice. For the same reason urinary frequency may also occur. The usual dose of methenamine mandelate is 0.5 to 1 g three times a day.

In addition to methenamine mandelate (Mandelamine), the hippurate salt of methenamine (Hiprex) is also available.

Nalidixic acid (NegGram), a relatively new drug, is chemically unrelated to other urinary antiseptics.[2] It is well absorbed from the gastrointestinal tract and is largely excreted in the urine, in part as glucuronide.

Nalidixic acid is effective only against gram-negative bacteria such as *E. coli*, *Proteus*, and some strains of *Pseudomonas*, *Enterobacter*, and *Klebsiella*. Resistance to the drug develops readily. Nalidixic acid is ineffective against systemic infections because its activity is greatly reduced in the presence of proteins.

Nausea, vomiting, diarrhea, allergic reactions, and neurological disturbances may occur as a consequence of the administration of nalidixic acid.

Preparations of **nalidixic acid** (NegGram) include tablets of 250 and 500 mg.

Nalidixic acid

Oxolinic acid (Utibid) is a quinoline derivative, similar in indications and actions to nalidixic acid. It is effective in the treatment of gram-negative urinary tract infections caused by susceptible organisms. The drug may cause CNS side effects. It is available in 750 mg tablets.

REFERENCES

1 Bell, P. H., and Robin, R. O., Jr.: Studies in chemotherapy: a theory of the relation of structure to activity of sulfanilamide type compounds, J. Am. Chem. Soc. **64**:2905, 1942.

2 Carroll, G.: NegGram (nalidixic acid), a new antimicrobial chemotherapeutic agent, J. Urol. **90**:476, 1963.

3 Davis, B. D.: The binding of sulfonamide drugs by plasma proteins: a factor in determining the distribution of drugs in the body, J. Clin. Invest. **22**:753, 1943.

4 Draper, J. W.: Development of sulfonamides: historical account, Curr. Med. Digest **23**:855, 1965.

5 Knight, V., Draper, J. W., Brady, E. A., and Attmore, C. A.: Methenamine mandelate: antimicrobial activity, absorption and excretion, Antibiot. Chemother. (Basel) **2**:615, 1952.

6 Lehr, D.: Inhibition of drug precipitation in the urinary tract by the use of sulfonamide mixtures; sulfathiazole-sulfadiazine mixture, Proc. Soc. Exp. Biol. Med. **58**:11, 1945.

7 Lehr, D.: Comparative merits of 3,4-dimethyl-5-sulfanilamido-isoxazole (Gantrisin) and a sulfapyrimidine triple mixture (an evaluation of properties important at the bedside), Antibiot. Chemother. (Basel) **3**:71, 1953.

8 Poth, E. J., and Ross, C. A.: The clinical use of phthalylsulfathiazole, J. Lab. Clin. Med. **29**:785, 1944.

9 Richards, W. A., Riss, E., Kass, E. H., and Finland, M.: Nitrofurantoin: clinical and laboratory studies in urinary tract infections, Arch. Intern. Med. **96**:437, 1955.

10 Sanford, J. P.: Nitrofurantoin in extragenitourinary infections? Curr. Ther. Res. **2**:476, 1960.

11 Weinstein, I., Madoff, M. A., and Samet, C. A.: The sulfonamides, N. Engl. J. Med. **263**:793, 842, 1960.

12 White, M. G., and Asch, M. J.: Acid-base effects of topical mafenide acetate in the burned patient, N. Engl. J. Med. **284**:1281, 1971.

13 Woods, D. D.: Relation of p-aminobenzoic acid to mechanism of action of sulphanilamide, Br. J. Exp. Pathol. **21**:74, 1940.

14 Work, T. S., and Work, E.: The basis of chemotherapy, New York, 1948, Interscience Publishers, Inc.

REVIEWS

15 Appel, G. B., and Neu, H. C.: The nephro-toxicity of antimicrobial agents, N. Engl. J. Med. **296:**784, 1977.

16 Ballin, J. C.: Evaluation of a new topical agent for burn therapy, silver sulfadiazine (Silva-dene) J.A.M.A. **230:**1184, 1974.

17 Jones, S. R.: An approach to the management of urinary tract infection, Ration. Drug Ther. **13:**1, Nov., 1979.

18 Schiffman, D. O.: Evaluation of an anti-infec-tive combination: trimethoprim-sulfamethoxa-zole (Bactrim, Septra), J.A.M.A. **231:**635, 1975.

CHAPTER 53

Antibiotic drugs

Among the hundreds of compounds produced by microorganisms that have inhibitory action on other microorganisms, only a relatively small number have a favorable therapeutic index. These are the clinically useful antibiotics. In the present discussion, particular attention will be paid to the potency, antibacterial spectrum, metabolism, and mode of action of these various antibiotic drugs.

PENICILLIN

Penicillin is a highly effective bactericidal antibiotic which has very low toxicity. If it were not for penicillin allergy, the antibiotic would approach perfection for infections caused by susceptible organisms. Penicillin is obtained from cultures of *Penicillium chrysogenum*. The semisynthetic penicillins are made by modification of the mold product.

Penicillin is an organic acid. Its sodium, potassium, and procaine salts are commonly used. There are several other naturally occurring penicillins that differ from penicillin G in having a side chain other than benzyl. Some of these are penicillin F, dihydro F (amylpenicillin), and also K and X. None of these naturally occurring compounds has a significant advantage over penicillin G, and some, such as K, may be much less effective in vivo because of a high degree of plasma protein binding.

Although several biosynthetic penicillins have been prepared by adding various precursors of the side chain to the *Penicillium* culture medium, more recently a new procedure has opened up a field for the preparation of new penicillins. A key intermediate, 6-aminopenicillanic acid, is produced by fermentation, and new penicillins are prepared by adding various groups to this intermediate.

Penicillin has been completely synthesized through cooperative efforts of several groups of workers. Total synthesis is much too difficult for commercial production.

The available penicillins may be placed in several groups. Penicillin G, or benzylpenicillin, is the prototype. Semisynthetic penicillins, which have a broader antibacterial spectrum but are still susceptible to penicillinase, represent an important group. Other semisynthetic penicillins are resistant to penicillinase and are sometimes called *antistaphylococcal penicillins*.

Minor modifications of penicillin G yielded penicillin V, which is more acid resistant but has no great advantages over penicillin G.

The "broad spectrum" penicillins have a greater effect on many gram-negative organisms. They include ampicillin, amoxicillin, carbenicillin, and ticarcillin. This group is still susceptible to penicillinase.

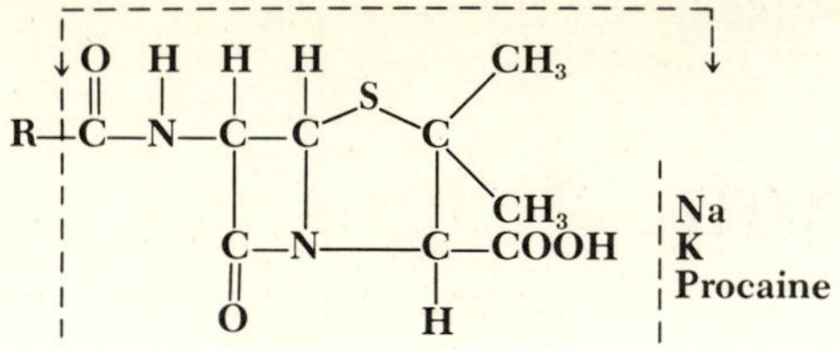

Basic penicillin structure

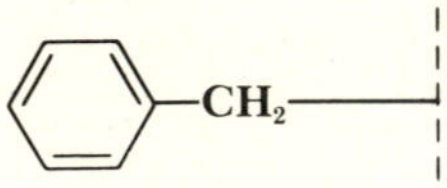

Na
K
Procaine

Penicillin G (benzylpenicillin)

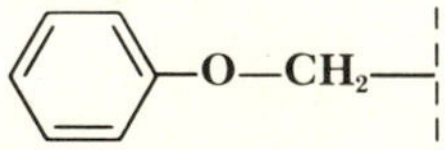

Penicillin V (phenoxymethylpenicillin)

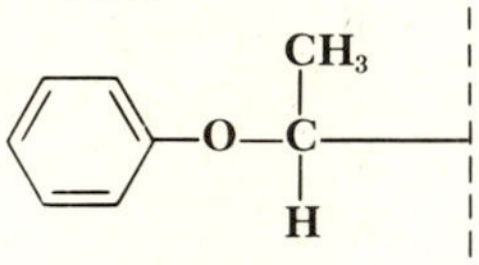

Phenethicillin (Syncillin)

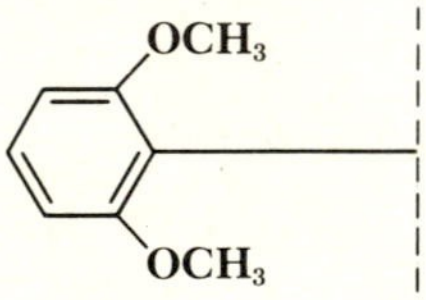

Methicillin (Staphcillin)

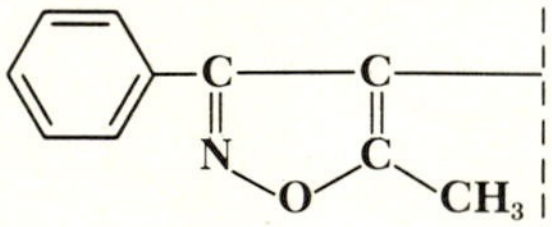

Oxacillin (Prostaphlin)

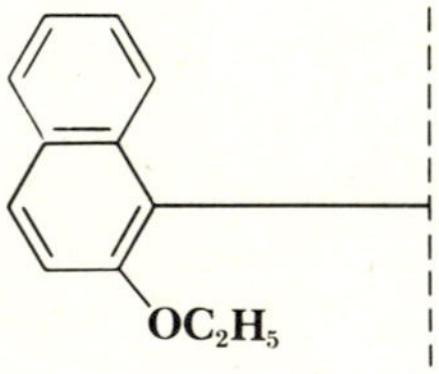

Nafcillin (Unipen)

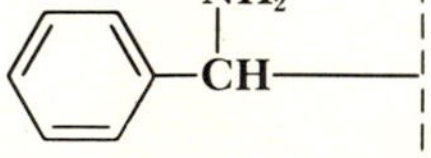

Ampicillin (Polycillin)

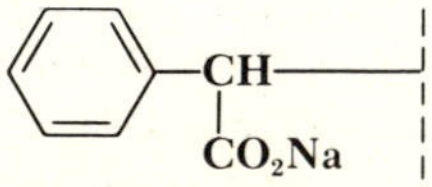

Carbenicillin (Pyopen)

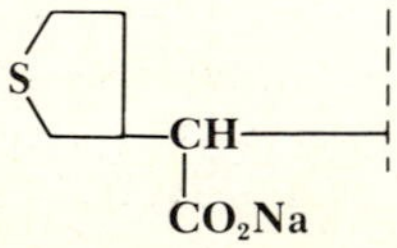

Ticarcillin (Ticar)

The penicillinase-resistant penicillins include oxacillin, cloxacillin, dicloxacillin, methicillin, and nafcillin.

Potency

Penicillin preparations are standardized on the basis of their growth-inhibition potency against test organisms such as *Bacillus subtilis* or staphylococci. Activity is expressed in units and is measured in comparison with a standard preparation by determining the zone of inhibition of bacterial growth on an inoculated agar plate. The amount of activity represented by 1 unit is sufficient to prevent multiplication of a susceptible organism such as *Bacillus subtilis* or certain staphylococci in as much as 20 to 50 ml of broth. One milligram of penicillin G represents 1667 units. This means that 1 unit is equivalent to 0.6 μg of penicillin G.

The enormous activity of penicillin may be appreciated from the fact that if 1 mg of the antibiotic were placed in about 5 gallons of broth, the growth of several susceptible organisms would be prevented by the resulting minute concentration of the antibiotic. By contrast, it would be necessary to add 2 to 20 g of a sulfonamide to this volume of culture medium to obtain similar growth inhibition.

Microorganisms inhibited by less than 1 unit of penicillin/ml may be considered moderately susceptible. The highly susceptible infective agents are usually inhibited by less than 0.1 unit/ml. Blood levels of 0.1 to 1.0 unit/ml can be achieved without difficulty in clinical practice.

Mode of action

Penicillin is a bactericidal antibiotic that inhibits the synthesis of the cell wall of susceptible bacteria. Its basic action is on a transpeptidase in bacteria.

The bactericidal activity of penicillin is quite different from that of the common disinfectants. Penicillin does not kill bacteria rapidly on contact. It apparently produces some alteration in the bacteria that makes them more susceptible to death and disruption. It has been established that rapidly multiplying bacteria are most susceptible to the killing effect of penicillin.

Pharmacokinetics

The absorption of penicillin G from the gastrointestinal tract is incomplete and variable. To obtain comparable blood levels it is usually necessary to administer five times as much of the antibiotic by the oral route as by intramuscular injection. The reasons for this incomplete absorption are inactivation of the drug by the gastric juice and, once it reaches the large intestine, by bacteria as well. Some of the newer penicillin preparations such as penicillin V are fairly resistant to an acid environment.

The absorption of penicillin following oral administration is greatly influenced by the presence of food in the stomach and the rate of gastric emptying. More predictable results are obtained if the drug is taken on an empty stomach.

Blood levels obtained following administration of 100,000 units of penicillin G sodium by various routes are shown in Fig. 53-1. It is clear that very transient high levels reaching 2 to 4 units/ml can be obtained by either the intravenous or intramuscular route. The same dose given orally produces a blood level of only about 0.4 units/ml, but demonstrable activity remains for a longer time.

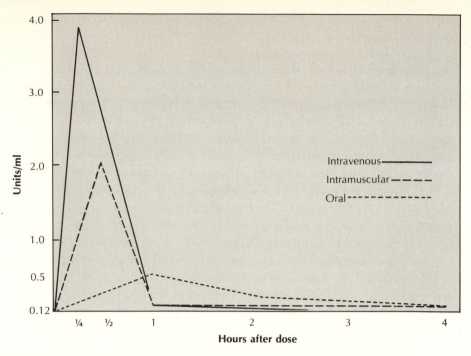

FIG. 53-1. Relative blood serum concentrations of penicillin following intravenous, intramuscular, and oral administration of 100,000 units of crystalline sodium penicillin G. (From Welch, H., et al.: Principles and practice of antibiotic therapy, New York, 1954, Medical Encyclopedia, Inc.)

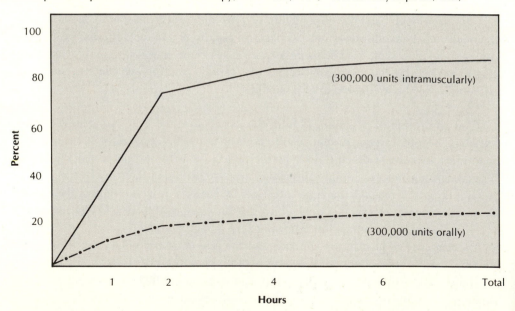

FIG. 53-2. Comparison of cumulative urinary excretion of penicillin following intramuscular and oral administration of crystalline sodium penicillin G. (From Welch, H., et al.: Principles and practice of antibiotic therapy, New York, 1954, Medical Encyclopedia, Inc.)

The rapid decline of penicillin blood levels results from rapid renal clearance of the antibiotic. It has been well established that penicillin is actively secreted by the renal tubules, apparently by the same mechanism as p-aminohippurate or iodopyracet (Diodrast). Drugs have been developed that can block this tubular secretory mechanism. One of these is probenecid (Benemid), which is quite effective. It is of little use in penicillin therapy, however, since it is just as easy to use larger doses of penicillin as to administer a second drug for the purpose of preventing its excretion. Probenecid, on the other hand, has an important clinical application as a uricosuric drug.

A number of repository preparations of penicillin are available for the purpose of producing sustained blood levels. Procaine penicillin G and benzathine penicillin G are two such preparations. With the latter preparation, demonstrable penicillin blood levels can be maintained for as long as 20 days. It is important to keep in mind, however, that demonstrable blood levels are often defined as 0.03 unit/ml or more. This low concentration of the antibiotic may not suffice in many infections, although it may be beneficial in prevention of streptococcal infections and prophylaxis of rheumatic fever.

Distribution of penicillin in the body is far from uniform. First, the antibiotic is partially bound to plasma proteins. Under normal circumstances it penetrates poorly into the cerebrospinal fluid, aqueous humor, and joint fluids. On the other hand, inflammation at these various sites greatly increases the permeability to penicillin.

The cumulative urinary excretion of sodium penicillin G following its oral and intramuscular administration is shown in Fig. 53-2. As much as 80% of the intramuscularly administered dose may be recovered in the urine in less than 4 hours. Only about 20% is usually recovered following the oral administration of the antibiotic. With oral administration, this difference results from lack of absorption of much of the administered dose.

The inherent toxicity of penicillin as determined in animal experiments is extremely low. In several animal species the acute toxicity of penicillin is so low that death from overdosage has been attributed to the cation rather than to penicillin itself.

Toxicity and hypersensitivity

Unfortunately, however, a significant percentage of the human population shows hypersensitivity reactions to penicillin. These reactions are of many different types, ranging from immediate anaphylactic reactions to late manifestations of the serum sickness type. It is believed that several hundred severe anaphylactic reactions have occurred following penicillin injections, many terminating fatally.

Hypersensitivity reactions are seen most often following topical use of penicillin and most rarely after oral administration. The incidence of such reactions has been estimated to vary from 1% to 8% in the general population.

Skin tests for the determination of penicillin allergy are unreliable and dangerous when penicillin G itself is injected in small quantities intracutaneously. On the other hand, preparations are available, at least for experimental purposes, in which penicilloylpolylysine (PPL) is suitable for testing allergy to the major determinant. Also, a mixture of penicillin, penicilloate, and other products is suitable for testing allergy to the minor determinants. Despite these refinements in diagnosing penicillin allergy, tests are not completely reliable. As a consequence, the history of previous reactions is very important, and even in the presence of a negative intradermal test, it is best to be prepared for the possibility of anaphylactic reaction whenever the antibiotic is injected.

In addition to hypersensitivity reactions, penicillin is capable of producing other adverse effects. Neural tissue may be susceptible to penicillin, particularly when the drug is injected intrathecally or applied directly to the surface of the brain. Convulsive phenomena have been noted following such procedures. There is seldom any reason for injecting penicillin intrathecally.

Broad-spectrum penicillins susceptible to penicillinase

Ampicillin (Penbritin, Omnipen, Polycillin) differs from penicillin G mainly in having a greater effect on many gram-negative microorganisms. Also the drug is more acid resistant and is absorbed better following oral administration. Ampicillin is effective in the treatment of urinary tract infections caused by *Escherichia coli* and *Proteus mirabilis* (susceptible strains). The antibiotic is also effective in the treatment of respiratory infections and meningitis caused by susceptible *Hemophilus* strains. Ampicillin may cause skin rash in 10% of patients, especially if the patient has infectious mononucleosis. Some rashes produced by ampicillin may not be allergic. Ampicillin is available in capsules, 250 and 500 mg. The sodium salt is available for intramuscular and intravenous administration.

Amoxicillin trihydrate (Amoxil, Larotid) differs from ampicillin only in producing somewhat higher serum concentrations, and it may be better absorbed in children.

Carbenicillin disodium (Geopen) differs from ampicillin in its greater activity against *Pseudomonas aeruginosa* and *Bacteroides fragilis*. Also it may be active against strains of *Hemophilus* and *Proteus* that are resistant to ampicillin. A special feature of carbenicillin is its high sodium content. Since 1 g of the antibiotic contains 6 mEq of sodium, large doses may cause sodium overload in renal and cardiac patients. Carbenicillin disodium (Geopen) should not be given orally, since it is not absorbed. **Carbenicillin indanyl sodium** (Geocillin) is available in tablets for oral administration but is not commonly used.

Ticarcillin disodium (Ticar) is closely related to carbenicillin and is available for intramuscular and intravenous use. It may have somewhat greater potency against the difficult gram-negative bacilli than carbenicillin.

Penicillins resistant to penicillinase

The penicillinase-resistant penicillins are very useful in the treatment of infections caused by organisms that are resistant to penicillin G, such as hospital-acquired staphylococcal infections. If the organism turns out to be susceptible to penicillin G, it is best to switch because of its lower cost and some other advantages. Although these penicillins are resistant to staphylococcal penicillinase, a few strains appeared, which developed "methicillin resistance" not based on penicillinase.

TABLE 53-1. Summary of current usage of penicillins and cephalosporins*

Agent generic name (trade name)	Spectrum of activity	Usual adult dosage (GI absorption)	Route	Mode of action (cidal or static)	Side effects
Ampicillin	Gram-positive (*not* resistant staph), gram-negative (especially *H. influenzae*)	0.25-0.5 g q6h 150-200 mg/kg/day	Oral Intramuscular Intravenous	Cidal	GI, skin rash (especially in patients with infectious mono), fever, rate ↑ SGOT, anaphylactoid reactions, convulsions (with excessively rapid IV)
Carbenicillin (Pyopen, Geopen)	Gram-positive (*not* resistant staph), gram-negative (especially *Pseudomonas, Proteus, E. coli, Enterobacter, H. influenzae*, not *Klebsiella*)	5.0 g q4h given over 2 hour period (nonabsorbed)	Intravenous	Cidal	Similar to other penicillins, ↑ SGOT, nausea, neutropenia, hemolytic anemia, convulsions (high dose in patients with renal failure), possible abnormalities in coagulation tests (high dose in patients with uremia) [Note: 4.7 mEq (108 mg) Na+/g], possible hypokalemia
Cephalothin (Keflin)	Gram-positive, gram-negative (especially *E. coli, P. mirabilis*), *not* enterococci, indole positive *Proteus, Pseudomonas*	0.5-3.0 g q6h (nonabsorbed)	Intramuscular Intravenous	Cidal	Rash, fever, eosinophilia, ↑ SGOT, neutropenia, anaphylactoid reactions, convulsions (high dose in patients with renal failure), positive Coombs test, thrombocytopenia, false positive "Clinitest," phlebitis
Cephaloridine (Loridine)	Gram-positive (variable against resistant staph), gram-negative (especially *E. coli, P. mirabilis*)	0.5-1.0 g q6-8h (nonabsorbed)	Intramuscular Intravenous	Cidal	Rash, eosinophilia, acute tubular necrosis, ↑ SGOT, neutropenia, anaphylactoid reactions, rare nausea and vomiting
Cephalexin (Keflex)	Gram-positive (not enterococci variable against resistant staph and *Neisseriae*), gram-negative (urinary infections due to most *E. coli, P. mirabilis*, and some *Klebsiella*; variable against *Salmonella* and *Shigella*)	0.25-0.5 g q6h	Oral	Cidal	Similar to other cephalosporins

Continued.

*Courtesy Dr. Jay P. Sanford, Washington, D.C.

TABLE 53-1. Summary of current usage of penicillins and cephalosporins—cont'd

Agent generic name (trade name)	Spectrum of activity	Usual adult dosage (GI absorption)	Route	Mode of action (cidal or static)	Side effects
Cefazolin (Ancef, Kefzol)	Similar to cephalothin	0.25 g q8h to 1.0 g q6h	Intramuscular, Intravenous	Cidal	Rash (uncommon), ↑ SGOT, ↑ alkaline phosphatase
Methicillin (Staphcillin, Dimocillin)	Gram-positive, especially staph	1-2 g q6h (nonabsorbed)	Intramuscular, Intravenous	Cidal	Similar to penicillin G plus eosinophilia, leukopenia, nephrotoxicity, Coombs positive hemolytic anemia
Oxacillin (Prostaphlin or Resistopen)	Gram-positive, especially staph	0.5-1.0 g q4-6h	Oral, Intramuscular, Intravenous	Cidal	Occasional GI, fever, skin rash, asymptomatic ↑ SGOT, ↓ hemoglobin, neutropenia; transient hematuria (infants)
Dicloxacillin (Dynapen, Pathocil, Veracillin)	Gram-positive, especially staph	0.125-0.5 g q6h ac	Oral	Cidal	Similar to cloxacillin
Nafcillin (Unipen)	Gram-positive, especially staph	0.25-1.0 g q6h ac; 0.5-1.0 g q4-6h	Oral, Intramuscular, Intravenous	Cidal	GI, fever, skin rash, asymptomatic ↑ SGOT
Hetacillin	Same as ampicillin	0.225 g q6h	Oral	Cidal	Same as ampicillin
Penicillin G	Gram-positive, gram-negative, E. coli, P. mirabilis, H. influenzae; Shigella and Salmonella in high concentration	Usual dose 600,000 to 1 million U; Large dose 10-12 million U; Usual dose 1 million U (1 g) before meals	Intramuscular, Intravenous, Oral	Cidal	Anaphylactoid reactions, drug fever, skin rashes, Coombs positive hemolytic anemia; Skin rashes, convulsions (high dose, especially in renal failure); GI—uncommon
Benzathine penicillin G (Bicillin)		600,000 to 1 million U	Intramuscular	Cidal	As above, plus local reactions

Methicillin was the first penicillinase-resistant penicillin and is still used. However, nafcillin is the most potent antibiotic in this group.

Methicillin sodium (Staphcillin) is administered intramuscularly or intravenously, and the drug is quite unstable in solution. Its only advantage is in infections caused by staphylococci that are resistant to penicillin G. The antibiotic may have some nephrotoxic potential.

Nafcillin sodium (Unipen, Nafcil) may be administered orally, intramuscularly, or intravenously. It is more potent than methicillin, it may penetrate the spinal fluid better, and it is largely excreted in the bile.

Oxacillin sodium (Prostaphlin, Bactocill) is very similar in actions and indications to nafcillin. It may be given orally or parenterally. **Cloxacillin sodium** (Tegopen, Cloxapen) and **Dicloxacillin sodium** (Dynapen, Dycill) are very similar to oxacillin and are available in capsules for oral administration.

CEPHALOSPORINS

The cephalosporins are β-lactam antibiotics obtained originally from a *cephalosporium* mold. These antibiotics have the same mechanism of action as the penicillins, but differ in antibacterial spectrum, in resistance to β-lactamase, and also in pharmacokinetics. Whereas the penicillins are derivatives of 6-aminopenicillanic acid, the cephalosporins are derivatives of 7-aminocephalosporanic acid. The related cephamycins have a 7-α-methoxy group, which may increase their resistance to β-lactamases.

The antibacterial spectrum of the cephalosporins is similar to that of the penicillinase-resistant penicillins, except that they are less effective against *Hemophilus influenzae*, and they are ineffective against *Pseudomonas*, several species of *Proteus*, *Klebsiella*, *B. fragilis*, and enterococci.

Because of their broad antibacterial spectrum and resistance to β-lactamase, the cephalosporins are being greatly overused in clinical situations in which the penicillins would be just as effective and less costly. For example, the cephalosporins do not penetrate well into the cerebrospinal fluid even in meningitis and they do not enter ocular fluids well.

The cephalosporins are eliminated both by glomerular filtration and tubular secretion. Probenecid prolongs the half-life of these drugs as does renal impairment. The cephalosporins may cause bone marrow depression and some of them, particularly cephaloridine, may cause renal tubular necrosis.

The cephalosporins are best classified on the basis of their mode of administration. The *orally administered* members of the group include **cephalexin monohydrate** (Keflex), **cephaloglycin dihydrate** (Kafocin), **cefaclor** (Ceclor), and **cefadroxil monohydrate** (Duricef). The *parenteral* cephalosporins include **cephalothin sodium** (Keflin), **sterile cephapirin sodium** (Cefadyl), **Cephacetrile sodium** (Celospor), **sterile cefazolin sodium** (Ancef, Kefzol), **cefamandole nafate** (Mandol), and the cephamycin **cefoxitin sodium** (Mefoxin). Finally, **cephradine** (Anspor, Velosef) can be administered either orally or parenterally.

Comparison of cephalosporins

The increasing number of cephalosporins are basically similar in their indications and uses. A physician could become familiar with one oral and one parenteral drug without having to learn about all members of the group. It should be remembered that these antibiotics should not be considered drugs of first choice in most infections, although they may be very useful in the prevention of infections in surgery. However, for this indication, the cephalosporins should not be given for prolonged periods before and after surgery.

Cephalothin and cephapirin are not significantly different as regards pharmacokinetics, potency, and indications. Cefazolin gives higher serum levels, although it is bound to proteins to a greater extent and has a serum half-life of 1.8 hours compared to 0.5 hour for cephalothin. It is also claimed to penetrate human tissues, such as bone and bile more effectively, although it does not penetrate into the cerebrospinal fluid.

The newer cephalosporins, cefamandole and cefoxitin (a cephamycin), may have somewhat greater effectiveness in certain gram-negative bacillary infections but are less active against penicillinase-producing staphylococci. Cefoxitin is the most active drug in this class against *B. fragilis*.

There is clearly a clinical equivalence between cephalexin and cephradine, and cephalothin and cephapirin. The newer cephalosporins, cefamandole and cefoxitin, should be reserved for situations in which they offer clear-cut advantages.

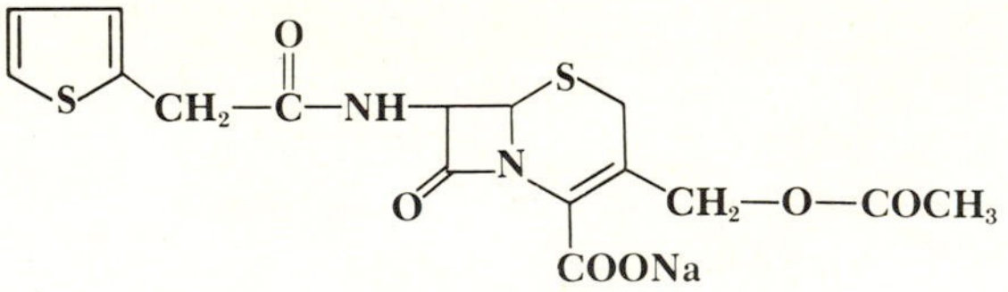

Cephalothin

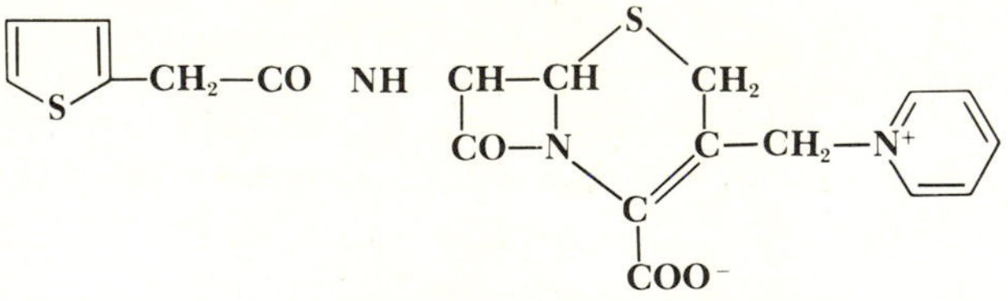

Cephaloridine

AMINOGLYCO-SIDES

The aminoglycoside antibiotics—streptomycin, neomycin, kanamycin, gentamicin, and tobramycin—are bactericidal drugs, which are indicated for the treatment of serious infections caused by many gram-negative bacilli and some gram-positive organisms. However, for the latter indications penicillin and the cephalosporins may be preferable. The aminoglycosides have a broad antibacterial spectrum, but streptococci, pneumococci, clostridia, *Bacteroides*, and fungi are usually resistant. The essential features of several aminoglycosides are shown in Table 53-2.

TABLE 53-2. Summary of characteristics of aminoglycosides*

Agent generic name (trade name)	Spectrum of activity	Usual adult dosage (GI absorption)	Route	Mode of action (cidal or static)	Side effects
Streptomycin	Gram-positive, gram-negative, TBC	0.5-2.0 g/day (nonabsorbed)	Intramuscular	Cidal	Vestibular damage, auditory damage, drug fever, neuromuscular blockade, skin rash, circumoral paresthesias with flushing
Neomycin	Similar to kanamycin				
Kanamycin (Kantrex)	Gram-positive, gram-negative, TBC; especially staph-resistant	15 mg/kg/day divided q6h (nonabsorbed)	Intramuscular Intravenous	Cidal	Ototoxicity (auditory), nephrotoxicity, neuromuscular blockade, skin rash (rare)
Gentamicin (Garamycin)	Gram-positive, gram-negative (both *Proteus* and *Pseudomonas*)	0.8-5.0 mg/kg/day divided q8h (nonabsorbed)	Intramuscular Intravenous	Cidal	Nephrotoxicity (protein ↑ BUN), vestibular toxicity, fever, skin rash: avoid concurrent use with ethacrynic acid

*Courtesy Dr. Jay P. Sanford, Washington, D.C.

The aminoglycosides include streptomycin, gentamicin, kanamycin, neomycin, tobramycin, paromomycin, and spectinomycin. The most commonly used antibiotic in this group is gentamicin. **General features**

The aminoglycosides are not absorbed well following oral administration. For that reason they are generally administered intramuscularly or intravenously except in the case of neomycin and paromomycin, which have some usefulness in decreasing the intestinal flora. The aminoglycosides are not greatly bound to serum proteins and are well distributed in the body. However, their penetration into the spinal fluid may not be good enough for some therapeutic purposes. The aminoglycosides are excreted by glomerular filtration without tubular reabsorption.

The aminoglycosides are ototoxic and nephrotoxic and may cause neuromuscular blockade. Ototoxicity reflects itself in vestibular and auditory disturbances by damage to the sensory receptors, such as the hair cells in the cochlea. Whereas streptomycin and neomycin primarily affect vestibular function, kanamycin has relatively greater auditory toxicity. These drugs may cause dose-related changes in vestibular and auditory function, ranging from disturbances in equilibration and tinnitus to permanent deafness.

Nephrotoxicity may range from proteinuria to severe azotemia but is usually reversible. Since the aminoglycosides are excreted by the kidney, preexisting renal damage calls for caution and readjustment of dosage schedules.

The neuromuscular blocking effect of the aminoglycosides may lead to apnea, particularly in *myasthenia gravis* or with certain general anesthetics and neuromuscular blocking agents. Intravenous calcium gluconate is effective in antagonizing neuromuscular effects of the aminoglycosides and neostigmine may be useful.

Resistance develops rapidly to the antibacterial action of streptomycin and more slowly to the other aminoglycosides. Resistance to one aminoglycoside does not necessarily mean resistance to all. Plasmids mediate resistance in most cases. They induce the production of enzymes that acetylate or phosphorylate the aminoglycoside. These enzymes may be specific for some but not all of the aminoglycosides. For example, some organisms, such as the *Pseudomonas*, may be resistant to gentamicin but may be susceptible to amikacin.

Streptomycin   Streptomycin, discovered in 1944,[50] differs from penicillin in being an organic base rather than an acid. It is not absorbed from the gastrointestinal tract, has a much broader antibacterial spectrum although a generally lower potency, and has direct toxic effects in the mammal. At present the main usefulness of this antibiotic is in the treatment of tuberculosis and in combination with penicillin, in which the synergism between the two drugs may be of great importance in selected cases.

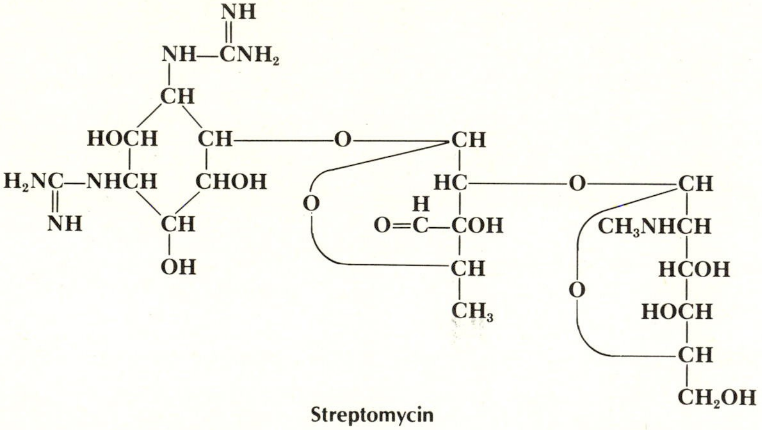

Streptomycin

Gentamicin and Tobramycin   Gentamicin sulfate (Garamycin) and tobramycin sulfate (Nebcin) are very similar chemically and pharmacologically. Their main difference is the greater potency of tobramycin against *Pseudomonas aeruginosa*.

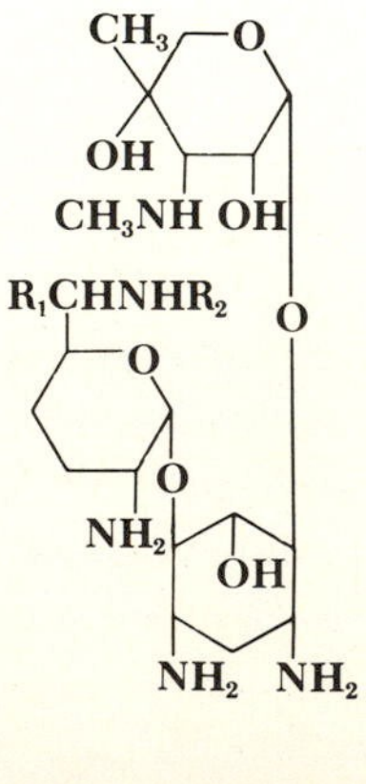

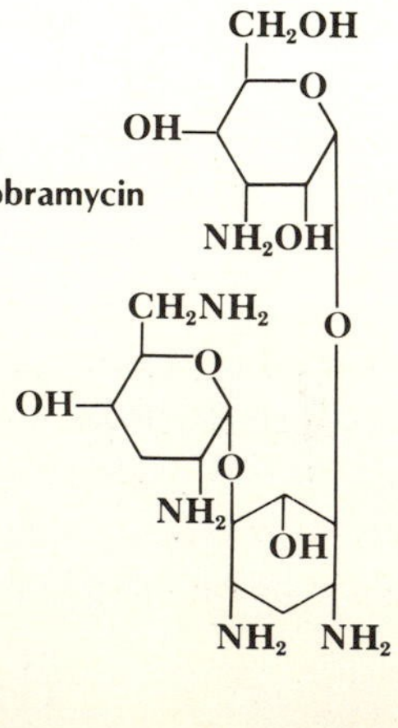

The major usefulness of gentamicin and tobramycin is in the treatment of systemic infections caused by susceptible gram-negative bacteria. Streptococci, pneumococci, anaerobic bacteria, and fungi are resistant. In the clinical use of these drugs, renal elimination, nephrotoxicity, ototoxicity, and neuromuscular dysfunction should be taken into consideration. In addition, gentamicin should not be mixed with carbenicillin or heparin.

Gentamicin sulfate (Garamycin) is available in solutions containing 20 mg/ml and in disposable syringes. Tobramycin sulfate (Nebcin) is available in solutions containing 10 or 40 mg/ml and in disposable syringes. The dosage for adults with normal renal function of either drug is 3 to 5 mg/kg daily in divided doses administered intramuscularly or intravenously.

Amikacin sulfate (Amikin) is a chemically modified semisynthetic aminoglycoside. The chemical modification confers resistance to the inactivating effect of enzymes that are capable of destroying the activity of gentamicin and tobramycin. Amikacin is actually a derivative of kanamycin. The drug is available for the treatment of infections caused by gram-negative bacteria in solutions containing 50 and 250 mg/ml for intramuscular and intravenous administration.

Neomycin sulfate (Mycifradin sulfate) is quite toxic and should be used only topically or orally. When given orally, only a small percentage of the dose is absorbed, and reduction of intestinal flora may be beneficial in the treatment of hepatic coma.

Kanamycin sulfate (Kantrex) may be useful in the treatment of gram-negative bacillary infections, but many resistant strains have appeared and gentamicin is generally preferred. Oral administration may be useful for reduction of ammonia production by the intestinal flora.

Paromomycin may be used orally for the treatment of intestinal amebiasis. It is discussed on p. 681.

Other aminoglycosides

The tetracyclines are broad-spectrum bacteriostatic antibiotics, which inhibit protein synthesis in bacteria by blocking the combination of aminoacyl transfer ribonucleic acid (RNA) with messenger RNA. These antibiotics are highly effective in the treatment of brucellosis, *Mycoplasma pneumoniae*, and cholera, and they may be useful as alternatives in many infections in which the drug of choice cannot be used. Being bacteriostatic, the tetracyclines occasionally interfere with the killing effect of a bactericidal antibiotic such as penicillin.

The three tetracycline antibiotics, **chlortetracycline** (Aureomycin), **oxytetracycline** (Terramycin), and **tetracycline** were discovered as a result of extensive screening experiments on antibiotics produced by soil organisms. These drugs are characterized by a wide antibacterial spectrum, effectiveness of oral administration, and a very favorable therapeutic index. They are essentially bacteriostatic drugs, except in very high concentrations. Their use may in some cases modify the infection rather than eradicate it completely. Their characteristics are summarized in Table 53-3.

TETRACYCLINES

TABLE 53-3. Summary of characteristics of tetracyclines*

Agent generic name (trade name)	Spectrum of activity	Usual adult dosage (GI absorption)	Route	Mode of action (cidal or static)	Side effects
Tetracycline, chlortetracycline, oxytetracycline	Gram-positive, gram-negative, including *Bacteroides*, *Chlamydiae* (LGV), *M. pneumoniae, Rickettsiae.* Oxytetracycline—TBC	0.25-0.5 g q6h 0.2-0.6 g/day 0.5-1.0 g q12 h	Oral Intramuscular Intravenous	Static	GI, skin rash, anaphylactoid reactions (rare), deposition in teeth, negative N balance, hepatotoxicity, enamel agenesis, benign ↑ CSF pressure (outdated drug—Fanconi syndrome)
Demeclocycline (Declomycin)	Gram-positive, gram-negative, *Mycoplasma pneumoniae, Chlamydiae*	0.15-0.3 g q6h	Oral	Static	GI, skin rash, deposition in teeth, negative N balance, *phototoxicity, hepatotoxicity,* benign ↑CSF pressure, *oncholysis,* anaphylactoid reactions
Minocycline (Minocin)	Gram-positive, gram-negative, *Chlamydiae*	100 mg q 12 h	Oral	Static	Similar to other tetracyclines
Doxycycline (Vibramycin)	Gram-positive, gram-negative, *M. pneumoniae, Chlamydiae*	0.1 g q12h on 1st day, then 0.1 g/day	Oral	Static	Similar to other tetracyclines, phototoxicity less than demethylchlortetracycline, probably greater than tetracycline
Methacycline (Rondomycin)	Gram-positive, gram-negative, *Chlamydiae*	0.15 g q6h	Oral	Static	Similar to other tetracyclines

*Courtesy Dr. Jay P. Sanford, Washington, D.C.

Tetracycline is a true broad-spectrum antibiotic and for that reason it is probably overused. Such excessive use has led to the development of many resistant strains of bacteria and to superinfections, which in some series have been as high as 20% of patients. In general, broad-spectrum agents are more conducive to superinfections than are antibiotics having a narrow spectrum.

Tetracycline hydrochloride is widely used in the treatment of infections caused by *Mycoplasma pneumoniae*, or chlamydiae, in cholera, in various infections related to the respiratory tract such as mucoviscidosis, in rickettsial infections, and in the management of skin infections such as acne and many others.

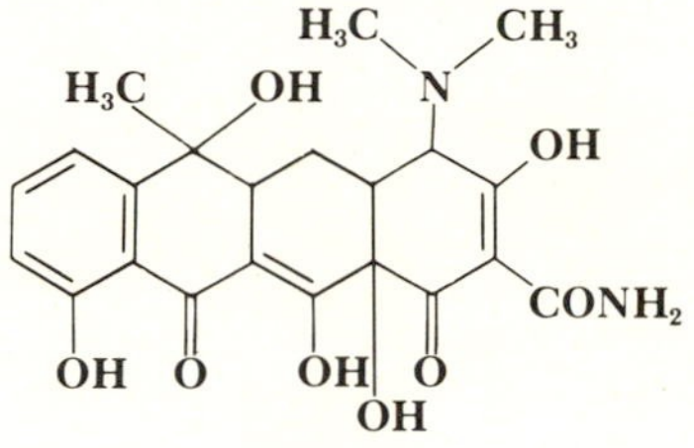

Tetracycline

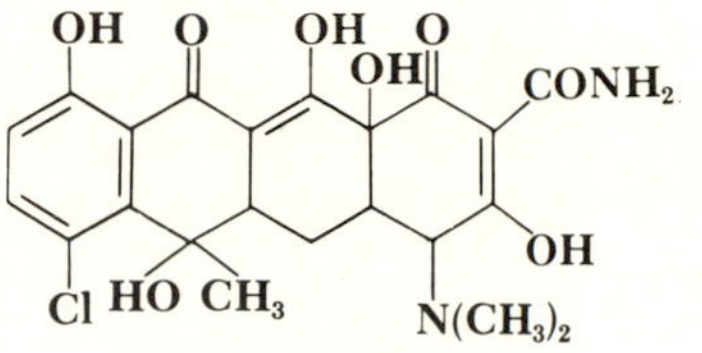

Chlortetracycline

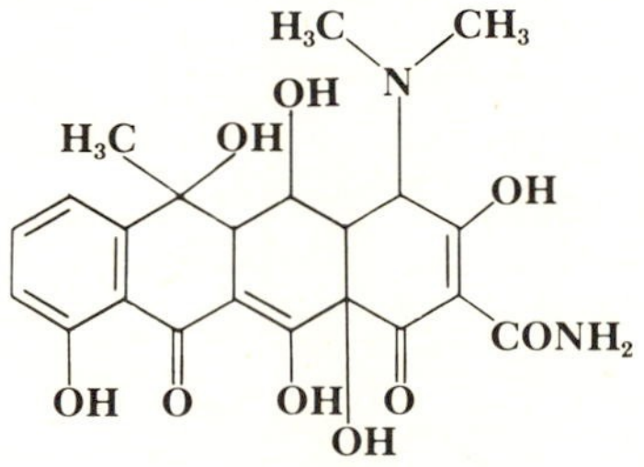

Oxytetracycline

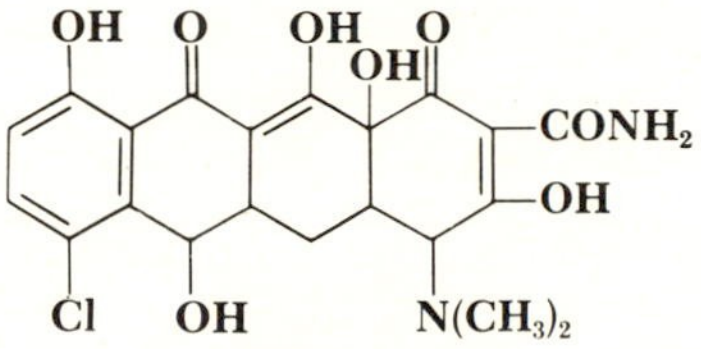

Demeclocycline

In addition to the three well-known tetracycline antibiotics, other derivatives have been introduced. **Demeclocycline** (Declomycin) was introduced a few years ago. Although certain advantages have been claimed for this drug, some cases of photosensitization have been reported following its use. Its ultimate status in relation to the other tetracyclines cannot be stated at present **Methacycline** (Rondomycin) resembles demeclocycline in its pharmacology. **Doxycycline monohydrate** (Vibramycin monohydrate) differs from other tetracyclines in that less frequent administration is effective because the drug is less readily excreted. It may cause phototoxicity. **Rolitetracycline** (Syntetrin) is a very soluble derivative of tetracycline and is suitable for parenteral administration. It may be injected intravenously or intramuscularly.

Another slowly excreted member of the tetracycline family is **minocycline** (Minocin). The slowly excreted tetracyclines, such as demeclocycline, methacycline, and minocycline, may accumulate in the body and produce toxicity when renal function is impaired. Doxycycline is slowly excreted also but appears to be safer in renal failure.

Problem 53-1. The causative agent in a stubborn urinary tract infection was found to be most susceptible to the tetracyclines. The physician selected doxycycline because of the convenience of twice-daily administration. Was this a good choice? No, because doxycycline is not excreted in the urine to the same extent as some other tetracyclines.[42]

Pharmacokinetics

All these drugs are absorbed rapidly but incompletely from the gastrointestinal tract. Calcium salts and gastric antacids prevent their absorption. Variable amounts may remain in the large intestine, and the bacterial flora of the intestinal contents may be altered considerably. The development of serious staphylococcal gastroenteritis during therapy with one of the tetracyclines has been attributed to the phenomenon of *superinfection*, with micrococci producing exotoxin.

Oral administration of 250 mg of tetracycline will produce a serum level of about 0.7 μg/ml in less than 2 hours (Fig. 53-3). This level will decline very gradually to about half this value in approximately 12 hours. This slow decline may be explained by the low renal clearance of the drug. During the first 12 hours only about 10% to 20% of the dose appears in the urine.

The drug is widely distributed in the various tissues and probably penetrates into cells, but its level in the cerebrospinal fluid is less than in plasma. Probably as a consequence of its chelating properties, tetracycline tends to localize in bones and teeth, where it may be detected by its fluorescence.[43] Tetracycline fluorescence is widespread but tends to disappear from normal tissues, except from bones and teeth, in about 24 hours. It tends to remain in inflammatory tissue somewhat longer, whereas it clings to neoplastic tissue for a surprisingly long time.

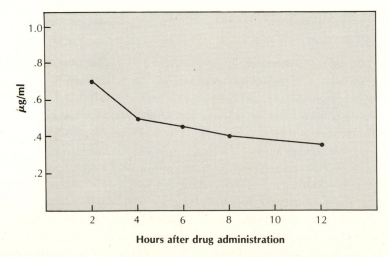

FIG. 53-3. Average serum concentration following oral administration of 0.25 g of tetracycline. (From Welch, H., et al.: Principles and practice of antibiotic therapy, New York, 1954, Medical Encyclopedia, Inc.)

Problem 53-2. Inhibition of gastrointestinal absorption of tetracycline by gastric antacids is generally attributed to chelation. Would sodium bicarbonate interfere with the absorption of the antibiotic, and if so, by what mechanism? In an experimental study of this problem, it was found that sodium bicarbonate interferes with the dissolution of tetracycline contained in capsules and thus interferes with absorption.

Adverse effects caused by tetracyclines include nausea, vomiting, enterocolitis, stomatitis, and superinfections. Phototoxicity may occur after the administration of demeclocycline (Declomycin).   *Adverse effects*

Administration of the tetracyclines in large doses has produced liver damage in patients, as proved by liver biopsy. Recent evidence suggests that tetracycline in large doses produces a negative nitrogen balance and probably exerts an antianabolic action. Interference with protein synthesis may be the basis of these effects. A similar action may explain the mechanism of its action against bacteria.

Chloramphenicol (Chloromycetin) is a broad-spectrum antibiotic having an antibacterial spectrum and potency very similar to those of the tetracyclines. It is not effective, however, against *Entamoeba histolytica* but is more effective than the tetracyclines in the treatment of typhoid fever.   **CHLORAM-PHENICOL**

It may be seen from the structural formula of chloramphenicol that this antibiotic is a derivative of nitrobenzene.

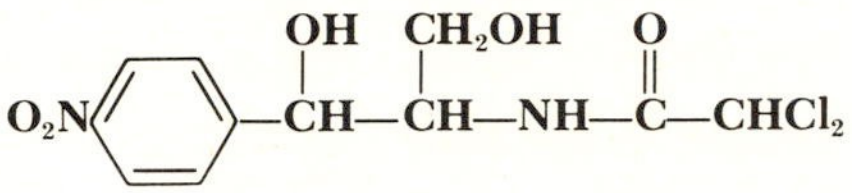

Chloramphenicol

The drug is well absorbed from the gastrointestinal tract. It is largely metabolized in the body, so that only about 10% of an administered dose appears in the urine in the unchanged form.

The mode of action of chloramphenicol is not completely understood. The drug is largely bacteriostatic. Considerable evidence indicates that it interferes with protein synthesis in bacteria and also in human protein-synthesizing systems, at least as demonstrated with human bone marrow cells in tissue culture. Chloramphenicol attaches to the bacterial ribosomes (50S subunits) and prevents the binding of amino acids, thus interfering with the growth of the peptide chain.

The acute toxicity of chloramphenicol in experimental animals is about the same as that of the tetracyclines. In clinical usage many minor side effects such as gastrointestinal disturbances, glossitis, skin rash, and superinfection may occur. These are similar to the effects produced by the tetracyclines. On the other hand, it is generally recognized that chloramphenicol has a much greater tendency than have commonly used antibiotics to produce blood dyscrasias such as aplastic anemia. Although the incidence of this serious toxic effect is small, it is sufficient to make physicians very cautious in the use of chloramphenicol. Chloramphenicol is partic-   *Toxicity* ularly dangerous in infants, in whom it can lead to a symptom complex often referred to as the "gray syndrome."

The gray syndrome occurs in premature and newborn infants when chloramphenicol is administered during the first few days of life. Symptoms consist of cyanosis, vascular collapse, and elevated chloramphenicol levels in the blood. The syndrome results from lack of development of glucuronyl transferase in the liver, which normally detoxifies the antibiotic by changing it to the glucuronide.[62]

Since chloramphenicol can cause fatal aplastic anemia in rare cases, it should not be used if there is a suitable alternative. At the same time the antibiotic is not contraindicated if an infection is severe and the drug appears to be the best by susceptibility tests.

Chloramphenicol sodium succinate, a water-soluble derivative, is available for parenteral administration.

POLYPEPTIDE ANTIBIOTICS

Bacitracin, polymyxin, and colistin are discussed as a group for two reasons. First, all three are nephrotoxic when administered systemically in large enough doses. Second, they are used mostly for special purposes and only rarely as systemic chemotherapeutic agents.

Bacitracin

Bacitracin, a mixture of polypeptides, was first isolated from cultures of a gram-positive bacillus. Its name was derived from Tracy, the name of the patient from whom the bacillus was isolated.

The antibacterial spectrum of bacitracin is remarkably similar to that of penicillin. It is particularly effective against gram-positive organisms, those of the *Neisseria* group, and spirochetes.

The main usefulness of bacitracin is in treating infections of the skin and mucous membranes, where it can be applied topically. When used by intramuscular injection, renal tubular damage regularly occurs in patients or experimental animals if large enough doses are used.

The activity of bacitracin is expressed in a unit that represents 26 μg of a standard preparation. For topical use, ointments containing 500 units/g of base are available.

Bacitracin is valuable for topical application and, compared to penicillin, has the great advantage of seldom causing sensitivity reactions. The drug is not absorbed from the gastrointestinal tract.

Polymyxins, including colistin

Polymyxin B is one of a serious of polypeptide antibiotics produced by *Bacillus polymyxa*, a soil bacillus. This antibiotic has a potent bactericidal effect on gram-negative bacilli. Unfortunately, when administered to patients in daily doses exceeding 4 mg/kg, it is likely to cause renal tubular damage. This appears to be a direct toxic effect, readily demonstrable in experimental animals.

The main usefulness of polymyxin is for topical application. Many preparations for available for this purpose, and the drug is generally combined with either bacitracin or neomycin in order to widen the antibacterial spectrum. The polymyxins are useful in the treatment of severe urinary tract infections.

The systemic use of polymyxin is hazardous, and the daily dose should not exceed 3 to 4 mg/kg in adults.

In addition to nephrotoxic action, systemic use of polymyxin can produce CNS effects such as vertigo and paresthesia.

Polymyxin B is not absorbed significantly from the gastrointestinal tract and may occasionally be used by mouth for intestinal chemotherapy. When the drug is applied to open wounds, absorption may take place and the total quantity applied in a day should not exceed 3 to 4 mg/kg.

Colistin is a polypeptide antibiotic very similar in antibacterial spectrum and toxicity to polymyxin B. Although some investigators believe that the drug is less neurotoxic and is not as likely to produce paresthesia, others question the superiority of this drug over polymyxin B.[45] It is available as sodium colistimethate (Coly-Mycin), used in daily doses of 2 to 5 mg/kg by intramuscular injection.

Since penicillin and the broad-spectrum antibiotics became available, several important additional discoveries have been made in the fight against gram-positive organisms, such as the introduction of erythromycin, the discovery of newer antibiotics effective against resistant micrococci (staphylococci), and the development of the newer penicillins.

NEWER ANTI-BIOTICS AGAINST GRAM-POSITIVE ORGANISMS

Erythromycin (Ilotycin), a macrolide antibiotic, was isolated from a strain of *Streptomyces*. It is an organic base having a molecular weight of about 700. This antibiotic is particularly effective against gram-positive microorganisms, although gonococci, *Hemophilus* organisms, and the large viruses of the lymphogranuloma venereum group are somewhat affected by it. Its antibacterial spectrum is between that of penicillin and of the tetracyclines, but the gram-negative bacilli such as *Escherichia coli* and *Salmonella* organisms are not inhibited by it. Its mode of action appears to be largely bacteriostatic, since it has a true killing effect only at very high concentrations. Erythromycins are among the safest antibiotics commonly used for respiratory infections, particularly in patients allergic to penicillin. Erythromycins should not be used in serious staphylococcal infections or in the treatment of gonococcal infections because better drugs are available.

Gastric juice tends to destroy erythromycin, but enteric-coated preparations and the erythromycin stearate are well absorbed. It is given in doses of 0.5 g every 6 hours, and blood levels of 2 μg/ml or more can be obtained. Many gram-positive organisms are inhibited by levels below this amount.

Erythromycin estolate (Ilosone) is stable in acid, is well absorbed, and is excreted in lesser amounts in bile. Thus, when taken with food, it gives faster, higher, and longer lasting blood levels than comparable doses of erythromycin. Cholestatic jaundice has been reported following the use of this drug and other esters of erythromycin. Although this occurs rarely, caution is necessary in its use.

In addition to erythromycin estolate (Ilosone), the antibiotic is also available as

erythromycin base (Ilotycin), the stearate, **erythromycin ethylsuccinate** (Pedia-mycin), **erythromycin gluceptate** (Ilotycin Gluceptate), and **erythromycin lacto-bionate** (Erythrocin Lactobionate). In general the erythromycin base is rapidly destroyed by gastric juice and the stearate is more stable but is not absorbed as well as the esters.

Vancomycin hydrochloride (Vancocin hydrochloride) is a glycopeptide that is highly toxic but bactericidal against gram-positive cocci. It should only be used orally to treat staphylococcal enteritis and in severe infections caused by gram-positive cocci when other antibiotics may be ineffective or the patient is allergic to them. Vancomycin can cause permanent deafness and fatal uremia.

Novobiocin (Albamycin) has a narrow antibacterial spectrum, being effective against gram-positive cocci. The main disadvantage of this antibiotic is the high incidence of adverse reactions, probably based on sensitization. Skin rashes, fever, and blood dyscrasias are caused in such a high percentage of patients that novobiocin should probably never be used.

Lincomycin (Lincocin) is structurally unrelated to previously discussed antibiotics. Its antibacterial spectrum resembles that of erythromycin. It is effective against gram-positive organisms, *Neisseria*, and *Bacteroides*. It is administered by mouth, intramuscularly, or intravenously. Its usual adult dose is 0.5 g every 6 to 8 hours. Side effects from lincomycin include gastrointestinal manifestations, skin rashes, and anaphylactoid reactions.

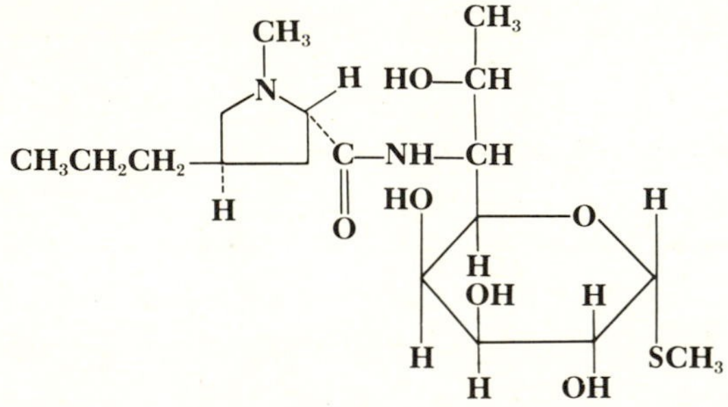

Lincomycin

Clindamycin (Cleocin) is closely related to lincomycin structurally. In fact, it differs only in a chloro substitution of the 7-hydroxyl group. The spectrum of activity of the drug includes gram-positive organisms (not *Neisseria* or enterococci), *Actinomyces*, and *B. fragilis*. The drug is administered by mouth in a usual adult dose of 150 to 450 mg every 6 hours. The drug may be either bactericidal or bacteriostatic and acts by inhibiting protein synthesis in the 50 S subunit of the ribosome. Adverse effects caused by clindamycin include gastrointestinal manifestations, neutropenia, eosinophilia, rashes, and elevated serum glutamic-oxaloacetic transaminase (SGOT) levels.

Although clindamycin has produced excellent results in the treatment of anaerobic infections,[66] severe hemorrhagic colitis has occurred in some patients following the use of the antibiotic. This serious complication may limit the usefulness of clindamycin.

Clindamycin hydrochloride (Cleocin hydrochloride) is available in capsules, 75 and 150 mg. Clindamycin palmitate is available in granules for suspension, 75 mg/5 ml. Clindamycin phosphate (Cleocin phosphate) is available in injectable solutions containing 150 mg/ml.

Nystatin (Mycostatin) and **amphotericin B** (Fungizone) are also called *polyene* antibiotics. This name refers to the fact that these antibiotics contain a large ring with a conjugated double-bond system. There is evidence to indicate that the polyene antibiotics injure the membrane of the fungi, perhaps by complexing with sterols that occur in these membranes. Because of this interaction, sterols protect yeasts against the action of these antibiotics. Bacterial membranes are not injured by the polyenes. On the other hand, the hemolytic anemia sometimes caused by the polyene antibiotics may be a consequence of injury of the red cell membrane, which is known to contain cholesterol.

Nystatin is effective against *Candida albicans* and some other fungi. It appears to be useful against those monilial infections that can be reached by topical application. The drug is inactivated by gastric juice, and no systemic effects can be expected when it is administered orally although it has been incorporated in tetracycline preparations.

Amphotericin B appears to be the most effective antibiotic against deep-seated mycotic infections.[47] The usefulness of the antibiotic has been demonstrated against histoplasmosis, cryptococcosis, blastomycosis, and coccidiodomycosis. It has also proved to be effective in systemic infections caused by *Candida albicans*.[38]

The drug is administered intravenously but can cause thrombophlebitis at the site of injection and may also produce some renal damage, skin rash, and gastrointestinal upset. Test doses of 1 to 5 mg are injected first. If there is no untoward reaction, these may be followed by daily doses of 20 to 50 mg. Although amphotericin B is obviously a dangerous drug, its use may be justified in severe systemic fungous infections. Its intravenous LD_{50} in mice is of the order of 5 mg/kg.

The drug is poorly absorbed from the intestine.

Griseofulvin represents an interesting development in the treatment of certain dermatomycoses. The antibiotic is produced by a *Penicillium* mold. When given orally for long periods of time, it is apparently incorporated into the skin, hair, and nails and exerts a fungistatic activity against various species of *Microsporum*, *Trichophyton*, and *Epidermophyton*. Prolonged administration is necessary because ringworm of the skin may require several weeks for improvement. In fungal infections of the nails, treatment may have to be continued for several months. The most common side effects consist of gastric discomfort, diarrhea, and headache. Urticaria and skin rash may also occur.

Griseofulvin

TABLE 53-4. Summary of antifungal drugs and their side effects*

Type of infecting fungi	Site of infection	Antifungal agent	Route of administration	Dosage	Side effects and comments
Candida species	Superficial	Amphotericin B or nystatin	Topical	Not applicable	Apply 3 or 4 times daily for 7 to 14 days; with vaginitis, daily or twice daily for 14 days. Side effects: essentially none
	Intestinal	Nystatin (Mycostatin)	Oral	500,000 U 3 times daily for 7 to 14 days	Side effects: essentially none; large doses, occasionally GI distress and diarrhea
	Systemic—not endocarditis	Amphotericin B (Fungizone)	Intravenous	Initial dose 0.25 mg/kg intravenous over 6 hours (suspend in 5% glucose solution, NOT saline), then increase stepwise to 1 mg/kg administration daily or 3 times/wk; total dose 0.5 to 1.0 g	If administered rapidly, convulsions, anaphylaxis, hypotension, ventricular fibrillation or cardiac arrest; phlebitis, fever, nausea, vomiting, anorexia, metallic taste, abdominal pain, nephrotoxicity, anemia, hypokalemia, ↓ urinary 17OH corticoids
		or flucytosine (Ancobon)	Oral	50-150 mg/kg/day	GI distress (nausea, vomiting, diarrhea), leukopenia
	Systemic—endocarditis	Amphotericin B	Intravenous	As above	Removal of prosthesis or primary surgery usually required
Dermatophytes	Intradermal and hair	Griseofulvin (Fulvicin, Grifulvin, Grisactin)	Oral	12.5 mg/kg or 500 mg/day in adults	Photosensitivity, urticaria, GI upset, fatigue, leukopenia (rare); interferes with coumarin drugs; increases blood and urine prophyrins, therefore should not be used in patients with porphyria. Adjunct treatment: tolnaftate (Tinactin) or Desenex 2 to 3 times daily
	Onychomycosis	Griseofulvin	Oral	12.5 mg/kg or 500 mg/day in adults for 6 to 12 months	

Fungi causing deep mycoses: Actinomycosis		Penicillin G or ampicillin or tetracycline	10,000 to 20,000 U/kg 50 mg/kg 25 mg/kg	See Tables 53-1 and 53-3
Nocardia		Sulfonamide—rapid-acting and/or cycloserine (Seromycin)	1.0 g q4h	See Table 52-2
		Sulfamethoxazole-trimethoprim	Oral, 15 mg/kg	See Table 54-1
Sporotrichosis	Cutaneous and lymphatic	Potassium iodide, saturated solution		
Histoplasmosis, coccidioidomycosis, systemic sporotrichosis, aspergillosis, mucormycosis, chromablastomycosis	Systemic	Amphotericin B	See Candida, systemic, not endocarditis	Total dosage variable, but usually 2.5 g or more
Blastomycosis	Systemic	Amphotericin B or 2-hydroxystilbamidine	See Candida, systemic, not endocarditis	
Cryptococcosis	Systemic	Amphotericin B or flucytosine	See Candida, systemic, not endocarditis	

*Courtesy Dr. Jay P. Sanford, Washington, D.C.

Griseofulvin (Fulvicin, Grifulvin V, Grisactin) is available in tablet form containing 125, 250, or 500 mg.

Several other antifungal agents are available, mostly for topical application. These include candicidin, miconazole, clotrimazole, flucytosine, haloprogin, tolnaftate, iodochlorhydroxyquin, and undecylenic acid.

Candicidin (Candeptin, Vanobid) is a polyene antibiotic available in ointments and capsules or tablets to be inserted in the vagina.

Miconazole nitrate (Monistat, Micatin) is an imidazole derivative, which may act on the fungal plasma membrane. Although the drug can be used intravenously for the treatment of infections caused by *Candida albicans*, *Cryptococcus*, and *Aspergillus*, its main usefulness is its topical application for dermatophytosis and candidal infections.

Clotrimazole (Lotrimin) is related to miconazole and is used primarily as a topical fungicide in the form of creams or vaginal tablets.

Flucytosine (Ancobon) is a simple fluorinated compound available for the treatment of systemic infections caused by *Candida* or *Cryptococcus neoformans*. Although the drug is less toxic than amphotericin B, it may cause blood dyscrasias and CNS toxicity. Flucytosine (Ancobon) is available in 250 and 500 mg capsules.

Haloprogin (Halotex) is a synthetic topical antifungal agent used for the treatment of skin infections caused by a variety of fungi.

Tolnaftate (Tinactin) is a synthetic topical, somewhat selective antifungal agent. Although it is effective in epidermophytosis, it does not eliminate candidal organisms. The drug is not adequate for fungal infections of the nails, scalp, and soles.

Iodochlorhydroxyquin (clioquinol; Vioform) is useful in epidermophytosis. The drug has antibacterial effects also. It should be used topically on the skin, avoiding areas around the eyes.

Undecylenic acid is a harmless topical agent for mild epidermophytosis.

ANTIVIRAL AGENTS

Several developments have taken place in the chemotherapy of viral diseases during the last few years (Table 53-5). The inhibitor of nucleic acid synthesis, idoxuridine, has produced spectacular results by topical application in herpetic keratitis, and the new drug amantadine has provided a new approach to the prevention of influenza A_2 infections. Amantadine blocks the penetration of the virus into the host cell.[15] In addition to these approaches, there is great interest in the stimulation of interferon production by synthetic polyanions of defined composition such as pyran copolymer.[19]

Idoxuridine (5-iodo-2'-deoxyuridine; IDU; Stoxil) is a pyrimidine analog that blocks the synthesis of nucleic acids. It is applied topically in a 0.1% solution to the conjunctiva every 1 to 2 hours in the treatment of herpetic keratitis caused by the herpes simplex virus. This is an important therapeutic advance because herpetic keratitis can lead to blindness. No effective treatment existed prior to the introduction of idoxuridine. Unfortunately the drug is ineffective by systemic administration, probably because of rapid destruction. Nevertheless, the drug has been used sys-

TABLE 53-5. Summary of currently used antiviral drugs*

Drug	Indication	Usual adult dosage	Route	Side effects	Comments
Amantadine (Symmetrel)	Prophylaxis of influenza A; possible therapy of influenza A in elderly or chronically ill patients if seen less than 20 hr after onset of illness	100 mg bid	Oral	Jitteriness, inability to concentrate, insomnia, tremors, confusion, depression, and hallucinations; incidence generally at a low level and is dose-related	Primary reliance on prevention of influenza A infections remains with immunization
5-lodo-2'-deoxyuridine, idoxuridine (IDUR, Stoxil)	Severe herpes simplex virus infections (encephalitis, generalized diseases of newborn)	Total dose 430 mg/kg given over a 5 day period (always less than 30 g)	Intravenous	Leukopenia, thrombocytopenia, stomatitis, alopecia, fingernail loss, and occasionally jaundice; nausea and vomiting can occur during infusion	IDUR poorly soluble and pH must be adjusted to 8.2-8.6 before drug goes into solution (3 to 8 g/1000 ml D5W); filter sterilize before use
	Herpes simplex keratitis		Topical		
Cytosine arabinoside (Ara-C, Cytosar)	Progressive varicella-zoster virus infections in compromised host; primary varicella pneumonia in adult	100 mg/M²/day for 3 to 5 days; 24-hour infusion	Intravenous	Leukopenia, thrombocytopenia, anemia with reticulocytopenia, and megaloblastoid changes; chromosomal changes acutely; anorexia, nausea, and vomiting occur	
Adenine arabinoside (Ara-A)	Severe herpes simplex virus infections (encephalitis, generalized diseases of newborn); progressive cytomegalovirus pneumonia in compromised host	As above	As above	As above	Current information insufficent to determine whether IDUR or Ara-C is first drug of choice
	Investigational in herpes simplex encephalitis and mucocutaneous infections	10-15 mg/kg/day	Intravenous	Nausea, anemia	
Methisazone	Progressive vaccinia (vaccinia necrosum)	Initial dose 200 mg/kg followed by 8 doses of 50 mg/kg at 6-hour intervals	Oral	Anorexia, nausea, and vomiting; hepatotoxicity	

*Courtesy Dr. Jay P. Sanford, Washington, D.C.

temically in the treatment of herpes simplex encephalitis and varicella-zoster infections. Some of the toxic effects of idoxuridine are bone marrow depression, alopecia,
gastric ulcers, loss of fingernails, and hepatotoxicity.

Amantadine (Symmetrel) is a new synthetic drug of unusual structure that inhibits the penetration of certain viruses into the host cell. In vitro it is effective
against influenza and rubella viruses. In humans its effectiveness as a chemoprophy-
lactic measure against influenza A_2 (Asian) virus has been demonstrated. Amantadine
reduced the number of clinical illnesses and also diminished the serological response
to influenza infection. Mice could be protected against several strains of influenza
A_2 virus even when treatment was delayed as much as 72 hours after inoculation.[20]

Amantadine is available in capsules containing 100 mg of the drug and also as a
syrup. The adult daily dose is 200 mg.

Although amantadine appears to be quite nontoxic on the basis of animal experiments, it can produce CNS stimulation and even convulsions when given in large
doses. Nervousness, dizziness, hallucinations, and even grand mal convulsions have
been associated with the use of the drug in humans. These adverse reactions are not
common, however, and are more likely to occur following the administration of
large doses.

Amantadine is a new approach to viral diseases. Its ultimate place in chemo-
prophylaxis in comparison with immunization procedures is a matter of debate.[15]
Amantadine has some therapeutic effect in parkinsonism (p. 158).

Idoxuridine   **Amantadine**

Methisazone, or n-methylisatin-β-thiosemicarbazone, shows some therapeutic
promise against the poxyviruses such as smallpox and complications of vaccination.

Vidarabine (Vira-A) or adenine arabinoside inhibits DNA viruses, such as herpes
simplex, and varicella agents. Topically, vidarabine may be used for the treatment
of ocular herpes simplex, although results in genital herpes infections have been
poor. Vidarabine may be administered intravenously for the treatment of herpes
encephalitis. For intravenous infusion vidarabine (Vira-A) is available as a suspension containing 200 mg of the drug. Systemic use may cause many adverse effects
and should be undertaken only in grave illnesses.

Acyclovir is an important investigational agent, which is active against herpes
virus infections.[68] It is a nucleoside analog, 9-(2-hydroxymethyl) guanine. Cells
infected with herpes simplex phosphorylate the drug much faster than uninfected

cells. This phosphorylation yields acycloguanosine triphosphate, which inhibits preferentially virus-specified DNA polymerase.

Investigational antiviral agents include immunopotentiating compounds, such as **levamisole** and **methisoprinol** (Isoprinosine), and other antimetabolites, such as 2-deoxyglucose or purine and pyrimidine analogs.

Interferon inducers represent a novel approach to antiviral chemotherapy. Interferon is an antiviral protein produced by cells as a consequence of virus infections. Not only viruses but also bacteria and their products are capable of inducing the formation of interferon by the cells of the host.[19] More recently, it has been shown that chemically defined substances such as a polyanionic pyran copolymer or double-stranded RNA from a synthetic source can also act as interferon inducers. Early trials in human beings and animals indicate that these synthetic materials may induce demonstrable serum interferon levels.[19]

Clinical experience with chemotherapeutic agents in a wide variety of infections allows certain generalizations regarding the best choice. These will be summarized, based on a more extensive report.[41] There may be exceptions to these recommendations in individual cases in which susceptibility tests reveal resistance of the causative agent to a drug that ordinarily would be a good choice (Table 53-6).

CLINICAL PHARMACOLOGY OF ANTIBACTERIAL AGENTS
Selection of a chemotherapeutic agent

With the availability of effective weapons against infection, it is inexcusable not to cure an infection that would be curable with optimal treatment. Some of the causes of failure of anti-infective therapy are unavoidable. Others, however, may be iatrogenic.

Causes of failure of antibacterial therapy

Some of the causes of failure are as follows:
Incorrect clinical or bacteriological diagnosis
Improper selection of drugs
Improper method of administration or inadequate dose
Futile prophylaxis
Alteration in bacterial flora and superinfection
Inaccessible lesion
Drug resistance
Deficiency in host defenses
Drug toxicity and hypersensitivity

The possible effects of antibiotics on the gastrointestinal tract are of two types. They may alter the bacterial flora or they may have direct toxic effects unrelated to the bacterial flora.[33]

Gastrointestinal effects of antibiotics

Alteration of the bacterial flora is deliberately sought when antibiotics are used prior to bowel surgery. The nonabsorbable antibiotics such as neomycin, kanamycin, and certain sulfonamides have often been employed for this purpose. Despite some enthusiastic proponents of such a prophylactic measure, many investigators believe that it has no advantages over the preoperative cleansing of the bowel.

TABLE 53-6. Drugs of choice for various infections

Causative agent	Drugs
Gram-positive	
Streptococcus pyogenes	Penicillin; erythromycin; a cephalosporin
Streptococcus viridans *	Penicillin with streptomycin; ampicillin; vancomycin
Enterococcus*	Penicillin with streptomycin; vancomycin with streptomycin
Pneumococcus	Penicillin; erythromycin; tetracycline
Staphylococcus aureus	
Penicillinase-producing	Oxacillin; nafcillin; cloxacillin; others based on susceptibility such as a cephalosporin, erythromycin, lincomycin, vancomycin
Nonpenicillinase-producing	Penicillin; erythromycin; a cephalosporin; lincomycin
Clostridium	Penicillin; erythromycin; tetracycline
Corynebacterium diphtheriae	Penicillin; erythromycin; tetracycline
Actinomyces	Penicillin with tetracycline; sulfonamides
Gram-negative	
Neisseria meningitidis	Penicillin; sulfonamides; tetracycline
Neisseria gonorrhoeae	Penicillin; tetracycline; erythromycin
Salmonella	Chloramphenicol; ampicillin
Shigella	Tetracycline; ampicillin
Escherichia coli *	Ampicillin; kanamycin; tetracycline
Enterobacter *	Kanamycin; tetracycline
Klebsiella *	A cephalosporin; kanamycin; chloramphenicol; polymyxin B; colistimethate
Brucella	Tetracycline; chloramphenicol
Hemophilus influenzae	Ampicillin; chloramphenicol
Hemophilus ducreyi	Tetracycline; sulfonamides
Bordetella pertussis	Ampicillin; tetracycline
Pseudomonas *	Polymyxin B; colistimethate; gentamicin
Proteus *	Kanamycin; neomycin; chloramphenicol (penicillin for *Proteus mirabilis*)
Bacteroides	Clindamycin; chloramphenicol; tetracycline
Miscellaneous	
Fusobacterium (Vincent's angina)	Penicillin; erythromycin; tetracycline
Treponema pallidum	Penicillin; erythromycin; tetracycline
Leptospira	Penicillin; tetracycline
Rickettsia	Tetracycline; chloramphenicol
Psittacosis-lymphogranuloma group	Tetracycline; chloramphenicol
Histoplasma capsulatum	Amphotericin B
Candida	Amphotericin B; nystatin
Cryptococcus	Amphotericin B
Coccidioides	Amphotericin B
Blastomyces	Amphotericin B
Microsporum and *Trichophyton*	Griseofulvin

*Susceptibility tests may be essential.

Staphylococcal enterocolitis has occurred in patients who received oxytetracycline, neomycin, multiple antibiotics, or preoperative bowel antisepsis.

Candidiasis is commonly seen in patients who receive long-term treatment with broad-spectrum antibiotics. The number of yeasts in the stools can be diminished by the simultaneous use of nystatin, but it is not certain that the gastrointestinal symptoms are caused by the yeasts. The condition improves if the antibiotic is discontinued.

Prophylaxis of hepatic coma is an indication for the use of neomycin, kanamycin, or paromomycin, a closely related drug. The mode of action of these antibiotics in the prevention of hepatic coma is explained by their inhibitory effect on ammonia production in the intestine.

Malabsorption syndrome may result from the continued oral administration of neomycin. Changes in the jejunal mucosa and interference with the absorption of fat, glucose, D-xylose, iron, and vitamin B_{12} have been demonstrated.

Liver disease may be induced by some antibiotics. Large doses of intravenously administered tetracycline are quite hepatotoxic. Erythromycin estolate and triacetyl-oleandomycin can produce an obstructive hepatitis. Novobiocin can increase serum bilirubin in newborns by inhibiting the enzyme glucuronyl transferase.

Effectiveness and safety of antibiotic therapy depend on several host factors that will be summarized briefly.

Host factors in antibiotic therapy

Defense mechanisms of the host have much to do with the success or failure of treatment. Debilitating diseases or the administration of large doses of corticosteroids or immunosuppressant drugs may interfere with antibiotic therapy.

The age of the patient influences both the effectiveness and the safety of antibiotic therapy. Infants in the first month of life excrete penicillin more slowly, presumably because of less developed tubular secretory mechanism. Older infants and children require larger doses of penicillin than adults. Tetracycline may be deposited in tooth enamel and dentin and perhaps also in the bones of children. Chloramphenicol can cause the "gray syndrome" when given to infants during the first month of life.

Undeveloped glucuronide conjugation by the liver makes chloramphenicol more hazardous.

Pregnancy is a contraindication to the use of many drugs. Tetracyclines can cause dental defects in the fetus.

Liver disease may be aggravated by chloramphenicol, the tetracyclines, novobiocin, and erythromycin. *Defective renal function* would cause the accumulation of sulfonamides, tetracycline, and other antibiotics that are largely cleared by the kidney. *Urinary obstructions* in any part of the urinary tract are a most important host factor in making the eradication of the infection very difficult.

Pharmacogenetic defects such as glucose-6-phosphate dehydrogenase deficiency may predispose an individual to hemolytic anemia from various antimicrobial drugs such as sulfamethoxypyridazine, sulfadimethoxine, sulfisoxazole, nitrofurantoin, and chloramphenicol.

TABLE 53-7. Elimination and dose intervals of antimicrobial agents*

			Dose intervals	
Drug	Route of elimination	Normal half-life (hr)	Normal	Moderate renal failure
Cephalothin	Renal Hepatic	0.5-0.85	q6h	q6h
Chloramphenicol	Hepatic (renal)	2.5	q6h	q6h
Colistimethate	Renal	2	q12h	q36-60h
Erythromycin	Hepatic	1.5	q6h	q6h
Gentamicin	Renal	2.5	q8h	q12-24h
Isoniazid	Renal Hepatic	2-4	q8h	q12h
Kanamycin	Renal	3-4	q8h	q24-72h
Lincomycin	Hepatic	4.5	q6h	q6h
Nitrofurantoin	Renal	0.5	q8h	Avoid
Aminosalicylic acid	Renal Hepatic	1	q8h	Avoid
Ampicillin	Renal Hepatic	1.5	q6h	q6h
Carbenicillin	Renal Hepatic	1.5	q6h	q6h
Methicillin	Renal Hepatic	0.5	q4h	q4h
Oxacillin	Renal Hepatic	0.5	q6h	q6h
Penicillin G	Renal (hepatic)	0.5	q8h	q8h
Streptomycin	Renal	2.5	q12h	q24h
Sulfisoxazole	Renal	3-4	q6h	q8-12h
Tetracycline	Renal Hepatic	6-8	q6h	q24-48h

*Modified from Bennett, W. M., et al.: Ann. Intern. Med. **86**:754, 1977.

REFERENCES

1 Abraham, E. P.: The cephalosporins, Pharmacol. Rev. **14**:473, 1962.

2 Abraham, E. P.: The chemistry of new antibiotics, Am. J. Med. **39**:692, 1965.

3 Adams, H. R.: Neuromuscular blocking effect of aminoglycoside antibiotics in non-human primates, J. Am. Vet. Med. Assoc. **163**:613, 1973.

4 Ambrose, C. T., and Coons, A. H.: Studies on antibody production. VIII. Inhibitory effect of chloramphenicol on synthesis of antibody in tissue culture, J. Exp. Med. **117**:1075, 1963.

5 Andriole, V. T., and Kravetz, H. M.: The use of amphotericin B in man, J.A.M.A. **180**:269, 1962.

6 Baldwin, D. S., Levine, B. B., McCluskey, R. T., and Gallo, G. R.: Renal failure and interstitial nephritis due to penicillin and methicillin, N. Engl. J. Med. **279**:1245, 1968.

7 Barr, W. H., Adir, J., and Garrettson, L.: Decrease of tetracycline absorption in man by sodium bicarbonate, Clin. Pharmacol. Ther. **12**:779, 1971.

8 Bodey, G. P., Rodriquez, V., and Stewart, D.: Clinical pharmacological studies of carbenicillin, Am. J. Med. Sci. **257**:185, 1969.

9 Bodey, G. P., and Terrell, L. M.: In vitro activity of carbenicillin against gram-negative bacilli, J. Bacteriol. **95**:1587, 1968.

10 Brown, B. C., Price, E. V., and Moore, M. B.:

Penicilloyl-polylysine as an intradermal test of penicillin sensitivity, J.A.M.A. **189**:599, 1964.

11 Bryson, V., and Demerec, M.: Bacterial resistance, Am. J. Med. **18**:723, 1955.

12 Busfield, D., Child, K. J., and Tomich, E. G.: An effect of phenobarbitone on griseofulvin metabolism in the rat, Br. J. Pharmacol. **22**: 137, 1964.

13 Butler, W. T.: Pharmacology, toxicity and therapeutic usefulness of amphotericin B, J.A.M.A. **195**:371, 1966.

14 Caldwell, J. R., and Cluff, L. E.: The real and present danger of antibiotics, Ration. Drug Ther. **7**:1, 1973.

15 Council on Drugs: The amantadine controversy, J.A.M.A. **201**:372, 1967.

16 Cutler, R. E., Gyselynck, A. M., Fleet, W. P., and Forrey, A. W.: Correlation of serum creatinine concentration and gentamicin half-life, J.A.M.A. **219**:1037, 1972.

17 Dowling, H. F.: Present status of therapy with combinations of antibiotics, Am. J. Med. **39**: 796, 1965.

18 Dubos, R. J.: Studies on a bactericidal agent extracted from a soil bacillus: preparation of the agent. Its activity in vitro, J. Exp. Med. **70**:1, 1939.

19 Editorial: Interferon induction, N. Engl. J. Med. **277**:1316, 1967.

20 Eggers, H. J., and Tamm, I.: Antiviral chemotherapy, Annu. Rev. Pharmacol. **6**:231, 1966.

21 Feingold, D. S.: Antimicrobial chemotherapeutic agents: the nature of their action and selective toxicity, N. Engl. J. Med. **269**:900, 957, 1963.

22 Frimpter, G. W., Timpanelli, A. E., Eisenmenger, W. J., Stein, H. S., and Ehrlich, L. I.: Reversible "Fanconi syndrome" caused by degraded tetracycline, J.A.M.A. **184**:111, 1963.

23 Gale, E. F.: Mechanisms of antibiotic action, Pharmacol. Rev. **15**:481, 1963.

24 Gill, A. F., and Hoof, E. W.: Changing patterns of bacterial resistance to antimicrobial drugs, Am. J. Med. **39**:780, 1965.

25 Grieco, M. H.: Cross-allergenicity of the penicillins and cephalosporins, Arch. Intern. Med. **119**:141, 1967.

26 Hinman, A. R., and Wolinsky, E.: Nephrotoxicity associated with the use of cephaloridine, J.A.M.A. **200**:724, 1967.

27 Isaacs, A., and Lindenmann, J.: Virus interference. I. Interferon, Proc. R. Soc. Lond. [Biol.] **147**:258, 1957.

28 Jao, R. L.: and Jackson, G. G.: Gentamicin sulfate: a new antibiotic against gram-negative bacilli, J.A.M.A. **189**:817, 1964.

29 Jawetz, E., and Gunnison, J. B.: Antibiotic synergism and antagonism: an assessment of the problem, Pharmacol. Rev. **5**:175, 1953.

30 Koch-Weser, J., and Gilmore, E. B.: Benign intracranial hypertension in an adult after tetracycline therapy, J.A.M.A. **200**:345, 1967.

31 Kunin, C. M.: Clinical pharmacology of the new penicillins. I. The importance of serum protein binding in determining antimicrobial activity and concentration in serum, Clin. Pharmacol. Ther. **7**:166, 1966.

32 Kunin, C. M.: Clinical pharmacology of the new penicillins. II. Effect of drugs which interfere with the binding to serum proteins, Clin. Pharmacol. Ther. **7**:180, 1966.

33 Kunin, C. M.: Effects of antibiotics on the gastrointestinal tract, Clin. Pharmacol. Ther. **8**: 495, 1967.

34 Kunin, C. M., and Finland, M.: Clinical pharmacology of the tetracycline antibiotics, Clin. Pharmacol. Ther. **2**:51, 1961.

35 Lederberg, J.: Bacterial protoplasts induced by penicillin, Proc. Natl. Acad. Sci. **42**:574, 1956.

36 Levison, M. E., Johnson, W. D., Thornhill, T. S., and Kaye, D.: Clinical and in vitro evaluation of cephalexin, J.A.M.A. **209**:1331, 1969.

37 Lewis, C. N., Putnam, L. E., Hendricks, F. D., Kerlan, I., and Welch, H.: Chloramphenicol (Chloromycetin) in relation to blood dyscrasias, with observations on other drugs, Antibiot. Chemother. **2**:601, 1952.

38 Louria, D. B., and Dineen, P.: Amphotericin B in treatment of disseminated moniliasis, J.A.M.A. **174**:273, 1960.

39 McCormack, R. C., Kaye, D., and Hook, E. W.: Resistance of Group A streptococci to tetracycline, N. Engl. J. Med. **267**:323, 1962.

40 McCuistion, C. H., Jr., Lawlis, M. G., and Gonzalez, B. B.: Toxicological studies and effectiveness of griseofulvin in dermatomycosis, J.A.M.A. **171**:2174, 1959.

41 Med. Lett. **5**:17, 1963.

42 Med. Lett. **14**:4, 1972.

43 Owen, L. N.: Fluorescence of tetracyclines in bone tumours, normal bone, and teeth, Nature **190**:500, 1961.

44 Park, J. T., and Strominger, J. L.: Mode of action of penicillin: biochemical basis for the mechanism of action of penicillin and for its toxicity, Science **125**:99, 1957.

45 Petersdorf, R. G.: Colistin—a reappraisal, J.A.M.A. **183**:123, 1963.

46 Pollock, A. A., Berger, S. A., Richmond, A. S., Simberkoff, M. S., and Rahal, J. J.: Amikacin therapy for serious gram-negative infection, J.A.M.A. **237**:562, 1977.

47 Procknow, J. J., and Loosli, C. G.: Treatment of deep mycoses, Arch. Intern. Med. **101:**765, 1958.

48 Rollo, I. M.: Antibacterial chemotherapy, Annu. Rev. Pharmacol. **6:**209, 1966.

49 Sabath, L. D., Elder, H. A., McCall, C. E., and Finland, M.: Synergistic combinations of penicillins in the treatment of bacteriuria, N. Engl. J. Med. **277:**232, 1967.

50 Schatz, A., Bugie, E., and Waksman, S. A.: Streptomycin, a substance exhibiting antibiotic activity against gram-positive and gram-negative bacteria, Proc. Soc. Exp. Biol. Med. **55:** 66, 1944.

51 Schimpff, S., Satterlee, W., Young, V. M., and Serpick, A.: Empiric therapy with carbenicillin and gentamycin for febrile patients with cancer and granulocytopenia, N. Engl. J. Med. **284:** 1061, 1971.

52 Sidell, S., Burdick, R. E., Brodie, J., Bulger, R. J., and Kirby, W. M. M.: New antistaphylococcal antibiotics, Arch. Intern. Med. **112:** 21, 1963.

53 Smith, D. H.: The current status of R factors, Ann. Intern. Med. **67:**1337, 1967.

54 Steer, P. L., Marks, M. I., Klite, P. D., and Eickhoff, T. C.: 5-Fluorocytosine: an oral antifungal compound, Arch. Intern. Med. **76:** 15, 1972.

55 Strominger, J. L., and Tipper, D. J.: Bacterial cell wall synthesis and structure in relation to the mechanism of action of penicillins and other antibacterial agents, Am. J. Med. **39:**708, 1965.

56 Turk, M., Belcher, D. W., Ronald, A., Smith, R. H., and Wallace, J. F.: New cephalosporin antibiotic—cephaloridine, Arch. Intern. Med. **119:**50, 1967.

57 Utz, J. P.: Antimicrobial therapy in systemic fungal infections, Am. J. Med. **39:**826, 1965.

58 Waksman, S. A.: Neomycin: nature, formation, isolation, and practical application, New Brunswick, N.J., 1953, Rutgers University Press.

59 Walters, E. W., Romansky, M. J., and Johnson, A. C.: Lincomycin. In Laboratory and clinical studies: antimicrobial agents and chemotherapy, Ann Arbor, Mich., 1963, American Society for Microbiology.

60 Weinstein, L., Kaplan, K., and Chang, T.: Treatment of infections in man with cephalothin, J.A.M.A. **189:**829, 1964.

61 Weinstein, M. J., Luedemann, G. M., Oden, E. M., Wagman, G. H., Rosselet, J. P., Marquez, J. A., Coniglio, C. T., Charney, W., Herzog, H. L., and Black, J.: Gentamicin, a new antibiotic complex from Micromonospora, J. Med. Chem. **6:**463, 1963.

62 Weiss, C. F., Glazko, A. J., and Weston, J. K.: Chloramphenicol in the newborn infant: a physiological explanation of its toxicity when given in excessive doses, N. Engl. J. Med. **262:**787, 1960.

63 Yaffe, S. J.: Antibiotic dosage in newborn and premature infants, J.A.M.A. **193:**818, 1965.

REVIEWS

64 Allen, J. C.: The treatment of acute bacterial meningitis in the adult, Ration. Drug Ther. **13:**1, Sept., 1979.

65 Finegold, S. M.: Antimicrobial therapy of anaerobic infections: a status report, Hosp. Pract., Oct., 1979, p. 71.

66 Gorbach, S. L., and Thadepalli, H.: Clindamycin in pure and mixed anaerobic infections, Arch. Intern. Med. **134:**87, 1974.

67 Guernsey, J. M.: The use of antimicrobial drugs in patients with acute abdominal disease, Ration. Drug Ther. **8:**1, Sept. 1974.

68 Hirsch, M. S., and Swartz, M. N.: Antiviral agents, N. Engl. J. Med. **302:**903, 949, 1980.

69 International symposium on gentamicin, a new aminoglycoside antibiotic, J. Infect. Dis. **119:** 341, 1969.

70 Jones, S. R.: An approach to the management of urinary tract infection, Ration. Drug Ther. **13:** 1, Nov. 1979.

71 Pittinger, C. B., and Adamson, R.: Antibiotic blockade of neuromuscular function, Annu. Rev. Pharmacol. **12:**169, 1972.

72 Sack, R. B.: Enterotoxigenic *Escherichia coli* —an emerging pathogen, N. Engl. J. Med. **295:**893, 1976 (editorial).

73 Schoenfield, L. J.: Biliary excretion of antibiotics, N. Engl. J. Med. **284:**1213, 1971.

74 Seneca, H.: Biological basis of chemotherapy of infections and infestations, Philadelphia, 1971, F. A. Davis Co.

74a Smith, J. W.: Proper use of antibiotics, Tex. Med. **73:**1, 1977.

75 Stevens, D. A.: Drugs for systemic fungal infections, Ration. Drug Ther. **13:**1, May, 1979.

76 Weinstein, L.: Some principles of antimicrobial therapy, Ration. Drug. Ther. **11**(3):1, 1977.

77 Wise, R.: New penicillin—present and future, J.A.M.A. **232:**493, 1975.

CHAPTER 54

Drugs used in treatment of tuberculosis

The primary drugs in the treatment of tuberculosis are *isoniazid, ethambutol,* and *rifampin.* Secondary drugs include *streptomycin, aminosalicylic acid, ethionamide, capreomycin, kanamycin, pyrazinamide,* and *viomycin.*

Isoniazid and rifampin are the most effective drugs. Streptomycin is used infrequently because it must be administered parenterally, it is toxic, and there is rapid development of bacterial resistance. Aminosalicylic acid is still used in children, but it has considerable gastrointestinal toxicity. The secondary drugs are generally more toxic than members of the primary group but may have importance in selected cases (Table 54-1).

Combinations of drugs are necessary in the treatment of tuberculosis except when prophylaxis is desired. The purpose of combinations is to prevent the development of resistant tubercle bacilli.

ISONIAZID

The potent effect of isoniazid on the tubercle bacillus was discovered somewhat by accident as the result of routine screening of chemical intermediates in the synthesis of thiosemicarbazones.

Isoniazid is remarkably potent against the tubercle bacillus. It inhibits growth in the test tube at concentrations of less than 1 μg/ml. Its mechanism of action is not known, but it is of interest that pyridoxal antagonizes its neurotoxic effect without preventing its antibacterial action. It is also possible that the drug is incorporated into nicotinamide-containing coenzymes in mycobacteria. Some of the CNS effects of isoniazid have been attributed to interference with enzymes that require pyridoxal.

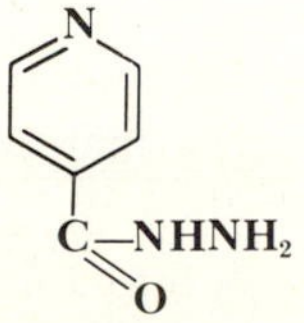

Isoniazid

Isoniazid is rapidly absorbed from the gastrointestinal tract. It is widely distributed in the body and penetrates efficiently into the cerebrospinal fluid. Its metab-

TABLE 54-1. Current antituberculous agents and side effects*

	Usual dosage†	Route	Side effects, toxicity, and precautions
Primary agents			
Isoniazid (INH)	3-5 mg/kg/day, usually 300 mg/day	Oral (intramuscular available)	Peripheral neuropathy (less than 1%); pyridoxine 50 to 100 mg daily will reduce this incidence; other neurological sequelae include convulsions, optic neuritis, toxic encephalopathy, psychosis, muscle twitching, dizziness, and alterations of sensorium (all rare); allergic skin rashes, fever, hepatitis (less than 1%); blood dyscrasias (rare)
Ethambutol	25 mg/kg/day for 2 months, then 15 mg/kg/day	Oral (intravenous available)	Optic neuritis with decreased visual acuity, central scotomas, and loss of green and red perception; peripheral neuropathy and headache (rare); rashes (rare); monthly evaluation of visual acuity, with greater than 10% loss considered significant, usually reversible if drug is discontinued
Rifampin	600 mg/day (single dose)	Oral	Although toxicity is uncommon, the following have been reported: gastrointestinal irritation, drug fever, skin rash, mental confusion, thrombocytopenia, leukopenia, transient abnormalities in liver function (SGOT, alkaline phosphatase). Interferes with some chemical determinations of bilirubin (false elevation); eosinophilia (rare); avoid in first trimester of pregnancy; discolors urine a brownish color. Increases requirement for coumarin-type anticoagulants.

*Courtesy Dr. Jay P. Sanford, Washington, D.C.
†Adult dosages only.

olism is not completely known, but acetylation is one of the important processes of biotransformation. The acetyl derivative and some of the original drug are cleared by the kidney.

Genetically conditioned differences in the ability to acetylate isoniazid are good examples of pharmacogenetics. Persons who show low acetylating ability maintain higher blood levels and may be more subject to the toxic effects of the drug.[7] More than 80% of patients are slow acetylators, and neurotoxicity is more common in this group. On the other hand, hepatotoxicity may be more common in the small group of fast acetylators.

Isoniazid is administered in doses of 3 to 4 mg/kg once a day. Larger doses have been used in tuberculous meningitis. Oral administration is preferred, but parenteral routes of administration can also be used.

Adverse effects caused by isoniazid include peripheral neuritis, hepatic necrosis, arthritic reactions, and hematological disturbances. Neurotoxicity is treated with large doses of pyridoxine.

TABLE 54-1. Current antituberculous agents and side effects—cont'd

	Usual dosage	Route	Side effects, toxicity, and precautions
Secondary agents			
p-Aminosalicylic acid (PAS) (Na^+ or K^+ salt)	10-12 g/day (200 mg/kg/day)	Oral	Gastrointestinal irritation (10% to 15%); goitrogenic action (rare); depressed prothrombin activity (rare); G6PD-mediated anemia (rare); drug fever, rashes, hepatitis, myalgia, arthralgia; Na^+ or K^+ must be taken into account in those with heart failure or renal insufficiency; give medication with meals or antacids
Ethionamide	500-750 mg/day (10-15 mg/kg/day)	Oral	Gastrointestinal irritation (up to 50% on large dose); goiter; peripheral neuropathy (rare); convulsions (rare); changes in affect (rare); difficulty in diabetes control; rashes, hepatitis; purpura; stomatitis; give drug with meals or antacids; 50 to 100 mg pyridoxine/day concomitantly; SGOT monthly
Pyrazinamide (PZA)	25 mg/kg/day (maximum 2.5 g/day)	Oral	Hyperuricemia (with or without symptoms); hepatitis (not over 2% if recommended dose not exceeded); gastric irritation; photosensitivity (rare); SGOT monthly; serum uric acid periodically, or if symptomatic gouty attack occurs
Cycloserine	750-1000 mg/day (15 mg/kg/day)	Oral	Convulsions, psychoses (5% to 10% of those receiving 1.0 g/day); headache; somnolence; hyperreflexia; increased CSF protein and pressure; contraindicated in epileptics; 100 mg pyridoxine (or more) daily should be given concomitantly
Kanamycin	1.0 g 3 or 4 times/wk (or 0.5 g daily)	Intramuscular	Ototoxicity (largely hearing loss); vertigo less common; nephrotoxicity; neuromuscular blockade; paresthesias; eosinophilia; drug fever; rashes; anaphylactoid reactions (rare); periodic renal functional assessments; audiograms when indicated
Viomycin	1.0 g 3 or 4 times/wk (or 0.5 g daily)	Intramuscular	Similar to kanamycin; hypocalcemia and hypokalemia; edema
Experimental agent			
Capreomycin (experimental)	1.0 g/day (15 mg/kg/day)	Intramuscular	Similar to kanamycin and viomycin

Drug interactions are significant. Rifampin increases the hepatic toxicity of isoniazid. Phenytoin toxicity is increased by isoniazid by interference with the metabolism of the antiepileptic drug. Adjustments of doses are necessary.

Resistance to isoniazid develops rapidly, and the combination with another effective drug delays the development of resistance.

Although the administration of vitamin B_6 may prevent neurotoxicity of isoniazid, there is no reason to believe that the effect of the drug on mycobacteria involves interference with this vitamin, since mycobacteria can synthesize B_6. Furthermore, pyridoxal phosphate does not prevent the effect of isoniazid on the tubercle bacillus.[7]

Isoniazid is available in 50, 100, and 300 mg tablets. There are also syrups and solutions for intramuscular administration.

Ethambutol hydrochloride (Myambutol) is highly effective in combination with other drugs in the treatment of tuberculosis. It has largely replaced aminosalicylic acid.

Ethambutol is absorbed rapidly from the gastrointestinal tract and is excreted mostly unchanged by the kidney. The drug does not cross the blood-brain barrier but may do so in meningitis.

Adverse effects of ethambutol are limited largely to ocular toxicity, which is dose dependent. Ocular toxicity manifests itself in loss of visual acuity and alterations in color perception. These manifestations are reversible and are not commonly experienced if dosage is limited to 15 to 25 mg/kg in one dose each day. It is believed that zinc deficiency may increase the ocular toxicity of ethambutol.

Ethambutol hydrochloride (Myambutol) is available in 100 and 400 mg tablets.

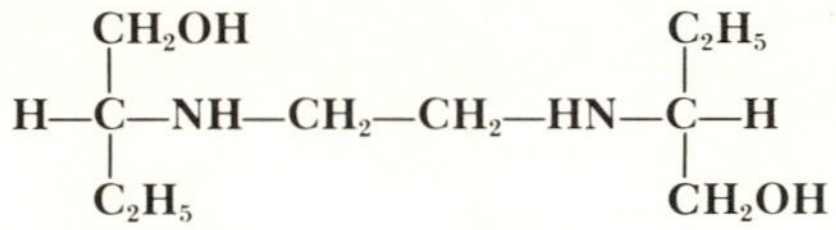

$$CH_2OH \qquad\qquad C_2H_5$$
$$H-\underset{\underset{C_2H_5}{|}}{\overset{\overset{|}{}}{C}}-NH-CH_2-CH_2-HN-\underset{\underset{CH_2OH}{|}}{\overset{\overset{|}{}}{C}}-H$$

Ethambutol

Rifampin is a semisynthetic derivative of rifamycin B produced by *Streptomyces mediterranei*. The drug is highly effective in the treatment of tuberculosis.[3,10,11] The antibacterial spectrum of rifampin is broad, since it includes both gram-positive and gram-negative organisms. Its therapeutic efficacy in the elimination of meningococcal carriers has been demonstrated.[2] Rifampin inhibits deoxyribonucleic acid (DNA)–dependent RNA polymerase,[4] the bacterial enzyme being more susceptible than its mammalian counterpart. After oral administration of 600 mg of rifampin, blood levels of 8 μg/ml are attained in less than 2 hours.[2] Serum antibacterial activity is often present in 12 hours.[10] Combinations of isoniazid and rifampin are highly effective in the treatment of tuberculosis.[10]

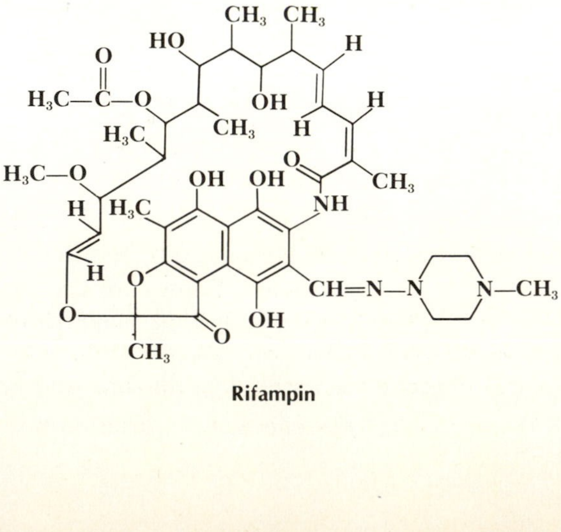

Rifampin

The development of rifampin may be considered a major advance in antituberculosis chemotherapy. It is of great value in patients with drug-resistant infections. Since resistance develops to rifampin, it is imperative to use it in combination with another antituberculous agent.

Rifampin is absorbed well from the gastrointestinal tract and is widely distributed through the body fluids, including the cerebrospinal fluid. The drug is metabolized in the liver and is excreted mostly in the bile. Some of its metabolites appear in the urine and cause a reddish discoloration.

Although most patients tolerate rifampin well, it may cause some adverse effects and numerous drug interactions. Adverse effects include abdominal symptoms, leg cramps, hepatotoxicity, and hypersensitivity with an influenza-like disease. Drug interactions are numerous. Rifampin increases the hepatotoxicity of isoniazid and decreases the effectiveness of oral anticoagulants and oral contraceptives. Aminosalicylic acid may interfere with the absorption of rifampin.

Rifampin acts on many bacteria and viruses in addition to being tuberculocidal. Since resistance develops rapidly to rifampin, its use is not recommended for infections other than tuberculosis.

Rifampin (Rifadin, Rimactane) is available in 300 mg capsules. It is administered in doses of 10 to 20 mg/kg daily in a single dose.

OTHER DRUGS

A number of drugs are viewed as alternatives to the previously discussed agents or secondary agents in the treatment of tuberculosis. Because of their frequent and serious side effects, this use should be limited to severe infections in which the less hazardous drugs may be ineffective.

Streptomycin was the first effective drug in the treatment of tuberculosis. Because it must be administered intramuscularly and because of its numerous toxic effects (p. 643) and the development of resistance, the drug is used only in selected cases of tuberculosis at present. It is most useful in combination with other drugs in the early months of therapy, in patients who cannot take oral medications, and in intermittent therapy. Occasionally, streptomycin is administered twice a week with other agents given daily. The dose of streptomycin is 20 mg/kg once daily for 2 or 3 weeks. Very often the drug is given less frequently but for longer periods. Streptomycin sulfate is available as a powder and in solution for injection containing 400 mg/ml or 500 mg/ml.

_p_-Aminosalicylic acid. The discovery of the usefulness of _p_-aminosalicylic acid (PAS) in the treatment of tuberculosis was a consequence of fundamental studies on the effect of various substances, including salicylic acid, on the oxygen uptake of the tubercle bacillus.[1] Salicylic acid was found to increase the oxygen consumption of virulent tubercle bacilli, and it became of interest to study the effect of related drugs.

_p_-Aminosalicylic acid inhibits growth of virulent tubercle bacilli at concentrations as low as 1 μg/ml. It has no effect on virulent saprophytic mycobacteria. In patients the drug is less effective than streptomycin and must be administered in very large doses, even up to 15 to 20 g/day. The great value of the drug results from the fact that it delays development of resistance to other tuberculostatic drugs.

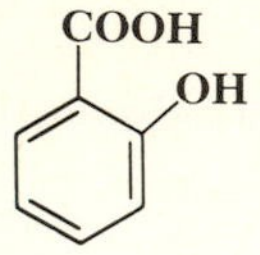

COOH
OH

Salicylic acid

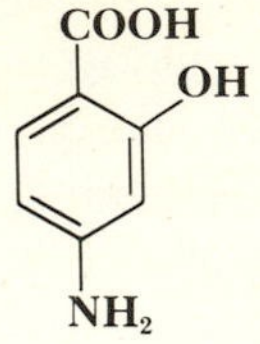

COOH
OH

NH$_2$

p-Aminosalicylic acid

The adverse effects of p-aminosalicylic acid consist of gastrointestinal disturbances, occasional skin rash, and, rarely, hepatic damage and interference with thyroid function.

The inhibitory effect of p-aminosalicylic acid on the tubercle bacillus is antagonized by p-aminobenzoic acid, a finding that suggests that its mode of action may be related to antagonism to this growth factor.

Ethionamide (Trecator) is a pyridine derivative, as is isoniazid. It is used in the treatment of tuberculosis in doses of 0.5 to 1 g/day. It is less effective than isoniazid.

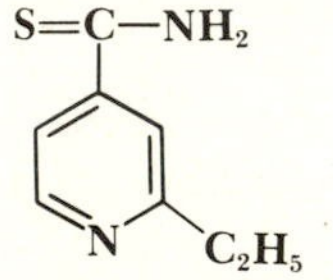

S=C—NH$_2$

N   C$_2$H$_5$

Ethionamide

Cycloserine (Oxamycin, Seromycin) has been somewhat effective in treatment of tuberculosis in combinations with other drugs. Unfortunately it is neurotoxic. It is administered by mouth in doses of 250 mg daily. Frequent side effects such as nausea, vomiting, hypotension, and peripheral neuritis limit the usefulness of cycloserine.

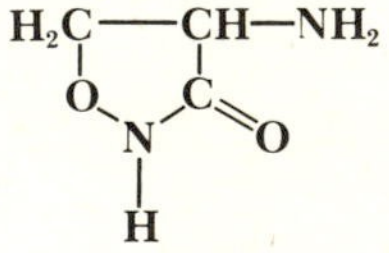

H$_2$C——CH—NH$_2$

O   C
N   O
H

Cycloserine

The mechanism of action of cycloserine involves competition for D-alanine as a precursor of some cell wall component.[5] As a consequence, the drug induces protoplast formation. Despite its neurotoxicity, cycloserine has some usefulness as a second-line drug in the treatment of tuberculosis and also in some urinary infections.

Cycloserine is well absorbed from the gastrointestinal tract, is widely distributed in the body, and penetrates well into the spinal fluid. It is excreted mostly unchanged into the urine, although part is metabolized.

Viomycin, a polypeptide antibiotic, is also somewhat effective against the tubercle bacillus but causes renal and auditory damage.

Pyrazinamide (pyrazinoic acid amine) is an analog of nicotinamide. It is inhibitory to the tubercle bacillus when administered in large doses, 3 g/day. It can cause hepatic damage and retention of uric acid.

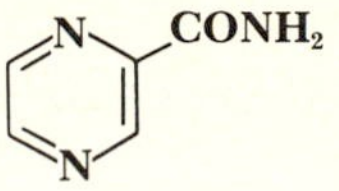

$$N\text{---}CONH_2$$

Pyrazinamide

Capreomycin sulfate (Capastat Sulfate) is a polypeptide antibiotic related to viomycin. Renal damage and ototoxicity limit the usefulness of this drug. **Kanamycin sulfate** (Kantrex) is not very useful in the treatment of tuberculosis. It must be administered parenterally and it can cause severe eighth nerve damage.

The most common atypical mycobacteria are susceptible to a combination of isoniazid and ethambutol, with rifampin as the secondary drug.

DRUGS FOR ATYPICAL MYCOBACTERIAL INFECTIONS

REFERENCES

1 Bernheim, F.: The effect of various substances on the oxygen uptake of the tubercle bacillus, J. Bacteriol. 41:387, 1941.

2 Deal, W. B., and Sanders, E.: Efficacy of rifampin in treatment of meningococcal carriers, N. Engl. J. Med. 281:641, 1969.

3 Editorial: Rifampin—a major new chemotherapeutic agent for the treatment of tuberculosis, N. Engl. J. Med. 280:615, 1969.

4 Hartmann, G., Honikel, K. O., Knüsel, F., and Neusch, J.: The specific inhibition of DNA-directed RNA synthesis by rifamycin, Biochim. Biophys. Acta 145:843, 1967.

5 Hoeprich, P. D.: Alanine: cycloserine antagonism, Arch. Intern. Med. 112:405, 1963.

6 Mitchell, R. S.: Control of tuberculosis, N. Engl. J. Med. 276:842, 905, 1967.

7 Robson, J. M., and Sullivan, F. M.: Antituberculosis drugs, Pharmacol. Rev. 15:169, 1963.

8 Ruiz, R. C.: D-Cycloserine in the treatment of tuberculosis resistant to standard drugs, study of 116 cases, Dis. Chest 45:181, 1964.

9 Skolnick, J. L., Stoler, B. S., Katz, D. B., and Anderson, W. H.: Rifampin, oral contraceptives and pregnancy, J.A.M.A. 236:1382, 1976.

10 Vall-Spinosa, A., Lester, W., Moulding, T. Davidson, P. T., and McClatchy, J. K.: Rifampin in the treatment of drug-resistant *Mycobacterium tuberculosis* infections, N. Engl. J. Med. 283:616, 1970.

11 Verbist, L., and Gyselen, A.: Antituberculous activity of rifampin in vitro and in vivo and the concentrations obtained in human blood, Am. Rev. Respir. Dis. 98:923, 1968.

REVIEWS

12 Brewin, A.: The treatment of tuberculosis, Ration. Drug Ther. 10:1, Oct. 1976.

12a Buechner, H. A.: The medical management of tuberculosis, Ration. Drug. Ther. 14:1, Oct. 1980.

13 Goldstein, M. S.: The rational treatment of tuberculosis today, Hosp. Formulary, Feb., 1977, p. 78.

14 Kagan, B. M.: Antimicrobial therapy, ed. 2, Philadelphia, 1974, W. B. Saunders Co.

15 Moulding, T., and Davidson, P. T.: Tuberculosis. I. Drug therapy, Drug Ther., Jan. 1974.

CHAPTER 55

Drugs used in treatment of leprosy

The most effective drugs in the treatment of leprosy are the sulfones. **Dapsone** (Avlosulfon) is most commonly used and is preferred to **sulfoxone** (Diasone) because of better absorption.

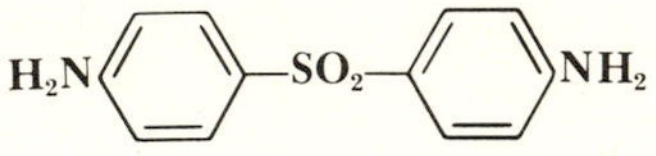

$$H_2N-\bigcirc-SO_2-\bigcirc-NH_2$$

4,4′-Diaminodiphenylsulfone

It is believed that the mode of action of these sulfones is similar to that of the sulfonamides, since *p*-aminobenzoic acid tends to antagonize their bacteriostatic activities. It is not known why these compounds have greater effectiveness than do the sulfonamides against leprosy.

With sulfone treatment, greatest improvement is noted in the ulcerative lesions. Nasal obstruction improves in 3 to 6 months. Bacteria disappear very slowly, and even after 5 years of treatment 50% of lepromatous patients continue to have positive smears.[2] Ethambutol and rifampin may be effective in the treatment of leprosy.[4]

An investigational drug **clofazimine** (Lamprene) appears to be as effective in leprosy as dapsone. It may be especially valuable in patients who have become resistant to treatment with sulfones. Clofazimine (Lamprene) is available in 100 mg capsules as an investigational drug.

REFERENCES

1 Bushby, S. R. M.: The chemotherapy of leprosy, Pharmacol. Rev. **10:**1, 1958.

2 Smith, J. W.: Leprosy, Tex. Med. **67:**58, 1971.

3 Trautman, J. R.: The management of leprosy and its complications, N. Engl. J. Med. **273:** 756, 1965.

4 U.S. Leprosy Panel: Rifampin Therapy of lepromatous leprosy, A. M. J. Trop. Med. Hyg. **24:**475, 1975.

CHAPTER 56

Antiseptics and disinfectants

There are many drugs that are useful in decreasing the bacterial flora when applied directly to the skin, infected wounds, instruments, or excreta. These locally effective drugs have a low enough therapeutic index to make them unsuited as systemic chemotherapeutic agents.

GENERAL CONCEPT

Antiseptics are drugs that are applied to living tissues for the purpose of killing bacteria or inhibiting their growth. *Disinfectants* are bactericidal drugs that are applied to nonliving materials. Other terms related to antiseptics and disinfectants that are commonly misused are as follows:

germicide Anything that destroys bacteria but not necessarily spores.
fungicide Anything that destroys fungi.
sporicide Anything that destroys spores.
sanitizer An agent that reduces the number of bacterial contaminants to a safe level, as may be judged by public health requirements.
preservative An agent or process that prevents decomposition by either chemical or physical means.

Disinfectants were used long before the discovery of bacteria. The first germicides used were deodorants, since foul odors were associated with disease. Chlorinated soda was used on infected wounds as early as 1825 (Labarraque), and its use was recommended at about the same time for the purification of drinking water.

BRIEF HISTORY

Phenol was used also as a deodorant and later as an antiseptic for infected wounds. Lister (1867) is usually credited with the introduction of phenol into surgery, but it was actually used long before the nature of infections was understood.

The use of alcohol was delayed for many years because Koch (1881) had reported that it did not kill anthrax spores. The superior germicidal properties of 70% alcohol were established by Beyer (1912).

Tincture of iodine was introduced into the *United States Pharmacopeia* in 1830, but it was not used extensively until the Civil War.

The importance of cleansing the hands with chlorine-containing solutions for the prevention of puerperal fever was clearly demonstrated by Semmelweis. This clinician, while working as an assistant at the Lying-in Hospital in Vienna, made some shrewd observations on the cause of puerperal fever. The ward where he worked was used for the training of medical students. Semmelweis noted that the mortality on the ward was lower when the medical students were on vacation. This

673

observation by itself could have had many different explanations. He also noted, however, the odor from the autopsy room whenever the students were present. He suspected that the students were carrying "decomposing organic matter" from the autopsy room to the delivery room. He proved his hypothesis when cleansing of the students' hands with a solution of chloride and lime resulted in a marked reduction in mortality from puerperal sepsis. (For a detailed history see Reddish.[3])

POTENCY OF ANTISEPTICS

Prior to the discovery of chemotherapeutic agents there was much preoccupation with the development of more and more potent antiseptics. Much effort was expended in synthesizing new compounds that could kill bacteria rapidly at high dilutions. The new antiseptics were generally compared with phenol, and the ratio of the dilutions necessary for killing test organisms in vitro was called the *phenol coefficient*. These efforts were so successful that antiseptics were synthesized that were hundreds of times more potent than phenol in killing bacteria in less than 10 minutes.

In retrospect, much of this effort was misdirected. Any drug that can kill bacteria in a few minutes is bound to have toxic effects on mammalian tissues. It is not surprising that even the most potent antiseptics were completely incapable of curing a systemic bacterial infection because the testing method used for their development was designed for *potency* and not for a favorable *therapeutic index*. The discoverers of Prontosil decided to test every compound against a systemic infection in mice. The sulfonamides and penicillin would never have been discovered by testing methods such as the use of the phenol coefficient. Not only the phenol coefficient but all tools for the evaluation of antiseptics are poor. It is not surprising that the field is dominated by empiricism and greatly influenced by fashion.

COMMONLY USED ANTISEPTICS AND DISINFECTANTS
Phenols

Phenol is a caustic substance that precipitates proteins. In a 1:90 dilution it can kill many bacteria in less than 10 minutes. Phenol has considerable systemic toxicity and is absorbed from denuded surfaces or burned areas. It can cause convulsions and renal damage.

Many derivatives of phenol find application as antiseptics or disinfectants. Saponated solutions of cresol (Lysol), resorcinol, and thymol have some medicinal uses, but the most widely used phenol derivative is hexachlorophene, which is incorporated into soaps and creams. In a 3% solution, hexachlorophene causes a marked reduction of bacterial counts on the skin without being irritating. Soaps containing hexachlorophene are generally used for preoperative scrubbing of the surgeon's hands and for antisepsis of the patient's skin.

The safety of hexachlorophene preparations, particularly for bathing newborn infants, has been seriously questioned. Such infants absorb some of the drug through the skin when the bath contains 3% of the antiseptic. Although no obvious toxicity has been demonstrated in human infants, newborn monkeys washed daily for 90 days with 3% solutions of hexachlorophene showed mean plasma levels of 2 to 3 μg/ml and developed brain lesions.[2] The Food and Drug Administration now advises against the use of 3% hexachlorophene for total body bathing. Such a product is still considered effective as a bacteriostatic skin cleanser and possibly effective in the treatment of staphylococcal skin infection. Evidence is lacking for the effectiveness and safety of hexachlorophene as an "aid to personal hygiene."

Halogen compounds

Tincture of iodine containing 2% iodine is often used for the preoperative preparation of the skin. The tincture stains the skin and is irritating to some individuals.

Povidone-iodine is a complex of polyvinylpyrrolidone and iodine. It releases iodine slowly and is claimed to be less irritating than tincture of iodine.

Sodium hypochlorite and chloramine T

Sodium hypochlorite and chloramine T release chlorine. They were popular at one time for the cleansing of infected wounds.

Halazone, tetraglycine hydroperiodide (Globaline), and aluminum hexaurea sulfate triiodide (Hexadine S) are among the compounds that are used for water disinfection by means of halogen release.

Oxidizing agents

Hydrogen peroxide, 3%, releases "nascent" oxygen in the presence of catalase in the tissues. Probably its only value lies in its ability to remove foreign material by means of the oxygen bubbles it forms. Other oxidizing antiseptics are potassium permanganate, zinc peroxide, and sodium perborate.

Alcohols and aldehydes

Ethyl alcohol is most bactericidal at 70% concentration by weight (78% by volume). It is commonly used as a skin antiseptic.

Isopropyl alcohol is at least as good an antiseptic as ethyl alcohol. It may be used as a 50% solution, but it is quite active when concentrated.

Formaldehyde in 40% concentration in formalin is used for the disinfection of instruments and excreta. It probably kills bacteria by combining with their proteins.

Surface-active compounds

Surface-active compounds have both hydrophilic and hydrophobic groups. They tend to accumulate in interfaces and probably disturb bacterial cell membranes that contain lipids. The surface-active antiseptics are of two types: anionic and cationic.

Anionic antiseptics. Various soaps and detergents such as sodium lauryl sulfate and sodium ethasulfate are antibacterial largely against gram-positive organisms. They are not nearly as important as the cationic antiseptics.

Cationic antiseptics. The hydrophilic group is usually a quaternary ammonium. Common representatives are benzalkonium (Zephiran), cetylpyridinium (Ceepryn), and benzethonium (Phemerol).

The cationic surface-active antiseptics are more potent at a higher pH. Their activity is decreased by soaps. In general they kill both gram-positive and gram-negative organisms, with some exceptions in the latter category.

The cationic antiseptics such as benzalkonium are commonly used for antisepsis of the skin and disinfection of instruments. The phenol coefficient of these compounds is very high, up to 500, but is reduced in the presence of pus and organic matter in general.

Metal-containing antiseptics   Mercuric chloride in a 1:1000 solution has been used widely as a skin antiseptic. It undoubtedly combines with SH groups in bacteria. Yellow mercuric oxide ointment, 1%, is used in the treatment of conjunctivitis.

The organic derivatives of mercury have been widely used as skin antiseptics. Some popular preparations are thimerosal (Merthiolate), nitromersol (Metaphen), and merbromin (Mercurochrome). These antiseptics are largely bacteriostatic.

Silver nitrate in a 1% solution has been traditionally applied to the eyes of newborn infants to prevent ophthalmia neonatorum caused by gonococci. This practice is being replaced by the application of penicillin in the conjunctival sac of the newborn infant.

Zinc salts are mild antiseptics and also astringents. Zinc sulfate ointment is used in some types of conjunctivitis, and zinc oxide ointment is a traditional remedy in the treatment of a variety of skin diseases. Calamine lotion USP contains mostly zinc oxide, with a small amount of ferric oxide. Phenolated calamine lotion USP also contains 1% phenol.

Nitrofurans   Nitrofurazone (Furacin) has been used in the form of ointments and solutions at a concentration of 0.2%. Although quite effective against both gram-positive and gram-negative organisms, it can cause skin sensitization in many patients.

Acids   Benzoic acid and salicylic acid have been used for many years as fungistatic agents. Whitfield's ointment is a mixture of 6% benzoic acid and 3% salicylic acid. It is commonly used for the treatment of fungal infections of the feet. Undecylenic acid (Desenex) is widely used in the treatment of "athlete's foot" and other fungal infections of the skin.

Mandelic acid and methenamine, used as urinary antiseptics, are discussed on p. 630.

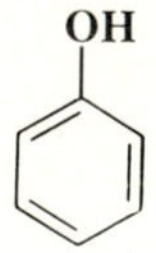

Phenol

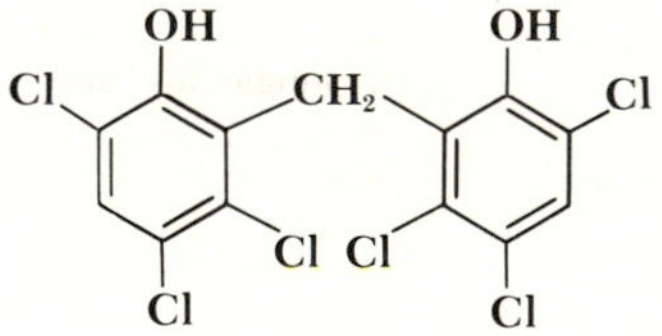

Hexachlorophene

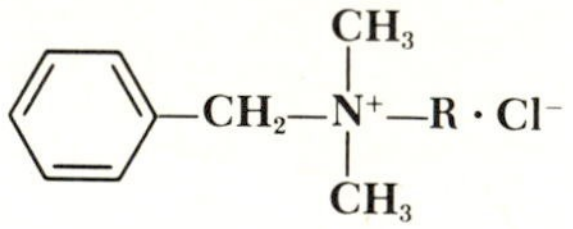

Benzalkonium chloride

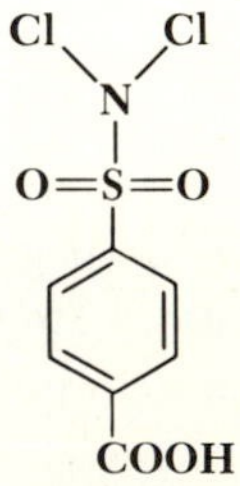

Halazone

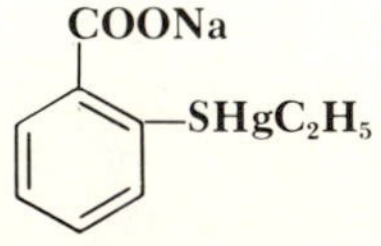

Thimerosal

With the development of powerful chemotherapeutic agents, the indications for the use of antiseptics have declined. They are unquestionably useful for reducing the bacterial counts on the skin, both on the surgeon's hands and on the patient. They generally have no place in the treatment of fresh wounds or infected wounds, where cleansing with saline is most important. Deeply infected wounds call for systemic chemotherapy.

INDICATIONS AND USES OF ANTISEPTICS

There is no general agreement on the most effective antiseptics. Some authorities consider the iodophors and chlorhexidine (Hibiclens) most effective. The iodophors release iodine slowly and are not as irritating as tincture of iodine. Chlorhexidine (Hibiclens) in a 4% solution is highly effective as a surgical scrub. Ethyl alcohol as a 70% aqueous solution is an efficient bactericidal agent. Isopropyl alcohol is somewhat more bactericidal than ethyl alcohol. Benzalkonium chloride (Zephiran) is an effective antiseptic, but some gram-negative bacteria resist its action. Hexachlorophene (pHisoHex) has several disadvantages. Its action is delayed, it is ineffective against several gram-negative organisms, and its absorption in infants can cause systemic toxicity.

Experimental studies indicate that alcohol is an excellent rapidly acting skin antiseptic. Hexachlorophene does not kill bacteria as rapidly. Much of the benefit of hexachlorophene is attributed to the film it leaves on the skin after repeated applications.

The skin cannot be completely sterilized. Cleansing, facilitated by surface-active agents such as the anionic or cationic surfactants, removes the superficial bacterial flora, which probably contains most of the pathogenic organisms. Alcohol is also excellent for preoperative preparations of the skin, but mild tincture of iodine and organic mercurials still have some advocates.

REFERENCES

1 Dineen, P.: Local antiseptics. In Modell, W., editor: Drugs of choice 1980-1981, St. Louis, 1980, The C. V. Mosby Co.

2 FDA Drug Bulletin, Dec., 1971.

3 Reddish, G. F., editor: Antiseptics, disinfectants, fungicides and chemical and physical sterilization, Philadelphia, 1957, Lea & Febiger.

CHAPTER 57

Drugs used in treatment of amebiasis

Amebiasis is caused by the protozoon *Entamoeba histolytica*. It occurs sporadically or in epidemics, the latter often following contamination of a water supply with sewage.

Entamoeba histolytica has two principal phases in its life cycle: the *trophozoite* and the *cystic*. The trophozoite is motile and can penetrate into the intestine, eventually reaching the liver. Ingested cysts liberate trophozoites in the intestine and cause the intestinal and extraintestinal forms of amebiasis.

From a therapeutic standpoint the amebicides can be divided into intestinal and extraintestinal drugs. The former are often poorly absorbed from the intestine and are used primarily for eradicating the infection at that site. Most antiamebic drugs belong to this category and cannot be relied on for eradication of the trophozoites in the liver or lungs. On the other hand, metronidazole, emetine, and chloroquine are effective in the extraintestinal forms of the disease.

Drugs useful in the treatment of intestinal amebiasis include, in addition to metronidazole and emetine, the antibiotics tetracycline or paromomycin, iodoquinol, and the obsolete arsenicals such as carbarsone.

Paromomycin is amebicidal, whereas tetracycline alters the bacterial flora with an indirect effect on the amebae.

ALKALOIDS OF IPECAC—EMETINE

Emetine is obtained from the dried root of *Cephaelis ipecacuanha*, or ipecac. The crude preparation has been used for centuries in treatment of dysentery, although it is only effective against amebic and not bacillary enteric infections. As early as 1912, emetine was used by intramuscular injection in treatment of amebiasis. The drug is still useful in efforts at eradication of the extraintestinal trophozoites. Emetine is useful also in controlling symptoms in acute amebiasis but is not curative.

The alkaloid is directly amebicidal at high dilutions in vitro. It exerts similar effects on trophozoites localized in tissues. It has a marked symptomatic effect in acute amebic dysentery but cannot be relied on for eradication of *Entamoeba histolytica* within the intestinal contents. As a consequence, if used alone, it would convert the acute form of the disease into the chronic or carrier phase.

678

TABLE 57-1. Antiamebic and some other antiprotozoal drugs of choice

Infecting organism	Drug of choice	Usual dosage	Route	Side effects and alternative agents
Entamoeba histolytica				
Intestinal (nondys- enteric)	Iodoquinol (diiodohy- droxyquin; Diodoquin)	650 mg tid — 21 days	Oral	Nausea, abdominal cramps, rash
Intestinal (dysen- teric)	Metronidazole (Flagyl)	750 mg tid — 10 days	Oral	Local pain electrocardiographic changes, arrhythmias, periph- eral neuropathy
Extraintestinal	Metronidazole (Flagyl)	750 mg tid — 10 days	Oral	Nausea, headache, diarrhea; alternatives: emetine or chloroquine
Giardia lamblia	Quinacrine hy- drochloride	100 mg tid — 5 days	Oral	CNS effects, yellow staining of skin and sclerae, urticaria, blood dyscrasias; alternative: metronidazole
Balantidium coli	Tetracycline	500 mg tid — 7 days	Oral	
Trichomonas vaginalis	Metronidazole (Flagyl)	250 mg tid — 10 days	Oral	Nausea, headache, diarrhea, rash, paresthesias

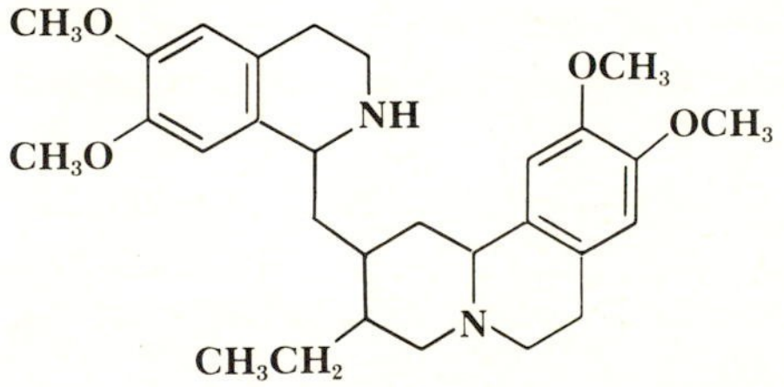

Emetine

The mechanism of action of emetine involves inhibition of protein synthesis in the parasites and in mammalian cells but not in bacteria. The related dihydroemetine dihydrochloride is available only from the Center for Disease Control, Atlanta. It may be somewhat less cardiotoxic than emetine.

Emetine is a toxic drug. Its main toxic action is manifest on cardiac and skeletal muscle. A dosage schedule of 65 mg/day for 10 days can be tolerated by most adults, but even on this dosage there may occur electrocardiographic changes such as T-wave inversion. Emetine is a cumulative drug, and its administration should not be continued beyond 10 days.

IODOQUINOL

Iodoquinol (diiodohydroxyquin; Yodoxin) is an intestinal amebicide that may be useful in combination with other drugs in the treatment of various forms of amebiasis. It may be used alone in asymptomatic carriers. The related drug, iodochlorhydroxy- quin, has caused an epidemic of subacute myelo-optic neuropathy (SMON) in Japan and is not used in this country. In rare cases iodoquinol can also cause SMON, but its most common adverse effects are related to gastrointestinal symptoms.

Iodoquinol (Yodoxin) is available in 210 mg tablets. The drug is also available generically. The usual dose for adults is 650 mg three times daily for up to 3 weeks.

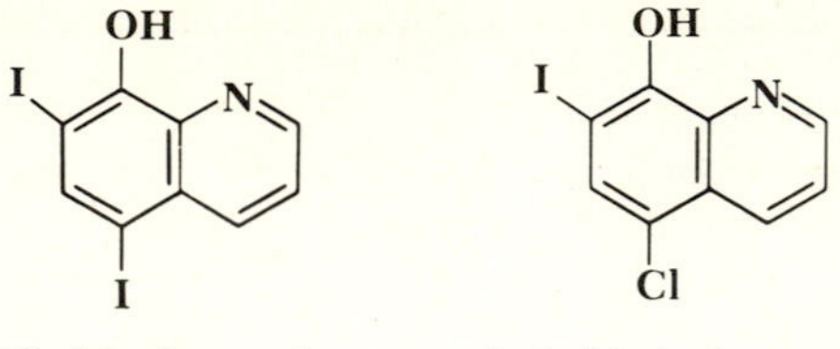

Diiodohydroxyquin   **Iodochlorhydroxyquin**

ARSENICALS   The organic arsenicals carbarsone and glycobiarsol are intestinal amebicides, which have become obsolete because more effective and less toxic drugs are available.

Carbarsone, or p-ureidobenzenearsonic acid, is a pentavalent arsenical that has been used in the treatment of amebiasis for many years. Its effectiveness is comparable to that of the iodoquinolines. Since the drug is absorbed from the gastrointestinal tract, arsenic poisoning may occur, and most experts advise against its use in the presence of liver damage.

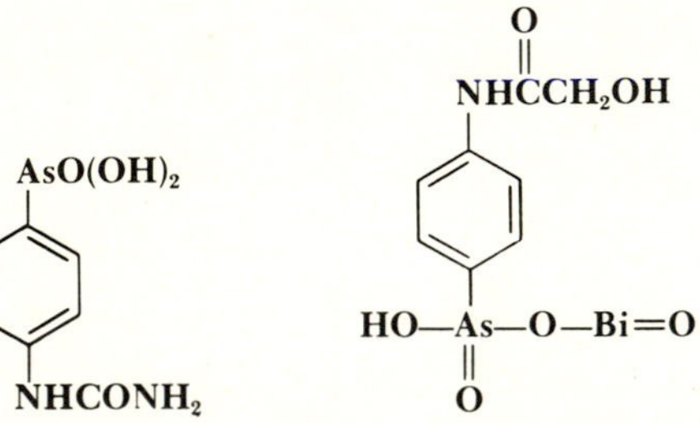

Carbarsone   **Glycobiarsol**

Another arsenical, **glycobiarsol** (Milibis), contains both arsenic and bismuth. It is not well absorbed from the gastrointestinal tract and is very effective against the intestinal ameba, although no action can be expected against trophozoites in the tissues. Thus, in hepatic amebiasis, additional amebicides such as chloroquine or emetine are necessary.

AMINOQUINO-   Chloroquine (Aralen) is a well-known antimalarial compound that is highly con-
LINES—   centrated in the liver[5] and is highly effective in treatment of amebic hepatitis and
CHLOROQUINE   amebic abscess of the liver. Its introduction as an extraintestinal amebicide was a most important therapeutic development in view of the many side effects and cardiotoxicity encountered with emetine, the only other effective extraintestinal antiamebic compound.

Chloroquine cannot be expected to eradicate the intestinal form of *Entamoeba histolytica*, and concomitant medication with an intestinal amebicide such as iodo-quinol is mandatory.

The recommended dosage of chloroquine is 0.25 g four times daily for 2 days, followed by 0.25 g twice daily for 2 weeks. Other dosage schedules have also been recommended. Additional information on chloroquine is included in Chapter 59.

ANTIBIOTICS

Early work with the antibacterial drugs has shown that patients with intestinal amebiasis improve more rapidly when these drugs are added to the usual antiamebic regimen. Later the tetracyclines, erythromycin, bacitracin, and paromomycin were found to be quite effective against intestinal forms of the disease.

The antibiotics may be useful as therapeutic adjuncts in amebiasis but are not effective enough to be used without some other amebicide. Paromomycin (Humatin) and erythromycin are directly amebicidal, whereas the tetracyclines act by modifying the bacterial flora and influence the amebae indirectly.

DRUGS USED IN TREATMENT OF TRICHOMONIASIS

Many amebicidal drugs have a killing effect on *Trichomonas vaginalis* also. Most of them such as carbarsone, glycobiarsol, and iodochlorhydroxyquin are effective only when applied topically. In contrast, the relatively new drug **metronidazole** (Flagyl) is highly effective in the treatment of *Trichomonas* infections when given orally. The drug is administered in 250 mg doses two or three times a day by mouth, usually for 10 days. Metronidazole may cause gastrointestinal symptoms, ataxia, vertigo, hematological complications such as leukopenia, and secondary monilial infection. Metronidazole may cause a disulfiram-like reaction when alcohol is ingested. The drug is contraindicated in pregnant women.

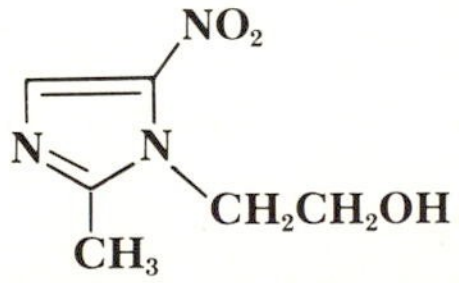

Metronidazole

Metronidazole (Flagyl) is also effective in the treatment of *Giardia* infections. There is some concern over its carcinogenicity in animals.

REFERENCES

1 Anderson, H. H.: Newer drugs in amebiasis, Clin. Pharmacol. Ther. **1**:78, 1960.

2 Balamuth, W., and Lasslo, A.: Comparative amoebicidal activity in some compounds related to emetine, Proc. Soc. Exp. Biol. Med. **80**:705, 1952.

3 Berberian, D. A., Dennis, E. W., and Pipkin, C. A.: The effectiveness of bismuthoxy *p*-N-glycolylarsanilate (Milibis) in the treatment of the intestinal amebiasis, Am. J. Trop. Med. **30**:613, 1950.

4 Clark, D., Solomons, E., and Siegal, S.: Drugs for vaginal trichomoniasis, Obstet. Gynecol. **20**:615, 1962.

5 Conan, N. J., Jr.: The treatment of hepatic amebiasis with chloroquine, Am. J. Med. **6**:309, 1949.

6 Most, H., and Van Assendelft, F.: Laboratory and clinical observations of the effect of terramycin in treatment of amebiasis, Ann. N.Y. Acad. Sci. **53**:427, 1950.

7 Sikat, P., Heemstra, J., Brooks, R., and Yankton, S. D.: Metronidazole chemotherapy for Trichomonas vaginalis infections, J.A.M.A. **182**:904, 1962.

REVIEWS

8 Kean, B. H.: The treatment of amebiasis, a recurrent agony, J.A.M.A. **235**:501, 1976.

9 Most, H.: Treatment of common parasitic infections of man encountered in the United States (second of two parts), N. Engl. J. Med. **287**:698, 1972.

10 Powell, J. S.: Therapy of amebiasis, Bull. N.Y. Acad. Med. **47**:469, 1971.

11 Wittner, M., and Rosenbaum, R. M.: Role of bacteria in modifying virulence of *Entamoeba histolytica*, Am. J. Trop. Med. Hyg. **19**:755, 1970.

CHAPTER 58

Anthelmintic drugs

Worm infections represent the most common parasitic diseases of humans. It has been estimated that in various parts of the world more than 800 million persons are infected with helminths.

A number of drugs have been used in the treatment of helminthiasis, largely on an empirical basis. Some of the early anthelmintics were highly toxic, whereas in recent years much more attention is being paid to the safety of such medications.

The drugs of choice for various helminthiases are shown in Table 58-1.

INDIVIDUAL ANTHELMINTICS Piperazine salts

Piperazine citrate (Antepar) forms piperazine hexahydrate, which is effective in the treatment of infections caused by *Ascaris* and *Enterobius*. However, pyrantel pamoate (Antiminth) is preferred for *Ascaris*, and mebendazole (Vermox) or pyrantel pamoate (Antiminth) is preferred for *Enterobius* infections.

Piperazine salts are well tolerated, although they may cause gastrointestinal symptoms and allergic reactions. Piperazine citrate should not be used in renal and hepatic insufficiency or in epileptic patients, since it may induce seizures. When used in large doses, the drug may cause CNS manifestations.

Piperazine citrate is available in a syrup containing 500 mg/5 ml or in 250 and 500 mg tablets. The oral dose for ascariasis in adults is 3.5 g once daily for 2 days. For pinworm infections the drug is given for 7 days in doses of 65 mg/kg daily, but not more than 2.5 g in 24 hours.

Studies on the mode of action of piperazine indicate that it causes paralysis of susceptible worms by a selective effect on the myoneural junction. The curare-like action is very weak on mammalian muscles, but worms appear to be much more susceptible.

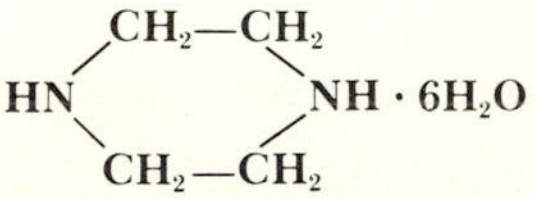

Piperazine hexahydrate

Hexylresorcinol

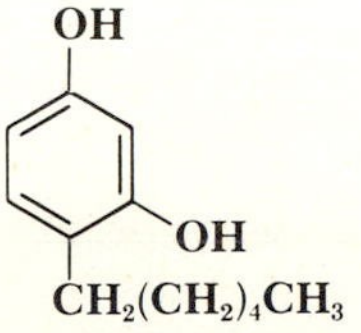

Hexylresorcinol

Hexylresorcinol was perhaps the first anthelmintic developed by a systematic in vitro screening method.[10] It is still valuable in the treatment of *Trichuris* infections, but mebendazole or thiabendazole is preferred. *Text continued on p. 688.*

TABLE 58-1. Summary of anthelmintic drugs*

Infecting organism	Drug of choice	Usual dosage	Route	Side effects and comments
Nematodes—intestinal				
Trichuris trichiura	Mebendazole (Vermox)	100 mg bid—q2 days	Oral	Diarrhea, usually 75% cure
	or			
	Hexylresorcinol	Up to 500 ml of 0.2% solution	Rectal	
Enterobius vermicularis (pinworm)	Mebendazole (Vermox)	100 mg single dose	Oral	Diarrhea, 90% cure
	or			
	Pyrvinium pamoate (Povan)	5 mg/kg single dose	Oral	Red stools, vomiting, diarrhea, photosensitivity
	or			
	Pyrantel pamoate	10 mg/kg single dose	Oral	Mild symptoms in 20%, somnolence, nausea, diarrhea
Ascaris lumbricoides	Mebendazole (Vermox)	100 mg bid—3 days	Oral	Mild symptoms in 20%, somnolence, nausea, diarrhea
	or			
	Pyrantel pamoate	10 mg/kg single dose	Oral	Mild symptoms in 20%, somnolence, nausea, diarrhea
Necator americanus (hookworm)	Mebendazole (Vermox)	100 mg bid—3 days		Mild symptoms in 20%, somnolence, nausea, diarrhea
	or			
	Pyrantel pamoate	10 mg/kg—3 days		Mild symptoms in 20%, somnolence, nausea, diarrhea
				Usually only available in soft gelatin capsules as a veterinary drug
	Bephenium hydroxy-naphthoate (Alcopar)	5.0 g (2.5 g of base) bid for 3 days	Oral	Nausea, vomiting, diarrhea
Ancylostoma duodenale	Bephenium hydroxy-naphthoate (Alcopar)	5.0 g (2.5 g of base) bid for 3 days	Oral	See *Necator americanus*
Trichostrongylus orientalis	Piperazine citrate	See *Ascaris lumbricoides*		
	or			
	Thiabendazole	See *Trichuris trichiura*		
	or			
	Bephenium hydroxy-naphthoate	See *Ancylostoma duodenale*		
Strongyloides stercoralis (strongyloidiasis)	Thiabendazole	25 mg/kg bid—2 days	Oral	Side effects: see *Trichuris trichiura*; alternative: pyrvinium pamoate (see *Enterobius vermicularis* for dosage)

Nematodes—extraintestinal

Organism (disease)	Drug	Dosage	Route	Side effects/remarks
Wuchereria bancrofti or Wuchereria (Brugia) malayi (filariasis)	Diethylcarbamazine (Hetrazan, Notezine, Banocide)	2 mg/kg tid—21 days	Oral after meals	Fever, malaise, vertigo, urticaria, headache, nausea, vomiting, inflammatory reactions of lymph nodes
Onchocerca volvulus (onchocerciasis)	Suramin (Naphuride, Bayer 205, Antrypol, Germanin) plus	Initial dose of 0.2 g to test for idiosyncrasy, then 1.0 g at weekly intervals for 5 weeks	Intravenous	See Trypanosoma rhodesiense; also fever, headache, muscle and joint pains; when possible all tumors should be excised
	Diethylcarbamazine (Hetrazan, Notezine, Banocide)	25 mg daily for 3 days, then 50 mg daily for 3 days, then 100 mg daily for 3 days, then 150 mg daily for 12 days	Oral	See Wuchereria; severe allergic reactions often require antihistamines or corticosteroids
Loa loa (eyeworm disease)	Diethylcarbamazine	2 mg/kg tid—21 days	Oral	See Wuchereria; also calabar swellings may appear; pruritus, arthralgia; allergic reactions often require antihistamines or corticosteroids
Acanthocheilonema perstans (acanthocheilonemiasis, dipetalonemiasis)	Diethylcarbamazine	See Wuchereria		
Dracunculus medinensis (dracunculiasis, guinea worm)	Niridazole (Ambilhar)	25 mg/kg daily—7 days	Oral	Vomiting, headache, dizziness, and ECG changes; rare instances of loss of consciousness, convulsions, psychosis
Trichinella spiralis (trichinosis)	Thiabendazole (Mintezol)	25 mg/kg bid—5 to 7 days	Oral	Side effects: see Trichuris trichiura; palliative measures include corticosteroids
Cutaneous Larva migrans (creeping eruption, Ancylostoma braziliense, dog and cat hookworms)	Thiabendazole (Mintezol)	25 mg/kg bid—2 days, repeat in 3 to 7 days if active lesions persist	Oral	Side effects: see Trichuris trichiura
Visceral Larva migrans (Toxocara canis, toxocariasis)	Thiabendazole (Mintezol)	25 mg/kg bid until symptoms subside or toxicity precludes further treatment	Oral	Side effects: see Trichuris trichiura

*Courtesy Dr. Jay P. Sanford, Washington, D.C.

Continued.

TABLE 58-1. Summary of anthelmintic drugs—cont'd

Infecting organism	Drug of choice	Usual dosage	Route	Side effects and comments
Trematodes				
Schistosoma haematobium (genitourinary bilharziasis)	Niridazole (Ambilhar)	25 mg/kg daily—7 days	Oral	Side effects: see *Dracunculus* *Alternative:* stibophen (Fuadin); in 50-75 kg person—1.5 ml intramuscularly 1st day; 3.5 ml 2nd day; 5.0 ml 3rd day; then 5.0 ml on alternate days of 18 injections total of 100 ml. Side effects: nausea, vomiting, arthralgia *Or alternative:* lucanthone hydrochloride (Miracil D, Nilodin), 10 to 20 mg/kg for 8 to 20 days. Some use it only in children less than 16 years. Side effects: nausea, vomiting, yellow skin, vertigo, restlessness, headache, confusion, and tremor
Schistosoma mansoni (intestinal bilharziasis)	Niridazole (Ambilhar)	25 mg/kg—7 days	Oral	Side effects: see *Dracunculus* *Alternatives:* see *S. haematobium*
Schistosoma japonicum (Oriental schistosomiasis)	Antimony potassium tartrate—0.5% solution	Total dose 360 ml; 8, 12, 16, 20, 24, 28 ml on alternate days, then 28 ml on alternate days to total dose	Intravenous	Nausea, vomiting, epigastric distress, conjunctivitis, peripheral neuritis, dizziness, faintness, precordial distress, ST-T wave changes on ECG; arthralgia and myalgia; paroxysmal coughing with injection; vascular collapse and death
Clonorchis sinensis (liver fluke)	Chloroquine phosphate (Aralen, Resochin)	0.5 g bid—3 days then 0.5 g daily for 30 days	Oral	Side effects: see Malaria, *Plasmodium vivax*
Fasciola hepatica (sheep liver fluke disease)	Emetine hydrochloride	30 mg daily—18 days	Intramuscular	Side effects: see *Entamoeba histolytica*, dysenteric, intestinal
Paragonimus westermani (lung fluke)	Bithional (Actamer, Bitin)	30 to 50 mg/kg every other day for 10 to 15 doses	Oral	Diarrhea, abdominal pain, nausea, vomiting, occasional urticaria

Cestodes

Parasite	Drug	Dosage	Route	Comment/Side effects
Diphyllobothrium latum (fish tapeworm)	Niclosamide (Cestocide, Yomesan)	1.0 g, then 1 hour later 1.0 g	Oral—chewed	Nausea, abdominal pain, diarrhea, pruritus
	or			
	Quinacrine hydrochloride (Atabrine)	0.1 g every 10 min to total of 0.8 g	Oral	Comment: 2 hours after last dose, administer saline purge. Side effects: nausea, vomiting, transient dizziness, yellowish discoloration of skin
Taenia saginata (beef tapeworm)	Same as *Diphyllobothrium latum*			*Alternative:* Oleoresin of aspidium, 4 to 8 g plus 8 g of acacia in water, one-half early in morning, the rest 1 hour later. Side effects: headache, vertigo, gastroenteritis, abdominal pain, diarrhea, nausea, vomiting, visual disturbances
Taenia solium (pork tapeworm)	Quinacrine hydrochloride (Atabrine)	See *Diphyllobothrium latum*		*Alternative:* Oleoresin of aspidium—see *Taenia saginata*
Hymenolepis nana (dwarf tapeworm)	Quinacrine hydrochloride (Atabrine)	0.1 g every 10 min to total of 0.5 g	Oral	See *Eiphyllobothrium latum*
	or			
	Niclosamide	1.0 g, then 1 hour later 1.0 g	Oral—chewed	See *Diphyllobothrium latum*
Echinococcus granulosus (echinococcosis)	None	—	—	Complete surgical excision of cyst

Pyrvinium pamoate   Pyrvinium pamoate (Povan) is a cyanine dye, which is effective in the treatment of pinworm infections when administered in a single dose. Although it is effective, mebendazole or pyrantel pamoate is preferred. Pyrvinium pamoate is not absorbed significantly from the gastrointestinal tract. It may cause gastrointestinal symptoms, and it stains the stool red.

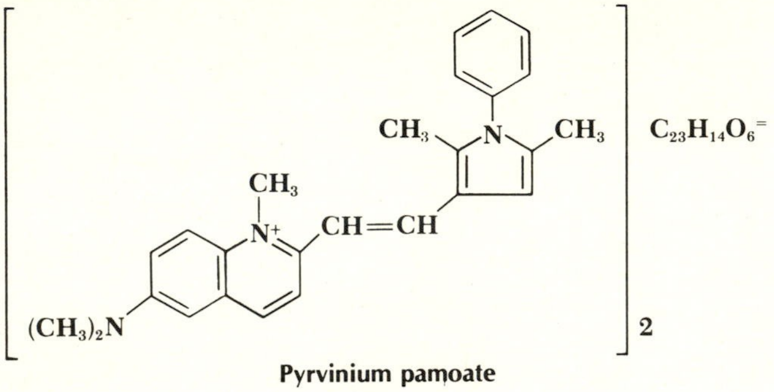

Pyrvinium pamoate

The cyanine dyes may exert an inhibitory effect on the oxidative metabolism of a number of helminths. Respiration and glycolysis of various worms are inhibited by these dyes.

Pyrvinium pamoate is administered in a single dose of 5 mg/kg. It is used in the treatment of *Enterobius* infection.

Bephenium hydroxy-naphthoate   Bephenium hydroxynaphthoate (Alcopar) is a quaternary ammonium compound, which is the best drug for treating hookworm infections.[8] The drug is absorbed only to a slight extent, and with the exception of some gastrointestinal adverse effects it appears to be of low toxicity. This drug is not available in the United States.

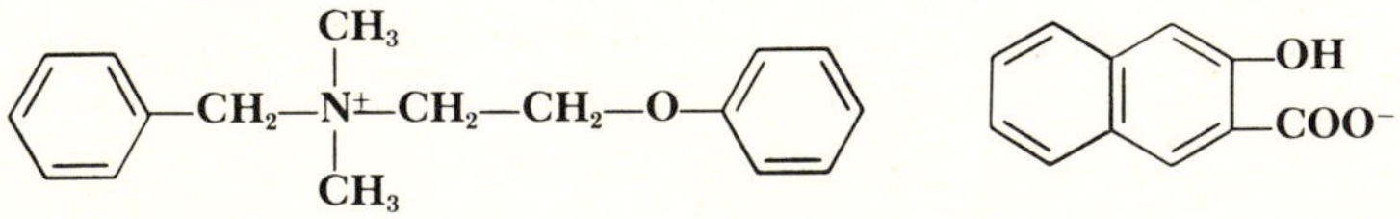

Bephenium hydroxynaphthoate

Tetrachloroethylene   The use of tetrachloroethylene in the treatment of hookworm infections is an outgrowth of the similar use of carbon tetrachloride. The latter is effective but is markedly toxic to the liver. When fats are avoided in the diet, tetrachloroethylene is absorbed to a much lesser extent from the gastrointestinal tract. It is much less toxic than carbon tetrachloride, probably because of lack of absorption.

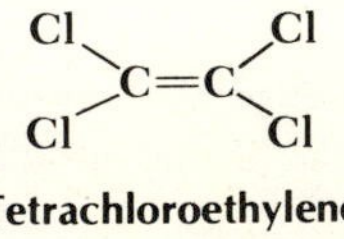

Tetrachloroethylene

In mixed *Ascaris* and hookworm infections tetrachloroethylene may cause the *Ascaris* to migrate. It is generally recommended that the *Ascaris* infection be treated first with pyrantel pamoate (Antiminth).

Pyrantel is effective in the treatment of infections caused by *Ascaris* and pinworm when given in a single large dose. The drug is also effective in the treatment of hookworm infections but is ineffective against *Trichuris*.

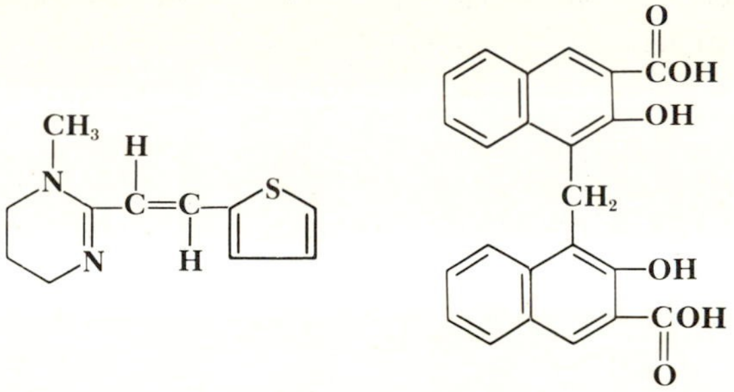

Pyrantel pamoate

Pyrantel pamoate

Adverse effects caused by pyrantel are largely gastrointestinal, headache, drowsiness, and skin rashes.

Pyrantel pamoate (Antiminth) is available as an oral suspension, 250 mg/5 ml.

Quinacrine

The antimalarial drug quinacrine (Atabrine) is effective in the treatment of tapeworm infections. However, niclosamide (Yomesan) is the preferred drug for infections caused by tapeworms.

The drug is sometimes administered by duodenal intubation, which assists in preventing side effects. Administration of sodium bicarbonate with divided doses of quinacrine is favored by some authorities in an effort to counteract the nausea and vomiting commonly associated with large doses.

Thiabendazole

Thiabendazole is the drug of choice in the treatment of infections caused by *Strongyloides stercoralis*. It is also effective in the treatment of pinworm infections, in cutaneous larva migrans (creeping eruption), and in hookworm infections. Results in trichinosis appear promising[16] but not conclusively established. The drug is also used in whipworm infections and in *Dracunculus medinensis* infections.

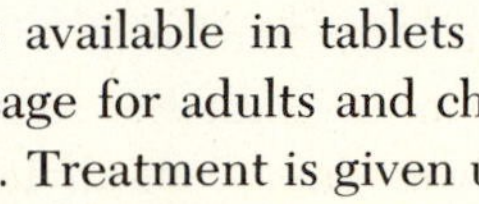

Thiabendazole

Adverse effects resulting from the use of thiabendazole are transient and dose related. They are gastrointestinal, chills, angioedema, tinnitus, and hypotension.

Thiabendazole (Mintezol) is available in tablets (chewable), 500 mg, and oral suspensions, 500 mg/5 ml. Dosage for adults and children is 25 mg/kg twice daily after meals. Maximal dose is 3 g. Treatment is given usually for 1 or 2 days, depending on the causative agents of the disease.

Mebendazole   Mebendazole (Vermox) is a broad-spectrum anthelmintic, which is effective against hookworms and *Ascaris* infections. Since it is effective in the treatment of several other worm infections, it is often used in mixed infections.

Mebendazole (Vermox) is available in 100 mg chewable tablets. One tablet is given twice a day for 3 days, although enterobiasis may respond to a single dose.

Niclosamide   Niclosamide is effective in the treatment of large and small tapeworm infections. The drug causes the worm segments to disintegrate. For this reason, if used in the treatment of *Taenia solium* infections, it should be followed by a cathartic in 1 to 2 hours.

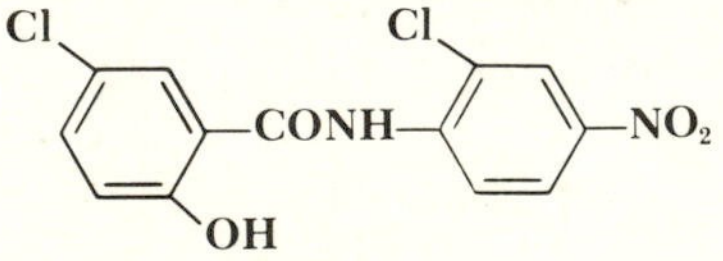

Niclosamide

Niclosamide (Yomesan) is available in tablets, 500 mg. Dosage for adults and children over 8 years of age is two doses of 1 g each 1 hour apart.

DRUGS USED IN TREATMENT OF SCHISTOSOMIASIS AND FILARIASIS
Antimony compounds   Various antimony compounds are effective in the treatment of schistosomiasis.[13] Antimony potassium tartrate (tartar emetic) is quite effective, but it is more toxic than stibophen (Fuadin), which is preferred by many. Stibophen is administered intramuscularly in 5 ml doses of a 6.3% solution, starting with smaller doses of 1.5 to 3.5 ml the first 2 days. A course of treatment consists of 20 injections on alternate days. Tartar emetic is still the drug of choice in *Schistosoma japonicum* infections, stibophen having little effect in this species.

The toxic effects of antimony compounds are abdominal disturbance, headache, fainting, skin rash, and electrocardiographic changes. Hepatitis and renal damage have also been observed.

Diethylcarbamazine   Diethylcarbamazine citrate (Hetrazan), a piperazine derivative, is effective for the treatment of filarial infestations caused by *Wuchereria bancrofti*, *Onchocerca volvulus*, and *Loa loa*. The usual dose is 2 mg of the citrate/kg three times a day for 7 to 21 days.

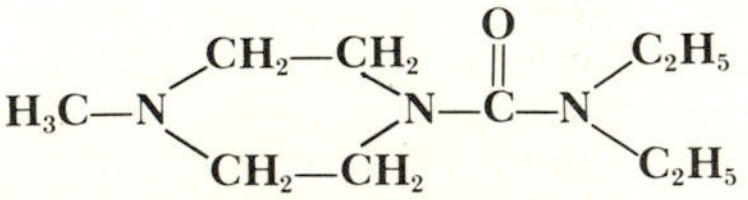

Diethylcarbamazine

The exact mode of action of this drug is not known. Although it contains piperazine, this compound by itself is ineffective in filariasis. The main effect in humans consists of disappearance of the microfilariae of *W. bancrofti* from the circulation. It is believed that the adult worms are killed or sterilized by the drug. The destruction of the microfilariae of *O. volvulus* by diethylcarbamazine can produce severe allergic manifestations.

Niridazole is probably the drug of choice in the treatment of *Schistosoma hematobium* infections. The drug may also be effective against *S. mansoni* and *S. japonicum* and *Dracunculus medinensis*. The drug should not be given to patients with liver disease or neuropsychiatric or convulsive disorders. Adverse effects of niridazole include gastrointestinal disturbances, arrhythmias, and neuropsychiatric disturbances. The drug may produce hemolytic anemia in patients with glucose-6-phosphate dehydrogenase deficiency.

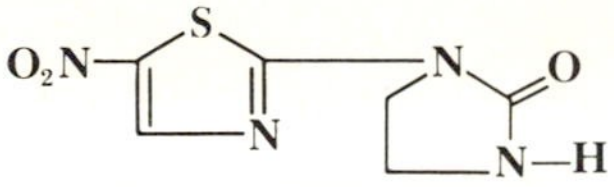

Niridazole

Niridazole

Niridazole (Ambilhar) is available in tablets, 500 mg. The drug must be obtained from the Center for Disease Control, Atlanta. Dosage for adults and children consists of 25 mg/kg daily in two divided doses for 5 to 7 days.

Suramin (Bayer 205) is effective against the adult worm of onchocerciasis. The drug must be injected intravenously, the usual dose for adults being 20 mg/kg once a week.

Suramin

In addition to suramin and diethylcarbamazine, a number of antimonials and arsenicals are also used in treatment of filariasis, with some favorable results. Their unpleasant side effects and the necessity of many injections represent disadvantages in the general use of drugs containing antimony and arsenic.

Some remarkably toxic compounds were used at one time in the treatment of helminthiasis. They will be mentioned only to emphasize the fact that they are dangerous and obsolete. Some of these are carbon tetrachloride, oil of chenopodium, santonin, and pelletierine.

OLDER AND OBSOLETE ANTHELMINTICS

REFERENCES

1 Brown, H. W.: The actions and uses of anthelmintics, Clin. Pharmacol. Ther. 1:87, 1960.
2 Brown, H. W.: The treatment of four common parasitic infections, Pharmacol. Phys. 3(1): 1969.
3 Bueding, E., and Swartzwelder, C.: Anthelmintics, Pharmacol. Rev. 9:329, 1953.
4 Bumbalo, T. S., Fugazzotto, D. J., and Wyczalek, J. V.: Treatment of enterobiasis with pyrantel pamoate, Am. J. Trop. Med. Hyg. 18:50, 1969.
5 Campbell, W. C., and Cuckler, A. C.: Thiabendazole in the treatment of and control of parasitic infections in man, Tex. Rep. Biol. Med. 27(Supp. 2):665, 1969.
6 Carr, P., Pichardo Sarda, M. E., and Nunez,

A.: Anthelmintic treatment of uncinariasis, Am. J. Trop. Med. 3:495, 1954.
7 Dunn, T. L.: Effect of piperazine derivatives on certain intestinal helminths, Lancet 1:592, 1955.
8 Goodwin, L. G., Jayewardene, L. G., and Standen, O. D.: Clinical trials with bephenium hydroxynaphthoate (Alcopar) against hookworm in Ceylon, Br. Med. J. 2:1572, 1958.
9 Katz, R., Ziegler, J., and Blank, H.: The natural course of creeping eruption and treatment with thiabendazole, Arch. Dermatol. 91:420, 1965.
10 Lamson, P. D., Caldwell, E. L., Brown, H. W., and Ward, C. B.: Hexylresorcinol in treatment of human ascariasis, Am. J. Hyg. 13:568, 1931.

11 Mansour, T. E.: The pharmacology and biochemistry of parasitic helminths, Adv. Pharmacol. **3:**129, 1964.

12 Miller, M. J., Krupp, I. M., Little, M. D., and Santos, C.: Mebendazole: an effective anthelmintic for trichuriasis and enterobiasis, J.A.M.A. **230:**1412, 1974.

13 Most, H.: Treatment of schistosomiasis, Am. J. Trop. Med. **4:**455, 1955.

14 Most, H.: Treatment of the more common worm infections, J.A.M.A. **185:**874, 1963.

15 Saz, H. J., and Bueding, E.: Relationships between anthelmintic effects and biochemical and physiological mechanisms, Pharmacol. Rev. **18:**871, 1966.

16 Stone, O. J., Stone, C. T., Jr., and Mullins, J. F.: Thiabendazole—probable cure for trichinosis, J.A.M.A. **187:**536, 1964.

17 Swartzwelder, J. C.: Intestinal helminthiases and their treatment, J. Louisiana Med. Soc. **111:**394, 1959.

18 Thompson, P.: Parasite chemotherapy, Annu. Rev. Pharmacol. **7:**77, 1967.

REVIEWS

19 Botero, D.: Chemotherapy of human intestinal parasitic diseases, Annu. Rev. Pharmacol. Toxicol. **18:**1, 1978.

20 Desowitz, R. S.: Antiparasite chemotherapy, Annu. Rev. Pharmacol. **11:**351, 1971.

21 Drugs for parasitic infections, Med. Lett. **20:** 17, 1978.

22 Drugs for parasitic infections, Med. Lett. **16:** 5, 1974.

23 Most, H.: Treatment of common parasitic infections of man encountered in the United States, N. Engl. J. Med. **287:**495, 1972.

CHAPTER 59

Antimalarial drugs

For centuries malaria was treated with cinchona bark, and until fairly recently the cinchona alkaloid, quinine, was the most generally employed antimalarial drug. Since World War II, very important developments have taken place in this field. Much more effective drugs have been developed, and new concepts concerning antimalarial therapy have evolved.

The malarial parasite is a protozoan organism of the genus *Plasmodium*. Of four species of *Plasmodium* that infect human beings, three are important. These are *Plasmodium falciparum, Plasmodium vivax*, and *Plasmodium malariae*. The fourth, *Plasmodium ovale*, is numerically unimportant. Other plasmodia also occur in animals, and some of these have been important in antimalarial screening studies.

The insect vector is the female *Anopheles* mosquito. Public health measures directed at eradication of the mosquito are of great importance. It is unlikely, however, that such efforts will be completely successful. The other approach to the problem of malaria is chemotherapy.

The life cycle of the malarial parasite has been divided into several phases: (1) sporozoite phase, (2) primary tissue phase, (3) asexual blood phase, (4) sexual phase, and (5) secondary tissue phase, which, however, does not occur in *P. falciparum* infections.

The major new concept of great importance in therapy is recognition of the importance of the primary and secondary tissue phases, which are commonly referred to as the exoerythrocytic cycle of the malarial parasite. The liver is the only organ in which exoerythrocytic stages have been demonstrated.

The *Anopheles* mosquito inoculates *sporozoites* into the bitten person. The various antimalarial agents have no effect on sporozoites, which remain in the bloodstream for a very short time and are localized in various tissues such as the liver.

From this primary tissue localization the parasite penetrates into red cells, where it is first seen as a *trophozoite*, which develops into the mature *schizont*. When the parasitized red cell bursts, it releases *merozoites*, and a malarial chill occurs. Certain modified trophozoites develop into *gametocytes*. These sexual forms represent the link between the human being and the mosquito and are important in the perpetuation of the disease in an area. Fertilization takes place in the mosquito, and sporozoites eventually appear in its salivary glands, ready for the next person who may be bitten.

PRESENT CONCEPTS OF MALARIA

693

TREATMENT OF MALARIA

The classification of antimalarial drugs is based on the various stages of the life cycle of the *Plasmodium*. Drugs that cure a clinical attack by eliminating the asexual forms are known as *schizonticides*. They include chloroquine (Aralen), amodiaquine hydrochloride (Camoquin), quinine sulfate (Quine), hydroxychloroquine (Plaquenil), and pyrimethamine (Daraprim). Tetracycline and combinations of a sulfonamide with pyrimethamine are effective also.

Radical cure implies the elimination of both the asexual forms and the exoerythrocytic forms of the malarial parasite from the body. In falciparum malaria the usual schizonticides may be sufficient to achieve radical cure, since no exoerythrocytic forms are left after treatment. In vivax malaria primaquine must be added to the treatment to obtain a radical cure.

Clinical prophylaxis can be achieved by the schizonticide chloroquine administered in a 300 mg dose once a week. Individuals receiving clinical prophylaxis may have to take primaquine after returning from an area where malaria is prevalent. *Causal prophylaxis* involves the use of primaquine, and because of the toxicity of this drug, there is no general agreement on the need for causal prophylaxis (Table 59-1).

Chloroquine

Chloroquine (Aralen), a 4-aminoquinoline derivative, was first synthesized in Germany in 1934. It was considered too toxic on the basis of a few tests in human beings and was discarded. A closely related compound was used by the French in North Africa in World War II and appeared quite effective and well tolerated. Subsequently a larger series of related compounds was synthesized in the United States, and extensive studies soon showed that chloroquine was the most satisfactory in the group.

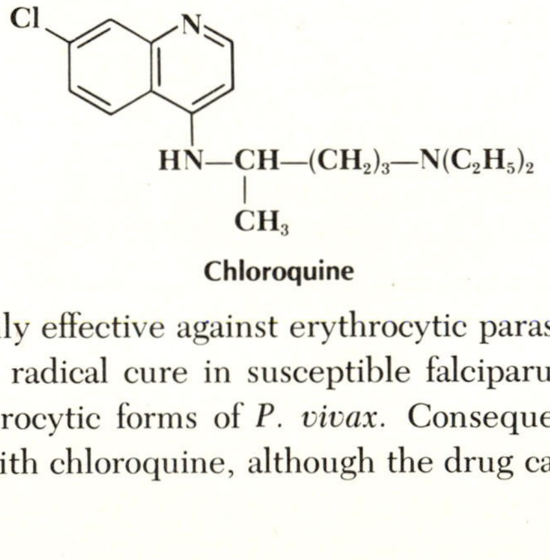

$$HN—CH—(CH_2)_3—N(C_2H_5)_2$$
$$|$$
$$CH_3$$

Chloroquine

Antimalarial activity

Chloroquine is highly effective against erythrocytic parasites. It is a suppressive drug that can produce radical cure in susceptible falciparum malaria but will not eliminate the exoerythrocytic forms of *P. vivax*. Consequently, relapses occur in vivax malaria treated with chloroquine, although the drug can terminate the clinical attacks very efficiently.

Metabolism

Chloroquine is rapidly and almost completely absorbed from the gastrointestinal tract. Its distribution is such that some tissues such as liver may contain more than 500 times as much of the drug as does plasma. This affinity for the liver suggested its use in hepatic amebiasis.

Chloroquine may occasionally be injected by the intramuscular route. However, this is seldom necessary. For intramuscular injection, chloroquine hydrochloride is given in a dose of 250 mg. For other uses see p. 680.

TABLE 59-1. Summary of drugs used in the treatment of malaria*

Infecting organism	Drug of choice	Usual dosage	Route	Side effects and comments
Malaria				
Acute attack due to *P. vivax, P. malariae, P. ovale,* "chloroquine-sensitive" *P. falciparum*	Chloroquine phosphate (Aralen, Resochin) plus	1 g (600 mg base), then 0.5 g in 6 hours, then 0.5 g daily for 2 days. (Total dose 2.5 g)	Oral	Pruritus, vomiting, headache, skin eruption, depigmentation of hair, partial alopecia, hemolytic anemia, leukopenia, thrombocytopenia, rare deafness, retinal damage
	Primaquine phosphate	26.3 mg (15 mg base) daily for 14 days	Oral	Hemolytic anemia in G6PD defect, neutropenia, GI, rare CNS symptoms, hypertension, arrhythmias
Acute attack due to *P. falciparum* (chloroquine-resistant strains — S.E. Asia, S. America)	Quinine sulfate plus	650 mg tid — 10 days	Oral	Arrhythmias, tinnitus, hypotension, headache, nausea, abdominal pain, visual disturbance, blood dyscrasia
	Pyrimethamine (Daraprim) plus	25 mg every 12 hours for 3 days	Oral	Megaloblastic anemia, blood dyscrasia, rare rash, convulsions, shock
	Sulfadiazine	500 mg qid — 5 days	Oral	See Table 52-2 for side effects. *Alternative:* Dapsone (Avlosulfon), 25 mg daily for 28 days
Prophylaxis and suppression	Chloroquine phosphate plus	500 mg (300 mg base) once weekly, continued for 6 weeks after last exposure	Oral	As above
	Primaquine phosphate	26.3 mg (15 mg base) daily for 14 days after last exposure in endemic area	Oral	As above

*Courtesy Dr. Jay P. Sanford, Washington, D.C.

Toxicity

Studies in human volunteers have shown that the toxicity of chloroquine is quite low when suppressive doses are employed. In larger doses dizziness, blurring of vision, headache, diarrhea, and epigastric distress have been reported. These symptoms disappear when the dosage is decreased. Retinopathy and corneal deposits may also occur[9] and may result in blindness.

Resistance to chloroquine

Chloroquine-resistant *P. falciparum* has been encountered with increasing frequency in South America, Southeast Asia, and Africa.[2,5] Such strains have created a serious problem in South Vietnam since 1965. While combined chloroquine-quinine therapy was usually effective, a very high percentage of patients, more than 40%, had relapses within 2 weeks. Several new drug combinations have been introduced to meet this problem.

One of these combinations is quinine with tetracycline. Also quinine with pyrimethamine and a sulfonamide are effective in the treatment of chloroquine-resistant falciparum malaria. This may be the only use for quinine in malaria.

Amodiaquin
Amodiaquin (Camoquin) is similar to chloroquine as an antimalarial. It is given by mouth in doses of 0.6 g daily as a suppressive antimalarial or 1.8 g in divided doses the first day, followed by 0.6 g/day for 2 or 3 days for clinical control.

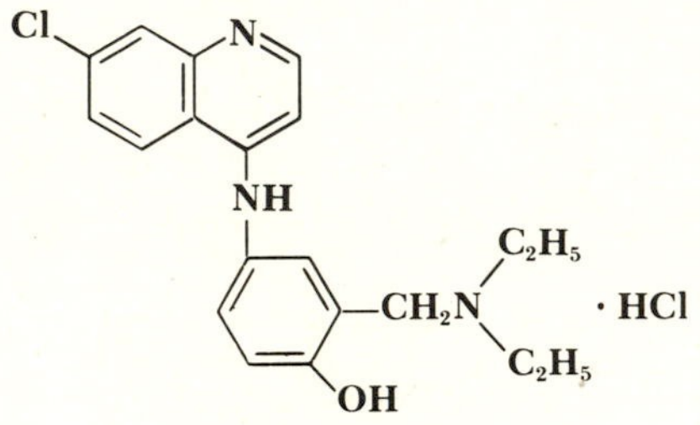

Amodiaquin hydrochloride

Hydroxychloroquine
Hydroxychloroquine sulfate (Plaquenil) is a 4-aminoquinoline, which is very similar to chloroquine without significant advantages over the parent drug.

Primaquine
Certain 8-aminoquinolines have the ability to destroy exoerythrocytic malarial parasites. Primaquine is at present considered to be the most effective representative of this group of antimalarial drugs.

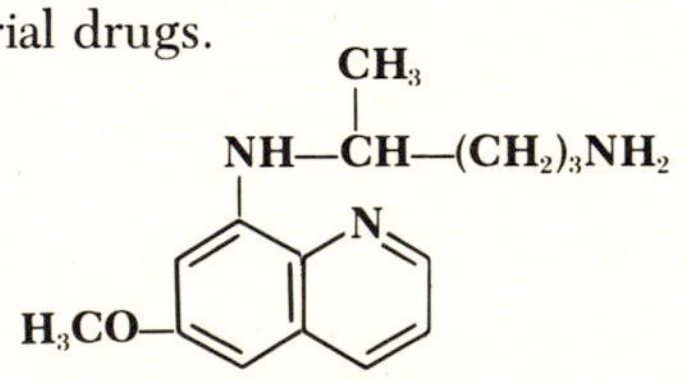

Primaquine

The development of primaquine is a late consequence of studies on the synthetic antimalarial drug pamaquine (Plasmochin). It was shown as early as 1925 that this drug was lethal to gametocytes, although it was not safe enough for complete elimination of the asexual forms from the blood. The drug was tried in some areas in combination with quinine for the purpose of controlling malaria by eliminating the gametocytes. There was an indication during these trials that the relapse rate in vivax malaria was reduced. This finding suggested an important property of the 8-aminoquinolines. Pamaquine was fairly toxic and did not appear promising. On the other hand, when related 8-aminoquinolines were synthesized during World War II, several were found to be safer than pamaquine. Pentaquine was first used as a curative antimalarial drug but was superseded by primaquine because the latter was found to be less toxic.

Primaquine is useful in producing radical cure in *P. vivax* infections because of its effect on the exoerythrocytic stages. It is also effective against the exoerythrocytic forms of *P. falciparum*. It has some activity against the asexual forms of these parasites, but this activity is not high enough to make it an efficient suppressive as well as curative drug. For this reason primaquine is usually given in combination with a suppressive antimalarial drug.

Antimalarial activity

Clinical trials in vivax malaria have shown that concomitant administration of chloroquine as a suppressive, coupled with 15 mg primaquine/day for 14 days, will often achieve a radical cure. In a comparable group receiving chloroquine alone, the relapse rate was 39%.[1]

Primaquine is rapidly absorbed from the gastrointestinal tract. In contrast with chloroquine, however, it is also rapidly metabolized and excreted. Its tissue fixation is very slight, and the drug is altered and excreted in less than 24 hours.

Metabolism

Although primaquine is generally well tolerated at the recommended therapeutic dosages, some patients may complain of anorexia, nausea, abdominal cramps, and other vague symptoms. There may be depression of the activity of the bone marrow, with leukopenia and anemia. The effects on the blood, including some methemoglobinemia, are aggravated by concomitant use of quinacrine.

Toxicity

Hemolytic anemia that follows primaquine therapy is related to an interesting genetic abnormality. It is more likely to occur in dark-skinned races.[10] The red cells of susceptible persons show a defect in the mechanisms that protect hemoglobin against denaturation. The reduced glutathione (GSH) content of such cells was as low as 50 mg/100 ml as compared with 75 mg/100 ml in normal cells. The metabolic error in primaquine-sensitive red cells appears to be a deficiency of glucose-6-phosphate dehydrogenase.[6] These GSH-deficient red cells are also sensitive to acetanilid, sulfanilamide, phenylhydrazine, sulfoxone, and acetophenetidin (p. 68).

Pyrimethamine is an inhibitor of dihydrofolate reductase of malarial parasites. Resistance to its action develops rapidly, and for this reason the drug is only used for prophylaxis and for the treatment of *P. falciparum* malaria, which is resistant to chloroquine.

Pyrimethamine

The discovery of the potent antimalarial drug pyrimethamine (Daraprim) was the result of observations on the similarities between the antimalarial drug chlorguanide and certain folic acid antagonists such as the 2,4-diamino-5-substituted pyrimidines. One of these antimetabolites was found to have antimalarial activity in animals, and soon many others were tested. Pyrimethamine is a member of this series.

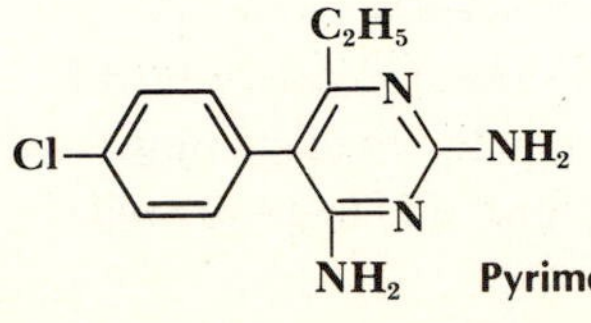

Pyrimethamine

Toxicity   Pyrimethamine appears to be quite safe when administered in doses of 25 to 50 mg once or twice a week.[7] Megaloblastic anemia of a transient nature has occurred in some persons following the use of pyrimethamine.[12] This action may be related to metabolic antagonism to folic acid or folinic acid. Pyrimethamine blocks the enzyme dihydrofolic acid reductase.

Pyrimethamine is related to trimethoprim; however, the latter has a greater affinity for bacterial dihydrofolic acid reductase.

The drug is not recommended for treatment of the acute attack because it is slow-acting. Although it has remarkable gametocidal activity against some strains of *P. falciparum*, it is ineffective against others. Resistant strains have become common.

Trimethoprim   Trimethoprim is a synthetic diaminopyrimidine compound related to pyrimethamine. Both inhibit dihydrofolate reductase. Trimethoprim is synergistic with sulfonamides, which is to be expected since it acts sequentially with the latter in blocking the synthesis of folic acid in bacteria. For the same reason pyrimethamine and sulfonamides may be synergistic in the treatment of malaria.[11] Trimethoprim in combination with sulfamethoxazole is being used in the treatment of some bacterial infections (p. 627).

Other antimalarial drugs   **Quinine** has been the traditional antimalarial remedy that has been gradually replaced by newer drugs. It is a suppressive drug and will not cure vivax malaria. Even as a suppressive, it is not nearly as efficient as chloroquine or other newer antimalarial drugs. The drug has become very important again in the treatment of chloroquine-resistant falciparum malaria.

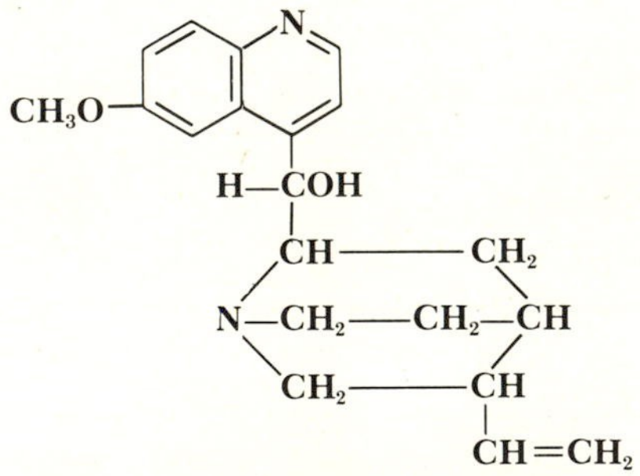

Quinine

The adult dose of quinine sulfate is 1 g three times daily. The drug is rapidly absorbed, and most of it is metabolized, about 10% being excreted unchanged in the urine and the remainder in the form of metabolic products. Metabolism and excretion are both rapid, and no cumulation occurs when quinine sulfate is given daily for long periods of time. In a patient who cannot take or tolerate oral quinine, the drug may be injected as the dihydrochloride by slow intravenous drip. For this purpose 650 mg of quinine is dissolved in 300 ml of saline solution.

Quinine can produce a variety of toxic effects, some of which are known by the collective name *cinchonism*. Headache, nausea, tinnitus, and visual disturbances can occur. Allergic skin rashes and asthmatic attacks have also been reported.

Quinine has other uses in medicine. It is given occasionally for the relief of leg cramps, as a diagnostic test for myasthenia gravis, in the treatment of myotonia congenita, and as a sclerosing agent.

Quinacrine (Atabrine) is a yellow acridine derivative. It was at one time an important antimalarial, but chloroquine has so many advantages over quinacrine that the latter is gradually being abandoned in treatment of malaria.

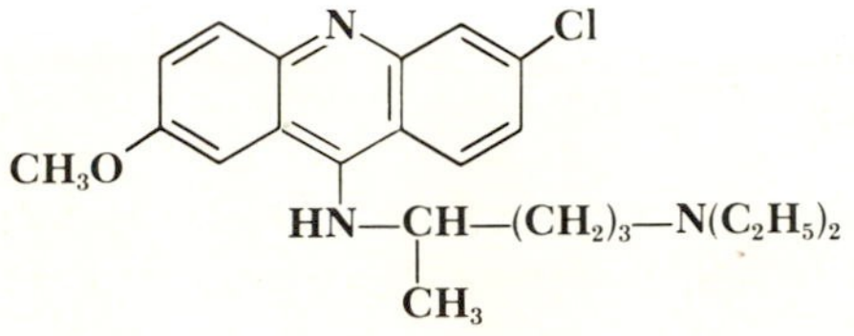

Quinacrine

Quinacrine is probably more valuable at present for purposes other than antimalarial therapy. It is important in the treatment of certain tapeworm infestations.

Chlorguanide (Paludrine) was synthesized in England during World War II. It is a suppressive antimalarial drug. Its action may be related to metabolic antagonism to folic acid, perhaps because of a metabolic product of this compound. The suppressive effect of chlorguanide is somewhat slow in onset.

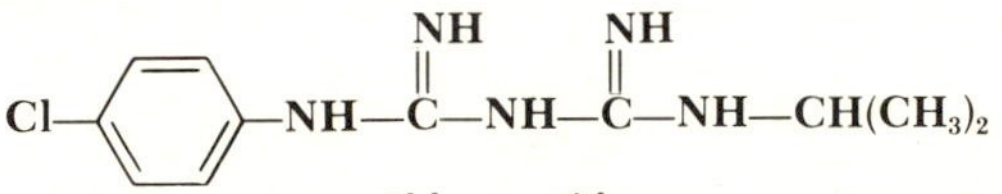

Chlorguanide

Perhaps the greatest disadvantage of this drug has to do with development of resistance by plasmodia. Studies on the chemical relationship between chlorguanide and folic acid antagonists were directly responsible for the development of pyrimethamine. A chlorguanide derivative appears promising as a long-term suppressant when injected as pamoate salt.

Cycloguanide pamoate (Camolar), an insoluble salt of a chlorguanide derivative, is remarkable in that a single intramuscular injection exerts a protective effect for several months. This prolonged effect is a consequence of its extremely slow absorption from muscle. Cycloguanide pamoate may play an important role in eradication of malaria in some parts of the world, provided that its continued use does not reveal serious adverse effects. The drug is not yet generally available.

REFERENCES

1 Alving, A. S., et al.: Korean vivax malaria: curative treatment with pamaquine and primaquine, Am. J. Trop. Med. **2:**970, 1953.

2 Bartelloni, P. J., Sheehy, T. W., and Tigertt, W. D.: Combined therapy for chloroquine-resistant *Plasmodium falciparum* infection, J.A.M.A. **109:**173, 1967.

3 Beutler, E.: The hemolytic effect of primaquine and related compounds: a review, Blood
14:103, 1959.

4 Beutler, E.: Drug-induced blood dyscrasias,
J.A.M.A. 189:143, 1964.

5 Blount, R. E.: Management of chloroquine-
resistant falciparum malaria, Arch. Intern.
Med. 119:557, 1967.

6 Carlson, P. E., Flanagan, C. L., Ickes, C. E.,
and Alving, A. S.: Enzymatic deficiency in
primaquine-sensitive erythrocytes, Science
124:484, 1956.

7 Coatney, G. R., Myatt, A. V., Hernandez, T.,
Jeffery, G. M., and Cooper, W. C.: The protective and therapeutic effects of pyrimethamine (Daraprim) against Chesson strain vivax
malaria, Am. J. Trop. Med. 2:777, 1953.

8 Elslager, E. F., and Thompson, P. E.: Parasite
chemotherapy, Annu. Rev. Pharmacol. 2:193,
1962.

9 Henkind, P., and Rothfield, N. F.: Ocular abnormalities in patients treated with synthetic
antimalarial drugs, N. Engl. J. Med. 269:433,
1963.

10 Hockwald, R. S., Arnold, J., Clayman, C. B.,
and Alving, A. S.: Status of primaquine: Toxicity of primaquine in Negroes, J.A.M.A. 149:
1568, 1952.

11 Hunsicker, L. G.: The pharmacology of antimalarials, Arch. Intern. Med. 123:645, 1969.

12 Myatt, A. V., Hernandez, T., and Coatney, G.
R.: Studies in human malaria: the toxicity of
pyrimethamine (Daraprim) in man, Am. J.
Trop. Med. 2:788, 1953.

13 Rieckmann, K. H.: Determination of the drug
sensitivity of *Plasmodium falciparum*, J.A.M.A.
217:573, 1971.

14 Schellenberg, K. A., and Coatney, G. R.: The
influence of antimalaria drugs on nucleic acid
synthesis in *Plasmodium gallinaceum* and *Plasmodium berghei*, Biochem. Pharmacol. 6:143,
1961.

15 Schnitzer, R. J., and Hawking, F., editors: Experimental chemotherapy, vol. 1, New York,
1963, Academic Press, Inc.

16 Sheehy, T. W., and Dempsey, H.: Methotrexate therapy for *Plasmodium vivax* malaria,
J.A.M.A. 214:109, 1970.

17 Sheehy, T. W., Reba, R. C., Neff, T. A., Gaint-
ner, J. R., and Tigertt, W. D.: Supplemental
sulfone (dapsone) therapy; use in treatment of
chloroquine-resistant falciparum malaria, Arch.
Intern. Med. 119:561, 1967.

18 Thompson, P. E.: Parasite chemotherapy,
Annu. Rev. Pharmacol. 7:77, 1967.

19 Van Dyke, K., Lantz, C., and Szustkiewicz,
C.: Quinacrine: mechanisms of antimalarial
action, Science 169:492, 1970.

REVIEWS

20 Drugs for parasitic infections, Med. Lett. 20:
17, 1978.

21 Most, H.: Treatment of common parasitic infections of man encountered in the United
States (second of two parts), N. Engl. J. Med.
287:698, 1972.

CHAPTER 60

Drugs used in chemotherapy of neoplastic disease

Although not as impressive as antimicrobial chemotherapy, the search for pharmacological approaches to neoplastic diseases has made some impressive gains. Actual cures have been obtained with drugs in the treatment of choriocarcinoma, Hodgkin's disease, and acute lymphocytic leukemia. Prolongation of survival can be achieved in a large number of malignant diseases by chemotherapy, although the quality of life is often impaired. The cancer chemotherapeutic agents are generally toxic, and their use requires considerable skill.

The current emphasis in cancer chemotherapy is on combinations. Such combinations take into account the phase of the cell cycle affected by the drug, synergistic effects, and prevention of drug resistance.

The cell cycle is divided into several portions. The resting phase is designated as G_0. The G_1 phase ends with a sudden increase in RNA synthesis, which signals the beginning of the S phase. During the S phase there is a marked increase in DNA synthesis, which ceases when the cells enter the short G_2 phase that ends with the mitotic process.

The cancer chemotherapeutic agents may be *cell cycle–specific* or *cell cycle–nonspecific*. Cells that are in a resting state do not respond to cell cycle–specific agents. However, they may respond to alkylating agents or to other drugs that combine directly with DNA.

The antileukemic activity of the nitrogen mustards was discovered during World War II. The discovery was an outgrowth of earlier observations on the leukopenic effect of mustard gas (bis[2-chloroethyl]sulfide). As a result of this discovery, the less toxic nitrogen mustards (bis[chloroethyl]amines) and eventually many other alkylating agents were introduced into chemotherapy of neoplastic diseases.[6]

The development of folic acid antagonists and other antimetabolites as potential antitumor agents originated from observations on the role of folic acid in white cell production. It seemed reasonable that compounds structurally related to folic acid could inhibit white cell production, and this was indeed demonstrated.

These observations stimulated interest in other metabolic antagonists as possible chemotherapeutic agents, and eventually several purine, pyrimidine, and amino acid antagonists were discovered. Nucleic acid biosynthesis has been the chief target of the chemotherapeutic approach.[9]

GENERAL CONCEPT

DEVELOPMENT OF ANTINEOPLASTIC CHEMOTHERAPY

INACTIVATION OF NUCLEIC ACIDS

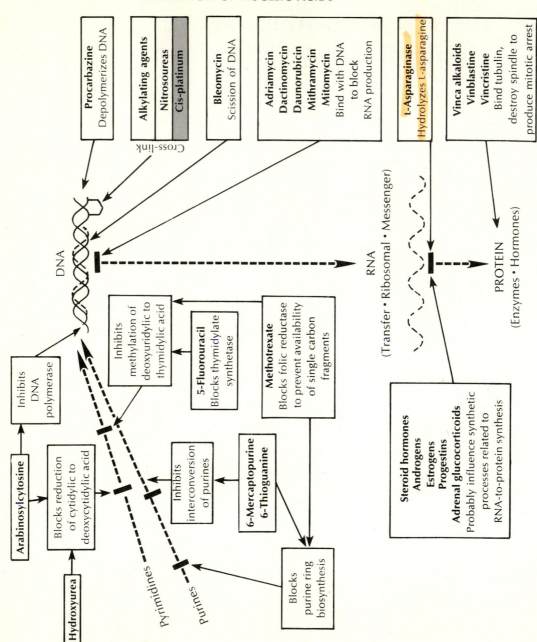

BIOSYNTHESIS OF NUCLEIC ACIDS

FIG. 60-1. Mechanism of action of antineoplastic drugs. (From Goldberg, R. S., and Krakoff, I., Hosp. Formulary, Oct., 1979, p. 891. Reprint from Hospital Formulary. © 1980, Harcourt Brace Jovanovich, Inc.)

The drugs currently employed in the management of malignant diseases fall **CLASSIFICATION** into the following categories:

Alkylating agents
    Mechlorethamine hydrochloride
      (Mustargen)
    Chlorambucil (Leukeran)
    Cyclophosphamide (Cytoxan)
    Melphalan (Alkeran)
    Thiotepa
    Busulfan (Myleran)
    Carmustine (BiCNU)
    Lomustine (CeeNU)
Antimetabolites
    Methotrexate
    Cytarabine (Cytosar)
    Fluorouracil (Adrucil)
    Mercaptopurine (Purinethol)
    Thioguanine

Hormones
    Adrenal corticosteroids
    Estrogens
    Antiestrogens
    Androgens
Antibiotics
    Bleomycin sulfate (Blenoxane)
    Dactinomycin (Cosmegen)
    Doxorubicin hydrochloride (Adriamycin)
    Mithramycin (Mithracin)
    Mitomycin (Mutamycin)
Miscellaneous
    Vinblastine sulfate (Velban)
    Vincristine sulfate (Oncovin)
    Hydroxyurea (Hydrea)
    Procarbazine hydrochloride (Matulane)
    Cisplatin (Platinol)
    Mitotane (Lysodren)

The mechanism of action of the various cancer chemotherapeutic agents is shown in Fig. 60-1.

The alkylating agents are highly reactive agents that transfer alkyl groups to **ALKYLATING** important cell constituents by combining with amino, sulfhydryl, carboxyl, and **AGENTS** phosphate groups. They are *cell cycle–nonspecific*, being capable of combining with cells at any phase of their cycle. It is believed that they alkylate DNA and, more specifically, guanine. This basic action may explain the preferential toxicity of these compounds for rapidly multiplying cells (Table 60-1).

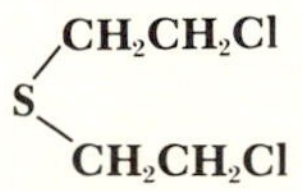

$$S \begin{cases} CH_2CH_2Cl \\ CH_2CH_2Cl \end{cases}$$

Sulfur mustard

$$CH_3N \begin{cases} CH_2CH_2Cl \\ CH_2CH_2Cl \end{cases}$$

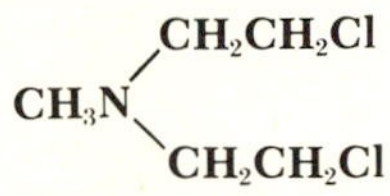

Nitrogen mustard

Mechlorethamine hydrochloride (nitrogen mustard; Mustargen) must be injected intravenously because the compound is highly reactive. More recently, attempts have been made to inject the drug intra-arterially close to the tumor. It is believed that the action of mechlorethamine hydrochloride lasts only a few minutes and that it disappears from the blood very rapidly.

The dose of mechlorethamine hydrochloride is 0.1 to 0.2 mg/kg/day for 4 days, injected intravenously. The drug can cause venous thrombosis, severe vomiting, and delayed depression of the bone marrow. In toxic doses mechlorethamine hydro-

TABLE 60-1. Dosage and toxicity of alkylating agents

Drug	Route of administration	Usual dose	Toxic effects
Mechlorethamine hydrochloride	Intravenous	0.1 mg/kg/day	Nausea and vomiting; bone marrow depression and bleeding; venous thrombosis
Chlorambucil	Oral	0.1-0.2 mg/kg/day	Bone marrow depression and bleeding
Cyclophosphamide	Intravenous	4 mg/kg/day	Nausea and vomiting; bone marrow depression and bleeding; alopecia may occur
	Oral (maintenance)	1-3 mg/kg/day	
Thiotepa	Oral	5-10 mg/day	Bone marrow depression and bleeding
	Intravenous	0.2 mg/kg	Nausea and vomiting; bone marrow depression and bleeding
Busulfan	Oral	2-8 mg/day	Bone marrow depression and bleeding

Nitrogen mustard **Ethyleneimmonium intermediate**

Cyclophosphamide

Busulfan

Melphalan

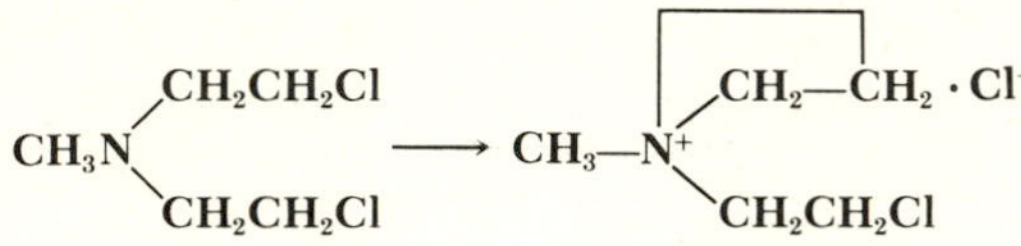

chloride can cause involution of lymphatic tissues and the thymus, ulcerations of gastrointestinal mucosa, convulsions, and death.

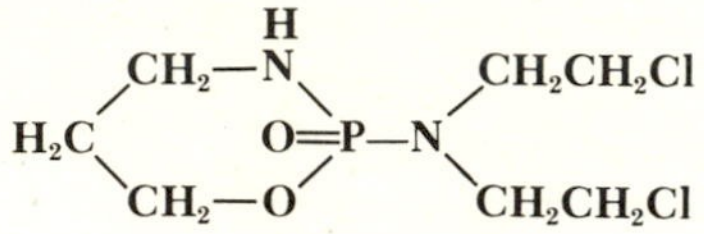

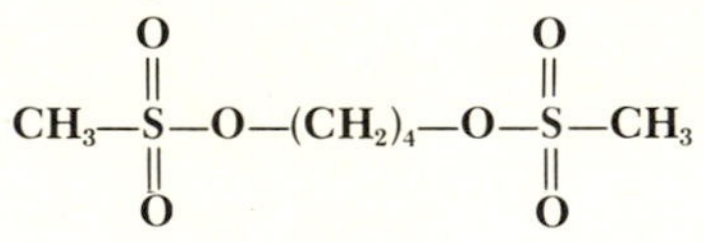

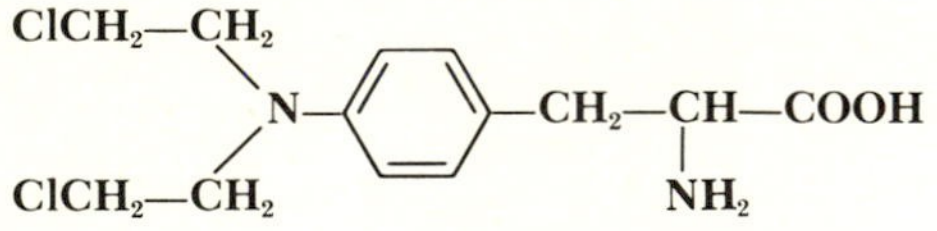

The main indication for mechlorethamine hydrochloride (Mustargen) is in the treatment of Hodgkin's disease and lymphomas, but the drug may be useful in other malignancies also.

Other alkylating agents have the advantage over mechlorethamine in that they can be administered orally.

Chlorambucil (Leukeran) is used primarily in chronic lymphocytic leukemia, Hodgkin's disease, multiple myeloma, and primary macroglobulinemia. **Cyclophosphamide** (Cytoxan) is a widely used cytotoxic drug, which is metabolically activated in the liver. The drug is generally useful in the treatment of lymphomas, acute lymphocytic leukemia in children, multiple myeloma, and some solid tumors, such as those of the ovary and breast, neuroblastoma, and others. Cyclophosphamide is commonly used as an immunosuppressive agent in a variety of diseases. Hemorrhagic cystitis is a characteristic toxic effect of cyclophosphamide. **Melphalan** (Alkeran) is a phenylalanine derivative of nitrogen mustard. It has been used in the treatment of multiple myeloma and some solid tumors, such as those of the ovary, testis, and breast. Occasionally the drug is infused intra-arterially for the regional treatment of certain tumors. **Thiotepa** is used parenterally in the treatment of carcinoma of the ovary and breast. **Busulfan** (Myleran) is used mainly in the treatment of chronic myelocytic leukemia, since the drug has a selective effect on granulocytes.

Carmustine (BiCNU) and **lomustine** (CeeNU) are nitrosoureas that alkylate DNA and RNA.

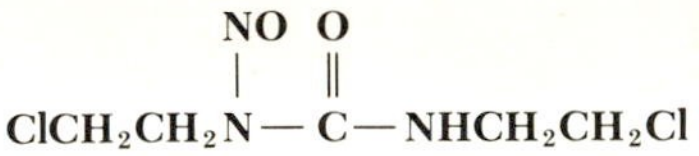

$$\underset{\text{Carmustine}}{ClCH_2CH_2N-\overset{\overset{NO}{|}}{\underset{}{C}}\overset{\overset{O}{\|}}{-}NHCH_2CH_2Cl}$$

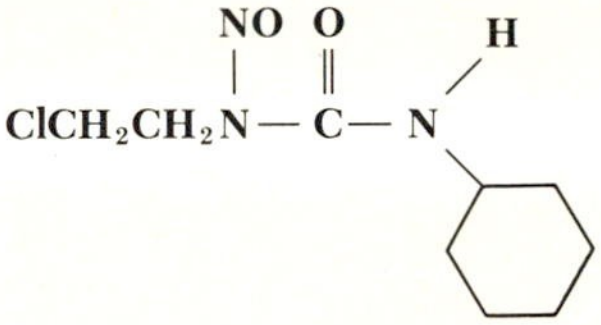

$$\underset{\text{Lomustine}}{ClCH_2CH_2N-C-N}$$

Lomustine may have additional effects on DNA synthesis. An important characteristic of the nitrosoureas is their lipid solubility, which allows them to cross the blood-brain barrier and exert an effect on brain tumors.

The folic acid antagonists inhibit nucleic acid synthesis by blocking the enzyme dihydrofolate reductase. **Methotrexate,** formerly known as amethopterin, is effective in the treatment of acute leukemias of children and lymphomas and may be curative in women with choriocarcinoma. In combination with other agents, methotrexate may be useful in the treatment of some solid tumors such as carcinoma of the breast, ovary, and colon. Methotrexate produces many toxic effects such as nausea, vomiting, diarrhea, alopecia, aphthous stomatitis, skin rash, and bone marrow depression. Leucovorin calcium, within a few hours after overdosage, may serve as an antidote. Methotrexate is available in tablets containing 2.5 mg, and methotrexate sodium in a powder for injection, 5 and 50 mg.

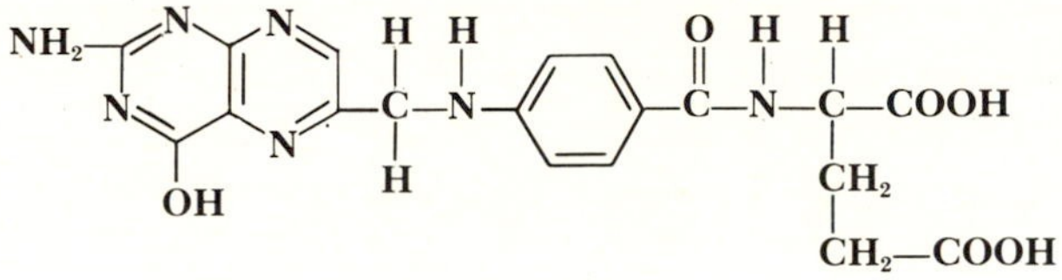

ANTIMETABOLITES
Folic acid antagonists

Folic acid (pteroylglutamic acid)

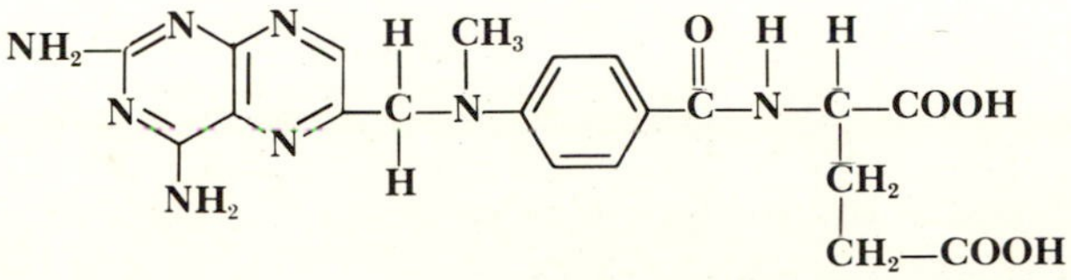

Methotrexate

The most important purine antagonist, mercaptopurine, acts by several mechanisms. First, it is converted to the ribonucleotide. As such it competes with

Purine antagonists

enzymes that convert hypoxanthine ribonucleotide (inosinic acid) to adenine and xanthine ribonucleotides. In addition, mercaptopurine is converted into 6-methyl mercaptopurine and its ribonucleotide. This metabolite ties up the enzyme that synthesizes phosphoribosylamine, which is required for RNA and DNA synthesis.

Thioguanine is also metabolized to the ribonucleotide, which enters the pathway of nucleic acid synthesis substituting for guanine. Thus "fraudulent" polynucleotides that block nucleic acid synthesis are produced.

Mercaptopurine is effective in the treatment of acute lymphocytic and chronic myelocytic leukemias. Its toxic manifestations include bone marrow depression, gastrointestinal disturbances, and jaundice. Allopurinol was originally developed for the purpose of blocking the metabolism of mercaptopurine by xanthine oxidase. Mercaptopurine (Purinethol) is obtainable in tablets containing 50 mg.

Thioguanine is an antimetabolite similar to mercaptopurine with essentially the same indications and adverse effects.

Azathioprine, a derivative of mercaptopurine, has become widely used as an immunosuppressive drug in organ transplantation. Bone marrow depression, oral lesions, gastrointestinal disturbances, alopecia, and intercurrent infections are some of the toxic effects of azathioprine. Azathioprine (Imuran) is available in tablets containing 50 mg. Azathioprine is much more useful as an immunosuppressant than in cancer chemotherapy. It splits in the body to 6-mercaptopurine.

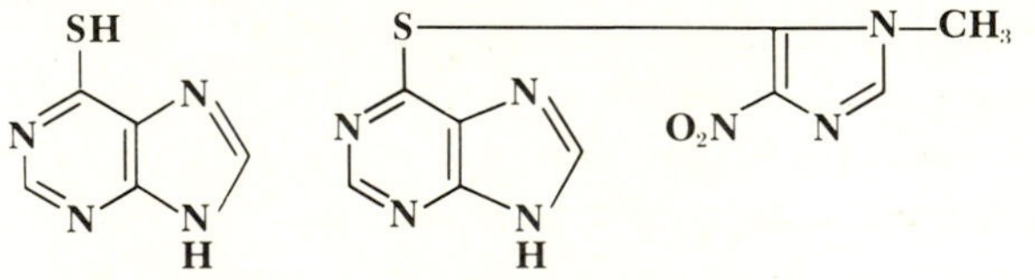

Mercaptopurine   Azathioprine

Pyrimidine antagonists   **Fluorouracil** is a pyrimidine antimetabolite of some usefulness in the treatment of carcinoma of the colon, breast, ovary, pancreas, and liver. It is a highly toxic drug, producing the same sort of disturbances as mercaptopurine and also hyperpigmentation and photosensitization. The drug is available as a solution, 50 mg/ml, for intravenous injection. Fluorouracil is also available for topical application as Efudex solution or cream. The solution contains 2% or 5% fluorouracil, the cream 5%.

Fluorouracil is converted to the ribonucleotide, which may be reduced to 5-fluoro-2'-deoxyuridine-5'-phosphate (F-dUMP). This enzymatic product inhibits thymidylate synthetase, which is involved in the production of deoxyuridylic acid (dUMP).

Cytarabine (cytosine arabinoside; Cytosar) is a pyrimidine antagonist that differs from deoxycytidine (cytosine deoxyriboside) in containing arabinose rather than deoxyribose. It is converted to the nucleotide, which then blocks the conversion of cytidine nucleotide to deoxycytidine nucleotide. It also prevents the formation of DNA by blocking the incorporation of deoxycytidine triphosphate.

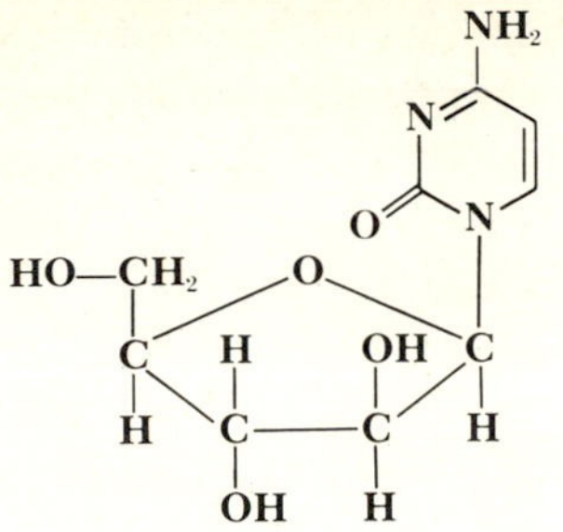

Cytarabine

Cytarabine must be injected intravenously, since it is not effective after oral administration. It finds some usefulness in the treatment of acute lymphocytic and acute myelocytic leukemias. It is also of interest as a possible antiviral agent (p. 657).

Steroid hormones such as estrogens, androgens, and corticosteroids are useful **HORMONAL** in some neoplastic diseases. The estrogens include diethylstilbestrol and ethinyl **AGENTS** estradiol. Androgens that are widely used, particularly in the treatment of carcinoma of the breast, include testosterone propionate, fluoxymesterone, and the recently introduced calusterone (Methosarb). The most widely used corticosteroid is prednisone, which is effective in various lymphomas and some other malignancies.

The progestogens include medroxyprogesterone (Provera), hydroxyprogesterone (Delalutin), and megestrol acetate (Megace). The progestogens are sometimes effective in renal and endometrial carcinomas.

Estrogens, alone with castration and other measures, are used in treatment of prostatic carcinoma. Both androgens and estrogens have been employed in management of advanced mammary carcinoma. The choice depends on the age of the patient. Estrogens are used in women well past the menopause, whereas androgens may be helpful in patients who are still menstruating. The main benefit obtained from this type of treatment is reduction of pain related to metastatic lesions in the bones.

The *rationale* for the use of the estrogens and androgens is the belief that prostatic and mammary carcinoma are to some extent "hormone-dependent."

The adverse effects of the estrogens (diethylstilbestrol) are gastrointestinal symptoms, hypercalcemia, edema, uterine bleeding, and feminization in males. The adverse effects expected from large doses of androgens (testosterone propionate) in the treatment of advanced mammary carcinoma are virilization, edema, and hypercalcemia.

Tamoxifen citrate (Nolvadex) is an antiestrogen, which apparently competes with estradiol for the estrogen receptor. The drug is not a steroid. Its main usefulness is in carcinoma of the breast in postmenopausal and also premenopausal women. Carcinoma of the breast is also being treated with this antiestrogen.

RADIOACTIVE
ISOTOPES

Radioactive phosphorus (^{32}P) is used in the treatment of polycythemia vera and also in chronic leukemias. It has a biological half-life of about 8 days in humans. It is handled just like normal phosphorus, being incorporated into nucleic acids and deposited in bone. It emits β rays that exert a destructive effect on the rapidly multiplying cells in which it is concentrated. ^{32}P is administered in doses of about 1 mCi daily for 5 days. Either the oral or intravenous route may be used, and the doses are not greatly different.

Radioactive iodine (^{131}I), radioactive gold (^{198}Au), and other isotopes are not as useful as ^{32}P. Nevertheless, ^{131}I has some limited application in metastatic thyroid carcinoma. Colloidal ^{198}Au has been tried in the treatment of lymphomas and in neoplastic diseases involving serous cavities. Its uses are largely experimental.

ANTIBIOTICS

Bleomycin sulfate (Blenoxane) binds to DNA and has been found useful in the treatment of squamous cell carcinomas of the head and neck. Also, this drug has some usefulness in treatment of testicular tumors and malignant lymphomas. Although bleomycin is not a depressant of the bone marrow, it can cause an unusual toxic manifestation—pulmonary fibrosis.

Dactinomycin (actinomycin D; Cosmegen) is a toxic antibiotic that combines with DNA and blocks RNA production. It is effective in the treatment of choriocarcinoma of women, Wilms' tumor, and testicular carcinoma. The drug causes bone marrow depression and gastrointestinal toxicity.

Doxorubicin hydrochloride (Adriamycin) is an anthracycline antibiotic that combines with DNA and is cell cycle–specific, inhibiting the S phase preferentially. Doxorubicin is useful in the treatment of a variety of acute leukemias such as Hodgkin's disease and neuroblastoma. The drug is combined with cisplatin in the treatment of tumors of the bladder and testicular and ovarian carcinoma. Bone marrow depression is common and a characteristic toxic effect is cardiotoxicity. Tissue necrosis is severe in case of extravasation.

Mithramycin (Mithracin) is a toxic antibiotic that inhibits DNA-dependent RNA synthesis. In addition to its effect in testicular tumors, the drug has an effect on calcium metabolism, probably by acting on osteoclasts. Among numerous toxic effects, thrombocytopenia, bleeding, and gastrointestinal manifestations are most common.

Mitomycin (Mutamycin) is a toxic antibiotic, which is an alkylating agent that combines with DNA. The drug is used occasionally when other alkylating agents are ineffective. It causes severe bone marrow depression, gastrointestinal toxicity, and renal toxicity.

MISCELLANEOUS
ANTINEOPLASTIC
AGENTS

Vinblastine (Velban) is an alkaloid obtained from the periwinkle plant *(Vinca)*. It has antineoplastic activity, presumably as a consequence of mitotic arrest. Its toxic effects, commonly seen also with other antimetabolites, include nausea and vomiting, leukopenia, and alopecia. It is administered intravenously in doses of 0.1 to 0.15 mg/kg daily. Other alkaloids related to vinblastine are also being investigated. It is quite effective in the treatment of Hodgkin's disease and choriocarcinoma.

Vincristine (Oncovin) is a *Vinca* alkaloid that is particularly effective in the treatment of acute leukemia in children and Wilms' tumor. Nausea, vomiting, leukopenia, neurotoxic effects, and alopecia are toxic effects of the *Vinca* alkaloids. Vincristine is a spindle toxin.

L-Asparaginase is an enzyme that is effective in the treatment of human leukemia. Apparently some malignant cells require exogenous asparagine, but normal cells synthesize their own. The discovery of L-asparaginase as an antineoplastic agent resulted from observations[12] on the suppressive effect of guinea pig serum, now known to contain L-asparaginase, on experimental leukemias. The drug is still experimental but is of great interest because it exploits a basic metabolic difference between normal and malignant cells.

Procarbazine (Matulane) is a synthetic methylhydrazine derivative that finds some usefulness in the treatment of generalized Hodgkin's disease. The drug has numerous adverse effects ranging from gastrointestinal symptoms, bone marrow depression, monoamine oxidase (MAO)–inhibitory action, and disulfiram-like effects. Procarbazine is available in capsules, 50 mg.

Hydroxyurea (Hydrea) may be useful in patients with chronic myelocytic leukemia when there is no response to busulfan. Bone marrow depression is its most serious adverse effect. The drug is available in capsules, 500 mg.

Mitotane (Lysodren) is a synthetic compound related to DDT that has specific toxicity for the adrenal gland. The drug is available in 500 mg tablets.

CHOICE OF DRUGS IN CANCER CHEMOTHERAPY

In addition to the use of surgery and radiation, various drugs may be effective in the treatment of malignancies. In fact, chemotherapy is considered the primary method of treatment in the following conditions: choriocarcinoma of the female, Wilms' tumor, acute and chronic leukemias, multiple myeloma, and polycythemia vera.

As a general rule, the drugs of choice for various malignancies change rapidly in the light of statistics accumulated by cancer chemotherapy study groups. This is particularly true for possible synergistic combinations.

Chronic myelocytic leukemia responds to a number of drugs. In order of preference they are busulfan, chlorambucil, and mercaptopurine. It is believed that the drugs are as effective as irradiation and can be substituted for each other as resistance develops.

Chronic lymphocytic leukemia may be treated with irradiation or drugs when the disease becomes progressive. Chlorambucil is preferred by many experts. In resistance cases, corticosteroids may be useful, and among these prednisone in large doses is favored by many.

Acute leukemias of children respond well to antimetabolites such as methotrexate. The acute lymphoblastic leukemias are also responsive to corticosteroids and vincristine. Other drugs are being used also, but nitrogen mustards are ineffective. In acute myeloblastic and monocytic leukemias, mercaptopurine has been found useful; cytarabine has been effective in causing remissions in acute granulocytic leukemias of adults.

Hodgkin's disease and *lymphosarcoma* are often treated with chlorambu-

TABLE 60-2. Dosage and toxicity of some antimetabolites, antibiotics, hormones, and *Vinca* alkaloids*

Drug	Route of administration	Usual dose	Toxic effects
Antimetabolites			
Methotrexate	Oral and intravenous	2.5 mg daily for leukemia 10-30 mg daily for choriocarcinoma	Stomatitis, enteritis, bone marrow depression, alopecia, skin rash; leucovorin is a useful antidote if given within a few hours after methotrexate
Fluorouracil	Intravenous	15 mg/kg daily for 4 days	Stomatitis, enteritis, leukopenia, hemorrhages
Mercaptopurine	Oral	2.5 mg/kg daily	Stomatitis, enteritis, jaundice, bone marrow depression
Antibiotic			
Actinomycin D	Intravenous	75 μg/kg total dose in 5 days	Vomiting, stomatitis, enteritis, leukopenia, alopecia
Hormones			
Diethylstilbestrol	Oral	1-5 mg three times/day	Nausea, vomiting, feminization, hypercalcemia
Fluoxymesterone	Oral	10 mg three times/day	Masculinization, hirsutism, fluid retention, hypercalcemia
Prednisone	Oral	1 mg/kg daily	Cushing-type effects
***Vinca* alkaloids**			
Vinblastine	Intravenous	0.10-0.15 mg/kg weekly	Nausea, vomiting, stomatitis, leukopenia, alopecia
Vincristine	Intravenous	0.02-0.05 mg/kg weekly	Nausea, vomiting, neurotoxic effects, leukopenia, alopecia

*Based on data from several sources.

cil, mechlorethamine hydrochloride, methotrexate, vinblastine, and corticosteroids. Occasional favorable response is obtained but no definite prolongation of life.

Multiple myeloma responds to the alkylating agents such as cyclophosphamide or melphalan. Prednisone is useful also, as is vincristine.

Choriocarcinoma is most effectively treated with methotrexate or in resistant cases with actinomycin D. Vinblastine may be useful when the two preferred agents become ineffective.

Regional cancer chemotherapy by means of intra-arterial nitrogen mustards or methotrexate with folinic acid is being used with some favorable results in selected patients.

Malignant effusions are often treated with mechlorethamine instillations, although quinacrine solutions may also be effective.

Certain combinations of chemotherapeutic agents have shown distinct advantages, particularly in the treatment of Hodgkin's disease and lymphomas. The combination designated as MOPP consists of mechlorethamine, Oncovin (vincristine sulfate), procarbazine, and prednisone. COP refers to the combined use of cyclophosphamide, Oncovin, and prednisone. There is every reason to believe that other drugs, such as adriamycin and the nitrosoureas, may become important in combination chemotherapy. Another combination that has been used widely is known as CAM. It consists of cyclophosphamide, cytarabine, and methotrexate.

Drug combinations

REFERENCES

1 Ansfield, F. J., Schroeder, J. M., and Curreri, A. R.: Five years' clinical experience with 5-fluorouracil, J.A.M.A. **181:**295, 1962.

2 Busch, H., and Lane, M.: Chemotherapy, Chicago, 1967, Year Book Medical Publishers, Inc.

3 Cortes, E. P., Holland, J. F., Wang, J. J., and Sinks, L. F.: Doxorubicin in disseminated osteosarcoma, J.A.M.A. **221:**1132, 1972.

4 DeVita, V. T., and Rall, D. P.: Pharmacologic aspects of the chemotherapy of solid tumors, Pharmacol. Phys. **2**(9):1, 1968.

5 Farber, S.: Chemotherapy in the treatment of leukemia and Wilms' tumor, J.A.M.A. **198:**826, 1966.

6 Goodman, L. S., Wintrobe, M. M., Dameshek, W., Goodman, M. J., Gilman, A., and McLennan, M. T.: Nitrogen mustard therapy, J.A.M.A. **132:**126, 1946.

7 Heidelberger, C.: Cancer chemotherapy with purine and pyrimidine analogues, Annu. Rev. Pharmacol. **7:**101, 1967.

8 Hersh, E. M., Whitecar, J. P., McCredie, K. B., Bodey, G. P., and Freireich, E. J.: Chemotherapy, immunocompetence, immunosuppression and prognosis in acute leukemia, N. Engl. J. Med. **285:**1211, 1971.

9 Hitchings, G. H.: A quarter century of chemotherapy, J.A.M.A. **209:**1339, 1969.

10 Hitchings, G. H., and Elion, G. B.: Chemical suppression of the immune response, Pharmacol. Rev. **15:**365, 1963.

11 Hoover, R., Gray, L. A., Cole, P., and MacMahon, B.: Menopausal estrogens and breast cancer, N. Engl. J. Med. **295:**401, 1976.

12 Kidd, J. G.: Regression of transplanted lymphomas induced *in vivo* by means of normal guinea pig serum. I. Course of transplanted cancers of various kinds in mice and rats given guinea pig serum, horse serum or rabbit serum, J. Exp. Med. **98:**565, 1953.

13 Miller, E. C., and Miller, J. A.: Mechanisms of chemical carcinogenesis: nature of proximate carcinogens and interactions with macromolecules, Pharmacol. Rev. **18:**805, 1966.

14 Oliverio, V. T., and Zubrod, C. G.: Clinical pharmacology of the effective antitumor drugs, Annu. Rev. Pharmacol. **5:**335, 1965.

15 Penman, S.: Ribonucleic acid metabolism in mammalian cells, N. Engl. J. Med. **276:**502, 1967.

16 Pitot, H. C.: Some biochemical aspects of malignancy, Annu. Rev. Biochem. **35:**335, 1966.

17 Rundles, R. W.: Triethylene melamine (TEM) therapy in malignant diseases, GP **9:**75, 1954.

18 Santos, G. W.: The pharmacology of immunosuppressive drugs, Pharmacol. Phys. **2**(8):1, 1968.

19 Selawry, O. S., and Hananian, J.: Vincristine treatment of cancer in children, J.A.M.A. **183:**741, 1963.

20 Schnider, B. I., and Gold, C. L.: Recent developments in cancer chemotherapy, Med. Ann. D.C. **28:**637, 1959.

REVIEWS

21 Cancer chemotherapy, Med. Lett. **20:**81, 1978.

22 Chabner, B. A., Myers, C. E., Coleman, N., and Johns, D. G.: The clinical pharmacology of antineoplastic agents, N. Engl. J. Med. **292:**1159, 1975.

23 DeVita, V. T., and Schein, P. S.: The use of drugs in combination for the treatment of cancer, N. Engl. J. Med. **288:**998, 1973.

24 Folkman, J.: Tumor angiogenesis: therapeutic implications, N. Engl. J. Med. **285:**1182, 1971.

25 Haskell, C. M., and Cline, M. J.: The treatment of acute leukemia, Ration. Drug Ther. **8:**1, 1974.

26 Honeycutt, W. M., Jansen, T., and Dillaha, C. J.: Topical antimetabolites and cytostatic agents, Cutis **6:**63, 1970.

27 Huggins, C.: The hormone-dependent cancers, J.A.M.A. **186:**481, 1963.

28 Krakoff, I. H.: Cancer chemotherapeutic agents, CA **23:**208, 1973.

29 Lokich, J. J.: Managing chemotherapy-induced bone marrow suppression in cancer, Hosp. Pract., Aug., 1976, p. 61.

30 Marsh, J. C., and Mitchell, M. S.: Chemotherapy of cancer, Drug Therapy, Jan., 1974.

31 Miller, E.: The metabolism and pharmacology of 5-fluorouracil, J. Surg. Oncol. **3:**309, 1971.

32 Oswalt, C. E., and Cruz, A. B.: Cancer chemotherapeutic agents, Tex. Med. **73:**57, 1977.

33 Stone, M. J.: Recent advances in oncology, Dallas Med. J., Sept., 1978, p. 406.

SECTION TEN

Principles of immunopharmacology

CHAPTER 61

Principles of immunopharmacology

The control of disease by immunological means has two objectives: the production of *desired immunity* and the elimination of *undesired immune reactions*. The first of these objectives is achieved by *immunization procedures* rather than drugs. For this reason, discussions of immunopharmacology are more concerned with the chemical basis of *undesired* immune reactions and their possible elimination by means of drugs.

The impressive developments in clinical immunology with emphasis on various classes of lymphocytes have not been matched by corresponding advances in the pharmacological approach. In treating immunological disorders, physicians rely largely on corticosteroids, immunosuppressive agents, and replacement of deficiencies.

The basic mechanisms of immunological injury are anaphylactic mechanisms, cytolytic mechanisms, immune complex disorders, and delayed hypersensitivity reactions. In actual practice, physicians deal with autoimmune diseases, allograft rejections, immune complex problems, and erythroblastosis fetalis. There are other immunological disorders that are difficult to classify.

Several groups of drugs have been used clinically for the purpose of suppressing the immune response. Following are the most important: **IMMUNOSUPPRESSIVE AGENTS**

1. Corticosteroids
2. Cytotoxic drugs
   a. Antimetabolites: mercaptopurine and azathioprine (Imuran)
   b. Alkylating agents: cyclophosphamide (Cytoxan) and nitrogen mustard
   c. Folic acid antagonists: methotrexate

In addition to these drugs, radiation and antilymphocytic serum (ALS) are also potent immunosuppressive agents.

There is general agreement on certain features of the mode of action of the immunosuppressive drugs,[25] which can be summarized as follows: *Mode of action*

1. The cytotoxic drugs tend to destroy replicating cells. They have been classified as *cell cycle drugs* and *noncycle drugs*. The cell cycle drugs destroy *only* rapidly multiplying cells, whereas the noncycle drugs are injurious to nonreplicating cells as well. The antimetabolites and folic acid antagonists act only on dividing cells; the alkylating agents, being noncycle drugs, cause depletion in the total number of small lymphocytes.

2. Immunosuppressive agents inhibit the primary immune response more readily than an established immune state or an anamnestic response. Their main effect on antibody synthesis is exerted during the time when the antigen converts its clone of lymphocytes to antibody-producing cells.

3. Various components of the immune response are not equally affected by all suppressive drugs. Delayed hypersensitivity and IgG synthesis can be inhibited selectively. For example, mercaptopurine and antilymphocyte serum can inhibit the development of delayed hypersensitivity without blocking IgG synthesis.[1]

4. The goal of immunosuppressive therapy is the development of drug-induced immune tolerance to specific antigens, with conservation of other immunological capabilities.

5. Immunosuppressive drugs have many adverse effects. These are not unexpected because immune processes are important defenses against infections and may play a role in protecting the individual against neoplastic cells as well.

EFFECTOR MECH-ANISMS AND MEDIATORS IN IMMUNE INJURY

Several types of immune injury are recognized, each having characteristic effector mechanisms. Some of the latter are (1) anaphylaxis, (2) cytolysis, (3) immune-complex reactions, and (4) delayed hypersensitivity.

Anaphylactic mechanisms

The antibody in anaphylactic reactions is largely of the IgE type, which attaches itself to cells such as mast cells and leukocytes. When exposed to the antigen, the sensitized mast cells release vasoactive mediators, among which histamine appears the most important. The slow-reacting substance (SRS), an acidic lipid, may not originate from mast cells. In the rat[14] it is released by polymorphonuclear leukocytes. Serotonin is probably not present in human mast cells.

The release of histamine from human basophils or mast cells does not require complement when these cells are sensitized by IgE antibodies. On the other hand, if antibodies are prepared against mast cells, they will attack these cells and cause histamine release by a cytolytic mechanism that requires complement.

Cytolytic mechanisms

Cytolytic mechanisms are involved in the pathogenesis of various types of hemolytic anemia, thrombocytopenia, and leukopenia. The antigen may be a constituent of the cell, such as the Rh factor, or a drug attached to the cell. The antibodies are of the IgE variety except for the cold hemagglutinins (IgM). Complement is not required for cytolysis except when cold agglutinins are involved.

Immune-complex mechanisms

Immune-complex mechanisms are most clearly seen in acute and chronic glomerulonephritis and in serum sickness. Soluble antigen-antibody complexes may be deposited in the glomerular basement membranes where they activate the complement system. Leukotactic factors are generated, which attract polymorphonuclear leukocytes. The release of lytic enzymes from leukocytic lysosomes leads to digestion of the basement membrane.[2] There are variations on this theme. The antibodies

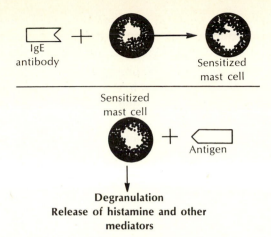

FIG. 61-1. Schema of mediator release caused by interaction of cell-bound IgE antibody and antigen.

may be directed against the basement membrane. In other instances the continued deposit formation leads to membranous glomerulonephritis.

The antibodies involved in immune-complex disease are of the IgG and IgM type, and complement plays an important role in the immunological injury.

The clinical condition that is a prime example of delayed hypersensitivity is *contact dermatitis.* Similar mechanisms are involved also in the rejection of grafts and in the tuberculin reaction.

Delayed hypersensitivity mechanisms

No humoral antibodies are involved in this type of reaction. Instead, sensitized small lymphocytes are responsible for recognizing the antigen. In addition, large numbers of nonsensitized mononuclear cells that accumulate at the site over a period of 24 to 48 hours act as the "inflammatory cells." The slow accumulation of these cells explains the delayed nature of the reaction. The mechanism of their accumulation may be related to the observation that sensitized lymphocytes exposed to the antigen in vitro release a factor (migration-inhibition factor) that causes macrophages to stick to capillary tubes, thus preventing their migration. There are other mediators of delayed hypersensitivity, such as lymphotoxin.[7] The role of the so-called lymph node–permeability factor is questionable and nonspecific.

Anaphylactic mechanisms are not susceptible to cytotoxic drugs for a number of reasons. These reactions depend on preformed antibodies, and the reactions are of the immediate type. Although it is possible that long-continued administration of cytotoxic drugs would have some effect, the toxicity of these agents precludes their prolonged administration.

Drug effects on immune injury

The therapeutic approaches to anaphylactic injury are aimed at (1) the development of blocking antibodies by hyposensitization, (2) inhibition of the release of vasoactive mediators, and (3) prevention of the effect of the mediators such as histamine.

The widely employed hyposensitization procedures are believed to increase the formation of blocking antibodies (IgG) that may bind the allergen. It is possible that other mechanisms are also involved. In the rapid desensitization to an antigen such as a serum in an individual known to be hypersensitive to it, there must clearly be other mechanisms involved than the production of blocking antibodies.

Disodium cromoglycate (Intal) is a chroman derivative that is claimed to inhibit the release of vasoactive mediators caused by interaction of antigen with reaginic antibodies.[14] When administered by inhalation, it exerts some therapeutic effect in asthma, which is demonstrable statistically in controlled series. That it is not a powerful therapeutic agent is indicated by some conflict of opinion about its efficacy.

$$\text{NaOOC} \quad \text{O} \quad \text{O—CH}_2\text{—CH—CH}_2\text{—O} \quad \text{O} \quad \text{COONa}$$

Disodium cromoglycate

Of great interest are observations indicating that histamine release from human leukocytes and animal mast cells is inhibited by drugs that are expected to raise intracellular cyclic AMP levels. Isoproterenol and theophylline, widely used in the treatment of asthma, have an inhibitory activity on histamine release by allergens from human leukocytes.[6] Although the relative importance of their action on release processes in relation to their bronchodilator action is impossible to state under clinical conditions, these observations have stimulated much research on the role of the β-adrenergic system in the allergic diathesis.[20]

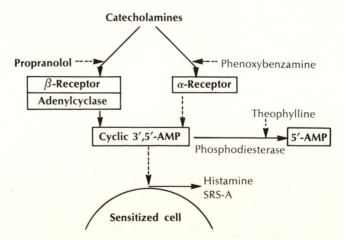

FIG. 61-2. Inhibitory effect of cyclic 3',5'-AMP on mediator release and the influence of some drugs. Broken arrow indicates an inhibitory effect.

There is not much known about drug effects on cytolysis. On the other hand, drugs may act at several sites in immune-complex disease. Immunosuppressive drugs may reduce the antibody levels and lower the number of granulocytes. It is of great interest that agranulocytic animals do not develop glomerulonephritis despite the presence of complexes in the circulation. Corticosteroids are employed in the treatment of glomerulonephritis. Their action is attributed to stabilization of granulocytic lysosomes, which are believed to play an important role in damaging the basement membrane of the glomeruli. Theoretic approaches to immune-complex disease include also the use of decomplementing agents. A glycoprotein extracted from cobra venom depletes the third component of complement,[11] a finding of great experimental interest.

Delayed hypersensitivity is suceptible to several drugs. The immunosuppressive drugs such as the antimetabolites have important effects on the nonsensitized inflammatory cells. This is understandable, since the inflammatory cells are short-lived and have very active nucleic acid metabolism.[19]

There is commonly an overlap in the anti-inflammatory and immunosuppressive effects of various drugs. For example, the corticosteroids have both actions. Mercaptopurine treatment reduces the number of mononuclear cells at inflammatory sites[16] in animal experiments.

The simplest way to explain the overlap is to consider that the immune injury leads to inflammation as a consequence of the activity of "inflammatory" cells. Drugs that reduce the number of these cells or inhibit their activities may exert both anti-inflammatory and apparent immunosuppressive effects. The cytotoxic drugs inhibit the multiplication of cells, whereas the milder anti-inflammatory drugs may exert more subtle effects on the inflammatory cells or may block the actions of their products. *Theoretically*, the anti-inflammatory drugs may block the effects of leukotactic factors on inflammatory cells, or they may inhibit the elaboration of mediators by these cells. They may also block the action of the mediators. No simple theory such as that of lysosomal stabilization[23] is sufficient to account for the vast differences in the spectrum of activity of the various types of anti-inflammatory drugs (p. 543).

IMMUNOSUPPRESSIVE AND ANTI-INFLAMMATORY DRUG ACTIONS

From the foregoing discussion it should be clear that some types of immune injury may be ameliorated by drug therapy. Some of the examples will be discussed briefly.

Rh hemolytic disease of the newborn is prevented very successfully by Rh_0 (D) immune globulin (RhoGAM). It is used for the passive immunization of the mother to prevent the formation of antibodies. It is injected within 72 hours after birth of an RH_0-positive (D-positive or D^u-positive) baby to a mother who is negative with respect to these factors.

Acute glomerulonephritis is often treated with corticosteroids (prednisone) and occasionally with other immunosuppressive agents. The same is true for idiopathic thrombocytopenic purpura and autoimmune hemolytic anemia.

CLINICAL APPLICATIONS

Renal transplantation has been greatly aided by the availability of azathioprine (Imuran), prednisone, and antilymphocytic serum (ALS). These drugs are used also in the transplantation of other organs.

The usefulness of drugs in the management of allergic and rheumatic diseases has been commented on in Chapters 20 and 31.

REFERENCES

1 Borel, Y., and Schwartz, R. S.: Inhibition of immediate and delayed hypersensitivity by 6-mercaptopurine, J. Immunol. 92:754, 1965.

2 Dixon, F. J.: The pathogenesis of glomerulonephritis, Am. J. Med. 44:493, 1968.

3 Gowans, J. L., and McGregor, D. D.: Immunological activities of lymphocytes, Prog. Allergy 9:1, 1965.

4 Ishizaka, K.: The identification and significance of gamma E, Hosp. Pract. 4:70, 1969.

5 Johnson, A. R., and Moran, N. C.: Inhibition of the release of histamine from rat mast cells: the effect of cold and adrenergic drugs on release of histamine by compound 48/80 and antigen, J. Pharmacol. Exp. Ther. 175:632, 1970.

6 Lichtenstein, L. M.: Mechanism of allergic histamine release from human leukocytes. In Austen, K. F., and Becker, E. L., editors: Biochemistry of the acute allergic reactions, Philadelphia, 1967, F. A. Davis Co.

7 Mackaness, G. B., and Blanden, R. V.: Cellular immunity, Prog. Allergy 11:89, 1967.

8 Makinodan, T., Santos, G. W., and Quinn, R. P.: Immunosuppressive drugs, Pharmacol. Rev. 22:189, 1971.

9 Medawar, P.: Antilymphocyte serum: its properties and potentials, Hosp. Pract. 4:26, 1969.

10 Mota, I.: The mechanism of anaphylaxis. I. Production and biological properties of "mast cell sensitizing" antibody, Immunology 7:681, 1964.

11 Muller-Eberhard, H. J.: Chemistry and reaction mechanisms of complement, Adv. Immunol. 8:1, 1968.

12 Norman, P. S.: The clinical significance of IgE, Hosp. Pract., Aug., 1975, p. 41.

13 Novack, S. N., and Pearson, C. M.: Cyclophosphamide therapy in Wegener's granulomatosis, N. Engl. J. Med. 284:938, 1971.

14 Orange, R. P., and Austen, K. F.: Pharmacologic dissociation of immunologic release of histamine and slow-reacting substance of anaphylaxis in rats, Proc. Soc. Exp. Biol. Med. 129:836, 1968.

15 Orange, R. P., Valentine, M. D., and Austen, K. F.: Antigen-induced release of slow-reacting substance of anaphylaxis in rats prepared with homologous antibody, J. Exp. Med. 127:767, 1968.

16 Page, A. R., Condie, R. M., and Good, R. A.: Effect of 6-mercaptopurine on inflammation, Am. J. Pathol. 40:519, 1962.

17 Parker, C. W.: Control of lymphocyte function, N. Engl. J. Med. 295:1180, 1976.

18 Piper, P. J., and Vane, J. R.: Release of additional factors in anaphylaxis and its antagonism by anti-inflammatory drugs, Nature 223:29, 1969.

18a Reinherz, E. L.: Current concepts in immunology, N. Engl. J. Med. 303:370, 1980.

19 Schwartz, R. S.: Therapeutic strategy in clinical immunology, N. Engl. J. Med. 280:367, 1969.

20 Szentivanyi, A.: The beta adrenergic theory of the atopic abnormality in bronchial asthma, J. Allerg. 42:203, 1968.

21 Uhr, J. W., and Moller, G.: Regulatory effects of antibody on antibody formation, Adv. Immunol. 8:81, 1968.

22 Ward, P. A., and Zwaifler, M. J.: Complement-derived leukotactic factors in inflammatory synovial fluids of humans, J. Clin. Invest. 50:606, 1971.

23 Weissmann, G.: Structure and function of lysosomes, Rheumatology 1:1, 1967.

24 Weissmann, G.: Lysosomal mechanisms of tissue injury in arthritis, N. Engl. J. Med. 286:141, 1972.

25 Winkelstein, A.: Principles of immunosuppressive therapy, Bull. Rheum. Dis. 21:627, 1971.

Poisons and antidotes

CHAPTER 62

Poisons and antidotes

A poison is generally defined as a compound that in relatively small quantities and by a chemical action can cause death or disability. According to this definition, there is essentially no difference between a drug and a poison. In large enough doses any drug can cause death or disability.

Toxicology is the science of poisons and poisonings. It may be considered a branch of pharmacology, since the latter discipline also deals with the adverse effects of drugs. A practical reason for the existence of a separate discipline has to do with the fact that many highly specialized procedures are used for laboratory diagnosis of poisonings. These require special laboratories staffed by properly trained toxicologists.

The diagnosis of poisoning is often difficult. It is based on the history, physical examination or pathological changes, and laboratory procedures. The investigation should include personal, occupational, and family history. Physical examination and pathological changes may be quite characteristic for certain types of poisoning. In many instances, however, laboratory procedures are essential to make a definitive diagnosis.

An increasingly important problem is that the physician may know the trade name of a preparation that caused the poisoning without knowing the chemical nature of the compounds contained in such a preparation. The development of poison control centers, where extensive files are maintained on the composition of various chemical and pharmaceutical preparations, may be an important step in helping the physician in poisoning cases.

In general, treatment of poisoning is based on removal of the poison, administration of antidotes, and symptomatic management.

Removal of orally administered poisons may be of great importance if the patient is seen within a few hours after swallowing the noxious agent.

Several procedures are available for emptying the stomach. Gastric lavage is widely used, but its effectiveness is not as great as generally believed. Considerable amounts of a poison may remain in the stomach despite gastric lavage. The use of emetic drugs is of considerable value in poisoning cases.

DIAGNOSIS OF POISONING

PRINCIPLES OF TREATMENT

Emetics   The two drugs that are recommended for the induction of vomiting in poisoning cases are apomorphine and syrup of ipecac. Cupric sulfate is effective also, but its use may be hazardous.

Apomorphine hydrochloride is injected by the subcutaneous route in a dose of 0.1 mg/kg. It induces vomiting within a few minutes by an action on the chemoreceptor trigger zone in the medulla. The emetic effect of the drug is prevented by the phenothiazine antiemetics. Apomorphine may cause respiratory depression, which may be antagonized by the narcotic antagonists. Apomorphine hydrochloride NF is available in tablets containing 6 mg to be prepared for hypodermic use.

Contraindications to the use of apomorphine include shock, coma, advanced age, and ingestion of corrosive substances and probably petroleum distillates.

Ipecac syrup is administered orally in a dosage of 20 ml for adults and 15 ml in children over 1 year of age. The emetic effectiveness increases if ingestion of the drug is followed by 200 ml of water. Ipecac acts locally and also on the chemoreceptor trigger zone. It usually induces vomiting within 20 to 30 minutes. Pediatricians recommend having syrup of ipecac available in the home, since the drug may be very useful in poisonings in children. Ipecac syrup is a USP preparation. Just as other emetics, syrup of ipecac is contraindicated in comatose patients and after the ingestion of corrosive poisons or petroleum distillates. Activated charcoal adsorbs and inactivates ipecac, and the two should not be administered simultaneously.

ANTIDOTES   Antidotes are used for prevention of absorption of the poison and for inactivating it or opposing its action following absorption. Antidotes are usually classified as chemical or physiological. The former actually combine with the poison, whereas the latter oppose its actions.

Until recently, chemical antidotes could serve only for inactivation of the poison in the stomach. Important developments have taken place in recent years in the field of systemically active chemical antidotes. The most important examples are dimercaprol, calcium disodium edetate, and penicillamine. Protective agents against radiation may also be viewed as antidotes against free radicals produced by radiation. An example of such a drug is 2-aminoethylisothiuronium (AET).

For inactivation of poisons in the gastric contents, one of the most widely used compounds is tannic acid, which can precipitate certain metals and alkaloids. Strong tea will precipitate strychnine, cinchona alkaloids, apomorphine, and also, to a slight extent, cocaine. Salts of zinc, cobalt, copper, mercury, lead, and nickel are also precipitated by strong tea.

Milk and egg white are useful in treatment of poisoning caused by mercuric chloride and phenols. Administration of these antidotes should be followed by gastric lavage to prevent slow absorption of the bound poison.

Adsorbents such as activated charcoal may also be useful. Following administration of adsorbents, a saline cathartic may be advantageous. Magnesium sulfate or sodium sulfate may be antidotal in poisoning resulting from barium or lead.

The development of the chemical antidotes dimercaprol and calcium disodium edetate, which are effective against metal poisons even after they are absorbed, represents a brilliant feat of pharmacological research.

Dimercaprol (BAL) was developed during World War II in Great Britain.[24] It was the outgrowth of studies directed at finding effective antidotes against the arsenic-containing vesicant lewisite. It was known previously that arsenicals combine with sulfhydryl groups, and when the effect of arsenicals on the sulfhydryl content of keratin was investigated, it was found that each atom of the metal combined with two of these thiol groups. This fact suggested that a dithiol with adjacent sulfhydryl groups might be efficient as an antidote. A number of such compounds were synthesized, and dimercaptopropanol, known at present as dimercaprol, was found to be most effective.

Dimercaprol

$$\begin{array}{l} \text{CH}_2\text{—SH} \\ | \\ \text{CH—SH} \\ | \\ \text{CH}_2\text{—OH} \end{array}$$

Dimercaprol

The greater antidotal action of dithiols, when compared with cysteine and other monothiols, is related to the fact that the former produce a ring structure of great stability in combination with the metal.

Dimercaprol is effective in the treatment of poisoning by compounds of mercury, arsenic, and gold. Its usefulness is not certain in antimony and bismuth poisoning. Dimercaprol should not be used in the treatment of poisoning caused by cadmium, iron, or selenium. In the case of cadmium, it has been shown that dimercaprol complexes are more toxic than the metal by itself. The drug is not recommended for the treatment of lead poisoning because calcium disodium edetate is much more effective. It may have some usefulness, however, in the management of lead encephalopathy.

There are two major therapeutic objectives in the use of dimercaprol. First, *Therapeutic objectives* the antidote can protect essential enzymes in the tissues from circulating metallic poisons by forming stable combinations with the poisonous agent. A second objective is to promote the excretion of the metal in the form of its dimercaprol complexes and thereby decrease the quantity of the poison in the body. Depending on the interval between the poisoning and the institution of the treatment, one or the other of these objectives may be more important.

Dimercaprol is rapidly metabolized in the body. When a dose of as much as 3 *Metabolism* mg/kg is administered every 4 hours, there is no cumulative toxicity. Liver damage increases the toxicity of dimercaprol. The drug is contraindicated in severe renal insufficiency also, although metabolic inactivation is more important than renal excretion in its disposition.

Toxicity and hypersensitivity

Dimercaprol is a potentially dangerous drug. Even doses of less than 100 mg/kg can cause swift death in animals. It is believed that in these high concentrations the drug inhibits metal-containing enzymes that are essential in cellular respiration.

Adverse effects of dimercaprol include pain at the site of injection, weakness, nausea, salivation, elevation of blood pressure, coma, and convulsions. Large doses may cause vascular collapse as a consequence of capillary damage. Alkalinization of the urine is claimed to protect against dissociation of the dimercaprol-metal complex and nephrotoxicity.

Preparations

Dimercaprol (BAL) is available in peanut oil for injection, 100 mg/ml. Dosage varies from 3 to 5 mg/kg intramuscularly for the initial injection. Administration is repeated one to four times daily, depending on the nature and severity of the poisoning.

Calcium disodium edetate and disodium edetate

Ethylenediamine tetraacetic acid and its salt disodium edetate are powerful chelating agents that form a highly stable complex with calcium. Despite the high stability of the chelate, calcium is displaced from it by lead, zinc, chromium, copper, cadmium, manganese, and nickel. Calcium disodium edetate is useful primarily in the treatment of lead poisoning.

Disodium edetate (Endrate) is quite dangerous when injected intravenously, since it chelates calcium and may lead to hypocalcemia that may be fatal. It has been used for lowering serum calcium concentrations in various clinical conditions, but this should be done only by experts.

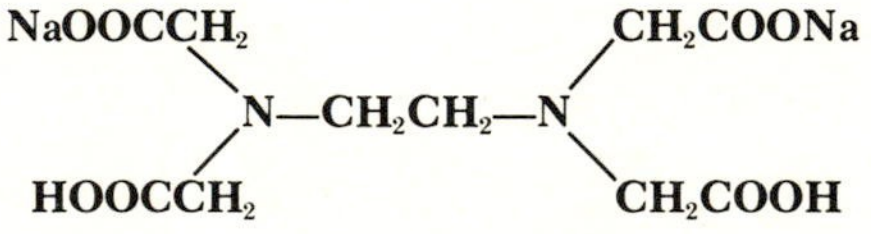

Disodium edetate

Calcium disodium edetate is administered by intravenous drip for 2 or 3 days in the treatment of lead poisoning. It promotes the renal excretion of the lead chelate, which is demonstrable within a few hours and becomes maximal in 1 or 2 days. Increased lead excretion may have diagnostic importance in lead encephalopathy when the diagnosis is uncertain. For diagnostic purposes the drug may be injected by the intramuscular route. Oral administration of calcium disodium edetate for the treatment of lead poisoning is not effective and may even be hazardous.

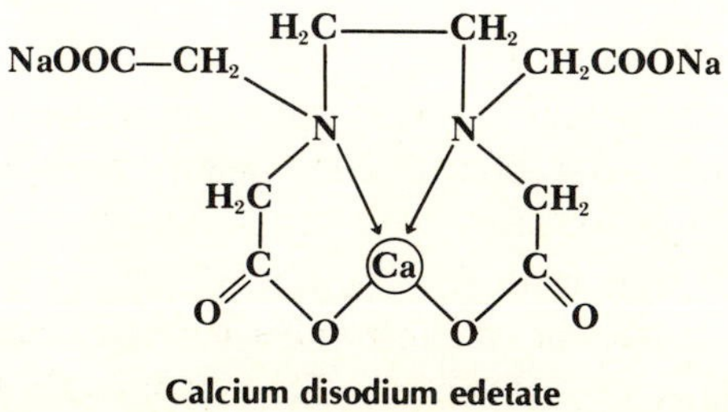

Calcium disodium edetate

Metabolism

In contrast to dimercaprol, calcium disodium edetate is not metabolized in the body and is excreted as a soluble metal complex in the urine.

Adverse effects

Adverse effects of calcium disodium edetate include renal damage, hypersensitivity reactions, and transient bone marrow depression.

Preparations

Calcium disodium edetate (Calcium Disodium Versenate) is available as a solution, 200 mg/ml in 5 ml containers, to be diluted for intravenous infusion. Disodium edetate (Endrate) is prepared as a solution for injection, 150 mg/ml in 20 ml containers.

Penicillamine

Penicillamine (Cuprimine) and its acetyl derivatives can chelate copper and other metals. It is used at the present time for removal of copper in hepatolenticular degeneration (Wilson's disease). Penicillamine chelates not only copper but other metals such as mercury, lead, and iron. Since other antidotes are more effective, the drug is recommended only for the removal of copper.

For an action unrelated to metal chelation, penicillamine has some usefulness in cystinuria because it forms soluble complexes with cystine and facilitates its excretion in a soluble form.

Adverse effects of penicillamine are renal damage, leukopenia, agranulocytosis, eosinophilia, and a decrease in serum iron levels.[34]

Penicillamine (Cuprimine) is available in capsules containing 250 mg. Dosage for adults is 250 mg four times daily, with gradual increase but not to exceed a daily dose of 4 to 5 g.

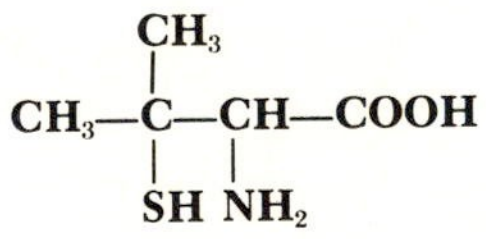

CH3
CH3—C—CH—COOH
SH NH2

Penicillamine

CH3
CH3—C—CH—COOH
H
SH N
COCH3

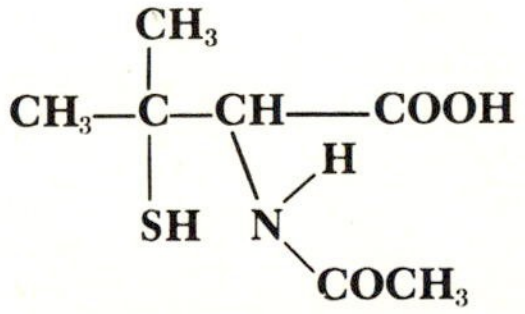

N-Acetylpenicillamine

Deferoxamine mesylate

Deferoxamine mesylate (Desferal) is a chelating agent used in the treatment of iron poisoning and for the removal of iron from the body (p. 596). The drug may be injected intramuscularly or by intravenous infusion. It has great affinity for iron in the ferric form. The drug is toxic and should not be used unless the severity of the poisoning justifies it. Deferoxamine mesylate (Desferal) is available as a powder for injection, 500 mg.

ESSENTIAL FEATURES OF CERTAIN POISONINGS

The toxic effects of the five drugs most commonly causing drug intoxication in the adult are summarized in Table 62-1. The essential features of some other poisonings are discussed in this section.

Scopolamine and atropine intoxication

Scopolamine intoxication is not uncommon because the drug is contained in some proprietary hypnotic preparations (Sominex). The symptoms induced by scopolamine

TABLE 62-1. Essential features of common poisons*

Drug	Oral fatal dose (estimated)	Lethal blood levels (estimated)	Effects	Therapy
Barbiturates				
Short-acting	3 g	3.5 mg/100 ml	Respiratory depression, hypotension, renal shutdown, hypothermia, pneumonia	Respiratory assistance, diuresis, dialysis
Long-acting	5 g	8.0 mg/100 ml		
Glutethimide	10 g	3.0 mg/100 ml	Apnea, mydriasis, hypotension, flaccid paralysis	Gastric lavage, respiratory assistance, diuresis, dialysis
Salicylates	10-20 g	50 mg/100 ml	Hyperventilation, respiratory alkalosis, metabolic acidosis (later), hypoprothrombinemia	Alkaline diuresis, vitamin K, dialysis
Phenothiazines	50 mg/kg of chlorpromazine or equivalent	Unknown	Miosis, irritability	Supportive control of convulsions
Meprobamate	12 g	Unknown	Hypotension, respiratory depression, coma	Respiratory assistance, dialysis

*Based on data from Castell, D. O., and Morrison, C. C.: Res. Phys. **13:**66, 1967.

and atropine have been discussed (p. 153). They include delirium, dilated pupils, tachycardia, dry mouth and skin, and hyperirritability. Injection of 10 to 30 mg of methacholine has no effect on salivation, sweating, or activity of the intestinal tract.

Treatment consists of sponging for high temperature and sedation for convulsions.

Bromide intoxication

The toxic dose is about 30 g or a blood level of 200 mg/100 ml. The drug is cumulative. Delirium, mental confusion, respiratory depression, and hypotension should suggest the possibility of bromide intoxication. Treatment is based on the administration of solutions containing sodium chloride.

Ethylene glycol intoxication

Ethylene glycol is contained in antifreeze preparations. Its lethal dose is about 100 ml. Ethylene glycol is metabolized to oxalate. Acidosis occurs and methemoglobinemia may be present. The symptoms vary according to the stage of intoxication. In the first stage, hyperactivity of the central nervous system (CNS) followed by coma is characteristic. In the second stage, cardiac and pulmonary signs with tachypnea, cyanosis, and possibility of pulmonary edema predominate. The third stage is characterized by renal failure with the deposition of calcium oxalate crystals in the renal tubules. Diagnosis is facilitated when such crystals are found in the urine. Treatment is based initially on gastric lavage and the administration of sodium lactate or bicarbonate for acidosis and methylene blue for methemoglobinemia.[21] Dialysis may be quite useful for removal of the poison and treatment of renal failure. Ethyl alcohol is claimed to compete with liver enzymes that metabolize ethylene glycol, but its use is still experimental.[21]

Carbon monoxide, a colorless and odorless gas, has a great affinity for hemoglobin. The resulting carboxyhemoglobin is unavailable for oxygen transport. The affinity of carbon monoxide for hemoglobin may be 200 to 300 times as great as that of oxygen. As a consequence, inhalation of even low concentrations of the gas can produce markedly elevated levels of carboxyhemoglobin. Serious toxic effects results when 40% of hemoglobin has been changed to carboxyhemoglobin.

Carbon monoxide poisoning

The symptoms of carbon monoxide poisoning consist of impairment of vision, headache, tachycardia, hyperpnea, and eventually coma and death when about 60% of the hemoglobin is in the form of carboxyhemoglobin. The skin shows characteristic cherry-red cyanosis resulting from the red color of carboxyhemoglobin.

Treatment consists of transferring the patient to fresh air, giving artificial respiration, and administering 100% oxygen.

The cyanide ion has a great affinity for respiratory enzymes. Its rapid lethal action probably results from inactivation of the enzyme cytochrome oxidase, which is very susceptible to this poison.

Cyanide poisoning

The lethal effect of hydrocyanic acid is extremely rapid, and the opportunities for treatment hardly exist. When potassium or sodium cyanide are ingested, the lethal dose appears to be 50 to 100 mg, and the rapidity of the lethal effect depends on the dose swallowed and the speed of gastroinestinal absorption, which is in turn influenced by the nature of the gastric contents.

In acute cyanide poisoning, death occurs suddenly, usually with terminal convulsions. In less severe cases gastrointestinal disturbances may be present, with or without convulsions. There is no agreement on the existence of chronic cyanide poisoning. Workers exposed to cyanide in industry may complain of a variety of gastrointestinal and neurological symptoms. Dermatitis also occurs.

Cyanide poisoning can be treated very effectively if there is opportunity for almost immediate therapy after the poison has been swallowed. In addition to gastric lavage for removal of unabsorbed cyanide, therapy is aimed at binding and inactivating the poison.

It has been shown that methemoglobin has great affinity for cyanide, forming cyanmethemoglobin.[5] Methemoglobin can be produced by inhalation of amyl nitrite and intravenous injection of about 300 mg of sodium nitrite in a 3% solution. If this is followed by intravenous injection of sodium thiosulfate, 12.5 to 25 g in a 25% solution, it is possible to protect the individual against several lethal doses of cyanide. This combined treatment could protect dogs against as many as 20 lethal doses of sodium cyanide.

Other measures such as artificial respiration and vasoconstrictors are also important, and the antidotes may have to be given repeatedly if symptoms recur.

Heavy metal poisoning   Poisoning caused by heavy metals is characterized by gastrointestinal disturbances, dermatological manifestations, peripheral neuritis, blood dyscrasias, and lethargy.

The heavy metals, in general, have an affinity for sulfhydryl groups, which are essential in many enzyme systems. Although the symptoms of metal intoxication depend on the particular metal, as a generalization it may be stated that the kidneys, gastrointestinal tract, and brain are commonly affected.

The insidiousness of metal poisoning is well exemplified by the current concern with the environmental effects of mercury. This metal was considered quite inert in its elemental form until recently. It was generally believed that if mercury were discharged into water it would settle and remain quite harmless at the bottom. In 1960 it was reported that 111 people died or suffered neurological damage in Minamata, Japan, as a consequence of eating shellfish contaminated by mercury discharged into the bay by a plastics manufacturer. Swedish studies have shown that metallic mercury can be changed by bacteria into methyl mercury that can enter the food cycle and become concentrated a thousandfold in fish. In 1970 high levels of mercury were discovered in fish in the United States. This creates considerable concern because the organic mercurials may accumulate in the vital organs of human beings.

Arsenicals containing trivalent arsenic were widely used in the treatment of syphilis in the recent past. Neoarsphenamine and oxophenarsine (Mapharsen) were most important. Toxic effects from administration of trivalent arsenicals consists of nitritoid reactions, liver damage, neuritis, and bone marrow depression. The antidote is dimercaprol.

Pentavalent arsenicals such as tryparsamide were also used in some types of syphilis. Carbarsone is still used by mouth in the treatment of amebiasis. On a weight basis, the pentavalent compounds are much less toxic than the trivalent arsenicals. They are only moderately well absorbed from the intestine and are slowly changed in the body to trivalent arsenicals. Dimercaprol is the best antidote for poisoning caused by any arsenical.

Bismuth compounds have also been used in the treatment of syphilis. Bismuth subsalicylate in oil given by intramuscular injection was popular but is now obsolete. Bismuth subcarbonate is sometimes used by mouth in doses of 1 to 3 g in the treatment of diarrhea. It is not absorbed significantly from the intestine. Bismuth subnitrate was also employed for this purpose but was abandoned because nitrite poisoning with methemoglobinemia could occur as a consequence of bacterial action on bismuth subnitrate. Bismuth poisoning is characterized by stomatitis and by renal and hepatic damage. Dimercaprol is of questionable value as an antidote.

Mercurials are now obsolete for the treatment of syphilis. They are still used as diuretics and as disinfectants and antiseptics. Mercurial poisoning is characterized by stomatitis, kidney damage to the point of anuria, and damage to the intestinal mucosa. The antidote is dimercaprol. The environmental role of mercury is of great current concern.

Antimonials such as antimony potassium tartrate (tartar emetic) and stibophen (Fuadin) are still used in the treatment of schistosomiasis and some other tropical diseases. The toxicity of antimony is similar to that of arsenic. Dimercaprol is of questionable antidotal value in cases of poisoning caused by these metals.

Thallium is employed as a rodenticide and ant poison. Ingestion leads to serious poisoning, of which loss of hair is a characteristic feature. The usual metal-binding antidotes are ineffective in thallium poisoning.

Lead poisoning

Lead poisoning is usually a chronic occupational disease. Acute poisoning, characterized by encephalopathy, is a rare disorder and may occur in children and also in young adults who are exposed to a large dose of lead compounds. Dimercaprol in combination with calcium disodium edetate may be useful as an antidote.

The toxic levels of lead in the serum are 1.3 mg/L.

The most common symptoms and signs in lead poisoning are abdominal pain (lead colic), weakness, gingival lead line, pyorrhea, and muscle weakness of the extensors of the wrists. In addition, anemia, porphyrinuria, and stippling of erythrocytes can be demonstrated, and vague cerebral disturbances occur.

The smooth muscle contraction in lead colic is generally attributed to an effect of lead on this tissue. Some studies indicate that lead has a profound influence on porphyrin metabolism, and it is of interest that in porphyria abdominal pain is common. Coproporphyrin III has been found in large quantities in the urine of patients with lead poisoning.[19]

The most important drug in treatment of lead poisoning is calcium disodium edetate. Prior to the introduction of this drug, treatment of lead poisoning was dominated by certain concepts of induced deposition of lead in bones and mobilization of lead from these storage sites (so-called *deleading*).

Oral prophylactic treatment with chelating agents such as edetate disodium calcium or penicillamine for the prevention of lead poisoning in industrial workers is not recommended.[34] Such treatment is ineffective and may have adverse effects on serum iron, copper, magnesium, and zinc levels. In the case of penicillamine, long-term treatment may cause renal damage, leukopenia, eosinophilia, and decreased iron levels.

Miscellaneous poisons

Chlorinated hydrocarbon insecticides. Various chlorinated hydrocarbons are used as insecticides. Some of these are chlorophenothane (DDT), chlordane, hexachlorocyclohexane (lindane), dieldrin, and others. These insecticides may be absorbed when ingested. Being lipid soluble, they can penetrate through the skin. They are stored in body fat. Large doses of these compounds produce convulsions and death. Smaller amounts may cause tremors and hyperirritability.

Although the acute toxicity of the chlorinated insecticides is not very great (their lethal dose being of the order of 50 to 300 mg/kg in animals), there is some concern over the cumulation of these compounds in body fat and their possible adverse chronic effects on health and/or environment. The cumulation of these compounds in body fat is not unlimited, since their slow degradation eventually will keep up with their entry into the body. As a consequence, the concentration in human fat has become stabilized at levels of about 10 parts per million of DDT and metabolites. The effect of these insecticides on the environment, however, may be considerable, affecting not only insects but also birds that feed on the insects.

Organophosphorus compounds. The organophosphorus compounds are used as insecticides. Their ability to inhibit cholinesterase and the antidotal action of atropine and pralidoxime are discussed in Chapter 11.

Organic solvents. The complex aliphatic hydrocarbons contained in kerosene, gasoline, and industrial solvents may cause anesthesia and respiratory depression when inhaled in high concentrations. They may also cause acute pneumonitis when swallowed.

The halogenated aliphatic hydrocarbons can also act as anesthetics and may cause death as a consequence of respiratory depression and cardiovascular collapse. In addition, most halogenated hydrocarbons can damage the liver and the kidneys. Carbon tetrachloride is an important cause of hepatic damage. Evidence is increasing that this is a direct action on the liver cells.

It is of great interest that mammalian tissues can reduce carbon tetrachloride to chloroform to some extent.[3] Also, chloroform is reduced to methylene chloride, at least in vitro. There may be a connection between the hepatotoxicity of the alkyl halides and their metabolic handling.

Nicotine. Nicotine is used as an insecticide. Its poisonous properties are characterized by nausea, vomiting, and initial rise of blood pressure caused by ganglionic stimulation and norepinephrine release, followed by ganglionic paralysis with fall of blood pressure. Death results from respiratory paralysis. Thromboangiitis and tobacco amblyopia have been attributed to chronic nicotine poisoning.

Treatment of nicotine poisoning is supportive, with emphasis on artificial respiration. There is no specific antidote for nicotine.

REFERENCES

1 Adams, D. A., Goldman, R., Maxwell, M. H., and Latta, H.: Nephrotic syndrome associated with penicillamine therapy of Wilson's disease, Am. J. Med. **36**:330, 1964.

2 Arena, J. M.: Treatment of some common household poisonings, Pharmacol. Phys. **3**(9): 1, 1969.

3 Butler, T. C.: Reduction of carbon tetrachloride in vivo and reduction of carbon tetrachloride and chloroform in vitro by tissues and tissue constituents, J. Pharmacol. Exp. Ther. **134**: 311, 1961.

4 Castell, D. O., and Morrison, C. C.: Common adult poisons, Res. Phys. **13**:66, 1967.

5 Chen, K. K., and Rose, C. L.: Nitrite and thiosulfate therapy in cyanide poisoning, J.A.M.A. **149**:113, 1952.

6 Clemmesen, C.: Treatment of narcotic intoxication. Results and principles of the "Scandinavian" method, especially concerning stimulation, Danish Med. Bull. **10**:132, 1963.

7 Done, A. K.: Clinical pharmacology of systemic antidotes, Clin. Pharmacol. Ther. **2**: 750, 1961.

8 Done, A. K.: Pharmacologic principles in the treatment of poisoning, Pharmacol. Phys. **3**(7): 1, 1969.

9 Foreman, H., Finnigan, C., and Lushbaugh, C. C.: Nephrotoxic hazard from uncontrolled edathamil calcium-disodium therapy, J.A.M.A. **160**:1042, 1956.

10 Gosselin, R. E., and Smith, R. P.: Trends in the therapy of acute poisonings, Clin. Pharmacol. Ther. **7**:279, 1966.

11 Hollister, L. E.: Overdoses of psychotherapeutic drugs, Clin. Pharmacol. Ther. **7**:142, 1966.

12 Kehoe, R. A.: Misuse of edathamil calcium-disodium for prophylaxis of lead poisoning, J.A.M.A. **157**:341, 1955.

13 Lamanna, C., and Carr, J. C.: The botulinal, tetanal, and enterostaphylococcal toxins: a review, Clin. Pharmacol. Ther. **8**:286, 1967.

14 Mandelbaum, J. M., and Simon, N. M.: Severe methyprylon intoxication treated by hemodialysis, J.A.M.A. **216**:139, 1971.

15 Medved, L. I., and Kagan, J. S.: Toxicology, Annu. Rev. Pharmacol. **6**:293, 1966.

16 Milthers, E.: Poisoning in childhood, Danish Med. Bull. **10**:132, 1963.

17 Modell, W.: Drug-induced diseases, Annu. Rev. Pharmacol. **5**:285, 1965.

18 Murphy, J. V.: Intoxication following the ingestion of elemental zinc, J.A.M.A. **212**:2119, 1970.

19 Parkinson, E. S., and Cholak, J.: Problems in the analysis of urinary coproporphyrin III, Indust. Hyg. Quart. **13**:158, 1952.

20 Penneys, N. S., Israel, R. M., and Indgin, S. M.: Contact dermatitis due to 1-chloroacetophenone and chemical mace, N. Engl. J. Med. **281**:413, 1969.

21 Peterson, D. I., Peterson, J. E., Hardinge, M. G., and Wacker, W. E. C.: Experimental treatment of ethylene glycol poisoning, J.A.M.A. **186**:955, 1963.

22 Russell, F. E.: Pharmacology of animal venoms, Clin. Pharmacol. Ther. **8**:849, 1967.

23 Sherlock, S.: Hepatic reactions to therapeutic agents, Annu. Rev. Pharmacol. **5**:429, 1965.

24 Stocken, L. A., and Thompson, R. H. S.: Reactions of British anti-lewisite with arsenic and other metals in living systems, Physiol. Rev. **29**:168, 1949.

25 Von Oettingen, W. F.: Poisoning: a guide to clinical diagnosis and treatment, Philadelphia, 1958, W. B. Saunders Co.

26 Zavon, M. R., Hine, C. H., and Parker, K. D.: Chlorinated hydrocarbon insecticides in human body fat in the United States, J.A.M.A. **193**:181, 1965.

27 Zbinden, G.: Experimental and clinical aspects of drug toxicity, Adv. Pharmacol. **2**:1, 1963.

REVIEWS

28 Almeyda, J., and Levantine, A.: Cutaneous reactions to cardiovascular drugs, Br. J. Dermatol. **88**:313, 1973.

29 Arena, J. M.: Poisoning—treatment and prevention, J.A.M.A. **232**:1272, 1975.

30 Berman, L. B.: The art and science of clinical toxicology, J.A.M.A. **240**:265, 1978.

31 Caranasos, G. J., Stewart, R. B., and Cluff, L. E.: Drug-induced illness leading to hospitalization, J.A.M.A. **228**:713, 1974.

32 Dimijian, G. G., and Radelat, F. A.: Evaluation and treatment of the suspected drug user in the emergency room, Arch. Intern. Med. **125**:162, 1970.

33 Hurwitz, A., and Klaassen, C.: The treatment of poisoning, Ration. Drug Ther. **14**:1, March, 1980.

34 Lilis, R., and Fischbein, A.: Chelation therapy in workers exposed to lead, J.A.M.A. **235**:2823, 1976.

35 Maher, J. F.: Nephrotoxicity of drugs and chemicals, Pharmacol. Phys. **4**:1, 1970.

36 Nunez, L. J.: Current and future trends in environmental toxicology, Clin. Toxicol. Consultant **1**:65, 1979.

37 Pathak, M. A., and Fitzpatrick, T. B.: Photosensitivity caused by drugs, Ration. Drug Ther. **6**:1, 1972.

38 Schreiner, G. E.: Dialysis of poisons and drugs—annual review, Trans. Am. Soc. Artif. Organs **16**:544, 1970.

SECTION TWELVE

Drug interactions

CHAPTER 63

Drug interactions

Discussions on drug interactions often begin with frightening statistics on the large number of drugs taken by most patients and the dire consequences that may result from drug interactions. What is usually not mentioned is the justification for using several drugs concomitantly in many patients, the beneficial nature of many drug interactions, and the uncritical manner in which many supposedly adverse drug interactions are reported in the literature.

The uninitiated could get the impression when examining large and complex tables of drug interactions that the problem is not only vast but is almost beyond the ability of the physician to handle. What is often not recognized is that the majority of interactions listed in such tables are trivial and create no problems to the physician, who adjusts dosages to the patient's needs and is alert to any adverse effects.

The clinically significant drug interactions can be minimized by avoiding combinations of drugs known to be incompatible according to the current pharmacological literature and tables of drug interactions such as the one presented in this chapter. It should be possible to develop systems in hospital pharmacies that would prevent the dispensing of incompatible drugs. Ultimately, however, it is the physician's familiarity with the current clinical literature and understanding of the mechanisms underlying drug interactions that are more likely to prevent their occurrence.

Adverse drug reactions based on drug interactions are not always iatrogenic. Self-medication with over-the-counter drugs may be a contributing factor. In addition, environmental contaminants such as the chlorinated insecticides (DDT) may stimulate drug metabolism by hepatic microsomal enzymes and could conceivably contribute to unusual reactions to drugs.

MECHANISMS UNDERLYING ADVERSE EFFECTS OF DRUG INTERACTIONS

A drug may influence the effect of another drug by several different mechanisms. The influences may be exerted on (1) intestinal absorption, (2) competition for plasma protein binding, (3) metabolism or biotransformation, (4) adrenergic neuronal uptake, (5) action at the receptor site, (6) renal excretion, and (7) alteration of electrolyte balance.

Intestinal absorption

Antacids that contain calcium, magnesium, or aluminum interfere with the absorption of tetracycline, which forms a chelate with the metals. Aluminum-containing antacids interfere with the absorption of phosphate. Carbonates and phytates (cereals) prevent the absorption of iron. Cholestyramine may interfere with the absorption of phenylbutazone, warfarin,[56] and thyroxine.

Antacids may influence drug absorption also by changing the lipid-soluble non-ionized moiety of weak acids and bases in the gastrointestinal tract. It should be recalled (p. 21) that the lipid-soluble, nonionized fraction is much better absorbed. Because of this, antacids would be expected to diminish the absorption of weak acids such as phenylbutazone, nitrofurantoin, sulfonamides, and some barbiturates and oral anticoagulants.

Other gastrointestinal drug interactions may be of clinical significance. Antibiotics that alter the bacterial flora in the intestine may decrease the formation of vitamin K and thus increase the anticoagulant action of the coumarins. Folate deficiency may result from the use of drugs which inhibit the intestinal conjugase that breaks down the polyglutamate portion of the naturally occurring folic acid. By this mechanism, megaloblastic anemia may result in some patients after the use of phenytoin or triamterene. Mineral oil may interfere with the absorption of vitamin D.

Direct chemical interactions may occur not only in the gastrointestinal tract but also when drugs are mixed for intravenous infusions. Unstable drugs such as methicillin or levarterenol should not be mixed with other drugs without consideration of possible direct drug interactions. Carbenicillin inactivates gentamicin when mixed for intravenous infusion.

Competition for plasma protein binding

Many drugs are bound to plasma proteins to varying degrees, and the bound fraction fails to exert pharmacological effects. For example, two antibiotics having the same potency in a protein-free culture medium will have vastly different clinical effectiveness if their affinities for plasma proteins differ greatly.[3,47]

Certain drugs compete for the same binding sites on plasma proteins. As a consequence, one drug may displace another, thus increasing the latter's free fraction and pharmacological effectiveness. Tolbutamide can be displaced from its plasma binding by dicumarol, resulting in severe hypoglycemia.[46,71,75] Chloral hydrate increases the anticoagulant action of warfarin because its metabolite, trichloroacetic acid, competes with the anticoagulant for plasma protein binding.[69]

Metabolism or biotransformation

The inhibition of the metabolism of one drug by another is a well-established mechanism of enhanced drug effect.[11] By their enzyme-inhibiting action, the anticholinesterases enhance the actions by acetylcholine, succinylcholine, and some other choline esters. Allopurinol inhibits xanthine oxidase and thus increases the plasma levels of mercaptopurine and azathioprine. The monoamine oxidase (MAO) inhibitors have caused severe reactions by preventing the destruction of tyramine in the body.[31,56,72]

Many drugs can accelerate their metabolism and also that of other drugs by induction of hepatic microsomal enzymes (p. 38). Phenobarbital accelerates the metabolism of coumarin anticoagulants, phenytoin, griseofulvin, cortisol, estrogens, androgens, and progesterone. In addition to the barbiturates, glutethimide, phenytoin, and the chlorinated hydrocarbon insecticides such as DDT are enhancers of drug metabolism (p. 38).

Enzyme induction by phenobarbital and other drugs leads to a decreased effectiveness of drugs and may also result in catastrophes when the inducer is discontinued without changing the dose of the second drug. For example, if phenobarbital is suddenly discontinued without lowering the dosage of a coumarin anticoagulant, severe hemorrhagic episodes may develop (Fig. 4-3).

Adrenergic neuronal uptake

Amphetamine and guanethidine are transported by the same mechanism across the adrenergic neuronal membrane. Because of this, amphetamine may prevent the antihypertensive action of guanethidine. The tricyclic antidepressants have a "cocaine-like" blocking effect on the amine uptake mechanism and may nullify the antihypertensive effect of guanethidine by preventing its uptake into the adrenergic neuron.[34,50,55,56]

Action at the receptor site

The numerous examples of additive effects or various antagonisms resulting from action at the receptor site do not represent great problems if the drugs are administered by persons well versed in pharmacology (p. 67).

Renal excretion

There are several interesting examples of drug interactions resulting from an influence on renal tubular reabsorption. The best example, of course, is the inhibition of penicillin excretion by probenecid. Interference in the uricosuric action of probenecid by small doses of salicylates and the promotion of phenobarbital clearance after sodium bicarbonate administration are other examples of one drug influencing the renal excretion of another.

Acidification of the urine after the oral administration of ammonium chloride or alkalinization following sodium bicarbonate may have a demonstrable effect on the renal clearance of several drugs, but the quantitative importance of such knowledge in therapeutics is not great except in phenobarbital poisoning.

Alteration of electrolyte balance

A drug may alter the concentration of many different constituents of the body, thus influencing the action of another drug. Some of the best examples originate from the area of fluid and electrolyte balance. Hypokalemia caused by the thiazide diuretics promotes arrhythmias when digitalis compounds are employed. Ammonium chloride administration reestablishes the effectiveness of mercurial diuretics when blunted by metabolic alkalosis.

The sudden release of catecholamines by reserpine may precipitate arrhythmias in a patient who has been receiving digitalis therapy. A patient treated with MAO inhibitors is vulnerable to drugs such as amphetamine that cause release of catecholamines from nerve endings because the concentration of the catecholamines at these stores is elevated and more is available for release.

**INTERACTIONS IN
VARIOUS DRUG
CATEGORIES**

Most drug interactions present themselves in therapeutics as either an enhanced or diminished drug effect. The enhanced drug effects may manifest themselves as idiosyncratic responses that may occasionally have catastrophic consequences (Table 63-1).

Diminished responses resulting from drug interactions are generally not very dramatic. It can happen, however, that manipulations of dosage necessitated by drug interactions may have serious consequences when one of the drugs is discontinued without simultaneous adjustment of the dosage of the other drug. For example, chloral hydrate stimulates the metabolism of several coumarin anticoagulants.[19] If the dosage of the coumarin is increased over a period of several days and then chloral hydrate is suddenly discontinued, the anticoagulant effect may become excessive and bleeding will follow. But the interactions of chloral hydrate with the oral anticoagulants may be more complex than previously thought. The metabolic product of chloral hydrate, trichloroacetic acid, interferes with the binding of warfarin to plasma proteins. Increased anticoagulation may result,[69,84] which is the opposite of the interaction resulting from increased metabolism of dicumarol just described.

The clinically significant drug interactions are listed in Table 63-2 along with their probable mechanisms. The table is only a quick survey, and for details the original references should be consulted.

**SIGNIFICANCE OF
ADVERSE DRUG
REACTIONS**

Some drug interactions such as those in Table 63-1 may be life-threatening, whereas others are unimportant and require only a simple adjustment in the dosage. An important determinant of the seriousness of an interaction is the therapeutic margin of the drugs involved. With anticoagulants, oral hypoglycemic drugs, digitalis, and antiarrhythmic drugs the margin of safety is not great, and relatively small changes in plasma concentration resulting from drug interactions could have catastrophic effects. On the other hand, drugs with great margins of safety do not cause

TABLE 63-1. Clinically observed adverse effects based on drug interactions

Major symptoms	Drugs involved
Hypertensive crisis	MAO inhibitors + Tyramine (cheese)
	MAO inhibitors + Methamphetamine
Hemorrhagic episodes	Warfarin + Phenylbutazone
	Warfarin + Phenyramidol
Respiratory paralysis	Neomycin + Succinylcholine
	Neomycin + Ether
Hypoglycemic reaction	Tolbutamide + Phenylbutazone
	Tolbutamide + Sulfisoxazole
Cardiac arrhythmias	Digitalis + Chlorothiazide
	Digitalis + Reserpine

TABLE 63-2. Clinically significant drug interactions

First drug	Second drug(s)	Possible result	Mechanism*
Analgesics			
Aspirin	Anticoagulant	Enhanced anticoagulation	2
	Sulfonylureas	Enhanced hypoglycemia	2
	p-Aminosalicylate	PAS toxicity	2
	Probenecid	Decreased uricosuria	8
Phenylbutazone	Anticoagulant	Enhanced anticoagulation	2
	Sulfonylurea	Enhanced hypoglycemia	2, 3
	Estrogen, androgen	Decreased hormonal effects	3
Phenyramidol	Anticoagulant	Enhanced anticoagulation	3
Morphine	Phenothiazine	Enhanced analgesia	7
Meperidine	Atropine	Enhanced atropine effect	7
Propoxyphene	Amphetamine	Enhanced amphetamine effect	7
Anticoagulants			
Coumarin drugs	Aspirin, acetaminophen, clofibrate, phenylbutazone, indomethacin, methyldopa, methylphenidate, quinidine	Enhanced anticoagulation	2
	Barbiturates, glutethimide, griseofulvin, meprobamate	Decreased anticoagulant effect	3
	Chloral hydrate	Increased or decreased anticoagulant effect	2, 3
	Vitamin K	Decreased anticoagulant effect	7
Heparin	Polymyxin	Incompatibility in intravenous solution	10
Antimicrobials			
Aminoglycosides	d-Tubocurarine	Enhanced tubocurarine effect	7
Cephalothin	Barbiturates, erythromycin, tetracycline	Incompatibility in intravenous solution	10
Chloramphenicol	Barbiturates, phenytoin	Enhanced sedation	3
	Anticoagulants	Enhanced anticoagulation	3
	Penicillin	Antibiotic antagonism (some infections)	7
	Diphtheria or tetanus toxoid	Decreased immune response	11
Furazolidone	Amphetamine, methyldopa, sympathomimetics, tyramine	Hypertension, excitement	3
Griseofulvin	Phenobarbital	Decreased phenobarbital effect	3
Penicillin G	Sulfonamides, tetracycline	Antibiotic antagonism (some infections)	7
Polymyxin B	d-Tubocurarine, succinylcholine	Muscle paralysis	7
Sulfonamides	Aspirin, phenylbutazone	Sulfonamide toxicity	2
	Anticoagulants	Enhanced anticoagulation	2
	Sulfonylureas	Enhanced hypoglycemia	2
Tetracycline	Antacids	Decreased absorption	1

*Mechanisms: 1 = interference with gastrointestinal absorption; 2 = plasma protein binding competition; 3 = metabolism or biotransformation; 4 = enzyme induction; 5 = adrenergic neuronal uptake; 6 = depletion of catecholamines at adrenergic neuron; 7 = action at receptor site or related to end-organ response; 8 = renal excretion; 9 = alteration of electrolyte balance; 10 = direct combination; 11 = inhibition of protein synthesis. *Continued.*

TABLE 63-2. Clinically significant drug interactions—cont'd

First drug	Second drug(s)	Possible result	Mechanism
Antihistamines			
Antihistaminic drugs	Alcohol, reserpine, phenothiazines	Enhanced sedation	7
	Atropine	Enhanced atropine effects	7
Anticonvulsants			
Phenytoin	Dicumarol, chloramphenicol, methylphenidate, phenyramidol	Enhanced phenytoin effect	3
	Phenobarbital	Decreased phenytoin effect	3
Antidepressants			
MAO inhibitors	Tyramine, amphetamine, levodopa, methyldopa, sympathomimetics	Hypertension, excitement	3
Tricyclic drugs	Guanethidine	Decreased guanethidine effect	5
	MAO inhibitor	Enhanced MAO inhibitor toxicity	7
	Phenothiazines, antianxiety drugs	Additive effect	7
Antihypertensives			
Guanethidine	Sympathomimetics, amphetamine	Hypertensive crisis	5
	Levarterenol	Enhanced levarterenol effect	5
	Tricyclic antidepressants	Decreased guanethidine effect	5
Methyldopa	Sympathomimetics	Decreased methyldopa effect	7
Pargyline (same as MAO inhibitors)	MAO inhibitors	Decreased methyldopa effect	3
Reserpine	Sympathomimetics, tricyclic drugs	Decreased reserpine effect	7
	Indirect sympathomimetics, metaraminol	Decreased metaraminol effect	6
	Anesthetic	Hypotension	6
	Levarterenol	Enhanced levarterenol effect	7
Antineoplastic agents			
Mercaptopurine	Allopurinol	Enhanced mercaptopurine effect	3
Methotrexate	Aspirin, sulfonamides	Enhanced methotrexate toxicity	2
Digitalis			
Digitalis preparations	Thiazides, calcium	Digitalis toxicity	9
	Reserpine	Arrhythmias	7
	Phenobarbital	Decreased digitalis effect	4
Diuretics			
Thiazides	Digitalis	Digitalis toxicity	9
	Antihypertensive drugs	Enhanced antihypertensive effect	7
	Sulfonylureas	Antagonism of hypoglycemia	7
	Curare drugs	Enhanced curare effects	9
Mercurials	Ammonium chloride	Enhanced diuresis	9
	Alkalinizing agents	Decreased diuresis	9
Ethacrynic acid	Aminoglycosides	Ototoxicity	7

TABLE 63-2. Clinically significant drug interactions—cont'd

First drug	Second drug(s)	Possible result	Mechanism
Antianxiety and antipsychotic drugs			
Benzodiazepines	Alcohol, hypnotics, phenothiazines, tricyclic antidepressants	Enhanced sedation	7
Phenothiazines	Alcohol, hypnotics, narcotics, antihistamines, tricyclic antidepressants	Enhanced sedation	7
	Antihypertensives	Enhanced antihypertensive effect	7
	Convulsants	Lowered convulsive threshold	7
Hormones			
Insulin	Oral hypoglycemics, propranolol, MAO inhibitors	Enhanced hypoglycemic effect	7
Corticosteroids	Barbiturates, phenytoin, antihistamines	Decreased corticosteroid effect	4
Estrogens, progestogens	Androgens	Antagonism of androgen anticancer effect	7
	Clofibrate	Decreased hypocholesterolemic effect	3
Hypnotics			
Phenobarbital	Anticoagulants, phenytoin, griseofulvin, hypnotics, corticosteroids	Decreased drug effects	4
	Alcohol, phenothiazines, antianxiety drugs	Enhanced sedation	7
Chloral hydrate	Alcohol	Enhanced sedation	7
	Anticoagulant	Increased or decreased anticoagulant effect	2, 3
Uricosuric agents			
Probenecid	Aspirin, ethacrynic acid	Decreased uricosuria	7
	Penicillin	Enhanced penicillin levels	7

serious problems as a consequence of drug interactions. This principle should be kept in mind when examining large tables of drug interactions.

REFERENCES

1 Aggeler, P. M., O'Reilly, R. A., Leong, L., and Kowitz, P. E.: Potentiation of anticoagulant effect of warfarin by phenylbutazone, N. Engl. J. Med. **276**:496, 1967.
2 Antilitz, A. M., Tolentino, M., and Kosai, M. F.: Effect of butabarbital on orally administered anticoagulants, Curr. Ther. Res. **10**:70, 1968.
3 Anton, A. H.: The relation between the binding of sulfonamides to albumin and their antibacterial efficacy, J. Pharmacol. Exp. Ther. **129**:282, 1960.
4 Asatoor, A. M., Levi, A. J., and Milne, M. D.: Tranylcypromine and cheese, Lancet **2**:733, 1963.
5 Blackwell, B.: Hypertensive crisis due to monoamine-oxidase inhibitors, Lancet **2**:849, 1963.
6 Blackwell, B., Marley, E., and Ryle, A.: Hypertensive crisis associated with monoamine-oxidase inhibitors, Lancet **1**:722, 1964.

7 Brachfeld, J., Wirthshafter, A., and Wolfe, S.: Imipramine-tranylcypromine incompatibility; near-fatal toxic reaction, J.A.M.A. **186:**1172, 1963.

8 Bressler, R.: Combined drug therapy, Am. J. Med. Sci. **255:**89, 1968.

9 Brodie, B. B.: Displacement of one drug by another from carrier or receptor sites, Proc. R. Soc. Med. **58:**946, 1965.

10 Brodie, B. B.: Physiochemical and biochemical aspects of pharmacology, J.A.M.A. **202:**600, 1967.

11 Burns, J. J., and Conney, A. H.: Enzyme stimulation and inhibition in the metabolism of drugs, Proc. R. Soc. Med. **58:**955, 1965.

12 Busfield, D., Child, K. J., Atkinson, R. M., and Tomich, E. G.: An effect of phenobarbitone on blood-levels of griseofulvin in man, Lancet **2:**1042, 1963.

13 Carter, S. A.: Potentiation of the effect of orally administered anticoagulants by phenyramidol hydrochloride, N. Engl. J. Med. **273:**423, 1965.

14 Catalano, P. M., and Cullen, S. I.: Warfarin antagonism by griseofulvin, Clin. Res. **14:**266, 1966.

15 Chen, W., Vrindten, P. A., Dayton, P. G., and Burns, J. J.: Accelerated aminopyrine metabolism in human subjects pretreated with phenylbutazone, Life Sci. **1:**35, 1962.

16 Christensen, L. K., Hansen, J. M., and Kristensen, M.: Sulphaphenazole-induced hypoglycaemic attacks in tolbutamide-treated diabetics, Lancet **2:**1298, 1963.

17 Conney, A. H.: Pharmacological implications of microsomal enzyme induction, Pharmacol. Rev. **19:**317, 1967.

18 Cucinell, S. A., Conney, A. H., Sansur, M., and Burns, J. J.: Drug interactions in man. I. Lowering effect of phenobarbital on plasma levels of bishydroxycoumarin (Dicumarol) and diphenylhydantoin (Dilantin), Clin. Pharmacol. Ther. **6:**420, 1966.

19 Cucinell, S. A., Odessky, L., Weiss, M., and Dayton, P. G.: The effect of chloral hydrate on bishydroxycoumarin metabolism, J.A.M.A. **197:**366, 1965.

20 Cullen, S. I., and Catalano, P. M.: Griseofulvin-warfarin antagonism, J.A.M.A. **199:**582, 1967.

21 Dayton, P. G., Tarcan, Y., Chenkin, T., and Weiner, M.: The influence of barbiturates on coumarin plasma levels and prothrombin response, J. Clin. Invest. **40:**1797, 1961.

22 Domino, E. F., Sullivan, T. S., and Luby, E. D.: Barbiturate intoxication in a patient treated with a MAO inhibitor, Am. J. Psychiatry **118:**941, 1962.

23 Eisen, M. J.: Combined effect of sodium warfarin and phenylbutazone, J.A.M.A. **189:**64, 1964.

24 Elis, J., Laurence, D. R., Mattie, H., and Prichard, B. N. C.: Modification by monoamine oxidase inhibitors of the effect of some sympathomimetics on blood pressure, Br. Med. J. **2:**75, 1967.

25 Ellenhorn, M. J., and Sternad, F. A.: Problems of drug interactions, J. Am. Pharmacol. Assoc. **6:**62, 1966.

26 Field, J. B., Ohta, M., Boyle, C., and Remer, A.: Potentiation of acetohexamide hypoglycemia by phenylbutazone, N. Engl. J. Med. **277:**889, 1967.

27 Fowler, T. J.: Some incompatibilities of intravenous admixtures, Am. J. Hosp. Pharm. **24:**450, 1967.

28 Fox, S. L.: Potentiation of anticoagulants caused by pyrazole compounds, J.A.M.A. **188:**320, 1964.

29 Garrettson, L. K., Perel, J. M., and Dayton, P. G.: Methylphenidate interaction with both anticonvulsants and ethyl biscoumacetate, J.A.M.A. **207:**2053, 1969.

30 Gessner, P. K.: Antagonism of the tranylcypromine-meperidine interaction by chlorpromazine in mice, Eur. J. Pharmacol. **22:**187, 1973.

31 Gillette, J. R.: Biochemistry of drug oxidation and reduction by enzymes in hepatic endoplasmic reticulum, Adv. Pharmacol. **4:**219, 1966.

32 Goldberg, L. I.: Monamine oxidase inhibitors, J.A.M.A. **190:**456, 1964.

33 Goss, J. E., and Dickhaus, D. W.: Increased bishydroxycoumarin requirements in patients receiving phenobarbital, N. Engl. J. Med. **273:**1094, 1965.

34 Gulati, O. D., Dave, B. T., Gokhale, S. D., and Shah, K. M.: Antagonism of adrenergic neuron blockade in hypertensive subjects, Clin. Pharmacol. Ther. **7:**510, 1966.

35 Hansen, J. M., Kristensen, M., Skovsted, L., and Christensen, L. K.: Dicoumarol-induced diphenylhydantoin intoxication, Lancet **2:**265, 1966.

36 Hodge, J. V., Nye, E. R., and Emerson, G. W.: Monoamine-oxidase inhibitors, broad beans, and hypertension, Lancet **1:**1108, 1964.

37 Horwitz, D., Goldberg, L. I., and Sjoerdsma, A.: Increased blood pressure responses to dopamine and norepinephrine produced by monoamine oxidase inhibitors in man, J. Lab. Clin. Med. **56:**747, 1960.

38 Horwitz, D., Lovenberg, W., Engelman, K.,

and Sjoerdsma, A.: Monoamine oxidase inhibitors, tyramine, and cheese, J.A.M.A. **188**:1108, 1964.

39 Hunninghake, D. B., and Azarnoff, D. L.: Drug interactions with warfarin, Arch. Intern. Med. **121**:349, 1968.

40 Hussar, D. A.: Therapeutic incompatibilities: drug interactions, Am. J. Pharmacol. **139**:215, 1967.

41 Jawetz, E.: The use of combinations of antimicrobial drugs, Annu. Rev. Pharmacol. **8**:151, 1968.

42 Kane, F. J., and Taylor, T. W.: A toxic reaction to combined Elavil-Librium therapy, Am. J. Psychiatry **119**:1179, 1963.

43 Kinoshita, F. K., Frawley, J. P., and DuBois, K. P.: Quantitative measurement of induction of hepatic microsomal enzymes by various dietary levels of DDT and toxaphene in rats, Toxicol. Appl. Pharmacol. **9**:505, 1966.

44 Koch-Weser, J.: Quinidine-induced hypoprothrombinemic hemorrhage in patients on chronic warfarin therapy, Ann. Intern. Med. **68**:511, 1968.

45 Krakoff, I. H.: Clinical pharmacology of drugs which influence uric acid production and excretion, Clin. Pharmacol. Ther. **8**:124, 1967.

46 Kristensen, M., and Hansen, J. M.: Potentiation of the tolbutamide effect of dicumarol, Diabetes **16**:211, 1967.

47 Kunin, C. M.: Clinical pharmacology of the new penicillins. II. Effect of drugs which interfere with binding to serum proteins, Clin. Pharmacol. Ther. **7**:180, 1966.

48 Landauer, A. A., Milner, G., and Patman, J.: Alcohol and amitriptyline effects on skills related to driving behavior, Science **163**:1467, 1969.

49 Lees, F., and Burke, C. W.: Tranylcypromine, Lancet **1**:13, 1963.

50 Leishman, A. W. D., Mathews, H. C., and Smith, A. J.: Antagonism of guanethidine by imipramine, Lancet **1**:112, 1963.

51 MacDonald, M. G., and Robinson, D. S.: Clinical observations of possible barbiturate interference with anticoagulation, J.A.M.A. **204**:97, 1968.

52 MacDonald, M. G., Robinson, D. S., Sylvester, D., and Jaffe, J. J.: The effects of phenobarbital, chloral betaine, and glutethimide administration on warfarin plasma levels and hypoprothrombinemic responses in man, Clin. Pharmacol. Ther. **10**:80, 1969.

53 Mannering, G. J.: Significance of stimulation and inhibition of drug metabolism in pharmacological testing. In Burger, A., editor: Selected pharmacological testing methods, New York, 1968, Marcel Dekker, Inc.

54 Mason, A.: Fatal reaction associated with tranylcypromine and methylamphetamine, Lancet **1**:1073, 1962.

55 Mitchell, J. R., Arias, L., and Oates, J. A.: Antagonism of the antihypertensive action of guanethidine sulfate by desipramine hydrochloride, J.A.M.A. **202**:973, 1967.

56 Morelli, H. F., and Melmon, K. L.: The clinician's approach to drug interactions, Calif. Med. **109**:380, 1968.

57 Nour-Eldin, F., and Lewis, F. J. W.: Tolerance to phenindione of patients with different thromboembolic disorders, Acta Haematol. **32**:338, 1964.

58 Oakley, D. P., and Lautch, H.: Haloperidol and anticoagulant treatment, Lancet **2**:1231, 1963.

59 Odell, G. B.: Studies in kernicterus. I. The protein binding of bilirubin, J. Clin. Invest. **38**:823, 1959.

60 Olesen, O. V.: The influence of disulfiram and calcium carbimide on the serum diphenylhydantoin, Arch. Neurol. **16**:642, 1967.

61 Oliver, M. F., Roberts, S. D., Hayes, D., Pantridge, J. F., Suzman, M. M., and Bersohn, I.: Effect of atromid and ethyl chlorophenoxyisobutyrate on anticoagulant requirements, Lancet **1**:143, 1963.

62 Owens, J. C., Neely, W. B., and Owen, W. R.: Effect of sodium dextrothyroxine in patients receiving anticoagulants, N. Engl. J. Med. **266**:76, 1962.

63 Penlington, G. N.: Droperidol and monoamineoxidase inhibitors, Br. Med. J. **1**:483, 1966.

64 Pettinger, W. A., Soyangco, F. G., and Oates, J. A.: Inhibition of monoamine oxidase in man by furazolidone, Clin. Pharmacol. Ther. **9**:442, 1968.

65 Pyörälä, K., and Kekki, M.: Decreased anticoagulant tolerance during methandrostenolone therapy, Scand. J. Clin. Lab. Invest. **15**:367, 1963.

66 Remmer, H., Estabrook, R. W., Schenkman, J., and Greim, H.: Reaction of drugs with microsomal liver hydroxylase: its influence on drug action, Naunyn Schmiedeberg Arch. Pharmacol. Pharm. Exp. Pathol. **259**:98, 1968.

67 Robinson, D. S., and MacDonald, M. G.: The effect of phenobarbital administration on the control of coagulation achieved during warfarin therapy in man, J. Pharmacol. Exp. Ther. **153**:250, 1966.

68 Schrogie, J. J., and Solomon, H. M.: The anticoagulant response to bishydroxycoumarin. II. The effect of D-thyroxine, clofibrate, and nor-

ethandrolone, Clin. Pharmacol. Ther. **8:**70, 1967.

69 Sellers, E. M., and Koch-Weser, J.: Potentiation of warfarin-induced hypoprothrombinemia by chloral hydrate, N. Engl. J. Med. **283:**828, 1970.

70 Shapiro, S., Redish, M. H., and Campbell, H. A.: The prothrombinopenic effect of salicylate in man, Proc. Soc. Exp. Biol. Med. **53:**251, 1943.

71 Silverman, W. A., Anderson, D. H., Blanc, W. A., and Crozier, D. N.: A difference in mortality rate and incidence of kernicterus among premature infants allotted to two prophylactic antibacterial regimens, Pediatrics **18:**614, 1956.

72 Sjöqvist, F.: Psychotropic drugs. II. Interaction between monoamine oxidase (MAO) inhibitors and other substances, Proc. R. Soc. Med. **58:** 967, 1965.

73 Solomon, H. M., and Schrogie, J. J.: The effect of phenyramidol on the metabolism of bishydroxycoumarin, J. Pharmacol. Exp. Ther. **154:** 660, 1966.

74 Solomon, H. M., and Schrogie, J. J.: Change in receptor site affinity: a proposed explanation for the potentiating effect of D-thyroxine on the anticoagulant response to warfarin, Clin. Pharmacol. Ther. **8:**797, 1967.

75 Solomon, H. M., and Schrogie, J. J.: The effect of various drugs on the binding of warfarin-^{14}C to human albumin, Biochem. Pharmacol. **16:** 1219, 1967.

76 Stowers, J. M., Constable, L. W., and Hunter, R. B.: A clinical and pharmacological comparison of chlorpropamide and other sulfonylureas, Ann. N.Y. Acad. Sci. **74:**689, 1959.

77 Vesell, E. S., and Page, J. G.: Genetic control of the induction of an hepatic microsomal drug metabolizing enzyme in man, J. Clin. Invest. **48:**2202, 1969.

78 Vigran, I. M.: Dangerous potentiation of meperidine hydrochloride by pargyline hydrochloride, J.A.M.A. **187:**953, 1964.

79 Vital Brazil, O., and Corrado, A. P.: The curariform action of streptomycin, J. Pharmacol. Exp. Ther. **120:**452, 1957.

REVIEWS

80 Azarnoff, D. L., and Hurwitz, A.: Drug interactions, Pharmacol. Phys. **4**(2):1, 1970.

81 Brater, D. C., and Morelli, H. F.: Cardiovascular drug interactions, Annu. Rev. Pharmacol. Toxicol. **17:**293, 1977.

82 Drug interactions that can affect your patients, Patient Care **4:**91, 1970.

83 Hansten, P. D.: Drug interactions, Philadelphia, 1979, Lea & Febiger.

84 Koch-Weser, J., and Sellers, E. M.: Drug interactions with coumarin anticoagulants, N. Engl. J. Med. **285:**487, 547, 1971.

85 Melmon, K. L.: Preventable drug reactions—causes and cures, N. Engl. J. Med. **284:**1361, 1971.

86 Seller, E. M., and Koch-Weser, J.: Kinetics and clinical importance of displacement of warfarin from albumin by acidic drugs, Ann. N.Y. Acad. Sci. **179:**213, 1971.

Prescription writing and drug compendia

CHAPTER 64

Prescription writing and drug compendia

A prescription is a written order given by a physician to a pharmacist. In addition to the name of the patient and that of the physician, the prescription should contain the name or names of the drugs ordered and their quantities, instructions to the pharmacist, and directions to the patient.

The art of prescription writing has been declining in modern medicine as a result of several developments. Most of the preparations are compounded today by pharmaceutical companies, and the pharmacist's role in most cases consists only of dispensing. Also, the practice of writing long, complicated prescriptions containing many active ingredients, adjuvants, correctives, and various vehicles has been abandoned in favor of using single pure compounds. Even when combinations of several active ingredients are desirable, the pharmaceutical companies often have available several forms of suitable combinations. It may be said that this practice deprives the physician of the opportunity to adjust the various components of a mixture to the individual requirements of the patient. The custom of prescribing trademarked mixtures also has other disadvantages. The physician may be so accustomed to prescribing a mixture of drugs by a trade name that he may not be quite certain about the individual components of it, some of which may be unnecessary or undesirable in a given case.

Drugs may be prescribed by their official names, which are listed in the *United States Pharmacopeia* (USP) or *National Formulary* (NF); by their nonofficial generic names, or *United States Adopted Name* (USAN); or by a manufacturer's trade name. The designation USAN has been recently coined for generic or nonproprietary names adopted by the American Medical Association–United States Pharmacopeia Nomenclature Committee in cooperation with the respective manufacturers. Adoption of USAN names does not imply endorsement of the product by the American Medical Association Council on Drugs or by the United States Pharmacopeia.

There is considerable advantage to prescribing drugs by their official or generic names. This often allows the pharmacist to dispense a more economical product than a trademarked preparation of one company. It would also eliminate the expense of each pharmacy's maintaining a multiplicity of very similar preparations, a saving that could ultimately benefit the patient.

PRESCRIPTION WRITING

On the other hand, the physician may have reasons for prescribing one manufacturer's product. This is often the only way to be certain that the preparation given to the patient will be exactly what is intended, not only in its active ingredients but even to the point of its appearance and taste. A child who is accustomed to the flavor of a certain vitamin mixture may refuse to swallow a similar product if its taste is different. Also, there are some childlike adults who pay much attention to the physical properties and taste of products to which they are accustomed.

Although it is not generally appreciated by physicians, absorption of a drug from the gastrointestinal tract may vary greatly, depending on the manufacturing process used in the preparation of a tablet or capsule. For example, chloramphenicol capsules made by various manufacturers may produce quite different blood levels. The whole problem of generic equivalence needs to be reexamined.

On the whole, the use of generic names is more common in teaching hospitals than in general practice. There is much discussion at present concerning the relative advantages of prescribing by generic names rather than by trade names. The outcome of this debate should be of great interest in medical economics.

Parts of prescription

Traditionally a prescription is written in a certain order and consists of four basic parts:

1. *Superscription*—This is simply ℞, the abbreviation for *recipe*, the imperative of *recipere*, meaning "take thou."

2. *Inscription*—This represents the ingredients and their amounts. If a prescription contains several ingredients in a mixture, it is customary to write them in the following order: (1) basis or principal ingredient, (2) adjuvant, which may contribute to the action of the basis, and (3) corrective, which may eliminate some undesirable property of the active drug or the vehicle, which is the substance used for dilution.

3. *Subscription*—This contains directions for dispensing. Often is consists only of *M.*, the abbreviation for *misce*, meaning "mix."

4. *Signature*—This is often abbreviated as *Sig.* and contains the directions to the patient, such as "Take one teaspoonful three times a day before meals." The signature should indicate whether the medicine is intended for external application and whether it has some special poisonous properties. Wherever possible, instructions of a general nature, such as "take as directed," should be avoided since the patient may misunderstand verbal directions given by the physician.

In addition to the basic parts of a prescription, it should have the patient's name and the physician's signature, followed by the abbreviation M.D.

Modern trends in prescription writing

The parts of the prescription described in the previous paragraphs represent a tradition that is undergoing considerable change. Latin, even in the form of abbreviations, is not really necessary. Its main purpose in the past was to conceal from the patient the nature (and often worthlessness) of a drug. At the present time, prescriptions are written in English. Even such abbreviations as *M.* or *Sig.* may be avoided. It is also advisable to avoid as much as possible the use of the decimal point and state the number of milligrams in a dose instead of using the decimal fraction of a gram.

There are other interesting trends in prescription writing.[2] Much confusion results from the fact that the name of a drug is not spelled out on the label, and therefore the patient knows only that he is taking some sort of pills having certain physicial characteristics. The busy physician wastes much time trying to identify medications given to his patients by other physicians. It may not be an exaggeration to say that drug treatment in some instances may be truly double-blind.

To avoid this unsatisfactory development, some physicians ask the pharmacist to name the drug on the label, indicating their wish by checking an appropriate box on the prescription form. They also indicate in another box the number of allowable refills.

Until recently, prescriptions for narcotic drugs were regulated by the Harrison Anti-Narcotic Act and the drug abuse control amendments of 1965. These regulations have been replaced by the Federal Controlled Substances Act of 1970 and the regulations issued by the Director of the Federal Bureau of Narcotics and Dangerous Drugs. The new regulations became effective May 1, 1971. The drugs controlled by the Act are placed in five categories, or schedules:

Prescriptions and the Federal Controlled Substances Act

Schedule I. Hallucinogenic substances and some opiates for which there is no current accepted medical use.

Schedule II. Drugs of high abuse potential, such as most narcotics of the former Class A group, amphetamines, some closely related compounds, and some barbiturates.

Schedule III. Depressants such as some barbiturates, nalorphine, straight paregoric, certain amphetamine combination drugs, and narcotics of former Class B group.

Schedule IV. Chloral hydrate, meprobamate, paraldehyde, and some long-acting barbiturates. (Generally, the abuse potential for drugs in this schedule is lower than for the representatives of the previous schedules.)

Schedule V. Paregoric combination preparations and other drugs and compounds for which the abuse potential is lower than for members of schedule IV.

All prescriptions for controlled drugs (schedules II to V) must contain the full name and address of the patient, full name, address, and DEA (Drug Enforcement Administration) number of the prescribing doctor, signature of the prescribing doctor, and date. Prescriptions for schedule II drugs are not refillable. Schedules III and IV drugs may be refilled up to five times within 6 months of initial issuance if so authorized by the prescribing physician. Prescriptions for schedule V drugs may be refilled as authorized by the prescribing physician.

Two examples of prescriptions are shown on p. 752.

Typical prescriptions

Authoritative information on drugs can be found in the *United States Pharmacopeia* and the *National Formulary* as well as in many textbooks of pharmacology.

DRUG COMPENDIA

John Doe, M.D.
555 Medical Arts Building
City
Telephone: 361-4282

Name   David Smith   Date   May 9, 1981
Address   201 Hall Street   Age   37

℞

      Tetracycline USP, 250 mg
      Dispense twenty capsules
      Label: Take one capsule four times a day

Reg. No. _____   John Doe, M.D.

John Doe, M.D.
555 Medical Arts Building
City
Telephone: 361-4282

Name   David Smith   Date   May 9, 1981
Address   201 Hall Street   Age   37

℞   g or ml

      Ammonium chloride   12
      Terpin hydrate elixir, to make   120
      M.
      Label: Take one teaspoonful in half glass
              of water for cough every 4 hours
              if necessary

Reg. No. _____   John Doe, M.D.

The *United States Pharmacopeia* and the *National Formulary* are referred to as official publications. The official position of these compendia is based on the Federal Food, Drug and Cosmetic Act of 1938, which recognizes them as "official compendia."

The *United States Pharmacopeia* was first published in 1820. It and the *National Formulary* became official in 1906, when they were so designated by the first Food and Drug Act. The *United States Pharmacopeia* is revised by physicians, pharmacists, and medical scientists who are elected by delegates to the United States Pharmacopeial Convention. The delegates originate from schools of medicine and pharmacy, from medical and pharmaceutical societies, and from some departments of the government.

The *United States Pharmacopeia* is published every 5 years. For a drug to be included there must be good evidence for its therapeutic merit or its pharmaceutical necessity.

The *National Formulary* is compiled by a board of the American Pharmaceutical Association. It is published every 5 years, and only drugs of demonstrated therapeutic value are included.

AMA Drug Evaluations 1980 is a valuable source of information on most drugs that are available in the United States. It is particularly useful in checking on currently accepted therapeutic practices and available preparations.

If physicians could limit their use of drugs to those that are listed in the *United States Pharmacopeia* or those that have been recommended by *AMA Drug Evaluations 1980*, they would be protected against unfounded claims or the power of advertising. When a new drug represents a great therapeutic advance, physicians may be unable to wait for such authoritative reviews. They must often rely on the written or verbal statements of recognized experts in the field. In any case, they should not depend solely on the advertising literature or drug circulars and package inserts.

REFERENCES

1 Cutting, W.: A note on names, Clin. Pharmacol. Ther. **5**:569, 1963.
2 Friend, D. G.: Principles and practices of prescription writing, Clin. Pharmacol. Ther. **6**:411, 1965.
3 Ingelfinger, F. J., and Elia, J. J.: Prescription and proscription, N. Engl. J. Med. **285**:1199, 1971.

Appendixes

Drug blood concentrations

The concentration of drugs in the blood is of interest in clinical medicine and medicolegal situations. The tabular presentation of drug blood concentrations on pp. 758-761 is intended as a source of information and as a guide to the available literature. It should be recognized that the figures given are often based on a few cases and are subject to change as more information accumulates. Furthermore, the significance of blood concentrations depends on numerous factors, and the table should be consulted with full recognition of the role of modifying influences.

IMPORTANCE OF DRUG SERUM CONCENTRATIONS

The determination of drug serum concentrations is not important when the pharmacological effects of the drug can be easily monitored. For example, in the use of coumarin anticoagulants or antihypertensive drugs, the effects of the drugs provide a good indication for adequacy of serum levels and dosage. On the other hand, there are drugs that are used prophylactically, such as phenytoin, quinidine, and others, which provide therapeutic problems in the absence of knowledge of their serum concentrations. The determination of phenytoin in the serum is useful also for revealing noncompliance with the physician's instructions.

The relationship between serum concentration and its pharmacological effect is complicated by numerous factors such as (1) tolerance, (2) drug interactions, (3) the underlying disease, (4) protein binding, and (5) active metabolites.

The role of tolerance, drug interactions, and underlying disease in modifying the relationship between serum concentration and drug effect is easily understood. The importance of protein binding and the role of active metabolites are not always appreciated.

The role of protein binding is illustrated by the following problem.

Problem A. The therapeutic concentration of phenytoin is 20 mg/L. It is about 95% bound to serum albumin. In the case of uremia, hypoalbuminemia, or the presence of other drugs that displace phenytoin from its binding site, the bound fraction could go down to 90%. What will be the effect on the free drug fraction and the potential toxicity of phenytoin? If the total phenytoin concentration in the serum is reported to be 20 mg/L, the free fraction will be 2 mg, which is twice as much as it would be with normal albumin binding and could be toxic.[20]

□ Much of this information has been compiled and kindly provided by Dr. Charles L. Winek, Chief Toxicologist, County of Allegheny, and Professor of Toxicology, Duquesne University.

The complicating effect of active metabolites is demonstrated in the case of propranolol. This drug is metabolized to 4-hydroxy-propranolol, which is an active β blocker. If one knows the serum concentration of propranolol, it still may not be possible to state the intensity of β blockade. Other complicating factors may result from the application of radioimmunoassays. In a few instances the biological activity—usually of an endogenous compound—and the concentration as measured by radioimmunoassay do not correlate well.

DEFINITION OF BLOOD CONCENTRATIONS

therapeutic blood concentration The concentration of drug in blood, serum, or plasma after therapeutically effective dosage in humans. The values in the table are generally those reported with oral administration of the drug.

toxic blood concentration The concentration of drug in blood, serum, or plasma associated with serious toxic symptoms in humans.

lethal blood concentration The concentration of drug in blood, serum, or plasma that has been reported to cause death or is so far above therapeutic or toxic concentrations that it might cause death in humans.

• • •

The following table gives the therapeutic, toxic, and lethal blood concentrations of a large number of drugs.

Drug and chemical blood concentrations*

Compound	Therapeutic or "normal" concentration	Toxic concentration	Lethal concentration
Acetaminophen (Tylenol)	10-20 mg/L	400 mg/L	1500 mg/L
Acetazolamide (Diamox)	10-15 mg/L	—	—
Acetohexamide (Dymelor)	21-56 mg/L		—
Acetone		200-300 mg/L	550 mg/L
Aluminum	0.13 mg/L	—	—
Ammonia	500-1700 mg/L		—
Aminophylline (Theophylline)	10-20 mg/L		—
Amitriptyline (Elavil)	50-200 μg/L	400 μg/L	10-20 mg/L
Amphetamine	20-30 μg/L	—	2 mg/L
Arsenic	0.0-20 μg/L	1.0 mg/L	15 mg/L
Barbiturates			
Short-acting	1 mg/L	7 mg/L	10 mg/L
Intermediate-acting	1-5 mg/L	10-30 mg/L	30 mg/L
Phenobarbital	~10 mg/L	40-60 mg/L	80-150 mg/L
Barbital	~10 mg/L	60-80 mg/L	100 mg/L
Benzene	—	Any measurable	0.94 mg/L
Beryllium	Tissue levels generally used (lung and lymph)	—	—

From Winek, C. L.: Tabulation of therapeutic, toxic and lethal concentrations of drugs and chemicals in blood, Clin. Chem. **22**:832, 1976.

*Some common brand names that may be more familiar than the generic name, alternative forms (e.g., aminophylline/theophylline), and the like are given parenthetically.

†McBay reports much lower values.

Drug and chemical blood concentrations—cont'd

Compound	Therapeutic or "normal" concentration	Toxic concentration	Lethal concentration
Boron (boric acid)	0.8 mg/L	40 mg/L	50 mg/L
Bromide	50 mg/L	0.5-1.5 g/L	2 g/L
Brompheniramine (Dimetane)	8-15 μg/L	—	—
Cadmium	0.1-0.2 μg/L	50 μg/L	—
Caffeine	—	—	>100 mg/L
Carbamazepine (Tegretol)	2 mg/L	8-10 mg/L	—
Carbon monoxide	1% saturation of Hb	15-35% saturation of Hb	50% saturation of Hb
Carbon tetrachloride	—	20-50 mg/L	
Carisoprodol (Rela, Soma)	10-40 mg/L	—	—
Chloral hydrate (Noctec)	10 mg/L	100 mg/L	250 mg/L
Chloroform	—	70-250 mg/L	390 mg/L
Chlordiazepoxide (Librium)	1.0-3.0 mg/L	5.5 mg/L	20 mg/L
Chlorpheniramine	—	20-30 mg/L	—
Chlorpromazine (Thorazine)	0.5 mg/L	1-2 mg/L	3-12 mg/L
Chlorpropamide (Diabinese)	30-140 mg/L	—	—
Chlorprothixine (Taractan)	0.04-0.3 mg/L	—	—
Codeine	25 μg/L	—	—
Copper	1-1.5 mg/L	5.4 mg/L	—
Cyanide	0.15 mg/L	—	>5 mg/L
DDT	13 μg/L	—	—
Desipramine (Norpramin)	0.59-1.4 mg/L	—	10-20 mg/L
Dextropropoxyphene (Darvon)	50-200 μg/L	5-10 mg/L	57 mg/L†
Diazepam (Valium)	0.5-2.5 mg/L	5-20 mg/L	>50 mg/L
Dieldren	1.5 μg/L	—	—
Digitoxin	20-35 μg/L	—	320 μg/L
Digoxin	0.6-1.3 μg/L	2-9 μg/L	—
Dinitro-o-cresol	—	30-40 μg/L	75 mg/L
Diphenhydramine (Benadryl)	5 mg/L	10 mg/L	—
Divinyl oxide	—	—	700 mg/L
Doxepin (Sinequan)	—	—	>10 mg/L
Ethanol	—	1.5 g/L	>3.5 g/L
Ethchlorvynol (Placidyl)	5 mg/L	20 mg/L	150 mg/L
Ethinamate (Valmid)	5-10 mg/L	—	—
Ethosuximide (Zarontin)	25-75 mg/L	—	—
Ethyl chloride	—	—	400 mg/L
Ethyl ether	0.9-1.0 g/L	—	1.4-1.89 g/L
Ethylene glycol	—	1.5 g/L	2-4 g/L
Fluoride	0.5 mg/L	—	2 mg/L
Glutethimide (Doriden)	0.2 mg/L	10-80 mg/L	30-100 mg/L
Gold (sodium aurothiomalate)	3-6 mg/L	—	—
Halothane (Fluothane)	—	—	200 mg/L
Hydrogen sulfide	—	—	0.92 mg/L
Hydromorphone (Dilaudid)	—	—	0.1-0.3 mg/L
Imipramine (Tofranil)	0.05-0.16 mg/L	0.7 mg/L	2 mg/L
Iron	500 mg/L (erythrocytes)	6 mg/L (serum)	—
Isopropanol	—	3.4 g/L	—
Lead	0.05-1.3 mg/L	1.3 mg/L	—
Lidocaine	2 mg/L	6 mg/L	—

Continued.

Drug and chemical blood concentrations—cont'd

Compound	Therapeutic or "normal" concentration	Toxic concentration	Lethal concentration
Lithium	4.2-8.3 mg/L	13.9 mg/L	13.9-34.7 mg/L
LSD (lysergic acid diethylamide)	—	1-4 µg/L	—
Magnesium	0.8-1.3 mmol/L	—	0.5 mmol/L
Manganese	0.15 mg/L	4.6 mg/L	—
Meperidine (Demerol)	600-650 µg/L	5 mg/L	30 mg/L
Meprobamate	10 mg/L	100 mg/L	200 mg/L
Mercury	60-120 µg/L	—	—
Methadone	480-860 µg/L	2 mg/L	>4 mg/L
Methamphetamine	—	5 mg/L	40 mg/L
Methanol	—	200 mg/L	>890 mg/L
Methapyrilene	2 µg/L	30-50 mg/L	>50 mg/L
Methaqualone (Quaalude)	5 mg/L	10-30 mg/L	>30 mg/L
Methsuximide (Celontin)	2.5-7.5 mg/L	—	—
Methylene chloride	—	—	>280 mg/L
Methylenedioxyamphetamine (MDA)	—	—	4-10 mg/L
Methyprylon (Noludar)	10 mg/L	30-60 mg/L	100 mg/L
Morphine	0.1 mg/L	—	0.05-4 mg/L
Nickel	0.41 mg/L	—	—
Nicotine	—	10 mg/L	5-52 mg/L
Nitrofurantoin (Furadantin)	1.8 mg/L	—	—
Nortriptyline (Aventyl)	1.2-1.6 µg/L	5 mg/L	13 mg/L
Orphenadrine	—	2 mg/L	4-8 mg/L
Oxalate	2 mg/L	—	10 mg/L
Papaverine	1 mg/L	—	—
Paraldehyde	50 mg/L	200-400 mg/L	500 mg/L
Paramethoxyamphetamine (PMA)	—	—	2-4 mg/L
Pentazocine (Talwin)	0.14-0.16 mg/L	2-5 mg/L	10-20 mg/L
Perphenazine (Trilafon)	—	1 mg/L	—
Phencyclidine	—	<0.5 mg/L	1.0 mg/L
Phenmetrazine	—	—	4 mg/L
Phensuximide (Milontin)	10-19 mg/L	—	—
Phenylbutazone (Butazolidin)	100 mg/L	—	—
Phenytoin (Dilantin)	5-22 mg/L	50 mg/L	100 mg/L
Phosphorus	Concentration in tissues usually used	—	—
Primidone (Mysoline)	10 mg/L	50-80 mg/L	100 mg/L
Probenecid (Benemid)	100-200 mg/L	—	—
Procainamide	6 mg/L	10 mg/L	—
Prochlorperazine (Compazine)	—	1 mg/L	—
Promazine (Sparine)	—	1 mg/L	—
Propoxyphene	50-200 µg/L	5-20 mg/L	57 mg/L
Propranolol (Inderal)	0.025-0.2 mg/L	—	8-12 mg/L
Propylhexedrine (Benzedrex)	—	—	2-3 mg/L
Quinidine	3-6 mg/L	10 mg/L	30-50 mg/L
Quinine	—	—	12 mg/L
Salicylate (acetylsalicylic acid)	20-100 mg/L	150-300 mg/L	500 mg/L
Strychnine	—	2 mg/L	9-12 mg/L
Sulfadiazine	80-150 mg/L	—	—
Sulfadimethoxine (Madribon)	80-100 mg/L	—	—

Drug and chemical blood concentrations—cont'd

Compound	Therapeutic or "normal" concentration	Toxic concentration	Lethal concentration
Sulfaguanidine	30-50 mg/L	—	—
Sulfanilamide	100-150 mg/L	—	—
Sulfisoxazole (Gantrisin)	90-100 mg/L	—	—
Theophylline	20-100 mg/L	—	—
Thioridazine (Mellaril)	1-1.5 mg/L	10 mg/L	20-80 mg/L
Tin	0.12 mg/L	—	—
Tolbutamide (Orinase)	53-96 mg/L	—	—
Toluene	—	—	10 mg/L
Tribromoethanol	—	—	90 mg/L
Trichloroethane	—	—	0.01-1 g/L
Trimethobenzamide (Tigan)	1.0-2.0 mg/L	—	—
Warfarin	1.0-10 mg/L	—	—
Zinc	0.68-1.36 mg/L	—	—
Zoxazolamine (Flexin)	3-13 mg/L	—	—

REFERENCES

1 Beller, G. A., Smith, T. W., Abelmann, W. H., Haber, E., and Hood, W. B.: Digitalis intoxication: a prospective clinical study with serum level correlations, N. Engl. J. Med. **284**:989, 1971.

2 Berkowitz, B. A., Aslin, J. H., Shnider, S. M., and Way, E. L.: Relationship of pentazocine plasma levels to pharmacological activity in man, Clin. Pharmacol. Ther. **10**:320, 1969.

3 Clarke, E. G. C.: Isolation and identification of drugs in pharmaceuticals, body fluids, and postmortem material, London, 1969, The Pharmaceutical Press.

4 Collom, W. D.: Personal communication, 1969.

5 Cravey, R. H., and Baselt, R. C.: Methamphetamine poisoning, J. Forensic Sci. Soc. **8**:110, 1968.

6 Curry, A.: Poison detection in human organs, ed. 2, Springfield, Ill., 1969, Charles C Thomas, Publisher.

7 Dayton, P. G., Yu, T. F., Chen, W., Berger, L., West, L. A., and Gutman, A. B.: The physiological disposition of probenecid, including renal clearance, in man, studied by an improved method for its estimation in biological material, J. Pharmacol. Exp. Ther. **140**:278, 1963.

8 Fatteh, A. J.: Therapeutic serum concentrations of meperidine (Demerol), Forensic Med. **11**:120, 164.

9 Fochtman, F. W., and Winek, C. L.: Therapeutic serum concentration of meperidine (Demerol), J. Forensic Sci. **14**:213, 1969.

10 Gwilt, J. R., Robertson, A., and McChesney, E. W.: Determination of blood and other tissue concentrations of paracetamol in dog and man, J. Pharm. Pharmacol. **15**:440, 1963.

11 Hausner, E. P., Shafer, C. L., Corson, M., Johnson, O., Trujillo, T., and Langham, W.: Clinical evaluation of dicumarinyl derivatives with metabolic study of radioactively labeled anticoagulants in animals, Circulation **3**:171, 1951.

12 Hollister, L. E., and Kosek, J. C.: Sudden death during treatment with phenothiazine derivatives, J.A.M.A. **192**:1035, 1965.

13 Koch-Weser, J., and Klein, S. W.: Procainamide dosage schedules, plasma concentrations and clinical effects, J.A.M.A. **215**:1454, 1971.

14 Lillehei, J. P.: Aminophylline: oral vs. rectal administration, J.A.M.A. **205**:530, 1968.

15 Loughridge, L. W.: Peripheral neuropathy due to nitrofurantoin, Lancet **2**:1133, 1962.

16 McBay, A. J.: Chemical findings in poisonings, N. Engl. J. Med. **274**:1257, 1966.

17 McBay, A. J.: Personal communication, 1967.

18 McBay, A. J.: Toxicological findings in fatal poisonings, Clin. Chem. **19**:361, 1973.

19 Ohio Chemical: Historical and clinical data on the inhalation anesthetic agents, Madison, Wis., 1966.

20 Reidenberg, M. M.: Protein binding of diphenylhydantoin and desmethylimipramine in plas-

ma from patients with poor renal function, N. Engl. J. Med. **285**:264, 1971.

21 Roche Laboratories: Product reference manual, Nutley, N.J.

22 Shand, D. G., Nuckolls, E. M., and Oates, J. A.: Propranolol plasma levels in adults, Clin. Pharmacol. Ther. **11**:112, 1970.

23 Sheldon, J., Anderson, J., and Stoner, L.: Serum concentration and urinary excretion of oral sulfonylurea compounds: relation to diabetic control, Diabetes **14**:362, 1965.

24 Thomson, P. D., Rowland, M., and Melmon, K. L.: Influence of heart failure, liver disease, and renal failure on the disposition of lidocaine in man, Am. Heart J. **82**:417, 1971.

25 Weikel, J. H.: J. Am. Pharmacol. Assoc. **47**: 477, 1958.

26 Yates, C. M., Todrick, A., and Tait, A. C.: Aspects of the clinical chemistry of desmethylimipramine in man, J. Pharm. Pharmacol. **15**: 432, 1963.

REVIEWS

27 Koch-Weser, J.: Serum drug concentrations as therapeutic guides, N. Engl. J. Med. **287**:227, 1972.

28 Winek, C. L.: Tabulation of therapeutic, toxic and lethal concentrations of drugs and chemicals in blood, Clin. Chem. **22**:832, 1976.

Comparison of selected effects
of commonly abused drugs

Some selected effects of commonly abused drugs are summarized in the table shown on pp. 764-767. This table is intended for quick reference only. Greater detail on the subject is available in Chapter 31 dealing with contemporary drug abuse.

Drug category	Physical dependence	Characteristics of intoxication
Opiates (see p. 342 for classification)	Marked	Analgesia with or without depressed sensorium; pinpoint pupils (tolerance does not develop to this action); patient may be alert and appear normal; respiratory depression with overdose
Barbiturates	Marked	Patient may appear normal with usual dose, but narrow margin between doses needed to prevent withdrawal symptoms and toxic dose is often exceeded and patient appears "drunk," with drowsiness, ataxia, slurred speech, and nystagmus on lateral gaze; pupil size and reaction normal; respiratory depression with overdose
Nonbarbiturate sedatives Glutethimide (Doriden)	Marked	Pupils dilated and reactive to light; coma and respiratory depression prolonged; sudden apnea and laryngeal spasm common
Antianxiety agents* ("minor tranquilizers")	Marked	Progressive depression of sensorium as with barbiturates; pupil size and reaction normal; respiratory depression with overdose
Ethanol	Marked	Depressed sensorium, acute or chronic brain syndrome, odor on breath, pupil size and reaction normal
Amphetamines	Mild to absent	Agitation, with paranoid thought disturbance in high doses; acute organic brain syndrome after prolonged use; pupils dilated and reactive; tachycardia, elevated blood pressure, with possibility of hypertensive crisis and CVA; possibility of convulsive seizures
Cocaine	Absent	Paranoid thought disturbance in high doses, with dangerous delusions of persecution and omnipotence; tachycardia; respiratory depression with overdose
Marihuana	Absent	Milder preparations: drowsy, euphoric state with frequent inappropriate laughter and disturbance in perception of time or space (occasional acute psychotic reaction reported); stronger preparations such as hashish: frequent hallucinations or psychotic reaction; pupils normal, conjunctivas injected (marihuana preparations frequently adulterated with LSD, tryptamines, or heroin)
Psychotomimetics LSD, STP, tryptamines, mescaline, morning glory seeds	Absent	Unpredictable disturbance in ego function, manifest by extreme lability of affect and chaotic disruption of thought, with danger of uncontrolled behavioral disturbance; pupils dilated and reactive to light

Modified from Dimijian, G. G.: Drug Ther. **1:**7, 1971.

*Meprobamate (Equanil), chlordiazepoxide (Librium), diazepam (Valium), ethchlorvynol (Placidyl), and

Characteristics of withdrawal	"Flashback" symptoms	Masking of symptoms of illness or injury during intoxication
Rhinorrhea, lacrimation, and dilated, reactive pupils, followed by gastrointestinal disturbances, low back pain, and waves of gooseflesh; convulsions not a feature unless heroin samples were adulterated with barbiturates	Not reported	An important feature of opiate intoxication, due to analgesic action, with or without depressed sensorium
Agitation, tremulousness, insomnia, gastrointestinal disturbances, hyperpyrexia, blepharoclonus (clonic blink reflex), acute brain syndrome, major convulsive seizures	Not reported	Only in presence of depressed sensorium or after onset of acute brain syndrome
Similar to barbiturate withdrawal syndrome, with agitation, gastrointestinal disturbances, hyperpyrexia, and major convulsive seizures	Not reported	Same as in barbiturate intoxication
Similar to barbiturate withdrawal syndrome, with danger of major convulsive seizures	Not reported	Same as in barbiturate intoxication
Similar to barbiturate withdrawal syndrome, but with less likelihood of convulsive seizures	Not reported	Same as in barbiturate intoxication
Lethargy, somnolence, dysphoria, and possibility of suicidal depression; brain syndrome may persist for many weeks	Infrequently reported	Drug-induced euphoria or acute brain syndrome may interfere with awareness of symptoms of illness or may remove incentive to report symptoms of illness
Similar to amphetamine withdrawal	Not reported	Same as in amphetamine intoxication
No specific withdrawal symptoms	Infrequently reported	Uncommon with milder preparations; stronger preparations may interfere in same manner as psychotomimetic agents
No specific withdrawal symptoms; symptomatology may persist for indefinite period after discontinuation of drug	Commonly reported as late as 1 year after last dose	Affective response or psychotic thought disturbance may remove awareness of, or incentive to report, symptoms of illness

ethinamate (Valmid).

Continued.

Drug category	Physical dependence	Characteristics of intoxication
Phencyclidine	Unknown	Disinhibition, agitation, confusion, chaotic thought disturbance, unpredictable behavior, hypertension, meiosis, respiratory collapse, cardiovascular collapse, death
Anticholinergic agents	Absent	Nonpsychotropic effects such as tachycardia, decreased salivary secretion, urinary retention, and dilated, nonreactive pupils plus depressed sensorium, confusion, disorientation, hallucinations, and delusional thinking
Inhalants†	Unknown	Depressed sensorium, hallucinations, acute brain syndrome; odor on breath; patient often with glassy-eyed appearance

†The term "inhalant" is used to designate a variety of gases and highly volatile organic liquids, including the sprayed into the nasopharynx (droplet transport required) and substances that must be ignited prior to

Characteristics of withdrawal	"Flashback" symptoms	Masking of symptoms of illness or injury during intoxication
No specific withdrawal symptoms	Occasionally reported	Same as in LSD intoxication
No specific withdrawal symptoms; mydriasis may persist for several days	Not reported	Pain may not be reported as a result of depression of sensorium, acute brain syndrome, or acute psychotic reaction
No specific withdrawal symptoms	Infrequently reported	Same as in anticholinergic intoxication

aromatic glues, paint thinners, gasoline, some anesthetic agents, and amylnitrite. The term excludes liquids administration (such as marihuana).

APPENDIX C

Half-lives of drugs in normal subjects

Drug	Half-life (hours)						Major route of elimination
	<1.0 ± 0.5	2 ± 0.5	4 ± 1.5	12 ± 6	24 ± 6	>30	
Acetaminophen		X					Hepatic
Acetazolamide			X				Renal
Acetylsalicylic acid	X						Renal (hepatic)
Allopurinol							Renal
Amantadine				X			Renal
Amikacin		X					Renal
Amiloride			X				Renal
p-Aminosalicylic acid	X						Renal (hepatic)
Amobarbital					X		Hepatic
Amoxicillin	X						Renal
Amphetamine				X			Hepatic (renal)
Amphotericin B					X		Nonrenal
Ampicillin	X						Renal (hepatic)
Antipyrine				X			Hepatic
Atropine					X		Renal (hepatic)
Aurothiomalate sodium						X	Renal
Barbital						X	Renal
Bupivacaine		X					Hepatic
Calcitonin	X						—
Carbamazepine						X	Hepatic
Carbenicillin	X						Renal (hepatic)
Cefazolin		X					Renal
Cephalexin	X						Renal
Cephalothin	X						Renal (hepatic)
Chloramphenicol		X					Hepatic (renal)
Chlordiazepoxide				X			Hepatic
Chlorpromazine					X		Hepatic
Chlorpropamide						X	Hepatic (renal)
Chlortetracycline			X				Renal (hepatic)
Clindamycin		X					Hepatic (renal)
Cloxacillin	X						Hepatic (renal)
Colchicine	X						Renal (hepatic)
Colistimethate			X				Renal
Cortisone	X						Hepatic
Cyclophosphamide			X				Hepatic (renal)

☐ Modified from Bennett, W. M., et al.: Ann. Intern. Med. **86**:754, 1977; and Pagliaro, L. A., and Benet, L. Z.: J. Pharmacokinet. Biopharm. **3**:353, 1975.

Drug	Half-life (hours)						Major route of elimination
	<1.0 ± 0.5	2 ± 0.5	4 ± 1.5	12 ± 6	24 ± 6	>30	
Cycloserine				X			Renal
Cytarabine		X					Nonrenal
Dapsone					X		Renal
Desipramine					X		Hepatic
Diazepam						X	Hepatic (renal)
Diazoxide					X		Renal
Dicloxacillin	X						Renal (hepatic)
Dicumarol					X		Nonrenal
Digitoxin						X	Hepatic (renal)
Digoxin						X	Renal (non-renal)
Diphenoxylate		X					Hepatic
Doxycycline				X			Renal (hepatic)
Ephedrine			X				Renal (hepatic)
Ethambutol			X				Renal
Ethosuximide						X	Hepatic (renal)
Furosemide	X						Renal
Gentamicin		X					Renal
Glutethimide				X			Hepatic
Griseofulvin				X			—
Guanethidine						X	Renal (non-renal)
Haloperidol					X		Renal (hepatic)
Heparin		X					Nonrenal
Hydralazine			X				Hepatic (renal)
Hydrocortisone	X						Hepatic
Indomethacin		X					Hepatic (renal)
Insulin	X						Nonrenal
Isoniazid		X					Hepatic (renal)
Kanamycin		X					Renal
Lidocaine		X					Hepatic (renal)
Lincomycin			X				Hepatic (renal)
Lithium					X		Renal
Meperidine			X				Hepatic (renal)
Meprobamate				X			Hepatic (renal)
6-Mercaptopurine	X						Hepatic
Methacycline				X			Hepatic (renal)
Methadone				X			Hepatic (renal <21%)
Methaqualone				X			Hepatic
Methicillin	X						Renal (hepatic)
Methimazole				X			Renal
Methyltestosterone			X				Hepatic
Minocycline				X			Hepatic
Minoxidil			X				Nonrenal
Morphine		X					Hepatic
Nafcillin	X						Hepatic (renal)
Nalidixic acid	X						Renal (hepatic)
Nitrofurantoin	X						Renal
Nitroglycerin	X						Hepatic
Nortriptyline					X		Hepatic
Oxacillin	X						Renal (hepatic)

Continued.

Drug	Half-life (hours)						Major route of elimination
	<1.0 ± 0.5	2 ± 0.5	4 ± 1.5	12 ± 6	24 ± 6	>30	
Oxyphenbutazone						X	Hepatic
Oxytetracycline				X			Renal (hepatic)
Penicillin G	X						Renal
Pentazocine			X				Hepatic
Pentobarbital						X	Hepatic
Phenacetin	X						Hepatic
Phenobarbital						X	Hepatic (renal)
Phenylbutazone						X	Hepatic
Phenytoin					X		Hepatic (renal)
Pralidoxime	X						Hepatic (renal)
Prednisolone		X					Hepatic
Probenecid				X			Nonrenal (renal)
Procainamide		X					Renal (hepatic)
Propoxyphene			X				Hepatic (renal >23%)
Propranolol			X				Hepatic
Propylthiouracil	X						Renal
Pseudoephedrine			X				Renal
Quinidine			X				Nonrenal (renal 12% to 36%)
Reserpine							Nonrenal
Rifampicin			X				Hepatic
Salicylic acid			X				Renal (hepatic)
Spectinomycin		X					Renal
Streptomycin		X					Renal
Sulfadiazine				X			Renal
Sulfamethoxazole				X			Renal
Sulfamethoxypyrida-zine					X		Renal
Sulfinpyrazone			X				Hepatic
Sulfisoxazole			X				Renal
Testosterone		X					Hepatic
Tetracycline				X			Renal (hepatic)
Theophylline			X				Hepatic
Thiothixene						X	Hepatic
l-Thyroxine						X	Hepatic
Tobramycin		X					Renal
Tolbutamide				X			Hepatic
l-Triiodothyronine					X		Hepatic
Trimethoprim				X			Renal
Vancomycin			X				Renal
Warfarin						X	Nonrenal

Index